th edition

Clinical Imaging:

An Atlas of Differential Diagnosis

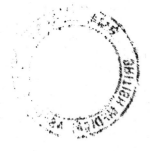

5 th edition

Clinical Imaging:

An Atlas of Differential Diagnosis

Ronald L. Eisenberg, MD
Associate Professor Radiology
Harvard Medical School
Radiologist
Beth Israel Deaconess Medical Center
Boston, Massachusetts

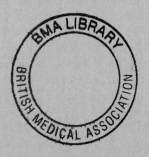

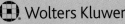
Wolters Kluwer | Lippincott Williams & Wilkins
Health
Philadelphia • Baltimore • New York • London
Buenos Aires • Hong Kong • Sydney • Tokyo

Acquisitions Editor: Brian Brown
Product Manager: Ryan Shaw
Vendor Manager: Alicia Jackson
Senior Manufacturing Manager: Benjamin Rivera
Senior Marketing Manager: Angela Panetta
Design Coordinator: Stephen Druding
Production Service: Spearhead Global, Inc.

Library of Congress Cataloging-in-Publication Data

Eisenberg, Ronald L.
    Clinical imaging : an atlas of differential diagnosis / Ronald L. Eisenberg. — 5th ed.
        p. ; cm.
    Includes bibliographical references and index.
    ISBN-13: 978-0-7817-8860-1 (alk. paper)
    ISBN-10: 0-7817-8860-9 (alk. paper)
    1. Diagnostic imaging—Atlases. 2. Diagnostic imaging—Handbooks, manuals, etc. 3. Diagnosis, Differential—Atlases.
4. Diagnosis, Differential—Handbooks, manuals, etc. I. Title.
    [DNLM: 1. Diagnostic Imaging—Atlases. 2. Diagnosis, Differential—Atlases. WN 17 E36c 2010]
    RC78.7.D53E36 2010
    616.07′54—dc22

                                                                                          2009015308

Care has been taken to confirm the accuracy of the information presented and to describe generally accepted practices. However, the authors, editors, and publisher are not responsible for errors or omissions or for any consequences from application of the information in this book and make no warranty, expressed or implied, with respect to the currency, completeness, or accuracy of the contents of the publication. Application of the information in a particular situation remains the professional responsibility of the practitioner.

The authors, editors, and publisher have exerted every effort to ensure that drug selection and dosage set forth in this text are in accordance with current recommendations and practice at the time of publication. However, in view of ongoing research, changes in government regulations, and the constant flow of information relating to drug therapy and drug reactions, the reader is urged to check the package insert for each drug for any change in indications and dosage and for added warnings and precautions. This is particularly important when the recommended agent is a new or infrequently employed drug.

Some drugs and medical devices presented in the publication have Food and Drug Administration (FDA) clearance for limited use in restricted research settings. It is the responsibility of the health care provider to ascertain the FDA status of each drug or device planned for use in their clinical practice.

To purchase additional copies of this book, call our customer service department at (800) 638-3030 or fax orders to (301) 223-2320. International customers should call (301) 223-2300.

Visit Lippincott Williams & Wilkins on the Internet: at LWW.com. Lippincott Williams & Wilkins customer service representatives are available from 8:30 am to 6 pm, EST.

10 9 8 7 6 5 4 3 2 1

CCS1009

To Zina, Avlana, and Cherina

CONTENTS

PREFACE to the first edition

Pattern recognition leading to the development of differential diagnoses is the essence of radiology. Both the practicing radiologist faced with the reality of daily film reading and the senior resident taking the oral board examination are usually unaware of the underlying disease when they are presented with a specific finding for which they must suggest a differential diagnosis and a rational diagnostic approach. This book offers differential diagnoses for a broad spectrum of radiographic patterns, not only in conventional radiography but also in ultrasound and computed tomography. Added to these lists of differential possibilities are descriptions of the specific imaging findings to be expected for each diagnostic entity as well as differential points to aid the reader in arriving at a precise diagnosis. A wealth of illustrations is provided to point out the often subtle differences in appearance among conditions that can produce a similar overall radiographic pattern. Extensive cross referencing is provided to limit duplication and to permit the reader to find various radiographic manifestations of the same condition.

I must stress that this book in no way intends to supplant the current excellent textbooks in general radiology and imaging subspecialties. Rather, it is designed to complement these works by providing a handy reference for practicing radiologists and residents faced with the daily challenge of interpreting radiographic examinations.

PREFACE

The warm response from residents and practicing radiologists to the first four editions has been extremely gratifying. To reflect trends in diagnostic imaging, yet maintain the single-volume format, some sections on plain radiography have been eliminated to make room for new sections dealing with computed tomography and magnetic resonance imaging. Whenever appropriate, the lists of differential diagnoses from previous editions have been updated and new illustrations added.

I hope that this expanded volume will be even more successful than its predecessors in meeting the goal of providing a handy reference for practicing radiologists and residents faced with the increasingly complex daily challenge of interpreting radiographic examinations.

1

Chest Patterns

Localized Alveolar Pattern

Condition	Imaging Findings	Comments
Bacterial pneumonia		
Staphylococcus (Fig C 1-1)	Rapid development of extensive alveolar infiltrates, usually involving a whole lobe or even several lobes. Air bronchograms are infrequent because the acute inflammatory exudate fills the airways, leading to segmental collapse and a loss of volume.	Most frequently occurs in children, especially during the first year of life. In adults, usually affects hospitalized patients with lowered resistance or as a complication of a viral respiratory infection. A characteristic finding in childhood disease is the development of pneumatoceles, thin-walled cystic spaces in the parenchyma that typically disappear spontaneously within several weeks. Pleural effusion (or empyema) often occurs.
Streptococcus (see Fig C 17-3)	Indistinguishable from staphylococcal pneumonia. Homogeneous or patchy consolidation in a segmental distribution with a lower lobe predominance and often some loss of volume.	Uncommon condition that usually follows viral infections such as measles, pertussis, and epidemic influenza. Unlike staphylococcal infection, streptococcal pneumonia rarely causes the development of pneumatoceles. Early and rapid accumulation of empyema fluid was a characteristic feature before the advent of antibiotics.
Pneumococcus (Fig C 1-2)	Homogeneous consolidation that almost invariably abuts against a visceral pleural surface and almost always contains an air bronchogram.	Most commonly occurs in alcoholics and other compromised hosts. Cavitation and pleural reaction are rare. In children, may produce the so-called round or spherical pneumonia, in which a well-circumscribed spherical consolidation on both frontal and lateral views simulates a pulmonary or mediastinal mass (Fig C 1-3).

B

A

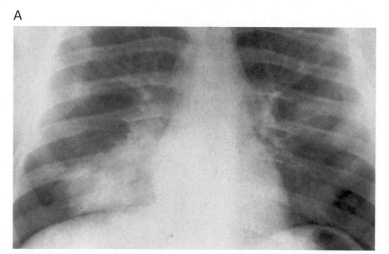
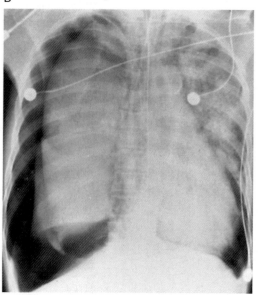

Fig C 1-1
Staphylococcal pneumonia. (A) Ill-defined bronchopneumonia at the right base. (B) In another patient, there is consolidation in the left upper lobe and entire right lung with a moderate right pneumothorax. The extensive consolidation presents further collapse of the right lung. The pneumothorax was due to the rupture of a pneumatocele, although no pneumatocele can be identified.

Condition	Imaging Findings	Comments
Klebsiella (Fig C 1-4)	Homogeneous parenchymal consolidation containing air bronchograms (simulates pneumococcal pneumonia). Primarily involves the right upper lobe. Typically induces a large inflammatory exudate, causing increased volume of the affected lobe and characteristic bulging of an adjacent interlobar fissure (see Fig C 15-1).	Most commonly develops in alcoholics and in elderly patients with chronic pulmonary disease. Unlike acute pneumococcal pneumonia, *Klebsiella* pneumonia causes frequent and rapid cavitation, and there is a much greater incidence of pleural effusion and empyema.

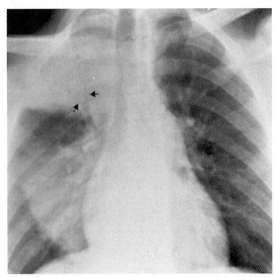

Fig C 1-2
Pneumococcal pneumonia. Homogeneous consolidation of the right upper lobe and the medial and posterior segments of the right lower lobe. Note the associated air bronchograms (arrows).

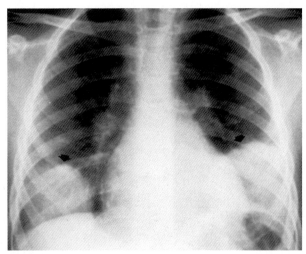

Fig C 1-3
"Spherical" pneumonia. Frontal view of the chest shows a rounded soft-tissue density in the posterolateral aspects of both lower lobes (arrows) with mild bilateral hilar prominence.[1]

A

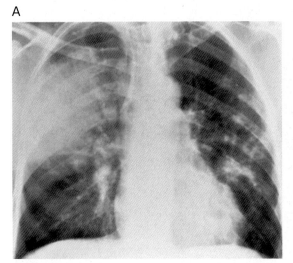

B

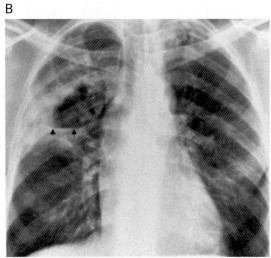

Fig C 1-4
***Klebsiella* pneumonia.** (A) Air-space consolidation involving much of the right upper lobe. (B) Progression of the necrotizing infection produces a large abscess cavity with an air-fluid level (arrows).

Condition	Imaging Findings	Comments
Other enteric gram-negative bacteria (Fig C 1-5)	Nonspecific, often inhomogeneous pattern of consolidation that most commonly affects the lower lobes. Cavitation is relatively common, and pleural effusion may occur.	*Escherichia coli*, *Serratia marcescens*, Enterobacteriaceae, *Proteus*, *Pseudomonas aeruginosa*, *Salmonella*, and *Brucella*. Most commonly develop in debilitated or immunocompromised patients.
Haemophilus influenzae (Fig C 1-6)	Nonspecific patchy pulmonary infiltrate that is often bilateral. May be unilateral lobar or segmental consolidation, simulating pneumococcal disease. Typically extensive pleural involvement that often appears out of proportion to the associated parenchymal infiltrate.	Serious infections primarily affect children under the age of 4 years and older patients who have undergone antibiotic therapy or who suffer from diseases that increase their general susceptibility to infection. This organism is the leading cause of epiglottitis (see Fig C 35-2), the second leading cause of childhood otitis media, and a common cause of childhood bacterial meningitis.
Haemophilus pertussis (whooping cough) (Fig C 1-7)	Various combinations of atelectasis, segmental pneumonia, and hilar lymph node enlargement. Coalescence of air-space consolidation contiguous to the heart produces a typical "shaggy heart" contour.	Although often considered to have been largely eradicated by immunization, immunity is apparently not lifelong, and pertussis has become a not uncommon cause of bronchitis in adults. Acute infection most frequently affects nonimmunized children younger than 2 years of age.
Tularemia (see Fig C 14-2)	Patchy consolidations that may be bilateral, multilobar, or both. Ipsilateral hilar adenopathy and pleural effusion occur in approximately half the cases.	Pneumonia represents hematogenous spread or inhalation of *Francisella tularensis*, which is usually transmitted to humans from infected animals (rodents, small mammals) or insect vectors.

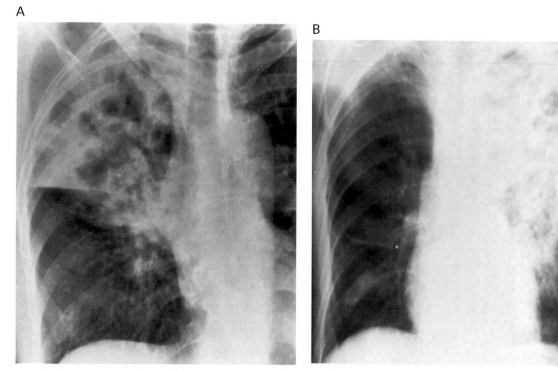

A   B

Fig C 1-5
Enteric gram-negative bacteria. (A) *Proteus.* (B) *Pseudomonas.*[2]

Condition	Imaging Findings	Comments
Yersinia pestis (see Figs C 2-13 and C 14-3)	Patchy segmental infiltration or dense lobar consolidation simulating pneumococcal pneumonia. Typically, there is enlargement of hilar and paratracheal lymph nodes and, often, pleural effusion.	The pneumonic type of plague causes severe pulmonary consolidation, necrosis, and hemorrhage and is usually fatal. This organism is still widespread among wild rodents.
Anthrax	Patchy parenchymal infiltrates that are usually associated with pleural effusion and mediastinal widening (lymph node enlargement and hemorrhagic mediastinitis).	Bacterial disease of cattle, sheep, and goats that primarily affects humans who inhale spores from infected animals or their products (eg, wool, hides).
Legionnaires' disease (Fig C 1-8)	Patchy or fluffy alveolar infiltrate that rapidly progresses to involve adjacent lobes and the contralateral side.	Acute gram-negative bacterial pneumonia that occurs in local outbreaks or as sporadic cases and may cause a fulminant, often fatal, pneumonia. Small pleural effusions are common, whereas cavitation and hilar adenopathy are unusual. Most patients respond well to erythromycin, though the radiographic resolution often lags behind the clinical response.

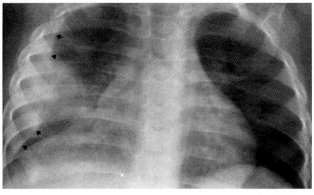

Fig C 1-6
***Haemophilus influenzae* pneumonia.** In addition to the ill-defined right lower lung consolidation, note the extensive pleural thickening or fibrinous exudate (arrows) that appears out of proportion to the associated parenchymal infiltrate.[3]

Fig C 1-7
Haemophilus pertussis. Bilateral central parenchymal infiltrates and linear areas of atelectasis obscure the normally sharp cardiac border to produce the shaggy heart contour.

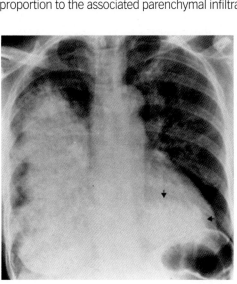

Fig C 1-8
Legionnaires' disease. There is extensive consolidation of much of the right lung, with a smaller area of infiltrate (arrows) at the left base.

Condition	Imaging Findings	Comments
Bacteroides (Fig C 1-9)	Patchy or confluent consolidation that is generally confined to the lower lobes. Cavitation and empyema are common.	Gram-negative anaerobic bacteria that are commonly found in the gastrointestinal and genital tracts. Pneumonia develops from aspiration of infected material or septic infarctions resulting from emboli arising in veins in the peritonsillar area or pelvis.
Fungal pneumonia Histoplasmosis (Fig C 1-10)	In the primary form, single or multiple areas of consolidation that are most often in the lower lung and associated with hilar lymph node enlargement.	Striking hilar adenopathy, which may cause bronchial compression, may develop without radiographic evidence of parenchymal disease. Although the findings simulate primary tuberculosis, pleural effusion rarely occurs with histoplasmosis.
Blastomycosis (Fig C 1-11)	Nonspecific patchy areas of air-space consolidation.	Cavitation and miliary nodules infrequently occur. Blastomycosis may appear as a solitary pulmonary mass that, when associated with unilateral lymph node enlargement, may mimic a bronchogenic carcinoma.

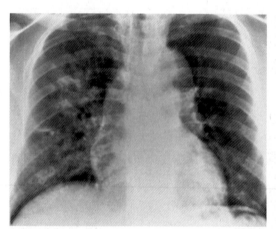

Fig C 1-9
***Bacteroides* pneumonia.** Patchy areas of consolidation primarily involve the middle and lower portions of the right lung.

A

B

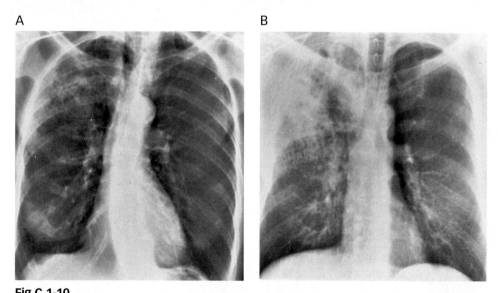

Fig C 1-10
Histoplasmosis. (A) Initial film demonstrates an ill-defined area of parenchymal consolidation in the right upper lobe. (B) One week later, there is a marked extension of the infiltrate, which now involves most of the upper half of the right lung.

Condition	Imaging Findings	Comments
Coccidioidomycosis (Fig C 1-12)	Pulmonary involvement usually begins as a fleeting area of patchy pneumonia that is often accompanied by ipsilateral hilar adenopathy and, less frequently, by pleural effusion.	Thin-walled cavities without surrounding reaction are suggestive of this organism (see Fig C 9-5).
Cryptococcosis (torulosis) (Fig C 1-13)	Segmental or lobar consolidation that most commonly occurs in the lower lobes.	More commonly produces a single, fairly well-circumscribed mass that is usually in the periphery of the lung and is often pleural based. Cavitation is relatively uncommon compared with its frequency in the other mycoses.
Actinomycosis/ nocardiosis (Figs C 1-14 and C 1-15)	Nonsegmental air-space consolidation (may resemble pneumonia or a tumor mass). Cavitation and empyema are common if not appropriately treated.	Extension of the infection into the pleura produces an empyema, which classically leads to osteomyelitis of the ribs and the formation of a sinus tract.

A

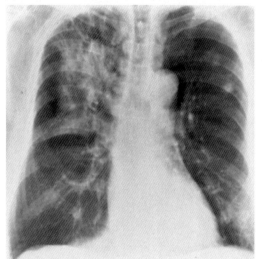

B

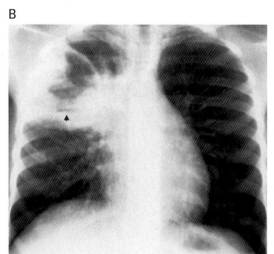

Fig C 1-11
Blastomycosis. (A) Patchy areas of air-space consolidation in the right upper lung associated with several nodules in the left upper lung. (B) In another patient, there is development of a right upper lobe cavity with thick walls and a faintly visible air-fluid level (arrow). There is an associated soft-tissue mass along the lateral wall of the cavity.[4]

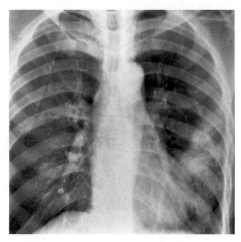

Fig C 1-12
Coccidioidomycosis pneumonia. Ill-defined area of patchy infiltrate in the left lower lung.

A

B

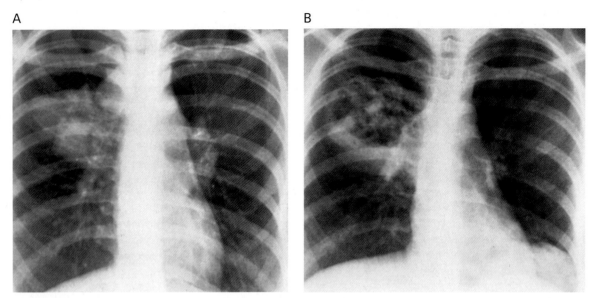

Fig C 1-13
Cryptococcosis. (A) Initial film demonstrates an air-space consolidation in the right upper lung. (B) With progression of the infection, the right upper lung pneumonia has cavitated, and a left lower lobe air-space consolidation has developed.

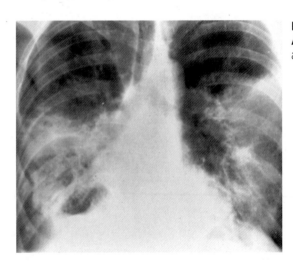

Fig C 1-14
Actinomycosis. Bilateral, nonsegmental air-space consolidation.

A

B

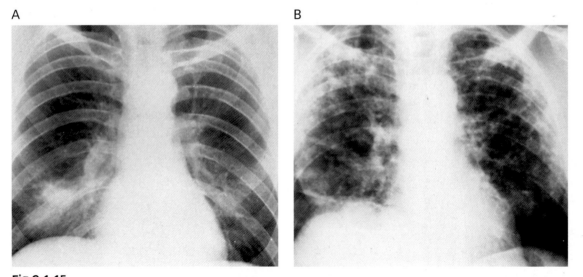

Fig C 1-15
Nocardiosis. (A) Initial chest radiograph demonstrates an area of nonspecific alveolar infiltrate in the right lower lobe. (B) Without appropriate therapy, infection spreads to involve both lungs diffusely with a patchy infiltrate and multiple small cavities.

Condition	Imaging Findings	Comments
Candidiasis	Patchy, segmental, homogeneous air-space consolidation.	Reflects hematogenous dissemination. Cavitation and hilar adenopathy may occur.
Aspergillosis (see Fig C 22-1)	Single or multiple areas of consolidation with poorly defined margins.	Almost always a secondary infection in which the fungus colonizes a damaged bronchial tree, pulmonary cyst, or cavity of a patient with underlying lung disease. The radiographic hallmark is a pulmonary mycetoma, a solid homogeneous rounded mass separated from the wall of the cavity by a crescent-shaped air space.
Mucormycosis (see Fig C 11-7)	Progressive severe pneumonia that is widespread and confluent and often cavitates.	Occurs in patients with diabetes or an underlying malignancy (leukemia, lymphoma). Usually originates in the nose and paranasal sinuses, where the infection may destroy the walls and create an appearance that simulates a malignant neoplasm.
Sporotrichosis (see Fig C 11-6)	Various nonspecific patterns (fibronodular infiltrates, cavitary nodular masses, chronic pneumonia). Hilar lymph node enlargement is common and may cause bronchial obstruction. Spread through the pleura into the chest wall may produce a sinus tract.	Chronic infection that is usually limited to the skin and the draining lymphatics. In rare instances, disseminated disease can involve the lungs and the skeletal system (extensive destructive arthritis with large-joint effusions).
Mycoplasma/viral infection (Figs C 1-16 and C 1-17)	Patchy air-space consolidation that is usually segmental and predominantly involves the lower lobes. Bilateral and multilobar involvement is common.	Initially, acute interstitial inflammation appears as a fine or coarse reticular pattern. Most infections are mild, though the radiographic signs are more extensive than might be expected from the physical examination.

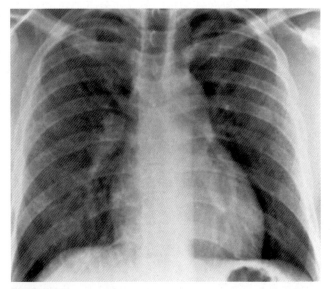

Fig C 1-16
***Mycoplasma* pneumonia.** Initial acute interstitial inflammation produces a diffuse fine reticular pattern.

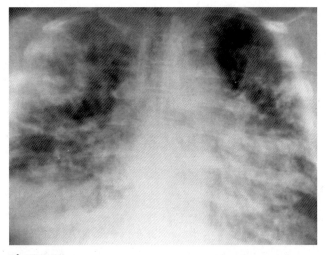

Fig C 1-17
Viral pneumonia. Diffuse peribronchial infiltrate with associated air-space consolidation obscures the heart border (shaggy heart sign). A patchy alveolar infiltrate is present in the right upper lung.

Condition	Imaging Findings	Comments
Mononucleosis	Nonspecific patchy air-space consolidation.	Generalized lymphadenopathy and splenomegaly are characteristic findings. Hilar lymph node enlargement, usually bilateral, can be demonstrated in approximately 15% of cases (see Fig C 11-1). Pneumonia is a rare complication.
Varicella	Extensive bilateral fluffy nodular infiltrate that tends to coalesce near the hilum and lung bases.	Healed varicella pneumonia classically appears as tiny miliary calcifications (see Fig C 17-5), scattered widely throughout both lungs, which develop several years after the acute infection.
Cytomegalovirus	In adults, rapid development of diffuse bilateral alveolar infiltrates that are most common in the outer third of the lungs.	Primarily involves patients with underlying reticuloendothelial disease or immunologic deficiencies, or those receiving immunosuppressive therapy (especially after renal transplantation). May be radiographically indistinguishable from *Pneumocystis carinii* pneumonia.
Rickettsial infection (Fig C 1-18)	Dense, homogeneous, segmental, or lobar consolidation simulating pneumococcal disease. Predominantly affects the lower lobes and may be bilateral.	Pneumonia develops in approximately half the patients with Q fever. Pleural effusion occurs in about one-third of the cases, whereas hilar involvement and small focal lesions are rare.
Parasitic pneumonia *Pneumocystis carinii* (Fig C 1-19; see Figs C 2-14 and C 4-19)	Initially, a hazy, perihilar granular infiltrate that spreads to the periphery and appears predominantly interstitial. In later stages, patchy areas of air-space consolidation with air bronchograms. Massive consolidation with virtually airless lungs may be a terminal appearance.	Common organism in immunosuppressed patients (especially those with AIDS and those treated for lymphoproliferative diseases or with renal transplants). Hilar adenopathy and significant pleural effusions are rare and should suggest an alternative diagnosis. Because the organism cannot be cultured and the disease it causes is usually fatal if untreated, an open-lung biopsy is often necessary if a sputum examination reveals no organisms in a patient suspected of having this disease.

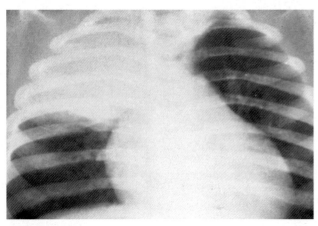

Fig C 1-18
Q fever. Right upper lobe air-space consolidation simulating pneumococcal pneumonia.

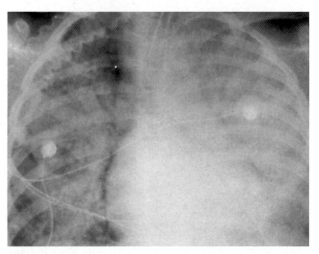

Fig C 1-19
***Pneumocystis carinii* pneumonia.** Severe, bilateral air-space consolidation with air bronchograms. The patient was undergoing immunosuppressive therapy for lymphoma and died shortly after this radiograph was made.

Condition	Imaging Findings	Comments
Amebiasis	Air-space consolidation in the right lower lobe that may be obscured by an extensive pleural effusion.	Usually arises from direct extension of hepatic infection through the right hemidiaphragm (occasionally may be of hematogenous origin).
Toxoplasmosis	Combined interstitial and alveolar disease, often with hilar lymph node enlargement.	Especially virulent organism in immunocompromised patients. Central nervous system involvement is common and may lead to a brain abscess.
Ascariasis (see Fig C 20-4)	Patchy or extensive areas of consolidation that are often bilateral.	Reflects an allergic response caused by larvae migrating through the lungs.
Cutaneous larva migrans (creeping eruption) (see Fig C 20-7)	Transient, migratory pulmonary infiltrates associated with lung and blood eosinophilia.	Pulmonary involvement develops in approximately half the patients about 1 week after the skin eruption caused by penetration and migration of the larvae of the dog and cat hookworm (Ancylostoma braziliense).
Strongyloidiasis (see Fig C 20-5)	Ill-defined patchy areas of air-space consolidation or fine miliary nodules.	Pulmonary manifestations occur during the stage of larval migration (in most patients, the chest radiograph remains normal).
Paragonimiasis (see Figs C 8-3 and C 11-9)	Patchy air-space consolidation that primarily involves the bases of the lungs. Characteristic finding is the "ring shadow," composed of a thin-walled cyst with a prominent crescent-shaped opacity along one side of its border.	Chronic infection of the lung caused by a trematode that is acquired by eating raw, or poorly cooked, infected crabs or crayfish. Although many patients with a heavy infestation are asymptomatic, others present with cough, pain, hemoptysis, and brownish sputum.
Tuberculosis Primary (Fig C 1-20)	In primary disease, a lobar or segmental air-space consolidation that is usually homogeneous, dense, and well defined. Associated enlargement of the hilar or mediastinal lymph nodes is very common (see Figs C 10-1 and C 10-2). Pleural effusion often occurs, especially in adults (see Fig C 33-1).	Primary tuberculosis may affect any lobe. The diagnosis cannot be excluded because the infection is not in the upper lobe. Although traditionally considered a disease of children and young adults, with the dramatic decrease in the prevalence of tuberculosis (especially in children and young adults), primary pulmonary disease can develop at any age.

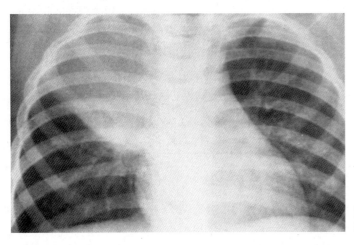

Fig C 1-20
Primary tuberculosis. Consolidation of the right upper lobe.

Condition	Imaging Findings	Comments
Secondary (reactivation)	Initially a nonspecific hazy, poorly marginated alveolar infiltrate that most commonly affects the upper lobes, especially the apical and posterior segments. Cavitation is common (see Fig C 9-3) and may result in bronchogenic spread characterized by multiple patchy infiltrates.	Bilateral (though often asymmetric) upper lobe disease is common and is almost diagnostic of reactivation tuberculosis. Because an apical lesion may be obscured by overlying clavicle or ribs, an apical lordotic view is often of value. Pleural effusion and lymph node enlargement are rare in secondary disease.
Atypical mycobacteria (see Fig C 11-4)	Often radiographically indistinguishable from primary tuberculosis, though pleural effusion and hilar adenopathy are much less common.	Often produces thin-walled cavities with minimal surrounding parenchymal disease. Patients with an atypical mycobacterial infection have a negative tuberculin test and do not respond to antituberculous therapy.
Postobstructive pneumonitis (Fig C 1-21)	Homogeneous increase in density corresponding exactly to a lobe or one or more segments, usually with a substantial loss of volume.	With slowly progressive, obstructive endobronchial processes such as bronchogenic carcinoma and bronchial adenoma, infection is frequent so that there may be only slight or moderate loss of volume. Pneumonitis, bronchiectasis, and abscesses that develop behind the obstruction are usually sufficient to counteract, at least partly, collapse induced by air absorption. The characteristic radiographic picture of "obstructive pneumonitis" should immediately suggest the presence of an obstructing endobronchial lesion. Nonneoplastic causes include mucoid impaction (hypersensitivity aspergillosis), aspirated foreign bodies, and the tracheobronchial form of amyloidosis.
Pulmonary infarct (Fig C 1-22)	Area of consolidation that most commonly involves the lower lobes and is often associated with pleural effusion and elevation of the ipsilateral hemidiaphragm. A highly characteristic, though uncommon, appearance is a pleural-based, wedge-shaped density that has a rounded apex (Hampton hump) and often occurs in the costophrenic sulcus. In many instances, an infarction produces a nonspecific parenchymal density that simulates an acute pneumonia.	Although it is often said that infarction invariably extends to a visceral pleural surface, this is of little diagnostic value, as most pneumonias have a similar appearance. The pattern of resolution of the consolidation is of value in distinguishing among acute inflammatory processes, pulmonary hemorrhage, edema, and frank necrosis. Pulmonary infarctions tend to shrink gradually while retaining the same general configuration seen on initial views (resorption of the perimeter of the infarct with preservation of the pleural base). In contrast, the resolution of pneumonia tends to be patchy and is characterized by a fading of the radiographic density throughout the entire involved area. Parenchymal hemorrhage and edema generally clear within 4 to 7 days; the resolution of necrotic lung tissue usually requires 3 weeks or more.

Condition	Imaging Findings	Comments
Pulmonary contusion Fig C 1-23 (see Figs C 6-14 and C 34-2)	Varies from irregular patchy areas of air-space consolidation to an extensive homogeneous density involving almost an entire lung.	Most common pulmonary complication of blunt chest trauma in which there is exudation of edema and blood into both the air spaces and the interstitium of the lung. In the absence of an appropriate clinical history of trauma or evidence of rib fractures, pulmonary contusion may be indistinguishable from pneumonia. Resolution typically occurs rapidly, with complete clearing within 2 weeks.

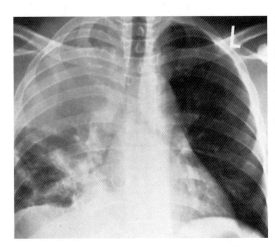

Fig C 1-21
Postobstructive pneumonitis. Homogeneous increased density involving the right upper lobe secondary to carcinoma of the lung. Patchy increased opacification at the right base is due to a combination of atelectasis and infiltrate secondary to extension of the tumor into neighboring bronchi.

A   B

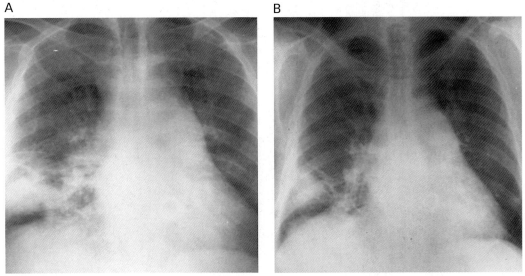

Fig C 1-22
Pulmonary infarction. (A) Chest film made 3 days after open-heart surgery demonstrates a very irregular opacity at the right base (pneumonia versus pulmonary embolization with infarction). (B) On a film made 5 days later, the consolidation is seen to have reduced in size yet to have retained the same general configuration as on the initial view. The diagnosis of pulmonary embolism was confirmed by a radionuclide lung scan.[5]

Condition	Imaging Findings	Comments
Lipoid pneumonia (Fig C 1-24)	Granular pattern of small, scattered alveolar densities that predominantly occur in the perihilar and lower lobe areas.	Caused by the aspiration of various vegetable, animal, or mineral oils into the lungs. As the oil is taken from the alveolar spaces by macrophages that pass into the interstitial space, a fine reticular pattern is produced. Infrequently appears as a granulomatous-lipoid mass that may be huge and may simulate bronchogenic carcinoma (see Fig C 6-15).
Lung torsion	Opacification of the affected lung develops if the torsion is not relieved and the vascular supply is compromised.	Rare complication of trauma that occurs almost invariably in children, presumably because of the easy compressibility of their thoracic cage. Torsion occurs through 180°, that the base of the lung comes to lie at the apex of the hemithorax and the apex at the base. The pulmonary opacification is due to exudation of blood into the air spaces and interstitial tissues.

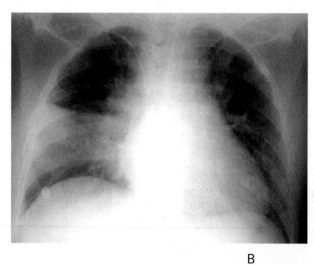

Fig C 1-23
Pulmonary hemorrhage. Consolidation of the middle lobe in a patient with AIDS-related Kaposi's sarcoma.[6]

B

A

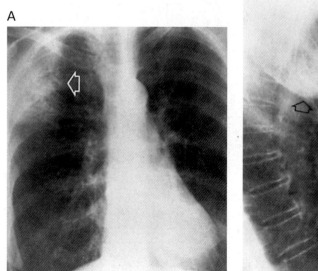
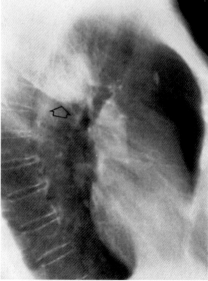

Fig C 1-24
Lipoid pneumonia. (A) Frontal and (B) lateral views demonstrate an air-space consolidation in the posterior segment of the right upper lobe (arrows). Note the prominence of interstitial reticular markings leading from the right hilum to the infiltrate.

Condition	Imaging Findings	Comments
Localized pulmonary edema (Fig C 1-25)	Nonsymmetric, atypical alveolar consolidation.	Most commonly occurs in patients with preexisting lung disease such as chronic emphysema. Unilateral pulmonary edema is most frequently related to dependency.
Bronchioloalveolar (alveolar cell) carcinoma (Fig C 1-26)	In the less common diffuse form, a pattern varying from poorly defined nodules scattered throughout both lungs to irregular pulmonary infiltrates, often with air bronchograms.	More frequently appears as a well-circumscribed, peripheral solitary nodule that often contains an air bronchogram (see Fig C 6-13) (never associated with solitary nodule caused by bronchogenic carcinoma or a granuloma). Although the margins of the tumor are usually well circumscribed, the mass may be poorly defined and simulate an area of focal pneumonia.

A B

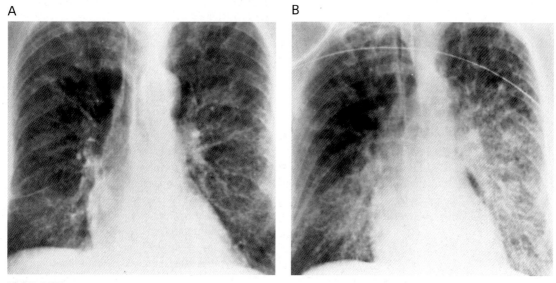

Fig C 1-25
Pulmonary edema in pulmonary emphysema. (A) Initial chest radiograph demonstrates a paucity of vascular markings in the right middle and upper zones along with increased interstitial markings elsewhere. (B) With the onset of congestive heart failure, there is patchy interstitial and alveolar edema that does not affect the segments in which the vascularity had been severely diminished.

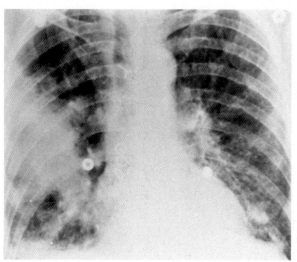

Fig C 1-26
Alveolar cell carcinoma. Patchy, ill-defined right-sided mass simulates an area of focal pneumonia.

Condition	Imaging Findings	Comments
Lymphoma	Patchy areas of parenchymal infiltrate that may coalesce to form a large homogeneous nonsegmental mass. Cavitation and pleural effusion may occur.	Pleuropulmonary involvement usually occurs by direct extension from mediastinal nodes along the lymphatics of the bronchovascular sheaths. At times, it may be difficult to distinguish a superimposed infection after radiation therapy or chemotherapy from the continued spread of lymphomatous tissue. However, any alveolar lung infiltrate in a patient with known lymphoma is more likely to represent an infectious than a lymphomatous process. Primary pulmonary lymphoma is rare and presents as a homogeneous mass that rarely obstructs the bronchial tree and thus almost invariably contains an air bronchogram. When most or all of a segment or lobe is involved, the appearance may simulate acute pneumonia.
Pseudolymphoma	Segmental consolidation extending outward from a hilum and containing an air bronchogram.	Rare benign condition that histologically closely resembles malignant lymphoma. Although apparently segmental, in most cases the consolidation stops short of the visceral pleura at the periphery of the lung.
Löffler's syndrome (idiopathic eosinophilic pneumonia) (see Fig C 18-1)	Transient, rapidly changing, nonsegmental areas of parenchymal consolidation associated with blood eosinophilia. The infiltrates are often located in the periphery of the lung, running more or less parallel to the lateral chest wall and simulating a pleural process.	A similar appearance can develop secondary to parasites (filariasis, ascariasis, cutaneous larva migrans), drug therapy (nitrofurantoin), and fungal infections (hypersensitivity bronchopulmonary aspergillosis). When caused by an identifiable extrinsic agent, the disease usually is acute and responds promptly to the removal of the offending organism or drug. When no obvious cause is detectable, the pulmonary consolidation and eosinophilia tend to be more prolonged and persistent, though there is usually a dramatic response to steroids.
Radiation pneumonitis (Fig C 1-27)	Patchy areas of irregular consolidation that are localized to the radiation port and are often associated with a considerable loss of volume.	Acute radiation pneumonitis is rarely detectable less than 1 month after the end of treatment and must be differentiated from bacterial pneumonia. The late or chronic stage of radiation damage is characterized by extensive fibrosis and loss of volume that may be difficult to distinguish from the lymphangitic spread of a malignant tumor.
Sarcoidosis (see Fig C 2-17)	Ill-defined densities that may be discrete or may coalesce into large areas of segmental consolidation. This pattern resembles an acute inflammatory process and may contain an air bronchogram.	Infrequent manifestation. More characteristic radiographic changes are a diffuse reticulonodular pattern and typical bilateral enlargement of hilar and paratracheal lymph nodes (see Figs C 11-6 and C 12-8).

Condition	Imaging Findings	Comments
Progressive massive fibrosis (pneumoconiosis) (see Figs C 8-9 and C 8-10)	Nonsegmental conglomerate masses that are usually bilateral and relatively symmetric and almost always restricted to the upper half of the lungs. They commonly develop in the mid-zone or periphery of the lung and tend to migrate later toward the hilum, leaving overinflated and emphysematous lung tissue between the consolidation and the pleural surface.	Caused by the confluence of numerous individual nodules in patients with advanced silicosis or coal-miner's pneumoconiosis. The conglomerate fibrotic lesions may cavitate as a result of central ischemic necrosis or tuberculous caseation.
Asbestosis/talcosis	In patients with extensive interstitial fibrosis, large conglomerate opacities may develop that are well or ill defined, are often multiple and nonsegmental, and predominantly involve the lower lung (in contrast to the upper lobe predominance of the conglomerate opacities in silicosis).	Pleural plaque formation, which may be massive and bizarre in shape, is characteristic of both conditions (see Figs C 32-4 and C 32-5). In asbestosis, there is often thin, curvilinear calcification of the diaphragmatic pleura, obscuration of the heart border (shaggy heart sign), and a high incidence of associated malignancy (bronchogenic carcinoma, mesothelioma).
Systemic lupus erythematosus	Nonspecific patchy infiltrate that is more commonly situated peripherally in the lung bases.	Often associated with bilateral pleural effusions and cardiac enlargement due to pericardial effusion (see Fig C 33-4).

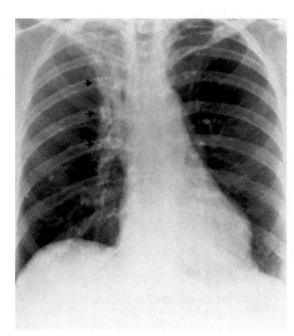

Fig C 1-27
Radiation pneumonitis. After postmastectomy radiation, a mass of fibrous tissue (arrows) extends from the right hilum to parallel the right border of the mediastinum.

Pulmonary Edema Pattern (Symmetric Bilateral Alveolar Pattern)

Condition	Comments
Cardiovascular disease causing pulmonary venous hypertension (Figs C 2-1 and C 2-2)	Most common cause of the pulmonary edema pattern. Usually associated with cardiomegaly (especially if the result of left ventricular failure); other cardiogenic causes include mitral valvular disease, left atrial myxoma, and the hypoplastic left heart syndromes. Noncardiogenic causes include disorders of the pulmonary veins (primary or secondary to mediastinal fibrosis or tumor), veno-occlusive disease, and anomalous pulmonary venous return. Unilateral pulmonary edema is probably most frequently related to dependency (Fig C 2-2). A patchy, asymmetric pattern may develop in patients with emphysema.
Renal failure/uremia (Fig C 2-3)	Causes include acute glomerulonephritis and chronic renal disease. Complex mechanism (left ventricular failure, decreased oncotic pressure, hypervolemia, increased capillary permeability). May produce a dense "butterfly" pattern.

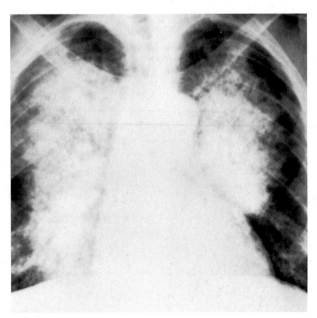

Fig C 2-1
Congestive heart failure. Diffuse bilateral symmetric infiltration of the central portion of the lungs along with relative sparing of the periphery produces the butterfly, or bat's wing, pattern. The margins of the edematous lung are sharply defined. The consolidation is fairly homogeneous and is associated with a well-defined air bronchogram on both sides.[7]

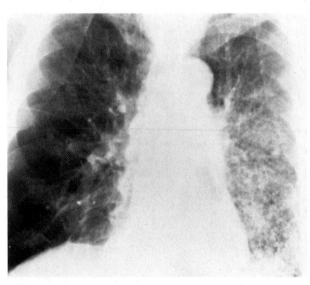

Fig C 2-2
Unilateral pulmonary edema due to dependency. Diffuse alveolar pattern is limited to the left lung.

Condition	Comments
Fluid overload/ overtransfusion (hypervolemia, hypoproteinemia) (Fig C 2-4)	A common cause of the pattern, particularly during the postoperative period and in elderly patients. Rapid clearing with appropriate treatment. The pulmonary edema pattern may also be the result of an incompatible blood transfusion.
Neurogenic/postictal (Fig C 2-5)	An often asymmetric pattern of pulmonary edema may develop after head trauma, seizures, or stroke. Related to increased intracranial pressure (typically disappears within several days after surgical relief). Normal heart size (if no underlying cardiac disease).

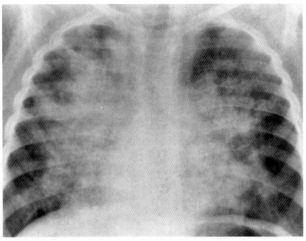

Fig C 2-3
Chronic renal failure. Typical perihilar alveolar densities producing the butterfly pattern of uremic lung. Unlike pulmonary edema due to congestive heart failure, in chronic renal failure the cardiac silhouette is of normal size.

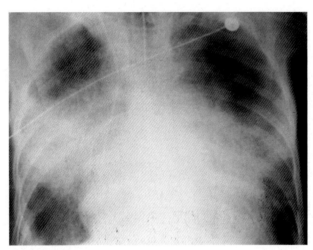

Fig C 2-4
Fluid overload. Pulmonary edema pattern developing in the postoperative period in an elderly patient. Note the endotracheal tube and pulmonary artery catheter.

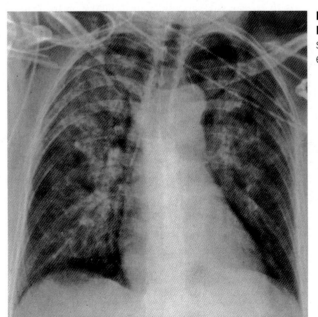

Fig C 2-5
Neurogenic pulmonary edema. Diffuse bilateral air-space consolidations with a heart of normal size and no evidence of pleural effusions or Kerley lines.[109]

Condition	Comments
Inhalation of noxious gases (Fig C 2-6)	Transient pulmonary edema pattern that develops within a few hours of exposure and clears within a few days (if not fatal). Causes include the inhalation of nitrogen dioxide (silo-filler's disease), sulfur dioxide, phosgene, chlorine, carbon monoxide, and hydrocarbon compounds.
Aspiration of gastric contents (Mendelson's syndrome)	Often an asymmetric pattern of pulmonary edema (depends on the position of the patient when aspiration occurred). Caused by vomiting related to anesthesia, seizure, or coma (alcohol or barbiturate poisoning, cerebrovascular accident). Grave prognosis unless immediate steroid and antibiotic therapy (then resolves in 7 to 10 days).
Near-drowning (Fig C 2-7)	No radiographic difference between fresh and saltwater aspiration. Complete resolution, usually in 7 to 10 days.
Aspiration of hypertonic contrast material	High osmotic force causes massive influx of fluid into the alveolar air spaces.
High altitude	Pulmonary edema pattern (often irregular and patchy) is a manifestation of mountain or altitude sickness. Rapid clearing after oxygen administration or return to sea level.
Transient tachypnea of newborn	Loss of definition of prominent vascular markings due to retained fetal lung fluid that clears rapidly in 1 to 4 days. Normal heart size. Predisposing factors include cesarean section, prematurity, breech delivery, and maternal diabetes.
Rapid re-expansion of lungs (post-thoracentesis)	Unilateral pulmonary edema pattern (unless both lungs re-expanded) that follows the rapid removal of large amounts of air or fluid from the pleural space.
Fat embolism (Fig C 2-8)	Develops 1 to 2 days after trauma (usually leg fractures). The radiographic resolution requires 7 days or longer. Absence of cardiomegaly, pulmonary venous hypertension, and interstitial edema differentiates this condition from cardiogenic edema.

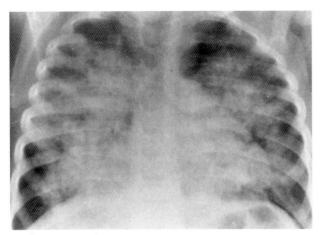

Fig C 2-6
Hydrocarbon poisoning. Diffuse pulmonary edema pattern, with the alveolar consolidation most prominent in the central portions of the lung.

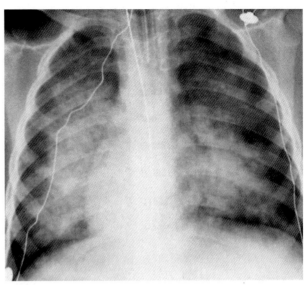

Fig C 2-7
Near-drowning. Diffuse pulmonary edema pattern.

A

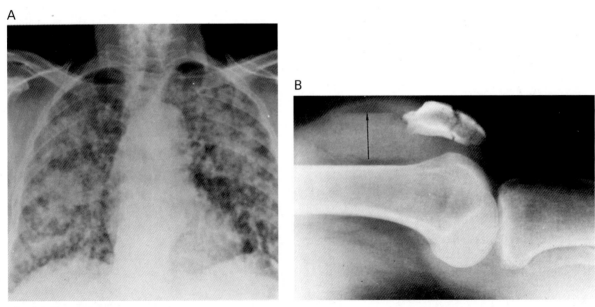

B

Fig C 2-8
Fat embolism. (A) Frontal chest radiograph made 3 days after a leg fracture demonstrates diffuse bilateral air-space consolidation due to alveolar hemorrhage and edema. Unlike cardiogenic pulmonary edema, the distribution in this patient is predominantly peripheral rather than central, and the heart is not enlarged. (B) Recumbent radiograph of the knee obtained with a horizontal beam demonstrates the characteristic fat-blood interface (arrow) in a large suprapatellar effusion. Marrow fat that enters torn peripheral vessels can be trapped by the pulmonary circulation and lead to diffuse alveolar consolidation.[8]

Condition	Comments
Amniotic fluid embolism (Fig C 2-9)	Diffuse air-space consolidation that is virtually indistinguishable from the appearance caused by other forms of acute pulmonary edema. The entrance of amniotic fluid containing particulate matter into the maternal circulation during spontaneous delivery or cesarean section can cause sudden and massive obstruction of the pulmonary vascular bed, leading to shock and often death. Because the condition is often rapidly fatal, radiographs are infrequently obtained; most of the rare nonfatal cases are incorrectly diagnosed.
Thoracic trauma (contused lung) (Fig C 2-10)	Alveolar edema pattern due to contusion or hemorrhage is the most common pulmonary complication of blunt chest trauma. The appearance is seldom symmetric (involvement is greater on the side of maximum impact). Unlike traumatic fat embolism, the radiographic changes of pulmonary contusion and hemorrhage are apparent soon after trauma and resolve rapidly (usually in 1 to 7 days).
Nontraumatic pulmonary hemorrhage (Figs C 2-11 and C 2-12)	Bilateral alveolar consolidation that may occur in patients with bleeding diatheses, idiopathic pulmonary hemosiderosis, Goodpasture's syndrome, polyarteritis nodosa, or Wegener's granulomatosis. There is usually clearing 2 to 3 days after a single bleeding episode, though reticular changes may persist much longer.

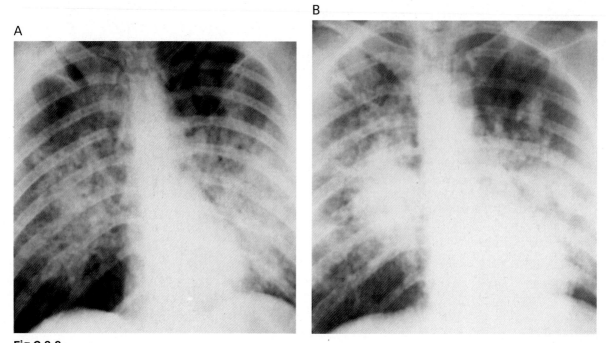

Fig C 2-9
Amniotic fluid embolism. (A) Initial film 6 hours after the onset of acute symptoms, showing heavy bilateral perihilar infiltrate. (B) Twelve hours later, the infiltrates have become more confluent in the perihilar zones.[9]

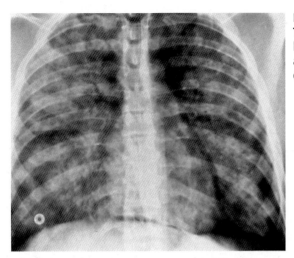

Fig C 2-10
Thoracic trauma. Continuous positive-pressure ventilation has caused diffuse interstitial emphysema, pneumothorax, and pneumoperitoneum to be superimposed on a pattern of diffuse alveolar opacities.

A   B

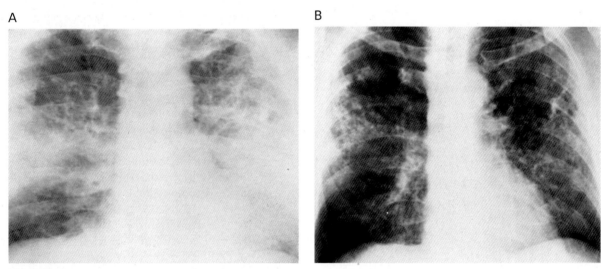

Fig C 2-11
Pulmonary hemorrhage. (A) Diffuse bilateral air-space consolidation developed in a patient receiving high-dose anticoagulant therapy. (B) With resolution of the hemorrhage, a reticular pattern is seen in the same distribution as the alveolar infiltrate.

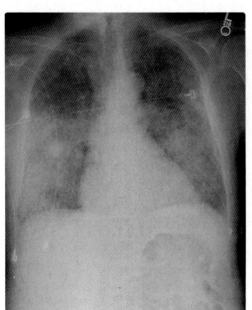

Fig C 2-12
Goodpasture's syndrome. Frontal chest film in a patient with massive pulmonary hemorrhage demonstrates extensive bilateral pulmonary consolidation, which is confluent in most areas. Note the normal heart size.

Condition	Comments
Acute radiation pneumonitis	Alveolar edema pattern is generally confined to the irradiated area. Rarely develops while the patient is receiving radiation therapy (radiographic changes are seldom apparent until at least 1 month after the end of treatment).
Narcotic abuse (Fig C 2-13)	Alveolar pulmonary edema pattern that may be unilateral due to gravitational influences. Most commonly a complication of heroin or methadone abuse. The radiographic findings may be delayed 6 to 10 hours after admission, and there is usually rapid resolution (1 to 2 days). The persistence of an edema pattern after 48 hours suggests aspiration or superimposed bacterial pneumonia.
Cocaine abuse (Fig C 2-14)	Both cardiogenic and noncardiogenic pulmonary edema have been reported in association with intravenous cocaine abuse and crack cocaine smoking and are common findings at autopsies of drug addicts. The pathogenesis of cocaine-induced pulmonary edema is complex and multifactorial. Myocardial ischemia and infarction, myocardial dysfunction, arrhythmia, and dilated cardiomyopathy may be contributing factors in cardiogenic edema. Damage to the pulmonary capillary endothelium with increased permeability may play a role in noncardiogenic edema.
Adult respiratory distress syndrome (ARDS) or "shock lung" (Fig C 2-15)	Bilateral pulmonary edema pattern that is typically delayed up to 12 hours after the clinical onset of respiratory failure. Severe, unexpected, life-threatening acute respiratory distress developing in a patient with no major underlying lung disease. Causes include sepsis, oxygen toxicity, disseminated intravascular coagulation, and cardiopulmonary bypass.

A   B

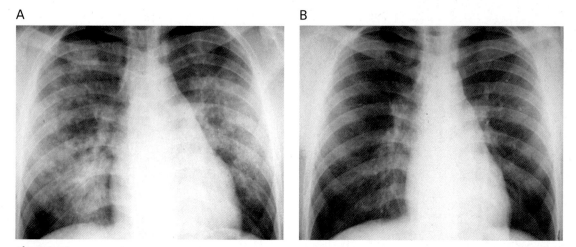

Fig C 2-13
Heroin abuse. (A) Initial radiograph obtained shortly after presentation to the emergency department reveals bilateral areas of increased opacity, a finding consistent with acute lung injury. (B) Follow-up study obtained two days later shows complete clearing of the areas of increased opacity. Such rapid clearing is common in heroin-induced lung injury.[10]

Condition	Comments
Pneumonia (Figs C 2-16 and C 2-17)	Bilateral alveolar infiltrates may develop after a broad spectrum of infections. The underlying organisms include bacteria, fungi, mycoplasma, viruses, malaria, and even worm infestation (almost invariably blood eosinophilia). In patients with AIDS, a butterfly pattern sparing the periphery of the lung is highly suggestive of *Pneumocystis carinii* pneumonia.

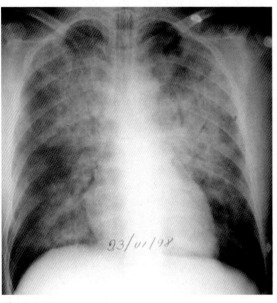

Fig C 2-14
Cocaine abuse. Extensive bilateral heterogeneous central and parahilar opacities representing cardiogenic pulmonary edema in a woman who presented with shortness of breath and chest pain after smoking crack cocaine.[11]

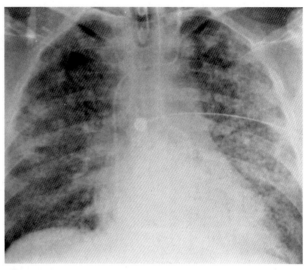

Fig C 2-15
Adult respiratory distress syndrome. Ill-defined areas of alveolar consolidation with some coalescence scattered throughout both lungs.

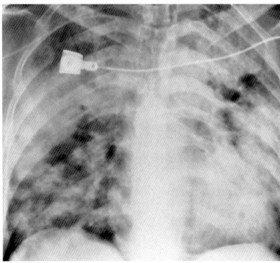

Fig C 2-16
Plague pneumonia. Diffuse air-space consolidation involves both lungs.

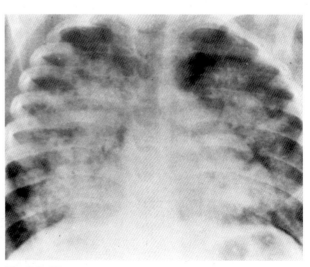

Fig C 2-17
Pneumocystis carinii **pneumonia in acquired immunodeficiency syndrome.** Diffuse bilateral pulmonary infiltrates.

Condition	Comments
Neoplasm	Symmetric bilateral alveolar infiltrates, usually associated with reticulonodular and linear densities, may develop in patients with alveolar cell carcinoma or lymphangitic metastases. Patients with lymphoma and leukemia may also develop bilateral alveolar infiltrates that predominantly involve the perihilar areas and lower lungs, though these findings are more often due to superimposed pneumonia, drug reaction, or hemorrhage than to the underlying malignancy itself.
Alveolar microlithiasis (Fig C 2-18)	Rare disease of unknown etiology characterized by the presence of a myriad of very fine micronodules of calcific density in the alveoli of the lungs of a usually asymptomatic person. Characteristic "black pleura" sign (due to contrast between the extreme density of the lung parenchyma on one side of the pleura and the ribs on the other side).
Alveolar proteinosis (Fig C 2-19)	Rare condition of unknown etiology characterized by the deposition in the air spaces of the lung of a somewhat granular material high in protein and lipid content. The bilateral and symmetric alveolar infiltrates are identical in distribution and character to those of pulmonary edema, though there is no evidence of cardiac enlargement or pulmonary venous hypertension. There is usually complete radiographic resolution, though it may occur asymmetrically and in a spotty fashion and may even be associated with the development of new foci of air-space consolidation in areas not previously affected.
Sarcoidosis (Fig C 2-20)	Infrequent manifestation (more commonly a diffuse reticulonodular pattern). Hilar and mediastinal lymph nodes are often enlarged.
Drug hypersensitivity/ allergy (penicillin)	Rapid development of an alveolar edema pattern.
Pulmonary embolism with infarction	Bilateral alveolar consolidation, primarily involving the lower zones, is a rare manifestation of extensive thromboembolism with infarction. Associated findings include enlarged central pulmonary arteries with rapid tapering, loss of lung volume (elevated hemidiaphragms), small pleural effusions, and a prominent azygos vein. The radiographic appearance is usually rather benign, considering the severity of the clinical symptoms.

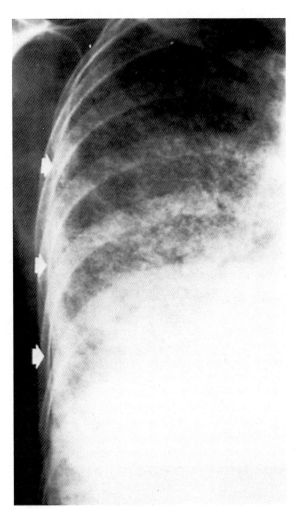

Fig C 2-18
Alveolar microlithiasis. Nearly uniform distribution of typical fine, sand-like mottling in the lungs. The tangential shadow of the pleura is displayed along the lateral wall of the chest as a dark lucent strip (arrows).[12]

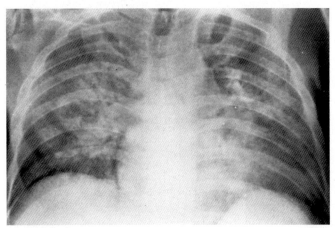

Fig C 2-19
Pulmonary alveolar proteinosis. Diffuse, bilateral air-space consolidation predominantly involves the central portions of the lung and simulates pulmonary edema. The patient was asymptomatic, and serial radiographs over several months showed little change.

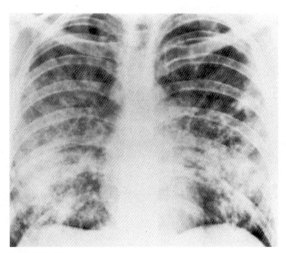

Fig C 2-20
Sarcoidosis. Diffuse reticular nodular and alveolar infiltrates.

Unilateral Pulmonary Edema Pattern

Condition	Comments
Ipsilateral pulmonary edema	
Rapid thoracentesis of large pleural effusion/ rapid evacuation of a pneumothorax (Fig C 3-1)	Typically occurs during the procedure or within 1 hour after it. Rapid re-expansion of the collapsed lung with a sudden increase in hydrostatic pressure and persistent high surface tension results in edema.
Prolonged lateral decubitus position (Fig C 3-2)	Gravity raises the hydrostatic pressure in the dependent lung, impairing circulation and affecting the production of surfactant. This mechanism may occur in some patients with methadone-induced edema who are found unconscious and lying on one side.
Pulmonary contusion (Fig C 3-3)	Direct damage to the pulmonary capillaries may cause not only intrapulmonary bleeding but also exudation of cells leading to edema. Blood products in the alveoli may also disrupt the surfactant system.

A   B

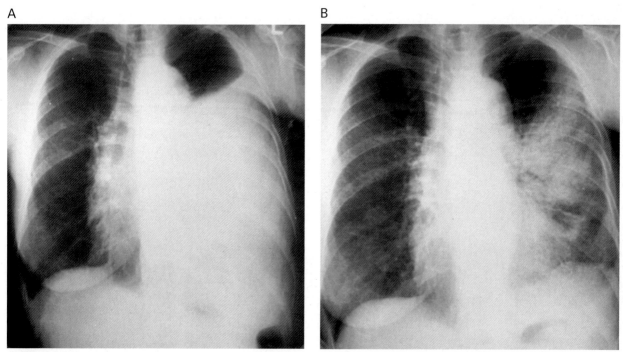

Fig C 3-1

Rapid thoracentesis. (A) Initial radiograph of an elderly woman with metastatic adenocarcinoma of the breast and a massive left pleural effusion. (B) Repeat examination taken 2 hours after the rapid removal of 2500 mL of fluid shows a left-sided pulmonary edema. The segment of left lung not compressed by effusion remains free of edema. Over the next 6 days, the edema resolved spontaneously.[13]

Condition	Comments
Postoperative systemic-to-pulmonary artery shunts (congenital heart disease)	Dramatic and almost immediate reaction resulting from increased blood flow to the side with the anastomosis. The Waterston and Blalock-Taussig procedures produce right-sided edema; the Potts procedure results in left-sided edema. In either case, increased blood flow causes high hydrostatic pressure. This results in increased venous pressure combined with pulmonary capillary damage and decreased surfactant, producing high surface tension.

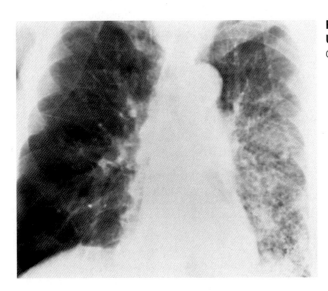

Fig C 3-2
Unilateral pulmonary edema due to dependency. The diffuse alveolar pattern is limited to the left lung.

A

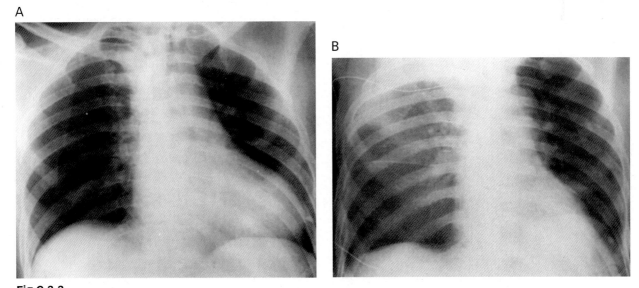

B

Fig C 3-3
Pulmonary contusion. (A) Admission chest radiograph shows several right rib fractures and an early right perihilar infiltrate. (B) Repeat examination shows right-sided post-traumatic pulmonary edema and capillary hemorrhage that developed the next day and persisted for a few weeks. An organized extrapleural hematoma is present in the right apex.[13]

Condition	Comments
Bronchial obstruction ("drowned lung")	Pulmonary edema in airless lung tissue peripheral to a totally obstructed bronchus is related to increased surface tension resulting from disruption of the alveolar lining layer caused by hypoxia due to loss of blood flow. This phenomenon usually clears within 1–24 hours after removal of the obstruction. Infection plays no role in this process.
Unilateral veno-occlusive disease	Congenital obstruction of pulmonary venous return or venous occlusion by primary or metastatic tumor causes edema, when the venous pressure rises higher than the colloid osmotic pressure of the blood.
Unilateral aspiration	Edema secondary to direct irritation of the alveolar lining layer with increased capillary permeability and an adverse effect on the surfactant system may develop unilaterally in patients after aspiration of freshwater or seawater, ethyl alcohol, kerosene, or gastric juices during anesthesia, a coma, or an epileptic seizure.
Central venous pressure catheter misdirected into a pulmonary artery	Rapid infusion of hypotonic saline stimulates neural reflexes and possibly a release of vasoactive substances resulting from a local decrease in colloid osmotic pressure.
Contralateral pulmonary edema	
Perfusion defects (Fig C 3-4)	Because an unperfused area cannot become edematous, contralateral pulmonary edema (ie, edema affecting only the normally perfused lung) can occur in such conditions as unilateral pulmonary emphysema with destruction of the capillary bed in the affected lung; congenital absence or hypoplasia of a pulmonary artery; Swyer-James syndrome; pulmonary thromboembolism involving an entire lung; and after lobectomy, in which the remaining lung becomes emphysematous on a compensatory basis and thus is underperfused.
Re-expansion of pneumothorax in a patient with left heart failure	Temporary compromise of perfusion of the previously collapsed lung due to increased pulmonary vascular resistance permits edema to occur only in the opposite lung.

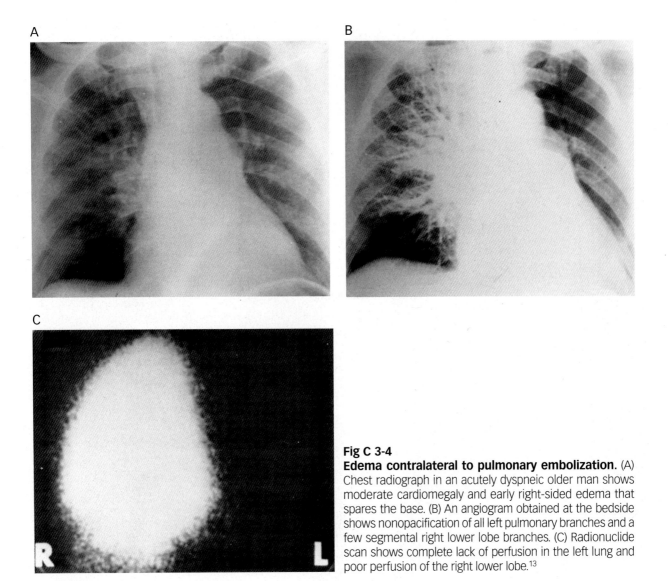

A

B

C

R   L

Fig C 3-4
Edema contralateral to pulmonary embolization. (A)
Chest radiograph in an acutely dyspneic older man shows
moderate cardiomegaly and early right-sided edema that
spares the base. (B) An angiogram obtained at the bedside
shows nonopacification of all left pulmonary branches and a
few segmental right lower lobe branches. (C) Radionuclide
scan shows complete lack of perfusion in the left lung and
poor perfusion of the right lower lobe.[13]

Diffuse Reticular or Reticulonodular Pattern

Condition	Comments
Lymphangitic metastases (Fig C 4-1)	More prominent in the lower lung zones and often associated with pleural effusion and enlargement of hilar or mediastinal lymph nodes. Most frequent primary tumor sites are the breast, stomach, thyroid, pancreas, larynx, cervix, and lung.
Lymphoma (Fig C 4-2)	Usually associated with hilar and mediastinal lymph node enlargement in Hodgkin's disease (often absent in non-Hodgkin's lymphoma). A similar pattern may occur in the terminal stages of leukemia.

A

B

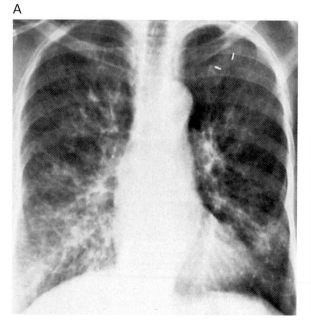
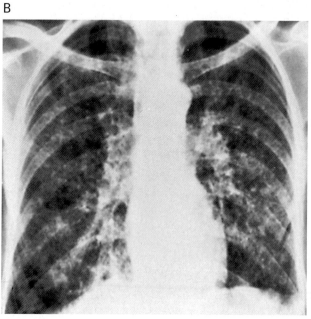

Fig C 4-1
Lymphangitic metastases. (A) Coarsened bronchovascular markings of irregular contour and poor definition primarily involve the right lower lung. Note the septal (Kerley) lines and the left mastectomy in this patient with carcinoma of the breast. (B) In this patient with metastatic carcinoma of the stomach, a superimposed nodular component representing hematogenous deposits produces a coarse reticulonodular pattern.

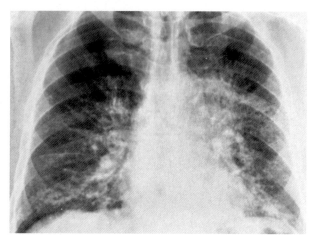

Fig C 4-2
Lymphoma. Diffuse reticular and reticulonodular changes, with striking prominence of the left hilar region.

Condition	Comments

Inorganic dust inhalation
(pneumoconiosis)

Silicosis
(Fig C 4-3)

Often more prominent in the middle and upper lung zones. Frequent enlargement of hilar lymph nodes ("eggshell" calcification is infrequent but almost pathognomonic). Other radiographic patterns include well-circumscribed nodular opacities and progressive massive fibrosis. In Caplan's syndrome, silicosis is associated with rheumatoid arthritis and rheumatoid necrobiotic nodules (see Fig C 7-7).

Asbestosis
(Fig C 4-4)

In the early stages, more prominent in the lower lung zones. The major radiographic abnormalities are pleural thickening, plaque formation, and calcification. A combination of parenchymal and pleural changes may partially obscure the heart border (shaggy heart sign). High incidence of mesothelioma (also bronchogenic and alveolar cell carcinoma).

Other inorganic dusts
(Figs C 4-5 to C 4-7)

Numerous conditions such as talcosis, berylliosis, coal-workers' pneumoconiosis, aluminum (bauxite) pneumoconiosis, and radiopaque dust causing dense nodules (siderosis [iron], stannosis [tin], baritosis [barium], antimony, and rare-earth compounds). Also occurs from talc (magnesium silicate) in intravenous drug abusers.

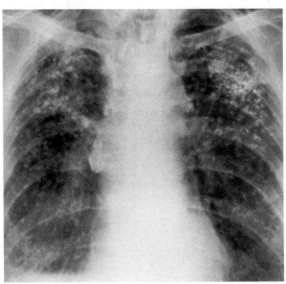

Fig C 4-3
Silicosis. Prominence of interstitial markings, upward retraction of the hila, and bilateral calcific densities that tend to conglomerate in the upper lobes.

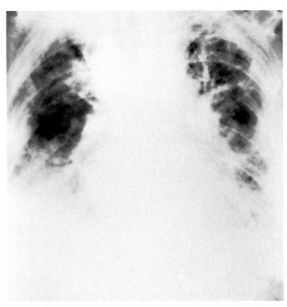

Fig C 4-4
Asbestosis. Severe disorganization of lung architecture with generalized coarse reticulation, which has become confluent in the right base and obliterates the right hemidiaphragm. There is marked pleural thickening, particularly in the apical and axillary regions. A spontaneous pneumothorax is on the left.[7]

Condition	Comments
Organic dust inhalation (Figs C 4-8 and C 4-9)	Late stage in such conditions as farmer's lung, bird-breeder's lung, silo-filler's disease (nitrogen dioxide), bagassosis (sugar cane), byssinosis (cotton), and mushroom-worker's lung.
Oxygen toxicity (Fig C 4-10)	Most commonly develops in infants undergoing long-term oxygen therapy for respiratory distress (has also been described in adults). Fibrosis, atelectasis, and focal areas of emphysema produce a "spongy" lung.

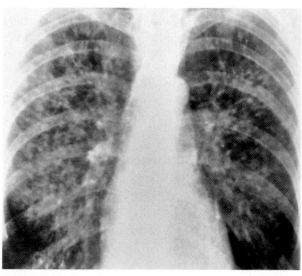

Fig C 4-5
Berylliosis. Diffuse reticulonodular pattern throughout both lungs, with relative sparing of the apices and bases.

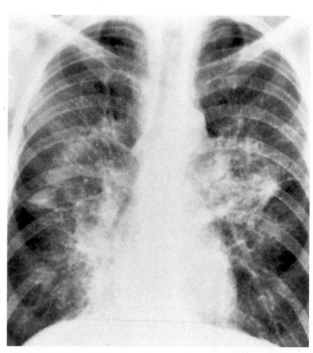

Fig C 4-6
Coal-workers' pneumoconiosis. Ill-defined masses of fibrous tissue in the perihilar region extend to the right base.

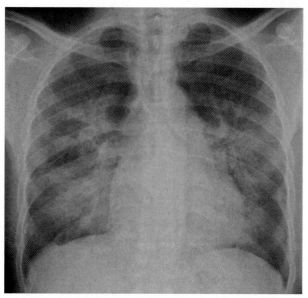

Fig C 4-7
Talc granulomatosis. File nodular opacities and areas of coalescence in an intravenous drug abuser.[11]

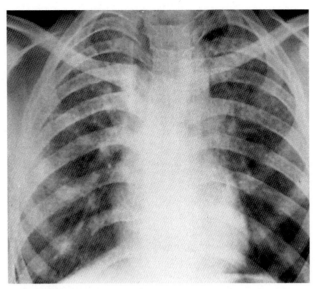

Fig C 4-8
Pigeon-breeder's lung. Diffuse reticulonodular infiltrate primarily involves the perihilar and upper lobe regions.

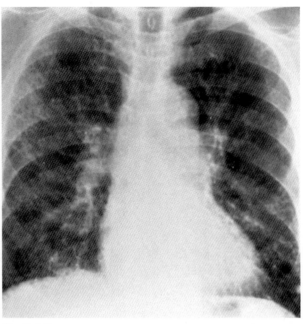

Fig C 4-9
Byssinosis. Prolonged exposure has resulted in irreversible pulmonary insufficiency and a diffuse reticular pattern.

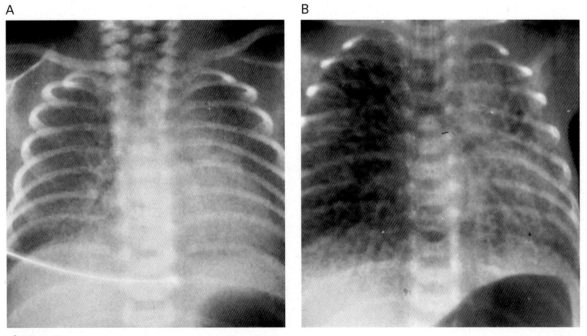

Fig C 4-10
Oxygen toxicity. (A) Initial chest radiograph of an infant demonstrates a typical granular parenchymal pattern with air bronchograms due to hyaline membrane disease. (B) After intensive oxygen therapy, multiple small round lucencies resembling bullae have developed, giving the lungs a sponge-like appearance.

Condition	Comments
Drug-induced pulmonary disease (Figs C 4-11 and C 4-12)	Allergic reaction to the drug with associated eosinophilia (nitrofurantoin) or toxic effect of a chemotherapeutic agent (busulfan, bleomycin, methotrexate).
Connective tissue disorders	
Scleroderma (see Fig C 5-5)	More prominent in the lung bases. Extrapulmonary findings include abnormal peristalsis of the esophagus and small bowel, erosion of the terminal tufts, and calcification in the fingertips.
Dermatomyositis/ polymyositis	More prominent in the lung bases. May have a coexisting primary malignancy elsewhere.
Rheumatoid disease (Fig C 4-13)	More prominent in the lung bases. Usually associated with evidence of rheumatoid arthritis.
Systemic lupus erythematosus	More prominent in the lung bases. Often has a coexisting pleural effusion.
Sjögren's syndrome	More prominent in the lung bases. Triad of keratoconjunctivitis sicca, xerostomia, and recurrent swelling of the parotid gland. Strong predominance in females. Changes in the joints resemble those of rheumatoid or psoriatic arthritis.
Chronic bronchitis (Fig C 4-14)	Coarse increase in interstitial markings ("dirty chest") that is often associated with emphysema and signs of pulmonary arterial hypertension.
"Small airways disease"	Inflammatory narrowing, mucous plugging, and fibrous obliteration of small airways of the lungs.

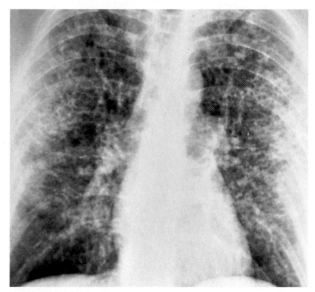

Fig C 4-11
Busulfan-induced lung disease. Severe coarse reticular pattern.

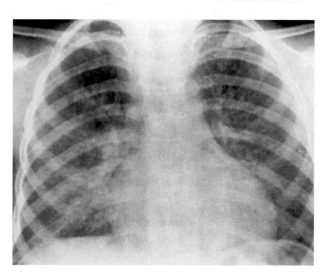

Fig C 4-12
Methotrexate-induced lung disease. Diffuse interstitial pattern with patches of alveolar consolidation in a child treated for myelogenous leukemia. After methotrexate therapy ended, there was rapid clinical and radiographic improvement.[14]

Condition	Comments
Acute bronchiolitis	More prominent in the lower lung zones and associated with severe overinflation of the lungs. Generally affects young children (under 3 years) and adults with pre-existing chronic respiratory disease. Bronchiolitis obliterans is the end stage of lower respiratory tract damage due to a variety of diseases.

A   B

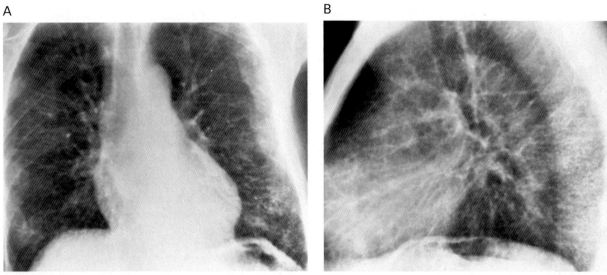

Fig C 4-13
Rheumatoid lung. (A) Frontal and (B) lateral views of the chest show diffuse thickening of the interstitial structures with prominent pleural thickening.

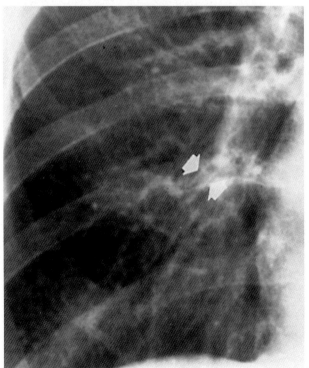

Fig C 4-14
Chronic bronchitis. Coned view of the right lower lung demonstrates a coarse increase in interstitial markings. The arrows point to the characteristic parallel-line shadows ("tramlines") outside the boundary of the pulmonary hilum.

Condition	Comments
Interstitial pulmonary edema (Fig C 4-15)	Loss of the normal sharp definition of pulmonary vascular markings (especially in the lower lung zones), perihilar haze, and thickening of the interlobular septa (Kerley-B lines). Also cardiomegaly and often redistribution of pulmonary blood flow from the lower to the upper lobes. Recurrent episodes of interstitial and alveolar edema and hemorrhage in patients with chronic left heart failure may result in the development of a coarse, often poorly defined reticular pattern that predominantly involves the middle and lower lung zones.
Infectious agents Tuberculosis (Fig C 4-16)	Localized or generalized prominence of interstitial structures reflects the healing phase in which tuberculous granulation tissue is replaced by fibrosis. The resulting scarring may result in considerable loss of volume.
Fungal infections (Fig C 4-17)	Localized or generalized prominence of interstitial structures may develop secondary to coccidioidomycosis, cryptococcosis, blastomycosis, and histoplasmosis.
Viral pneumonia (Fig C 4-18)	Generalized prominence of bronchovascular markings that may be a manifestation of various viral agents.

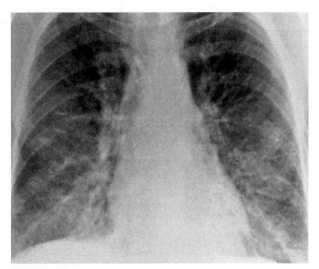

Fig C 4-15
Interstitial pulmonary edema. Edema fluid in the interstitial space causes a loss of the normal sharp definition of pulmonary vascular markings and a perihilar haze. At the bases, note the thin horizontal lines of increased density (Kerley-B lines) that represent fluid in the interlobular septa.

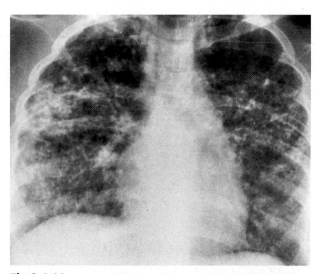

Fig C 4-16
Secondary tuberculosis. Diffuse interstitial fibrosis pattern.

Condition	Comments
Mycoplasma (Fig C 4-19)	More prominent in the lower lung zones. This appearance is less common than the localized form, in which a fine reticular infiltrate progresses rapidly to consolidation.

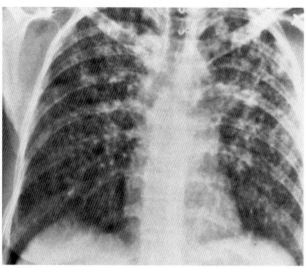

Fig C 4-17
Blastomycosis. Diffuse interstitial disease with upper lobe predominance. Note the volume loss in the upper lobe and the overdistention of the lower lobes along with the formation of bullae at the bases.[4]

A

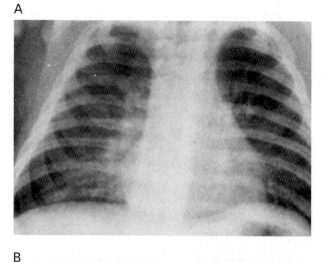

B

Fig C 4-18
Viral pneumonia. Diffuse interstitial infiltrates with perihilar haze in (A) a child and (B) an adult.

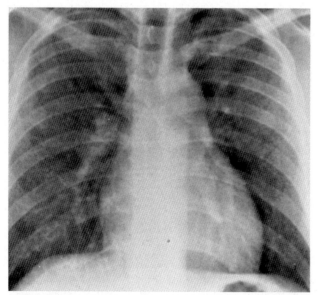

Fig C 4-19
Mycoplasma pneumoniae. Diffuse, fine reticular pattern represents acute interstitial inflammation. The radiographic pattern is indistinguishable from that of most viral pneumonias.

Condition	Comments
Pneumocystis carinii (Fig C 4-20)	More prominent in the perihilar areas. This pattern occurs in the early stages of the disease and is followed by patchy consolidations simulating pulmonary edema.
Schistosomiasis	Probably produced by migration of ova through vessel walls with subsequent reaction to these foreign bodies. Vascular obstruction may cause pulmonary hypertension (dilatation of central pulmonary arteries with rapid peripheral tapering).
Filariasis (see Fig C 18-6)	Tropical pulmonary eosinophilia. Patients with pulmonary disease usually do not have the characteristic cutaneous and lymphatic changes as in elephantiasis.
Toxoplasmosis	Early stage of the disease. Hilar lymph node enlargement is common.
Sarcoidosis (Figs C 4-21 and C 4-22)	Frequently associated with hilar and mediastinal lymph node enlargement, which often regresses spontaneously as the parenchymal disease develops.
Pulmonary Langerhans cell histiocytosis (Fig C 4-23)	More prominent in the upper lung zones. Most common cause of the coarse "honeycomb" pattern. Spontaneous pneumothorax is a frequent complication. Approximately one-third of patients are asymptomatic when initially diagnosed on a screening chest radiograph.

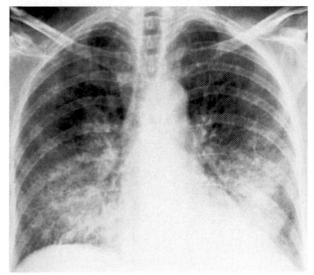

Fig C 4-20
Pneumocystis carinii. Diffuse reticular pattern in a patient with acute myelogenous leukemia. Note the early development of alveolar consolidations at the bases. A later film showed the typical pulmonary edema pattern.

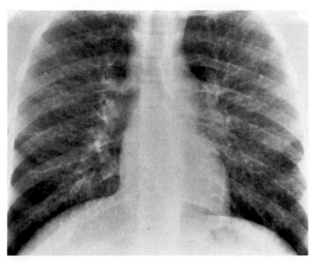

Fig C 4-21
Sarcoidosis. Diffuse reticulonodular pattern widely distributed throughout both lungs.

Condition

Cystic fibrosis (Fig C 4-24)

Comments

Coarse reticular pattern with overinflation of the lungs. Often segmental areas of consolidation or atelectasis due to pneumonia or bronchiectasis. Pulmonary fibrosis along the cardiac border may produce the shaggy heart appearance.

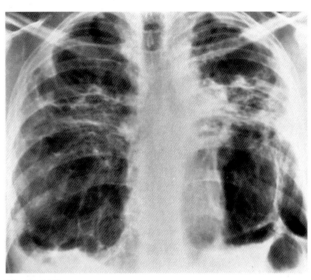

Fig C 4-22
Sarcoidosis. In end-stage disease, there is severe fibrous scarring, bleb formation, and emphysema.

A

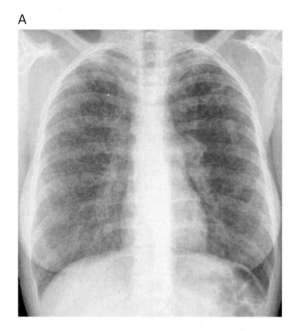

B

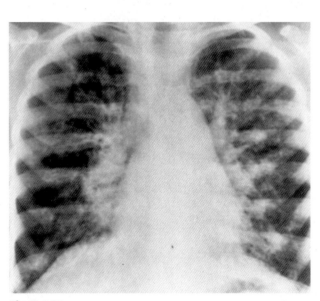

Fig C 4-24
Cystic fibrosis. Diffuse peribronchial thickening appears as a perihilar infiltrate associated with hyperexpansion and flattening of the hemidiaphragms.

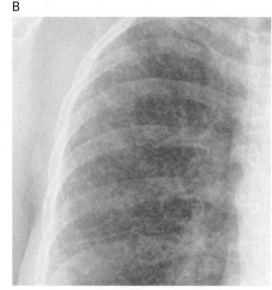

Fig C 4-23
Pulmonary Langerhans cell histiocytosis. (A) Frontal view shows widespread cystic changes in the lung and subsequent diffuse reticular opacities produced by the overlapping cysts. (B) Magnified view of the right upper lung shows the confluent superimposed lung cysts in detail.[15]

Condition	Comments
Dysautonomia (familial autonomic dysfunction; Riley-Day syndrome) (Fig C 4-25)	Appearance identical to that of cystic fibrosis. Often associated with patchy areas of pneumonia and atelectasis. An autosomal recessive condition, found almost exclusively in Jews, which causes widespread neurologic abnormalities.
Usual interstitial pneumonia (UIP) (Fig C 4-26)	Most commonly seen in patients with idiopathic pulmonary fibrosis. In the early stages, more prominent in the lower lung zones. Progressive volume loss on sequential studies.
Desquamative interstitial pneumonia (DIP) (Fig C 4-27)	More prominent in the lower lung zones. Progressive loss of lung volume on sequential studies. Spontaneous pneumothorax and pleural effusion may occur.
Idiopathic pulmonary hemosiderosis/ Goodpasture's syndrome	Often more prominent in the perihilar areas and the middle and lower lung zones. Initially represents a transition stage from acute air-space hemorrhage to complete resolution. Persistence of the reticular pattern after several bleeding episodes indicates irreversible interstitial fibrosis. Repeated pulmonary hemorrhage results in anemia and pulmonary insufficiency (also renal disease in Goodpasture's syndrome).

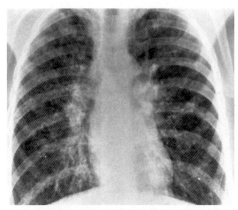

Fig C 4-25
Dysautonomia. Pattern identical to that of cystic fibrosis.

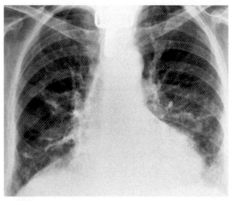

Fig C 4-26
Usual interstitial pneumonia. Diffuse, coarse reticulonodular pattern.

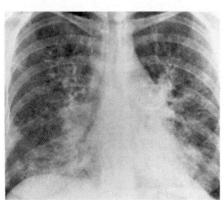

Fig C 4-27
Desquamative interstitial pneumonia.
Diffuse reticulonodular pattern indicating interstitial disease, combined with bibasilar air-space consolidation that obscures the borders of the heart.

Condition	Comments
Amyloidosis (Fig C 4-28)	More prominent in the lower lung zones. Hilar and mediastinal lymph nodes may be markedly enlarged (occasionally densely calcified).
Waldenström's macroglobulinemia	Rare lymphoproliferative disorder in which there is usually hepatosplenomegaly and palpable peripheral adenopathy.
Tuberous sclerosis	Diffuse interstitial fibrosis pattern with honeycombing that is more prominent in the lower lung zones. Chylous pleural effusion and pneumothorax are common. Sclerotic (occasionally lytic) bone lesions may occur.
Pulmonary lymphangiomyomatosis (Fig C 4-29)	Rare condition that produces a radiographic appearance identical to that of tuberous sclerosis. Part of a generalized syndrome characterized by an excessive accumulation of muscle in relation to extrapulmonary lymphatics.
Neurofibromatosis	Additional manifestations include skin nodules, multiple bullae, scoliosis, and mediastinal neurofibromas.
Niemann-Pick disease	Shows characteristic bone changes and splenomegaly.
Embolism from oily contrast material	Complication of lymphography. The fine reticular pattern usually clears within 72 hours.
Interstitial fibrosis secondary to pulmonary disease (see Fig C 1-26)	Common cause of localized or generalized interstitial thickening, though the offending agent is not always recognized. May be the sequela of recurrent infection, chronic aspiration, lung trauma, radiation, or thromboembolic disease.

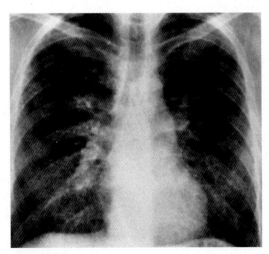

Fig C 4-28
Amyloidosis. Diffuse interstitial fibrosis pattern.

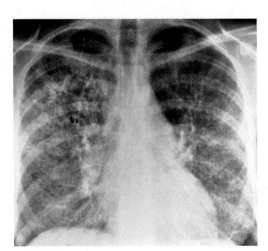

Fig C 4-29
Pulmonary lymphangiomyomatosis. Diffuse reticulonodular interstitial pattern throughout both lungs.

Honeycombing

Condition	Comments
Pneumoconiosis (Fig C 5-1)	Silicosis, asbestosis, berylliosis, coal-miner's lung, etc. Often associated with other radiographic manifestations (nodules, eggshell calcification, and progressive massive fibrosis in silicosis; pleural plaquing and calcification in asbestosis).
Sarcoidosis (Fig C 5-2)	Frequently associated with hilar and mediastinal lymph node enlargement, which often regresses spontaneously as the parenchymal disease develops.
Bronchiectasis (Fig C 5-3)	Irreversible dilatation of the bronchi related to a variety of causes, especially centrally obstructing lesions, infection or inflammation, congenital disorders, and pulmonary fibrosis.

A
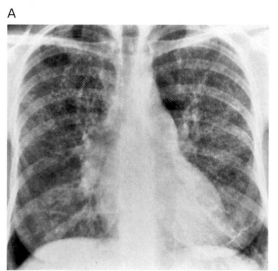
B
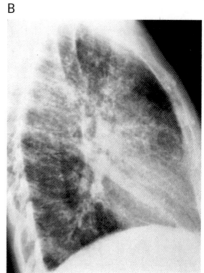

Fig C 5-1
Classic honeycomb pattern in pneumoconiosis. (A) Frontal and (B) lateral views.

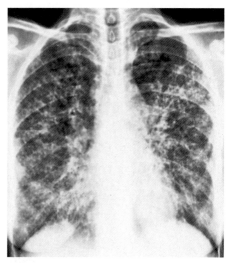

Fig C 5-2
Sarcoidosis. Coarse honeycomb pattern.
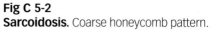

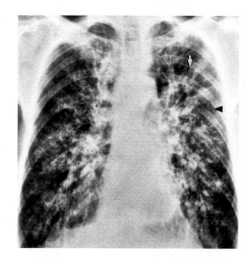

Fig C 5-3
Bronchiectasis (cystic fibrosis). Diffuse increase in interstitial markings radiating in a bronchovascular distribution with tramlines (arrows) and peribronchial cuffing (arrowhead).[16]

Condition	Comments
Idiopathic interstitial fibrosis (Hamman-Rich syndrome) (Fig C 5-4)	Usually most prominent at the bases and associated with progressive loss of lung volume. A similar diffuse interstitial fibrosis pattern may represent the end stage of a variety of pulmonary conditions, including chronic or recurrent pulmonary edema, the inhalation of noxious gases and organic dust, and drug therapy.
Pulmonary Langerhans cell histiocytosis (Fig C 5-5)	More prominent in the upper lung zones (sparing the bases). Spontaneous pneumothorax is a frequent complication.
Tuberculosis	Bronchiectasis and fibrosis may produce a localized honeycomb pattern in the upper lobes.
Connective tissue disorders (Fig C 5-6)	More prominent at the bases and usually associated with progressive loss of lung volume. Causes include scleroderma, rheumatoid lung, and dermatomyositis.
Ankylosing spondylitis	Rare manifestation that exclusively involves the upper lobes and resembles the fibrosis and bronchiectasis that may develop secondary to tuberculosis.
Desquamative interstitial pneumonia (DIP)	More prominent in the lower lung zones and associated with progressive loss of lung volume.

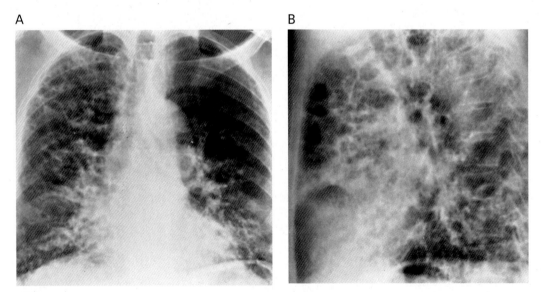

A   B

Fig C 5-4
Diffuse interstitial fibrosis. (A) Frontal and (B) lateral views of the chest demonstrate a coarse reticular pattern indicating pronounced fibrosis. Intervening small areas of lucency produce the appearance of a honeycomb lung, especially in the right upper lobe.

Condition	Comments
Amyloidosis (Fig C 5-7)	More prominent in the lower lung zones and often associated with hilar and mediastinal lymphadenopathy.
Neurofibromatosis (Fig C 5-8)	Additional manifestations include skin nodules, multiple bullae, scoliosis, and mediastinal neurofibromas.
Tuberous sclerosis	More prominent in the lower lung zones. Chylous pleural effusion and pneumothorax are common, and sclerotic (occasionally lytic) bone lesions may occur.
Niemann-Pick disease	Also characteristic bone changes and splenomegaly.
Lipoid pneumonia	Rare manifestation that usually involves a lower lobe.

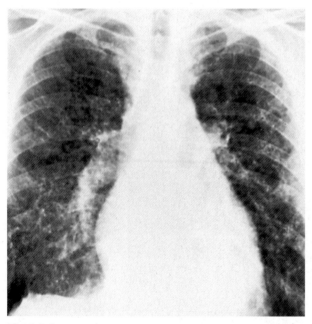

Fig C 5-5
Pulmonary Langerhans cell histiocytosis. Diffuse honeycomb pattern that is slightly more prominent in the upper lung zones.

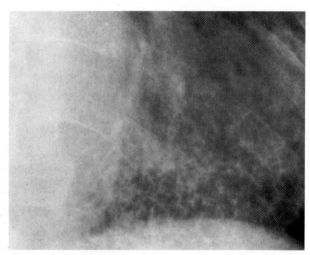

Fig C 5-6
Scleroderma. Coned view of the left lower lung demonstrates a honeycomb pattern, with small emphysematous areas combined with fibrosis and fine nodularity.

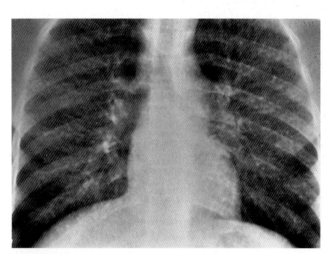

Fig C 5-7
Amyloidosis.

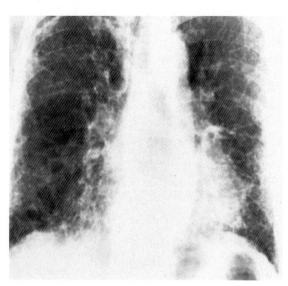

Fig C 5-8
Neurofibromatosis.

Solitary Pulmonary Nodule

Condition	Imaging Findings	Comments
Tuberculoma (Figs C 6-1 and C 6-2)	Round or oval, sharply circumscribed nodule that is seldom more than 4 cm in diameter. Central calcification and "satellite" lesions are common, as is calcification of hilar lymph nodes.	Primarily involves the upper lobes (especially the right). The draining bronchus may show irregular thickening or even frank stenosis.
Histoplasmoma (Figs C 6-3 and C 6-4)	Round or oval, sharply circumscribed nodule that is seldom more than 3 cm in diameter. Central calcification is common, and satellite lesions may occur.	Most frequently in the lower lobes. May be multiple and vary considerably in size. Often associated calcification of hilar lymph nodes.
Other fungal diseases (Fig C 6-5)	Usually a single, well-circumscribed nodule (may be multiple in coccidioidomycosis).	Actinomycosis, blastomycosis, coccidioidomycosis, cryptococcosis, and nocardiosis. Cavitation is common in actinomycosis, coccidioidomycosis, and nocardiosis. Empyema may complicate actinomycosis or nocardiosis.

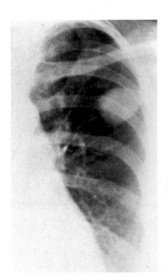

Fig C 6-1
Tuberculoma. Single smooth, well-defined pulmonary nodule in the left upper lobe. In the absence of a central nidus of calcification, this appearance is indistinguishable from that of a malignancy.

A

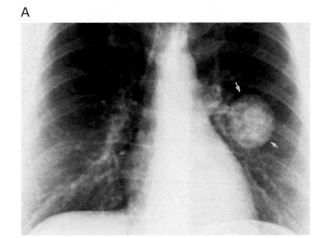

B

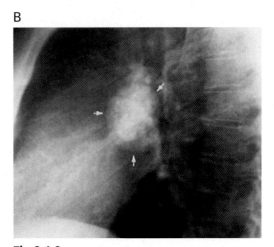

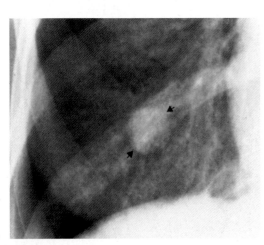

Fig C 6-3
Histoplasmoma. Solitary, sharply circumscribed granulomatous nodule (arrows) in the right lower lobe.

Fig C 6-2
Calcified tuberculoma. (A) Frontal and (B) lateral views of the chest show a large left lung soft-tissue mass (arrows) containing dense central calcification.

Condition	Imaging Findings	Comments
Echinococcal (hydatid) cyst (Fig C 6-6)	Solitary, sharply circumscribed, round or oval mass that tends to have a bizarre, irregular shape. Calcification is very rare.	Predilection for the lower lobes (especially the right). Communication with the bronchial tree causes an air-fluid level in the cyst (endocyst floats on the surface to produce the "water lily" sign [see Fig C 9-8] or "sign of the camalote") or the "crescent" sign (see Fig C 20-4) around its periphery.
Acute lung abscess (Fig C 6-7)	Round, often ill-defined mass that predominantly involves the posterior portions of the upper or lower lobes.	Bilateral in more than 60% of cases. Cavitation is very common (irregular, shaggy inner wall).

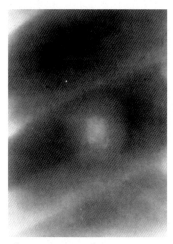

Fig C 6-4
Histoplasmoma. Characteristic central calcification in a solitary pulmonary nodule.

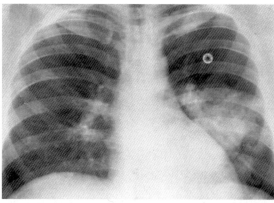

Fig C 6-5
Cryptococcosis. Single fairly well-circumscribed, mass-like consolidation in the superior segment of the left lower lobe.

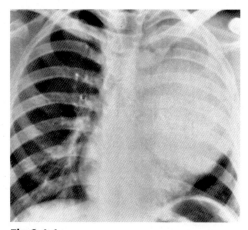

Fig C 6-6
Echinococcal cyst. Huge mass filling most of the left hemithorax.

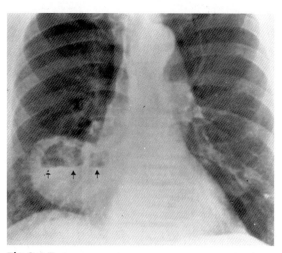

Fig C 6-7
Acute lung abscess. Large right middle lobe abscess containing an air-fluid level (arrows) in an intravenous drug abuser.

Condition	Imaging Findings	Comments
Bronchial adenoma (Fig C 6-8)	Solitary, round or oval, sharply circumscribed mass. Calcification and cavitation are very rare.	Approximately 25% appear as peripheral solitary nodules. The remaining 75% arise centrally in the bronchial lumen and cause segmental atelectasis or obstructive pneumonia. Hemoptysis occurs in more than half the patients.
Hamartoma (Figs C 6-9 and C 6-10)	Solitary, well-circumscribed, often lobulated mass. Popcorn calcification (multiple punctate calcifications in the lesion) is virtually diagnostic, but occurs in less than 10% of cases.	Serial examinations may show interval growth. An endobronchial lesion (10%) may cause segmental atelectasis or obstructive pneumonia.

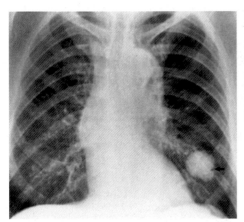

Fig C 6-8
Bronchial adenoma. Nonspecific solitary pulmonary nodule at the left base. Note the notched indentation of the lateral wall (arrow) of the mass. Although this "Rigler notch" sign was initially described as being pathognomonic of malignancy, an identical appearance is commonly seen in benign processes.

A   B

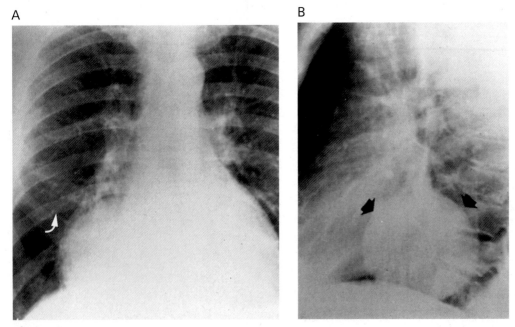

Fig C 6-9
Hamartoma. (A) Frontal view of the chest shows a large mass (arrow) in the right cardiophrenic angle; the mass mimics a pericardial cyst or herniation through the foramen of Morgagni, both of which tend to occur at this site. (B) Lateral view shows the mass to be posterior (arrows), effectively excluding the other diagnostic possibilities. The mass is indistinguishable from other benign or malignant processes in the lung.

Condition	Imaging Findings	Comments
Bronchogenic carcinoma (Fig C 6-11)	Ill-defined, lobulated, or umbilicated mass that usually exceeds 2 cm. Hilar and mediastinal lymph node enlargement is common, especially in oat-cell carcinoma.	Approximately 40% of solitary nodules are malignant. Bronchogenic carcinoma primarily involves the upper lobes with rare calcification and infrequent (2–10%) cavitation. Central or popcorn calcification virtually excludes a malignant lesion. The tumor almost invariably shows interval growth on serial films.
Hematogenous metastases (Fig C 6-12)	Single (25%) or multiple (75%) lesions that are generally well circumscribed with smooth or slightly lobulated margins and lower lobe predominance.	Represents approximately 5% of asymptomatic solitary pulmonary nodules. Calcification is rare (only in osteogenic sarcoma or chondrosarcoma). A malignant solitary pulmonary nodule is most likely a primary bronchogenic carcinoma in patients with carcinomas of the head and neck, bladder, breast, cervix, bile ducts, esophagus, ovary, prostate, or stomach. Conversely, patients with melanoma, sarcoma, or testicular carcinoma are more likely to have a solitary metastasis than a bronchogenic carcinoma.

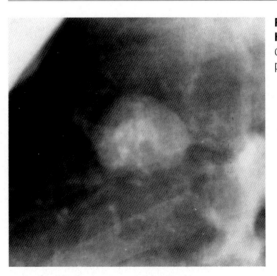

Fig C 6-10
Hamartoma. Well-circumscribed solitary nodule containing characteristic irregular scattered calcifications (popcorn pattern).

A   B

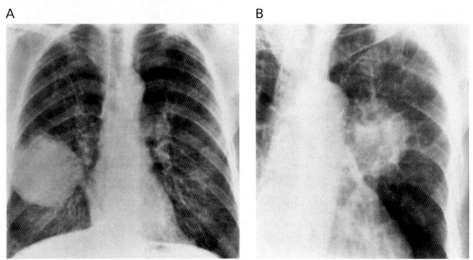

Fig C 6-11
Bronchogenic carcinoma. (A) Relatively well-defined mass. (B) Ill-defined solitary nodule.

Condition	Imaging Findings	Comments
Bronchioloalveolar (alveolar cell) carcinoma (Fig C 6-13)	Various patterns (smooth or lobulated, sharply circumscribed or ill defined).	Characteristic findings include an air bronchogram or bronchiologram in the mass and the "pleural tail" sign (linear strands extending from the lesion toward the pleura). The tumor tends to grow very slowly.
Non-Hodgkin's lymphoma	Single or, more commonly, multiple nodules that often have fuzzy outlines and strands of increased density extending into the adjacent lung.	May be a manifestation of primary or secondary disease. Hilar or mediastinal adenopathy is usually associated. Because the tumor rarely obstructs the bronchial tree (unlike carcinoma), air bronchograms often occur in the mass.
Multiple myeloma (plasmacytoma) (see Fig C 34-4)	Sharply circumscribed, extrapleural mass producing an obtuse angle with the chest wall.	Usually represents spread into the thorax of a primary rib lesion (therefore almost always a destructive process in one or more ribs).

A

B

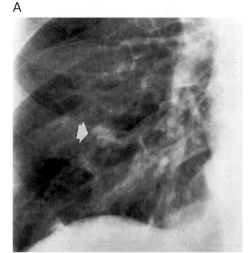
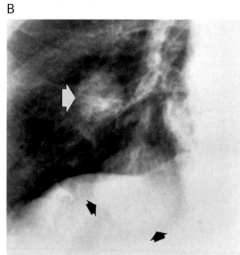

Fig C 6-12
Metastases. (A) Solitary metastasis (arrow). (B) Repeat examination 5 months later shows rapid growth of the previous solitary nodule (white arrow). There is a second huge nodule (black arrows) that was not appreciated on the previous examination because it projected below the right hemidiaphragm.

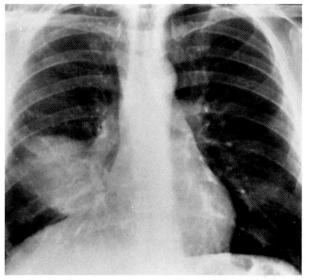

Fig C 6-13
Alveolar cell carcinoma. Large, well-circumscribed tumor mass.

Condition	Imaging Findings	Comments
Mesenchymal tumor	Usually solitary and well defined.	Rare tumor arising in the bronchial wall. May cause bronchial obstruction with peripheral atelectasis or obstructive pneumonia.
Carcinoid (Fig C 6-14)	Well-defined, round or ovoid mass that may have a lobulated margin.	Carcinoid tumors are sometimes located distal to segmental bronchi (peripheral carcinoids).
Pulmonary hematoma (Fig C 6-15)	Single or multiple, unilocular or multilocular, round or oval mass that may occasionally be huge. Usually in a peripheral subpleural location deep to the area of maximum trauma.	Results from hemorrhage into a pulmonary parenchymal laceration or a traumatic lung cyst. May communicate with the bronchial tree (air-fluid level). Generally shows a slow, progressive decrease in size (may persist for several months).
Lipoid pneumonia (Fig C 6-16)	Sharply circumscribed, smooth or lobulated mass that primarily occurs in the dependent portion of the lung. The lesion may have a shaggy border and simulate carcinoma.	Inflammatory reaction to aspirated oils (especially mineral oil). Characteristic streaky linear opacities may radiate outward from the periphery of the mass (interlobular septal thickening).

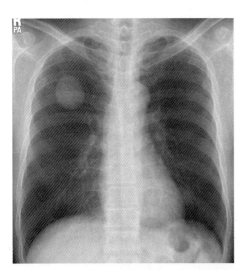

Fig C 6-14
Carcinoid. Well-defined round mass in the right upper lung.[17]

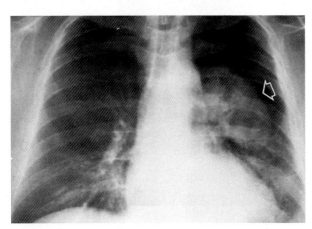

Fig C 6-15
Pulmonary hematoma. After a stab wound, a homoge-neous kidney-shaped opacity (arrow) developed in the supe-rior segment of the left lower lobe. There is blunting of the left costophrenic angle.

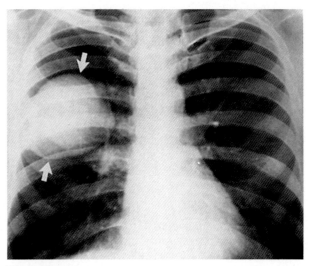

Fig C 6-16
Lipoid pneumonia. Sharply demarcated granulomatous-lipoid mass (arrows) simulating a neoplastic process.

Condition	Imaging Findings	Comments
Wegener's granulomatosis (see Fig C 9-14)	Round, solitary, or more commonly, multiple fairly well-circumscribed nodules that may simulate metastases.	Cavitation (thick walled with irregular shaggy inner margins) develops in about half the patients.
Rheumatoid necrobiotic nodule	Single or, more commonly, multiple smooth, well-circumscribed nodules that predominantly occur in a peripheral subpleural location.	Rare manifestation of rheumatoid lung disease that tends to wax and wane in relation to subcutaneous nodules. Cavitation is common (thick walled with smooth inner margins).
Bronchogenic cyst (see Figs C 23-3 and C 23-4)	Solitary round or oval, smooth, sharply circumscribed mass with a lower lobe predominance.	Approximately two-thirds of bronchogenic cysts are pulmonary (the rest are mediastinal). The cyst is homogeneous until a communication is established with contiguous lung (usually the result of infection).
Intralobar bronchopulmonary sequestration	Round, oval, or triangular mass that typically is well circumscribed and contiguous with the diaphragm (two-thirds of the cases are on the left).	Enclosed in visceral pleura of the affected lung. Although cystic, the mass appears homogeneous until a communication is established with contiguous lung (usually the result of infection). An intralobar sequestration is supplied by a systemic artery and drains via the pulmonary veins.
Extralobar bronchopulmonary sequestration (Fig C 6-17)	Well-defined, homogeneous mass that is related to the left hemidiaphragm (above or below it) in approximately 90% of cases.	Enclosed in its own visceral pleural layer (therefore seldom infected or air containing). An extralobar sequestration is supplied by a systemic artery (usually from the abdominal aorta) and drains via systemic veins (inferior vena cava or azygos system).

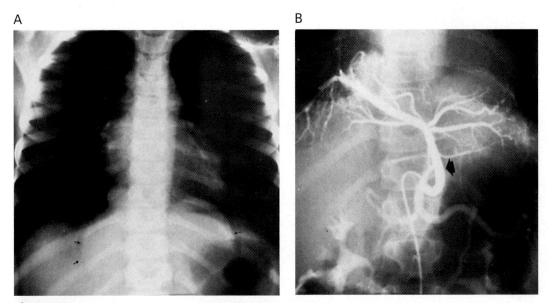

A   B

Fig C 6-17
Bilateral pulmonary sequestration. (A) Frontal view of the chest shows bilateral oval, slightly lobulated paravertebral masses (arrows) in the juxtadiaphragmatic region. (B) Selective angiogram of a large anomalous artery (arrow) arising from the celiac trunk shows several branches supplying the bilateral paravertebral masses. The venous drainage was via the pulmonary veins.[18]

Condition	Imaging Findings	Comments
Pulmonary arteriovenous fistula (Fig C 6-18)	Sharply defined, round or oval, often slightly lobulated lesion that predominantly involves the lower lobes.	Diagnosis requires identification of the feeding artery and the draining vein. Approximately one-third of the fistulas are multiple (arteriography of both lungs required if surgical resection is contemplated). About 50% of the patients have hereditary hemorrhagic telangiectasia (Rendu-Osler-Weber disease).
Mucoid impaction (Fig C 6-19)	Generally a finger-like mass, although it may have a Y- or V-shaped configuration when a bronchial bifurcation is plugged.	Affects patients with bronchospasm (plugs present in dilated proximal segmental bronchi) and a sensitivity to *Aspergillus fumigatus*. Almost always associated with asthma or pre-existing chronic bronchial disease. Usually transient, but may persist for months and even enlarge. Cavitation (lung necrosis) is rare.

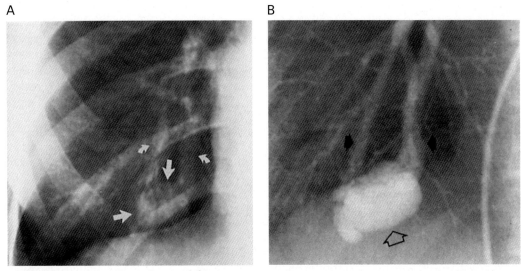

Fig C 6-18
Pulmonary arteriovenous fistula. (A) View of the right lung shows a round soft-tissue 8mass (straight arrows) at the left base. Feeding and draining vessels (curved arrows) extend to the lesion. (B) An arteriogram clearly shows the feeding artery and draining veins (closed arrows) associated with the arteriovenous malformation (open arrow).

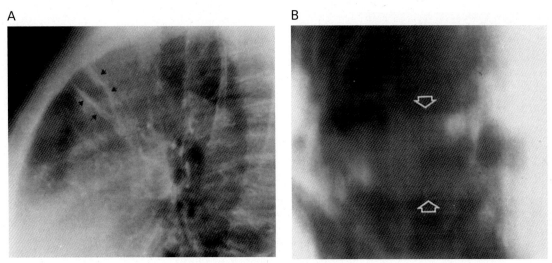

Fig C 6-19
Mucoid impaction. (A) V-shaped and (B) Y-shaped masses (arrows).

Condition	Imaging Findings	Comments
Congenital bronchial atresia	Smooth, sharply defined oval mass that has a strong predilection for the apicoposterior bronchus of the left upper lobe.	The mass consists of inspissated mucus that accumulates in the bronchus immediately distal to the point of obstruction. The lung parenchyma distal to the occlusion is overinflated because of collateral air drift. This very rare anomaly is usually asymptomatic and is discovered on a screening chest radiograph.
Pulmonary vein varix (Fig C 6-20)	Round or oval, lobulated, well-defined mass (may be multiple) involving the medial third of the lung.	Very rare congenital or acquired tortuosity and dilatation of a pulmonary vein just before its entrance into the left atrium. Typically, close association with adjacent pulmonary veins and often seen on only one of the orthogonal posterior and lateral views. Change in size and shape with Valsalva and Mueller maneuvers (as with arteriovenous fistulas).
Round pneumonia (Fig C 6-21)	Ranges from small dense mass to large ill-defined rounded opacity. The margins may be smooth, lobulated, or irregular or spiculated. Primarily involves the lower lobe.	Generally considered a disease of children, but may occur in adults. Often difficult to distinguish from bronchogenic carcinoma. Fewer than 20% demonstrate air bronchograms. Some patients present with no clinical symptoms, though they may give a history of cough and chills 1 week or longer previously.
Inflammatory pseudotumor	Solitary pulmonary nodule (or homogeneous consolidation) that may mimic a primary or metastatic neoplasm.	Probably represents a reparative process secondary to an unresolved pneumonia (though there is often no history of an acute respiratory illness).
Progressive massive fibrosis (PMF) (see Figs C 7-9 and C 7-10)	Large, often bilateral (but usually asymmetric), spindle-shaped mass in the upper half of the lungs. Typically arises near the periphery of the lung, with its lateral border (paralleling the rib cage) usually better defined than the medial edge. Tends to migrate toward the hila with time.	A manifestation of pneumoconiosis (especially silicosis or coal-miner's disease). Usually of homogeneous density unless there is cavitation (caused by ischemic necrosis or superimposed tuberculosis). May occasionally contain small calcifications (unlike bronchogenic carcinoma).

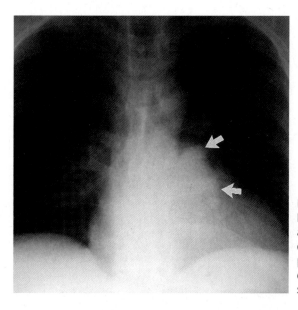

Fig C 6-20
Pulmonary vein varix. Frontal chest radiograph shows a round mass (arrows) inferior to the left hilum. The well-defined superior border and close association with the pulmonary veins inferiorly, as well as poor visualization on a lateral projection (not shown), are important features suggesting the diagnosis.[19]

A

B

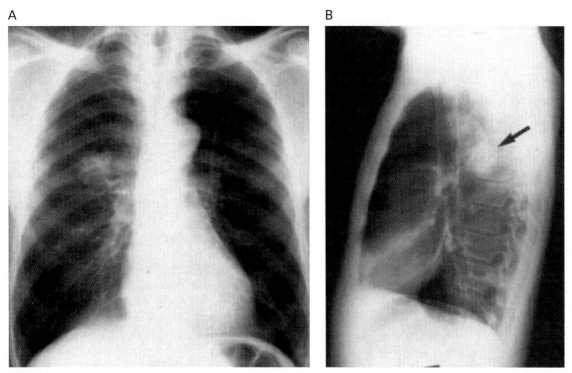

Fig C 6-21
Round pneumonia. Well-defined round mass (arrow) in the right mid-lung in posteroanterior (A) and lateral (B) chest radiographs that resolved completely after antibiotic therapy.[20]

Solitary Pulmonary Nodule on Computed Tomography

Condition	Comments
Benign versus malignant (Figs C 7-1 to C 7-3)	In general, the smaller the nodule, the more likely it is to be benign. About 80% of benign nodules are less than 2 cm in diameter. However, this does not exclude lung cancer, because about 15% malignant nodules are less than 1 cm in diameter and 40% are less than 2 cm. Although most nodules with smooth, well-defined margins are benign, approximately 20% of malignant nodules also have this appearance. A lobular contour implies uneven growth, which is associated with malignancy. However, this appearance can be seen in up to 25% of benign nodules. However, a nodule with an irregular, speculated margin with distortion of adjacent vessels (sunburst or corona radiate appearance) is likely to be malignant. When a benign lesion cavitates, the wall is typically smooth and thin (<4 mm), whereas those thick, irregular walls tend to be malignant. Although a substantial proportion of benign nodules are not calcified, the demonstration of central, diffuse solid, laminated, or popcorn calcification are reliable indicators of a benign cause.

Malignant calcification is usually diffuse and amorphous. Punctate calcification may also occur in lung cancer due to engulfment of a preexistent calcified granulomatous lesion or a metastasis (osteosarcoma or chondrosarcoma). Stability of a pulmonary nodule (>1 cm) for 2 years or more is a good sign of a benign process. The doubling time for most malignant nodules is between 30 and 400 days. Those that double either more rapidly or more slowly are typically benign. |

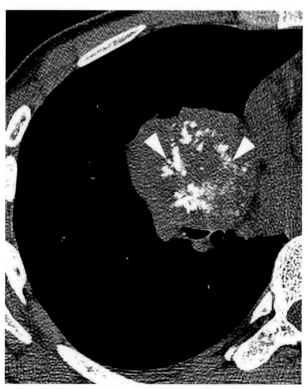

Fig C 7-1
Benign calcifications. Diffuse punctuate calcifications in a large (6 cm), lobulated carcinoid.[17]

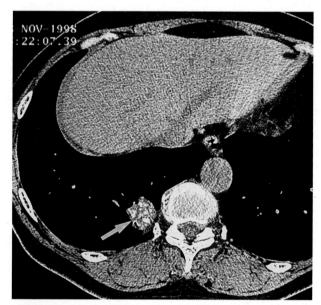

Fig C 7-2
Calcified metastasis mimicking hamartoma. Multiple punctuate calcifications in a mass (arrow) in the right lower lobe. A biopsy obtained because of prior resection of the rectum for a malignancy revealed a metastatic adenocarcinoma.[21]

Condition	Comments
Benign granuloma (Fig C 7-4)	Tuberculoma and histoplasmoma. Central calcification and "satellite" lesions are common, as is calcification of hilar lymph nodes. Tuberculomas primarily involve the upper lobes (especially the right); histoplasmomas are more common in the lower lobes.

A
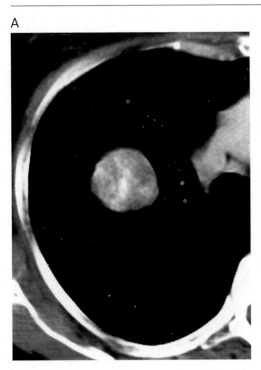

B
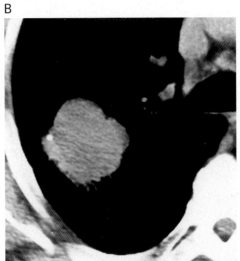

C
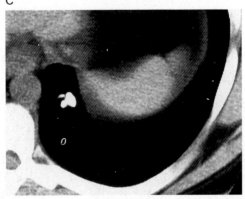

Fig C 7-3
Malignant calcification. (A) Amorphous calcification. (B) Peripheral punctuate calcification consistent with an "engulfed" granuloma. (C) Diffuse high-attenuation and lobulated contour in metastatic osteosarcoma.[22]

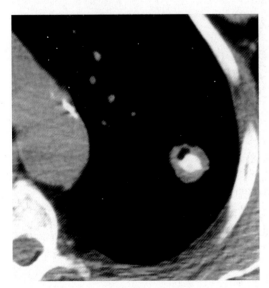

Fig C 7-4
Granuloma. Soft-tissue nodule with central calcification in an asymptomatic man. Note the eccentric calcification within the nodule.[22]

Condition	Comments
Other fungal diseases (Fig C 7-5 and C 7-6)	Actinomycosis, aspergillosis, blastomycosis, coccidiodomycosis, cryptococcosis, and nocardiosis. Cavitation is common in actinomycosis, coccidiodomycosis, and nocardiosis.
Echinococcal (hydatid cyst)	Frequently has a bizarre, irregular shape and rarely calcifies.
Acute lung abscess (Fig C 7-7)	Cavitation is very common (irregular, shaggy inner wall). Usually involves the posterior portions of the upper and lower lobes and is bilateral in more than 60% of cases.
Bronchial adenoma	About 25% appear as peripheral solitary nodules (the rest arise centrally in the bronchial lumen and cause segmental atelectasis or obstructive pneumonia)
Hamartoma (Figs C 7-8 and 7-9)	Popcorn calcification (multiple punctuate calcifications in the lesion) is virtually diagnostic, but occurs in less than 10% of cases. The presence of fat within a solitary pulmonary nodule is strongly suggestive of hamartoma (seen in about 50% of lesions and best seen on thin-section studies).
Hematoma	Results from hemorrhage into a pulmonary parenchymal laceration or a traumatic lung cyst. Usually in a peripheral subpleural location deep to the area of maximum trauma.

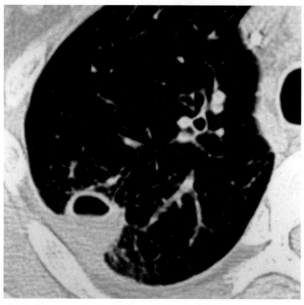

Fig C 7-5
Aspergillosis. Thin-walled cavitary nodule in the right lung of a patient with leukemia.[3]

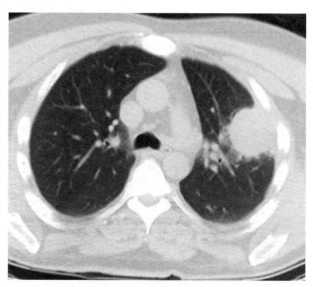

Fig C 7-6
Blastomycosis. Round, well-circumscribed left upper lobe mass with irregular borders in a heavy smoker. After a CT-guided biopsy was inconclusive, the patient underwent left upper lobectomy and mediastinal lymph node dissection for suspected lung carcinoma.[23]

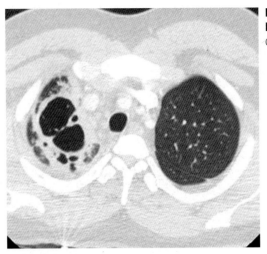

Fig C 7-7
Lung abscese (blastomycosis). Large apical thick-walled cavitary lesion in an acutely ill patient.[23]

A

B

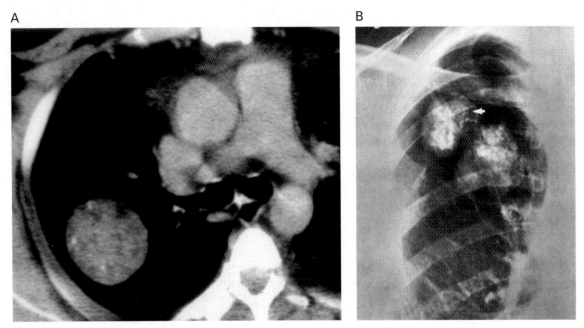

Fig C 7-8
Hamartoma. (A) Sharply marginated lesion with small focal areas of calcification and fat.[22] (B) Characteristic calcification of a hamartomatous nodule in another patient.[16]

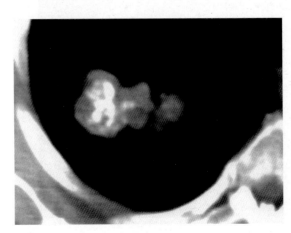

Fig C 7-9
Chondrohamartoma. Lobulated nodule with central popcorn-like in the right upper lobe (Reprinted from Bennett LL, Lesar MSL, Tellis. Multiple calcified chondrohamartomas of the lung: CT appearance. J Comput Assist Tomgr 9:180-182, 1985, cited in 24).

Condition	Comments
Lipoid pneumonia (Fig C 7-10)	Inflammatory reaction to aspirated oils (especially mineral oil) that primarily occurs in the dependent portion of the lung. The lesion may have a shaggy border and simulate malignancy.
Wegener's granulomatosis	Although more commonly multiple, there may be only a single nodule. The cavitation (thick walled with irregular shaggy inner margins) that develops in about half the patients may simulate malignancy.
Rheumatoid necrobiotic nodule	A single (more commonly multiple), often-cavitating nodule is a rare manifestation of rheumatoid lung disease.
Bronchopulmonary sequestration (Fig C 7-11)	Mass contiguous with the diaphragm. Intralobar sequestration drains via the pulmonary veins, while the extralobar type drains via systemic veins (inferior vena cava or azygos system).
Pulmonary arteriovenous fistula (Fig C 7-12)	Diagnosis requires identification of the feeding artery and the draining vein. About a third are multiple, and half are associated with hereditary hemorrhagic telangiectasia (Rendu-Osler-Weber disease).
Mucoid impaction (Fig C 7-13)	Usually a finger-like mass, although it may have a Y- or V-shaped configuration when a bronchial bifurcation is plugged. Affects patients with bronchospasm (plugs present in dilated proximal segmental bronchi) and a sensitivity to *Aspergillus fumigatus*.
Congenital bronchial atresia (Fig C 7-14)	Consisting of inspissated mucus that accumulates in the bronchus immediately distal to the point of obstruction, it has a strong predilection for the apical-posterior bronchus of the left upper lobe.

A

B

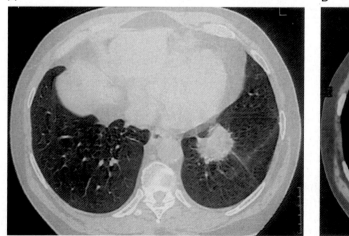
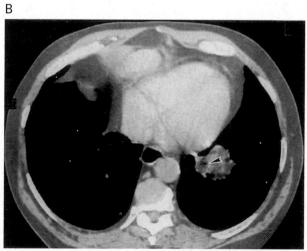

Fig C 7-10
Lipoid pneumonia. (A) Lung windowing shows a speculated mass in the left lower lobe. (B) Mediastinal windowing demonstrates that the mass contains fat attenuation, consistent with lipid deposits in the legion.

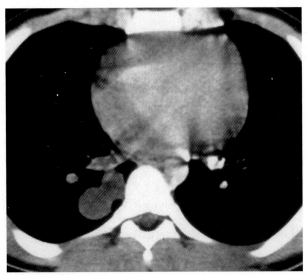

Fig C 7-11
Intralobar sequestration. Lobular, well-marginated nodule with homogeneous attenuation in the right lower lobe.[22]

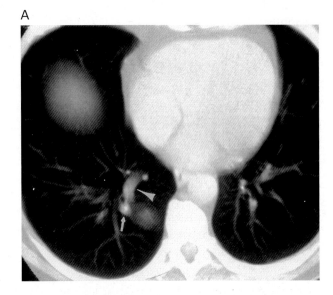
A

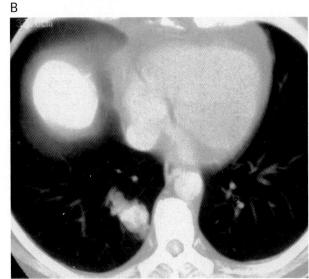
B

Fig C 7-12
Arteriovenous malformation. (A) Feeding artery (arrow) and an enlarged draining vein (arrowhead) associated with a right lower lung nodule. (B) Scan at a lower level shows the nidus of the malformation (Reprinted from Swensen SJ, Brown LR, Colby, et al. Lung nodule enhancement at CT: prospective findings. Radiology 201:447-455, 1996, cited in 24).

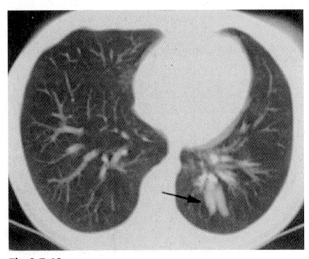

Fig C 7-13
Mucoid impaction. Characteristic V-shaped structure.[24]

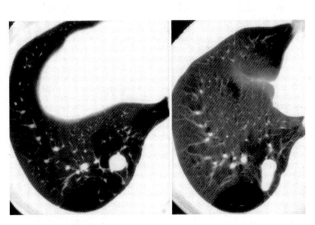

Fig C 7-14
Segmental bronchial atresia. Branching tubular area of increased attenuation in the right lower lobe as well as pulmonary parenchyma with lower-than-expected attenuation. This constellation of findings in teenager was considered so characteristic of segmental bronchial atresia that no further work-up was performed.[22]

Condition	Comments
Pulmonary vein varix	Very rare congenital or acquired tortuosity and dilatation of a pulmonary vein just before its entrance in the left atrium. Changes size and shape with Valsalva and Mueller maneuvers (as with arteriovenous fistulas).
Round pneumonia	Ranging from a small dense mass to a large, ill-defined rounded opacity, primarily in the lower lobe, it may be difficult to distinguish from malignancy. Some patients present with a history of cough and chills for 1 week or longer.
Inflammatory pseudotumor	Probably represents a reparative process secondary to an unresolved pneumonia (though there often is no history of an acute respiratory illness).
Amyloidoma (Fig C 7-15)	Limited form of amyloidosis that is usually misinterpreted as a neoplasm. Resection of the nodule is both diagnostic and curative.
Malignant Bronchogenic carcinoma (Fig C 7-16)	Primarily involves the upper lobes and almost invariably shows interval growth on serial studies. Usually an ill-defined, lobulated, or umbilicated mass that is generally more than 2 cm in diameter.
Hematogenous metastasis (Figs C 7-17 and C 7-18)	Single in about 25% of cases, metastases represent approximately 5% of asymptomatic pulmonary nodules. Calcification is rare (only in osteosarcoma or chondrosarcoma). A malignant solitary pulmonary nodule is most likely a primary bronchogenic carcinoma in patients with carcinomas of the head and neck, bladder, breast, cervix, bile ducts, esophagus, ovary, prostate, or stomach. Conversely, patients with melanoma, sarcoma, or testicular carcinoma are more likely to have a solitary metastasis than a primary lung cancer.

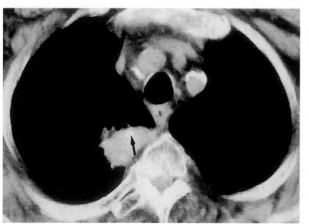

Fig C 7-15
Amyloidoma. Solid mass adjacent to the spine that contains amorphous calcification.[25]

A

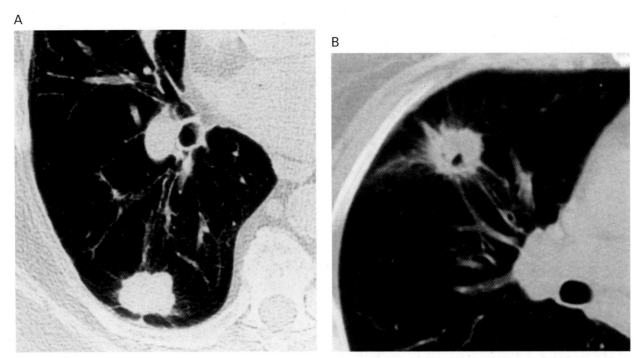

Fig C 7-16
Non–small cell cancer. (A) Lobulated and speculated nodule in the right lower lobe. (B) In another patient, there is eccentric cavitation within a speculated upper lobe nodule.[22]

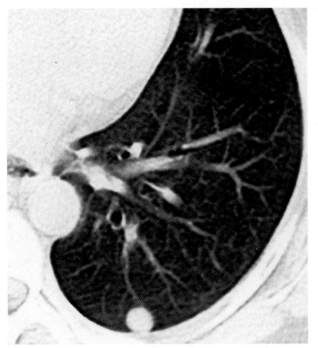

Fig C 7-17
Solitary metastasis. Smoothly marginated 1 cm peripheral nodule in a patient with bladder cancer.[22]

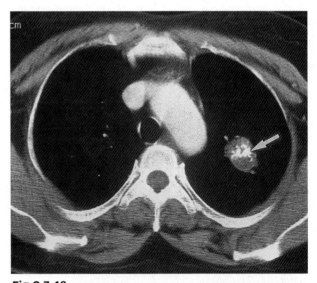

Fig C 7-18
Ossified metastasis. This left upper lobe nodule containing what appears to be dense calcification (arrow) proved to be a metastatic osteosarcoma.[21]

Condition	Comments
Bronchioloalveolar carcinoma (Fig C 7-19)	Smooth or lobulated, sharply circumscribed or ill-defined mass that tends to grow very slowly. Characteristic findings include an air bronchogram or bronchiologram in the mass and the "pleural tail" sign (linear strands extending from the lesion toward the pleura).
Non-Hodgkin's lymphoma	More commonly multiple and a manifestation of primary or secondary disease. There is usually associated hilar or mediastianal adenopathy. Because the tumor rarely obstructs the bronchial tree (unlike carcinoma), air bronchograms can often be detected within the mass.
Neuroendocrine tumor (Figs C 7-20 and C 7-21)	Up to 40% of carcinoids occur in the peripheral lung and present as solitary pulmonary nodules. They appear as round or ovoid, well-defined masses that may have slightly lobulated borders and usually show intense contrast enhancement. A punctuate or diffuse pattern of calcification or ossification can be seen in up to one-third of lesions on CT. Malignant neuroendocrine tumors usually show heterogeneous contrast enhancement due to intratumoral necrosis.
Plasmacytoma	Extrapleural mass that usually represents spread into the thorax of a primary rib lesion (therefore almost always a destructive process in one or more ribs).

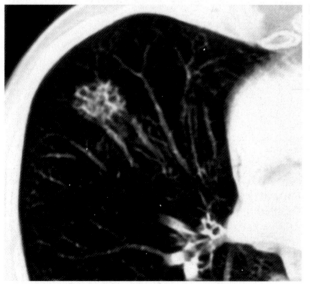

Fig C 7-19
Bronchioloalveolar carcinoma. Poorly marginated nodule in the right mid lung containing small focal areas of low attenuation, an appearance highly suggestive of bronchoalveolar cell carcinoma.[22]

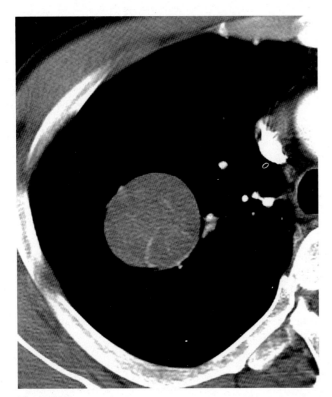

Fig C 7-20
Carcinoid. Well-defined, homogeneous mass in the right upper lobe.[17]

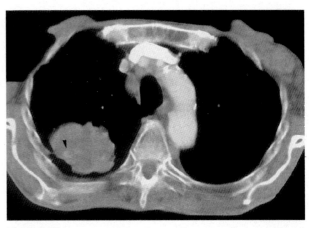

Fig C 7-21
Neuroendocrine carcinoma. Large mass containing punctuate calcifications (arrowhead) and low attenuation areas related to necrosis. Note the right paratracheal lymphadenopathy.[25]

Multiple Pulmonary Nodules

Condition	Imaging Findings	Comments
Pyogenic abscesses (Fig C 8-1)	Round, well-circumscribed masses (may have poor definition in the acute stage).	Cavitation (irregular, thick-walled) is very common. May reflect septic emboli in an intravenous drug addict.
Granulomatous infections (Figs C 8-2 and C 8-3)	Generally round or oval, well-circumscribed nodules. Irregular and poorly defined masses in *Pseudomonas*.	Histoplasmosis, tuberculosis, coccidioidomycosis, *Pseudomonas*. Calcification is common in histoplasmosis, tuberculosis, and coccidioidomycosis; cavitation is common in coccidioidomycosis and *Pseudomonas*.

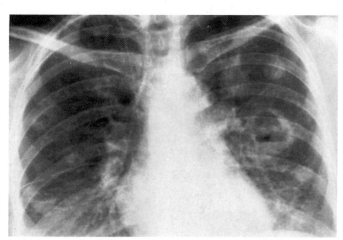

Fig C 8-1
Septic pulmonary emboli. Several round lesions, many with cavitation, are seen throughout the lungs in this intravenous drug abuser with staphylococcal tricuspid endocarditis.

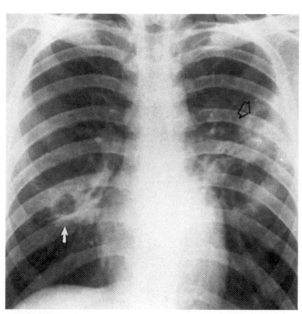

Fig C 8-2
Secondary tuberculosis. Bilateral cavitary lesions (arrows) with relatively thick walls.

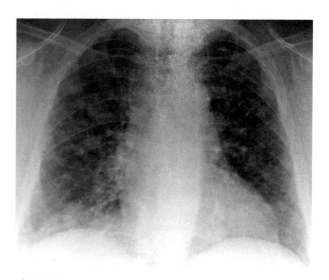

Fig C 8-3
Blastomycosis. Bilateral diffuse intermediate-sized nodules along with patchy consolidation at the lung bases.[24]

Condition	Imaging Findings	Comments
Viral infections (Figs C 8-4 and C 8-5)	Diffuse small, often ill-defined nodules throughout both lungs.	Varicella-zoster, cytomegalovirus (CMV), herpes simplex virus (HSV). Varicella (chickenpox) nodules often calcify 1 year or more after the initial infection (see Fig C 17-5).
Paragonimus westermani (Fig C 8-6)	Well-circumscribed cystic masses that have a predilection for the periphery of the lower lobes.	Characteristic appearance of multiple ring opacities or thin-walled cysts (may mimic cystic bronchiectasis).

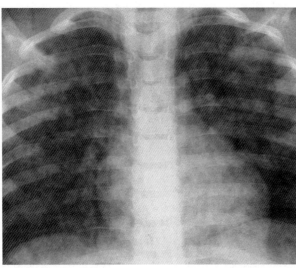

Fig C 8-4
Chickenpox pneumonia. Multiple ill-defined and occasionally confluent nodules throughout the lungs in a young child with severe combined immunodeficiency disease.[26]

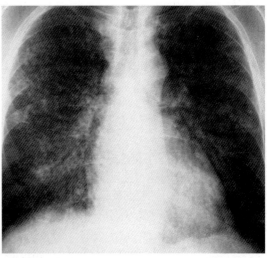

Fig C 8-5
CMV pneumonia. Multiple small, ill-defined nodules throughout the lungs that developed in a patient who had undergone a renal transplant 3 months earlier and was receiving immunosuppression therapy.[26]

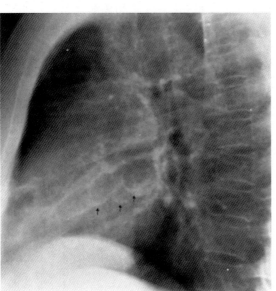

Fig C 8-6
Paragonimus westermani. Arrows point to a few of the multiple cysts in the right middle lobe. The cysts are thin walled, and most have a prominent crescent-shaped opacity along one side of their borders, the characteristic ring shadow of paragonimiasis.

Condition	Imaging Findings	Comments
Hematogenous metastases (Figs C 8-7 and C 8-8)	Various patterns (from diffuse micronodular shadows resembling miliary disease to multiple large, well-defined "cannonballs"). Tend to be more numerous in the lower lobes.	Nodules typically vary in size in the same patient. Calcification is rare but is virtually diagnostic of osteogenic sarcoma or chondrosarcoma. Cavitation occurs in approximately 4% and most commonly involves squamous cell neoplasms (also adenocarcinomas of the large bowel and sarcomas).
Bronchioloalveolar (alveolar cell) carcinoma (Fig C 8-9)	Poorly defined nodules scattered throughout both lungs.	Other presentations include a single well-circumscribed peripheral solitary nodule (see Fig C 6-13), focal "pneumonia" (see Fig C 1-25), and a miliary pattern (see Fig C 8-15).

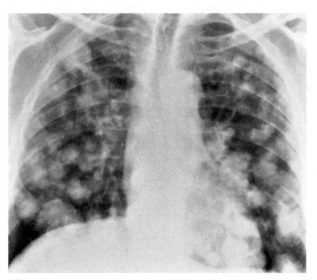

Fig C 8-7
Hematogenous metastases. Multiple well-circumscribed nodules scattered diffusely throughout both lungs.

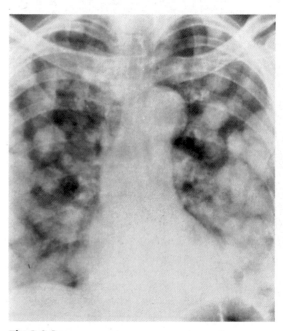

Fig C 8-8
Cannonball metastases in a patient with choriocarcinoma.

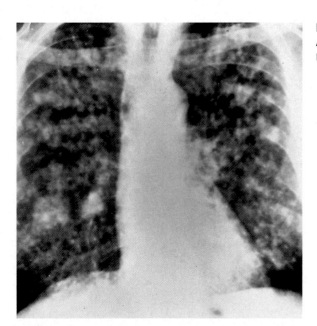

Fig C 8-9
Alveolar cell carcinoma. Multiple poorly defined nodules scattered throughout both lungs.

Condition	Imaging Findings	Comments
Papillomatosis of lung (see Fig C 11-18)	Round, sharply circumscribed nodules that frequently cavitate (often resembling advanced cystic bronchiectasis).	Usually associated with laryngeal or tracheal papillomas. Typically obstruct the airways, resulting in peripheral atelectasis and obstructive pneumonia.
Lymphoma	Multiple nodules that often have fuzzy outlines and are most numerous in the lower lobes.	Manifestation of secondary disease. Usually associated with mediastinal and hilar lymph node enlargement. Cyst-like lesions may simulate central cavitation.
Pulmonary arteriovenous fistulas (see Fig C 6-17)	Sharply defined, round or oval, often slightly lobulated nodules that predominantly involve the lower lobes. The lesions may change in size between the Valsalva and the Mueller maneuvers.	Diagnosis requires identification of the feeding artery and the draining vein. Approximately one-third of the fistulas are multiple (arteriography of both lungs required if surgical resection is contemplated). About 50% have hereditary hemorrhagic telangiectasia (Rendu-Osler-Weber disease).
Wegener's granulomatosis (see Fig C 11-14)	Round, fairly well-circumscribed nodules that may simulate metastases.	Cavitation (thick walled with irregular, shaggy inner margins) develops in approximately half the patients.
Rheumatoid necrobiotic nodules (Fig C 8-10)	Smooth, well-circumscribed nodules that predominantly occur in peripheral subpleural locations. Cavitation is common (thick walled with smooth inner margins).	Rare manifestation of rheumatoid lung disease that tends to wax and wane in relation to the activity of the rheumatoid arthritis and the presence of subcutaneous nodules. May be associated with pneumoconiosis (Caplan's syndrome).
Amyloidosis	Multiple nodules that may cavitate and show calcification or ossification.	Discrete masses of amyloid may develop in the rare parenchymal form of the disease. The nodular parenchymal form of the disease has a better prognosis than the tracheobronchial (obstructive) or diffuse interstitial types (see Fig C 4-27).
Pulmonary hematomas (see Fig C 6-14)	Unilocular or multilocular, round or oval nodules that are occasionally huge. Usually in peripheral subpleural locations deep to areas of maximum trauma.	Result from hemorrhage into pulmonary parenchymal lacerations or traumatic lung cysts. May communicate with the bronchial tree (air-fluid level). Generally a slow, progressive decrease in size (may persist for several months).

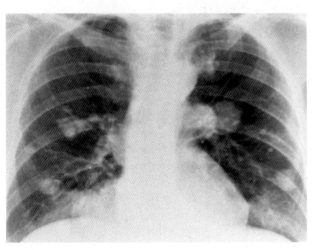

Fig C 8-10
Caplan's syndrome. Multiple well-circumscribed, rounded nodules of varying size in a patient with subcutaneous rheumatoid nodules.

Condition	Imaging Findings	Comments
Hamartomas (Fig C 8-11)	Characteristic popcorn calcification.	This most common benign tumor of the lung is usually solitary.
Sarcoidosis (Fig C 8-12)	Sharply circumscribed and widely distributed nodules that may simulate metastatic disease.	Rare manifestation. Usually associated with a reticulonodular pattern and often concomitant hilar and mediastinal adenopathy.
Pulmonary ossification	Small, densely calcified or ossified nodules throughout the lungs.	Primarily a manifestation of mitral stenosis (or other causes of elevated left atrial pressure).
Pneumoconiosis (progressive massive fibrosis) (Figs C 8-13 and C 8-14)	Conglomerate masses that predominantly involve the upper lobes and are usually irregular and ill defined with peripheral stranding.	Masses represent confluence of individual silicotic nodules, sometimes associated with superimposed tuberculous infection. They typically develop in the mid-zone or periphery of the lung and tend to migrate toward the hilum.
Polyarteritis	Poorly defined nodules that are often associated with patchy consolidations.	The pulmonary manifestations typically show progression and regression of lesions on serial films, reflecting the appearance of new lesions and the healing of old ones. The angiographic demonstration of multiple arterial aneurysms in one or more abdominal organs is considered virtually diagnostic of this disease.

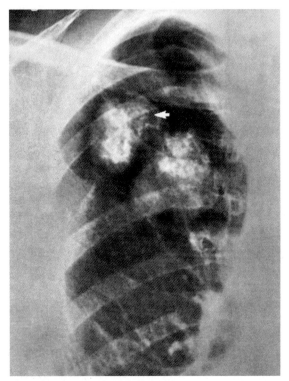

Fig C 8-11
Hamartomas. Characteristic calcification of the cartilaginous matrix (arrow).[16]

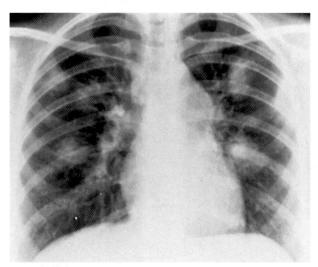

Fig C 8-12
Sarcoidosis. Patchy, ill-defined areas of air-space consolidation scattered throughout both lungs.

Condition	Imaging Findings	Comments
Pulmonary varices	Multiple, round, well-defined opacities that most commonly appear on lateral radiographs projecting posterior and inferior to the hilar structures.	Congenital or acquired tortuosity and dilatation of pulmonary veins just before their entrance into the left atrium. The varicosities change shape and size with the Valsalva and Mueller maneuvers (similar to arteriovenous fistulas).
Mucoid impactions (see Fig C 6-18)	Multiple (more commonly single), round, oval, or elliptical opacities caused by plugs in dilated bronchi.	Usually associated with hypersensitivity bronchopulmonary aspergillosis in patients with asthma or pre-existing chronic bronchial disease.

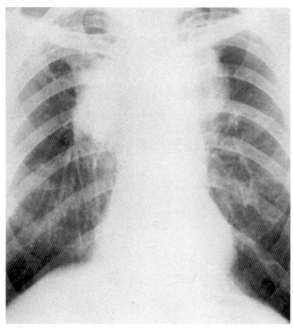

Fig C 8-13
Progressive massive fibrosis in silicosis. Nonsegmental areas of homogeneous density in both upper lobes.

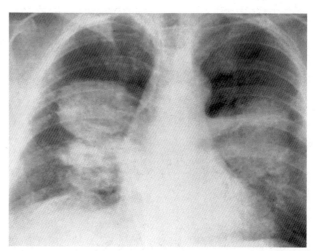

Fig C 8-14
Progressive massive fibrosis in silicosis. Large, irregular nodules in both perihilar regions.

Multiple Pulmonary Nodules on Computed Tomography

Condition	Imaging Findings	Comments
Pyogenic abscesses (Fig C 9-1)	Round, well-circumscribed masses (may have poor definition in the acute stage).	Cavitation (irregular, thick walled) is very common. May reflect septic emboli in an intravenous drug addict.
Granulomatous infections (Fig C 9-2)	Generally round or oval, well-circumscribed nodules.	Histoplasmosis, tuberculosis, coccidioidomycosis, and blastomycosis. Calcification is common in histoplasmosis, tuberculosis, and coccidioidomycosis; cavitation is common in coccidioidomycosis.
Hematogenous metastases (Figs C 9-3 and C 9-4)	Various patterns (from diffuse micronodular shadows resembling miliary disease to multiple large, well-defined "cannonballs"). Tend to be more numerous in the lower lobes.	Nodules typically vary in size in the same patient. Calcification is rare but is virtually diagnostic of osteogenic sarcoma or chondrosarcoma. Cavitation occurs in approximately 4% and most commonly involves squamous cell neoplasms (also adenocarcinomas of the large bowel and sarcomas).
Bronchioloalveolar (alveolar cell) carcinoma (Fig C 9-5)	Poorly defined nodules scattered throughout both lungs. Ground-glass opacification, with areas of increased density representing elements of adenocarcinoma.	BAC may also appear as a single well-circumscribed peripheral solitary nodule, Focal "pneumonia," a miliary pattern, or thin-walled cystic lesions.

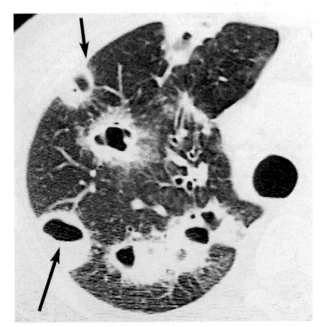

Fig C 9-1
Septic pulmonary emboli. Multiple cavitating nodules (*Nocardia*) in a young immunocompromised man. Note the feeding vessel sign (vessel leading directly to the nodule) in several nodules (arrows).[30]

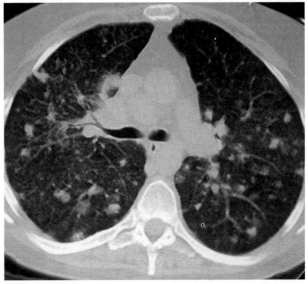

Fig C 9-2
Blastomycosis. Multiple intermediate-sized nodules in a patient with persistent and worsening symptoms of cough, chest pain, and fevers.[23]

Condition	Imaging Findings	Comments
Papillomatosis of lung (Fig C 9-6)	Round, sharply circumscribed nodules that frequently cavitate (often resembling advanced cystic bronchiectasis).	Usually associated with laryngeal or tracheal papillomas. Typically obstruct the airways, resulting in peripheral atelectasis and obstructive pneumonia.

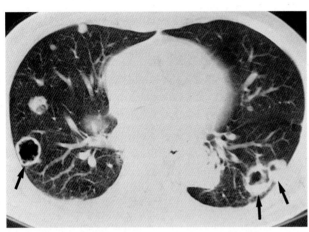

Fig C 9-3
Hematogenous metastases. Several cavitating nodules (arrows) in both lower lobes with irregular thickening of the walls in a patient with metastatic squamous cell cancer of the lungs.[22]

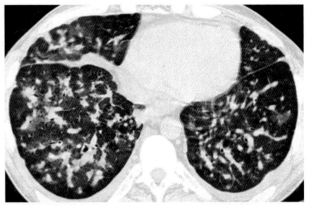

Fig C 9-4
Kaposi's sarcoma. Innumerable, bilateral, poorly defined peribronchovascular micronodules, some of which exhibit coalescence.[6]

A

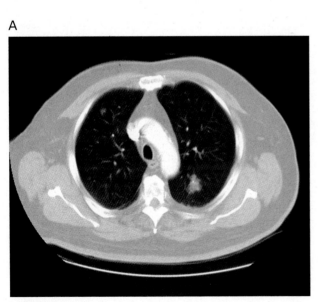

B

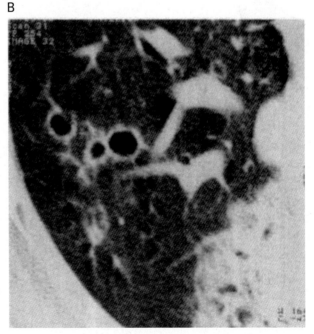

Fig C 9-5
Bronchioloalveolar carcinoma. (A) Ground-glass lesions bilaterally. The mass in the left lower lobe also contains solid elements, consistent with the diagnosis of bronchoialveolar carcinoma with adenocarcinoma features. (Courtesy of Diana Litmanovich, M.D., Boston) (B) Multiple thin-walled cystic lesions in the right lower lobe.[122]

Condition	Imaging Findings	Comments
Lymphoma (Fig C 9-7)	Multiple nodules that often have fuzzy outlines and are most numerous in the lower lobes.	Manifestation of secondary disease. Usually associated with mediastinal and hilar lymph node enlargement. Cyst-like lesions may simulate central cavitation.
Pulmonary arteriovenous fistulas	Sharply defined, round or oval, often slightly lobulated nodules that predominantly involve the lower lobes.	Diagnosis requires identification of the feeding artery and the draining vein. Approximately one-third of the fistulas are multiple (arteriography of both lungs required if surgical resection is contemplated). About 50% have hereditary hemorrhagic telangiectasia (Rendu-Osler-Weber disease).
Wegener's granulomatosis (Fig C 9-8)	Round, fairly well-circumscribed nodules that may simulate metastases.	Cavitation (thick walled with irregular, shaggy inner margins) develops in approximately half the patients.

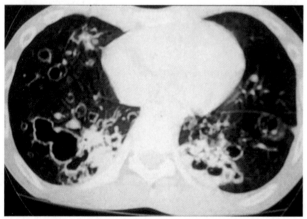

Fig C 9-6
Pulmonary papillomatosis. Multiple cavitating lung nodules, some of which contain air-fluid levels.[25]

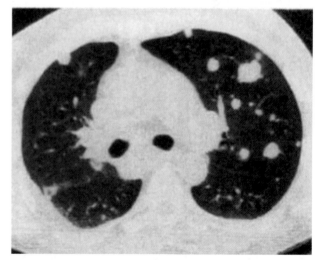

Fig C 9-7
Lymphoma. Multiple pulmonary nodules on a study obtained 10 months after cardiac transplantation.[123]

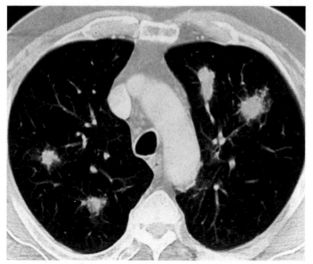

Fig C 9-8
Wegener's granulomatosis. Multiple irregular nodules in a peribronchovascular distribution.[109]

Condition	Imaging Findings	Comments
Rheumatoid necrobiotic nodules (Fig C 9-9)	Smooth, well-circumscribed nodules that predominantly occur in peripheral subpleural locations. Cavitation is common (thick walled with smooth inner margins).	Rare manifestation of rheumatoid lung disease that tends to wax and wane in relation to the activity of the rheumatoid arthritis and the presence of subcutaneous nodules. May be associated with pneumoconiosis (Caplan's syndrome).
Amyloidosis	Multiple nodules that may cavitate and show calcification or ossification.	Discrete masses of amyloid may develop in the rare parenchymal form of the disease.
Pulmonary hematomas	Unilocular or multilocular, round or oval nodules that are occasionally huge. Usually in peripheral subpleural locations deep to areas of maximum trauma	Result from hemorrhage into pulmonary parenchymal lacerations or traumatic lung cysts. May communicate with the bronchial tree (air-fluid level). Generally a slow, progressive decrease in size (may persist for several months).
Sarcoidosis (Fig C 9-10)	Sharply circumscribed and widely distributed nodules that may simulate metastatic disease.	Rare manifestation. Usually associated with a reticulonodular pattern and often concomitant hilar and mediastinal adenopathy.
Pneumoconiosis (progressive massive fibrosis) (Fig C 9-11)	Conglomerate masses that predominantly involve the upper lobes and are usually irregular and ill defined with peripheral stranding.	Masses represent confluence of individual silicotic nodules, sometimes associated with superimposed tuberculous infection. They typically develop in the mid-zone or periphery of the lung and tend to migrate toward the hilum.

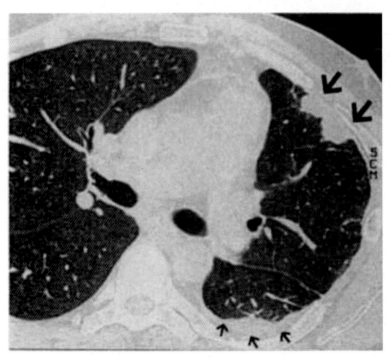

Fig C 9-9
Rheumatoid necrobiotic nodules. Two large, pleural-based nodules (large arrows) are seen at the level of the left upper lobe. The nodules are associated with marked posterior left-sided pleural thickening (small arrows).[147]

Condition	Imaging Findings	Comments
Talc injection (Fig C 9-12)	Irregular nodular in the middle and upper areas of the lungs that may coalesce to form conglomerate masses that resemble progressive massive fibrosis. Diffuse small nodules may be the first manifestation of talc-induced lung disease.	Talc (magnesium silicate) is an insoluble filler used in several oral medications to bind the active medicinal agent within the individual tablets. When oral medications are crushed, dissolved, and injected intravenously, talc particles embolize small pulmonary vessels and may then migrate into the pulmonary interstitium, where they induce a foreign-body reaction and fibrosis.
Polyarteritis	Poorly defined nodules that are often associated with patchy consolidations.	The pulmonary manifestations typically show progression and regression of lesions on serial films, reflecting the appearance of new lesions and the healing of old ones.
Mucoid impactions	Multiple (more commonly single), round, oval, or elliptical opacities caused by plugs in dilated bronchi.	Usually associated with hypersensitivity broncho-pulmonary aspergillosis in patients with asthma or pre-existing chronic bronchial disease.

A   B

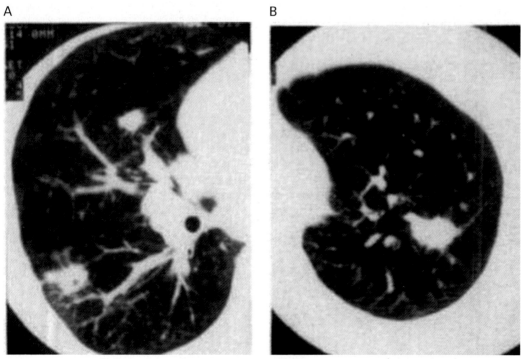

Fig C 9-10
Sarcoidosis. Two images show parenchymal nodules of high attenuation involving both lungs.[148]

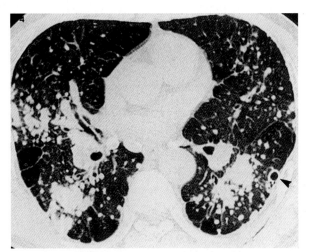

Fig C 9-11
Progressive massive fibrosis. Conglomerate masses and adjacent small nodules in coal workers' pneumoconiosis. The arrowhead points to a thoracostomy tube that was placed in the left hemithorax for a pneumothorax.[149]

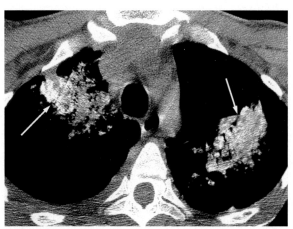

Fig C 9-12
Talc-induced lung disease. Bilateral irregular nodular areas of high attenuation in the upper lobes.[10]

Miliary Nodules*

Condition	Comments
Tuberculosis (Fig C 10-1)	Hematogenous dissemination that almost invariably leads to a dramatic febrile response with night sweats and chills. There may be minimal symptoms in severely debilitated patients, especially elderly persons and those receiving steroids.
Fungal diseases (Figs C 10-2 and C 10-3)	Hematogenous dissemination, most commonly of histoplasmosis but also coccidioidomycosis, blastomycosis, and candidiasis. May represent the healing phase of the acute epidemic form of histoplasmosis.
Disseminated hematogenous metastases (Fig C 10-4)	Most commonly thyroid carcinoma ("snowstorm"), which may remain unchanged for a long time because of the very low grade of malignancy. Other causes include trophoblastic disease, bone sarcomas, renal cell carcinoma, and, infrequently, melanoma and carcinomas of the breast and gastrointestinal tract.
Bronchioloalveolar (alveolar cell) carcinoma (Fig C 10-5)	Other presentations include a well-circumscribed, peripheral solitary nodule (see Fig C 6-13), focal "pneumonia" (see Fig C 1-25), and multiple poorly defined nodules (see Fig C 7-6).

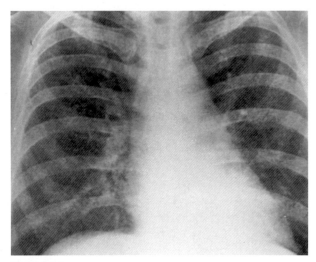

Fig C 10-1
Tuberculosis.

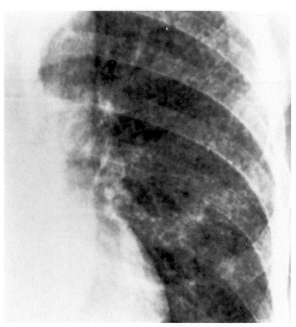

Fig C 10-2
Coccidioidomycosis. Coned view of the left lung shows a diffuse pattern of fine nodules simulating miliary tuberculosis.

*Diffuse fine nodules less than 5 mm in diameter

A

B

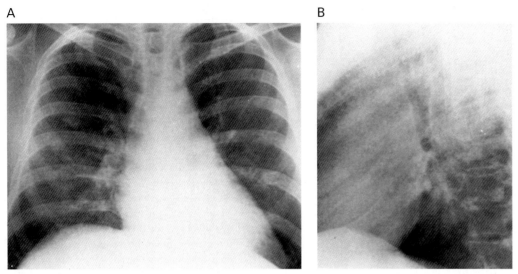

Fig C 10-3
Histoplasmosis. (A) Frontal and (B) lateral views.

B

A

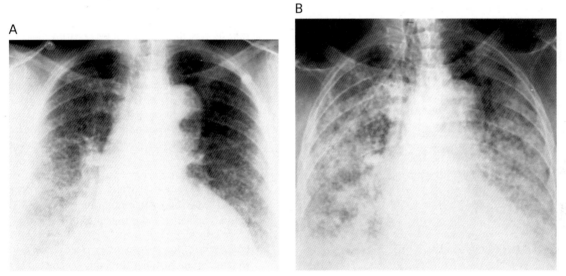

Fig C 10-4
Metastatic thyroid carcinoma. (A) Multiple fine miliary nodules scattered throughout both lungs. (B) At a later stage, there is a coarser miliary pattern.

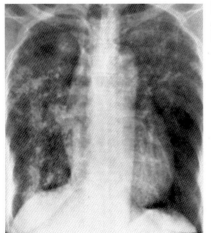

Fig C 10-5
Alveolar cell carcinoma. Miliary pattern diffusely involving both lungs represents bronchogenic spread.

Condition	Comments
Pneumoconiosis (Figs C 10-6 and C 10-7)	Silicosis, coal-workers' pneumoconiosis, and berylliosis. The nodules represent localized areas of fibrosis (or the summation of linear shadows).
Pulmonary Langerhans histiocytosis	Early active stage of the disease. The nodules represent individual granulomatous foci.
Sarcoidosis (see Fig C 14-8)	Associated bilateral and symmetric hilar adenopathy is virtually pathognomonic (though the adenopathy classically regresses as the parenchymal disease progresses).
Allergic alveolitis (farmer's lung)	Allergy involving the alveolar wall due to a variety of noninvasive fungi. Represents the subacute or chronic phase of the illness.
Viral pneumonia (Fig C 10-8)	Primarily chickenpox pneumonia (adults more than children). May heal with the development of multiple calcified nodules (as in histoplasmosis).
Alveolar microlithiasis (see Fig C 2-15)	Diffuse, very fine micronodules of calcific density that are usually asymptomatic. Characteristic black pleura sign (due to contrast between the extreme density of the lung parenchyma on one side of the pleura and the ribs on the other side).
Pulmonary hemosiderosis (Fig C 10-9)	Develops in patients with long-standing severe mitral stenosis who have had multiple episodes of hemoptysis.
Amyloidosis	Rare manifestation in which amyloid infiltrates almost every alveolar septum and is deposited around capillaries and within interstitial tissue.
Bronchiolitis obliterans	End result of lower respiratory tract damage in which the bronchioles become obstructed by organizing exudate and polypoid masses of granulation tissue.
Oil embolism	Complication of lymphography (lipid material in the extravascular interstitial tissue).
Interstitial fibrosis	Early stage before the development of the more classic reticulonodular and reticular patterns.
Niemann-Pick disease	Rare lipid storage disease. The miliary nodule pattern (and early age of onset) is a differential point from Gaucher's disease.
Parasitic disease (Fig C 10-10)	Schistosomiasis, filariasis.
Listeriosis (Fig C 10-11)	Rare bacterial disease that primarily occurs as an intrauterine infection with a high mortality rate, or as a disease of the newborn.

Condition	Comments
Rheumatoid disease	Miliary pattern occurs in the early "subacute" stage of the disease before the development of the more characteristic diffuse interstitial pulmonary fibrosis.
Wegener's granulomatosis	Rare manifestation representing a diffuse granulomatous reaction occurring around vessels. The small fine nodules usually develop in combination with larger, more ill-defined densities that often cavitate.

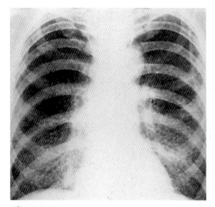

Fig C 10-6
Silicosis.

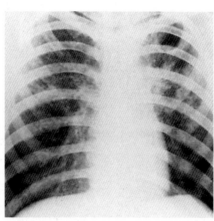

Fig C 10-7
Coal-workers' pneumoconiosis.

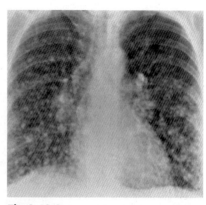

Fig C 10-8
Chickenpox pneumonia. Bilateral, coarse miliary infiltrates distributed diffusely throughout both lungs.

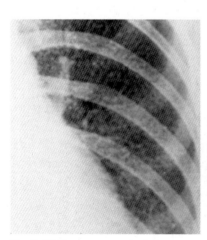

Fig C 10-9
Pulmonary hemosiderosis.[27]

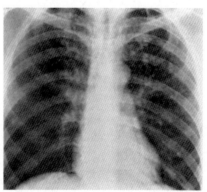

Fig C 10-10
Schistosomiasis. Perivascular granulomas produce small nodular and linear densities that are distributed diffusely throughout the lungs in a miliary pattern simulating tuberculosis.

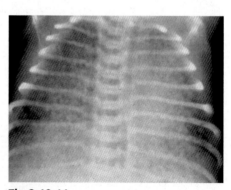

Fig C 10-11
Listeriosis. Diffuse miliary pattern of coarse, irregular granular densities is distributed throughout both lungs.

Cavitary Lesions of the Lungs

Condition	Imaging Findings	Comments
Bacterial lung abscess (Fig C 11-1)	Generally a thick-walled cavity with a shaggy inner lining.	Most frequently *Staphylococcus*, *Klebsiella*, *Pseudomonas*, and *Proteus*. An empyema is commonly associated. Multiple cavities often occur with anaerobic organisms.
Pneumatocele (Fig C 11-2)	Thin-walled cystic space (may be multiple).	Develops in approximately 50% of children with staphylococcal pneumonia. Results from a check-valve obstruction of the communication between a peribronchial abscess and the bronchial lumen.

A   B

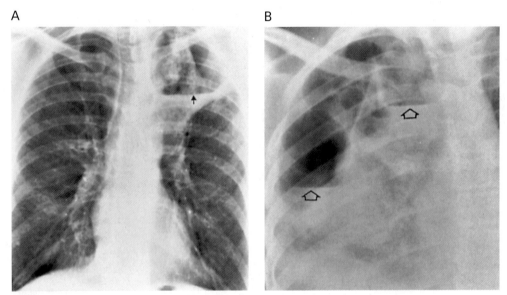

Fig C 11-1
Bacterial lung abscess. (A) *Proteus* pneumonia. Large, thick-walled left upper lobe abscess with an air-fluid level (arrow) and an associated infiltrate. (B) *Staphylococcal pneumonia.* Multiple lung abscesses with air-fluid levels (arrows) associated with diffuse air-space consolidation and a large pleural effusion.

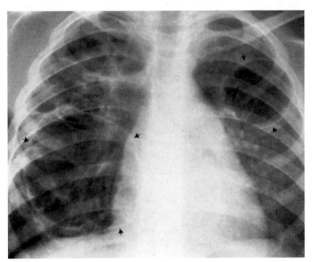

Fig C 11-2
Pneumatocele. Residual thin-walled cystic spaces (arrows) in the pulmonary parenchyma many years after a childhood staphylococcal pneumonia.

Condition	Imaging Findings	Comments
Mycobacteria (Figs C 11-3 and C 11-4)	Wall of the cavity is usually of moderate thickness and has a generally smooth inner lining.	Cavitation (often multiple) tends to be a more prominent feature of atypical mycobacterial disease than of *Mycobacterium tuberculosis*. Tuberculous cavities predominantly involve the apical and posterior regions of the upper lobes and the posterior segments of the lower lobes. Thin-walled cavities may persist after chemotherapy in the absence of acute disease.

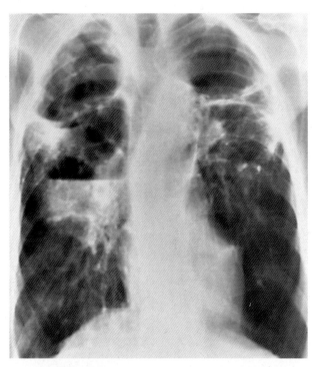

Fig C 11-3
Tuberculosis. Multiple large cavities with air-fluid levels in both upper lobes. Note the chronic fibrotic changes and upward retraction of the hila.

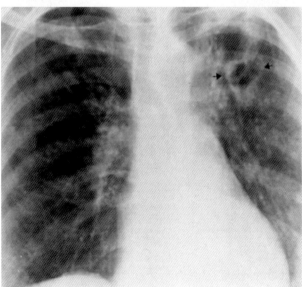

Fig C 11-4
Atypical mycobacteria. Cavitary lesion (arrows) in the left upper lobe. The wall of the cavity is mildly irregular, and there is minimal parenchymal disease

Condition	Imaging Findings	Comments
Fungal lung abscess (Figs C 11-5 to C 11-7)	Single or multiple cavities, most of which are thick walled (coccidioidomycosis tends to produce a very thin-walled lesion).	Pleural effusion and extension into the chest wall are common in actinomycosis and nocardiosis. Histoplasmosis typically involves the apical and posterior segments of the upper lobes (indistinguishable from tuberculosis), whereas coccidioidomycosis is characteristically located in the anterior segment. Candidiasis, aspergillosis, sporotrichosis, and mucormycosis are essentially limited to debilitated patients and those with underlying diseases (diabetes mellitus, lymphoma, leukemia).

B

A

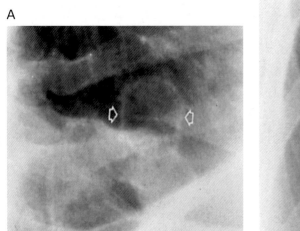
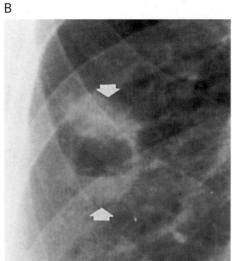

Fig C 11-5
Coccidioidomycosis. (A) Thin-walled cavity (arrows). (B) Irregular, thick-walled cavity with surrounding infiltrate (arrows).

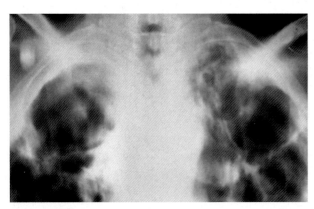

Fig C 11-6
Sporotrichosis. Frontal tomogram shows extensive bilateral upper lobe cavities.[15]

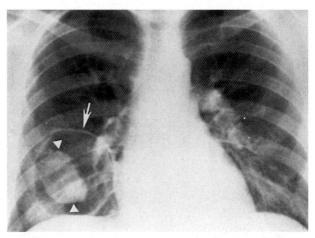

Fig C 11-7
Mucormycosis. Large thin-walled cavity (arrow) containing a smooth, elliptical, homogeneous mass (arrowheads) representing a fungus ball.

Condition	Imaging Findings	Comments
Amebic lung abscess	Thick-walled cavity with a ragged inner lining.	Almost always in the right lower lobe and associated with a right pleural effusion (organisms from a liver abscess enter the thorax by direct extension via the right hemidiaphragm).
Hydatid cyst (*Echinococcus granulosus*) (Fig C 11-8)	Thin-walled cavity, typically with a lower lobe predominance.	Rupture of the cyst into a bronchus results in part or all of its liquid contents being expelled into the bronchial system, producing the characteristic "meniscus sign" and "water lily sign" (irregularity of the air-fluid layer caused by collapsed cyst membranes). A hydropneumothorax may also occur.
Paragonimus westermani (Fig C 11-9)	Thin-walled cysts (ring shadows) that are generally multiple and have a predilection for the periphery of the lower lobes.	Typically a crescent-shaped opacity along one aspect of the inner lining. May mimic cystic bronchiectasis.

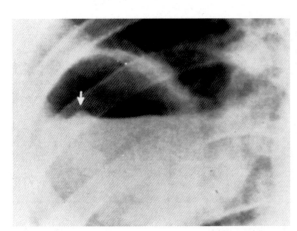

Fig C 11-8
Water lily sign in pulmonary echinococcal cyst. The endocyst membranes (arrow) are floating on the surface of fluid in a ruptured hydatid cyst.[28]

A

B

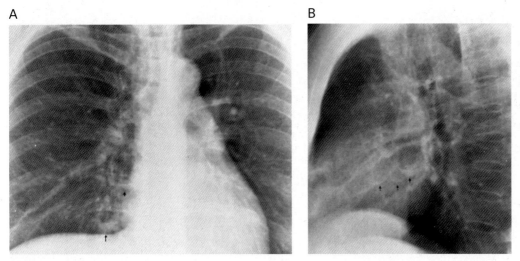

Fig C 11-9
Paragonimiasis. (A) Frontal and (B) lateral chest radiographs demonstrate multiple cysts (arrows) in the right middle lobe. The cysts are thin walled, and most have a prominent crescent-shaped opacity along one side of their borders, the characteristic ring shadow of paragonimiasis.

Condition	Imaging Findings	Comments
Pneumocystis carinii (Fig C 11-10)	Single or multiple thin-walled cavities.	Primarily seen in patients with AIDS.
Bronchogenic carcinoma (Fig C 11-11)	Generally a thick-walled cavity with an irregular, nodular inner lining (occasionally a thin-walled cavity simulating a bronchogenic cyst).	Cavitation in 2% to 10% of cases, most commonly in peripheral squamous cell tumors of the upper lobes. Multiple primaries are very rare.
Hematogenous metastases (Fig C 11-12)	Thin- or thick-walled cavities may develop in a few or multiple metastatic nodules. Most commonly involves upper lobe lesions.	Cavitation in approximately 4% of cases. Most commonly involves squamous cell neoplasms (also adenocarcinomas of the large bowel and sarcomas).
Hodgkin's disease	Single or multiple thick-walled cavities with irregular inner linings.	Cavitation typically develops in peripheral parenchymal consolidations (most often in the lower lobes). Usually, enlargement of mediastinal and hilar lymph nodes is also seen.
Septic embolism (Figs C 11-13 and C 11-14)	Generally thin-walled cavities (less commonly thick walled with shaggy inner linings).	Almost always multiple with lower lobe predominance. A wide variation in size may reflect recurrent showers of emboli.
Silicosis	Thick-walled cavity with an irregular inner lining. Often multiple with strong upper lobe predominance.	Generally a background of nodular or reticulonodular disease and associated hilar lymph node enlargement. Cavitation in conglomerate lesions is more often the result of superimposed tuberculosis than ischemic necrosis. Cavitation also occurs in coal-workers' pneumoconiosis.
Wegener's granulomatosis (Fig C 11-15)	Usually multiple thick-walled cavities with irregular inner linings (may eventually become thin-walled cystic spaces).	Cavitation eventually occurs in approximately half of patients. With treatment, the cavitary lesions may disappear or heal with scar formation.

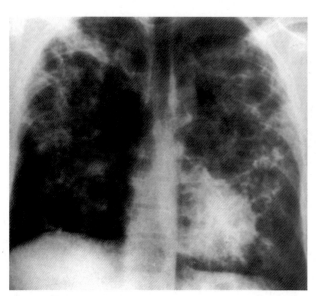

Fig C 11-10
Pneumocystis carinii. Innumerable thin-walled cavities.[29]

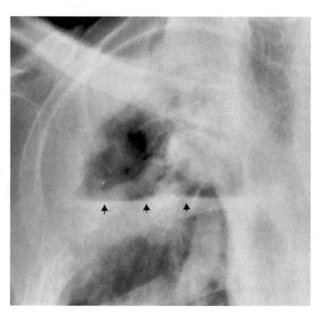

Fig C 11-11
Bronchogenic carcinoma. Large cavitary right upper lobe mass with an air-fluid level (arrows) and associated rib destruction.

Condition	Imaging Findings	Comments
Rheumatoid necrobiotic nodule	Thick-walled cavity with a smooth inner lining (may become thin-walled and even disappear with remission of the arthritis).	Often multiple and generally in a peripheral subpleural location (most often the lower lobe). May be associated with pleural effusion or spontaneous pneumothorax.

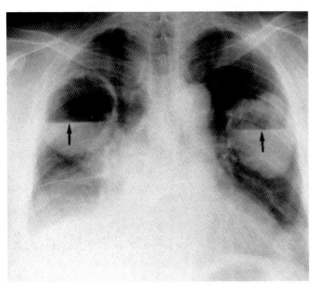

Fig C 11-12
Hematogenous metastases. Extensive cavitation with air-fluid levels (arrows) of squamous cell carcinoma on a film obtained after two cycles of chemotherapy.[22]

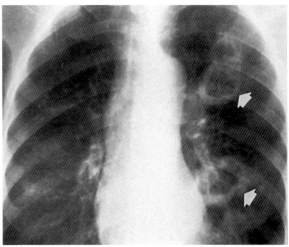

Fig C 11-13
Septic pulmonary emboli. Large cavity lesions (arrows) in the left lung of an intravenous drug abuser with septic thrombophlebitis.

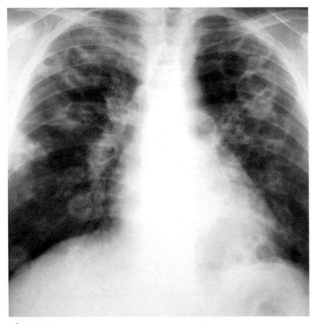

Fig C 11-14
Septic pulmonary emboli. Multiple cavitary nodules throughout both lungs representing *Nocardia* septic emboli in an intravenous drug abuser with AIDS.[30]

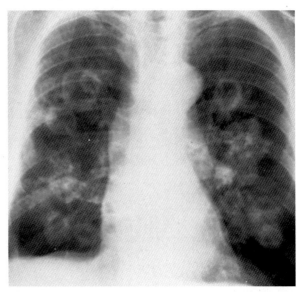

Fig C 11-15
Wegener's granulomatosis. Multiple thick-walled cavities with irregular, shaggy inner linings.

Condition	Imaging Findings	Comments
Cystic bronchiectasis (Fig C 11-16)	Multiple thin-walled cavities with lower lobe predominance. Often a tiny air-fluid level at the bottom of the ring shadow.	Cavities represent severely dilated segmental bronchi. Generally a considerable loss of volume in the affected region.
Bleb/bulla (Fig C 11-17)	Very thin-walled cystic space. Usually multiple with upper lobe predominance.	Air-fluid levels develop with infection. Often radiographic evidence of diffuse pulmonary emphysema.
Traumatic lung cyst	Single or several thin-walled cavities that may contain air-fluid levels.	Typically occurs in a peripheral subpleural location immediately underlying the point of maximum injury.
Sarcoidosis	Cystic lesions developing on a background of diffuse reticulonodular pulmonary disease.	Very uncommon manifestation (should suggest superimposed tuberculosis or fungal disease). A mycetoma may occur in a cavitary lesion.
Intralobar bronchopulmonary sequestration	Thin- or thick-walled cystic mass that is often multilocular or multiple.	Almost invariably arises contiguous to the diaphragm (two-thirds are on the left). May be obscured by pneumonia in the surrounding parenchyma.
Bronchogenic cyst	Solitary thin-walled cystic mass that may contain an air-fluid level.	Approximately 75% of bronchogenic cysts that are originally opaque and fluid filled eventually become air containing because of an infectious communication with the contiguous lung.
Congenital cystic adenomatoid malformation (see Fig C 15-7)	Multiple air-containing cysts scattered irregularly throughout a mass of soft-tissue density.	Expands the ipsilateral hemithorax (depresses the hemidiaphragm and shifts the mediastinum to the contralateral side). May occasionally be confused with a diaphragmatic hernia containing bowel loops. The malformation can often be detected by fetal ultrasound.

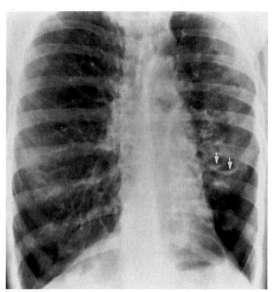

Fig C 11-16
Cystic bronchiectasis. Multiple cystic spaces, some with air-fluid levels (arrows), predominantly involve the left lung.

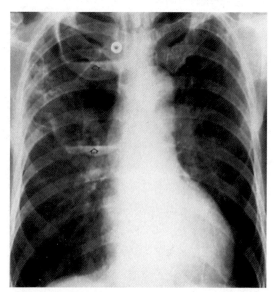

Fig C 11-17
Pulmonary emphysema. Large bullae in the right upper lung. The presence of air-fluid levels (arrows) in the cystic spaces indicates superimposed infection.

Condition	Imaging Findings	Comments
Cystic fibrosis (mucoviscidosis) (Fig C 11-18)	Thin-walled cystic lesions with or without air-fluid levels associated with diffuse, coarse, reticular changes, hyperinflation, and pulmonary arterial hypertension.	Ring shadows in this condition can be caused by cystic bronchiectasis, bullae, microabscesses, or honeycombing.
Papillomatosis (Fig C 11-19)	Multiple thin-walled cysts.	Laryngeal papillomatosis is a common disease in children that infrequently seeds distally in the tracheobronchial tree to produce excavating lesions in the lung.
Plombage (Fig C 11-20)	Plastic (lucite) spheres appear radiographically as multiple perfectly round, cavity-like lucencies.	Former therapy for pulmonary tuberculosis that consisted of filling of the extrapleural space with a sufficient volume of inert material to collapse the adjacent lung. The spheres are often not entirely watertight, so that a small amount of fluid may collect in each. On upright views, the resulting air-fluid levels can simulate cavitation and suggest the incorrect diagnosis of acute infection.

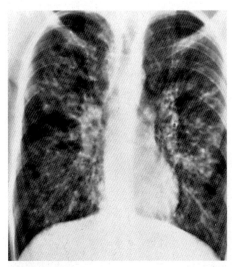

Fig C 11-18
Cystic fibrosis. Multiple small cysts superimposed on a diffuse, coarse, reticular pattern.

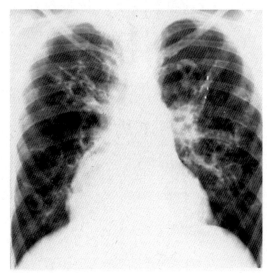

Fig C 11-19
Papillomatosis. Multiple thin-walled cystic lesions.

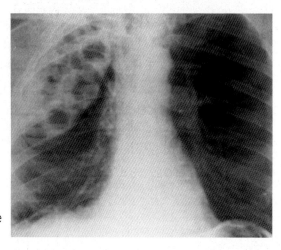

Fig C 11-20
Plombage. Air-fluid levels in the plastic spheres simulate cavitation.

Unilateral Hilar Enlargement

Condition	Comments
Inflammatory lymphadenopathy (Figs C 12-1 and C 12-2)	Histoplasmosis, tuberculosis, coccidioidomycosis. The hilar nodes often calcify and are usually associated with ipsilateral parenchymal disease.
Intrabronchial neoplasm	Hilar mass generally represents local nodal metastases (the endobronchial lesion itself usually produces only a minimal mass effect).
Metastatic neoplasm (Fig C 12-3)	Often bilateral, with involvement of mediastinal lymph nodes. In lymphangitic spread, there is generally a diffuse reticular or reticulonodular pattern.
Lymphoma	Primarily Hodgkin's disease, which often produces asymmetric bilateral hilar adenopathy. There may be pulmonary involvement or pleural effusion. The nodes may calcify after mediastinal irradiation.

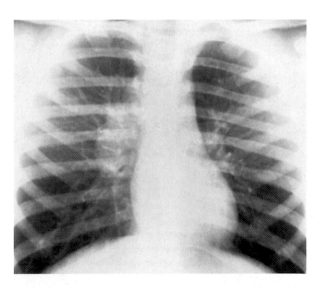

Fig C 12-1
Primary tuberculosis. Enlargement of right hilar nodes without a discrete parenchymal infiltrate.

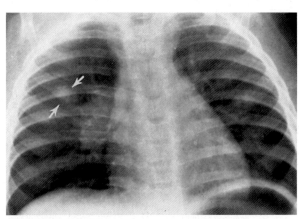

Fig C 12-2
Primary tuberculosis. The combination of a focal parenchymal lesion (arrows) and enlarged right hilar lymph nodes produces the classic primary complex.

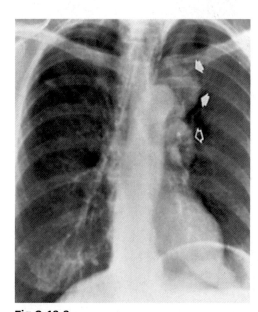

Fig C 12-3
Lymphadenopathy due to oat cell carcinoma of the lung. In addition to left hilar adenopathy (open arrow), there is enlargement of anterior mediastinal lymph nodes (closed arrows).

Condition	Comments
Valvular pulmonic stenosis (see Fig CA 15-6)	Poststenotic dilatation of the left pulmonary artery. There is usually enlargement of the right ventricle. Central dilatation of the right pulmonary artery also occurs, but the dilated segment is hidden in the mediastinum (left-sided enlargement is not due to the direction of the jet emanating from the constricted valve).
Pulmonary embolism (Fig C 12-4)	Result of vascular distention by bulk thrombus (not increased vascular resistance in the affected lung). The occluded vessel is often more sharply delineated than normal and may terminate suddenly ("knuckle" sign).
Pulmonary artery aneurysm	Congenital or posttraumatic.
Pulmonary artery coarctation	Poststenotic dilatation of the affected pulmonary artery.
Pulmonary arteriovenous fistula	Enlargement of hilar vessels is due to increased blood flow on the affected side. There is often evidence of single or multiple parenchymal nodules with characteristic feeding arteries and draining veins.
Normal variant (see Fig CA 15-1)	Prominence of the left pulmonary artery occurs in adults younger than 30 (especially women).
Narrowed or occluded pulmonary artery	Unilateral enlargement of the opposite hilum may develop in patients with carcinoma, Swyer-James syndrome, or congenital absence of the pulmonary artery.

A
B

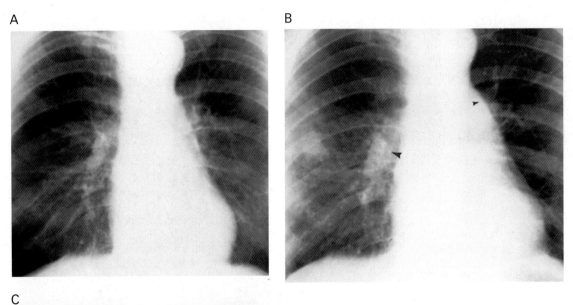

C

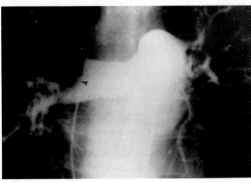

Fig C 12-4
Pulmonary embolism. (A) Baseline chest radiograph demonstrates normal-sized pulmonary arteries. (B) Enlargement of the main pulmonary artery (small arrow) and right pulmonary artery (large arrow) coincides with the onset of the patient's symptoms. (C) Arteriogram demonstrates multiple bilateral pulmonary emboli and a large right saddle embolus (arrow).

Bilateral Hilar Enlargement

Condition	Imaging Findings	Comments
Lymphadenopathy (Figs C 13-1 through C 13-6)	Bilateral enlargement of hilar nodes that may be associated with reticular or reticulonodular parenchymal disease.	Causes include infectious agents (especially tuberculosis, histoplasmosis, mycoplasma, and viral pneumonias), malignancy (carcinoma, lymphoma), silicosis, and sarcoidosis.
Congenital heart disease (see Fig CA 13-4)	Bilateral enlargement of pulmonary vessels that is usually associated with cardiomegaly.	Severe left-to-right shunts (atrial septal defect, ventricular septal defect, patent ductus arteriosus). Also cyanotic admixture lesions (transposition of great vessels, persistent truncus arteriosus).
Pulmonary arterial hypertension (Fig C 13-7)	Bilateral enlargement of central pulmonary arteries with rapid tapering and small peripheral vessels. Also cardiac enlargement (especially the right ventricle).	Primary or secondary to such conditions as widespread peripheral pulmonary emboli, Eisenmenger's syndrome (reversed left-to-right shunt), and chronic obstructive emphysema. Rare causes include metastases from trophoblastic neoplasms, immunologic disorders (Raynaud's phenomenon, rheumatoid disease), schistosomiasis, multiple pulmonary artery stenoses or coarctations, and vasoconstrictive diseases.

A
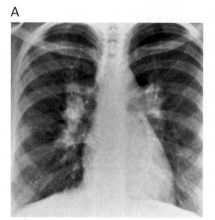
B
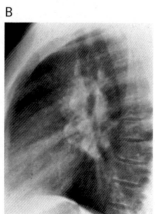

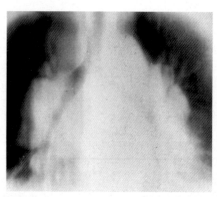

Fig C 13-1
Infectious mononucleosis. (A) Frontal and (B) lateral views of the chest demonstrate marked bilateral hilar adenopathy.

Fig C 13-2
Bronchogenic carcinoma. Tomography demonstrates bilateral bulky hilar adenopathy typical of oat cell carcinoma.

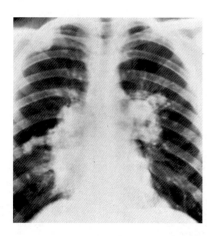

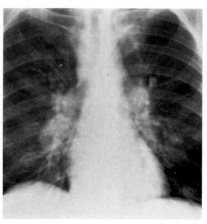

Fig C 13-3
Ossified metastases to hilar lymph nodes bilaterally from osteogenic sarcoma. There are also multiple parenchymal metastases.

Fig C 13-4
Lymphoma. Frontal view shows bilateral hilar adenopathy.

Condition	Imaging Findings	Comments
Pulmonary embolism	Bilateral enlargement of central pulmonary arteries. Usually obliteration of peripheral vessels and right-sided cardiac enlargement.	May reflect massive bilateral central emboli or widespread peripheral emboli.
Pulmonary venous hypertension	Bilateral enlargement of central pulmonary veins associated with cardiomegaly and cephalization of pulmonary blood flow.	Causes include left-sided heart failure and mitral stenosis.
Primary polycythemia	Generalized bilateral increase in central and peripheral pulmonary vascularity.	Increased blood volume produces prominence of the pulmonary vascular shadows, usually without the cardiomegaly associated with the increased pulmonary vascularity in patients with congenital heart disease. Intravascular thrombosis may cause pulmonary infarctions that appear as focal consolidations or bands of fibrosis.

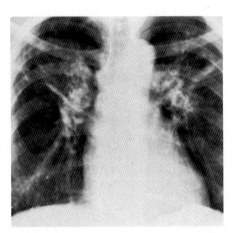

Fig C 13-5
Silicosis. Characteristic eggshell lymph node calcification associated with bilateral perihilar masses.

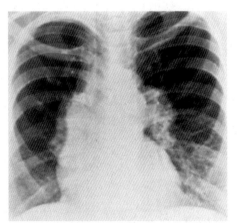

Fig C 13-6
Sarcoidosis. Prominent bilateral hilar adenopathy with a suggestion of enlarged nodes in the right and left paratracheal regions.

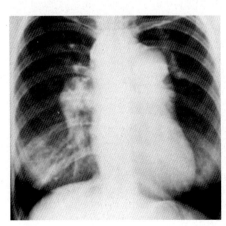

Fig C 13-7
Pulmonary arterial hypertension. Frontal chest film in a patient with atrial septal defect and Eisenmenger's physiology demonstrates a huge pulmonary outflow tract and central pulmonary arteries with abrupt tapering and sparse peripheral vasculature.[31]

Hilar and Mediastinal Lymph Node Enlargement

Condition	Imaging Findings	Comments
Primary tuberculosis (see Figs C 12-1 and C 12-2)	Enlarged hilar and paratracheal nodes that often calcify. Bilateral involvement in approximately 20% of cases.	Almost always associated with ipsilateral parenchymal disease (may even obscure the lymphadenopathy).
Histoplasmosis	Unilateral or bilateral enlargement of hilar, mediastinal, and, occasionally, intrapulmonary nodes.	Usually associated with parenchymal disease (often absent in children). The enlarged nodes may extrinsically obstruct the airways and cause distal infection or atelectasis. Calcification of nodes is common and may even lead to erosion into the bronchial lumen.
Coccidioidomycosis	Unilateral or bilateral enlargement of hilar or paratracheal nodes.	There may be associated parenchymal disease. Enlargement of paratracheal lymph nodes may indicate imminent dissemination.
Mycoplasma pneumoniae	Unilateral or bilateral enlargement of hilar nodes.	Common in children, rare in adults. Always associated with ipsilateral parenchymal disease.
Viral diseases (Fig C 14-1; see Fig C 13-1)	Hilar node enlargement that is often bilateral.	Psittacosis, infectious mononucleosis (also splenomegaly), rubeola, echovirus, varicella. Usually parenchymal involvement or increased bronchovascular markings.
Bacterial infections (Figs C 14-2 and C 14-3)	Various patterns of nodal enlargement.	Unilateral in pertussis (whooping cough) and tularemia (ipsilateral hilar enlargement in 25% to 50% of tularemic pneumonias); bilateral involvement in anthrax and plague.

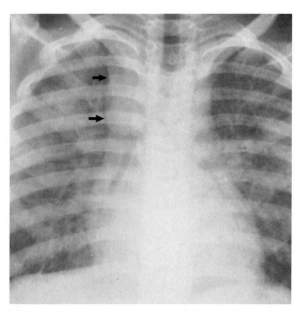

Fig C 14-1
Measles pneumonia. Diffuse, reticular interstitial infiltrate with a focal area of consolidation in the right upper lobe. Note the striking right hilar and mediastinal adenopathy (arrows).

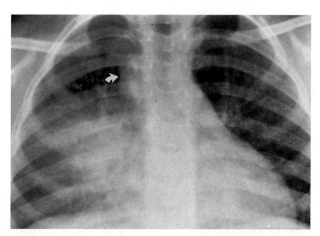

Fig C 14-2
Tularemia pneumonia. Air-space consolidation involving the right middle lobe and a portion of the right upper lobe. Note the right paratracheal nodal enlargement (arrow).

Condition	Imaging Findings	Comments
Bronchogenic carcinoma (Fig C 14-4)	Usually unilateral enlargement of hilar nodes.	Presenting sign in up to one-third of patients (primary carcinoma arising in a major hilar bronchus or metastasis from a small primary tumor in adjacent or peripheral parenchyma). Bulky, even bilateral, nodal enlargement suggests oat cell carcinoma.

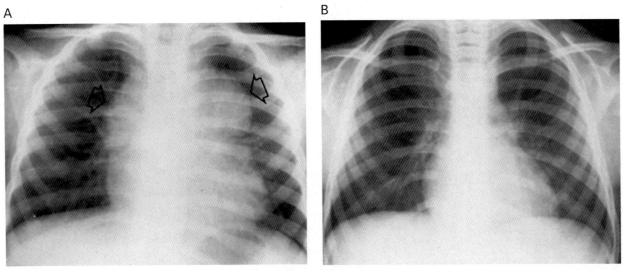

Fig C 14-3
Bubonic plague. (A) Initial film demonstrates massive enlargement of the mediastinal lymph nodes (arrows). (B) After chloramphenicol therapy, a repeat chest film demonstrates complete clearing of the lymphadenopathy.[32]

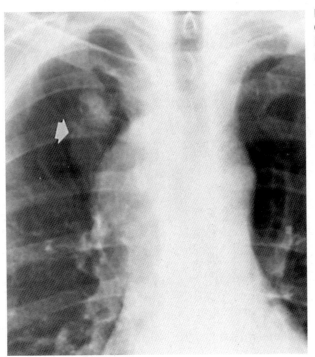

Fig C 14-4
Oat cell carcinoma. Prominent right mediastinal lymphadenopathy associated with an ill-defined primary malignant lesion (arrow).

Condition	Imaging Findings	Comments
Lymphoma (Figs C 14-5 and C 14-6)	Enlargement of all hilar and mediastinal nodes (the anterior mediastinal and retrosternal nodes are frequently affected). Typically bilateral but asymmetric (unilateral node enlargement is very rare).	Most common radiographic finding in Hodgkin's disease (visible on the initial chest films of ~50% of patients). Pulmonary involvement or pleural effusion occurs in about 30%. Calcification may develop in intrathoracic lymph nodes after mediastinal irradiation.
Leukemia (Fig C 14-7)	Symmetric enlargement of hilar and mediastinal nodes in approximately 25% of patients.	Lymphadenopathy occurs more commonly in lymphocytic than in myelocytic leukemia. There may also be pleural effusion and parenchymal involvement.
Metastases (lymphangitic spread)	Unilateral or bilateral enlargement of hilar or mediastinal nodes.	Usually associated with a diffuse reticular or reticulonodular pattern that predominantly involves the lung bases (see Fig C 4-1).

A   B

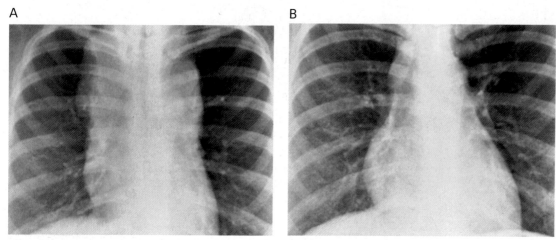

Fig C 14-5
Lymphoma. (A) Initial chest film demonstrates marked widening of the upper half of the mediastinum due to pronounced lymphadenopathy. (B) After chemotherapy, there is a marked decrease in the width of the upper mediastinum.

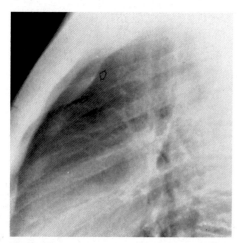

Fig C 14-6
Lymphoma. Lateral view of the chest shows subtle enlargement of a retrosternal (internal mammary) lymph node (arrows).

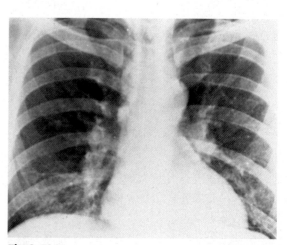

Fig C 14-7
Leukemia. Bilateral hilar and right paratracheal lymphadenopathy.

Condition	Imaging Findings	Comments
Silicosis (see Fig C 13-5)	Bilateral hilar node enlargement. Typical eggshell calcification (in approximately 10% of patients) is almost pathognomonic (occasionally occurs in sarcoidosis or radiated Hodgkin's disease) and can involve mediastinal, peritoneal, and retroperitoneal nodes.	Usually associated with a diffuse nodular or reticulonodular pattern throughout both lungs. A similar appearance may occur in chronic berylliosis.
Sarcoidosis (Fig C 14-8)	Bilaterally symmetric enlargement of hilar and paratracheal nodes develops in up to 90% of patients. The outer borders of the enlarged hila are usually lobulated.	Approximately half of patients have diffuse parenchymal disease. Nodal enlargement often resolves as the parenchymal disease develops, unlike lymphoma or tuberculosis. The bilateral symmetry is unlike tuberculosis, whereas the lack of retrosternal involvement is unlike lymphoma.
Pulmonary Langerhans cell histiocytosis	Symmetric enlargement of hilar and mediastinal nodes is a rare manifestation.	Early diffuse micronodular pattern that may become coarse in later stages. Lack of lymph node enlargement in a patient with diffuse interstitial pulmonary disease favors a diagnosis of histiocytosis X rather than sarcoidosis.
Idiopathic pulmonary hemosiderosis/ Goodpasture's syndrome	Symmetric enlargement of hilar nodes primarily occurs in the acute stage.	Episodes of pulmonary hemorrhage produce diffuse alveolar and interstitial disease.
Cystic fibrosis	Unilateral or bilateral hilar node enlargement is an uncommon finding.	Diffuse increase in pulmonary markings with hyperinflation and areas of atelectasis and bronchiectasis.
Bronchopulmonary amyloidosis	Symmetric enlargement of hilar and mediastinal nodes (may be densely calcified).	Rare manifestation of this plasma cell dyscrasia. Sometimes associated with diffuse pulmonary involvement.
Heavy-chain disease	Symmetric enlargement of mediastinal nodes.	Unusual manifestation of this rare plasma cell dyscrasia. Hepatosplenomegaly is common, whereas lung involvement is rare.
Drug-induced changes	Bilateral hilar or mediastinal lymph node enlargement.	May develop during diphenylhydantoin or trimethadione therapy.

B

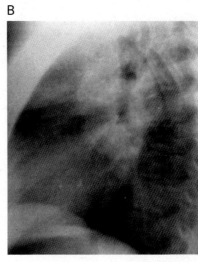

A

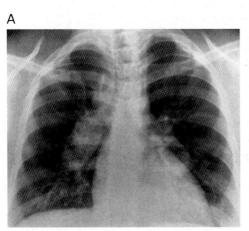

Fig C 14-8
Sarcoidosis. (A) Frontal and (B) lateral views of the chest demonstrate enlargement of the right hilar, left hilar, and right paratracheal lymph nodes, producing the classic 1-2-3 pattern of adenopathy.

Unilateral Lobar or Localized Hyperlucency of the Lung

Condition	Imaging Findings	Comments
Local obstructive emphysema	Localized hyperlucency of the lung associated with thin, attenuated vessels (predominantly involves the lower zones).	Approximately 50% of cases of emphysema have local rather than diffuse involvement radiographically. Affected zones show air trapping on expiration and overinflation at full lung capacity.
Bulla/bleb (Figs C 15-1 and C 15-2)	Sharply defined, air-containing spaces that are bounded by curvilinear, hairline shadows and vary in size from 1 cm to an entire hemithorax.	Predominantly unilateral. Unlike local obstructive emphysema, the vascular markings are absent rather than attenuated. Overinflation and air trapping usually occur.
Foreign body aspiration (see Fig C 31-3)	Segmental distribution with lower lobe predominance (especially on the right). Characteristic air trapping on expiratory films and often local oligemia.	Most common manifestation of foreign body aspiration. An opaque foreign body may be demonstrated.
Compensatory overaeration (Fig C 15-3)	Overinflation and oligemia of the remaining lobe(s).	Lobar collapse or agenesis causes overdistention of the normal portions of the lung.

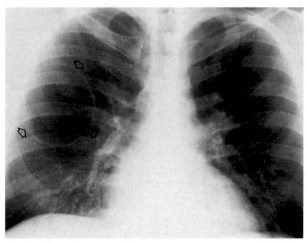

Fig C 15-1
Congenital emphysematous bulla. Large thin-walled air cyst (arrows) in the mid-portion of the right lung.

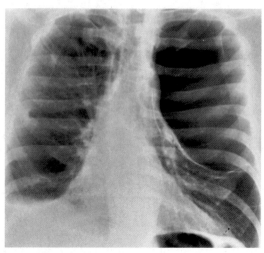

Fig C 15-2
Giant emphysematous bulla. The air-containing mass fills most of the left hemithorax.

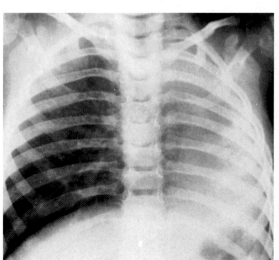

Fig C 15-3
Compensatory overaeration in agenesis of the left lung. There is virtually total absence of aerated lung in the left hemithorax. The right lung is markedly overinflated and has herniated across the midline. The entire mediastinum lies within the left hemithorax. The chest wall is asymmetric, and the ribs are somewhat close together on the left.

Condition	Imaging Findings	Comments
Pulmonary neoplasm	Segmental, lobar, or entire lung involvement. Air trapping on expiratory films.	Benign or malignant endobronchial neoplasms are a rare cause of unilateral or segmental hyperlucent lung (more commonly bronchial obstruction is complete and results in atelectasis or postobstructive pneumonia). Metastases to hilar lymph nodes occasionally compress a bronchus and cause oligemia.
Thromboembolic disease (Fig C 15-4)	Affected segment often shows moderate loss of volume but may still appear hyperlucent due to local oligemia (Westermark's sign).	Almost invariably associated with obstruction of a major lobar or segmental pulmonary artery. The affected artery is typically widened and is sharper than normal.

A

B

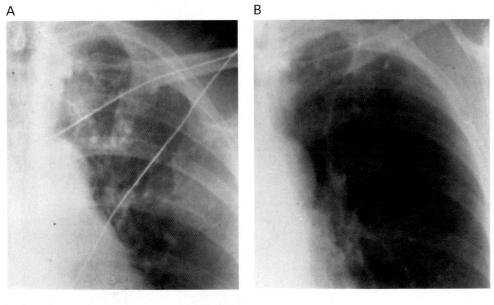

C

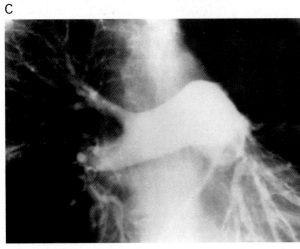

Fig C 15-4
Westermark's sign of pulmonary embolism. (A) Baseline chest radiograph demonstrates normal vascularity in the left upper lobe. (B) Striking hyperlucency of the left upper lobe coincided with the onset of the patient's symptoms. (C) Arteriogram performed on the same day the film in (B) was made shows an occluding clot in the left upper lobe and multiple emboli in the right lung.

Condition	Imaging Findings	Comments
Unilateral or lobar emphysema (Swyer–James syndrome) (Fig C 15-5)	Usually involvement of an entire lung (unilateral radiolucency), though a single lobe is occasionally affected. Air trapping during expiration (mediastinal shift toward the normal lung).	Probably results from acute pneumonia during infancy or childhood that causes bronchiolitis obliterans and an emphysema-like picture. The hilar and peripheral vessels are small.
Congenital lobar emphysema (Fig C 15-6)	Severe overinflation of a pulmonary lobe (especially the right upper or the right middle lobe).	Approximately one-third of cases apparent at birth (others noted several weeks later). Severe air trapping causes marked lobar enlargement, contralateral displacement of the mediastinum, and ipsilateral depression of the diaphragm.

A   B   C

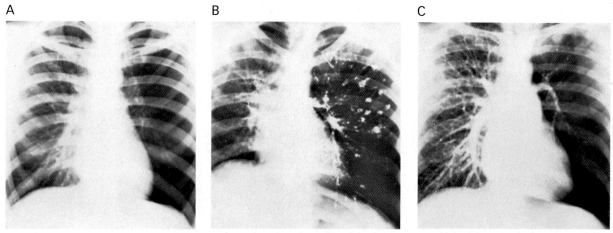

Fig C 15-5
Unilateral hyperlucent lung. (A) Frontal radiograph exposed at total lung capacity reveals a marked discrepancy in the radiolucency of the two lungs, with the left showing severe oligemia but normal lung volume. (B) Frontal radiograph at residual volume after bronchography demonstrates severe air trapping in the left lung and little change in volume from total lung capacity. Because the deflation of the right lung is normal, the mediastinum has swung sharply to the right. (C) A pulmonary arteriogram shows the discrepancy in blood flow to the two lungs. The left pulmonary artery is present, although diminutive, differentiating this appearance from congenital absence of the left pulmonary artery.[7]

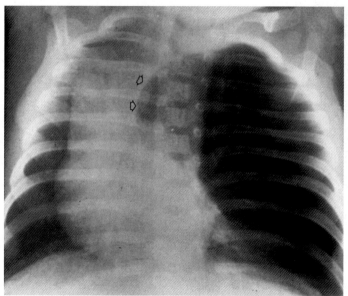

Fig C 15-6
Congenital lobar emphysema. Severe overdistension of the left upper lobe causes marked radiolucency of the left hemithorax along with depression of the ipsilateral hemidiaphragm and displacement of the mediastinum into the right hemithorax. The hyperinflated left upper lobe has herniated into the right side of the chest (arrows). Note the small and widely separated bronchovascular markings in the lucent left lung.

Condition	Imaging Findings	Comments
Cystic adenomatoid malformation (Fig C 15-7)	Usually appears as a mass composed of numerous air-containing cysts scattered irregularly throughout a soft-tissue density in a single lobe. Occasionally, a single air-filled cyst predominates, simulating infantile lobar emphysema.	Rare congenital anomaly consisting of an intralobar mass of disorganized pulmonary tissue that is classified as a hamartoma, though it is not neoplastic. If the malformation does not communicate with the bronchial tree, it contains only fluid and appears radiographically as a large pulmonary mass. The lesion expands the ipsilateral hemithorax by depressing the hemidiaphragm and shifting the mediastinum toward the contralateral side.
Hypogenetic lung syndrome (see Fig CA 8-8)	Small, often hyperlucent right lung associated with a small or absent pulmonary artery. May be associated with an anomalous draining vein that forms a broad, gently curved shadow descending to the diaphragm just to the right of the heart (scimitar sign).	Very rare anomaly in which the right lung is supplied partly or completely by systemic arteries (left-to-right shunt). Other cardiopulmonary anomalies are common.
Pulmonary branch stenosis	Ipsilateral lung is hypoplastic and has reduced volume, and there is an absent or diminutive hilum. No air trapping on forced expiration (unlike Swyer–James syndrome).	Very rare anomaly in which the involved lung is supplied by a hypertrophied bronchial circulation. The anomalous artery is usually on the side opposite the aortic arch (when on the left, there is a high incidence of associated cardiovascular anomalies).
Anomalous origin of left pulmonary artery from right pulmonary artery	Hyperlucent right lung due to air trapping and overinflation (anomalous vessel compresses the right main bronchus).	Very rare anomaly in which severe compression may collapse the lung. Compression of the trachea causes bilateral overinflation and air trapping on expiration. An esophagram shows pathognomonic posterior displacement of the esophagus and anterior displacement of the trachea by the interposed anomalous artery.

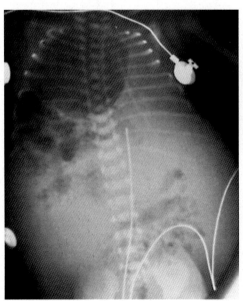

Fig C 15-7
Cystic adenomatoid malformation. Frontal radiograph of an infant's chest and abdomen at 1 hour of age demonstrates a large lucent mass in the right hemithorax with shift of the mediastinal structures to the left. In the lower right chest, the mass appears multicystic and resembles air-filled loops of bowel. Ascites is also present.[33]

Condition	Imaging Findings	Comments
Congenital bronchial atresia	Characteristic elliptical mass in the hilar region representing inspissated mucus distal to the point of atresia. May have a linear or branched pattern.	Very rare anomaly that most commonly involves the apicoposterior segment of the left upper lobe (can affect various segments). The bronchial tree peripheral to the point of obliteration is patent and air enters the affected segment by collateral air drift.
Tuberculosis	Overinflation and oligemia due to partial bronchial obstruction from ipsilateral hilar lymph node enlargement.	Primarily involves the anterior segment of an upper lobe or the medial segment of the middle lobe. May be the result of bronchostenosis from a tuberculous granuloma. Complete obstruction causes atelectasis.
Staphylococcal infection (pneumatocele) (see Fig C 11-2)	Characteristic thin-walled cystic spaces develop in approximately 50% of affected children. May be large and even fill an entire hemithorax. Often contain air-fluid levels.	Cystic spaces usually appear during the first week of a pneumonia and tend to disappear spontaneously within 6 weeks. Rare in adults. Probably results from check-valve obstruction of a communication between a peribronchial abscess and the bronchial lumen.
Hydrocarbon poisoning (Fig C 15-8)	Inhalation in children can lead to the formation of pneumatoceles simulating those in staphylococcal pneumonia.	Ingestion or inhalation of hydrocarbons is the leading cause of poisoning in children. Inhaled hydrocarbon initially produces perihilar infiltrates and pulmonary edema; ingested hydrocarbon is absorbed through the gastrointestinal tract and is carried by the bloodstream to the lungs, where it adds to the pulmonary injury.
Broncholith	Overinflation and oligemia due to partial bronchial obstruction from an endobronchial calcified mass.	Erosion of a calcified lymph node (usually from histoplasmosis) into the bronchial lumen.
Sarcoidosis	Hyperlucency of the lung due to air trapping and overinflation.	Rare cause. May be due to bronchial compression from enlarged nodes but more commonly results from endobronchial sarcoid deposits.

A B

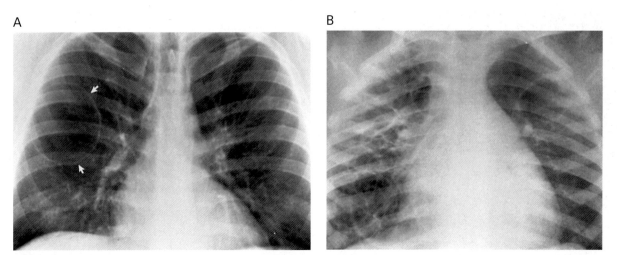

Fig C 15-8
Hydrocarbon poisoning. (A) Large thin-walled pneumatocele (arrows). (B) Multiple thin-walled pneumatoceles bilaterally but more marked on the right.

Condition	Imaging Findings	Comments
Nonpulmonary causes (normal vessels)		
Mastectomy	Unilateral hyperlucent lung. Absent breast shadow.	May be bilateral.
Absent pectoralis muscles (Fig C 15-9)	Unilateral hyperlucent lung.	Disparity in thickness of the supraclavicular soft tissues and axillary folds.
Faulty radiographic technique	Unilateral hyperlucent lung.	Most commonly due to patient rotation, which projects the soft tissues and the spine over one side of the chest while rotating them off the opposite, more lucent side (especially prominent in women with large pendulous breasts). Another cause is improper centering of the x-ray beam.

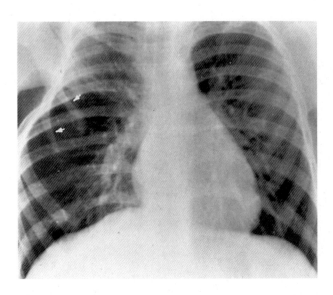

Fig C 15-9
Absence of the right pectoralis muscles. Asymmetry of the thoracic cage with hypoplasia of the anterior ribs (arrows). The lower portion of the right lung appears hyperlucent, whereas the apex seems comparatively opaque.

Bilateral Hyperlucent Lungs

Condition	Imaging Findings	Comments
Chronic obstructive emphysema (Fig C 16-1)	Severe hyperinflation (low, flat, or concave diaphragm; increased posteroanterior diameter of the chest; increased retrosternal space).	Marked attenuation and stretching (even virtual absence) of pulmonary vessels. Often evidence of pulmonary hypertension (enlargement of central pulmonary arteries with rapid peripheral tapering). The heart tends to be small and relatively vertical, and there are often single or multiple bullae. In α_1-antitrypsin deficiency, the emphysema predominantly involves the lower lobes.
Acute asthmatic attack (Fig C 16-2)	Severe overinflation of the lungs with air trapping. Characteristic tubular shadows ("tramlines") represent edema or thickening of bronchial walls.	Unlike emphysema, in this condition the vascular markings throughout the lungs are of normal caliber. Usually there is no radiographic abnormality between acute attacks.

A
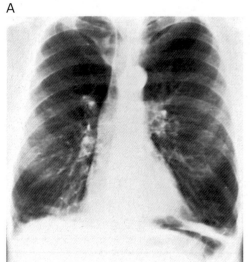
B
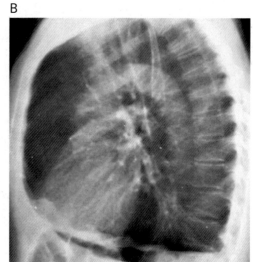

Fig C 16-1
Pulmonary emphysema. (A) Frontal and (B) lateral views of the chest demonstrate severe overinflation of the lungs along with flattening and even a superiorly concave configuration of the hemidiaphragms. There is also increased size and lucency of the retrosternal air space, an increase in the anteroposterior diameter of the chest, and a reduction in the number and caliber of peripheral pulmonary arteries.

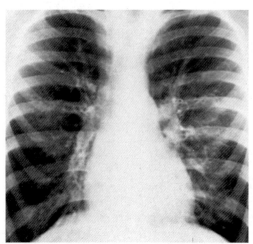

Fig C 16-2
Asthma. Frontal view of the chest demonstrating hyperexpansion of the lungs with depression of the hemidiaphragms, increased anteroposterior diameter of the chest and retrosternal air space, and prominence of the interstitial structures. The heart and pulmonary vascularity are normal.

Condition	Imaging Findings	Comments
Acute bronchiolitis	Severe overinflation of the lungs that is often associated with a reticulonodular pattern that predominantly involves the lower lobes.	Usually a viral infection of small airways that primarily affects children younger than the age of 3 years and is generally self-limited. May affect adults with pre-existing respiratory disease.
Bullous disease of the lung (Figs C 16-3 and C 16-4)	Multiple thin-walled, sharply demarcated, air-filled avascular spaces in the lung that most commonly occur in the upper lobes and may grow. Although there is overinflation as in chronic obstruction emphysema, there is no diffuse oligemia of the remaining pulmonary parenchyma.	Generally affects males, who remain asymptomatic until there is severe compression of the uninvolved lung parenchyma. Spontaneous pneumothorax from a ruptured bulla is a common complication.
Cystic fibrosis (mucoviscidosis) (Fig C 16-5)	Overinflation of the lungs associated with accentuation of interstitial markings and episodes of atelectasis and recurrent local pneumonia.	Obstruction of air passages by the tenacious mucus that is characteristic of this condition.
Diffuse infantile bronchopneumonia	Diffuse or patchy overinflation of the lungs that is usually associated with areas of consolidation and enlargement of peribronchial lymph nodes.	This pattern of bilateral pneumonia commonly complicates influenza, measles, or whooping cough. It may rarely occur with bacterial organisms.
Tracheal or laryngeal obstruction or compression	Overinflation of the lungs that may be associated with various tracheal abnormalities. Often recurrent pneumonias or evidence of parenchymal scarring from previous inflammatory disease.	Causes include vascular ring, tumor (squamous cell carcinoma, adenoid cystic carcinoma, osteochondroma, papilloma), tracheobronchomegaly (dilatation of deficient cartilage rings), relapsing polychondritis, localized tracheomalacia or stenosis (late complication of endotracheal intubation or tracheostomy), and saber-sheath trachea (narrowed coronal diameter due to chronic obstructive pulmonary disease).
Faulty radiographic technique	Bilateral "hyperlucent" lungs.	Overpenetrated film (especially portable radiographs and films on patients with very thin body habitus).

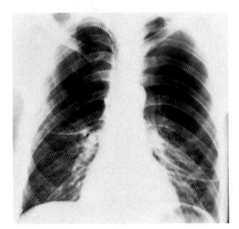

Fig C 16-3
Massive bilateral bullae. There is striking hyperlucency of both lungs.

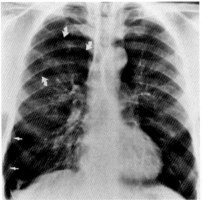

Fig C 16-4
Bullous emphysema. A small right pneumothorax (straight arrows) resulting from the rupture of a bulla. The curved arrows point to the walls of three of the multiple bullae in the upper portion of the right lung.

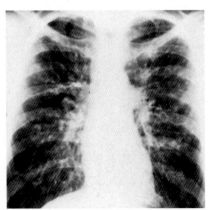

Fig C 16-5
Cystic fibrosis. Bilateral overinflation of the lungs associated with coarse interstitial markings.

Lobar Enlargement

Condition	Comments
Klebsiella pneumonia (Fig C 17-1)	Tends to form a voluminous inflammatory exudate that produces a homogeneous parenchymal consolidation (containing an air bronchogram) and bulging of an interlobar fissure. High frequency of abscess and cavity formation (rare in pneumococcal pneumonia).
Pneumococcal pneumonia	Appearance similar to *Klebsiella* pneumonia although cavitation is rare.
Haemophilus influenzae pneumonia (Fig C 17-2)	Most often develops in compromised hosts (chronic pulmonary disease, immune deficiency, alcoholism, diabetes).
Plague pneumonia	Hilar and paratracheal lymph node enlargement is common.
Tuberculous pneumonia	Manifestation of primary parenchymal involvement.
Lung abscess (Fig C 17-3)	Lobar expansion in an acute lung abscess (large mass, usually with cavitation) is probably related to air trapping by a check-valve mechanism in the communicating airway.
Bronchogenic carcinoma (Fig C 17-4)	Any large space-occupying mass that occupies a significant volume or is contiguous with a fissure.

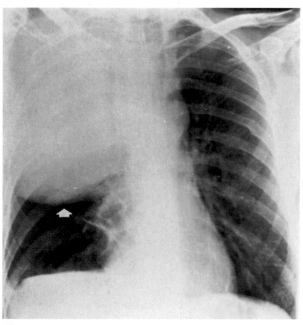

Fig C 17-1
***Klebsiella* pneumonia.** Downward bulging of the minor fissure (arrow) due to massive enlargement of the right upper lobe with inflammatory exudate.

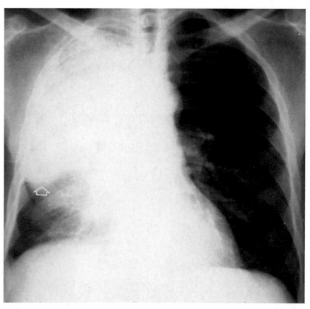

Fig C 17-2
***Haemophilus influenzae* pneumonia.** Acute lobar consolidation with downward bulging of the minor fissure (arrow) due to enlargement of the right upper lobe.[34]

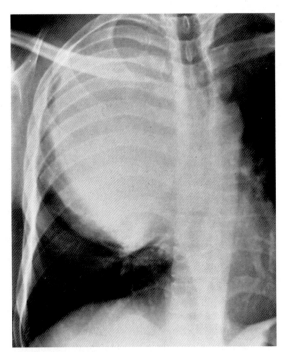

Fig C 17-3
Streptococcal pneumonia and empyema. A large
mottled opacity over the right upper lung represents
an extensive empyema that obscures the underlying
parenchymal pneumonia and produces an appearance
indistinguishable from that of lobar enlargement. The
patchy air densities in the empyema indicate communication with the bronchial tree.

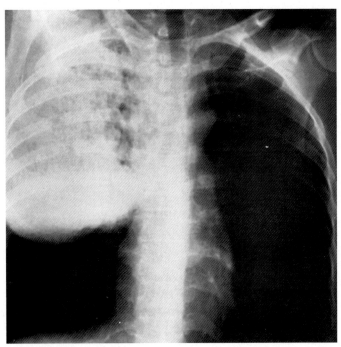

Fig C 17-4
Bronchogenic carcinoma. Appearance of massive lobar enlargement in a 30-year-old asymptomatic man.

Lobar or Segmental Collapse*

Condition	Imaging Findings	Comments
Bronchogenic carcinoma (Fig C 18-1)	Lobar collapse associated with a hilar mass (representing metastases to regional lymph nodes).	Because bronchial obstruction is a slowly progressive process, there is usually a distal infection with inflammatory exudate that prevents collapse once the bronchus is totally occluded. Characteristic Golden's S sign in right upper lobe collapse (upper laterally concave segment of the S is formed by the elevated minor fissure; lower medial convexity is caused by the tumor mass responsible for the collapse).
Bronchial adenoma (Fig C 18-2)	Lobar collapse.	Most common radiographic finding of a central adenoma. Collateral air drift may present complete collapse.
Foreign body	Lobar or segmental collapse. An opaque foreign body may be detectable.	In adults, collapse is usually associated with aspiration of food (eg, a large piece of meat). Bizarre variety of causes in children (who more commonly present with overaeration of the lung distal to the site of obstruction due to collateral air drift).

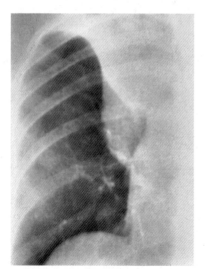

Fig C 18-1
Bronchogenic carcinoma. Typical reverse S-shaped curve (Golden's sign) representing collapse of the right upper lobe associated with malignant bronchial obstruction.

A

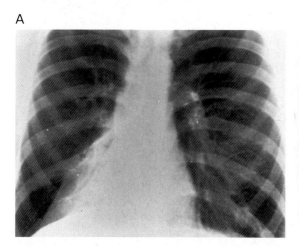

B

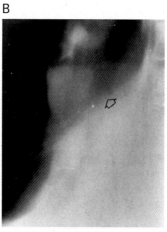

Fig C 18-2
Central bronchial adenoma.
(A) Frontal chest radiograph demonstrates a right lower lobe density with obscuration of the right hemidiaphragm and relative preservation of the right border of the heart, consistent with right lower lobe collapse. (B) Tomography shows an ill-defined mass causing a high-grade obstruction of the right lower lobe bronchus (arrow).

*See Figs C 18-6 through 18-11.

Condition	Imaging Findings	Comments
Malpositioned endotracheal tube (Figs C 18-3 and C 18-4)	Usually collapse of the left lung.	Advancing the tube too far (into the bronchus intermedius) occludes the left main-stem bronchus.
Mucous plug (Fig C 18-5)	Primarily segmental collapse.	Most common cause of small airway obstruction. Frequent complication of abdominal and thoracic surgery, anesthesia and respiratory depressant drugs, and infectious diseases (eg, tetanus) that produce respiratory depression and impaired clearance of tracheobronchial secretions.

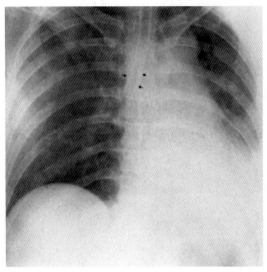

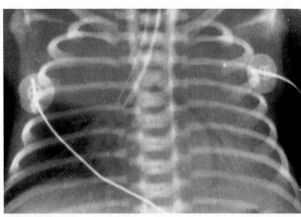

Fig C 18-4
Malpositioned endotracheal tube. Inordinately low position of the endotracheal tube in the bronchus intermedius causes collapse of the right upper lobe and the entire left lung.

Fig C 18-3
Malpositioned endotracheal tube. Collapse of the left lung, especially the left lower lobe, due to an endotracheal tube (arrows) in the right main-stem bronchus that effectively blocks the passage of air into the left bronchial tree.

A

B

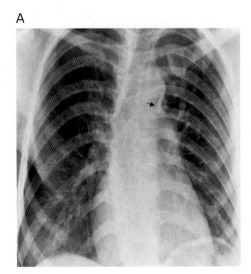

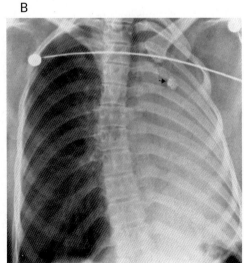

Fig C 18-5
Mucous plug in a paraplegic.
(A) Baseline radiograph is within normal limits. Note the calcified granuloma in the left perihilar region (arrow). (B) Complete collapse of the left lung after the lodging of a mucous plug in the left main-stem bronchus. Note the change in position of the calcified granuloma when the left lung collapses (arrow).

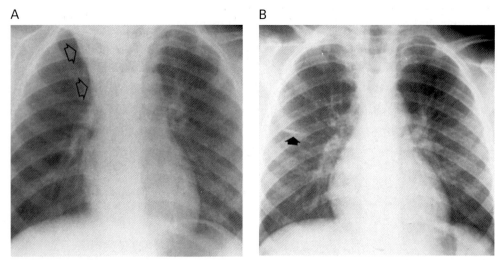

Fig C 18-6
Right upper lobe collapse. (A) Initial chest radiograph demonstrates the collapsed right upper lobe, which appears as a homogeneous soft-tissue mass (arrows) in the right apex along the upper mediastinum. (B) As the collapsed lobe expands, the soft-tissue has disappeared and the minor fissure (arrow) has reappeared.

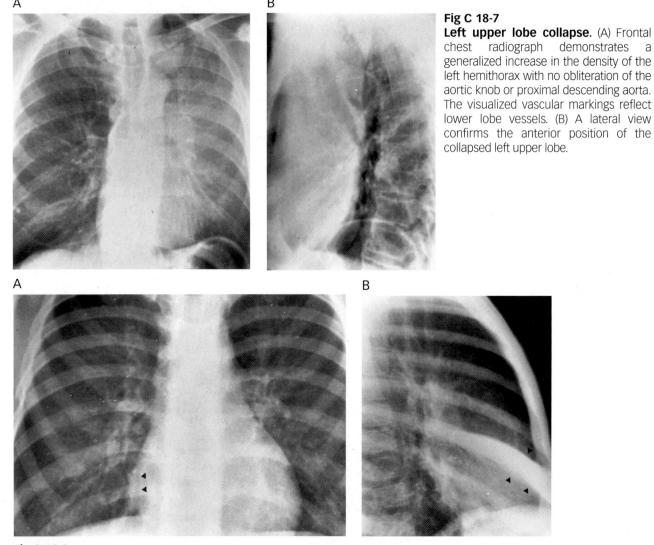

Fig C 18-7
Left upper lobe collapse. (A) Frontal chest radiograph demonstrates a generalized increase in the density of the left hemithorax with no obliteration of the aortic knob or proximal descending aorta. The visualized vascular markings reflect lower lobe vessels. (B) A lateral view confirms the anterior position of the collapsed left upper lobe.

Fig C 18-8
Right middle lobe collapse. (A) Frontal chest radiograph demonstrates minimal obliteration of the lower part of the right border of the heart (arrows). (B) Lateral view demonstrates collapse of the right middle lobe (arrows).

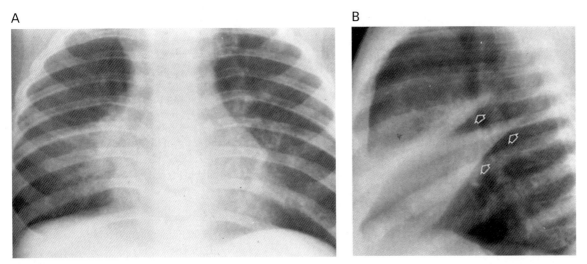

Fig C 18-9
Right middle lobe and lingular collapse. (A) Frontal chest radiograph demonstrates obliteration of the right and left borders of the heart. (B) Lateral view demonstrates collapse of both the right middle lobe and the lingula (arrows).

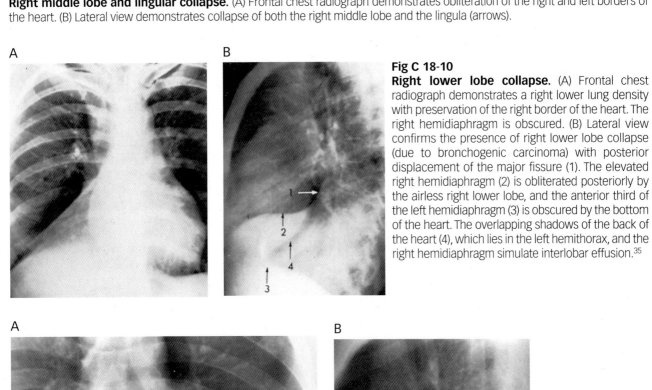

Fig C 18-10
Right lower lobe collapse. (A) Frontal chest radiograph demonstrates a right lower lung density with preservation of the right border of the heart. The right hemidiaphragm is obscured. (B) Lateral view confirms the presence of right lower lobe collapse (due to bronchogenic carcinoma) with posterior displacement of the major fissure (1). The elevated right hemidiaphragm (2) is obliterated posteriorly by the airless right lower lobe, and the anterior third of the left hemidiaphragm (3) is obscured by the bottom of the heart. The overlapping shadows of the back of the heart (4), which lies in the left hemithorax, and the right hemidiaphragm simulate interlobar effusion.[35]

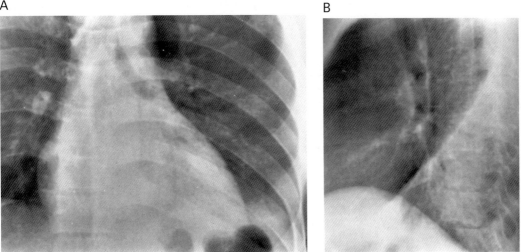

Fig C 18-11
Left lower lobe collapse. (A) Frontal chest radiograph demonstrates obliteration of the descending thoracic aorta and obscuration of much of the left hemidiaphragm. (B) Lateral view confirms the posterior portion of the collapsed left lower lobe.

Condition	Imaging Findings	Comments
Mucoid impaction	Segmental or subsegmental collapse.	Develops in patients with asthma and hypersensitivity (allergic) bronchopulmonary aspergillosis.
Bronchial metastases	Lobar or segmental collapse.	Most frequently renal cell carcinoma. Also breast carcinoma and melanoma.
Chronic obstructive pulmonary disease	Segmental or subsegmental collapse (also evidence of underlying disease).	Obstruction of small airways with the formation of small intraluminal mucous plugs (most commonly in acute exacerbations of asthma, chronic bronchitis, emphysema, and bronchiolitis obliterans).
Pneumonia	Segmental or subsegmental collapse.	Peribronchial inflammation may lead to small airway obstruction followed by collapse. Develops occasionally in bacterial, viral, and mycoplasma pneumonias.
Cystic fibrosis	Lobar, segmental, or subsegmental collapse superimposed on a coarse interstitial pattern.	Small airway obstruction due to excessively viscous mucus that is poorly cleared from the tracheobronchial tree.
Cardiac enlargement	Usually collapse of the left lower lobe.	Dilated left atrium (mitral stenosis, atrial septal defect).
Aortic aneurysm	Lobar or segmental collapse.	Extrinsic pressure on the bronchial tree.
Mediastinal neoplasm	Lobar or segmental collapse.	Extrinsic pressure on the bronchial tree.
Inflammatory bronchial stricture	Lobar, segmental, or subsegmental collapse. Usually evidence of an alveolar or interstitial infiltrate.	Most commonly because of tuberculosis (volume loss of the upper lobe). Also histoplasmosis and other granulomatous infections.
Fractured bronchus	Lobar or segmental collapse with characteristic rounded bronchial occlusion.	Result of severe thoracic trauma. Causes a pronounced collapse because it is sudden and complete.
Pulmonary embolism	Lobar or segmental collapse.	Unusual manifestation (precise mechanism unclear).
Bronchiectasis	Lobar or segmental collapse.	Caused by retained secretions in advanced disease. More commonly, there is only moderate volume loss.
Middle lobe syndrome	Collapse of the right middle lobe. The lymph node producing the compression may contain calcium.	Chronic process caused by quiescent granulomatous lymphadenitis (histoplasmosis, tuberculosis, occasionally silicosis). A similar process may involve other lobes or segments.

Condition	Imaging Findings	Comments
Lymphadenopathy	Lobar or segmental collapse.	Hilar adenopathy is often cited as the cause of collapse, although the volume loss probably reflects the underlying pathologic process (eg, primary bronchogenic carcinoma, tuberculosis). To support this view, sarcoidosis is associated with profound hilar adenopathy yet rarely causes any volume loss.
Radiation therapy	Lobar or segmental collapse (often a peculiar nonanatomic distribution of volume loss that coincides with the radiation port).	Late scarring may produce a substantial loss of volume superimposed on a characteristic interstitial pattern.
Broncholithiasis	Lobar or segmental collapse associated with intrabronchial calcification.	Results from erosion of a calcified lymph node into a bronchus.

Pulmonary Parenchymal Calcification

Condition	Imaging Findings	Comments
Histoplasmoma (Figs C 19-1 and C 19-2)	Central calcification that may be multiple or widespread.	Most common form of pulmonary calcification. Often associated with calcifications in regional lymph nodes and the spleen. Eccentric calcification in the mass may indicate a bronchogenic carcinoma growing around the histoplasmoma.
Other granulomatous infections (Fig C 19-3)	Central calcification that may be multiple or widespread.	Tuberculosis, coccidioidomycosis. There may be calcification of regional lymph nodes. Eccentric calcification in the mass may indicate a bronchogenic carcinoma growing around the granuloma.
Plasma cell granuloma (Fig C 19-4)	Fine or coarse calcification in a parenchymal nodule.	Common inflammatory pseudotumor of the lung that represents a benign proliferative response to pulmonary infection or injury. Occasionally the process is aggressive and encases bronchi or invades mediastinal structures, chest wall, or diaphragm.
Fungus ball	Various patterns of calcification of the mycelial mass may occur.	Scattered small nodules of calcification, a fine rim around the periphery of the mass, or an extensive process involving most of the mycelial ball.
Chickenpox (varicella) pneumonia (Fig C 19-5)	Tiny widespread calcifications.	Develops in adults 1 or more years after pulmonary chickenpox infection. The calcifications vary in size and number and predominate in the lower half of the lungs. No calcification of hilar lymph nodes (unlike histoplasmosis or tuberculosis).
Parasites	Multiple small pulmonary calcifications. May be solitary.	Paragonimiasis, schistosomiasis, cysticercosis, guinea worm, *Armillifer armillatus* (also in thoracic muscles or subcutaneous tissues).

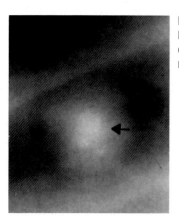

Fig C 19-1
Histoplasmoma. Central calcification (arrow) in a solitary pulmonary nodule.

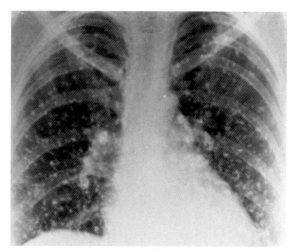

Fig C 19-2
Histoplasmosis. Diffuse calcifications in the lungs produce a snowball pattern.

Condition	Imaging Findings	Comments
Hypersensitivity bronchopulmonary aspergillosis (Fig C 19-6)	Calcification in fingerlike branching shadows with precise bronchial distribution.	Complex hypersensitivity reaction to the presence of aspergilli colonizing the bronchial tree that occurs almost exclusively in asthmatics. The dilated bronchi fill with mucoid material that can calcify. A similar appearance may be seen with mucoid impactions and bronchial atresia.

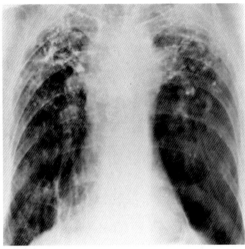

Fig C 19-3
Tuberculosis. Bilateral fibrocalcific changes at the apices. There is upward retraction of the hila.

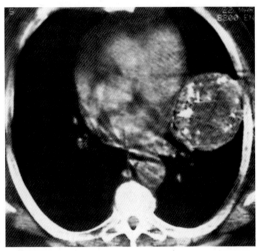

Fig C 19-4
Plasma cell granuloma. CT scan shows amorphous calcification in a large solitary mass in the lingula.[36]

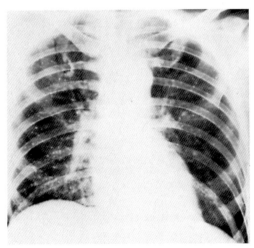

Fig C 19-5
Healed chickenpox pneumonia. Multiple tiny calcific shadows are scattered widely and uniformly throughout both lungs. This 42-year-old asymptomatic man had had florid chickenpox with acute pneumonia 15 years earlier.[7]

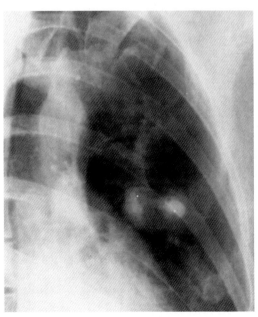

Fig C 19-6
Calcified mucoid impaction in bronchial atresia. (Courtesy of I. Ettman, MD.)[36]

Condition	Imaging Findings	Comments
Hamartoma (Fig C 19-7)	Single nodule with central calcification.	Popcorn-ball calcification is pathognomonic (but occurs in less than 10%).
Silicosis (Fig C 19-8)	Widespread small calcified nodules.	Punctate calcifications are reported to occur in silicotic nodules in up to 20% of cases. May also have characteristic eggshell lymph node calcification. A similar pattern may occur in pneumoconiosis.
Heavy metal inhalation	Widespread opaque nodules of metallic density.	Stannosis (tin), baritosis (barium), and antimony and rare-earth pneumoconioses.
Alveolar microlithiasis (see Fig C 2-15)	Widespread tiny, discrete, sand-like opacities of calcific density.	Tiny spherules of calcium phosphate in myriad alveoli and alveolar sacs. Black pleura sign (caused by the contrast between the extreme density of the lung parenchyma on one side of the pleura and the ribs on the other).
Pulmonary ossification	Widespread densely calcified or ossified nodules.	Manifestation of mitral stenosis (or other causes of elevated left atrial pressure). At up to 8 mm in size, usually much larger than the calcifications (up to 3 mm) of healed infectious diseases such as histoplasmosis or varicella.
Pulmonary osteopathia	Fine, branching, linear shadows of calcific density that usually involve a limited area of the lung.	Calcific density is often difficult to appreciate (since the shadows are very thin). Represents trabeculated bone along the bronchovascular distribution of the interstitial space.

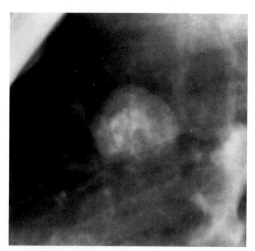

Fig C 19-7
Hamartoma. Pathognomonic popcorn-ball calcification in a solitary pulmonary nodule.

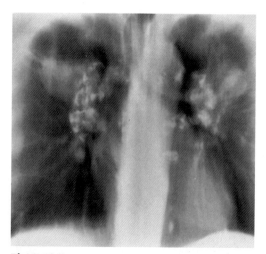

Fig C 19-8
Silicosis. Tomogram of the chest demonstrates characteristic eggshell lymph node calcification associated with bilateral perihilar masses.

Condition	Imaging Findings	Comments
Metastases (Fig C 19-9)	Calcification in multiple or widespread nodules.	Rare manifestation but virtually diagnostic of osteogenic sarcoma or chondrosarcoma. May very rarely be psammomatous calcification (thyroid, ovarian cystadenoma) or mucinous calcification (colloid carcinoma of the breast or gastrointestinal tract).
Bronchogenic carcinoma (Fig C 19-10)	Calcified nodule.	Very rare manifestation on plain chest radiographs, although occasionally calcification can be detected on CT.

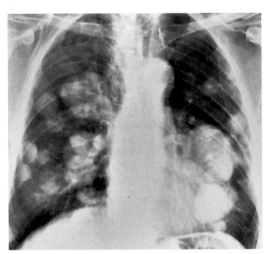

Fig C 19-9
Metastases from osteosarcoma.

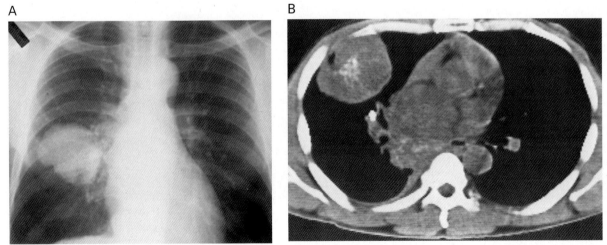

Fig C 19-10
Bronchogenic carcinoma. (A) Plain chest radiograph shows a large mass in the right upper lobe extending into the middle lobe. A second large lesion is evident in the azygoesophageal recess. (B) CT scan demonstrates dystrophic central calcification within the lesion and scattered calcifications in the mediastinal mass.[36]

Condition	Imaging Findings	Comments
Leiomyosarcoma (Fig C 19-11)	Calcified nodule.	Calcification presumably occurs in areas of ischemic tissue damage within the tumor.
Intrapulmonary teratoma	Mass with calcification or the pathognomonic presence of a tooth.	Extremely rare. The cystic nature of the lesion and collections of lipid material and calcification within it can be easily detected on CT.
Metabolic calcification (Fig C 19-12)	Widespread calcification.	Causes include primary or secondary hyperparathyroidism (especially chronic renal disease and maintenance hemodialysis), hypervitaminosis D, milk-alkali syndrome, and intravenous calcium therapy. Calcium tends to precipitate at sites of pneumonic exudation.
Broncholithiasis (Fig C 19-13)	Single or multiple parabronchial or endobronchial calcifications that often occur close to the proximal margin of an area of pulmonary collapse.	Results from erosion of a calcified lymph node or parenchymal focus into a bronchus. Fragments may lodge in the bronchus and cause obstruction or be expectorated.
Bronchial adenoma	Single calcified nodule.	Calcification and ossification are rare.
Amyloidosis (Fig C 19-14)	Calcification or ossification in solitary or multiple masses.	Very rare manifestation. Calcification may also occur in the tracheobronchial tree.
Pulmonary thrombus	Calcification in the region of a pulmonary artery.	Thrombi in the pulmonary arteries after embolism may rarely calcify.

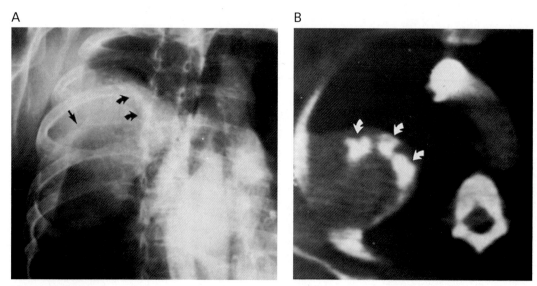

A   B

Fig C 19-11
Leiomyosarcoma. (A) Plain chest radiograph in a woman with a history of thymic irradiation in infancy and pleural decortication for pneumothorax shows a large right lung mass that extends to the chest wall and contains dense eccentric calcification (curved arrows). Note the rib destruction (straight arrow). (B) CT scan more clearly shows peripheral dense foci of eccentric calcification (arrows) within the mass. (Courtesy of Stephanie Flicker, MD.)[36]

Condition	Imaging Findings	Comments
Pulmonary arteriovenous fistula	Single or multiple calcifications.	Rare manifestation that is probably due to phleboliths. The feeding artery and draining vein can often be detected.
Bronchogenic cyst	Curvilinear calcification about the periphery of the mass.	Cyst wall calcification is rare.

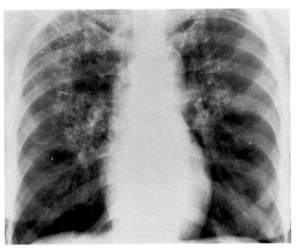

Fig C 19-12
Secondary hyperparathyroidism. Heterotopic calcification in a patient with chronic renal failure.

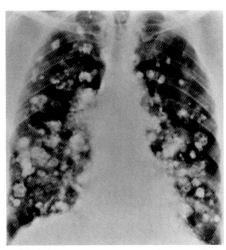

Fig C 19-13
Broncholithiasis. Innumerable calcified masses scattered throughout the lungs.

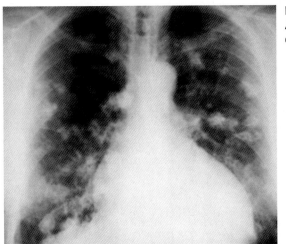

Fig C 19-14
Amyloidosis. Dystrophic calcification in nodular deposits in the lung.[36]

Pulmonary Disease with Eosinophilia

Condition	Imaging Findings	Comments
Acute idiopathic eosinophilic pneumonia (Löffler's syndrome) (Fig C 20-1)	Patchy parenchymal consolidation with blood eosinophilia.	Characteristic transitory and migratory pattern of ill-defined infiltrates that are nonsegmental in distribution and tend to involve the periphery of the lung. "Reversed pulmonary edema pattern" (involvement of the lung periphery in contrast to the perihilar or central distribution of pulmonary edema).
Chronic eosinophilic pneumonia	Patchy parenchymal consolidation with eosinophilic infiltration of the lung.	Pattern identical to that in Löffler's syndrome, except that the lesions tend to persist unchanged for weeks unless corticosteroid therapy is instituted. Blood eosinophilia occurs in most patients although it is not essential for the diagnosis.
Drug sensitivity (Figs C 20-2 and C 20-3)	Patchy nonsegmental, peripheral parenchymal consolidation with blood eosinophilia.	Sulfonamides, penicillin, isoniazid, and many other medications. Nitrofurantoin causes a diffuse reticular pattern. Withdrawal of the drug results in prompt disappearance of the clinical and radiographic manifestations.
Parasitic disease (Figs C 20-4 to C 20-8)	Patchy nonsegmental, peripheral parenchymal consolidation with blood eosinophilia.	Ascariasis, strongyloidiasis, tropical pulmonary eosinophilia (filariasis), ancylostomiasis (hookworm), visceral larva migrans (dog or cat roundworm), schistosomiasis. Amebiasis produces basilar consolidation (not peripheral) that may cavitate.
Hypersensitivity bronchopulmonary aspergillosis (Fig C 20-9)	Round, oval, or elliptical opacities (mucous plugs) that usually develop in segmental bronchi of the upper lobes. May have homogeneous consolidation. Blood eosinophilia.	Mucous plugs contain aspergilli and eosinophils. Usually a history of long-standing bronchial asthma. Involvement of several bronchi may produce a "cluster of grapes," or Y-shaped, shadow.

A   B   C

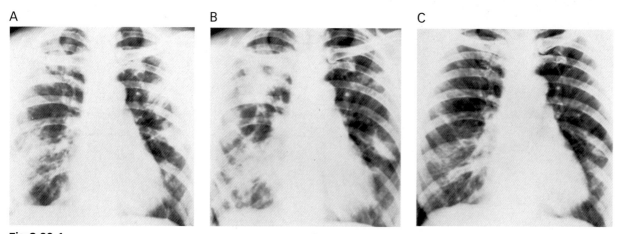

Fig C 20-1
Löffler's syndrome. (A) Initial frontal chest radiograph shows numerous bilateral areas of consolidation that have no precise segmental distribution. Note particularly the broad shadow of increased density along the lower axillary zone of the right lung. (B) One week later, the anatomic distribution of the consolidation has changed considerably, being more extensive in the right upper and lower lobes and less extensive in the left upper lobe. (C) One week later, after adrenocorticotropic hormone (ACTH) therapy, the radiographic abnormalities have completely resolved.[7]

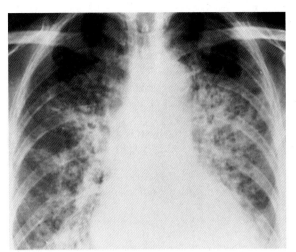

Fig C 20-2
Nitrofurantoin-induced lung disease. Mixed alveolar and interstitial pattern in an elderly woman who presented with progressive cough and dyspnea after the long-term use of nitrofurantoin for recurring urinary tract infections.[14]

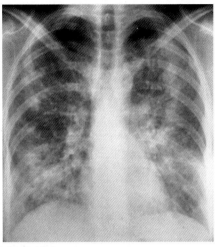

Fig C 20-3
Methotrexate-induced lung disease. The diffuse, bilateral, patchy densities were changeable and fleeting during the illness. The radiographic findings cleared completely after steroid therapy.[37]

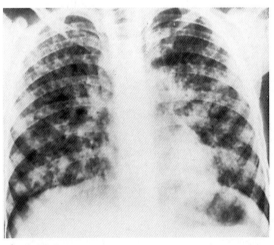

Fig C 20-4
Ascariasis. Extensive pulmonary infiltrates due to the presence of *Ascaris* larvae in the lungs.[38]

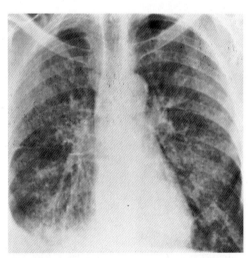

Fig C 20-5
Strongyloidiasis. Chest radiograph during the stage of larval migration shows a pattern of miliary nodules diffusely distributed throughout both lungs. There is also a large right pleural effusion.

Condition	Imaging Findings	Comments
Asthma (Fig C 20-10)	Hyperexpansion of the lungs with bronchial wall thickening (tubular shadows). Eosinophils in the sputum and slight blood eosinophilia.	Chest radiograph is often normal (especially in patients with mild disease and late age of onset). Increased incidence of pneumonia and atelectasis (mucous plugging or impaction).
Hypereosinophilic syndrome (eosinophilic leukemia)	Various patterns of eosinophilic infiltration of the pulmonary parenchyma.	Rare condition characterized by mature eosinophil infiltration of multiple organs. Occurs almost exclusively in males.
Wegener's granulomatosis (see Fig C 11-14)	Patchy parenchymal consolidation with minimal blood and tissue eosinophilia.	Almost invariably multiple and frequently cavitates.

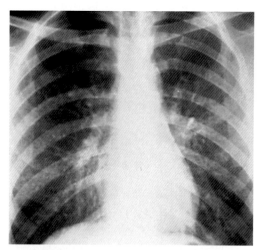

Fig C 20-6
Tropical pulmonary eosinophilia. Multiple small nodules with indistinct outlines produce a pattern of generalized increase in lung markings.[39]

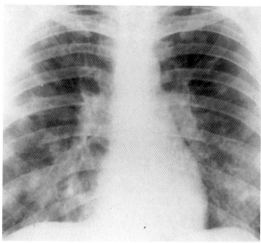

Fig C 20-7
Cutaneous larva migrans. Multiple small irregular areas of air-space consolidation widely scattered throughout both lungs.[40]

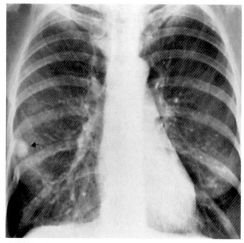

Fig C 20-8
Dirofilariasis. Well-circumscribed solitary pulmonary nodule (arrow) that is indistinguishable from a malignant coin lesion.

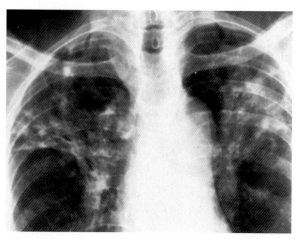

Fig C 20-9
Hypersensitivity bronchopulmonary aspergillosis. Patchy opacifications in segmental bronchi of the upper lobes in a patient with asthma and pronounced peripheral eosinophilia.

Condition	Imaging Findings	Comments
Allergic granulomatosis	Patchy parenchymal consolidation with considerable blood and tissue eosinophilia.	Granulomatous disease involving many organs and restricted to patients with a history of asthma. The consolidation is almost always multiple and frequently cavitates.
Polyarteritis nodosa	Fleeting nonsegmental patchy consolidation with tissue eosinophilia.	Hypersensitivity angiitis that typically involves the kidneys and may cause systemic hypertension. Other findings include pulmonary edema, accentuated interstitial markings, and miliary nodules.
Desquamative interstitial pneumonia (DIP) (Fig C 20-11)	Generalized reticular pattern with small numbers of eosinophils in the interstitium.	Progressive loss of lung volume on sequential studies. Spontaneous pneumothorax and pleural effusion may occur.
Coccidioidomycosis (Fig C 20-12)	Various patterns of pulmonary disease, often with significant blood eosinophilia.	May produce parenchymal consolidation, nodules (single, multiple, miliary) that may cavitate, and lymph node enlargement.

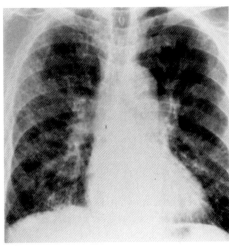

Fig C 20-10
Asthma. Recurrent pulmonary infections have led to the development of diffuse pulmonary fibrosis.

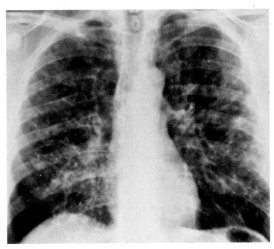

Fig C 20-11
Desquamative interstitial pneumonia. Generalized reticular pattern throughout both lungs.

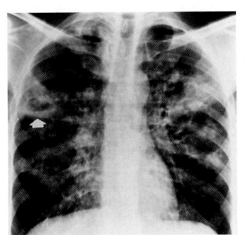

Fig C 20-12
Coccidioidomycosis. Patchy areas of air-space consolidation in both lungs. There is an air-fluid level (arrow) in a right upper lobe cavity abutting the minor fissure.

Skin Disorder Combined with Widespread Lung Disease

Condition	Imaging Findings	Comments
Systemic lupus erythematosus (see Figs C 36-4 and C 36-9)	Pericardial and pleural effusions. Nonspecific, poorly defined patchy areas of parenchymal consolidation that are usually in the lung bases and situated peripherally (probably reflect acute pneumonia). Fleeting basilar atelectasis may occur.	Cutaneous manifestations (in 80% of patients) include butterfly rash, discoid lupus, alopecia, and photosensitivity. Arthritis and arthralgia occur in approximately 95% of cases.
Sarcoidosis (Fig C 21-1)	Bilateral hilar and paratracheal adenopathy. Diffuse reticulonodular or fluffy alveolar pattern.	Cutaneous involvement (approximately 30% of cases) includes slightly raised, often purplish nodules (lupus pernio) that usually appear about the face, neck, shoulders, and digits. Large plaques resembling psoriasis may occur over the trunk or extremities.
Scleroderma (see Fig C 5-5)	Diffuse interstitial pattern that predominantly involves the lower lung zones.	Characteristic thickened and inelastic skin. Erosion of terminal phalangeal tufts with calcification in the fingertips.
Dermatomyositis	Diffuse interstitial pattern that predominantly involves the lung bases.	Cutaneous changes include puffiness of the face and an erythematous rash involving the neck, ears, chest, and shoulders. Bilateral and symmetric muscle weakness and diffuse subcutaneous and muscular calcification. Traditionally associated with an increased incidence of malignancy.
Rheumatoid arthritis (see Fig C 4-12)	Diffuse reticulonodular pattern, more prominent in the lung bases. Discrete nodular lesions (similar to subcutaneous nodules). Pleural effusion.	The hands are often cool and damp (reflecting autonomic nervous system dysfunction) and palmar erythema often occurs. In long-standing disease, the skin over the distal extremities often becomes atrophic and bruises easily. Nail-fold thrombi, small infarcts on the volar surface of the hands, digital gangrene, and ulcers of the lower part of the leg and ankle are manifestations of rheumatoid vasculitis.

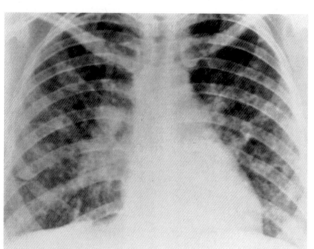

Fig C 21-1
Sarcoidosis. Diffuse reticulonodular pattern associated with hilar adenopathy.

Condition	Imaging Findings	Comments
Neurofibromatosis	Diffuse interstitial pulmonary fibrosis and bullae. Cutaneous nodules may project over the lungs.	Multiple fibromas and neuromas of the skin with café au lait spots. There may be posterior mediastinal masses and skeletal deformities (scoliosis and rib lesions).
Tuberous sclerosis (Fig C 21-2)	Diffuse interstitial fibrosis with honeycombing. Pneumothorax is common.	Cutaneous manifestations include adenoma sebaceum (acneform butterfly rash on the face) and subungual fibromas. Potato-like tumor masses also involve the brain, kidneys, and eyes.
Wegener's granulomatosis (see Fig C 11-14)	Multiple bilateral nodules. Thick-walled cavities in approximately half the cases.	Skin ulcerations and vesicular or hemorrhagic cutaneous lesions.
Hereditary hemorrhagic telangiectasis (Rendu–Osler–Weber disease)	Single or multiple pulmonary arteriovenous fistulas (prominent feeding artery and draining vein).	Cutaneous and mucous membrane telangiectasia.
Metastases from skin neoplasm	Multiple pulmonary nodules.	Melanoma (pigmented elevation), Kaposi's sarcoma (multiple bluish, hemorrhagic skin lesions). Often "bull's-eye" lesions in the gastrointestinal tract.
Mycosis fungoides	Various patterns (reticulonodular, multiple larger nodules, pleural effusion, enlargement of mediastinal lymph nodes).	Lymphomatous process that predominantly affects the skin (scaly cutaneous plaques or frank ulcerating tumors). Clinically resembles eczema or psoriasis and has a poor prognosis.
Lymphoma (see Figs C 13-4 and C 14-5)	Various patterns (reticulonodular, multiple larger nodules, enlargement of mediastinal lymph nodes).	Lymphomatous lesions in the skin are dermal or subcutaneous nodules that typically have a purple or red-brown color and are usually covered by relatively normal intact epidermis. Skin infiltrates may be the initial manifestation or may appear at any time during the course of the disease.
Erythema nodosum	Enlargement of hilar lymph nodes (usually bilateral). Occasional pulmonary infiltrates.	Acute skin eruption (especially of legs) consisting of symmetrically distributed, red, tender nodules. Associated with sarcoidosis. May represent an allergic reaction resulting from a variety of bacterial, chemical, and toxic agents.

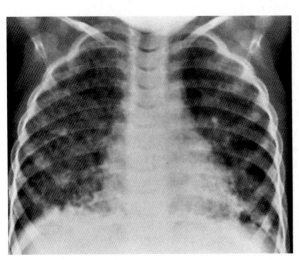

Fig C 21-2
Tuberous sclerosis. Diffuse interstitial fibrosis with honeycombing.

Condition	Imaging Findings	Comments
Fungal infections (Fig C 21-3)	Various patterns (parenchymal nodules, lymphadenopathy, pleural effusion).	Scaling macules and papules of the epidermis, hair, toenails, and fingernails. Certain fungi (especially *Candida* species) invade the epidermis when the skin is exposed to high humidity and becomes macerated (most commonly in the intertriginous areas under the breasts and in the umbilicus, groin, and axillae).
Pulmonary Langerhans cell histiocytosis (Fig C 21-4)	Diffuse coarse reticulonodular pattern (honeycomb lung). Pneumothorax is common.	Variety of skin lesions (may be the presenting sign), including scaly papules or vesicles, pruritic seborrheic or eczematous lesions in intertriginous areas, petechiae (due to perivascular infiltrates or thrombocytopenia), scaly or exudative eruptions of the scalp, and xanthomas.
Acquired immunodeficiency syndrome (AIDS)	Broad spectrum of pulmonary findings.	Variety of skin lesions of both infectious and noninfectious origins.
Chickenpox (Fig C 21-5)	Patchy, diffuse air-space pneumonia. In the healed phase, characteristic innumerable tiny widespread calcifications throughout both lungs.	Scarlatiniform rash with rapid development of typical vesicles and papules.
Measles (Fig C 21-6)	Reticular pattern in primary pneumonia. Segmental consolidation and atelectasis indicate bacterial superinfection.	Red maculopapular rash that breaks out first on the forehead; spreads downward over the face, neck, and trunk; and appears on the feet on the third day. Characteristic Koplik's spots (small, red, irregular lesions with blue-white centers) appear 1 to 2 days before the onset of the rash on the mucous membranes of the mouth and occasionally on the conjunctiva or intestinal mucosa.
Acanthosis nigricans	Increased incidence of bronchogenic carcinoma.	Bilateral, symmetric hyperkeratosis and hyperpigmentation of the skin (especially in the flexural and intertriginous areas). High incidence of abdominal malignancy (especially of the stomach).

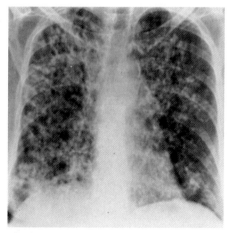

Fig C 21-3
Pulmonary candidiasis. Diffuse pattern of ill-defined nodules throughout both lungs.

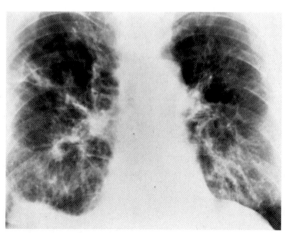

Fig C 21-4
Pulmonary Langerhans cell histiocytosis. Coarse reticular pattern diffusely involving both lungs.

Condition	Imaging Findings	Comments
Amyloidosis (Fig C 21-7)	Various patterns (intra-airway mass causing atelectasis or obstructive pneumonitis, parenchymal form with solitary or multiple masses, miliary form, lymphadenopathy, reticulonodular pattern).	Skin lesions are one of the most characteristic manifestations of amyloidosis and consist of slightly raised waxy papules or plaques that are usually clustered in the folds of the axillary, anal, or inguinal regions; the face and neck; or mucosal areas such as the ear or tongue. Gentle rubbing may induce bleeding into the skin, leading to purpura.
Hypersensitivity reaction (Fig C 21-8)	Various patterns depending on the stage of the condition.	Many forms of allergy, drug sensitivity, and parasitic infestation.
Burns	Various patterns (patchy pulmonary consolidation, atelectasis, pulmonary edema).	Cutaneous manifestations vary depending on the severity of the burn.
Bleeding disorders (see Fig C 2-11)	Alveolar infiltrates that may eventually produce interstitial fibrosis after repeated episodes of bleeding.	Spectrum of appearances—from extensive macules (ecchymoses) to tiny petechiae.

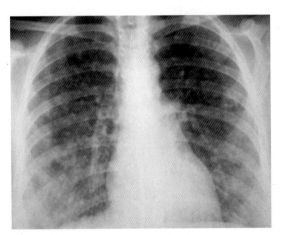

Fig C 21-5
Chickenpox pneumonia. Patchy, diffuse air-space consolidation.

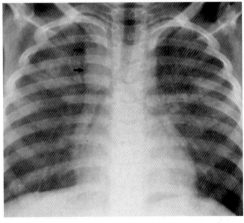

Fig C 21-6
Measles pneumonia. Diffuse, reticular interstitial infiltrate with a focal area of consolidation in the right upper lobe. Note the striking right hilar and mediastinal adenopathy (arrows).

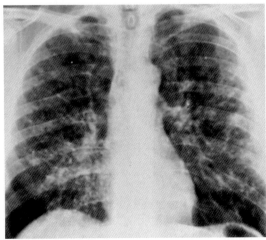

Fig C 21-7
Amyloidosis. Diffuse reticulonodular pattern.

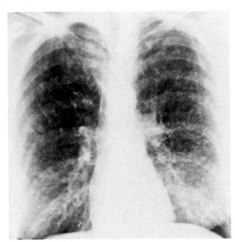

Fig C 21-8
Busulfan-induced lung disease. Diffuse coarse reticulonodular pattern.

Meniscus (Air-Crescent) Sign*

Condition	Comments
Aspergillus fungus ball (Figs C 22-1 through C 22-3)	Aspergillosis is the most common cause of this appearance. It generally develops in immunocompromised patients (especially those with disseminated malignancy).
Fungus ball of other etiology	Candidiasis, coccidioidomycosis, nocardiosis, and cryptococcosis.
Hydatid (echinococcal) cyst (Fig C 22-4)	Rupture between the pericyst and the exocyst permits the entry of air between these layers.

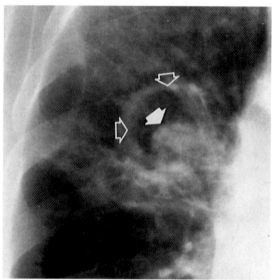

Fig C 22-1
Aspergillosis. A mycetoma (solid arrow) appears as a homogeneous rounded mass that is separated from the thick wall of the cavity by a crescent-shaped air space (open arrows).

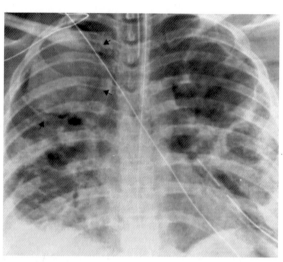

Fig C 22-2
Aspergillosis. Multiple cavities of various sizes are superimposed on a diffuse pulmonary infiltrate. A fungus ball almost fills the large cavity in the right upper lobe (arrows). A right pleural effusion is also seen in this patient with chronic lymphocytic leukemia.

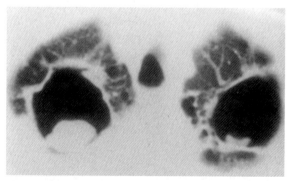

Fig C 22-3
Aspergillosis. Bilateral aspergillomas in an elderly man with residual tuberculosis. CT scan shows large cavities in the upper lobes containing fungus balls of different sizes.[41]

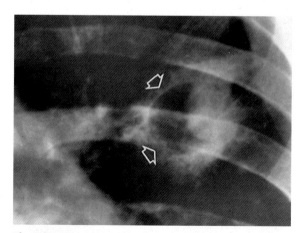

Fig C 22-4
Hydatid cyst. A crescent of air (arrows) is seen about the periphery of the echinococcal cyst.

*Lucent crescent along the inner border of a cavity or between a dense parenchymal lesion and surrounding lung structures.

Condition	Comments
Lung abscess with inspissated pus	Various infectious agents.
Neoplasm	Bronchogenic carcinoma, bronchial adenoma, sarcoma, and sclerosing hemangioma.
Granuloma	Tuberculous, fungal, or idiopathic.
Gangrene of lung	Large mass of necrotic lung in an abscess cavity. Most frequent in pneumococcal or *Klebsiella* pneumonia.
Intracavitary blood clot	Blood clot in a tuberculous cavity, infarct, or pulmonary laceration.

Anterior Mediastinal Lesions

Condition	Imaging Findings	Comments
Substernal thyroid (Fig C 23-1)	Sharply defined, smooth or lobulated mass that occurs in the superior portion of the mediastinum and may calcify.	Typically compresses the trachea or the esophagus or both. Occasionally occurs in the posterior mediastinum (almost exclusively on the right).
Thymoma (Figs C 23-2 and C 23-3)	Round or oval, smooth or lobulated mass that often calcifies and may protrude to one or both sides of the mediastinum. Usually arises near the junction of the heart and great vessels (displacing them posteriorly).	High fat content (relatively lucent on plain films and easily apparent on CT). As many as 25% to 50% of patients have myasthenia gravis (approximately 15% of patients with myasthenia gravis have thymic tumors). The normal thymus appears as an anterior mediastinal mass in neonates.

A   B

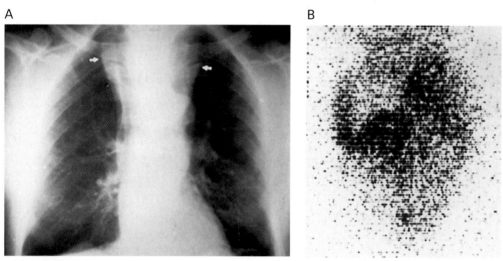

Fig C 23-1
Substernal thyroid. (A) Marked widening of the superior mediastinum to both sides (arrows) and severe deviation of the trachea to the right. (B) Iodine-131 scan shows increased uptake of the radionuclide in the area of the mass seen on the radiograph.[42]

A   B

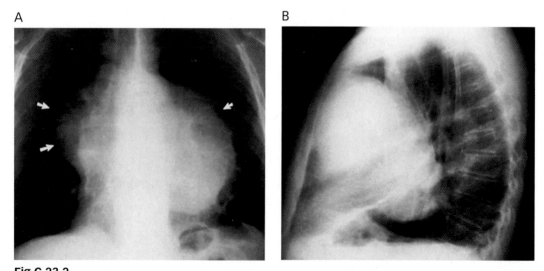

Fig C 23-2
Thymoma. (A) Frontal view shows a large bilateral lobulated mass (arrows) extending to both sides of the mediastinum. (B) Lateral view shows filling of the anterior precardiac space by a mass and posterior displacement of the left side of the heart.

Condition	Imaging Findings	Comments
Teratoma and other germinal cell neoplasms (Fig C 23-4)	Round or oval, smooth or lobulated mass that may protrude to one or both sides of the mediastinum.	Calcification (bone, teeth) or fat may occur in teratomas and dermoid cysts. Benign lesions tend to be smooth and cystic, whereas malignant lesions are often lobulated and solid.
Lymphoma (especially Hodgkin's)/leukemia (Fig C 23-5)	Enlargement of anterior mediastinal and retrosternal lymph nodes commonly occurs.	The presence of anterior mediastinal nodes in lymphoma is a differential point from sarcoidosis (which also affects hilar nodes but not nodes in the anterior compartment). There is often symmetric widening of the superior mediastinum on frontal views.

A
B

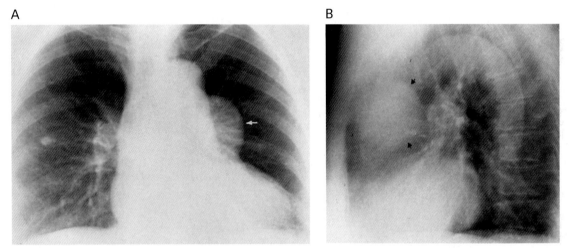

Fig C 23-3
Thymoma with myasthenia gravis. (A) Frontal and (B) lateral views of the chest demonstrate a large mass in the anterior mediastinum (arrows).

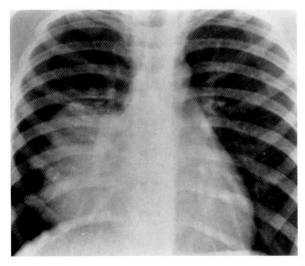

Fig C 23-4
Teratodermoid tumor. Large lobulated mass confluent with the right border of the heart.

Condition	Imaging Findings	Comments
Lymphangioma (hygroma)	Smooth or lobulated mass in the superior portion of the mediastinum.	Benign or invasive lesion that is often associated with a soft-tissue mass in the neck. Chylothorax may develop.
Mesenchymal tumor (Fig C 23-6)	Various patterns.	May be benign or malignant. A striking lucency suggests a lipoma or lipomatosis (steroid therapy). Phleboliths are diagnostic of a hemangioma.
Parathyroid tumor	Smooth or lobulated mass that may be too small to be detectable on plain films.	May displace the esophagus. There is often evidence of hyperparathyroidism in the thoracic spine.
Aneurysm of ascending aorta or sinus of Valsalva (Fig C 23-7)	Saccular or fusiform mass that tends to extend anteriorly and to the right.	May erode the sternum. Calcification is relatively uncommon.
Morgagni hernia (see Fig C 46-7)	Round or oval lower mediastinal mass that is almost invariably on the right.	Presence of gas-filled bowel (or contrast-filled colon from an enema) in the mass is diagnostic. The hernia appears as a homogeneous opacity if it is filled with liver or omentum (mimics a fat pad or a pericardial cyst).
Pericardial cyst (Fig C 23-8)	Round or lobulated, sharply demarcated lower mediastinal mass that is usually located in the right cardiophrenic angle.	Typically touches both the anterior chest wall and the anterior portion of the right hemidiaphragm. Usually asymptomatic.

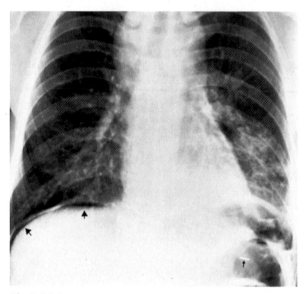

Fig C 23-5
Lymphoma. Diffuse widening of the upper portion of the mediastinum due to lymphadenopathy. There is an ill-defined lymphomatous parenchymal infiltrate at the left base. The metallic clip overlying the region of the spleen (small arrow) and the small amount of free intraperitoneal gas seen under the right hemidiaphragm (large arrows) are evidence of a recent exploratory laparotomy and splenectomy for staging of the lymphoma.

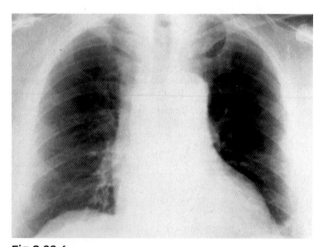

Fig C 23-6
Mediastinal lipomatosis. Generalized widening of the upper mediastinum.[43]

Condition	Imaging Findings	Comments
Mediastinal hemorrhage/hematoma	Uniform, symmetric widening of the mediastinum, especially the superior portion.	Generally a history of trauma, surgery, or dissecting aneurysm. A discrete hematoma may compress the superior vena cava and calcify. Any mediastinal compartment may be involved.
Mediastinitis (see Figs C 25-6 and C 25-7)	Generalized widening of the mediastinum, usually most evident superiorly. A lobulated paratracheal mass predominantly projecting to the right may develop in chronic disease.	Acute mediastinitis is most often because of esophageal rupture and may be associated with mediastinal air. Chronic mediastinitis (granulomatous or sclerosing) may calcify and compress vessels (especially the superior vena cava) or a major airway.
Benign lymphoid hyperplasia (Castleman's disease)	Solitary and sharply defined mass.	Although most common in the middle and posterior compartments, in the anterior mediastinum the lesion tends to be lobulated (suggesting a thymoma or teratoma).

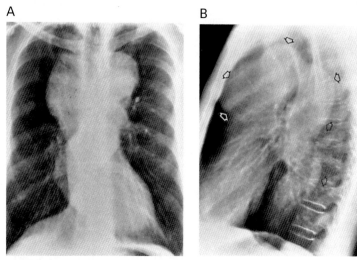

Fig C 23-7
Aneurysm of the thoracic aorta. (A) Frontal and (B) lateral views of the chest demonstrate marked dilatation of both the ascending and descending portions of the thoracic aorta (arrows, B), producing anterior and posterior mediastinal masses, respectively.

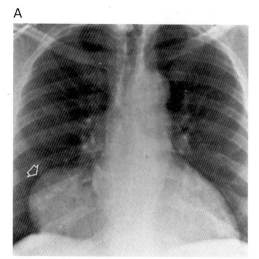

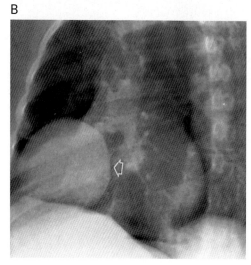

Fig C 23-8
Pericardial cyst. (A) Frontal and (B) oblique views demonstrate a smooth mass (arrows) in the right cardiophrenic angle.

Anterior Mediastinal Lesions on Computed Tomography

Condition	Comments
Fat density (–20 to –100 H) Lipomatosis	Frequent cause of generalized mediastinal widening. Excess fat deposition in the mediastinum may be associated with moderate obesity, steroid therapy, Cushing's syndrome, or diabetes or may be a normal variant in nonobese patients. Fat deposition localized to the superior portion of the anterior compartment may simulate a mass or aortic dissection.
Lipoma (Figs C 24-1 and C 24-2)	Benign collection of fatty tissue that is most common in the anterior mediastinum although it can also occur in the middle and posterior mediastina and adjacent to the diaphragm. Thymolipomas are anterior mediastinal masses that may be indistinguishable from lipomas. Liposarcomas are extremely rare, more commonly occur in the posterior mediastinum, generally have a higher density than benign fat, are inhomogeneous, and tend to show features of mediastinal invasion.

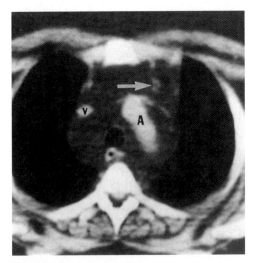

Fig C 24-1
Mediastinal lipomatosis. Abundant fat throughout the superior mediastinum that has a homogeneous attenuation similar to that of subcutaneous fat. (Arrow, residual thymic tissue or mediastinal lymph node; v, right innominate vein; A, aortic arch.)[44]

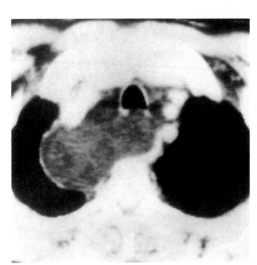

Fig C 24-2
Liposarcoma. Large, relatively inhomogeneous mass in the right side of the mediastinum. Note that the mass has a slightly higher attenuation than does the subcutaneous fat. The mass extended into the right side of the neck to involve the recurrent laryngeal nerve, paralyzing the right vocal cord.[44]

Condition	Comments
Omental hernia (Fig C 24-3)	Herniation of omental fat through a foramen of Morgagni's hernia can present as a localized fatty mass virtually indistinguishable from a lipoma.
Water density (0 to 15 H) Thymic cyst (Fig C 24-4)	True congenital thymic cysts are rare and originate from the thymopharyngeal duct. Although usually asymptomatic, large cysts can produce tracheal or cardiac compression. They are usually round and are frequently multiloculated. Hemorrhage into the cyst is common, and the cyst cavity often contains old blood, necrotic material, and cholesterol crystals so that its CT attenuation value may vary considerably from that of water. Cystic degeneration of a thymoma or thymic involvement by Hodgkin's disease or a germinoma may produce an indistinguishable CT appearance.

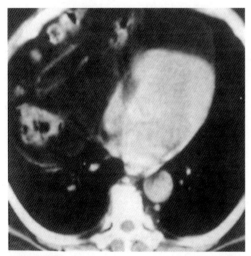

Fig C 24-3
Morgagni hernia. The right inferior mediastinal mass contains large bowel and omental fat. Focal eventration of the diaphragm can be differentiated from a Morgagni's hernia by the intact diaphragm in the former entity.[44]

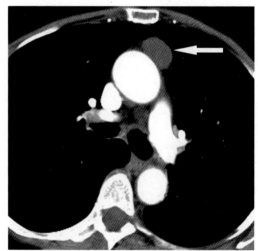

Fig C 24-4
Thymic cyst. Incidentally noted well-circumscribed mass of fluid attenuation (arrow).[45]

Condition	Comments

Soft-tissue density
(15 to 40 H)
  Thymoma/Thymic
  malignancy
  (Figs C 24-5 to C 24-8)

Wide variation of CT appearances with attenuation values varying from the low density of fat to soft-tissue density. Calcification is often visible in the mass. CT findings strongly suggestive of malignancy include extension of tumor into the mediastinum or lung parenchyma, pleural deposits (especially posteriorly and in the costophrenic angles) from transpleural seeding of tumor, and irregular pericardial thickening suggesting pericardial implants. Preservation of the low-density plane of cleavage representing fat between the tumor and mediastinal structures may be CT evidence of benignancy.

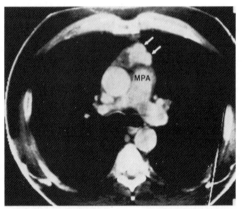

Fig C 24-5
Thymoma. Slightly lobulated mass (arrows) anterior to the main pulmonary artery (MPA) in a patient with myasthenia gravis.[46]

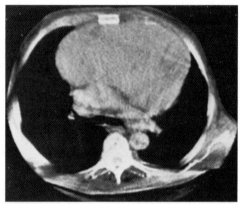

Fig C 24-6
Thymoma. Enormous soft-tissue mass in the anterior mediastinum with posterior displacement of other mediastinal structures. No difference in density can be seen between the mass and the heart behind it.

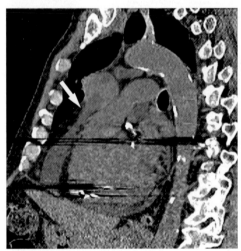

Fig C 24-7
Thymic carcinoma. Sagittal reformatted image shows that the anterior mediastinal mass is closely attached to the pericardium with loss of the fat plane (arrow) between the two entities, findings that suggest pericardial involvement. There is also a pericardial effusion.[45]

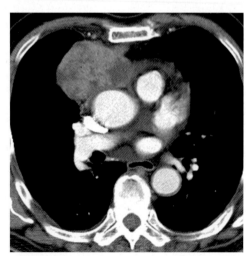

Fig C 24-8
Thymic carcinoid. Lobulated, heterogeneously enhancing mass. Loss of the fat plane between the mass and the pericardium suggests invasiveness.[45]

Condition	Comments
Thymic hyperplasia (Fig C 24-9)	Generalized enlargement of the thymus with preservation of its typical bilobed configuration.
Retrosternal thyroid (Fig C 24-10)	There is usually evidence of a connection between the mass and the thyroid gland in the neck. CT scans may show focal calcifications in the mass that are not detectable on plain chest radiographs. Multinodular goiters typically show a marked, rapid, and prolonged enhancement after the injection of intravenous contrast material.
Parathyroid tumor (Fig C 24-11)	Typically a small rounded mass that enhances more than muscle or lymph nodes but less than the great vessels.

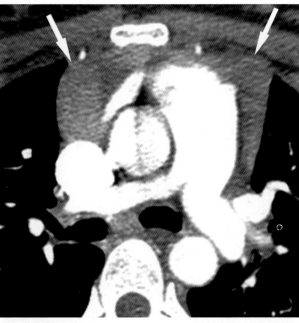

Fig C 24-9
Thymic hyperplasia. Bilobed, homogeneous soft-tissue lesion (arrows) in a patient with Graves' disease.[45]

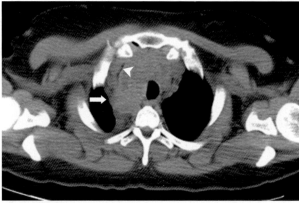

Fig C 24-10
Retrosternal goiter. Soft-tissue mass (arrow) extending into the anterior and middle mediastinum.[47]

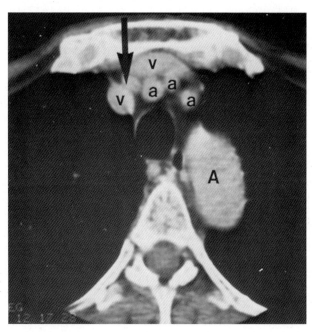

Fig C 24-11
Ectopic parathyroid adenoma. Small soft-tissue mass (arrow) in the anterior mediastinum. (A, aorta; a, major branches of the aorta; and v, brachiocephalic veins.)[48]

Condition	Comments
Teratoma and other germinal cell neoplasms (Fig C 24-12)	Solid teratomas are indistinguishable from other soft-tissue tumors. "Cystic" teratomas are not of homogeneous water density but rather appear as complex masses with components of fat, bone, and muscle density, reflecting their varied composition of tissues from all three germ layers. Cystic teratomas often demonstrate fat-fluid interfaces and may contain calcifications and soft-tissue nodules in the mass.
Lymphoma (Fig C 24-13)	Involvement of anterior mediastinal lymph nodes lying ventral to the aorta and superior vena cava. The presence of enlarged nodes in this region is a differential point from sarcoidosis that also affects hilar nodes (as does lymphoma) but not nodes in the anterior compartment.
Other neoplasms	Lymphangioma (hygroma), neurofibroma, other spindle cell tumors.
Mediastinitis/abscess	Suggested by the presence of bubbles of gas or a discrete cavity with a thick, shaggy wall.
Morgagni's hernia	A hernia containing fluid-filled bowel or part of the liver produces a mass of soft-tissue density.
Mediastinal hemorrhage/hematoma	Uniform, symmetric widening of the mediastinum (especially the superior portion) in a patient with a history of trauma, surgery, or dissecting aneurysm.

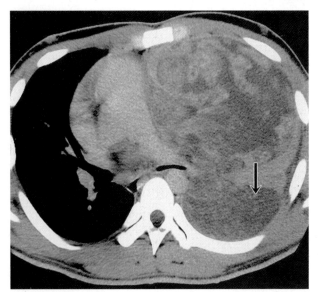

Fig C 24-12
Mixed germ cell tumor. Contrast scan shows a huge tumor that is primarily solid, thought there is a relatively large cystic component (arrow).[49]

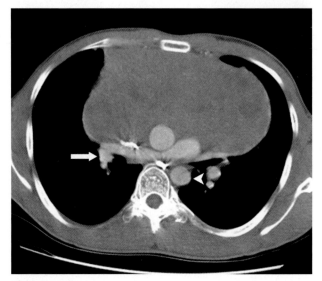

Fig C 24-13
Lymphoma. Large mass that fills the anterior mediastinum. Note that the lung interfaces with the hilar vessels (arrow) and aorta (arrowhead) are well preserved. Thus, on plain radiographs these middle mediastinal structures were clearly seen through the mass (hilum overlay sign), indicating that the lesion was either in the anterior or posterior portion of the mediastinum.[47]

Condition	Comments
Fibrosing mediastinitis (Fig C 24-14)	Rare benign proliferation of acellular collagen and fibrous tissue within the mediastinum. Although often idiopathic, many cases are thought to be the result of an abnormal immunologic response *Histoplasma capsulatum* infection. Fibrosing mediastinitis primarily affects the middle mediastinum.
Vascular/enhancing	Aneurysms, ectatic vessels.
Intrinsic high density (more than 90 H)	Retrosternal thyroid.

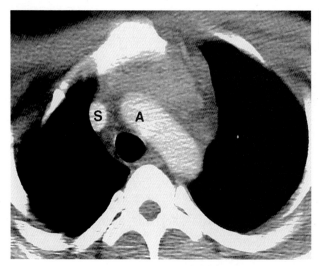

Fig C 24-14
Fibrosing mediastinitis. Soft-tissue attenuation mass in the anterior mediastinum. A, aorta; S, superior vena cava.)[50]

Middle Mediastinal Lesions

Condition	Imaging Findings	Comments
Lymph node enlargement (Fig C 25-1)	Unilateral or bilateral hilar and paratracheal masses.	Most commonly due to metastases, tuberculosis, histoplasmosis, lymphoma, pneumoconiosis, or sarcoidosis.
Aneurysm of aorta or major branch (Fig C 25-2)	Various patterns depending on the location of the aneurysm.	Transverse arch aneurysms typically obliterate the aorticopulmonary window and are symptomatic. Mural calcification is relatively common. Mediastinal masses may also be caused by pseudocoarctation of the aorta and by dilatation of the superior vena cava or azygos vein.

A

B

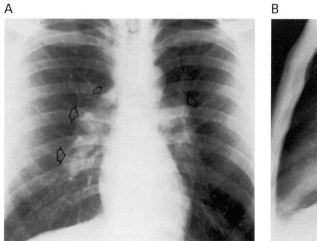
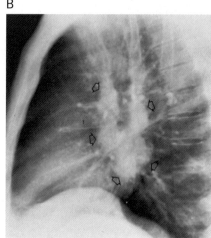

Fig C 25-1
Mediastinal lymphadenopathy in sarcoidosis. (A) Frontal and (B) lateral views of the chest demonstrate enlarged mediastinal lymph nodes (arrows).

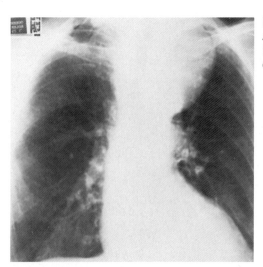

Fig C 25-2
Aneurysm of the left subclavian artery.
Left superior mediastinal widening in an elderly woman without chest symptoms.[43]

Condition	Imaging Findings	Comments
Bronchogenic cyst (Figs C 25-3 and C 25-4)	Round or oval, well-defined mass that is often lobulated and tends to mold itself to surrounding structures (because of its fluid contents).	Most commonly located just inferior to the carina. Often protrudes to the right and overlaps the right hilar shadow. Rarely communicates with the tracheobronchial tree.

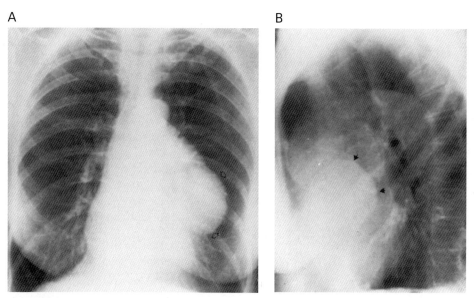

Fig C 25-3
Bronchogenic cyst. (A) Frontal and (B) lateral views of the chest demonstrate a smooth-walled, spherical mediastinal mass (arrows) projecting into the left lung and left hilum.

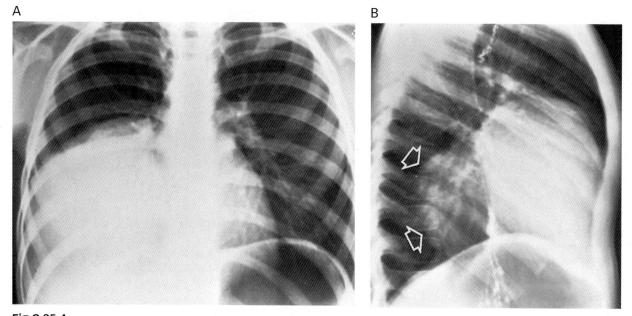

Fig C 25-4
Bronchogenic cyst. (A) Frontal and (B) lateral views of the chest demonstrate a huge middle mediastinal mass (arrows, B) protruding to the right and filling much of the lower half of the right hemithorax. The patient was asymptomatic.

Condition	Imaging Findings	Comments
Mediastinal hemorrhage/ hematoma (Fig C 25-5)	Uniform, symmetric widening of the mediastinum (especially the superior portion).	Generally a history of trauma, surgery, or dissecting aneurysm. A discrete hematoma may compress the superior vena cava and calcify.
Mediastinitis (Figs C 25-6 and C 25-7)	Generalized widening of the mediastinum, usually most evident superiorly. A lobulated paratracheal mass predominantly projecting to the right may develop in chronic disease.	Acute mediastinitis is most often due to esophageal rupture and may be associated with mediastinal air. Chronic mediastinitis (granulomatous or sclerosing) may calcify and compress vessels (especially the superior vena cava) or a major airway.
Pleuropericardial (mesothelial) cyst	Round, oval, or teardrop mass with smooth margins.	Fluid-filled cyst that is almost always asymptomatic and may change shape with respiration or alteration in body position. May also involve the anterior mediastinum.
Intrapericardial hernia (Fig C 25-8)	Gas-filled loops of bowel that lie alongside the heart and remain in conformity with the heart border on multiple projections (including decubitus views).	Extremely rare congenital or posttraumatic lesion that can contain (in decreasing order of frequency) omentum, colon, small bowel, liver, or stomach. Although often asymptomatic for long periods, most patients eventually present with cardiorespiratory or gastrointestinal complaints.
Benign lymphoid hyperplasia (Castleman's disease)	Smooth or lobulated solitary mass.	Rare condition that most often involves the posterior mediastinum.

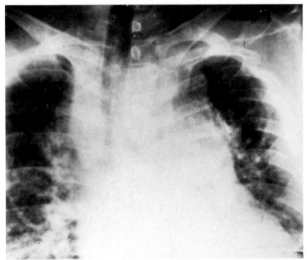

Fig C 25-5
Aortic transection. Frontal chest radiograph taken immediately after trauma demonstrates mediastinal widening, obscuration of the aorta, deviation of the trachea to the right, and downward displacement of the left main-stem bronchus.[51]

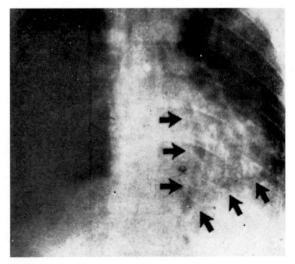

Fig C 25-6
Acute mediastinitis due to rupture of the esophagus. Plain radiograph demonstrates linear lucent shadows (arrows) that represent localized mediastinal emphysema and correspond to the fascial planes of the mediastinal and diaphragmatic pleurae in the region of the lower esophagus.[52]

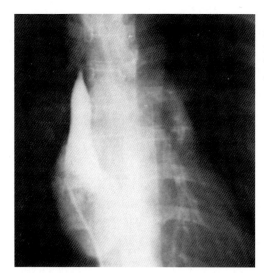

Fig C 25-7
Chronic sclerosing mediastinitis. Venogram shows smooth tapering of the lower portion of the superior vena cava. This 38-year-old woman had varicosities over her upper abdomen and lower chest.[52]

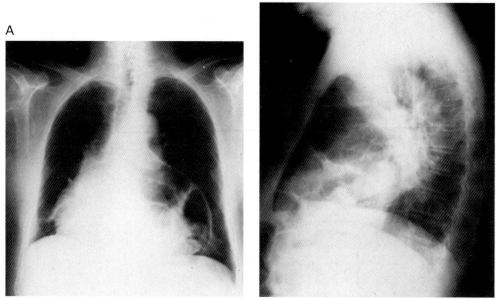

Fig C 25-8
Congenital intrapericardial hernia. (A) Frontal and (B) lateral views in an asymptomatic elderly man show loops of bowel in the chest conforming to the left pericardial border.[53]

Middle Mediastinal Lesions on Computed Tomography

Condition	Comments
Fat density (–20 to –100 H) Lipomatosis (Figs C 26-1 and C 26-2)	Extensive fat deposition in the mediastinum may be associated with moderate obesity, steroid therapy, Cushing's syndrome, or diabetes or may be a normal variant in nonobese patients.
Epicardial fat pad	Most common fatty mass in the thorax.
Pericardial lipoma	Localized collection of fat-density tissue (lipomas occur more commonly in the anterior mediastinum).

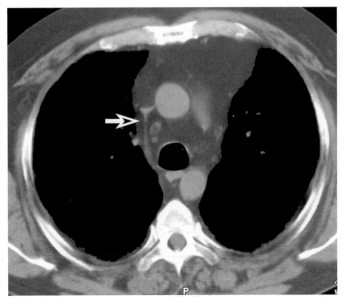

Fig C 26-1
Mediastinal lipomatosis. Diffuse fatty lesion with a mass effect on the superior vena cava and azygos vein.[54]

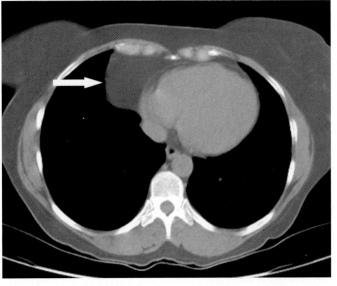

Fig C 26-2
Epicardial fat pad. Homogeneous fat attenuation (arrow) adjacent to the right border of the heart.[52]

Condition	Comments
Water density (0 to 15 H)	
Pericardial cyst (Fig C 26-3)	Smooth, thin-walled mass that most commonly occurs in the right cardiophrenic angle. Malleable lesion that may change shape when the patient is scanned in the prone or decubitus position. Easily differentiated from prominent epicardial fat pads or lipomas, which also present as cardiophrenic angle masses.
Bronchogenic cyst (Fig C 26-4)	Smooth, round, homogeneous mass that usually has a thin, imperceptible rim and does not show any change in attenuation after infusion of contrast material. May contain viscous mucoid or proteinaceous material that produces a higher attenuation in the range of a solid neoplasm.

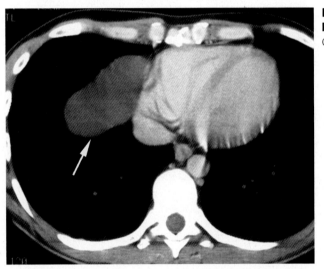

Fig C 26-3
Pericardial cyst. Contrast CT scan shows a thin-walled cyst of water attenuation (arrow).[55]

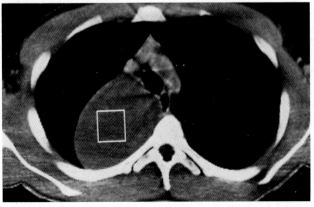

Fig C 26-4
Bronchogenic cyst. CT scan in a young man with an incidental upper respiratory infection shows a large right upper mediastinal mass extending from the right of the trachea to the posterior chest wall. The cyst had a uniform appearance and near-water density and extended vertically from the lower pole of the thyroid gland to the carina.[56]

Condition	Comments
Soft-tissue density (15 to 40 H) Lymphadenopathy (Figs C 26-5 to C 26-8)	Most commonly the result of metastases, lymphoma, granulomatous disease (tuberculosis, histoplasmosis), pneumoconiosis, or sarcoidosis.
Mediastinitis/abscess	Suggested by the presence of bubbles of gas or a discrete cavity with a thick, shaggy wall.

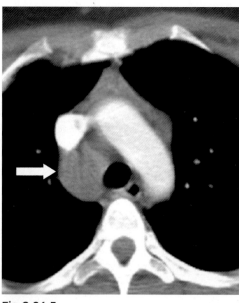

Fig C 26-5
Lymphadenopathy. The enlarged nodes (arrow) obliterate the air-soft tissue interface between the right lung and the tracheal wall (right paratracheal stripe).[52]

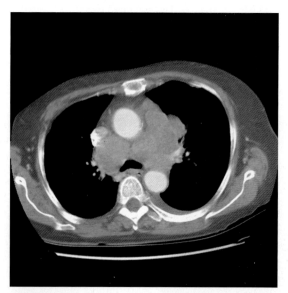

Fig C 26-6
Bronchogenic carcinoma. Soft-tissue mass within the aortopulmonary window and subcarinal space, a finding consistent with metastatic lymphadenopathy. There is also lymphadenopathy in the paratracheal region, which produced a thickened right paratracheal stripe on plain radiographs.[57]

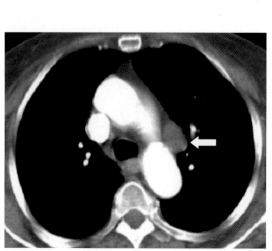

Fig C 26-7
Lymphoma. Enlarged nodes (arrow) obliterate the normal concave border of the interface between the left lung and the mediastinum constituting the aorticopulmonary window.[52]

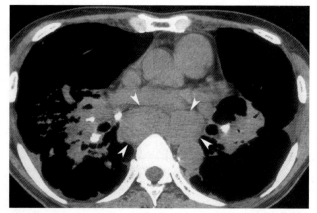

Fig C 26-8
Sarcoidosis. Diffuse bilateral mediastinal and hilar adenopathy. Calcification in the affected hilar nodes suggests a prolonged clinical course. Note the simultaneous presence of huge subcarinal nodes (arrowheads), an unusual finding in other granulomatous diseases such as tuberculosis.[58]

Condition	Comments
Mediastinal hemorrhage/ hematoma (See Fig C 56-11)	Uniform, symmetric widening of the mediastinum (especially the superior portion) in a patient with a history of trauma, surgery, or dissecting aneurysm.
Neoplasm (Fig C 26-9)	Variety of benign and malignant processes.
Fibrosing mediastinitis (Fig C 26-10)	Rare benign proliferation of acellular collagen and fibrous tissue within the mediastinum. Although often idiopathic, many cases are thought to be due to an abnormal immunologic response to Histoplasma capsulatum infection. Fibrosing mediastinitis most commonly involves the middle mediastinum, primarily in young patients, and presents with signs symptoms of obstruction or compression of the superior vena cava, pulmonary veins or arteries, central airways, or esophagus.
Vascular/enhancing (Figs C 26-11 to C 26-15)	Ectatic vessels, aneurysms, dissections, and congenital vascular anomalies.

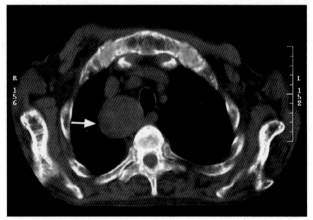

Fig C 26-9
Ectopic parathyroid adenoma. Large right paratracheal mass (arrow) with diffuse osteopenia from primary hyperparathyroidism.[57]

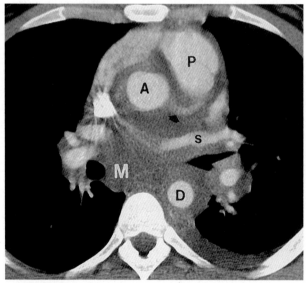

Fig C 26-10
Fibrosing mediastinitis. Soft-tissue mass diffusely infiltrates the mediastinum. There is a subcarinal mass (M), encasement of the left main coronary artery (arrow), and narrowing of the left superior pulmonary vein (S). (A, ascending aorta; D, descending aorta; P, main pulmonary artery.)[55]

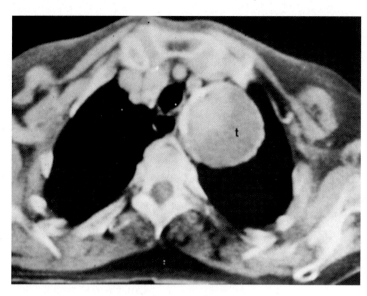

Fig C 26-11
Aneurysm of the left subclavian artery. Contrast-enhanced scan shows the large aneurysm partially filled with thrombus (t).[43]

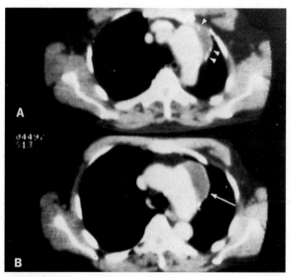

Fig C 26-12
Chronic traumatic aortic aneurysm. CT scans through (A) and slightly below (B) the aortic arch after the intravenous injection of contrast material demonstrate calcification in the wall of the aneurysm (arrowheads) and a large filling defect consisting of thrombus (arrow).

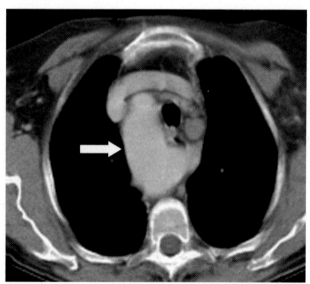

Fig C 26-13
Right-sided aortic arch. This vascular structure (arrow) caused loss of the normal right paratracheal stripe on plain radiographs.[52]

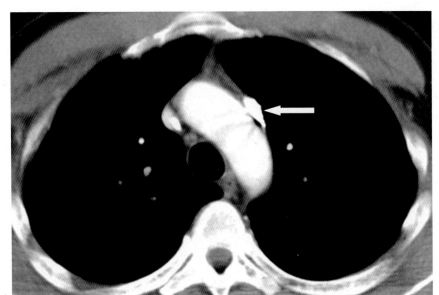

Fig C 26-14
Left-sided superior vena cava. CT scan at the level of the aortic arch shows the anomalous vessel (arrow), which drains into the coronary sinus.[52]

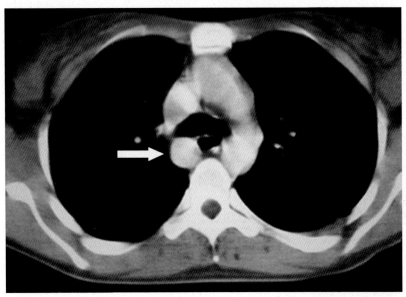

Fig C 26-15
Azygos continuation of the inferior vena cava. Enlargement of the azygos vein (arrow) that widened the inferior margin of the right paratracheal stripe on plain radiographs.[52]

Posterior Mediastinal Lesions

Condition	Imaging Findings	Comments
Neurogenic neoplasm (Fig C 27-1)	Sharply circumscribed, round or oval homogeneous mass that is usually unilateral and paravertebral.	Primarily neurofibromas and neurolemmomas in adults, ganglioneuromas and neuroblastomas in children. Chemodectomas (any mediastinal compartment) and pheochromocytomas are extremely rare. There may be associated rib or vertebral erosion, calcification, and a dumbbell appearance (part of the tumor is inside and part outside the spinal canal).
Spinal neoplasm	Rounded paravertebral mass with associated bone destruction.	Tumors include osteochondroma, aneurysmal bone cyst, chondrosarcoma, osteogenic sarcoma, Ewing's tumor, myeloma, and metastases. An extraosseous soft-tissue mass is a relatively infrequent finding.
Extramedullary hematopoiesis	Single or multiple (often bilateral), lobulated or smooth mass that generally occurs in the paravertebral region in the lower half of the thorax.	Usually associated with congenital hemolytic anemia. Splenomegaly (or a history of splenectomy) is common.
Aneurysm of descending aorta (Fig C 27-2)	Smooth or lobulated mass that typically projects from the posterolateral aspect of the aorta on the left side.	Frequently calcified and may become large enough to erode the vertebral column.

A
B

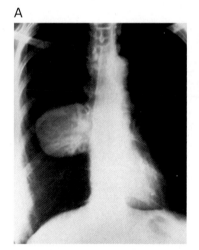
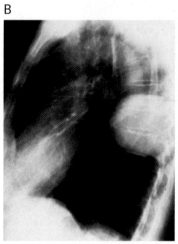

Fig C 27-1
Neurogenic tumor. (A) Frontal and (B) lateral views of the chest demonstrate a large right posterior mediastinal mass.[42]

A
B

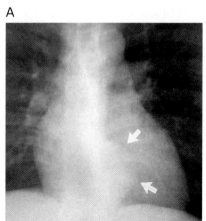
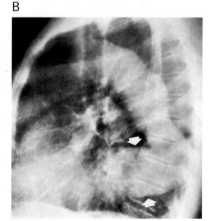

Fig C 27-2
Aneurysm of the descending aorta. (A) Frontal view of the chest demonstrates a localized bulging of the descending aorta (arrows). (B) Lateral view in another patient shows aneurysmal dilatation of the lower thoracic aorta (arrows). Note the marked tortuosity of the remainder of the descending aorta.

Condition	Imaging Findings	Comments
Bochdalek hernia (see Fig C 46-8)	Round or oval, retrocardiac mass that is usually unilateral (80% to 90% are on the left side).	Air-filled bowel loops in the mass are diagnostic. More commonly the hernia contains opaque omentum, liver, or spleen.
Hiatal hernia (Fig C 27-3)	Retrocardiac mass of variable size that usually contains an air-fluid level.	Diagnosis confirmed by esophagram. Rarely completely opaque (containing only omentum or liver).
Megaesophagus (Fig C 27-4)	Broad vertical opacity on the right side of the mediastinum that often contains an air-fluid level (especially in achalasia).	Causes of marked dilatation of the esophagus include achalasia, scleroderma, carcinoma, Chagas' disease, and inflammatory stenosis due to mediastinitis or recurrent esophagitis. May produce anterior bulging of the trachea.
Esophageal neoplasm	Smooth, rounded, usually unilateral mass.	Most commonly leiomyoma (may be fibroma or lipoma). Smooth compression of the esophageal lumen on barium swallow.

A   B

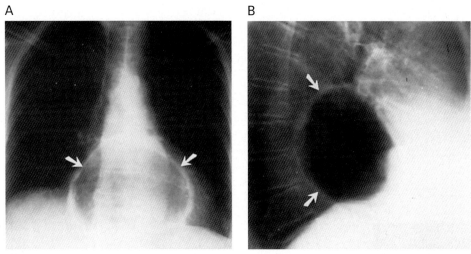

Fig C 27-3
Hiatal hernia. (A) Frontal and (B) lateral views of the chest demonstrate a huge air-filled hiatal hernia that appears as a posterior mediastinal mass (arrows).

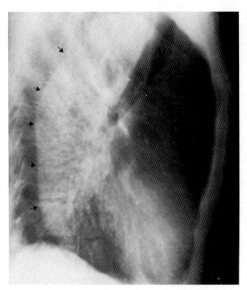

Fig C 27-4
Megaesophagus. Lateral chest film in a patient with achalasia shows a mixture of fluid and air density in the dilated esophagus (arrows).

Condition	Imaging Findings	Comments
Mediastinal hemorrhage/ hematoma	Uniform, symmetric widening of the mediastinum.	Generally a history of trauma, surgery, or dissecting aneurysm. A discrete hematoma may calcify.
Mediastinitis (see Figs C 25-6 and C 25-7)	Generalized widening of the mediastinum, usually more evident superiorly.	Acute mediastinitis is most often due to esophageal rupture and may be associated with mediastinal air. Chronic mediastinitis (granulomatous or sclerosing) may calcify.
Thyroid tumor (see Fig C 23-1)	Smooth or lobulated, well-defined mass that appears almost exclusively on the right.	Involves the superior portion of the mediastinum. Much more common in the anterior mediastinum.
Esophageal varices (Fig C 27-5)	Lobulated retrocardiac mass.	Usually a history of cirrhosis or variceal bleeding or other signs of portal hypertension.
Esophageal diverticulum (Zenker's)	Cyst-like structure in the superior mediastinum that often contains an air-fluid level.	Rarely large enough to be seen on chest radiographs. An esophagram is diagnostic.
Neurenteric cyst (Fig C 27-6)	Sharply defined, round or oval, lobulated, homogeneous mass.	Results from incomplete separation of the endoderm from the notochordal plate during early embryonic life. Often associated with a congenital defect of the thoracic spine and symptomatic in infancy.
Gastroenteric cyst	Sharply defined, round or oval mass in a paraspinal location. Tends to mold itself to the surrounding structures because of its fluid contents.	Represents failure of complete vacuolation of the originally solid esophagus to produce a hollow tube. Lined by esophageal, gastric, or small intestinal mucosa. May communicate with the gastrointestinal tract and contain air. Produces an extrinsic impression on the esophagus on barium studies.

A

B

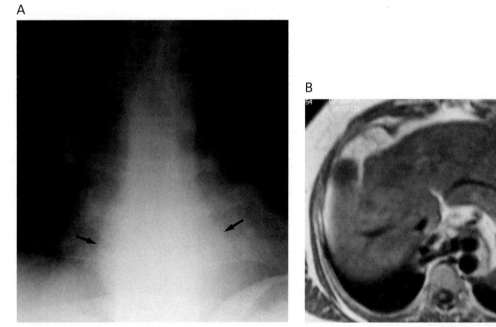

Fig C 27-5

Esophageal varices. (A) Frontal chest radiograph in a patient with severe cirrhosis shows a retrocardiac mass (arrows) that silhouettes the descending aorta and causes abnormal convexity of the azygoesophageal recess. (B) Corresponding MR image reveals extensive paraesophageal vascular channels consistent with varices.[19]

Condition	Imaging Findings	Comments
Meningocele (meningomyelocele)	Sharply defined, solitary or multiple, unilateral or bilateral mass.	Frequently associated with vertebral and rib anomalies. Usually communicates with the spinal subarachnoid space and fills on myelography.
Vertebral osteomyelitis (Fig C 27-7)	Bilateral fusiform mass in the paravertebral region.	Tuberculous and pyogenic infections usually cause vertebral erosion or destruction and often abscess formation in contiguous soft tissues.
Azygos continuation of the inferior vena cava (Fig C 27-8)	Irregular paravertebral mass representing the dilated azygos vein. No shadow of the inferior vena cava on lateral view.	Commonly associated with complex cardiac anomalies.

A
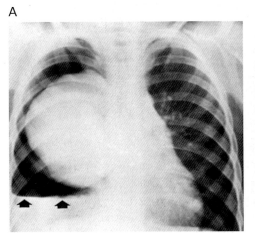

B
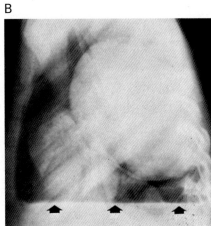

Fig C 27-6
Neurenteric cyst. (A) Frontal and (B) lateral views of the chest demonstrate a large, oval, homogeneous mass in the posterior mediastinum. Note the right hydropneumothorax (arrows) with a long air-fluid level that developed as a complication of a diagnostic needle biopsy.

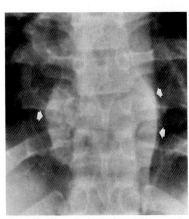

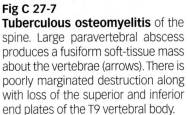

Fig C 27-7
Tuberculous osteomyelitis of the spine. Large paravertebral abscess produces a fusiform soft-tissue mass about the vertebrae (arrows). There is poorly marginated destruction along with loss of the superior and inferior end plates of the T9 vertebral body.

A
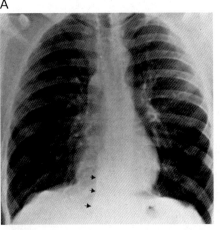

B
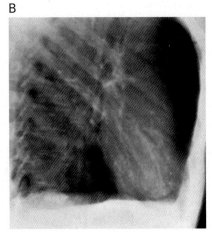

Fig C 27-8
Azygos continuation of the inferior vena cava. (A) On the frontal view, there is an irregular paravertebral mass (arrows). (B) Lateral view shows pulmonary vessels in the retrocardiac space but no shadow of the inferior vena cava.

Posterior Mediastinal Lesions on Computed Tomography

Condition	Comments
Fat density (−20 to −100 H)	
Omental hernia (Fig C 28-1A)	Herniation of omental fat through the foramen of Bochdalek.
Liposarcoma	Rare mediastinal tumor that occurs most commonly in the posterior mediastinum. Typically has a higher density than benign fat, is inhomogeneous, and shows features of mediastinal invasion.
Lipoma/lipomatosis	Homogeneously low attenuation values.
Extramedullary hematopoiesis	Generally occurs in the paravertebral region in the lower half of the thorax. More commonly produces a soft-tissue density.
Water density (0 to 15 H)	
Neurenteric cyst	Smooth, thin-walled mass. May contain viscous fluid with a density in the range of a solid tumor. Often associated with a congenital defect of the thoracic spine.
Gastroenteric cyst (Fig C 28-2)	Smooth, thin-walled mass. May contain viscous fluid with a density in the range of a solid tumor.
Bronchogenic cyst (Fig C 28-3)	Smooth, thin-walled mass. Up to 50% have attenuation higher than that of water as a result of the presence of milk or calcium, proteinaceous fluid, mucus, or blood debris within the cyst.
Meningocele (meningomyelocele)	Smooth, thin-walled mass. May contain viscous fluid with a density in the range of a solid tumor. Frequently associated with vertebral and rib anomalies.
Pancreatic pseudocyst (Fig C 28-4)	Rarely presents as a mass in the posterior or inferior mediastinum. CT can demonstrate extension of the mass through the retrocrural portion of the diaphragm.

A

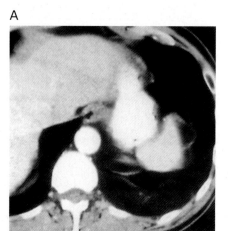

B

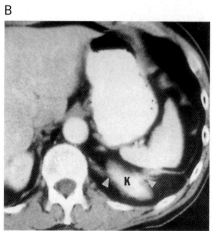

Fig C 28-1
Bochdalek hernia. (A) Intra-abdominal fat and (B) the top of the left kidney (K) extend through a posterior defect (arrowheads) in the left hemidiaphragm.[44]

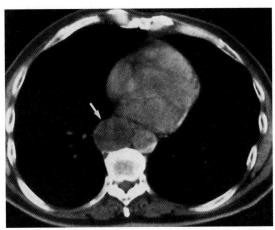

Fig C 28-2
Esophageal duplication cyst. Enhanced scan at the level of the left atrium in an asymptomatic elderly man reveals a cystic periesophageal mass (arrow) with an attenuation value of 12 HU.[59]

A

B

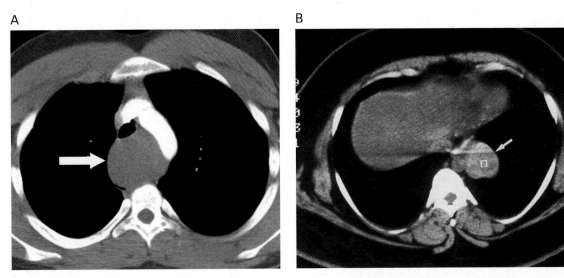

Fig C 28-3
Bronchogenic cyst. (A) Fluid-filled mass (arrow) in the posterior mediastinum.[52] (B) Unenhanced scan of the upper abdomen in an asymptomatic young man shows a high-attenuation (55 HU) periesophageal mass (arrow).[59]

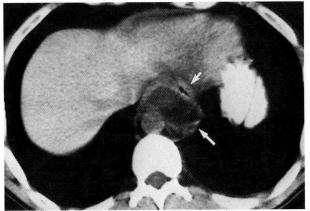

Fig C 28-4
Mediastinal pancreatic pseudocyst. Unenhanced scan of the upper abdomen in a young man with acute pancreatitis demonstrates a periaortic fluid collection (long arrow) displacing the esophagus (short arrow) anteriorly.[59]

Condition	Comments
Soft-tissue density (15 to 40 H)	
Neurogenic tumor (Fig C 28-5)	Variable attenuation values including a fatty appearance (without the fat-fluid interfaces seen in cystic teratomas) and a mixed pattern resulting from myxoid elements and vascular lakes. More vascular neural tumors (eg, paragangliomas) show dense homogeneous contrast enhancement, whereas neurolemmomas enhance to a lesser degree. Neurogenic tumors often originate from or extend into the corresponding neural foramen.
Hernia (Fig C 28-6; see Fig C 28-1B)	Hiatal hernia or Bochdalek's hernia (may contain an air-fluid level in the herniated bowel).

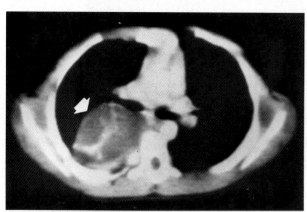

Fig C 28-5
Ganglioneuroma. Huge posterior mediastinal mass (arrow) with poor contrast enhancement.

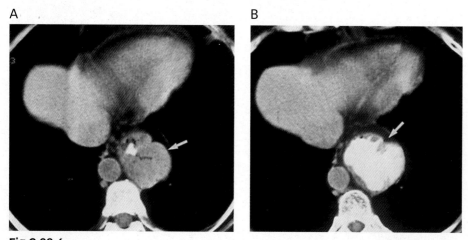

Fig C 28-6
Hiatal hernia. (A) Enhanced scan of the upper abdomen reveals a lower esophageal or periesophageal mass (arrow). (B) A repeat scan obtained after oral administration of additional contrast material demonstrates a better-distended hiatal sac with gastric folds (arrow).[59]

Condition	Comments
Mediastinitis/abscess/ infectious spondylitis (Figs C 28-7 and C 28-8)	Suggested by the presence of bubbles of gas or a discrete cavity with a thick shaggy wall. Osteolytic vertebral destruction can be seen in infectious spondylitis.
Spinal tumor (Fig C 28-9)	Primary or metastatic neoplasms can produce a paravertebral mass with osteolytic or osteoblastic vertebral changes.

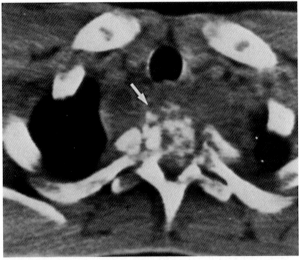

Fig C 28-7
Tuberculous spondylitis and paraspinal cold abscess.
Unenhanced scan obtained above the aortic arch shows a paravertebral mass that is destroying the vertebral body (arrow) and displacing the trachea anteriorly.[59]

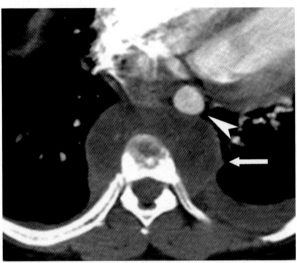

Fig C 28-8
Parspinal abscess. Soft-tissue mass (arrow) extending bilaterally that effaced the paraspinal lines (arrow). Arowhead indicates descending thoracic aorta.[52]

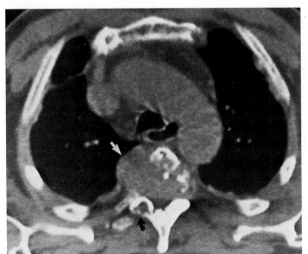

Fig C 28-9
Multiple myeloma. Unenhanced scan at the aortic arch level demonstrates a soft-tissue mass (white arrow) that is destroying the vertebral body and compromising the spinal canal. There are also associated osteolytic lesions of the posterior elements and adjacent ribs (black arrow).[59]

Condition	Comments
Mediastinal hemorrhage/hematoma (Fig C 28-10)	Uniform, symmetric widening of the mediastinum (especially the superior portion) in a patient with a history of trauma, surgery, or a dissecting aneurysm.
Extramedullary hematopoiesis (Fig C 28-11)	Generally occurs in the paravertebral region in the lower half of the thorax. May appear as a fat-density mass.
Lymphadenopathy (Fig C 28-12)	Posterior mediastinal (paraspinal) lymph nodes are considered enlarged if they exceed 6 mm in diameter (same criteria as for retrocrural nodes in the abdomen). Enlarged paraspinal nodes must not be mistaken for the azygos or hemiazygos veins, which are clearly tubular structures seen at multiple levels.
Bronchopulmonary sequestration	Congenital pulmonary malformation in which a portion of pulmonary tissue is detached from the remainder of the normal lung and receives its blood supply from a systemic artery. Typically appears as a sharply circumscribed mass in the posterior portion of a lower lobe (usually the left) contiguous to the diaphragm. May contain air or an air-fluid level if infection has resulted in communication with the airways or contiguous lung tissue.

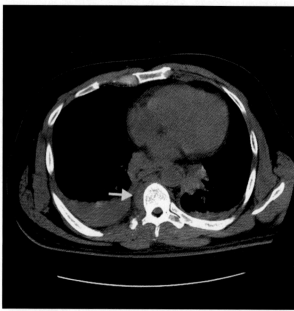

Fig C 28-10
Hematoma. Large mediastinal soft-tissue mass (arrow) from multiple right transverse process fractures of the lower thoracic spine. Note the associated right hemothorax.[63]

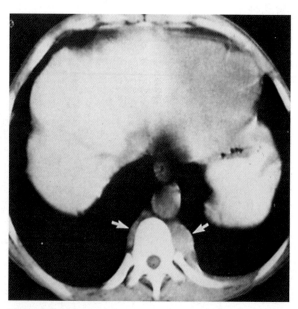

Fig C 28-11
Extramedullary hematopoiesis. Upper abdomen scan in a patient with homozygous sickle cell disease demonstrates bilateral, well-demarcated paravertebral soft-tissue masses (arrows) that are larger on the left. The diffuse increased attenuation of the liver reflects multiple blood transfusions.[59]

Condition	Comments
Esophageal carcinoma (Fig C 28-13)	May produce a large, bulky mass outside the esophagus. The obliteration of fat planes between the esophagus and neighboring structures can be a useful sign of extraesophageal spread if these planes were intact on a previous CT scan. However, clearly defined fat planes may not be seen in thin, cachectic patients or in patients who have had previous surgery or radiation therapy. Although the lack of fat planes in these patients is of uncertain significance, the presence of a fat plane rules out extension of tumor beyond the esophagus.
Esophageal dilatation (Fig C 28-14)	Esophageal motility disorders (achalasia, post-vagotomy syndrome, Chagas' disease, sclero-derma, presbyesophagus, diabetic and alcoholic neuropathy) and distal obstruction (benign or malignant stricture, compression by an extrinsic mass).

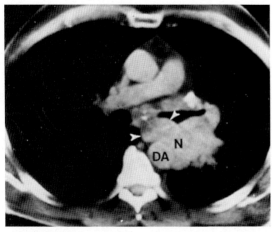

Fig C 28-12
Mediastinal spread from bronchogenic carcinoma. There is obliteration of the fat plane around the descending aorta (DA) by the adjacent neoplasm (N) in addition to extension of tumor deep into the mediastinum (arrowheads) behind the left main-stem bronchus and in front of the descending aorta.[46]

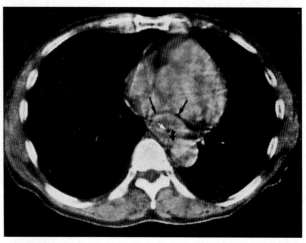

Fig C 28-13
Esophageal carcinoma. The circumferential mass of the bulky carcinoma (straight black arrows) fills the lumen of the esophagus (white arrow). Obliteration of the fat plane adjacent to the aorta (curved black arrow) indicates mediastinal invasion.

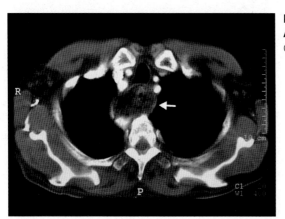

Fig C 28-14
Achalasia. Dilated esophagus (arrow) filled with food and contrast material.[63]

Condition	Comments
Intrathoracic goiter (Fig C 28-15)	One-fourth is posterior and occurs on the right side (left brachiocephalic vein and aortic arch prevent a goiter from the neck from descending on the left). Well-defined mass with anatomic contiguity with the cervical thyroid. Frequently focal calcification, relatively high attenuation, and rapid and prolonged contrast enhancement.
Vascular/enhancing (Figs C 28-16 to C 28-19)	Aneurysm or dissection of the aorta; dilatation of the azygos vein; esophageal varices; aortic arch and subclavian artery anomalies; pulmonary sling.

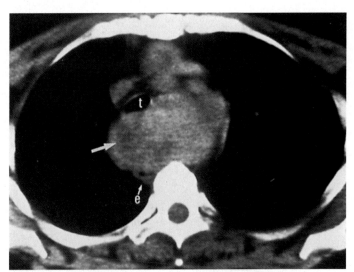

Fig C 28-15
Intrathoracic goiter. Enhanced scan above the aortic arch demonstrates a well-defined enhancing mass that displaces the esophagus (e), trachea (t), and major branches of the aortic arch and right brachiocephalic vein. There are areas of cystic degeneration (arrow) in the mass. Continuity with cervical thyroid tissue was seen on other images.[59]

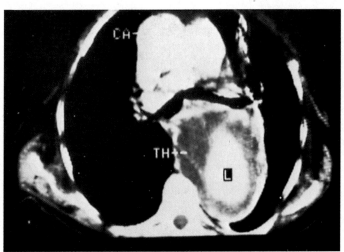

Fig C 28-16
Aneurysm of the descending aorta. Contrast-enhanced scan at a level just below the carina demonstrates a markedly dilated descending aorta (L) with a large mural thrombus (TH) surrounding the lumen of the descending aorta. Note also the markedly dilated ascending aorta (OA).

A

B

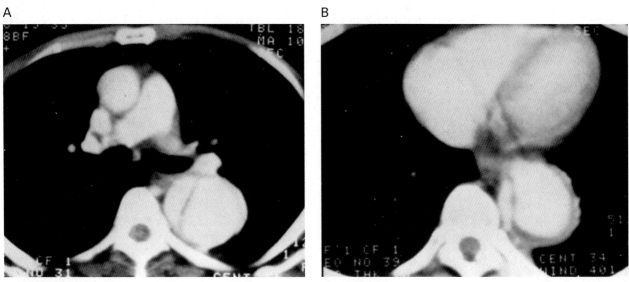

Fig C 28-17
Dissecting aneurysm. (A) Level of the pulmonary artery. (B) More caudal level.

A

B

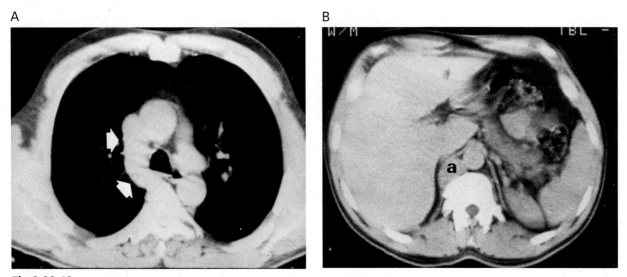

Fig C 28-18
Azygos continuation of the inferior vena cava. (A) The dilated azygos vein (arrows) produces a posterior mediastinal mass. (B) Upper abdominal CT scan shows the dilated azygos vein (a) in a retrocrural position adjacent to the aorta.

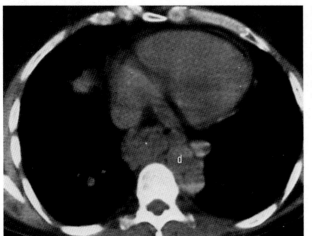

Fig C 28-19
Esophageal and periesophageal varices. Scan of the lower chest obtained during a drip infusion of contrast material shows that the esophagus is compressed by extensive periesophageal varices and is not adequately visualized. The descending aorta (d) is also surrounded by the periesophageal varices.[59]

Cystic Mediastinal Masses on Computed Tomography

Condition	Comments
Congenital bronchogenic cyst (Fig C 29-1)	Single, smooth, round or elliptical mass with an imperceptible wall. On CT, the cyst has a uniform attenuation value that varies depending on the contents from water to soft tissue and even to high attenuation if the cyst contains viscous mucoid or proteinaceous material. On T2-weighted MR images, the cyst has high signal intensity regardless of the nature of the cyst contents. Variable patterns of signal intensity can occur on T2-weighted scans because of variable cyst contents and the presence of protein, hemorrhage, or mucoid material.
Esophageal duplication cyst (Fig C 29-2)	Smooth, thin-walled mass with characteristics similar to a bronchogenic cyst. Many are asymptomatic, although they can cause dysphagia due to compression of the esophageal lumen. In pediatric patients, radionuclide scanning may show ectopic gastric mucosa within an esophageal duplication cyst.
Pericardial cyst (Fig C 29-3)	Similar in appearance to a bronchogenic cyst, pericardial cysts most commonly occur anteriorly in the right cardiophrenic angle. This asymptomatic, malleable lesion may change shape when the patient is scanned in the prone or decubitus position.
Neurenteric cyst	Similar in appearance to a bronchogenic cyst, it typically occurs posteriorly and is often associated with a congenital defect of the thoracic spine.
Meningocele (Fig C 29-4)	Herniation of the leptomeninges through an intervertebral foramen or a defect in a vertebral body. This paraspinal mass is frequently associated with neurofibromatosis, and there may be rib and vertebral abnormalities.
Lymphangioma (Fig C 29-5)	Rare malformation that usually appears as a smooth, lobulated mass that may mold to or envelop, rather than displace, adjacent mediastinal structures.

A

B

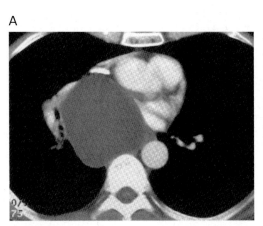
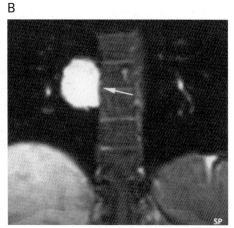

Fig C 29-1
Bronchogenic cyst. (A) Contrast CT scan shows a smooth mass with uniform water intensity and an imperceptible wall. (B) In another patient, coronal T1-weighted MR image shows a cyst with high–signal-intensity contents (arrow).[61]

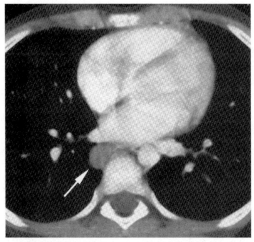

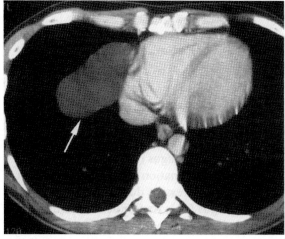

Fig C 29-2
Duplication cyst of the esophagus. Contrast CT scan shows a thin-walled cyst of water attenuation (arrow) adjacent to the esophagus.[61]

Fig C 29-3
Pericardial cyst. Contrast CT scan shows a thin-walled cyst of water attenuation (arrow).[61]

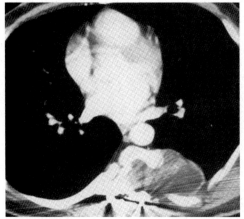

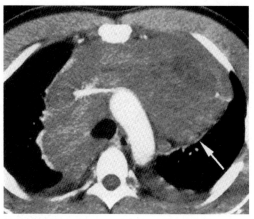

Fig C 29-4
Lateral thoracic meningocele. CT scan shows a low-attenuation mass protruding from the enlarged left intervertebral foramen.[61]

Fig C 29-5
Lymphangioma. Contrast CT scan shows a low-attenuation mass (arrow) that extends to all mediastinal compartments.[61]

Condition	Comments
Thymic cyst (Fig C 29-6)	Rare and usually asymptomatic, although large cysts can compress the trachea or esophagus. Acquired thymic cysts may develop in patients after radiation therapy for Hodgkin's disease, in association with thymic tumors, and after thoracotomy. Hemorrhage into the cyst is common, and the cyst cavity often contains old blood, necrotic material, and cholesterol crystals so that the CT attenuation value may vary considerably from that of water. Curvilinear calcification of the cyst wall occurs in a minority of cases.
Mature cystic teratoma (dermoid cyst) (Fig C 29-7)	Comprising at least two of the three germ cell layers, this lesion may contain elements reflecting ectoderm (skin, teeth, hair), mesoderm (bone, cartilage, muscle) and endoderm (bronchial and gastrointestinal epithelium, pancreatic tissue). It typically appears as a multilocular, heterogeneous mass with walls of varying thickness that may enhance. Soft tissue, fluid, fat, and calcium may be seen within the mass.
Neoplasm (cystic degeneration) (Figs C 29-8 and C 29-9)	Many tumors can undergo cystic degeneration and demonstrate mixed solid and cystic elements on CT or MR imaging. They include thymomas, Hodgkin's disease, germ cell tumors, mediastinal carcinoma, metastases to lymph nodes, neurofibromas, and nerve root tumors. Cystic degeneration of a solid mass is more likely to occur after radiation therapy or chemotherapy but may be seen prior to treatment. If the degeneration is extensive, the appearance may be indistinguishable from that of a congenital lesion.
Mediastinal pancreatic pseudocyst (Fig C 29-10)	A rare mass of the posterior mediastinum, CT can demonstrate extension of the lesion through the retrocrural portion of the diaphragm. The internal appearance of the cyst varies depending on the presence of hemorrhage or infection.
Mediastinal abscess	Uncommon lesion that is usually related to surgery (eg, median sternotomy), esophageal perforation, or spread of infection from an adjacent region. Sepsis may develop and the fatality rate is high. On CT, an abscess appears as a low-attenuation mass. In addition to clinical features, the presence of air bubbles within the lesion and contiguity or communication with an empyema or subphrenic abscess should permit differentiation from a true cyst or neoplasm.

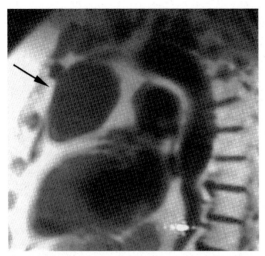

Fig C 29-6
Thymic cyst. Sagittal T1-weighted MR image shows a cyst of low-signal attenuation (arrow) in a thymic location.[61]

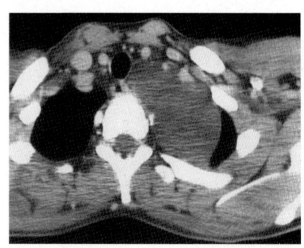

Fig C 29-7
Mature cystic teratoma. Contrast CT scan shows a heterogeneous anterior mediastinal mass with areas of fat (long arrow), calcification (short arrow), fluid attenuation, and thin soft-tissue septa.[61]

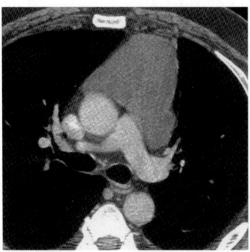

Fig C 29-8
Cystic thymoma. Contrast CT scan shows a thin-walled cystic lesion of water attenuation in a patient with a 2-month history of myasthenia.[61]

Fig C 29-9
Cystic schwannoma. Contrast CT scan shows a thin-walled mass of low attenuation in the paravertebral region.[61]

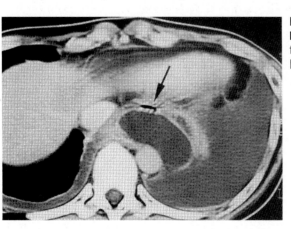

Fig C 29-10
Pancreatic pseudocyst. Contrast CT scan shows bilateral pleural effusions and a thin-walled periaortic cystic lesion that displaces the esophagus (arrow) anteriorly.[61]

Abnormality of the Azygoesophageal Recess on Computed Tomography

Condition	Comments
Normal appearance (Fig C 30-1)	
Lymph node enlargement Subcarinal nodes (Fig C 30-2)	Located in front and medial to the cranial part of the recess, these structures belong to the tracheobronchial lymph node group and drain the posterior mediastinum as well as the right middle lobe and both lower lobes.
Paraesophageal nodes	Located more posteriorly and caudally, these nodes drain the lower part of the esophagus. They may also be involved in bronchogenic carcinoma of the lower lobes as well as in lymphomas and testicular metastases.

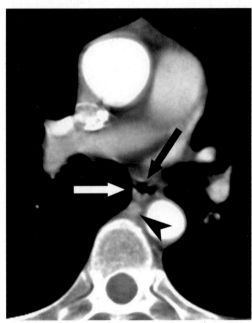

Fig C 30-1
Normal appearance. CT scan shows the azygoesophageal recess (white arrow) formed by the esophagus anteriorly (black arrow) and the azygos vein posteriorly (arrowhead). The azygoesophageal line seen on plain radiographs represents the interface between this recess and the lung.[52]

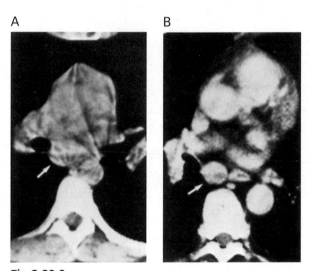

Fig C 30-2
Lymph node enlargement. (A) Enlargement of subcarinal lymph nodes (arrow) in a patient with malignant lymphoma produces reversal of the normal convexity at the level of the bronchus intermedius. The tumor cannot be delineated from mediastinal structures. (B) In a different patient with metastases from bronchogenic carcinoma of the right lower lobe, a scan obtained during the infusion of intravenous contrast material shows a distinct enlarged node (arrow) bulging into the recess at the level of the middle lobe bronchus.[60]

Condition	Comments
Vascular abnormalities	
Dilatation of the descending aorta (Fig C 30-3)	Elongation and unfolding of the aorta may push lung away from the azygoesophageal recess. Distortion of the recess may also be due to a congenital right-sided descending aorta.
Azygos vein dilatation	Collateral flow in the azygos vein system may result from obstruction of the superior vena cava or the inferior vena cava or from congenital absence of the hepatic segment of the inferior vena cava.
Left atrial enlargement	May bulge posteriorly into the azygoesophageal recess.
Esophageal varices	History of cirrhosis and other signs of portal hypertension.
Esophagogastric abnormalities	
Carcinoma of the esophagus (Fig C 30-4)	Increased thickness of the wall and periesophageal infiltration may distort the recess. This appearance may be enhanced by metastatic enlargement of periesophageal lymph nodes.

A

B

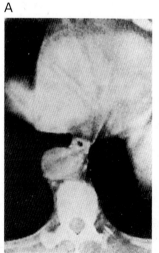
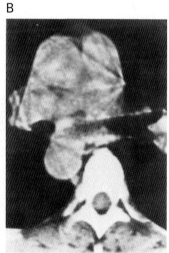

Fig C 30-3
Dilatation of the descending aorta. (A) The aorta pushes lung away from the azygoesophageal recess. (B) At the level of the bronchus intermedius in a patient with a right-sided descending aorta, the azygoesophageal recess is markedly distorted by the descending aorta's bulging toward the right lung.[60]

A

B

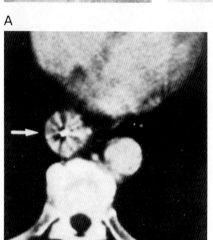
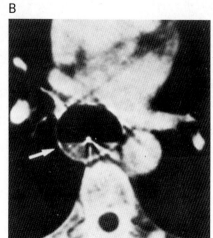

Fig C 30-4
Carcinoma of the esophagus. Feeding tube in lumen. (A) At a level corresponding to the ventricular cavities, there is thickening of the esophageal wall with reversal of the normal curvature of the azygoesophageal recess (arrow). (B) At the level of origin of the middle lobe bronchus, there is even more prominent bulging into the right lung because of prestenotic dilatation of the esophagus (arrow).[59]

Condition	Comments
Esophageal dilatation	Most commonly proximal to a stenotic tumor (may cause more prominent alteration in the azygoesophageal recess than that resulting from the primary tumor). Dilatation of the esophagus in achalasia may cause similar changes.
Hiatal hernia (Fig C 30-5)	Bulging into the right lung impinges on the recess.
Bronchogenic cyst (Fig C 30-6)	Most commonly located below the carina, where it may intrude into the azygoesophageal recess.
Pleural disorders Pleural thickening and effusion	Scans obtained in the right lateral position cause a shift of free pleural fluid that may permit a better demonstration of the mediastinal contour and the extent of pleural thickening.
Tumors (Fig C 30-7)	Primary (mesothelioma) or secondary tumors involving the mediastinal pleura may extend into the azygoesophageal recess.
Pulmonary disorders (Fig C 30-8)	Alteration of the azygoesophageal recess can be caused by atelectasis or consolidation that decreases the degree of aeration of the lung extending into it and thus obliterates the clear distinction between the mediastinum and lung.

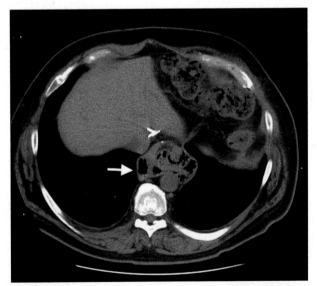

Fig C 30-5
Hiatal hernia. Large gas- and fluid-filled structure (arrow) that causes a rightward bulge of the distal azygoesophageal recess.[63]

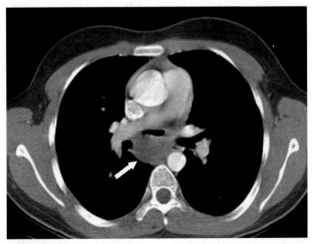

Fig C 30-6
Bronchogenic cyst. Subcarinal mass (arrow) producing an abnormal convexity of the azygoesophageal recess.[52]

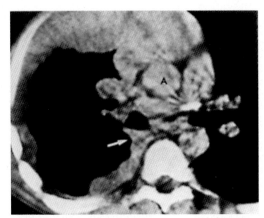

Fig C 30-7
Pleural mesothelioma. At the level of the right main bronchus, irregular pleural-based masses (arrow) that are most prominent anteriorly cause posterior displacement of the ascending aorta (A).[60]

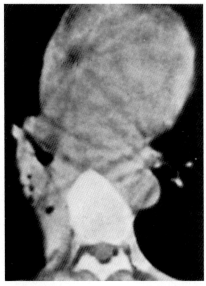

Fig C 30-8
Atelectasis. Collapse of the superior segment of the right lower lobe from bronchogenic carcinoma causes loss of demarcation between mediastinum and lung at the level of the middle lobe bronchus.[60]

Shift of the Mediastinum*

Condition	Comments
Decreased lung volume (shift to the affected side)	
Atelectasis	Increased opacification and elevation of the hemidiaphragm on the affected side.
Postoperative	Lobectomy, pneumonectomy. Elevation of the hemidiaphragm on the affected side and evidence of surgical clips.
Hypoplastic lung (see Fig C 15-3)	Increased opacification and elevation of the hemidiaphragm on the affected side. Small pulmonary artery and diminished pulmonary vascularity. Often an irregular reticular vascular pattern (dilated bronchial artery collaterals).

A   B

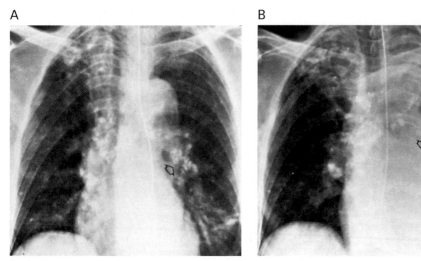

Fig C 31-1
Collapse of the left lung. (A) Initial examination showing old healed granulomatous disease. Note the position of the left infrahilar nodes (arrow). (B) Repeat chest film 2 days later shows opacification of the entire left hemithorax due to a mucus plug and a shift of the mediastinum to the affected side. Note the change in position of the left infrahilar calcifications (arrow).

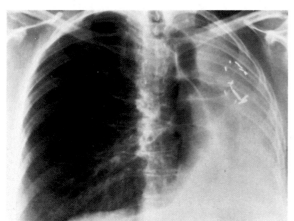

Fig C 31-2
Pneumonectomy. Opacification of the left hemithorax with multiple surgical clips. The trachea and other mediastinal contents are shifted to the affected side.

*See Figures C 31-1 and C 31-2

Condition	Comments
Increased lung volume (shift away from the affected side)	
Foreign body obstructing main-stem bronchus (Fig C 31-3)	Common cause of air trapping in children (ball-valve obstruction permits air to enter the lung but obstructs outflow). Ipsilateral hyperlucent lung with relatively opaque, but normal, contralateral lung.
Swyer–James syndrome (see Fig C 15-5)	Air trapping during expiration. Probably results from acute pneumonia during infancy or childhood that causes bronchiolitis obliterans and an emphysema-like appearance. Small hilar and peripheral vessels.
Congenital lobar emphysema (see Fig C 15-6)	In infants, the hyperlucent, hyperexpanded lobe frequently herniates through the mediastinum to compress normal lung and lead to serious respiratory insufficiency.
Bullous emphysema	Localized form of emphysema with characteristic large avascular lucent areas separated by thin linear densities.
Cystic adenomatoid malformation (see Fig C 15-7)	Complex foregut anomaly in infants consisting of multiple cystic structures (may become overdistended with air and cause mediastinal shift).

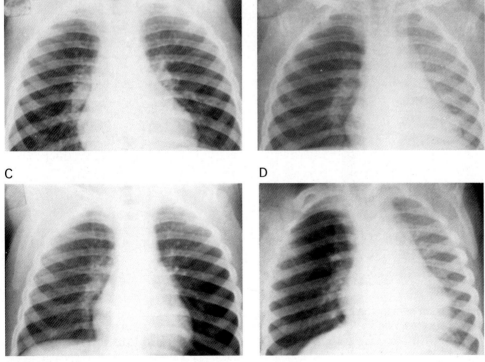

Fig C 31-3
Peanut in the right main-stem bronchus. (A) During inspiration, the lungs of this 2-year-old boy are well aerated. Air trapping in the right lung is seen during expiration (B) and with the right side down (C). The normal left lung is underaerated when that side is down (D).[61]

Condition	Comments
Bronchogenic cyst	In infants, a solitary air-filled mass with a connection to a partially obstructed bronchus causing a ball-valve mechanism (massive overdistention because air can enter but not leave the cyst).
Pulmonary/mediastinal masses	Infrequent cause of mediastinal shift to or away from affected side. Very large masses may shift the mediastinum to the contralateral side. Endobronchial lesions (eg, carcinoma) may cause ipsilateral atelectasis and shift of the mediastinum to the side of the mass.
Pleural space abnormalities (shift away from the affected side)	
Large unilateral pleural effusion (Fig C 31-4)	Mediastinal shift usually occurs only after almost the entire hemithorax is opaque.
Tension pneumothorax (Fig C 31-5)	Medical emergency that is the result of a leak of air from the lung into the pleural space. A shift of the mediastinum and depression of the diaphragm are frequently the first detectable signs. Total collapse of the lung may be a relatively late complication.

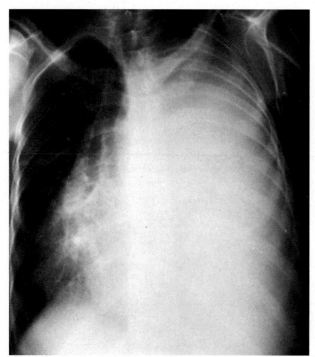

Fig C 31-4
Large unilateral pleural effusion. The left hemithorax is virtually opaque, and there is shift of the mediastinum to the right.

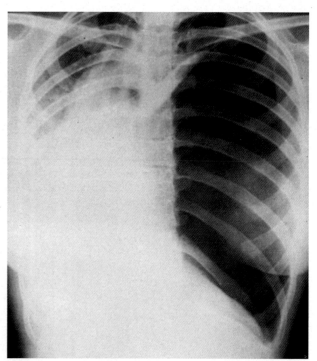

Fig C 31-5
Tension pneumothorax. The left hemithorax is completely radiolucent and lacks vascular markings. There is a dramatic shift of the heart and mediastinum to the right. The left hemidiaphragm is markedly depressed, and there is spreading of the left ribs.

Condition	Comments
Diaphragmatic hernia (Fig C 31-6)	Congenital or posttraumatic hernia that appears bubbly if it contains air-filled loops and opaque if it contains omentum, liver, or fluid-filled bowel.
Pleural masses	Metastatic tumor or malignant mesothelioma (ipsilateral lung may be completely opaque due to a massive pleural effusion).
Partial absence of pericardium	Striking shift of the heart to the left but no shift of other mediastinal structures (trachea, aorta).

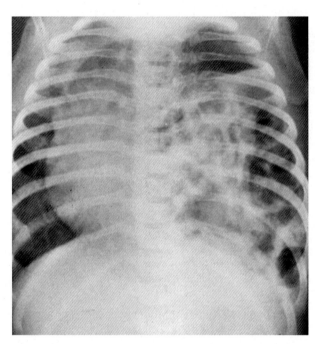

Fig C 31-6
Congenital diaphragmatic hernia. Multiple lucencies in the left chest due to gas-filled loops of bowel. The heart and mediastinal structures are shifted to the right.

Pneumomediastinum

Condition	Comments
Spontaneous pneumomediastinum (Figs C 32-1 and C 32-2)	Caused by rupture of marginally situated alveoli with passage of air through the interstitial tissues of the lung to the hilum and the mediastinum. Many patients have no evidence of underlying lung disease. Often precipitated by a sudden increase in intra-alveolar pressure.
Trauma to chest wall	Closed-chest trauma causes an abrupt increase in intrathoracic pressure. Rupture of alveoli into the perivascular sheaths in the interstitial tissue of the lung results in the passage of air to the hilum and the mediastinum.
Rupture of the esophagus (Fig C 32-3)	Most frequently occurs during episodes of severe vomiting (Boerhaave's syndrome), where the tear involves the lower 8 cm of the esophagus (relatively unsupported by connective tissue). The tear is classically vertical and involves the left posterolateral wall of the esophagus.
Bronchial or tracheal injury (Fig C 32-4)	Caused by trauma (shearing force) or a sudden increase in pressure against a closed glottis.

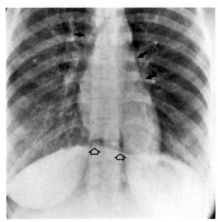

Fig C 32-1
Pneumomediastinum. In addition to bilateral elevation of the mediastinal pleura (closed arrows), there is a characteristic interposition of gas between the heart and the diaphragm that permits visualization of the central portion of the diaphragm in continuity with the lateral portions (open arrows).[62]

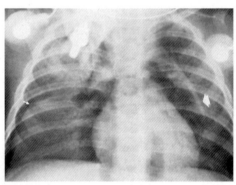

Fig C 32-2
Positive-pressure ventilation. After intubation and ventilation of a child with hydrocarbon poisoning, there is the development of a pneumomediastinum (large arrow) and pneumothorax (small arrow). Note that the stiffness of the lungs has prevented substantial collapse.

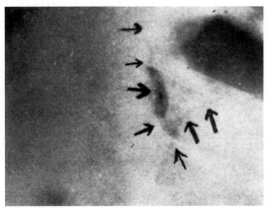

Fig C 32-3
Esophageal rupture. Linear lucent shadows (arrows) represent localized mediastinal emphysema and correspond to the fascial planes of the mediastinal and diaphragmatic pleurae in the region of the lower esophagus.[52]

Condition	Comments
Iatrogenic	Surgical procedures or instrumentation of the esophagus, trachea, bronchi, or neck. Also caused by overinflation during anesthesia and respiratory therapy.
Extension of gas from below the diaphragm	Retroperitoneal rupture of the duodenum or colon. Gas extends along the aorta or esophagus into the mediastinum.
Extension of gas from the neck (Fig C 32-5)	Trauma, surgical procedures, or perforating cervical lesions.
Tear of lung parenchyma	Leakage of air into the interstitial tissues followed by dissection toward the hilum and into the mediastinum. May be associated with birth trauma, anesthesia, resuscitation attempts, and the straining and coughing associated with pulmonary disease.
Hyaline membrane disease (Fig C 32-6)	Frequent complication, probably related to extension of pulmonary interstitial emphysema.
Asthma	Probably related to alveolar rupture secondary to increased pressure. Pneumomediastinum is more common in children, although it can occur in adults.

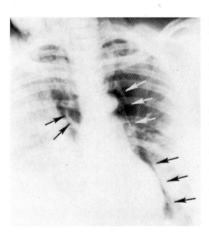

Fig C 32-4
Tracheobronchial injury. Frontal chest film made after blunt trauma to the upper chest that caused transection of both main-stem bronchi demonstrates free air in the mediastinum (upper black arrows) and through the fascial planes of the neck. The lucent zone (lower black arrows) along the left cardiac border simulates the pattern produced by a pneumopericardium or pneumothorax. However, the aortic arch is sharply circumscribed by air that extends around its cephalad and right lateral margins, at a level well above the pericardial reflection (white arrows). This clearly indicates that this air also is in the mediastinum and not confined to the pericardium or pleural space.[4]

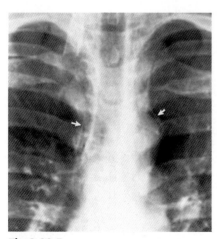

Fig C 32-5
Extension of gas from the neck. Pneumomediastinum (arrows) after cervical trauma (note the overlying surgical drain on the right).

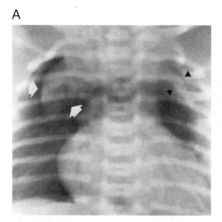

A

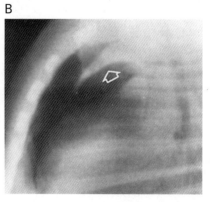

B

Fig C 32-6
Pneumomediastinum in an infant. (A) Elevation of both thymic lobes by mediastinal air (white arrows and black arrowheads) produces the angel's-wings sign. (B) Lateral projection shows the anterior mediastinal air lifting the thymus off the pericardium and great vessels (arrow).

Pleural-Based Lesion

Condition	Imaging Findings	Comments
Mesothelioma (Figs C 33-1 and C 33-2)	Solitary, sharply circumscribed, homogeneous (benign); irregular, scalloped or nodular mass (malignant).	Benign tumors may often be asymptomatic and curable by surgical resection. A diffuse malignant tumor is related to asbestos exposure and is often associated with a large pleural effusion that may obscure the underlying neoplasm.
Metastases (Fig C 33-3)	Single or multiple nodules.	Most common primaries are carcinomas of the bronchus, breast, ovary, and gastrointestinal tract. Actual metastatic deposits are often too small to be seen radiographically (CT is more sensitive). A large pleural effusion may be the only indication of pleural metastases.
Pleural fluid (loculated or interlobar) (Figs C 33-4 and C 33-5)	Smooth, sharply demarcated, homogeneous opacity.	Loculated fluid collections are caused by adhesions between contiguous pleural surfaces (tend to occur with or after pyothorax or hemothorax). An interlobar fluid collection generally results from cardiac decompensation and may simulate a neoplasm, although it tends to absorb spontaneously when the heart failure is relieved (vanishing or phantom tumor).
Pulmonary infarct	Homogeneous, wedge-shaped peripheral consolidation with its base contiguous to a visceral pleural surface.	Classic but uncommon manifestation of an infarct. An infarct has a rounded apex, convex toward the hilum (Hampton hump), whereas pleural thickening and free pleural fluid are generally concave toward the hilum.
Rib or chest wall lesion (see Fig C 34-4)	Extrapleural mass, often with destruction, fracture, or expansion of the underlying rib or sternum.	Primary or metastatic neoplasm, osteomyelitis, fracture with hematoma or callus.

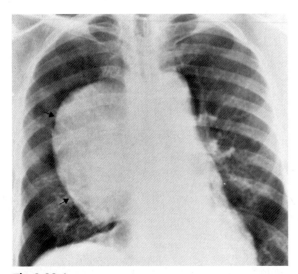

Fig C 33-1
Benign localized fibrous mesothelioma. Huge, homogeneous soft-tissue mass (arrows) arising from the mediastinal pleura and projecting into the right hemithorax. The patient had only mild underlying interstitial fibrosis and no pleural plaquing.

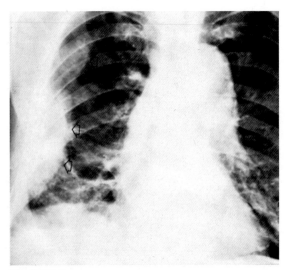

Fig C 33-2
Diffuse pleural mesothelioma. Multiple masses thicken the right pleura (arrows) in an elderly man with chronic asbestos exposure.[63]

Condition	Imaging Findings	Comments
Fibrin ball	Round, oval, or irregular mass that is most commonly located near the base of the lung.	Tumor-like collection that may develop in a serofibrinous pleural effusion and usually becomes evident after absorption of the effusion. May disappear spontaneously and rapidly or remain unchanged and mimic a solitary pulmonary nodule when viewed en face.
Pancoast tumor (superior sulcus tumor) (Fig C 33-6)	Apical mass, often with destruction of adjacent ribs.	Site of 6% of bronchogenic carcinomas. May be associated with Horner's syndrome. In the absence of bone destruction, the tumor may be identified only by asymmetry of presumed apical pleural thickening.

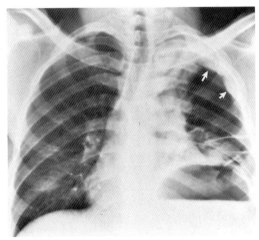

Fig C 33-3
Pleural metastases (arrows) from bronchogenic carcinoma. There is also elevation of the left hemidiaphragm because of phrenic nerve involvement and postobstructive atelectatic change secondary to the left perihilar lesion.

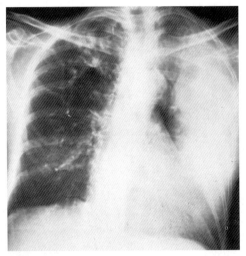

Fig C 33-4
Empyema. Large soft-tissue mass fills much of the left hemithorax.

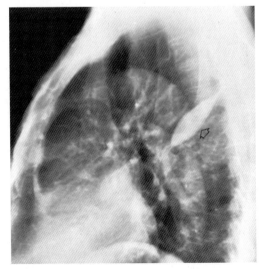

Fig C 33-5
Interlobar pleural fluid. Elliptical fluid collection (arrow) in the major fissure in a patient with cardiac decompensation.

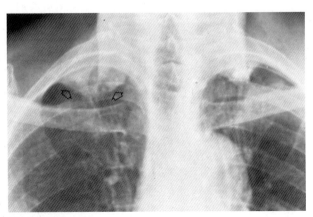

Fig C 33-6
Pancoast tumor. Increased opacification in the right apex (arrows). Although this appearance may simulate benign apical pleural thickening, the marked asymmetry and irregularity of the right apical mass should suggest the diagnosis of bronchogenic carcinoma.

Condition	Imaging Findings	Comments
Lipoma	Smooth, sharply circumscribed mass.	Rare lesion that may change shape during respiration (due to its relatively fluid contents). A large tumor occasionally erodes contiguous ribs.
Fungal infection (Fig C 33-7)	Peripheral mass, often with cavitation. May have associated rib destruction.	Actinomycosis, nocardiosis, blastomycosis, and torulosis.
Pulmonary granuloma	Smooth, sharply circumscribed mass that may contain central calcification.	Primarily histoplasmoma. Also other fungi and tuberculosis.
Rheumatoid nodule	Single or multiple nodules.	May have diffuse underlying interstitial fibrosis.
Lymphoma (Fig C 33-8)	Solitary nodule or diffuse tumor infiltration.	Although primary pleural lymphoma as the only site of malignancy is rare, lymphomatous involvement of the pleura may occur in association with mediastinal lymphadenopathy or pulmonary parenchymal lymphoma. The lymphomatous pleural deposits arise from lymphatic channels and lymphoid aggregates in the subpleural connective tissue below the visceral pleura. Associated pleural effusion is attributed to obstruction of lymphatic channels by mediastinal lymphadenopathy.

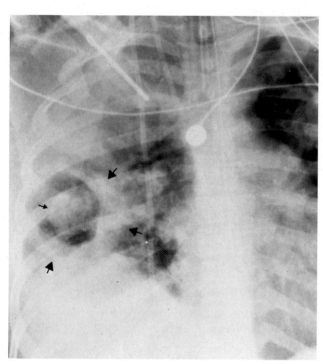

Fig C 33-7
Aspergillosis. Large peripheral thick-walled cavity (large arrows) that abuts the pleura and contains an intracavitary fungus ball (small arrow).

A   B

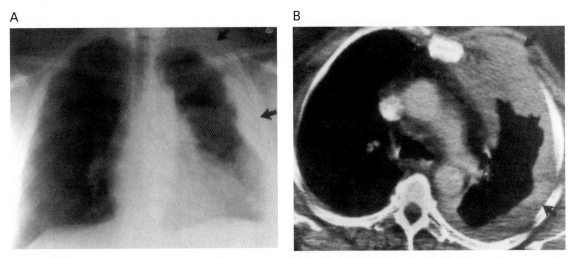

Fig C 33-8
Lymphoma. (A) Frontal chest radiographic shows irregular pleural thickening (arrows). (B) Concurrent CT scan demonstrates diffuse pleural thickening (arrows), greater than 1 cm in thickness, involving the left mediastinal and costal pleura.[64]

Extrapleural Lesion

Condition	Comments
Chest wall hematoma (Figs C 34-1 to C 34-3)	Usually a history of trauma and often evidence of a rib fracture. May also occur with sternal fractures (hematoma best seen on lateral view). Callus formation about an old rib fracture may be mistaken for a pulmonary nodule.

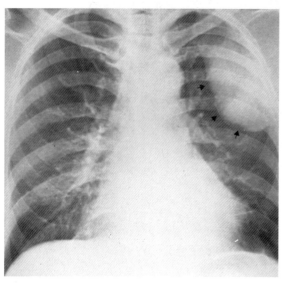

Fig C 34-1
Pulmonary hematoma. Large extrapleural density (arrows) over the left upper lobe.

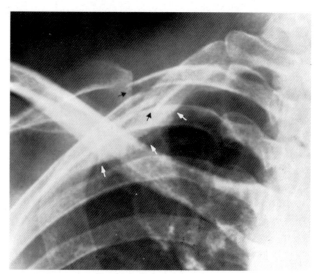

Fig C 34-2
Chest trauma. Small extrapleural hematoma (white arrows) associated with fractures of the first and second ribs (black arrows).

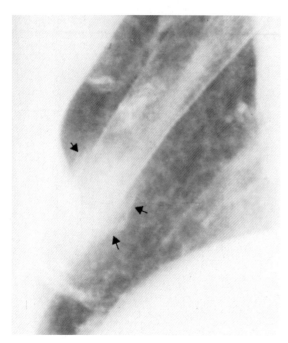

Fig C 34-3
Cough fracture. simulating a pulmonary nodule. A coned view of the right lower lung on a routine chest radiograph shows callus formation about a rib (arrows) in an asymptomatic person.

Condition	Comments
Rib neoplasm (Fig C 34-4)	Metastases and myeloma are the most common causes of an extrapleural mass associated with rib destruction in adults. Ewing's tumor and metastatic neuroblastoma are the most common causes in children.
Mediastinal, spinal, sternal, or subphrenic lesion (see Fig C 14-6)	Tumors, cysts, and inflammatory processes may produce extrapleural masses.
Chest wall infection	An extrapleural mass with rib destruction is most commonly a manifestation of actinomycosis (often with parenchymal infiltrate, pleural effusion, and even a cutaneous fistula). A similar pattern may also be due to nocardiosis, blastomycosis, aspergillosis, or, rarely, tuberculosis.
Extrapleural lipoma	Common chest wall lesion that may grow between ribs to present as both an intrathoracic and a subcutaneous mass. Characteristic fat density on CT.
Surgery or blunt trauma	Ruptured aneurysm, partial pleurectomy, sympathectomy, plombage, and mineral oil injection for the treatment of tuberculosis.
Congenital lobar agenesis	Missing lobe is often replaced by a chunk of extrapleural aureolar tissue that produces an anterior extrapleural mass paralleling the sternum. There is loss of the right heart border on frontal views.

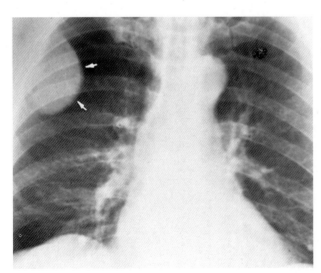

Fig C 34-4
Extramedullary myeloma. Large extrapleural mass (arrows) containing a proliferation of plasma cells.

Pleural Calcification

Condition	Imaging Findings	Comments
Organized hemothorax (Fig C 35-1)	Usually unilateral calcification of the visceral pleura (Fig C 35-1) in the form of a broad continuous sheet or multiple discrete plaques.	Typically extends from about the level of the mid-thorax posteriorly, coursing around the lateral lung margins in a generally inferior direction and roughly paralleling the major fissure. There is often evidence of healed rib fractures and a history of significant chest trauma.
Organized empyema (Fig C 35-2)	Usually unilateral calcification of the visceral pleura in the form of a broad continuous sheet or multiple discrete plaques.	Typically extends from about the level of the mid-thorax posteriorly, coursing around the lateral lung margins in a generally inferior direction and roughly paralleling the major fissure. Usually a history of severe pulmonary infection.
Old tuberculous empyema (Fig C 35-3)	Usually unilateral calcification of the visceral pleura in the form of a broad continuous sheet or multiple discrete plaques. May be bilateral (usually asymmetric).	Typically extends from about the level of the mid-thorax posteriorly, coursing around the lateral lung margins in a generally inferior direction and roughly paralleling the major fissure. Extensive apical parenchymal scarring or cavitary disease is virtually diagnostic.

A
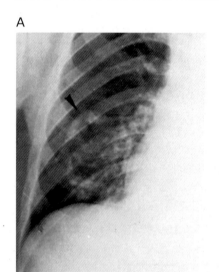

B
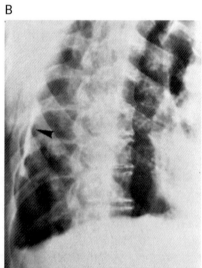

Fig C 35-1
Calcified thickened pleura. (A) The density in the lower lung (arrowhead) has a well-defined irregular border closely resembling a cavity. (B) An oblique view, however, shows a pathognomonic linear density (arrowhead) paralleling but separated from the chest wall.[65]

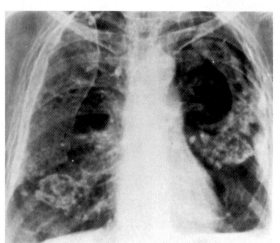

Fig C 35-2
Organized empyema. Bilateral broad continuous sheets of calcification overlie much of the lung surface.

Condition	Imaging Findings	Comments
Pneumoconiosis (Figs C 35-4 to C 35-6)	Usually bilateral plaques of calcification involving the parietal pleura, commonly along the diaphragm. There may sometimes be calcification in extensively thickened pleura along the lateral chest wall.	Most commonly caused by asbestosis. May also be due to other silicates (eg, talcosis). The diaphragmatic pleura are almost always extensively involved (unlike hemothorax or empyema). Extensive encasement of both lungs may occur. Basilar reticulonodular interstitial disease is highly suggestive, though often absent.

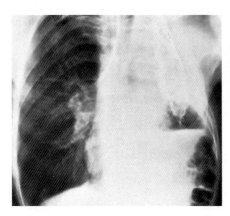

Fig C 35-3
Old tuberculous empyema. Broad sheet of calcification overlies much of the left hemithorax. Note the elevation of the left hemidiaphragm and retraction of the trachea to the left, all consistent with loss of volume due to the chronic granulomatous disease.

B

A

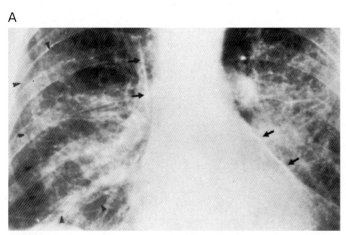

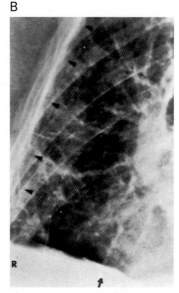

Fig C 35-4
Asbestosis. (A) Frontal view shows en face calcifications on the right (arrowheads) and linear calcifications in profile in the mediastinal reflection of the pleura on the right and in the pericardium on the left (transverse arrows). (B) A left oblique film shows linear pleural calcification in profile in the area of the central tendon of the right hemidiaphragm (arrows). The en face plaques in (A) now appear in profile as extensive linear calcifications (arrowheads) adjacent to anterior ribs.[66]

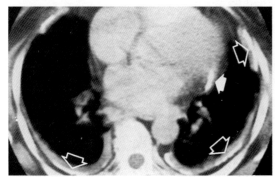

Fig C 35-5
Asbestosis. CT scan shows calcified pleural plaques along the lateral and posterior chest wall (open arrows) and adjacent to the heart (closed arrow).

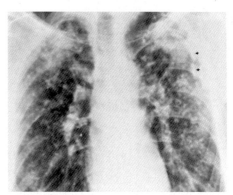

Fig C 35-6
Coal-workers' pneumoconiosis. Bilateral fibrous masses in the apices with upward retraction of the hila. Note the pleural calcification (arrows) in the left apex.

Pleural Effusion with Otherwise Normal-Appearing Chest

Condition	Imaging Findings	Comments
Tuberculosis (Fig C 36-1)	Serous exudate with low glucose content and predominantly lymphocytic reaction. Almost always unilateral.	Common manifestation of primary tuberculosis in adults (approximately 40%) but less frequent in children (10%). The patient may have a negative tuberculin test in early stages. Active pulmonary tuberculosis often develops if the effusion is not treated.
Other infections (Fig C 36-2)	Serous exudate that may be bilateral.	Bacteria, fungi (especially actinomycosis and nocardiosis), viruses, mycoplasma.
Thoracic lymphoma	Serosanguineous exudate that may be unilateral or bilateral.	Usually evidence of pulmonary or mediastinal lymph node involvement. Suggestive findings include hepatosplenomegaly and peripheral lymph node enlargement.
Metastatic carcinoma	Serous exudate with variable blood content and typically elevated glucose. Unilateral or bilateral.	Most common primary sites are breast, pancreas, stomach, ovary, and kidney. At times, a pleural effusion may be the only presenting finding.
Ovarian neoplasm (Meigs' syndrome)	Serous exudate that is more frequent on the right (may be left-sided or bilateral).	Most commonly an ovarian fibroma associated with ascites. Can also develop with other benign or malignant ovarian tumors. The effusion usually disappears after removal of the ovarian neoplasm.
Carcinoma of pancreas/ retroperitoneum	Serous exudate (pleural fluid negative for malignant cells).	Often no direct tumor involvement of the thorax. The effusion disappears after removal or treatment of the primary lesion.

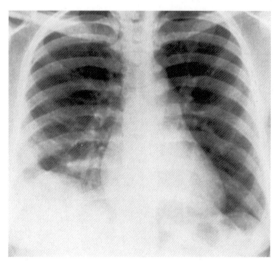

Fig C 36-1
Primary tuberculosis. Unilateral right tuberculous pleural effusion without parenchymal or lymph node involvement.

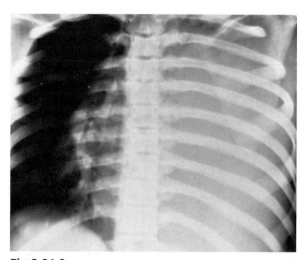

Fig C 36-2
Coccidioidomycosis. Complete homogeneous opacification of the left hemithorax. The massive pleural effusion must be associated with virtually complete collapse of the left lung as there is no contralateral shift of the mediastinal structures.

Condition	Imaging Findings	Comments
Pulmonary thromboembolic disease	Serosanguineous effusion that is most often unilateral.	Effusion is infrequently the sole manifestation of pulmonary embolism (may obscure small parenchymal abnormalities). The presence of fluid almost always indicates infarction.
Subphrenic abscess	Ipsilateral serous exudate.	More commonly associated with elevation and fixation of the hemidiaphragm and basal atelectasis (see Fig C 34-2). There may be gas or a mottled pattern of density in the subphrenic space.
Pancreatitis (Fig C 36-3)	Serous or serosanguineous exudate with a high amylase level. Predominantly left-sided (may be bilateral).	May occur in acute, chronic, or relapsing pancreatitis or with a pancreatic pseudocyst. Other manifestations include elevation of the hemidiaphragm and basal atelectasis.
Trauma	Varied composition (blood, chyle, or food after esophageal rupture).	Hemothorax complicating traumatic aortic rupture and effusion after esophageal perforation are almost always left-sided. The side of a chylothorax depends on the site of the thoracic duct rupture (see Fig C 38-1).
Abdominal surgery	Serous exudate.	Usually very small but may be detected in almost half the patients if lateral decubitus views are obtained.
Postmyocardial infarction syndrome (Dressler's syndrome)	Left-sided or bilateral transudate is the most common finding (80%) and may occur alone.	Characterized by fever and pleuropericardial chest pain that begins 1 to 6 weeks after acute myocardial infarction. Pericardial effusion or pulmonary infiltrates frequently occur (see Fig CA 22-2). Striking response to steroid therapy.

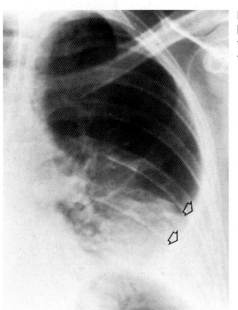

Fig C 36-3
Pancreatitis. Blunting of the normally sharp angle between the diaphragm and the rib cage (arrows) along with a characteristic upward concave border (meniscus) of the fluid level.

Condition	Imaging Findings	Comments
Cirrhosis with ascites	Transudate that is more often right-sided (may be on the left or bilateral).	Ascitic fluid probably enters the pleural space via diaphragmatic lymphatics (as in Meigs' syndrome). Usually evidence of ascites and other signs of cirrhosis.
Systemic lupus erythematosus (Fig C 36-4)	Serous exudate that is bilateral in approximately 50% of patients. The effusion is predominantly left-sided when unilateral. Tends to be small (occasionally massive).	Pleural effusion is an isolated abnormality in approximately 10% of cases. It is often associated with a pericardial effusion and usually clears without residua. Nonspecific cardiomegaly and pulmonary involvement develop in most patients.
Rheumatoid disease	Serous exudate with a predominance of lymphocytes and a low glucose level. Usually unilateral.	Occurs almost exclusively in men. May antedate the signs and symptoms of rheumatoid arthritis, but usually follows them. There is often no pulmonary evidence of rheumatoid disease.
Asbestosis	Serous or blood-tinged exudate that is usually bilateral and often recurrent.	More commonly occurs in association with pleural plaques and calcification.
Renal disease (Fig C 36-5)	Transudate or serous exudate.	Causes include nephrotic syndrome, acute glomerulonephritis, hydronephrosis, and uremic pleuritis.
Peritoneal dialysis	Serous exudate.	Probably the same underlying mechanism as with ascites. May be impossible to distinguish from a uremic effusion.

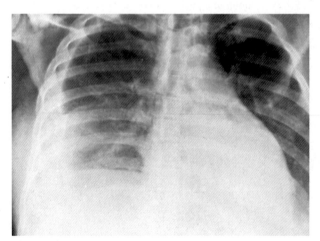

Fig C 36-4
Systemic lupus erythematosus. Large right pleural effusion in a young woman.

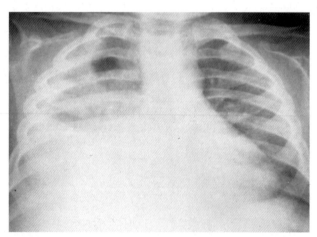

Fig C 36-5
Nephrotic syndrome. Diffuse cardiomegaly with a large right pleural effusion, which is situated both along the lateral chest wall and in a subpulmonic location.

Condition	Imaging Findings	Comments
Malposition of percutaneous central venous catheter (Fig C 36-6)	Unilateral collection of the fluid being instilled.	Results from perforation of the vessel either at the time of insertion of the catheter or later (gradual erosion of a relatively thin-walled intrathoracic vessel by the catheter tip).
Myxedema	Serous exudate.	More commonly causes a pericardial effusion.
Lymphedema	High protein content.	Results from hypoplasia of the lymphatic system.
Familial recurrent polyserositis (familial Mediterranean fever)	Serofibrinous exudate.	Familial disorder (Armenians, Arabs, non-Ashkenazic Jews) characterized by episodic acute attacks of abdominal and chest pain. Usually associated with arthritis and arthralgia.

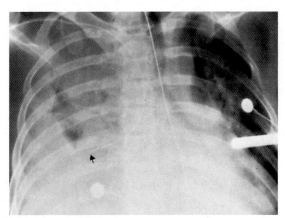

Fig C 36-6
Malposition of percutaneous central venous catheter. A right subclavian catheter, which was introduced for total parenteral nutrition, perforated the superior vena cava and eroded into the right pleural space. Note the tip of the catheter projecting beyond the right border of the mediastinum (arrow). The direct infusion of parenteral fluid into the pleural space has led to the development of a large right hydrothorax.

Pleural Effusion Associated with Other Radiographic Evidence of Chest Disease

Condition	Imaging Findings	Comments
Infectious agents (Fig C 37-1)	Various patterns of effusion and associated parenchymal disease.	Bacteria (especially staphylococcus, *Klebsiella*, tularemia), fungi (especially actinomycosis and nocardiosis), viruses, mycoplasma, and parasites (primarily amebiasis with liver abscess and ruptured hydatid cyst).
Subphrenic abscess (Fig C 37-2)	Ipsilateral effusion.	Usually elevation and fixation of the hemidiaphragm with basal atelectasis. There may be gas or a mottled pattern of density in the subphrenic space.
Bronchogenic carcinoma	Ipsilateral effusion in 10% to 15% of patients.	Commonly associated with obstructive pneumonia. There may be a peripheral mass (often contiguous to the visceral pleura) or hilar or mediastinal lymph node enlargement.
Lymphoma	Effusion in 15% to 30% of patients.	Typically enlargement of hilar and mediastinal nodes with single or multiple areas of consolidation. A similar pattern occurs in leukemia.
Metastases	Unilateral or bilateral effusion.	Multiple parenchymal nodules in hematogenous metastases; linear shadows in lymphangitic spread (there may also be lymph node enlargement).

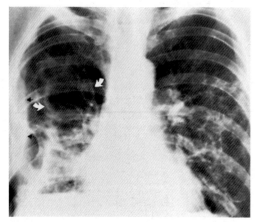

Fig C 37-1
Actinomycosis. Untreated infection led to the development of a large cavity (white arrows) with extension into the pleura to produce an empyema (black arrows). The right fifth posterior rib was partially resected during surgery, which revealed thickening of the pleura circumferentially around the right lower lobe.

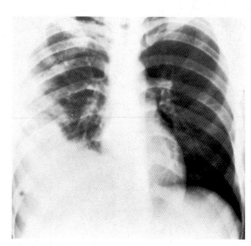

Fig C 37-2
Subphrenic abscess. Right pleural effusion and basilar atelectasis. Note the small bubbles of gas in the abscess.

Condition	Imaging Findings	Comments
Mesothelioma (Fig C 37-3)	Unilateral effusion that is often massive.	Characteristic finding in the diffuse malignant type. There is usually a diffuse peripheral mass contiguous with the pleura and a history of exposure to asbestos. Pleural effusion is rare in the localized benign form of mesothelioma.
Bronchiolar (alveolar cell) carcinoma	Effusion in approximately 10% of patients.	Various patterns of parenchymal disease (small nodule, massive consolidation, multiple disseminated nodules). It may be difficult to differentiate from metastatic neoplasm or disseminated lymphoma.
Multiple myeloma	Effusion is uncommon.	Single or multiple soft-tissue masses protruding into the thorax and arising from the ribs (with rib destruction) is almost pathognomonic. Rare primary chest wall tumors can present a similar pattern.
Pulmonary embolism and infarction (Fig C 37-4)	Effusion is usually small and unilateral.	Pulmonary changes vary from linear shadows to segmental consolidation. There is often elevation of the hemidiaphragm with basal atelectasis.

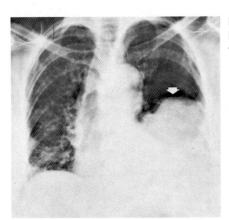

Fig C 37-3
Diffuse pleural mesothelioma. After thoracentesis, the top of a large mass is evident (arrow).[63]

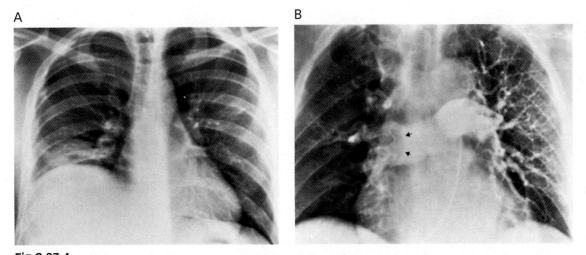

Fig C 37-4
Pulmonary embolism. (A) Plain chest radiograph demonstrates right basilar atelectasis associated with elevation of the right hemidiaphragm, representing a large subpulmonic pleural effusion. (B) Pulmonary arteriogram shows virtually complete obstruction of the right pulmonary artery (arrows).

Condition	Imaging Findings	Comments
Trauma (Fig C 37-5)	Blood (hemothorax), chyle (chylothorax), ingested food (esophageal rupture).	Traumatic aortic rupture and esophageal perforation are almost always left-sided. There may be evidence of fractured ribs, pulmonary or mediastinal hemorrhage, aortic aneurysm, pneumothorax, or pneumomediastinum.
Congestive heart failure (Fig C 37-6)	Effusion is frequently unilateral on the right but rarely on the left. May be bilateral.	Usually generalized cardiomegaly and clinical signs of cardiac decompensation. There may be an associated phantom tumor (fluid localized in an interlobar pleural fissure).
Constrictive pericarditis (Fig C 37-7)	Effusion is frequently unilateral on the right but rarely on the left. May be bilateral.	Effusion develops in approximately 50% of cases. Characteristic pericardial calcification.
Asbestosis	Effusion occurs in 10% to 20% of cases, is usually bilateral, and is often recurrent.	Usually pleural thickening or plaques that are often calcified. High incidence of associated bronchogenic carcinoma and mesothelioma.

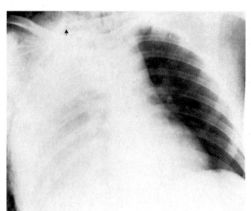

Fig C 37-5
Blunt trauma. There is almost complete homogeneous opacification of the right chest, reflecting a combination of a large hemothorax and underlying pulmonary contusion. The right first rib is fractured (arrow) and subcutaneous emphysema is present in the soft tissues of the right hemithorax.

A   B

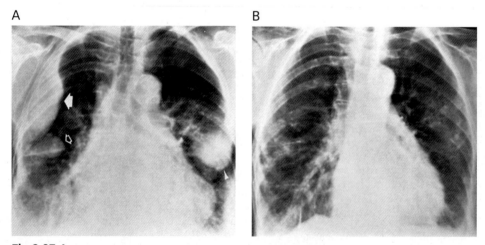

Fig C 37-6
Phantom tumors. (A) Frontal chest radiograph taken during an episode of congestive heart failure demonstrates marked cardiomegaly with bilateral pleural effusions. Note the fluid collections along the lateral chest wall (closed arrow), in the minor fissure (open arrow), and in the left major fissure (arrowhead). (B) With improvement in the patient's cardiac status, the phantom tumors have disappeared. Bilateral small pleural effusions persist.

Condition	Imaging Findings	Comments
Sarcoidosis (Fig C 37-8)	Effusion in 1% to 4% of patients.	Invariably associated with pulmonary disease. The effusion tends to clear within 2 months but may progress to chronic pleural thickening.
Systemic lupus erythematosus (Fig C 37-9)	Effusion in 35% to 75% of cases. Bilateral in half the cases, and predominantly left-sided when unilateral.	Often associated with cardiac enlargement (commonly because of pericardial effusion) and non-specific pulmonary changes (basal atelectasis or infiltrate).
Rheumatoid disease	Effusion is probably the most frequent manifestation in the thorax.	May be isolated or associated with a diffuse reticulonodular pattern that predominantly involves the bases.
Wegener's granulomatosis	Effusion is relatively common but is overshadowed by the pulmonary manifestations.	Single or multiple pulmonary nodules, often with cavitation (see Fig C 9-14) and frequently associated with renal disease.
Waldenström's macroglobulinemia	Effusion in approximately 50% of patients with lung involvement.	Diffuse reticulonodular pattern. Often hepatosplenomegaly and palpable peripheral adenopathy.
Drug-induced	Unilateral or bilateral effusions may occur.	Usually associated with a diffuse interstitial pattern. Causes include nitrofurantoin, hydralazine, and procainamide.

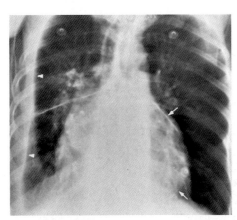

Fig C 37-7
Constrictive pericarditis. Lateral decubitus view of the chest demonstrates moderate enlargement of the cardiac silhouette and a large right pleural effusion (arrowheads). Note the calcified plaque (arrows) in the pericardium.

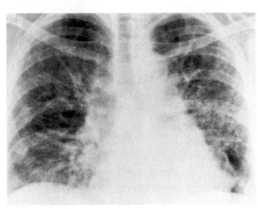

Fig C 37-8
Sarcoidosis. Small left pleural effusion in a patient with diffuse interstitial lung disease.

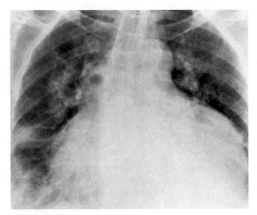

Fig C 37-9
Systemic lupus erythematosus. Bilateral pleural effusions, more marked on the right, with some streaks of basilar atelectasis. The massive cardiomegaly results from a combination of pericarditis and pericardial effusion.

Chylothorax

Condition	Comments
Iatrogenic (surgical injury to thoracic duct)	Most frequent cause of chylothorax. The thoracic duct crosses to the left of the spine between T5 and T7 and thus is particularly vulnerable to injury during surgery on the left hemithorax in the hilar region. A common complication particularly in children undergoing surgery for congenital heart disease.
Trauma to thoracic duct (Fig C 38-1)	Penetrating or nonpenetrating injuries (especially after a heavy meal when the duct is distended). There may be a fractured rib or vertebra, and several days may pass before the pleural fluid is detectable radiographically. An injury to the lower third of the thoracic duct produces a right-sided chylothorax. Rupture of the upper third causes left-sided fluid. Nonpenetrating trauma may be bilateral.
Tumor obstruction of thoracic duct (Fig C 38-2)	Most commonly caused by lymphoma or bronchogenic carcinoma. A right-sided chylothorax develops when the lower portion of the duct is invaded; left-sided involvement occurs when the upper half is affected. May also be bilateral.
Spontaneous chylothorax	One-third of the cases have no precipitating cause.

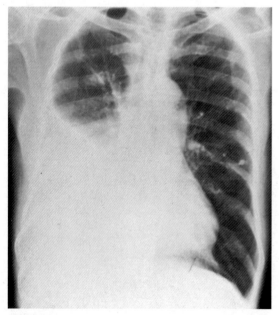

Fig C 38-1
Trauma to thoracic duct. A large volume of fluid in the right hemithorax obscures fractures of several lower right ribs.

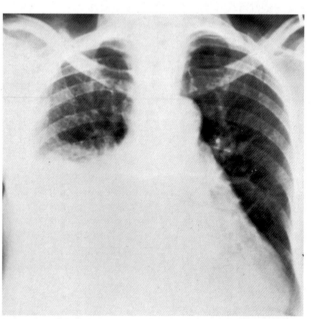

Fig C 38-2
Tumor obstruction of thoracic duct. Involvement of the lower portion of the thoracic duct by bronchogenic carcinoma. The large amount of chylous fluid obscures the underlying primary tumor.

Condition	Comments
Pulmonary lymphangiomatosis	Proliferation of smooth muscle obliterates the thoracic duct, resulting in chylothorax and chylous ascites.
Intrinsic thoracic duct abnormality	Atresia, tumor, or aneurysm with rupture of the thoracic duct.
Tuberculosis	Enlarged lymph nodes or paravertebral abscess may compress or erode the thoracic duct.
Filariasis	Nematode infection causing a peripheral lymphangitis that may ascend to involve the thoracic duct and cause perforation.

Pneumothorax

Condition	Comments
Spontaneous pneumothorax (Fig C 39-1)	Occurs most commonly in men in the third and fourth decades of life. Usually due to rupture of a pleural bleb (small cystic space generally situated over the lung apex).
Iatrogenic (Figs C 39-2 and C 39-3)	Complication of central line insertion, thoracentesis, tracheostomy, resuscitation or artificial ventilation, or a result of thoracotomy.

A

B

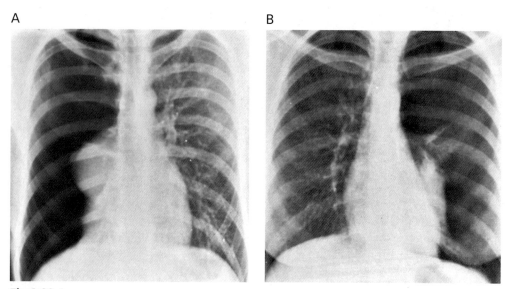

Fig C 39-1
Spontaneous pneumothorax. (A and B) Complete collapse of the lung in two different patients.

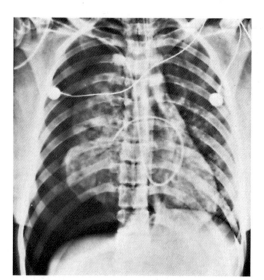

Fig C 39-2
Complication of pulmonary artery catheter insertion. A large right pneumothorax developed after puncture of the right pleura.[67]

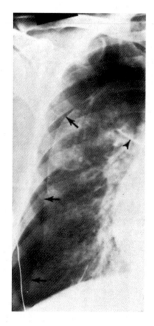

Fig C 39-3
Pneumothorax complicating nasoenteric tube placement. Large right-sided pneumothorax (black arrows) on a radiograph obtained immediately after removal of a feeding tube (arrowhead) from the pleural space.[68]

Condition	Comments
Trauma (Fig C 39-4)	May reflect laceration of the visceral pleura by fragments of a fractured rib.
Mediastinal emphysema	Pneumomediastinum and increased mediastinal pressure lead to the development of a unilateral or bilateral pneumothorax.
Hyaline membrane disease	Pneumothorax associated with air-space consolidation and interstitial emphysema is probably related to prolonged assisted ventilation. There may be an associated pneumomediastinum.
Interstitial lung disease (Fig C 39-5)	Pneumothorax associated with a diffuse reticulonodular pattern may occur in any cause of honeycomb lung (especially Langerhans cell histiocytosis), cystic fibrosis, hemosiderosis, and sarcoidosis.

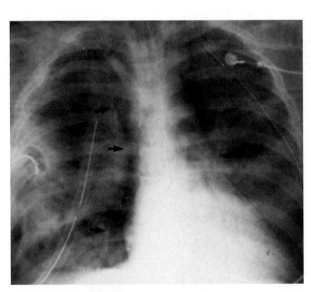

Fig C 39-4
Posttraumatic pneumothorax. Anteromedial pneumothorax (arrows) along with extensive air-space parenchymal disease.[69]

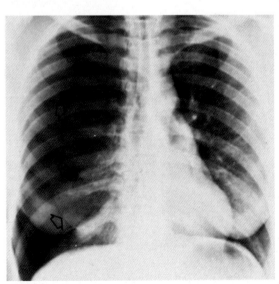

Fig C 39-5
Asthma. Severe coughing and straining during an acute attack led to the development of a large pneumothorax with substantial collapse of the right lung (arrows).

Condition	Comments
Infectious disease (Figs C 39-6 and C 39-7)	Pneumothorax associated with air-space consolidation may occur in acute bacterial pneumonia or in a bronchopleural fistula from tuberculosis, fungus, or other granulomatous disease. May also be caused by a ruptured pneumatocele in staphylococcal pneumonia in children.
Catamenial pneumothorax	Pneumothorax occurring coincidentally with menses in a woman with endometriosis.
Pneumoperitoneum	Passage of air upward through the diaphragm.
Pulmonary metastases	Pneumothorax associated with parenchymal nodules. Most commonly occurs in osteogenic and other types of sarcomas. A similar pattern may occur with Wilms' tumor and carcinomas of the pancreas and adrenals.

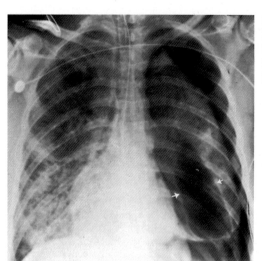

Fig C 39-6
Infectious disease. Moderate left pneumothorax in a patient with severe Pneumocystis pneumonia. Note the air in the pulmonary ligament (arrows) and the air bronchograms in the collapsed lung.

A   B

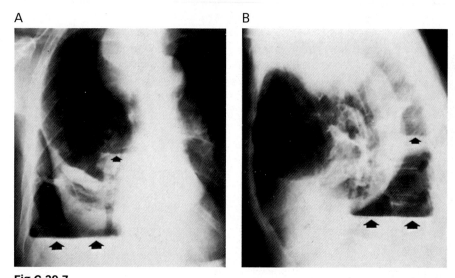

Fig C 39-7
Bronchopleural fistula. (A) Frontal and (B) lateral views of the chest demonstrate multiple air-fluid levels (arrows) in the right hemithorax. The large right superior mediastinal mass represented metastatic spread from a previously resected carcinoma of the right lung.

Condition	Comments
Pulmonary infarct	Pneumothorax is a rare complication that is probably caused by intermittent positive-pressure breathing or superimposed infection.
Adult respiratory distress syndrome (Fig C 39-8)	Pneumothorax associated with diffuse air-space consolidation in a patient treated with prolonged artificial ventilation.
Bauxite pneumoconiosis (Shaver's disease)	Spontaneous pneumothorax is a frequent complication of this occupational disorder in workers who process bauxite in the manufacture of corundum. A diffuse interstitial pulmonary fibrosis also may develop in workers who inhale fine aluminum powder.
Bronchopleural fistula (see Fig C 45-7)	Causes include lung abscess, empyema, malignant neoplasm (primary lung or esophagus or metastasis), radiation pneumonitis, and various types of suppurative or necrotizing pneumonia.

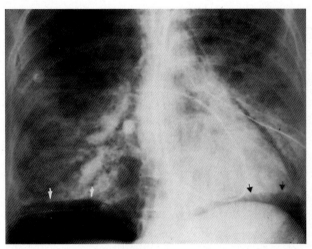

Fig C 39-8
Adult respiratory distress syndrome. Bilateral subpulmonary pneumothoraxes (arrows) in this patient with severe sepsis.[69]

Tracheal Mass/Narrowing

Condition	Imaging Findings	Comments
Adenoma (Fig C 40-1)	Round, sessile, smooth, sharply demarcated mass.	Cylindroma accounts for 40% of tracheal tumors. It tends to occur in the middle third, grows slowly, and metastasizes late (especially to bone and lung). Less frequent tumors are mucoepidermoid adenoma and carcinoid.
Tracheal carcinoma (Fig C 40-2)	Irregular, lobulated, or annular lesion.	Uncommon neoplasm that is most frequently of squamous cell origin (also adenocarcinoma and oat cell). Tends to invade mediastinal soft tissues and spread to lymph nodes and the esophagus. Hematogenous metastases to lung, bone, liver, and brain.
Extramedullary myeloma (Fig C 40-3)	Smooth intrinsic mass.	Abnormal plasma cell proliferation occasionally occurs outside the bone marrow. The vast majority occur in the head and neck—primarily in the nasal cavity, paranasal sinuses, and upper airway. Most patients with an extramedullary myeloma respond favorably to treatment and, even with local recurrences, may survive for many years.

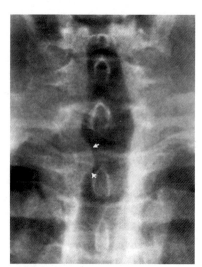

Fig C 40-1
Adenoma (arrows).

A

B

Fig C 40-2
Carcinoma of the trachea. (A) Lateral view of the chest shows an ill-defined soft-tissue density (arrows) in the tracheal air column. (B) A tomogram more clearly shows the mass (arrows).

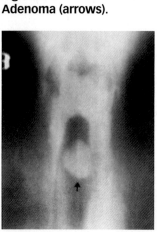

Fig C 40-3
Extramedullary myeloma. Proliferation of plasma cells forms a mass (arrow) in the trachea.[70]

Condition	Imaging Findings	Comments
Tracheal invasion from extrinsic tumor	Extrinsic mass.	Carcinomas of the thyroid, larynx, lung, and esophagus. A tracheoesophageal fistula may develop spontaneously or after radiation therapy.
Metastases (Fig C 40-4)	Solitary or multiple, sessile or pedunculated masses.	Metastases to the trachea are infrequent. The most common primary tumor is hypernephroma, followed by melanoma and carcinomas of the breast and colon.
Spindle cell tumor	Sessile, smooth, sharply demarcated mass.	Neurinoma, leiomyoma, fibroma, xanthoma, hemangioma. Malignant spindle cell tumors may be irregular but cannot be differentiated from benign tumors unless metastases are demonstrated.
Cartilaginous tumor	Smooth, sessile, well-circumscribed mass.	Chondroma, hamartoma.
Papillomatosis (Fig C 40-5)	Innumerable small nodules that may involve the entire trachea. Rarely, a single large papilloma.	Laryngeal papillomatosis is a common disease of children that may seed distally into the tracheobronchial tree and even cause bronchial obstruction. Infrequent pulmonary nodules typically excavate to produce multiple thin-walled cystic lesions (see Fig C 9-18).

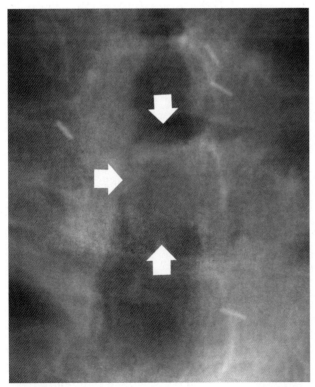

Fig C 40-4
Endobronchial metastasis. Soft-tissue mass in the trachea (arrow) representing a metastasis from cancer of the colon.[71]

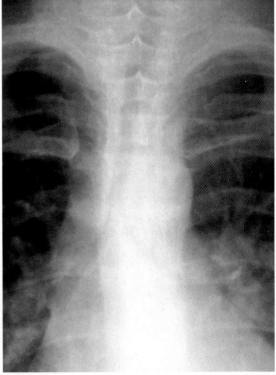

Fig C 40-5
Papillomatosis. Irregular narrowing throughout the trachea.[72]

Condition	Imaging Findings	Comments
Ectopic thyroid tumor	Smoothly rounded, often broad-based mass.	The ectopic thyroid tissue may undergo goitrous change or even become malignant. There may be a connecting bridge between the ectopic mass and the normally placed thyroid gland.
Intubation stricture (Figs C 40-6 and C 40-7)	Luminal narrowing of variable length.	Most commonly the result of tracheostomy. Also secondary to the use of endotracheal tubes (related to high-pressure cuffs).
Penetrating or blunt trauma	Often associated with subcutaneous emphysema, pneumomediastinum, pneumothorax, and fractures of the upper ribs.	If the original injury is not recognized, the healing process leads to luminal stenosis. An adjacent hematoma can cause an extrinsic impression and severely narrow the trachea.

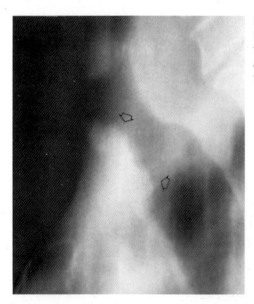

Fig C 40-6
Healing of tracheostomy stoma. Lateral tomogram demonstrates thickening of the anterior tracheal wall (arrows), secondary to fibrosis and granulation tissue, at the site of the stoma. This finding was of no functional significance.[73]

A

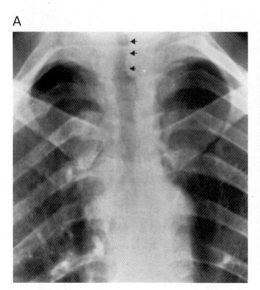

B

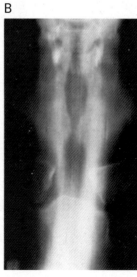

Fig C 40-7
Tracheal stenosis after intubation. (A) Plain chest radiograph demonstrates narrowing of the trachea (arrows) after prolonged intubation. (B) In another patient, a frontal tomogram shows a well-defined tubular area of tracheal narrowing at the tracheostomy cuff site.

Condition	Imaging Findings	Comments
Foreign body (Fig C 40-8)	Nonspecific filling defect in the airway.	Often difficult to detect and may require evidence of secondary aeration disturbances.
Amyloidosis (Fig C 40-9)	Diffuse narrowing of or nodular protrusions into the tracheal lumen.	Submucosal deposition of the proteinaceous amyloid material may result in obstructive hyperinflation, atelectasis, or recurrent pneumonia.
Tracheopathia osteoplastica (Fig C 40-10)	Multiple sessile nodular masses (often with rimming calcification).	Multiple submucosal osteocartilaginous growths along the inner surface of the trachea. The posterior membranous wall is typically spared, unlike the circumferential pattern in amyloidosis.

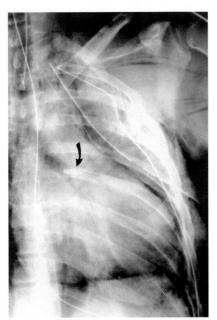

Fig C 40-8
Foreign body. Opaque filling defect (arrow) in the left upper lobe bronchus. This represented a tooth that was aspirated after the patient sustained multiple mandibular fractures following a motor vehicle accident.[71]

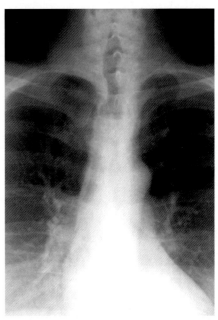

Fig C 40-9
Amyloidosis. Irregular narrowing of the trachea over a long segment.[72]

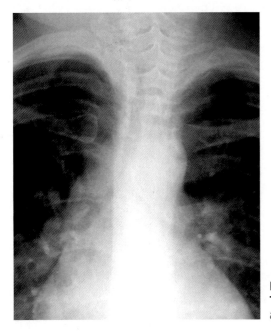

Fig C 40-10
Tracheobronchopathia osteochondroplastica. Narrowing and irregularity over a long segment of the trachea.[72]

Condition	Imaging Findings	Comments
Rhinoscleroma	Nodular masses or diffuse symmetric narrowing.	Chronic granulomatous disorder that primarily affects the nose, paranasal sinuses, and pharynx but may extend to involve the proximal and even the entire trachea. During the healing stage, the granulation tissue is replaced by fibrous tissue with resultant stenoses of the respiratory tract.
Sarcoidosis	Luminal narrowing or discrete nodules.	Usually supraglottic but may extend into the subglottic region or, rarely, into the distal trachea. Most patients have well-established sarcoidosis elsewhere.
Relapsing polychondritis (Fig C 40-11)	Diffuse, symmetric luminal narrowing (initially involves the larynx and the subglottic trachea).	Characteristic clinical syndrome of recurrent episodes of inflammation of the pinna of the ear and the nasal, laryngeal, and tracheal cartilages. Laryngeal and tracheal involvement (in 50% of cases) may result in airway obstruction or recurrent pneumonia.
Wegener's granulomatosis (Fig C 40-12)	Smooth luminal narrowing of variable length.	May rarely involve the subglottic larynx and proximal trachea, although much more common in the upper or lower respiratory tract.
Chronic obstructive pulmonary disease ("saber-sheath" trachea) (Fig C 40-13)	Narrowing of the coronal diameter of the intrathoracic trachea (to half that of the sagittal diameter or less).	The lateral walls of the trachea are usually thickened, and there is often evidence of ossification of the cartilaginous rings. The trachea abruptly changes to a normal rounded configuration at the thoracic outlet.

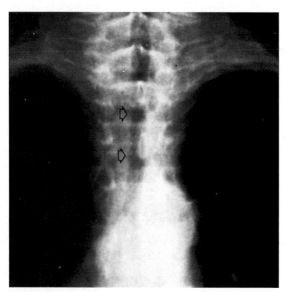

Fig C 40-11
Relapsing polychondritis. Narrowing of the trachea from the subglottic region to its bifurcation (arrows) in this patient with long-standing disease.[74]

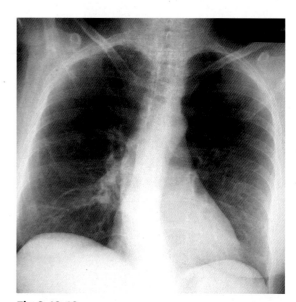

Fig C 40-12
Wegener's granulomatosis. Long segment of tracheal narrowing that extends from the subglottic space to the thoracic inlet.[72]

Condition	Imaging Findings	Comments
Fibrosing mediastinitis (Fig C 40-14)	Tracheal narrowing that is usually at the level of the carina and typically involves both main bronchi.	Rare benign proliferation of acellular collagen and fibrous tissue within the mediastinum. Although often idiopathic, many cases are thought to be due to an abnormal immunologic response to *Histoplasma capsulatum* infection. Affected patients are typically young and present with signs and symptoms of obstruction or compression of the superior vena cava, pulmonary veins or arteries, central airways, or esophagus.

A   B

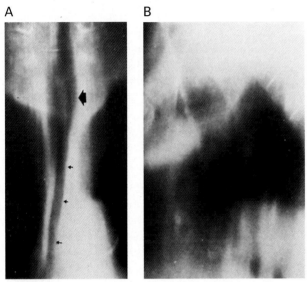

Fig C 40-13
Saber-sheath trachea. (A) Frontal and (B) lateral tomographic sections in a patient with chronic obstructive pulmonary disease demonstrate severe coronal narrowing of the intrathoracic trachea (small arrows) with an abrupt change to a more rounded cross-sectional shape at the thoracic outlet (large arrow). Calcific densities are present in the tracheal rings.[75]

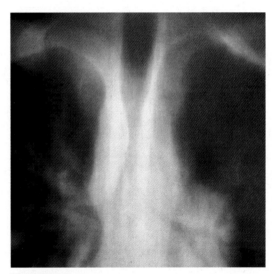

Fig C 40-14
Fibrosing mediastinitis. Diffuse narrowing of the trachea and both main bronchi and a soft-tissue mass encasing the distal trachea.[55]

Tracheobronchial Mass/Narrowing on Computed Tomography

Condition	Comments
Adherent mucus (Fig C 41-1)	Mucus usually can be differentiated from a true abnormality because of its low attenuation, "bubbly" appearance due to mixing with air, and occurrence along dependent portions of the airway. However, this may be difficult when mucus is thick and tenacious and adherent to nondependent portions of the airway. In such cases, repeating the examination after having the patient cough vigorously may demonstrate disappearance of the "lesion."
Hamartoma (Fig C 41-2)	The most common benign endobronchial tumor, it originates from a large bronchus, grows into the lumen, and causes bronchial obstruction before becoming large. Unlike parenchymal lesions, endobronchial hamartomas are often symptomatic because of airway obstruction, which can cause hemoptysis, cough, dyspnea, and obstructive pneumonia. In some masses containing fat or calcification, a specific diagnosis of hamartoma can be made.
Papilloma (Fig C 41-3)	Most common benign tracheobronchial neoplasm. The most common form of airway papilloma is juvenile laryngotracheal papillomatosis, in which multiple lesions develop secondary to infection with human papillomavirus. Solitary papilloma of the tracheobronchial tree is less common and is often associated with cigarette smoking. Although the condition is usually benign in children and may regress, in adults it can infiltrate and become malignant. Involvement of the distal airway can produce pulmonary nodules, which frequently cavitate.
Other benign tumors	Leiomyoma, lipoma, neurogenic tumor.
Inflammatory polyp	Thought to be related to some form of underlying irritation or inflammatory process (including foreign body and inhalation of hot or corrosive gas), this lesion typically occurs in the large airways.
Amyloid (Fig C 41-4)	More commonly, amyloidosis is a diffuse tracheobronchial disease causing diffuse mural thickening and luminal narrowing. Less commonly, solitary or multiple mural nodules are seen. Mural calcification may be evident on CT.

A B

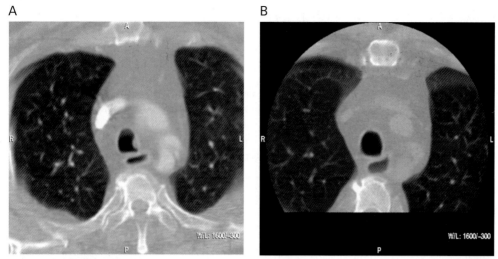

Fig C 41-1
Adherent mucus. (A) Initial study shows a 3-mm soft-tissue nodule (arrow) along the left lateral tracheal wall. (B) Repeat examination after the patient vigorously coughed shows that the nodule is no longer present and thus likely represented adherent mucus.[76]

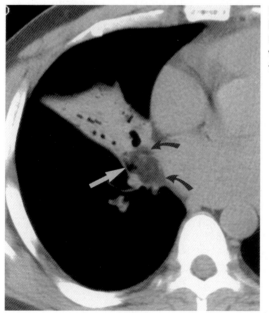

Fig C 41-2
Hamartoma. Endobronchial hamartoma. A mass (black arrows) of mixed fat (white arrow) and soft-tissue attenuation involves the right middle lobe bronchus, resulting in atelectasis of the right middle lobe.[76]

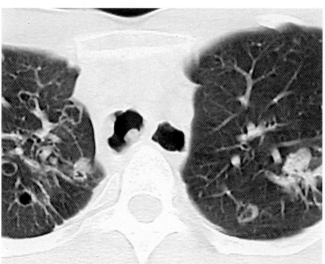

Fig C 41-3
Papillomatosis. Multiple nodules project into the tracheal lumen. There are also multiple papillomas in the lung parenchyma.[82]

Condition	Comments
Sarcoidosis (Fig C 41-5)	Endobronchial granulomas infrequently result in significant airway narrowing and lobar atelectasis.
Wegener's granulomatosis (Figs C 41-6 and C 41-7)	Focal or diffuse wall thickening and airway narrowing may be associated with calcification of the cartilaginous tracheal rings.
Tracheopathia osteochondroplastica (Fig C 41-8)	Idiopathic condition characterized by multiple sessile, submucosal osteocartilaginous nodules over a long segment of the trachea. Narrowing of long segments of the trachea and calcification of tracheal rings or multiple nodules are typically seen. In contrast to amyloid and relapsing polychondritis, tracheopathia osteochondroplastica spares the posterior membranous wall of the trachea.

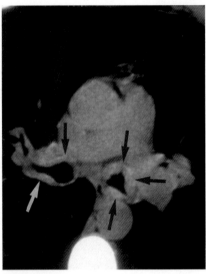

Fig C 41-4
Amyloidosis. Diffuse circumferential thickening of the bronchial walls bilaterally (arrows). Note the high-attenuation regions in the bronchial walls that likely represent calcification.[77]

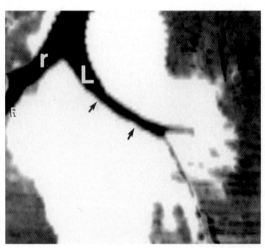

Fig C 41-5
Sarcoidosis. Coronal reformatted image shows diffuse narrowing of the left main bronchus (straight arrow) and its bifurcating branches surrounded by conglomerate mediastinal and left hilar adenopathy. Note occlusion of the left upper lobe bronchus (curved arrows) by the same process. L = left main bronchus; r = right main bronchus.[77]

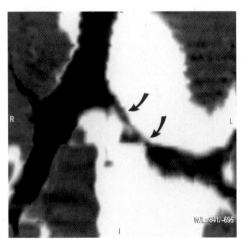

Fig C 41-6
Wegener's granulomatosis. Coronal reformatted image shows two focal strictures (arrows) in a diffusely narrowed left main bronchus.[77]

Condition	Comments
Primary malignant tumors (Figs C 41-9 to C 41-11)	Squamous cell carcinomas account for the majority of primary malignant tumors of the tracheobronchial tree. They typically occur in older patients with the risk factors of cigarette or alcohol abuse. These aggressive tumors with a poor prognosis appear as large, irregular tracheal masses. Most of the other malignant tumors are adenoid cystic carcinomas, which are less aggressive and have a better prognosis. Usually occurring during the third to fifth decades of life, they generally appear as focal polypoid endoluminal masses involving the posterolateral wall of the middle to lower third of the trachea.
Metastasis (Figs C 41-12 and C 41-13)	Infrequent occurrence that may result from direct involvement of the bronchial wall due to aspiration of tumor cells; lymphatic spread; hematogenous metastasis that causes a polypoid lesion inside the bronchial lumen; or tumor cells in the lymph nodes or lung parenchyma that surround the bronchus and grow along it, with some portion of the lesion invading through the bronchial wall. Primary malignancies with a tendency to metastasize to the airways include renal cell carcinoma, melanoma, adenocarcinoma, and sarcoma. Metastases typically appear as focal lesions of the airway; direct invasion from an adjacent source often produces more diffuse disease.
Miscellaneous tumors	Granular cell tumor, hemangioma, fibroma
Carcinoid (Figs C 41-14 and C 41-15)	Most carcinoids are primarily endobronchial lesions, and some small tumors are located entirely within the bronchial lumen. However, some display a dominant extraluminal component and a small endoluminal portion ("iceberg" lesion). CT provides anatomic localization of both the intra- and extraluminal portions.

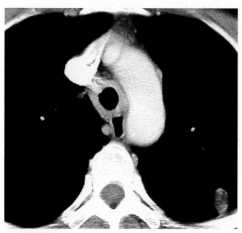

Fig C 41-7
Wegener's granulomatosis. Circumferential thickening of the tracheal mucosa.[2]

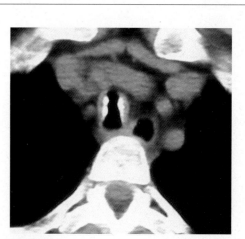

Fig C 41-8
Tracheobronchopathia osteochondroplastica.
Diffuse, irregular narrowing of the trachea with calcification of the lateral walls.[82]

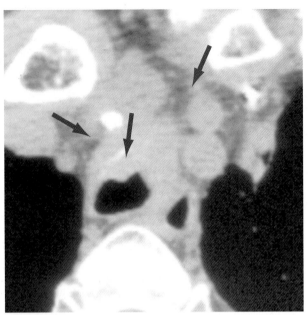

Fig C 41-9
Squamous cell carcinoma. Mass centered on the anterior and left lateral tracheal wall (curved arrows). Note that the lesion is disrupting the calcified tracheal ring (straight arrow).[76]

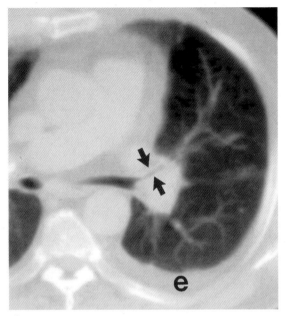

Fig C 41-10
Squamous cell carcinoma. Circumferential narrowing of the left upper lobe bronchus (arrows). e = effusion.[76]

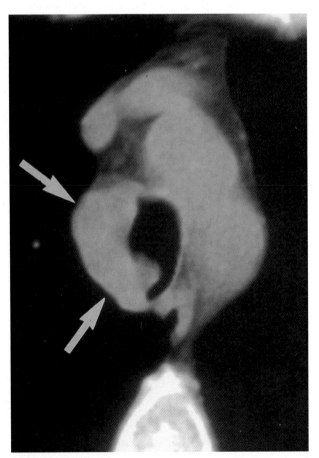

Fig C 41-11
Adenoid cystic carcinoma. Polypoid mass arising from the posterolateral wall of the trachea and protruding into the lumen.[76]

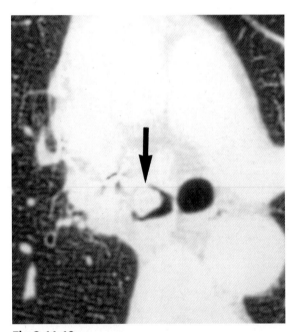

Fig C 41-12
Metastasis. An 8-mm soft-tissue mass (arrow) in the right main bronchus represents a metastasis from colon carcinoma.[76]

Condition	Comments
Infection (Figs C 41-16 and C 41-17)	Focal or diffuse airway lesions may be seen in tuberculosis, coccidioidomycois, histoplasmosis, aspergillosis, mucormycosis, and klebsiella. Endo-luminal masses of granulation initially produce irregular areas of stenosis. If untreated, this may lead to smooth fibrotic stenoses with associated distal pulmonary collapse or pneumonia. Prompt diagnosis and treatment can reverse or at lease improve the condition. Fibrosing mediastinis, usually due to histoplasmosis, can cause diffuse airway narrowing by extrinsic compression and appear as a calcified infiltrating mass. Rhinoscleroma is a chronic, progressive, granulomatous infection (caused by *Klebsiella rhinoscleromatis*) that affects the respiratory tract from the nose to the bronchi.

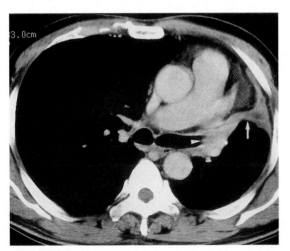

Fig C 41-13
Metastasis. Mass (arrowhead) in the orifice of the left upper lobe bronchus, representing a metastasis from renal cell carcinoma, causes collapse of the left upper lobe (arrow). (Courtesy of Jin Hwan Kim, MD, Department of Radiology, Chungnam National University, Taejeon, Korea.)[22]

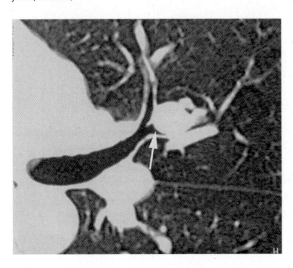

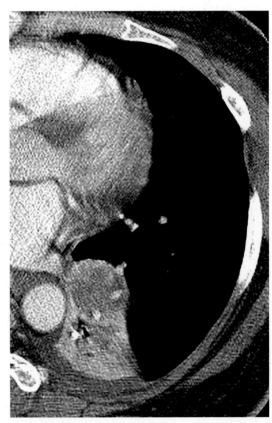

Fig C 41-15
Carcinoid. Endobronchial nodule (arrowhead) in the left basal trunk that causes atelectasis of the left lower lobe (arrow).[78]

Fig C 41-14
Carcinoid. Well-defined, round, partially endobronchial nodule (arrow) in the lateral subsegmental branch of the anterior segmental bronchus of the left upper lobe.[26]

Condition	Comments
Relapsing polychondritis (Figs C 41-18 and C 41-19)	Autoimmune connective tissue disease characterized by polyarthritis, aortitis or arteritis, uveal inflammation, and recurrent cartilage inflammation, especially of the ears, nose, larynx, and tracheobronchial tree (up to 70% affected individuals). This typically causes long-segment tracheobronchial strictures, mural thickening, and calcifications. Dynamic CT can demonstrate expiratory collapse of affected airways.
Foreign body aspiration (Fig C 41-20)	
Post-transplantation stenosis (Fig C 41-21)	Bronchial stenosis after lung transplantation reflects abnormal healing of the anastomosis. Improvements in surgical technique and drug therapy have cut the previous 50% incidence of post-transplantation airway complications to approximately 15%. Extraluminal gas and mucosal ulcerations are signs of anastomotic dehiscence, which occurs in the early postoperative period.
Fibrosing mediastinitis (Fig C 41-22)	Rare benign proliferation of acellular collagen and fibrous tissue within the mediastinum. Although often idiopathic, many cases are thought to be due to an abnormal immunologic response to *Histoplasma capsulatum* infection. Affected patients are typically young and present with symptoms of obstruction or compression of the superior vena cava, pulmonary veins or arteries, central airways, or esophagus.

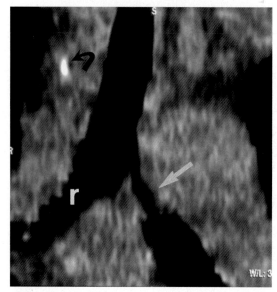

Fig C 41-16
Tuberculosis. Coronal reconstruction shows stenosis of a short focal segment (white arrow) of the left main bronchus. Note the calcification (arrow) of a mediastinal lymph node (black arrow). r = right main bronchus.[76]

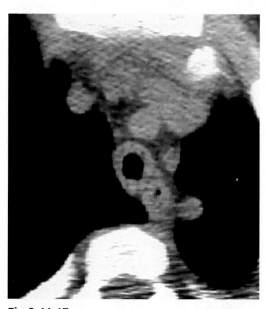

Fig C 41-17
Rhinoscleroma. Circumferential thickening of the trachea.[82]

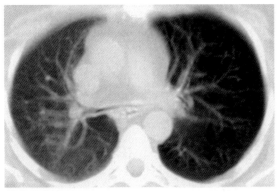

Fig C 41-18
Relapsing polychondritis. Expiratory scan shows abnormal collapse of the bronchi with air trapping in the left lung.[77]

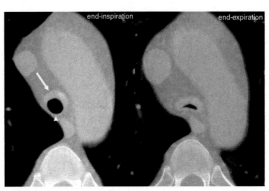

Fig C 41-19
Relapsing polychondritis. End-inspiration and end-expiration scans show dynamic collapse of the trachea with expiration (right). Note the calcification and thickening of the cartilaginous parts of the trachea (arrow), with sparing of the posterior wall (arrowhead).[82]

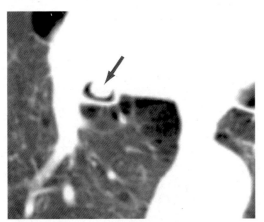

Fig C 41-20
Foreign body. Well-circumscribed mass in the bronchus intermedius (arrow).[76]

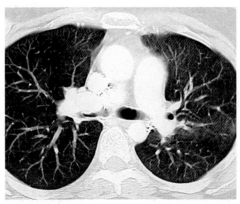

Fig C 41-21
Post-transplantation stenosis. Focal narrowing at the anastomotic site within the right lung in a patient who had undergone bilateral lung transplantation.[82]

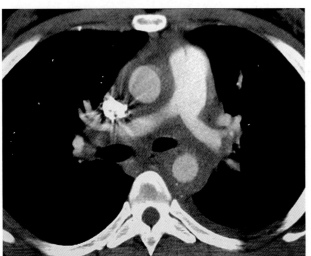

Fig C 41-22
Fibrosing mediastinitis. Mass of soft-tissue attenuation that diffusely infiltrates the mediastinum, encasing and narrowing the left main bronchus (*), ascending (A) and descending (D) aorta, proximal right (R) and left (L) pulmonary arteries, and esophagus (arrowhead).[55]

Broncholithiasis*

Condition	Comments

Erosion by and extrusion of a calcified adjacent lymph node (Figs C 42-1 and C 42-2)

By far the most common cause, it is usually associated with long-standing foci of necrotizing granulomatous lymphadenitis (especially tuberculosis). Nevertheless, the frequency of broncholithiasis complicating granulomatous infection is quite low. Broncholiths vary in size and are usually irregular, often possessing spur-like projections or sharp edges. It is thought that repeated physical impingement of calcified peribronchial lymph nodes on the bronchial wall during respiratory motion is responsible for broncholith formation. The most common sites are the proximal right middle lobe bronchus and the origin of the anterior segmental bronchus of the upper lobes because of airway anatomy and lymph node distribution.

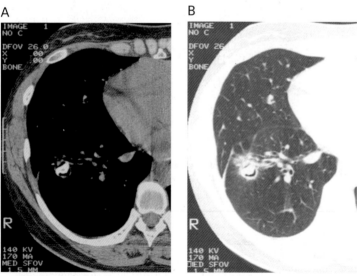

Fig 42-1
Extrusion of a calcified adjacent lymph node. CT scans with mediastinal (A) and lung (B) windows shows a calcified nodule within a dilated bronchus.[81]

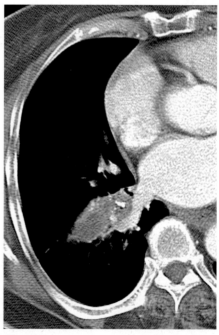

Fig 42-2
Extrusion of a calcified adjacent lymph node. Calcified nodule (arrowhead) in the anterior basal segment of the right lower lobe with secondary atelectasis.[79]

*The presence of calcified or ossified material within the bronchial lumen.

Condition	Comments
In situ calcification of aspirated foreign material/ aspiration of bone tissue (Figs C 42-3 and C 42-4)	Persistence of a noncalcified foreign body, such as a vegetable fiber, within a bronchus for a prolonged period can serve as a nidus for calcium deposition. Rarely, bone fragments or other radiopaque material may be aspirated
Erosion by and extrusion of calcified or ossified bronchial cartilage plate	Diffuse tracheobronchial calcification is commonly associated with advanced age. In rare cases, broncholithiasis can result from calcification of bronchial cartilage with subsequent sequestration of the calcified material into the bronchial lumen.
Disorders mimicking broncholithiasis Primary endobronchial infection with dystrophic calcification (Fig C 42-5)	Rarely, primary endobronchial fungus ball due to actinomycosis may calcify and result in the formation of a calcified endobronchial nodule.

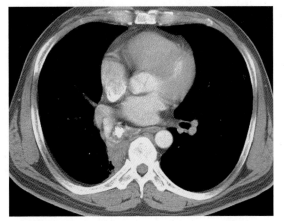

Fig 42-3
Calcification of an aspirated foreign body. The calcified nodule in the bronchus intermedius proved to be a vegetable fiber with dystrophic calcification. Note the atelectasis of the right lower lobe.[79]

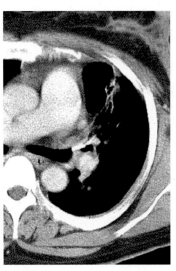

Fig 42-4
Aspiration of an opaque anchovy bone. Tubular calcified lesion at the orifice of the upper lobe bronchus (arrow).[79]

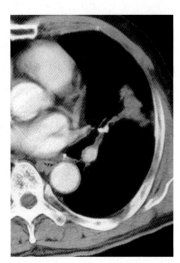

Fig 42-5
Endobronchial actinomycosis with dystrophic calcification. Calcified nodule within the bronchus of the lingular division of the left upper lobe (arrow) with peripheral atelectasis.[80]

Condition	Comments
Calcified endobronchial tumor (Figs C 42-6 and C 42-7)	Some calcification is often seen in central carcinoid tumors on CT examinations. When the tumor is totally ossified and situated within the bronchus, it simulates broncholithiasis. Although endobronchial hamartomas are rare, they can mimic broncholithiasis when they have a central cartilaginous core.
Tracheobronchial disease with mural calcification (Fig C 42-8)	Amyloid deposition may form a polypoid submucosal airway nodule with stippled calcification that mimics a broncholith. Protrusion into the lumen of a submucosal osteocartilaginous growth along the lateral wall of the trachea or main bronchus can also simulate broncholithiasis.

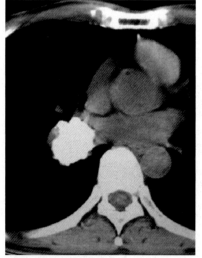

Fig 42-6
Carcinoid tumor. Sharply defined, totally ossified mass (arrow) that is centrally situated in the right lower lobe bronchus and produces abrupt bronchial obstruction.[79]

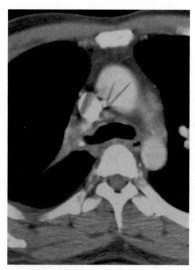

Fig 42-7
Hamartoma. Small calcified nodule obstructing the right upper lobe bronchus (arrow).[79]

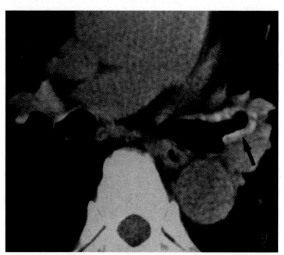

Fig 42-8
Amyloidosis. Localized thickening of the bronchial wall with calcification and partial intraluminal protrusion (arrows).[81]

Condition	Comments
Hypertrophied bronchial artery with intraluminal protrusion (Fig C 42-9)	The bronchial arteries become enlarged in such disorders as acute or chronic pulmonary infections, pulmonary thromboembolism, and chronic obstructive pulmonary disease. Protrusion of a hypertrophied bronchial artery into the lumen may mimic a broncholith on contrast-enhanced CT scans. Careful examination of images obtained above and below the abnormality or unenhanced CT may be required to confirm the vascular nature of the lesion.

A
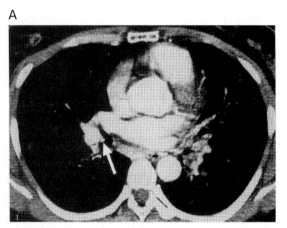

B
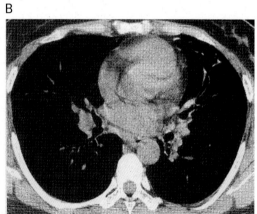

Fig 42-9
Hypertrophied bronchial artery. (A) Contrast-enhanced scan shows a high-attenuation nodular structure (arrow) at the bifurcation of the bronchus intermedius, which mimics broncholithiasis. (B) This unenhanced section scan reveals that the high-attenuation structure is not calcified.[82]

Retrotracheal Space Abnormalities

Condition	Comments
Vascular lesions Aberrant right subclavian artery (Fig C 43-1)	The aberrant vessel arises from the posterior portion of the aortic arch and crosses the mediastinum from left to right, posterior to the trachea and esophagus.
Aberrant left subclavian artery (Fig C 43-2)	The most common anomaly seen with a right-sided aortic arch, it is not associated with congenital heart disease. CT and MRI can differentiate this from a right-sided aortic arch with mirror-image branching, which is associated with a high prevalence of congenital heart disease.
Double aortic arch (Fig C 43-3)	One of the most common symptomatic anomalies of the aortic arch, it usually is apparent in infancy because of respiratory symptoms or difficulty in feeding related to tracheal or esophageal compression. The larger, higher, and more posterior right arch fuses with the left arch posteriorly to form a single descending aorta that is typically left-sided.
Aortic aneurysm (Fig C 43-4)	Can appear as a fusiform or saccular mass-like lesion that protrudes into the retrotracheal space. Complications include ulceration and rupture.
Esophageal lesions Atresia	Congenital incomplete formation of the tubular esophagus. It can manifest as an air-distended pouch or mass-like lesion (due to mucosal secretion) in the retrotracheal space that deforms the adjacent part of the trachea.

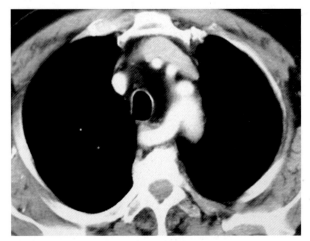

Fig C 43-1
Aberrant right subclavian artery. CT scan shows that the aberrant vessel arises as the last branch of a left-sided aortic arch posterior to the esophagus.[83]

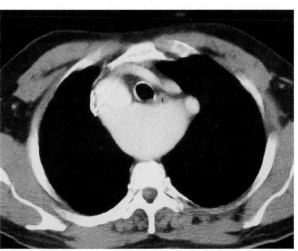

Fig C 43-2
Aberrant left subclavian artery with a right-sided aortic arch.[83]

Condition	Comments
Duplication cyst (Fig C 43-5)	Although most of these congenital lesions arise in the lower esophagus, one developing in the upper portion may appear as a mass in the retrotracheal space. Of water-attenuation on CT and with high signal intensity on T2-weighted MR images, they may have high signal intensity on T1-weighted images due to intracystic hemorrhage or proteinaceous debris.

A | B

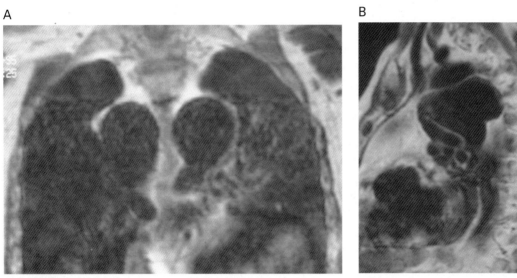

Fig C 43-3
Double aortic arch. (A) Coronal T1-weighted MR image shows the right and left aortic arches. (B) On a sagittal image, the retrotracheal space is obscured by both aortic arches.[83]

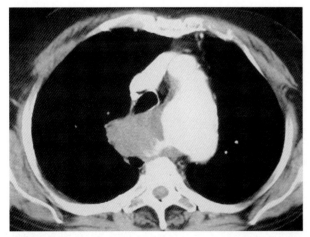

Fig C 43-4
Aneurysm of the transverse aortic arch. CT scan shows a penetrating atherosclerotic ulcer and a contained rupture or mediastinal hematoma.[83]

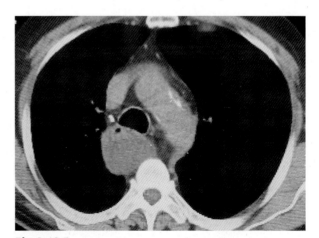

Fig C 43-5
Esophageal duplication cyst. CT scan shows a well-circumscribed mass with water attenuation adjacent to the esophagus. The appearance and location of the mass are typical for an esophageal duplication cyst in this asymptomatic young woman, in whom the lesion was an incidental finding on chest radiography.[83]

Condition	Comments
Zenker's diverticulum (Fig C 43-6)	Pulsion diverticulum in the upper esophagus that usually extends dorsally into the postcricoid area. If large, it can be detected in the retrotracheal space as a large air- or fluid-filled, mass-like lesion.
Achalasia	Dilatation of the esophagus due to inadequate relaxation of the lower esophageal sphincter can cause anterior displacement and bowing of the trachea by the fluid- or food-filled esophagus. Aspiration pneumonia is an associated complication
Tumors	Carcinoma can cause marked inhomogeneous thickening of the esophageal wall with infiltration extending to the posterior wall of the trachea. A leiomyoma can produce a smooth impression on the posterior wall of the trachea and anterior displacement of the airway.
Miscellaneous mediastinal masses Lymphatic malformation (Fig C 43-7)	Also known as lymphangioma, approximately 5% of these rare benign lesions occur in the mediastinum. Most are found in children over 2 years old (the site of 75% of lesions) and they can extend into the retrotracheal space. In adults, mediastinal lymphatic malformations are usually due to an incompletely resected childhood tumor. Although typically appearing as lobular, multicystic lesions, they may appear solid on CT or have high signal on T1-weighted MR images due to intracystic protein or hemorrhage.

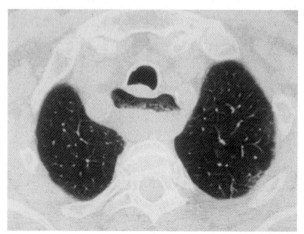

Fig C 43-6
Zenker's diverticulum. CT demonstrates a large retrotracheal diverticulum with an air-fluid level due to retained alimentary content.[83]

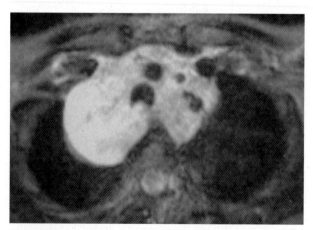

Fig C 43-7
Lymphatic malformation. Axial T2-weighted image shows a characteristic hyperintense lesion that surrounds, but does not displace, the trachea and great vessels. The tumor extends toward the anterior soft tissues of the chest wall.[83]

Condition	Comments
Hemangioma (Fig C 43-8)	Rare mediastinal tumor composed of large interconnecting vascular spaces with varying amounts of interposed stromal elements such as fat and fibrous tissue. The heterogeneous mass usually demonstrates rimlike peripheral contrast enhancement. Phleboliths are present in <10% of cases.
Thyroid goiter (Fig C 43-9)	Most thyroid masses in the mediastinum are caused by intrathoracic extension of neck masses. In approximately 20% of cases, the lesion extends posteriorly behind the esophagus and adjacent to the trachea to involve the retrotracheal space. On CT, the heterogeneous mass commonly contains areas of hemorrhage, necrosis, and calcification.
Hemorrhage (Fig C 43-10)	Complication of traumatic aortic injury or such iatrogenic procedures as placement of a central venous catheter. Posterior extension of mediastinal hemorrhage can produce a mass-like area in the retrotracheal space. In patients with aortic transaction, the trachea is typically displaced to the right.
Infection (Fig C 43-11)	Infection can spread to the retrotracheal space from contiguous structures such as the thoracic spine and paravertebral spaces, or caudad from the retropharyngeal and prevertebral spaces.
Acute mediastinitis (Fig C 43-12)	Diffuse inflammation or abscess formation in the retrotracheal space may result from rupture of the esophagus secondary to blunt thoracic trauma, foreign body impaction, or diagnostic or therapeutic endoscopic procedures. Esophageal fistulization related to esophageal carcinoma may also be a cause of mediastinal abscess

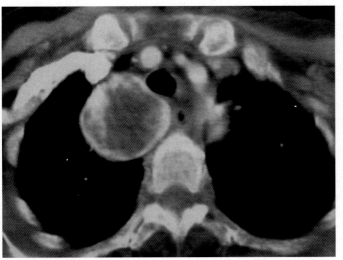

Fig C 43-8
Hemangioma. Contrast CT scan shows a well-defined mass with intense central and rim-like peripheral enhancement.[83]

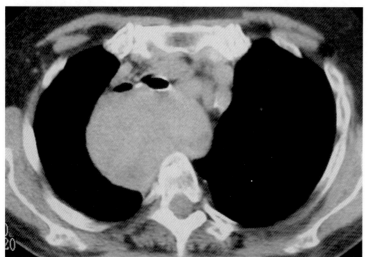

Fig C 43-9
Intrathoracic goiter. CT scan shows a well-defined, homogeneous soft-tissue mass that fills the retrotracheal space and displaces the trachea, esophagus, and supraaortic vessels anteriorly.[83]

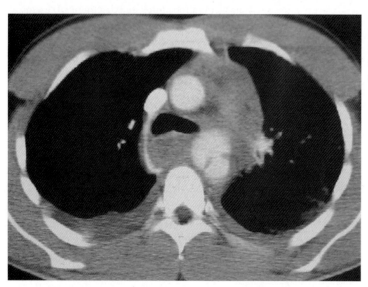

Fig C 43-10
Hematoma. Contrast CT scan shows a mediastinal hematoma in the retrotracheal space. There is a pseudoaneurysm (*) medial to the proximal descending thoracic aorta. Bilateral pleural effusions are also seen.[83]

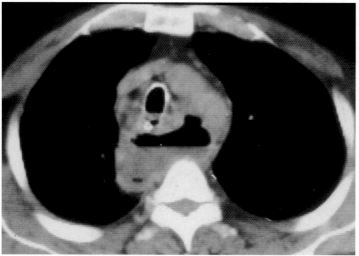

Fig C 43-11
Retropharyngeal infection with mediastinal abscess formation. CT scan shows widening of the middle mediastinum with a large abscess that fills the retrotracheal space and displaces the trachea and esophagus anteriorly. There is an air-fluid level within the abscess cavity.[83]

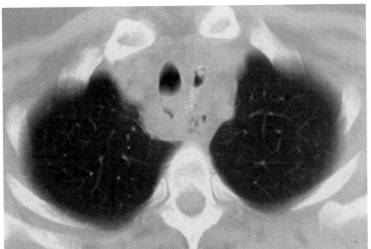

Fig C 43-12
Mediastinal abscess with fistulization. CT scan shows marked thickening of the esophageal wall. Air bubbles and a small amount of contrast material are seen within the retrotracheal space, reflecting the formation of a fistula (arrow).[83]

Upper Airway Obstruction in Children

Condition	Imaging Findings	Comments
Croup (Fig C 44-1)	Smooth tapered narrowing of the subglottic trachea.	Very common and usually mild.
Epiglottitis (Fig C 44-2)	Huge swelling of the epiglottis and aryepiglottic folds (fills the entire hypopharynx).	Much more uncommon and far more dangerous condition than croup. Caused by *Haemophilus influenzae.*
Foreign body (Fig C 44-3)	Opaque or nonopaque lesion that may involve the pharynx, larynx, or trachea.	Foreign body at the tracheal bifurcation is difficult to diagnose (causes symptoms of both upper and lower tract obstruction; prolonged and difficult inspiration and expiration on fluoroscopy).

A 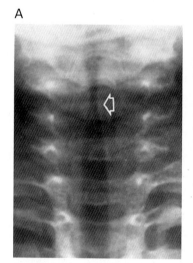   B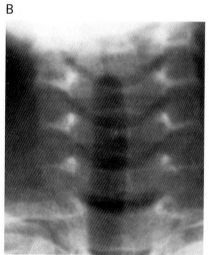

Fig C 44-1
Croup. (A) Smooth, tapered narrowing (arrow) of the subglottic portion of the trachea (gothic arch sign). (B) A normal trachea with broad shouldering in the subglottic region.

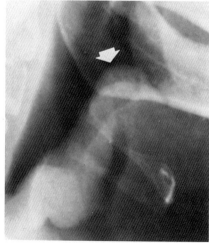

Fig C 44-2
Epiglottitis. Lateral radiograph of the neck demonstrates a wide, rounded configuration of the inflamed epiglottis (arrow).[84]

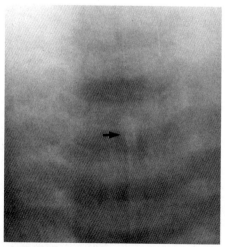

Fig C 44-3
Chicken bone in the glottis.[85]

Condition	Imaging Findings	Comments
Intrinsic mass (Fig C 44-4)	Single or multiple filling defects in the airway.	Tracheal hemangioma, fibroma, laryngeal papillomatosis, bronchial duplication cyst.
Extrinsic mass	Extrinsic impression on the airway.	Cystic hygroma, thyroglossal duct cyst, ectopic thyroid tissue, pulmonary or mediastinal mass, anomalous vessel.
Tracheal stricture	Diffuse or localized tracheal narrowing.	Posttraumatic, postoperative, postintubation. Primary congenital stenosis is exceedingly rare.
Vascular ring	Narrowing of the distal trachea.	Wide spectrum of anomalous vascular patterns (usually associated with a right-sided aortic arch). Often one or more impressions on the barium-filled esophagus.
Choanal atresia	Soft-tissue or bony obstruction. Usually no abnormality on plain radiographs.	Bilateral atresia causes severe respiratory distress in the newborn infant. The obstruction can be demonstrated after the introduction of a small amount of oily contrast material into the nostrils.
Enlarged tonsils and adenoids (Fig C 44-5)	Soft-tissue mass narrowing the airway in the nasopharynx and oropharynx.	May be gross hypertrophy without upper airway obstruction.

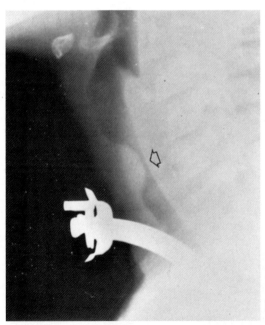

Fig C 44-4
Fibroma of the cervical trachea. Lateral view of the neck shows a sharply defined homogeneous soft-tissue density (arrow) arising from the upper anterior portion of the trachea. This 11-year-old boy had experienced dyspnea and inspiratory stridor for several years.[73]

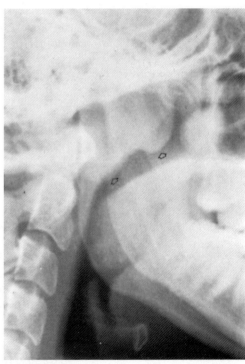

Fig C 44-5
Enlarged tonsils and adenoids. Marked impressions (arrows) on the upper airway.

Condition	Imaging Findings	Comments
Peritonsillar abscess	Soft-tissue mass in the region of the soft palate and hypopharynx.	
Pharyngeal airway obstruction by retroplaced tongue	Micrognathia associated with airway obstruction that varies between inspiratory and expiratory films.	Pierre Robin syndrome (cleft palate, micrognathia, retrodisplaced tongue); Möbius' syndrome (cranial nerve palsies often associated with micrognathia); extremely rare isolated micrognathia.
Esophageal atresia and tracheoesophageal fistula (Figs C 44-6 and C 44-7)	Blind air-filled upper esophageal pouch causing anterior displacement and compression of the tracheal air shadow.	Diagnosis confirmed by the looping of a radiopaque catheter (may inject a small amount of contrast material). Gas in the bowel indicates a distal tracheoesophageal fistula. Also H-type fistulas (cause recurrent aspiration).
Laryngomalacia	Downward displacement and buckling of the aryepiglottic folds in inspiration.	Aryepiglottic hypermobility (the larynx itself is structurally normal, but there is excessive relaxation of the supraglottic structures). The diagnosis is made fluoroscopically with the patient in the lateral position.
Tracheomalacia (Fig C 44-8)	Collapse of the trachea on expiration (may be focal or generalized).	Entity that is distinct from laryngomalacia, much less common, and due to weakening of the supporting cartilage and muscles of the trachea.
Congenital vocal cord paralysis (Fig C 44-9)	Unilateral or bilateral absence of normal movement of the vocal cords.	Life-threatening if bilateral (vocal cords tend to remain closed).

A

B

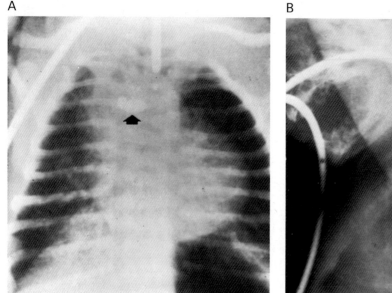
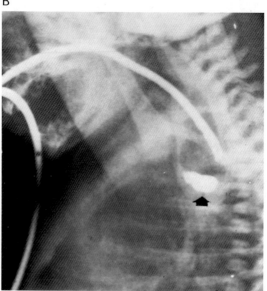

Fig C 44-6
Congenital tracheoesophageal fistula. Contrast material injected through a feeding tube demonstrates occlusion of the proximal esophageal pouch (arrows) in (A) frontal and (B) lateral projections. Note the air in the stomach.

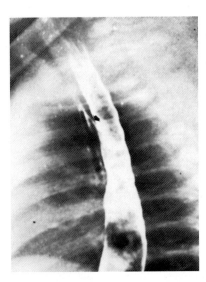

Fig C 44-7
Congenital tracheoesophageal fistula (type IV or
H, fistula). Note the sharp downward course of the fis-
tula from the trachea to the esophagus (arrow).

A   B

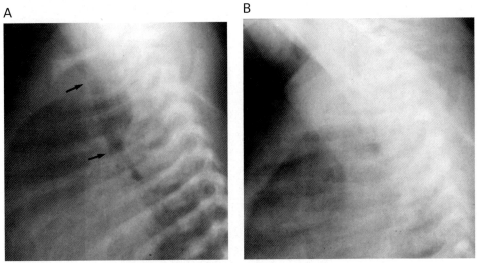

Fig C 44-8
Tracheomalacia. (A) Inspiratory view demonstrates a normal trachea (arrows). (B) On expiration, the tracheal air column is totally
obliterated.[85]

A   B

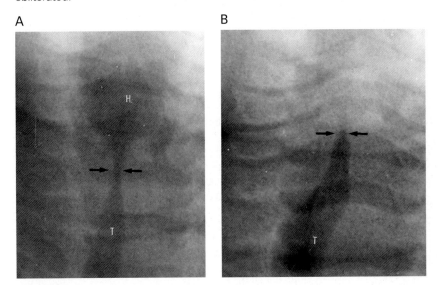

Fig C 44-9
Bilateral vocal cord paralysis. (A) Inspiratory view shows the typical midline apposition of the vocal cords (arrows). The hypopharynx (H) is overdistended. T = trachea. (B) On expiration, the vocal cords (arrows) remain in the midline, and the subglottic trachea (T) overdistends.[85]

Condition	Imaging Findings	Comments
Macroglossia	Enlarged tongue causing extrinsic impression on the airway.	May occur in hypothyroidism and in the Beckwith-Wiedemann syndrome (visceromegaly, omphalocele or umbilical hernia, pancreatic and adrenal hyperplasia, increased bone age, or neoplastic disease).
Laryngeal web (Fig C 44-10)	Narrowing of the air column.	Membranous stenosis in a glottic, supraglottic, or infraglottic position.
Diphtheria	Narrowing of the air column.	Extension of the characteristic membrane from the pharynx into the larynx, trachea, and even the bronchial tree can lead to increasing airway obstruction, cyanosis, and even death.

A

B

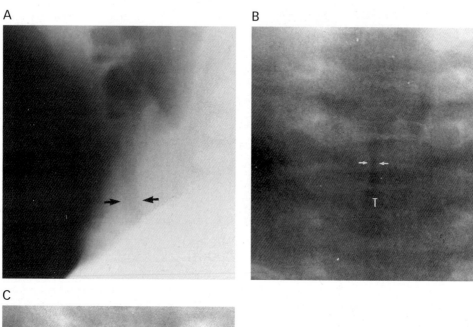

C

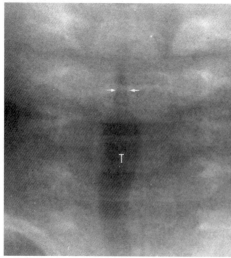

Fig C 44-10
Laryngeal web. (A) Inspiratory lateral view demonstrates an overdistended hypopharynx, an indistinct vocal cord area, and a mild paradoxically narrowed subglottic portion of the trachea (arrows). (B) Inspiratory frontal view demonstrates midline fixation of the cords (arrows) and subglottic narrowing of the entire trachea (T). (C) Expiratory view shows persistent fixation of the vocal cords (arrows) and overdistention of the subglottic trachea (T).[85]

Condition	Imaging Findings	Comments
Laryngospasm	Narrowing of the air column.	Life-threatening anaphylactic reactions occur seconds to minutes after the administration of a specific antigen (generally by injection, as with radiographic contrast material or less commonly by ingestion) and cause upper or lower airway obstruction, or both. Laryngeal edema may be experienced as a "lump" in the throat, hoarseness, or stridor, while bronchial obstruction is associated with a feeling of tightness in the chest or audible wheezing.

Widening of the Right Paratracheal Stripe
(5 Millimeters or More)

Condition	Comments
Tracheal disorders (see Fig C 40-5)	An abnormality of any of the layers of the trachea (mucosa, submucosa, cartilage rings) can widen the right paratracheal stripe. Conditions include benign and malignant tracheal tumors and diffuse tracheal narrowing (postintubation edema, tracheobronchitis, posttraumatic stenosis, relapsing polychondritis).
Causes of mediastinal widening (Fig C 45-1; see Figs C 14-4, C 14-5, and C 14-8)	Lymph node enlargement (sarcoidosis, metastases, lymphoma, tuberculosis, histoplasmosis); hemorrhage from blunt chest trauma; mediastinitis; intrathoracic goiter; and postsurgical changes from mediastinoscopy, cardiac surgery, and right radical neck dissection. Neurofibromatosis involving the right vagus nerve can also cause widening of the right paratracheal stripe.
Pleural disorders	Diseases that cause thickening of the parietal or visceral pleura or an increase in pleural fluid can widen the right paratracheal stripe. These include free or encapsulated pleural effusion, mesothelioma, and pleural thickening or fibrosis from any cause.
Miscellaneous disorders	Right upper lobe atelectasis, radiation fibrosis, polyarteritis nodosa, Wegener's granulomatosis, and desquamative interstitial pneumonia.

A   B

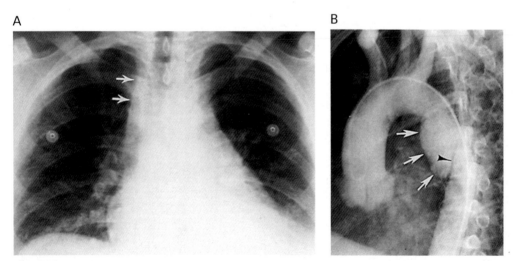

Fig C 45-1
Mediastinal hemorrhage secondary to blunt chest trauma. (A) Supine chest radiograph shows a right paratracheal stripe (arrows) measuring 1 cm in width. (B) Aortography in the same patient demonstrates a pseudoaneurysm at the level of the aortic isthmus (arrows). The arrowhead indicates an intimal flap.[86]

Elevated Diaphragm

Condition	Comments
Normal variant	Dome of the diaphragm tends to be approximately half an interspace higher on the right than on the left. In approximately 10% of individuals, the hemidiaphragms are at the same height or the left is higher than the right.
Eventration (Figs C 46-1 and C 46-2)	Unilateral hypoplasia of a hemidiaphragm (very rarely both) with the thinned, weakened musculature inadequate to restrain the abdominal viscera. Localized eventration primarily involves the anteromedial portion of the right hemidiaphragm, through which a portion of the right lobe of the liver bulges. In a posterior eventration, upward displacement of the kidney can produce a rounded mass. Total eventration occurs almost exclusively on the left. Eventrations may have paradoxical diaphragmatic motion (though more commonly seen in diaphragmatic paralysis).
Phrenic nerve paralysis (Fig C 46-3)	Unilateral or bilateral diaphragmatic elevation with characteristic paradoxical motion of the diaphragm (tends to ascend rather than descend with inspiration). Results from any process interfering with the normal function of the phrenic nerve (inadvertent surgical transection, primary bronchogenic carcinoma, or mediastinal metastases); intrinsic neurologic disease (poliomyelitis, Erb's palsy, peripheral neuritis, hemiplegia); injury to the phrenic nerve, thoracic cage, cervical spine, or brachial plexus; pressure from a substernal thyroid or aneurysm; or lung or mediastinal infection (paralysis may be temporary).

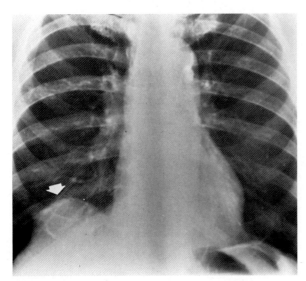

Fig C 46-1
Partial eventration. Of the right hemidiaphragm (arrow).

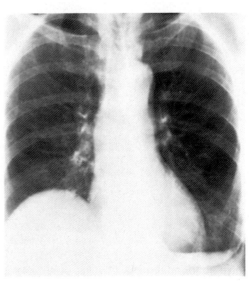

Fig C 46-2
Complete eventration. Of the right hemidiaphragm.

Condition	Comments
Increased intra-abdominal volume	Unilateral or bilateral diaphragmatic elevation in patients with ascites, obesity, or pregnancy.
Intra-abdominal inflammatory disease	Unilateral or bilateral diaphragmatic elevation. Most commonly due to subphrenic abscess. Also perinephric, hepatic, or splenic abscess; pancreatitis; cholecystitis; and perforated ulcer.
Intra-abdominal mass (Fig C 46-4)	Unilateral or bilateral diaphragmatic elevation caused by enlargement of the liver or spleen; abdominal tumor or cyst of the liver, spleen, kidneys, adrenals, or pancreas; or distended stomach or splenic flexure (left hemidiaphragm).

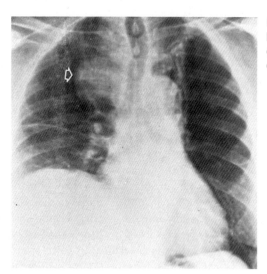

Fig C 46-3
Phrenic nerve paralysis. Primary bronchogenic carcinoma (arrow) involving the phrenic nerve causes paralysis of the right hemidiaphragm.

A   B

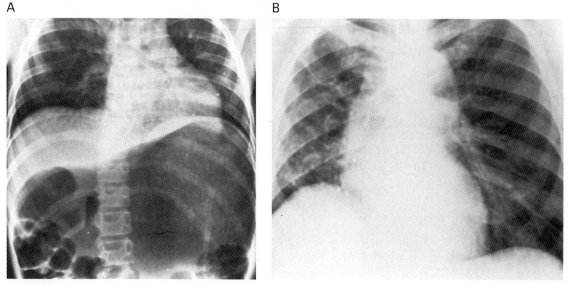

Fig C 46-4
Intra-abdominal mass. (A) Acute gastric dilatation causes diffuse elevation of both leaves of the diaphragm. (B) Huge syphilitic gumma of the liver produces elevation of the right hemidiaphragm.

Condition	Comments
Acute intrathoracic process (splinting of diaphragm) (Fig C 46-5)	Unilateral or bilateral diaphragmatic elevation due to chest wall injury, atelectasis, pulmonary infarct, or pleural disease (fibrosis, acute pleurisy).
Tumor or cyst of diaphragm	Very rare lesion that simulates unilateral diaphragmatic elevation.
Subpulmonic effusion (Fig C 46-6)	Closely simulates an elevated hemidiaphragm. On frontal views, the peak of the pseudodiaphragmatic contour is lateral to that of a normal hemidiaphragm (situated near the junction of the middle and lateral thirds rather than near the center).
Altered pulmonary volume	Unilateral or bilateral diaphragmatic elevation due to atelectasis (associated pulmonary opacity); postoperative lobectomy or pneumonectomy (rib defects, sutures, shift of the heart and mediastinum); hypoplastic lung (crowded ribs, mediastinal shift, absent or small pulmonary artery, sometimes the scimitar syndrome).
Diaphragmatic hernia (Figs C 46-7 and C 46-8)	Mimics unilateral diaphragmatic elevation on frontal views. Lateral views show the characteristic anterior location of Morgagni's hernia or the posterior position of Bochdalek's hernia.
Traumatic rupture of diaphragm (Figs C 46-9 and C 46-10)	Mimics unilateral diaphragmatic elevation. Injury to the right side causes herniation of the soft-tissue density of the liver into the right hemithorax. On the left, air-containing stomach and bowel herniate into the chest (may mimic diaphragmatic elevation if the bowel loops are filled with fluid).

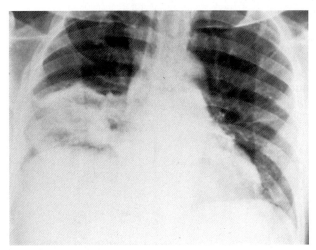

Fig C 46-5
Acute pneumonia. Elevation of the right hemidiaphragm due to splinting secondary to a right lower lung infiltrate.

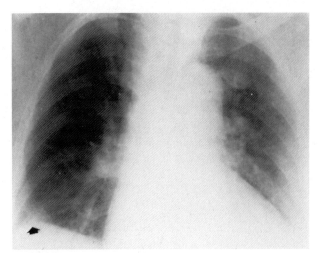

Fig C 46-6
Subpulmonic effusion. The peak of the pseudodiaphragmatic contour (arrow) is lateral to that of a normal hemidiaphragm.

A

B

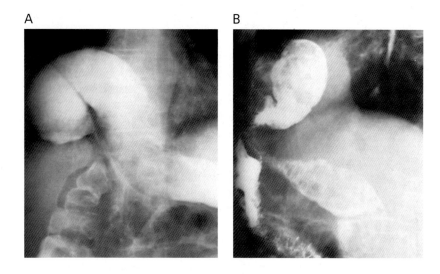

Fig C 46-7
Morgagni hernia. (A) Frontal and (B) lateral views demonstrate barium-filled bowel in a hernia sac that lies anteriorly and to the right.

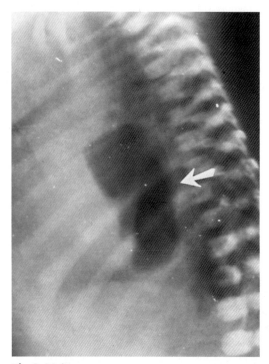

Fig C 46-8
Bochdalek hernia. Gas-filled loop of bowel (arrow) is visible posteriorly in the thoracic cavity.

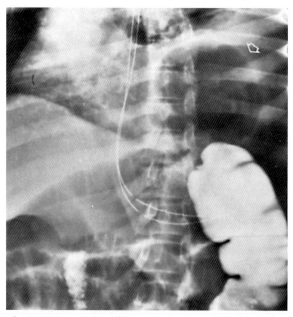

Fig C 46-9
Traumatic rupture of the diaphragm. Herniation of a portion of the splenic flexure (arrow), with obstruction to the retrograde flow of barium.

A

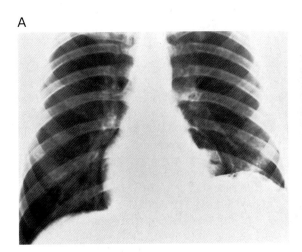

B

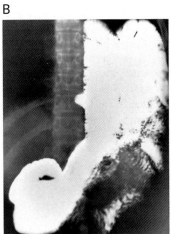

Fig C 46-10
Traumatic rupture of the diaphragm. (A) On a frontal projection, the radiographic appearance simulates eventration or paralysis of the left hemidiaphragm. (B) The administration of barium clearly demonstrates the herniation of bowel contents into the chest.

Interstitial Lung Disease on Computed Tomography*

Condition	Imaging Findings	Comments
Usual interstitial pneumonia (UIP) (Fig C 47-1)	Fine or coarse reticular opacities in the subpleural regions of the lung bases. Irregular pleural, vascular, and bronchial interfaces with normal parenchyma.	Most commonly seen in patients who have idiopathic pulmonary fibrosis (fibrosing alveolitis). Also occurs in patients with asbestosis and collagen vascular diseases, particularly rheumatoid arthritis and scleroderma.
Desquamative interstitial pneumonia (DIP) (Fig C 47-2)	Similar to UIP, although the fibrosis tends to be less severe.	Because the pathologic patterns of both UIP and DIP can often be seen in the same patient, it is probable that DIP represents the early stage and UIP the late stage of the same disease. The predominant pattern of ground-glass (rather than reticular) opacities is seen in nearly all patients, reflecting the presence of intra-alveolar macrophages and interstitial inflammation.
Cryptogenic organizing pneumonia (COP) (Fig C 47-3)	Patchy, unilateral or bilateral air-space consolidation and small nodular opacities with a predominantly subpleural distribution. Typical peribronchial thickening.	May be seen in several conditions, including viral and bacterial pneumonia, extrinsic allergic alveolitis, chronic eosinophilic pneumonia, and collagen vascular diseases. In most patients, however, no cause is found and the condition is referred to as *idiopathic* or *cryptogenic*.

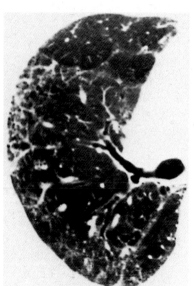

Fig C 47-1
Usual interstitial pneumonia. Scan at the level of the right upper lobe bronchus in a woman with idiopathic pulmonary fibrosis shows a reticular pattern and irregular interfaces predominantly in the subpleural lung regions.[87]

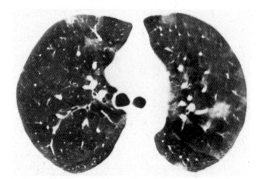

Fig C 47-2
Desquamative interstitial pneumonia. Scan at the carinal level shows patchy areas of airspace opacification ("ground-glass" density).[87]

Fig C 47-3
Cryptogenic organizing pneumonia. Air-space consolidation in the subpleural regions associated with peribronchial thickening (arrows).[87]

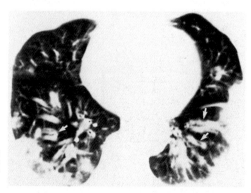

*Thickening of the interlobular septa producing a reticular, fine nodular, or reticulonodular pattern. Also thickening of fissures and visceral pleural surfaces. In late stages, coarse thickening around dilated cystic spaces (honeycombing).

Condition	Imaging Findings	Comments
Lymphangitic carcinomatosis (Fig C 47-4)	Uneven thickening of bronchovascular bundles and interlobular septa producing a virtually pathognomonic "beaded-chain" pattern.	Filling and expansion of lymphatics by tumor cells that is most common in carcinomas of the breast, lung, stomach, and colon. CT can demonstrate characteristic findings in patients with normal chest radiographs.
Pulmonary edema (Fig C 47-5)	Smooth thickening of interlobular septa.	Usually most evident in the lung periphery, where the septa appear as lines running perpendicular to the pleura.
Sarcoidosis (Fig C 47-6)	Irregular nodules or interstitial thickening along the bronchovascular bundles.	In late stages, fibrosis typically radiates from the hila to the middle and upper lung zones. Fibrotic distortion of lung parenchyma may be seen on CT before it is apparent on plain chest radiographs.
Asbestosis (Figs C 47-7 to C 47-9)	Interstitial abnormalities (parenchymal bands, thickened interlobular septa, and honeycombing) that typically have a subpleural distribution.	In patients with combined asbestos–cigarette smoke exposure, CT can play a major role in distinguishing emphysematous lung destruction from the peripheral interstitial changes of asbestosis. CT also may detect focal lung masses (cancer, round atelectasis) that are not visible on plain chest radiographs.

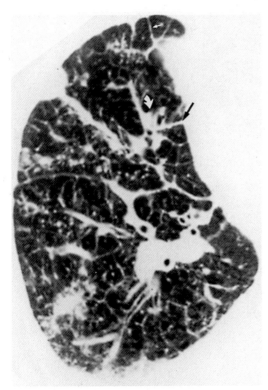

Fig C 47-4
Lymphangitic carcinomatosis. Scan through the right lower lung shows extensive abnormalities with thickening of the interlobular septa (straight arrows), major fissure, and bronchovascular bundles (curved arrow). There is also a pleural effusion.[87]

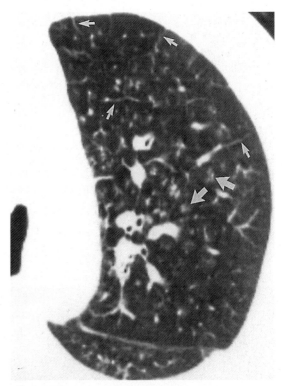

Fig C 47-5
Pulmonary edema. Thickening of the interlobular septa (small arrows) and ill-defined centrilobular opacities (large arrows). Note also the thickening of the peribronchovascular interstitium, with peribronchial cuffing.[88]

A

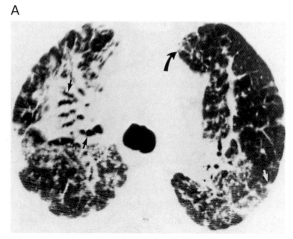

B

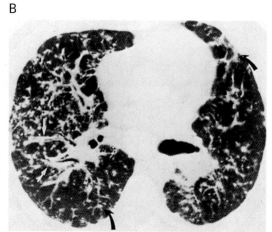

Fig C 47-6
Sarcoidosis. (A) Scan at the carinal level shows central conglomeration of fibrosis and ectatic bronchi (straight black arrows). Nodular thickening of the interlobular septa (curved arrow) and subpleural granulomas (white arrows) are also identified. (B) Scan through the lower lung zones demonstrates nodular thickening of the bronchovascular bundles (straight arrows) and interlobular septa (curved arrows).[87]

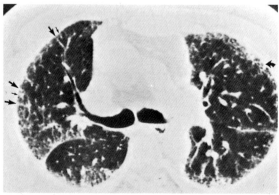

Fig C 47-7
Asbestosis. Supine scan shows moderate thickening of interlobular septal (arrows) and peribronchial (arrowheads) structures in the nondependent subpleural parenchyma. On the left, there is a suggestion of subpleural honeycombing (curved arrow). The interlobar fissures are thickened, and there is serration of the lung-pleural interface at sites of interstitial fibrosis, changes indicative of visceral pleural fibrosis.[89]

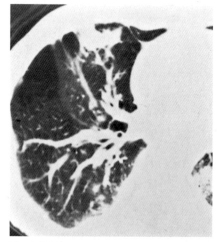

Fig C 47-8
Asbestosis. Scan through the right middle lobe shows an irregular mass with aerated lung interposed between it and the adjacent pleural thickening. A focal band of soft tissue can be seen in contact with the pleura. The mass was stable on serial radiographs and thus was considered to represent a variant of round atelectasis.[89]

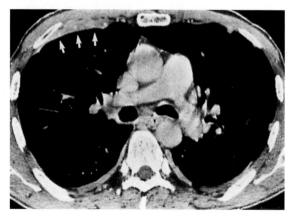

Fig C 47-9
Asbestosis. Moderate bilateral paraspinous and costal pleural thickening. Scattered calcifications are visible in the right anterior costal plaque (arrows).[89]

Condition	Imaging Findings	Comments
Other pneumoconioses (Fig C 47-10)	Fine nodular opacifications (1–10 mm) that usually are most numerous in the posterior aspect of the upper lung zones.	Silicosis, coal-workers' pneumonia, graphite pneumoconiosis, and talcosis. In severe disease, there is an increased number and size of the nodules with confluence.
Extrinsic allergic alveolitis (Fig C 47-11)	Fine nodular or reticulonodular pattern in the subacute stage. Bilateral areas of hazy increased density (ground-glass opacification) with preservation of underlying vascular markings may occur.	Hypersensitivity disease of the lungs caused by inhalation of antigens contained in certain organic dusts. In the acute stage, there is diffuse air-space consolidation that resolves to an interstitial pattern within a few days. Repeated exposure to the antigen may lead to acute and subacute changes superimposed on chronic fibrosis.
Pulmonary Langerhans cell histiocytosis (Fig C 47-12)	Small irregular nodules and cystic air spaces that diffusely involve the upper two-thirds of the lungs but characteristically spare the lower lung zones and the tips of the lingula and middle lobe.	Histologically an infiltrative lung disease of Langerhans cells. CT is better than plain chest radiographs in showing the structure and distribution of lung abnormalities. Nodules are typical of the early stages; cystic air spaces represent the late stage of disease.

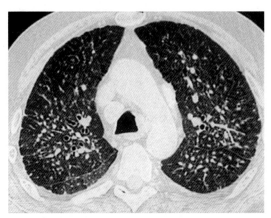

Fig C 47-10
Silicosis. Upper lobe distribution of small nodules.[90]

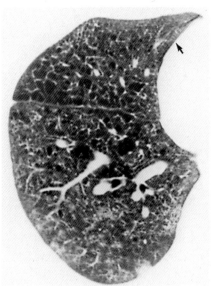

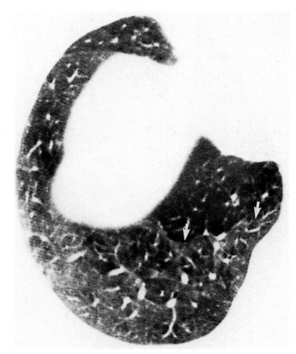

Fig C 47-11
Extrinsic allergic alveolitis. Bird-breeder's lung. Scan at the level of the right hemidiaphragm shows patchy areas of hazy interstitial density ("ground-glass" density; arrows) that typically do not obscure the underlying vascular markings.[87]

Fig C 47-12
Pulmonary Langerhans cell histiocytosis. Scan through the right lower lung zone shows cystic air spaces with thin walls. Characteristically the tip of the middle lobe (arrow) is spared.[87]

Condition	Imaging Findings	Comments
Lymphangiomyomatosis (Fig C 47-13)	Numerous thin-walled cystic air spaces of various sizes surrounded by relatively normal lung parenchyma.	Rare disease characterized by progressive proliferation of smooth muscle in the walls of bronchi, bronchioles, alveolar septa, pulmonary vessels, lymphatics, and pleura that leads to air trapping and the development of cystic air spaces. Seen only in women, almost all of whom are of childbearing age.
Radiation fibrosis (Fig C 47-14)	Reticular pattern. Often associated with volume loss, traction bronchiectasis, and pleural thickening that results in a sharp demarcation between normal and irradiated lung.	Late stage of radiation-induced lung injury, which develops gradually in patients with radiation pneumonitis when complete resolution does not occur. It evolves within the previously irradiated field, 6–12 months after radiation therapy, and usually becomes stable within 2 years after treatment.

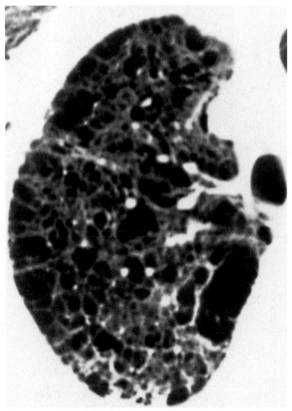

Fig C 47-13
Lymphangiomyomatosis. Scan through the right upper lobe shows numerous thin-walled cystic air spaces of various sizes. The patient also had pneumomediastinum and extensive subcutaneous emphysema.[5]

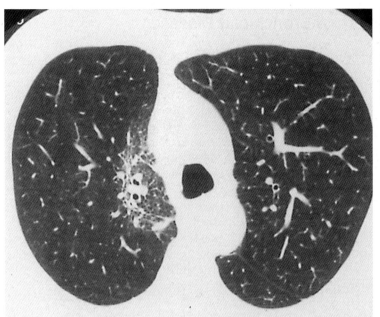

Fig C 47-14
Radiation fibrosis. HRCT performed 1 year after radiation therapy for lung carcinoma demonstrates a reticular pattern and ground-glass opacity in the medial aspect of the right upper lobe. Note the traction bronchiectasis due to fibrosis and the sharp demarcation between normal and irradiated lung.[88]

"Tree-in-Bud" Pattern of Bronchiolar Disease*

Condition	Comments

Endobronchial spread of infection
  Tuberculosis
  (Figs C 48-1 and C 48-2)
	Classic cause of the "tree-in-bud" pattern. This appearance suggests active and *contagious* disease, especially when associated with adjacent cavitary nodules within the lungs. The terminal tufts of the "tree-in-bud" pattern may represent lesions in the bronchioles and alveolar ducts, whereas the stalk may reflect a lesion affecting the last-order bronchus in the secondary pulmonary lobule. Associated findings on high-resolution CT include bronchial wall thickening, cavitation, pleural effusion, and lymphadenopathy with central necrosis

A

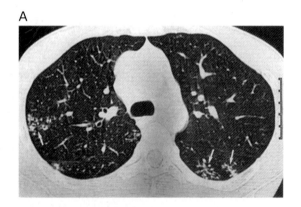

B

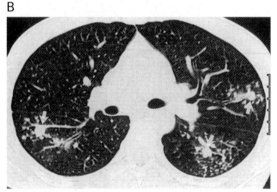

Fig C 48-1
Mycobacterium tuberculosis. (A) Multiple areas of the "tree-in-bud" pattern (arrows) in a young man from India with a multidrug-resistant strain. (B) More inferior image shows larger nodular opacities (arrows), representing extension of the granulomatous infection into adjacent alveoli. (B reprinted from ref. 62.)

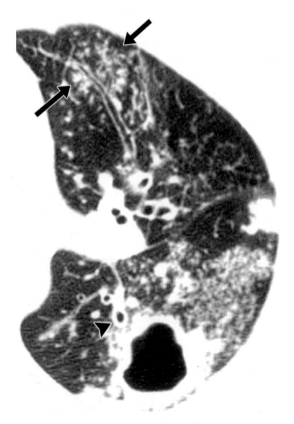

Fig C 48-2
Postprimary active tuberculosis. Thick-walled cavity and multiple peripheral small nodules and branching linear structures (arrows). Note the thickening of the bronchial walls (arrowhead).[91]

---

*Bronchial dilatation and filling by mucus, pus, or fluid, resembling a branching tree, and usually somewhat nodular in appearance, which is generally visible in the lung periphery and is indicative of airway disease.

Condition	Comments
Atypical mycobacterial and fungal infections (Figs C 48-3 to C 48-5)	May produce a pattern indistinguishable from that of tuberculosis, though without the upper lobe predominance.

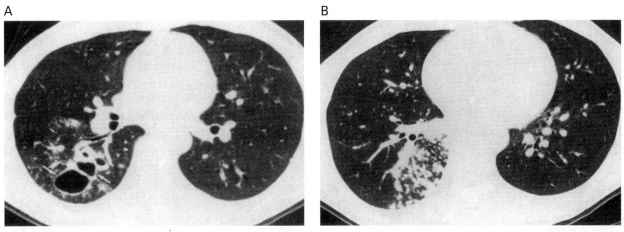

Fig C 48-3
Mycobacterium kansasii. (A) Cavitary lesions in the right upper lobe (arrows). (B) More inferior image shows the "tree-in-bud" pattern of endobronchial spread of infection. (B reprinted from ref. 56.)

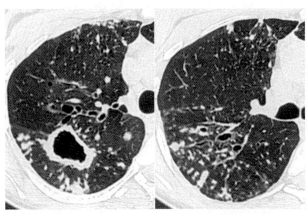

Fig C 48-4
***Mycobacterium avium-intracellulare* complex.** Multiple peripheral small nodules connected to branching linear opacities and a thick-walled cavity in the superior segment of the lower lobe. Note the thickening of the bronchial walls, bronchial dilatation, and mucus impaction.[91]

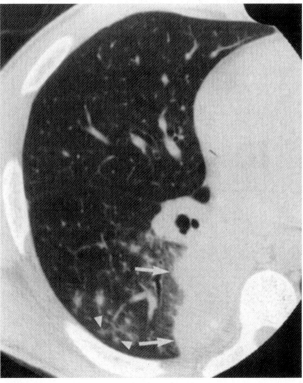

Fig C 48-5
Blastomycosis. Pulmonary consolidation (arrows) associated with endobronchial spread of fungus ("tree-in-bud," arrowheads) in the right lower lobe.[92]

Condition	Comments
Other bacterial infections (Fig C 48-6)	*Staphylococcus aureus* and *Haemophilus influenzae bronchiolitis* also can produce the "tree-in-bud" pattern.
Invasive pulmonary aspergillosis (Fig C 48-7)	Should be suggested when this pattern occurs in combination with a "halo" of ground-glass opacity in a patient with leukemia.
Viral infection (Figs C 48-8 and C 48-9)	Cytomegalovirus infection, which typically occurs in immunocompromised individuals, can cause thickening of the bronchovascular bundles and the "tree-in-bud" pattern. In infants and young children, this appearance may be due to bronchial wall thickening and dilatation related to respiratory syncytial virus.

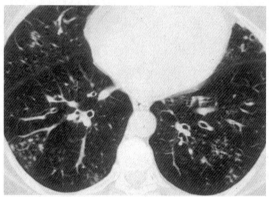

Fig C 48-6
Staphylococcus aureus bronchiolitis. Small peripheral centrilobular nodules and branching linear opacities in a patient with acquired human immunodeficiency syndrome.[91]

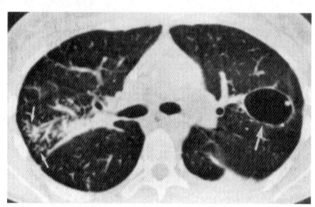

Fig C 48-7
Aspergillosis. Thin-walled cavity in the left upper lobe (large arrow) and "tree-in-bud" pattern in the right upper lobe (small arrows).[93]

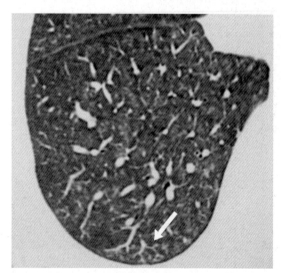

Fig C 48-8
Cytomegalovirus pneumonia. Centrilobular ground-glass opacities in addition to nodules and "tree-in-bud" opacities in a patient with chronic myelogenous leukemia who underwent bone marrow transplantation.[91]

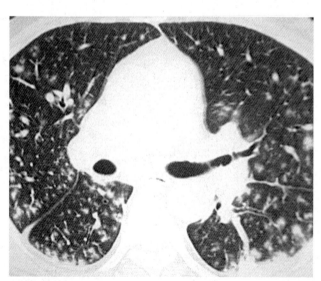

Fig C 48-9
Respiratory syncytial virus. Peripheral poorly defined centrilobular nodules and "tree-in-bud" opacities bilaterally in a patient with leukemia. Note the scattered lung nodules surrounded by halos of ground-glass attenuation.[91]

Condition	Comments
Allergic bronchopulmonary aspergillosis (Fig C 48-10)	Immune reaction results in damage to the bronchial wall, central bronchiectasis, and the formation of mucous plugs that contain fungus and inflammatory cells, producing the "finger-in-glove" sign of large airway impaction. Involvement of small airways causes the "tree-in-bud" pattern. Indirect signs of small airway disease include a mosaic pattern of lung attenuation and air trapping on expiratory scanning.
Cystic fibrosis (Fig C 48-11)	Abnormally low water content of airway mucus is at least partially responsible for decreased clearance of mucus, mucous plugging of small and large airways, and an increased incidence of bacterial airway infection. Bronchial wall inflammation progressing to bronchiectasis is eventually seen on HRCT, along with bronchial wall and peribronchial thickening and air trapping on expiratory scanning. Large amounts of bronchiolar secretions result in the "tree-in-bud" pattern.

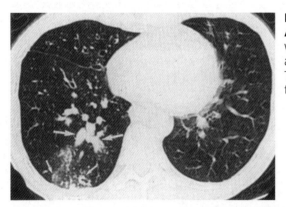

Fig C 48-10
Allergic bronchopulmonary aspergillosis. This woman with a history of asthma shows impaction of dilated large airways, producing the "finger-in-glove" sign (large arrows). There is also impaction of dilated small airways, producing the "tree-in-bud" pattern (small arrows).[93]

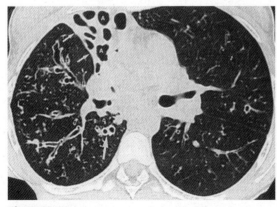

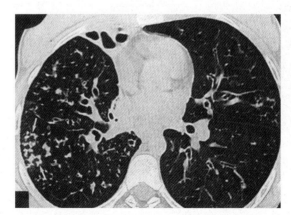

Fig C 48-11
Cystic fibrosis. (A) Dilated, thick-walled bronchi (large arrow), as well as collapse of the right middle lobe (small arrows), which contains dilated airways (A). (B) More inferior image shows the "tree-in-bud" pattern (arrows).[92]

Condition	Comments
Dyskinetic cilia syndromes (Fig C 48-12)	In these inherited abnormalities of ciliary structure and function, recurrent bronchial infections lead to bronchiectasis. Airway damage can extend to the smaller airways, resulting in bronchiolectasis, centrilobular opacities ("tree-in-bud" pattern), and air trapping.
Juvenile laryngotracheobronchial papillomatosis	Bronchiolar involvement by neoplasms is uncommon, but has been described with juvenile laryngotracheobronchial papillomatosis. Most frequently seen in adults, this condition is thought to be related to infection with the human papillomavirus. Papillomas may spread from the larynx to the bronchi and bronchioles and result in centrilobular nodules and the "tree-in-bud" appearance.
Aspiration (Fig C 48-13)	Aspiration of infected oral secretions or other irritant material can cause bronchiolar disease. In acute cases, extensive exudative bronchiolar disease may develop and result in a "tree-in-bud" pattern. Predisposing factors include structural abnormalities of the pharynx, esophageal disorders (achalasia, Zenker's diverticulum, hiatal hernia and reflux, esophageal carcinoma), neuorologic defects, and chronic illness.

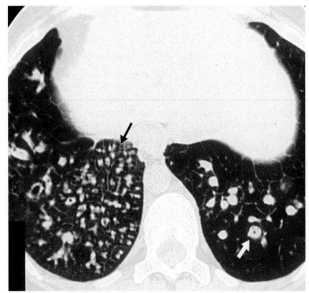

Fig C 48-12
Primary cilial dyskinesia. Bronchial (white arrow) and bronchiolar thickening with mucoid impaction and the "tree-in-bud" pattern (black arrow). Note the air trapping in the left lower lobe.[91]

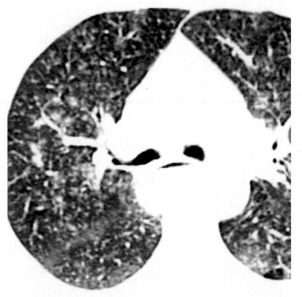

Fig C 48-13
Diffuse peribronchiolitis. Recurrent aspiration of foreign particles in a patient with achalasia. Multiple centrilobular areas of increased attenuation with a characteristic "tree-in-bud" appearance. Note the esophageal dilatation with an air-fluid level.[91]

Condition	Comments
Connective tissue disease (Fig C 48-14)	Rheumatoid arthritis and Sjögren syndrome may affect the small airways and produce the "tree-in-bud" pattern
Pulmonary intravascular tumor emboli (Figs C 48-15 and C 48-16)	Pulmonary intravascular tumor emboli are most commonly associated with cancers of the breast, liver, kidney, stomach, prostate and ovary. The "tree-in-bud" pattern due to tumor emboli may be caused either by filling of the centrilobular arteries with tumor cells or by a rare thrombotic microangiopathy, in which widespread fibrocellular intimal hyperplasia of small pulmonary arteries (carcinomatous arteritis) is initiated by tumor microemboli. Patients with pulmonary tumor emboli present with progressive dyspnea, cough, and signs of hypoxia and pulmonary hypertension.
Idiopathic Diffuse panbronchiolitis (Fig C 48-17)	Inflammatory lung disease of unclear etiology that is prevalent in Asia and represents a transmural infiltration of lymphocytes and plasma cells, with mucus and neutrophils filling the lumen of affected bronchioles. In addition to the "tree-in-bud" pattern appearance, there may be nodules, bronchiectasis, or large cystic opacities accompanied by dilated proximal bronchi.

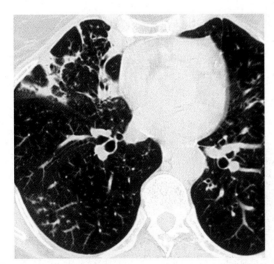

Fig C 48-14
Sjögren syndrome. Peripheral "tree-in-bud" patterns in the right lower lobe. Note the bronchial dilatation, bronchial wall thickening, and consolidation.[91]

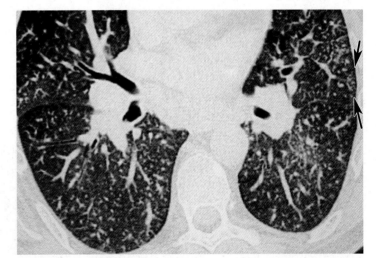

Fig C 48-15
Pulmonary intravascular tumor embolism. Multiple centrilobular nodules and branching lines with the "tree-in-bud" appearance (arrows), caused by tumor emboli from gastric adenocarcinoma.[91]

Condition	Comments
Cryptogenic organizing pneumonia (Fig C 48-18)	Irreversible fibrosis of small airway walls that narrows or obliterates the lumen. A common sequela of lung transplantation (representing chronic rejection) and bone marrow transplantation (in which it reflects chronic graft versus host disease), it also can result from collagen vascular disorders, inhalation of toxic fumes, and infection.

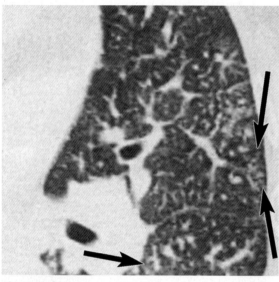

Fig C 48-16
Tumor emboli. Coned view at level of the left basal trunk shows multifocal "tree-in-bud" appearance (arrows) due by tumor emboli (thrombotic microangiopathy caused by metastatic gastric carcinoma).[35]

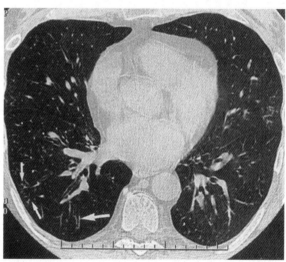

Fig C 48-17
Diffuse panbronchiolitis. Relatively mild case of dilated bronchioles (large arrow) and the "tree-in-bud" pattern (small arrows).[92]

A

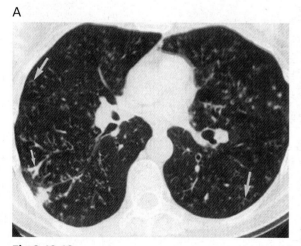

B

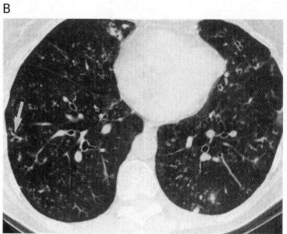

Fig C 48-18
Cryptogenic organizing pneumonia. (A) Nodular and linear branching opacities in a bronchiolar distribution (large arrows), as well as a "V-shaped" area of bronchiolar impaction (small arrow). (B) More inferior image shows the "tree-in-bud" pattern (arrow).[93]

Condition	Comments
Asthma (Fig C 48-19)	Diffuse obstructive lung disease with hyperactivity of the airways to a variety of stimuli and a high degree of reversibility (either spontaneously or as a result of treatment). In addition to the "tree-in-bud" pattern, HRCT findings include bronchiectasis, bronchial wall thickening, and areas of hyperlucency (resulting from decreased lung perfusion secondary to reflex vasoconstriction in hypoventilated areas as well as air trapping).

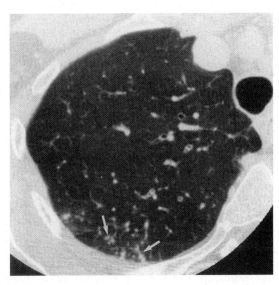

Fig C 48-19
Asthma. "Tree-in-bud" pattern in the posterior segment of the right upper lobe (arrows).[92]

Alveolar Lung Disease on Computed Tomography*

Condition	Imaging Findings	Comments
Bacterial pneumonia (Fig C 49-1)	Nonspecific alveolar pattern.	Although CT cannot suggest a specific organism, it can demonstrate that the pneumonia is more extensive than shown on plain chest radiographs. CT also can reveal a central tumor as the cause of pneumonia; show evidence of necrosis or abscess formation at an early stage; and detect pleural complications, such as pneumothorax, effusion, empyema, and bronchopleural fistula. In immunocompromised patients, CT may detect an early opportunistic infection of the lungs when plain chest radiographs are negative.
Tuberculosis Primary (Fig C 49-2)	Focal consolidation, often with hilar or mediastinal adenopathy and pleural effusion.	CT can show or confirm lymphadenopathy and subtle cavitation that is not visible on plain radiographs. It also can serve to guide bronchoscopy or biopsy.
Secondary (Fig C 49-3)	In addition to an alveolar pattern, cavitation is common. Atelectasis, lung scarring, and calcification often develop. Endobronchial dissemination of infection from rupture of a tuberculous cavity into the airway produces scattered ill-defined nodules or areas of more confluent opacifications surrounding small airways.	CT is of special value in patients with widespread abnormalities on plain radiographs, in whom it can detect cavities, identify areas of bronchiectasis, and distinguish pleural from adjacent parenchymal disease. In endobronchial dissemination, CT may reveal the cavity from which the infection spread into the airways.
Pneumocystis carinii pneumonia (Fig C 49-4)	Bilateral patchy consolidation or ground-glass pattern that often has a sharp demarcation between diseased and normal lung tissue.	Approximately 20% of patients have a more reticular pattern of disease. Thin-walled, air-filled lung cysts (especially apical and subpleural) occur in about 40% of patients and may cause a pneumothorax; thick-walled cavities usually indicate superinfection.

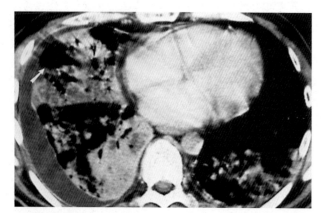

Fig C 49-1
***Legionella* pneumonia.** Central air bronchograms, abscess formation anteriorly (arrow), and accompanying pleural effusions.[94]

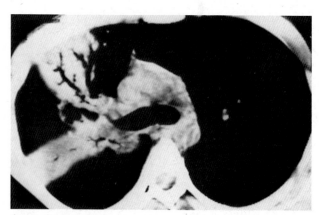

Fig C 49-2
Tuberculous pneumonia. Air bronchograms and accompanying hilar lymphadenopathy. (Courtesy of Junpei Ikezoe, MD.)[94]

*Rounded, often poorly defined nodules that are the same size as acini (6–10 mm) and can later coalesce to form larger lesions. Initially, there may be a ground-glass pattern (homogeneous slight increase in lung attenuation without obscuration of underlying vessels) as a small amount of fluid tends to layer against the alveolar walls and is indistinguishable from alveolar wall thickening in interstitial disease.

Condition	Imaging Findings	Comments
Invasive pulmonary aspergillosis (Fig C 49-5)	Single or multiple ill-defined nodules. Characteristic "halo sign" in which a zone of intermediate attenuation (hemorrhage and coagulative necrosis) surrounds a central dense fungal nodule.	More common in patients who are immunocompromised as a result of chemotherapy for lymphoma or leukemia or undergoing immunosuppressive therapy for organ transplantation than in those with AIDS. An "air-crescent" sign may develop late in the course of infection when the host's immune function begins to recover.
Other fungal infections	Various patterns of cavitary pneumonia or nodular disease.	Most frequently, *Cryptococcus neoformans*, which tends to disseminate to the brain and meninges.

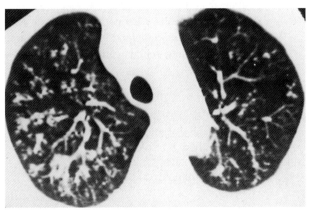

Fig C 49-3
Endobronchial spread of tuberculosis. Note the patchy peribronchial and peribronchiolar distribution of the nodular opacities. (Courtesy of Junpei Ikezoe, MD.)[94]

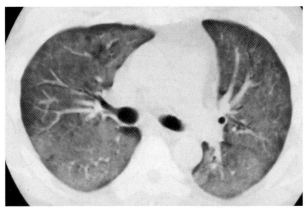

Fig C 49-4
***Pneumocystis carinii* pneumonia in AIDS.** Diffuse, bilateral ground-glass opacities with minimal peripheral sparing.[95]

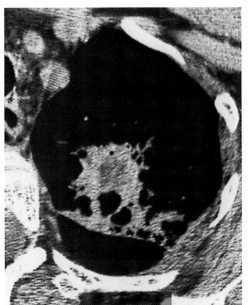

Fig C 49-5
Aspergillosis. Scan performed at the time of bone marrow recovery in a neutropenic chemotherapy patient shows a low-attenuation center that probably reflects early necrosis. The air-filled spaces near the lower border represent uninvolved emphysematous air spaces.[94]

Condition	Imaging Findings	Comments
Radiation pneumonitis (Fig C 49-6)	In early stages, a pattern of patchy opacifications that progresses to discrete and solid consolidation.	Usually limited to the radiation port, with a straight border between the irradiated opacified area and normal lung. Eventually leads to pulmonary fibrosis.
Pulmonary thromboembolism (Fig C 49-7)	Classically, a wedge-shaped peripheral opacification abutting the pleura with its apex directed toward the hilum.	May produce multiple peripheral nodules. A common and important finding is the presence of a feeding vessel leading to the lesion. Although this indicates the vascular origin of the process, a similar appearance can be seen with septic emboli and metastases.
Septic emboli (Fig C 49-8)	Multiple peripheral nodules, often with an evident feeding vessel.	Result from infectious particles reaching the lung from an infected heart valve, intravenous catheter, or injected debris. Persons at risk include drug abusers, immunocompromised patients, and those with indwelling venous catheters or prosthetic heart valves.

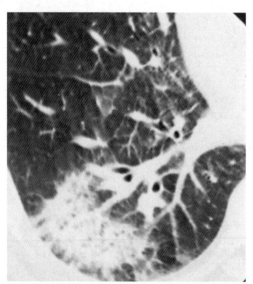

Fig C 49-6
Radiation pneumonitis. Two months after radiation therapy for tracheal carcinoma, localized air-space consolidation has developed in the right lower lobe. There is also interstitial disease that produces thickened intralobular septa centrally. Later scans showed the development of dense scarring.[94]

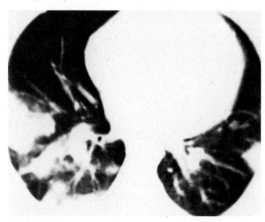

Fig C 49-7
Pulmonary thromboembolism. There are multiple rounded subpleural opacities, some of which have lung vessels leading to them. (Courtesy of Robert D. Tarver, MD.)[94]

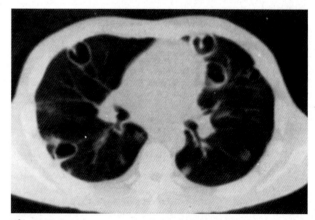

Fig C 49-8
Septic emboli. Multiple peripheral cavitating opacities. The vascular connections, particularly in the right middle lobe, indicate their hematogenous origin.[96]

Condition	Imaging Findings	Comments
Chronic eosinophilic pneumonia (Fig C 49-9)	Peripheral distribution of bilateral patchy consolidation.	Typically presents with subacute systemic and respiratory symptoms and blood eosinophilia.
Löffler's syndrome	Peripheral distribution of bilateral patchy consolidation.	Also associated with blood eosinophilia, though it differs from chronic eosinophilic pneumonia in that the air-space abnormalities are transient, resolving in some areas and reappearing in others over days.
Alveolar proteinosis (Fig C 49-10)	Bilateral, patchy, but usually symmetric air-space disease. Air bronchograms are surprisingly uncommon.	Plain radiographs may be strikingly abnormal despite the mild degree of respiratory impairment. There may be superimposed interstitial thickening that resolves after bronchopulmonary lavage and thus probably represents edema and cellular debris rather than fibrosis.

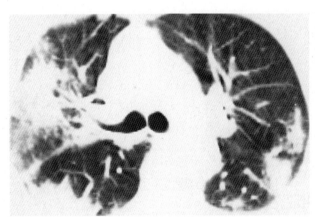

Fig C 49-9
Eosinophilic pneumonia. Bilateral patchy infiltrates with a peripheral distribution.[94]

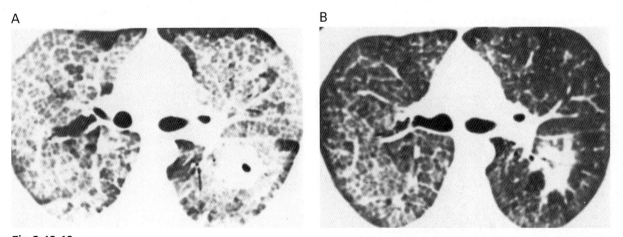

Fig C 49-10
Alveolar proteinosis. (A) Widespread air-space disease and superimposed reticular interstitial thickening. Note the nocardial abscess in the left lower lobe. (B) After bronchoalveolar lavage, the air-space and interstitial components have diminished.[97]

Condition	Imaging Findings	Comments
Bronchioloalveolar (alveolar cell) carcinoma (Fig C 49-11)	Widespread air-space disease that is often associated with prominent air bronchograms. CT attenuation in the affected lobe is typically less than that caused by pneumonia, reflecting the mucin content of the malignant cells and the air spaces.	Results from spread of tumor through the bronchioalveolar tree. Can involve an entire segment or lobe and even spread to the contralateral lung. After injection of contrast material, vessels within the affected lobe stand out against the low-attenuation background, producing the "angiogram sign" (not specific as it also can be seen in pulmonary edema, pulmonary infarction, and lipoid pneumonia).
Lipoid pneumonia (Fig C 49-12)	Posterior or lower lobe opacifications that may have low attenuation (reflecting aspiration of lipid material).	Results from chronic aspiration or inhalation of petroleum-based compounds or animal or vegetable oils (eg, in patients who use mineral oil as a laxative or who apply an oily compound to their lips or nose before going to bed).

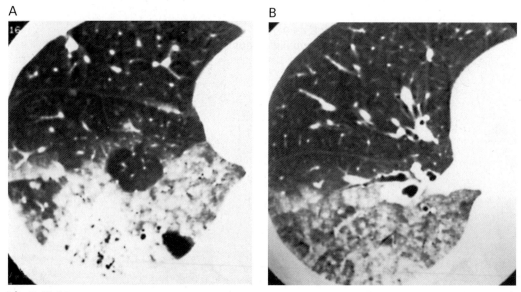

A   B

Fig C 49-11
Bronchioloalveolar carcinoma. (A) Widespread air-space filling with geographic margination. (B) Note the presence of air bronchograms. (Courtesy of David P. Naidich, MD.)[94]

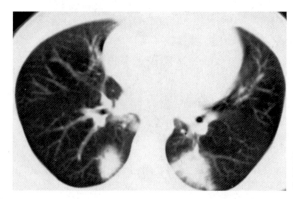

Fig C 49-12
Lipoid pneumonia. Characteristic dependent location of the consolidation.[94]

Condition	Imaging Findings	Comments
Alveolar sarcoidosis (Fig C 49-13)	Ill-defined opacifications that may be discrete or form larger areas of segmental consolidation. The pattern resembles an acute inflammatory process and may contain an air bronchogram.	Coalescence of small granulomas that results in encroachment on alveolar spaces that mimics air-space disease. More commonly a diffuse reticulonodular pattern and typical bilateral enlargement of hilar and paratracheal lymph nodes (see Figs C 13-6 and C 14-8).
Pulmonary contusion (Fig C 49-14)	Air-space consolidation that may be associated with rib or spine fractures, mediastinal or chest wall hematoma, and pneumothorax or hemothorax.	Most common chest injury resulting from blunt chest trauma. The shearing action on alveolar and capillary walls results in focal collections of hemorrhage and edema.
Pulmonary edema (Fig C 49-15)	Ground-glass, low-grade lung opacification or frank air-space consolidation.	Both cardiogenic and noncardiogenic edemas are reported to have a predominantly central distribution.

A

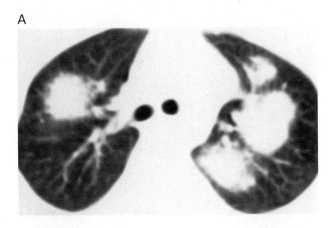

B

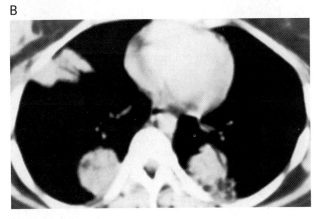

Fig C 49-13
Alveolar sarcoidosis. (A) Large central masses with partially well-defined and partially ill-defined margins. (B) More peripheral lesions with air bronchograms.[94]

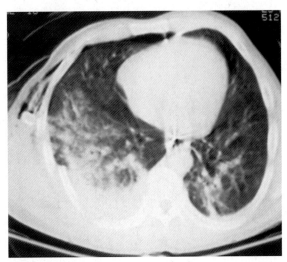

Fig C 49-14
Pulmonary contusion. There are accompanying hemothorax, rib fractures, subcutaneous emphysema, and pleural drain.[94]

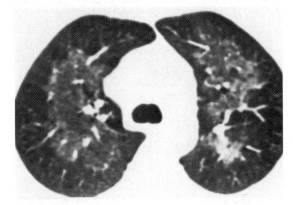

Fig C 49-15
Pulmonary edema. Central "ground-glass," low-grade lung opacification persists 3 weeks after myocardial infarction.[94]

Condition	Imaging Findings	Comments
Cocaine abuse/crack lung (Figs C 49-16 and C 49-17)	Variable degree of cardiomegaly, airspace disease and consolidation, interlobular septal thickening, and peribronchovascular edema.	Acute cardiac pulmonary edema, noncardiogenic edema due to increased permeability of damaged pulmonary capillary endothelium, and pulmonary eosinophilia.
Nontraumatic pulmonary hemorrhage (Fig C 49-18)	Widespread bilateral air-space consolidation.	May occur in patients with bleeding diatheses, idiopathic pulmonary hemosiderosis, Goodpasture's syndrome, polyarteritis nodosa, or Wegener's granulomatosis. There is usually clearing 2 to 3 days after a single bleeding episode, though reticular changes may persist much longer.

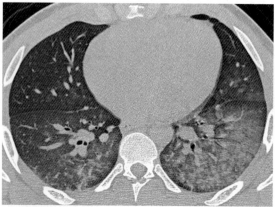

Fig C 49-16
Cocaine abuse. Acute pulmonary edema with bilateral heterogeneous opacities.[11]

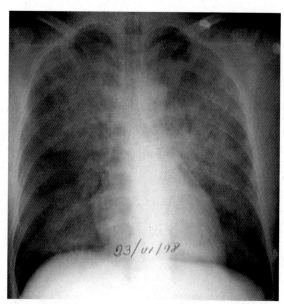

Fig C 49-17
Crack lung with pulmonary eosinophilia. Extensive bilateral heterogeneous central and peripheral opacities.

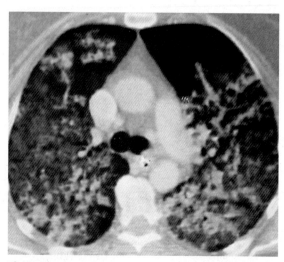

Fig C 49-18
Pulmonary hemorrhage. Widespread, patchy, and geographic air-space filling in this patient with necrotizing vasculitis.[94]

Condition	Imaging Findings	Comments
Metastases (Fig C 49-19)	Multiple, typically subpleural masses that are spherical or ovoid.	Identification of a pulmonary vascular connection to the nodule helps confirm its hematogenous origin. On CT, partial volume effects (creating the appearance of a connection with an adjacent vessel) can make a granuloma mimic a metastatic lesion if thin sections are not obtained.
Lymphoma (Fig C 49-20)	Nodular or patchy air-space disease that sometimes contains air bronchograms.	Seeding of the lung may result in a pattern indistinguishable from that of fungal infection. Lymphoma also can invade the lung directly from mediastinal or hilar lymph nodes.

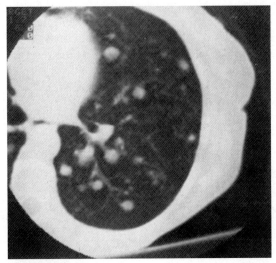

Fig C 49-19
Metastases. Multiple pulmonary nodules with vascular connections indicating their hematogenous origin.[96]

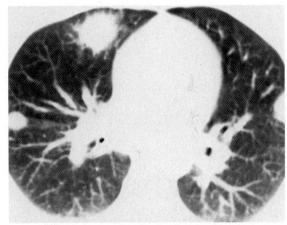

Fig C 49-20
Lymphoma. Multiple nodular opacities, some with well-defined and some with ill-defined margins. The major differential diagnostic consideration is fungal infection in this patient with Hodgkin's disease.[94]

Condition	Imaging Findings	Comments
Pulmonary lymphangitic carcinomatosis (Fig C 50-1)	Smooth or nodular thickening of the peribronchovascular interstitium and interlobular septa, with preservation of normal lung architecture at the lobular level. Hilar lymphadenopathy in approximately 50% of cases.	Tumor growth in the lymphatic system of the lungs occurs most commonly in patients with carcinomas of the breast, lung, stomach, pancreas, prostate, cervix, or thyroid. Although usually resulting from hematogenous spread to the lung, with subsequent interstitial and lymphatic invasion, it can occur because of direct lymphatic spread of tumor from mediastinal and hilar lymph nodes. Characteristic HRCT findings can be seen in patients with normal chest radiographs (which do not clearly visualize the peripheral lung regions where involvement tends to occur). In a patient with a known tumor and symptoms of dyspnea, HRCT findings typical of pulmonary lymphangitic carcinomatosis are usually considered diagnostic, and in clinical practice a lung biopsy is usually not performed.
Hematogenous metastases (Fig C 50-2)	Small discrete nodules that have a peripheral and basal predominance when limited in number, but a uniform distribution when there are innumerable lesions. Some nodules may appear to be related to small branches of pulmonary vessels.	Although HRCT may be used to characterize the distribution and morphology of lung nodules visible on chest radiographs in patients with hematogenous pulmonary metastases, conventional CT with contiguous slices is more valuable for detecting pulmonary metastases in patients with normal chest radiographs.

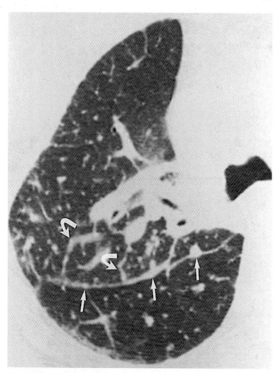

Fig C 50-1
Pulmonary lymphangitic carcinomatosis. Nodular thickening of the interlobular septa (curved arrows) and interlobar fissure (straight arrows).[88]

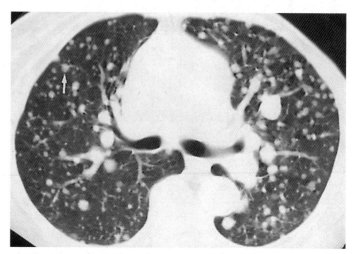

Fig C 50-2
Hematogenous metastases. Sharply defined nodules. Although some nodules (arrow) appear to be related to small vascular branches, most nodules lack a specific relationship to lobular structures and appear to be random in distribution. Note the subpleural nodules and lack of septal thickening.[88]

Condition	Imaging Findings	Comments
Bronchioloalveolar carcinoma (Fig C 50-3A, B)	Diffuse, patchy, or multifocal areas of consolidation that are peribronchovascular and contain air-bronchograms or air-filled cystic spaces. There may be extensive centrilobular air-space nodules or diffuse small nodules mimicking the appearance of hematogenous metastases.	Because fluid and mucus produced by the tumor is of low attenuation, bronchioalveolar carcinoma may demonstrate the "CT angiogram sign" (contrast-enhanced pulmonary vessels appearing denser than surrounding opacified lung). CT plays a crucial role in the initial evaluation of patients, as it can detect diffuse disease (indicating unresectability) in those who appear to have limited and potentially resectable lesions based on plain radiographs.
Kaposi's sarcoma (Fig C 50-4)	Irregular ("flamed-shaped") and ill-defined peribronchovascular nodules combined with peribronchovascular and interlobular septal thickening, pleural effusions, and lymphadenopathy.	Approximately 15% to 20% of patients with AIDS (almost all occurring in homosexual or bisexual men) develop Kaposi's sarcoma. Of these, pulmonary involvement occurs in about 20%. In most patients, the presence of typical nodules on CT and a parahilar distribution of abnormalities allow Kaposi's sarcoma to be distinguished from other thoracic complications of AIDS.

A   B

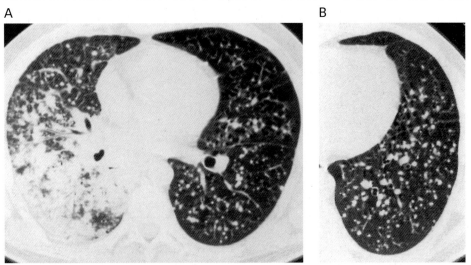

Fig C 50-3
Bronchioloaloveolar carcinoma. (A) Areas of consolidation in the right lower lobes, ill-defined nodules (some of which appear to be centrilobular), and multiple small, well-defined nodules. (B) Targeted view of the left lung shows numerous small nodules, at least some of which show a random distribution similar to hematogenous metastases. Note the presence of subpleural nodules.[88]

A   B

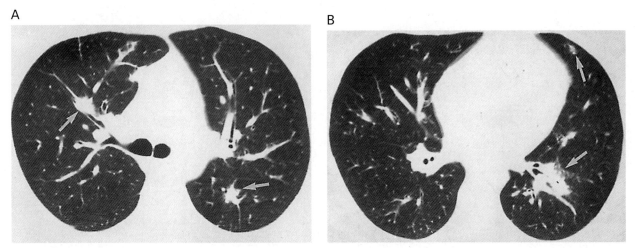

Fig C 50-4
Kaposi's sarcoma. (A, B) Ill-defined nodules (arrows) in the parahilar and peribronchovascular regions.[88]

Condition	Imaging Findings	Comments
Sarcoidosis (Fig C 50-5)	Small, sharply defined nodules that may be found in the peribronchovascular regions (adjacent to parahilar vessels and bronchi), adjacent to the major fissures, in the costal subpleural regions, within the interlobular septa, and in the centrilobular regions.	Nodules generally represent coalescent groups of microscopic granulomas, though they can reflect nodular areas of fibrosis. They may be numerous and distributed throughout both lungs, or be more localized to small areas in one or both lungs (often with an upper lobe predominance).
Inhalation disorders (Fig C 50-6)	Multiple small nodules in a centrilobular and subpleural location that are diffusely scattered throughout both lungs. In mild disease, they may be seen only in the upper lobes and have a posterior predominance.	Primarily silicosis and coal-workers' pneumoconiosis. Nodules infrequently occur in relation to thickened interlobular septa (as in pulmonary lymphangitic carcinoma or sarcoidosis). The development of irregular conglomerate masses (progressive massive fibrosis), indicating the presence of complicated disease, is always associated with a background of small nodules visible on HRCT.

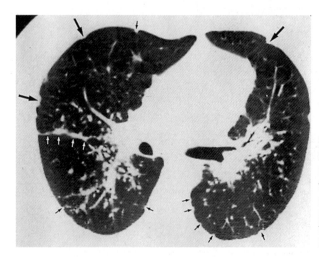

Fig C 50-5
Sarcoidosis. "Perilymphatic" distribution of numerous small nodules in relation to the parahilar, bronchovascular interstitium. The bronchial walls appear irregularly thickened. Subpleural nodules (small arrows) are seen bordering the costal pleural surfaces and right major fissure. This appearance is virtually diagnostic of sarcoidosis. Clusters of subpleural granulomas (large arrows) have been termed pseudoplaques.[88]

A

B

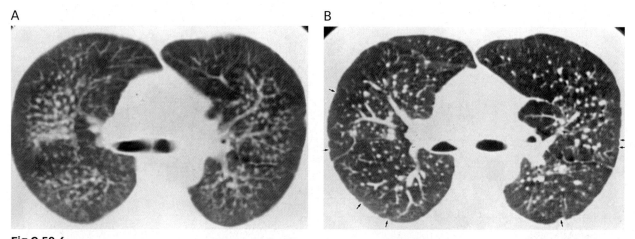

Fig C 50-6
Silicosis. (A) Conventional CT scan shows numerous lung nodules bilaterally, with relative sparing of the lung periphery. (B) HRCT at the same level more clearly defines the presence of subpleural nodules (small arrows). The nodules are smoothly marginated and sharply defined. The profusion of nodules is more easily evaluated on the conventional CT.[88]

Condition	Imaging Findings	Comments
Tuberculosis (Figs C 50-7 and C 50-8)	Ill-defined air-space nodules (reflecting endobronchial spread of infection) or small, well-defined nodules resulting from miliary or hematogenous spread of the disease.	Hilar and mediastinal lymph node enlargement is commonly seen in patients with active tuberculosis. HRCT may detect the presence of diffuse lung involvement when corresponding chest radiographs are normal or show only minimal or limited disease.
Atypical (nontuberculous) mycobacterial infections (Fig C 50-9)	Small or large nodules with areas of bronchiectasis, or patchy unilateral or bilateral air-space consolidation.	The presence of small nodules in areas of lung distant to the dominant focus of infection probably represents endobronchial spread of infection.

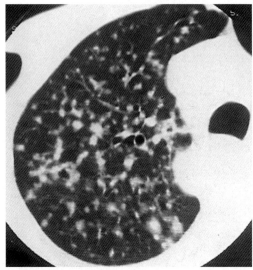

Fig C 50-7
Tuberculosis (endobronchial spread in reactivation disease). Typical appearance of numerous, diffuse, poorly defined nodules, some of which are perivascular and centrilobular.[88]

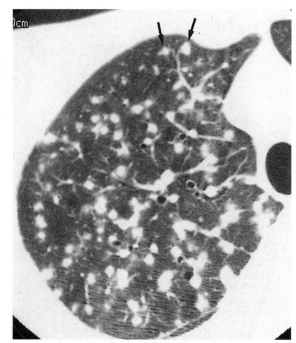

Fig C 50-8
Tuberculosis (miliary). Numerous well-defined 1–2-mm nodules diffusely distributed through the right lower lobe. Some nodules appear septal (arrows) or subpleural, whereas others appear to be associated with small feeding vessels, suggesting a hematogenous origin.[88]

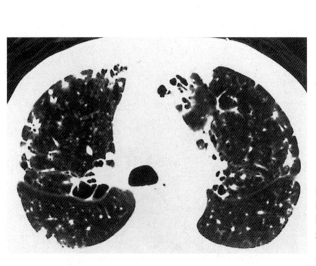

Fig C 50-9
Mycobacterium avium-intracellulare complex (MAC) infection. Characteristic findings of bronchiectasis and small nodules and clusters of nodules in the peripheral lung.[54]

Condition	Imaging Findings	Comments
Invasive pulmonary aspergillosis (Fig C 50-10)	"Halo" or ground-glass opacity surrounding focal dense parenchymal nodules.	The halo and central nodule are reported to reflect, respectively, a rim of coagulation necrosis or hemorrhage surrounding a central fungal nodule or infarct.
Septic embolism (Fig C 50-11)	Bilateral peripheral nodules in varying stages of cavitation.	Cavitary pulmonary nodules presumably result from septic occlusion of small peripheral arterial branches, resulting in the development of metastatic lung abscesses. A characteristic appearance is the finding of feeding vessels in association with the peripheral nodules.

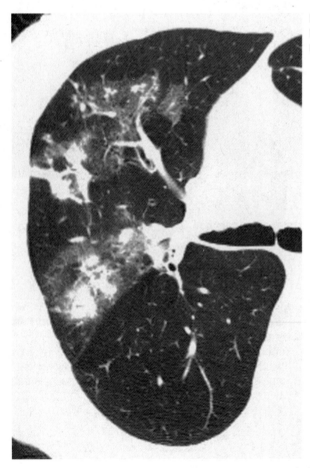

Fig C 50-10
Invasive pulmonary aspergillosis. Multiple pulmonary nodules are associated with the halo sign.[88]

A

B

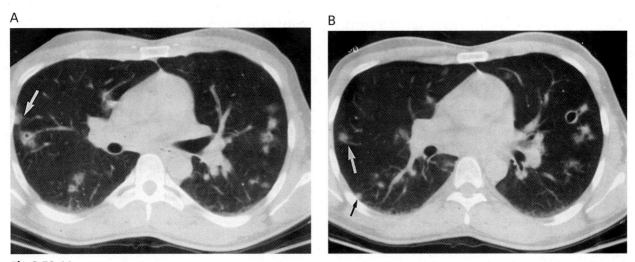

Fig C 50-11
Septic pulmonary emboli. (A, B) Scattered, mostly peripheral, poorly defined foci of air-space consolidation, many of which contain varying degrees of cavitation. Note that a number of these appear to be associated with "feeding" vessels (arrows), suggesting a hematogenous origin.[88]

Cystic Lung Disease on Computed Tomography

Condition	Imaging Findings	Comments
Emphysema (Figs C 51-1 and C 51-2)	Initially, scattered low-attenuation areas within the lung, easily separable from surrounding normal parenchyma despite the absence of clearly definable walls. With progression, whole zones of the lung become lucent, and there is often a decrease in the number and caliber of associated blood vessels.	Secondary findings that are frequently present include subpleural blebs and bullae and hyper-inflated lungs. Large bullae can compress and distort the underlying parenchyma, sometimes into bizarre configurations. CT is of special value in detecting otherwise unsuspected blebs and bullae in select high-risk populations, such as those with suspected α_1-antitrypsin deficiency or those who present with recurrent pneumothoraces.
Bronchiectasis (Fig C 51-3)	Dilated, thick-walled airways extending toward the lung periphery. With increasing severity, bronchi may become beaded and resemble a "string of pearls." In its most severe form, there may be discrete pulmonary cysts and the grouping of dilated bronchi to produce a "cluster of grapes" pattern.	The CT appearance varies depending on whether the bronchi course in a predominantly horizontal or vertical plane. When horizontal, dilated bronchi are seen along their length and produce parallel or "tram" lines. When vertical, dilated bronchi appear as thick-walled circular lucencies, almost always accompanied by adjacent pulmonary artery branches, which combine to produce a characteristic "signet ring" pattern.

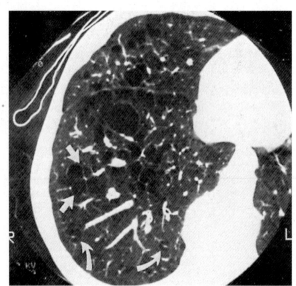

Fig C 51-1
Emphysema. There are scattered low-density cysts without clearly definable walls. Many appear to be aligned adjacent to peripheral vessels corresponding to lobular anatomy (straight arrows). Note that residual lobular vessels can still be identified within the center of some of these cysts (curved arrows).[98]

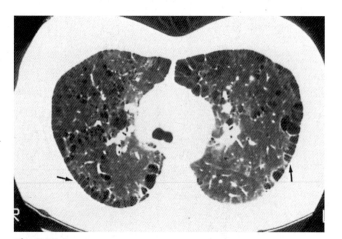

Fig C 51-2
Emphysema. Innumerable peripheral blebs and bullae diffusely involve both lungs. Septa separate individual bullae, resembling a stacked-coin appearance. These septa presumably account for the finding of prominent linear opacifications within the lungs ("dirty lung"). In addition to peripheral bullae, discrete areas of markedly low tissue attenuation without clearly definable walls also can be identified within the lung parenchyma. Note that the intervening lung parenchyma is normal and that the intrapulmonary vessels are well defined and have smooth contours.[98]

Condition	Imaging Findings	Comments
Usual interstitial pneumonia (UIP) (Fig C 51-4)	In severe disease, cystic spaces (measuring 2–4 mm) develop. In the final stages of disease, lung volume markedly decreases, and a characteristic pattern of honeycombing can be defined.	Most commonly related to idiopathic pulmonary fibrosis, a similar pattern can be seen in collagen vascular diseases (especially scleroderma and rheumatoid arthritis), pulmonary infections, and exposure to industrial inhalants (primarily asbestos).
Swyer-James syndrome (Fig C 51-5)	Diffuse emphysema (severe decreases in density of atelectatic involved lung segments), bronchiectasis, but patent central bronchi.	Presumably caused by an acute, possibly viral, bronchiolitis acquired in infancy or childhood that damages the terminal and respiratory bronchioles, so that subsequent normal development of the lung is impaired.

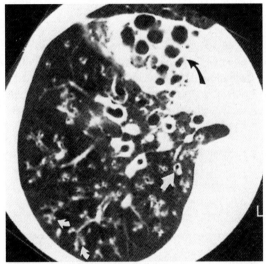

Fig C 51-3
Cystic bronchiectasis. Dilated, thick-walled bronchi lie adjacent to peripheral pulmonary artery branches, producing a signet ring appearance (arrows). Dilated bronchi within the atelectatic middle lobe resemble a cluster of grapes (curved arrow). Small, poorly defined centrilobular opacities seen peripherally represent fluid-filled distal airways (curved arrows).[98]

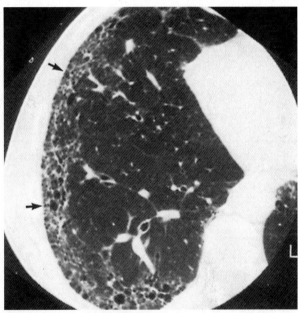

Fig C 51-4
Idiopathic pulmonary fibrosis. Coarse reticulation with variable-sized, thick-walled cysts producing a honeycombed appearance.[98]

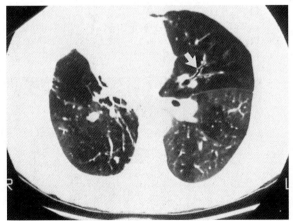

Fig C 51-5
Swyer-James syndrome. Diffuse emphysematous changes throughout both lungs associated with dilated bronchi (arrow). Sections through the central airways (not shown) showed no evidence of a central endobronchial lesion.[98]

Condition	Imaging Findings	Comments
Pulmonary Langerhans cell histiocytosis (Fig C 51-6)	Thin- and thick-walled irregular cystic spaces. With increasing severity, these cysts may develop bizarre, branching configurations mimicking bronchiectasis.	One study reported a predictable pattern of progression from small nodules, which cavitated to thick-walled cysts, and then to thin-walled cysts with eventual confluence.
Lymphangioleiomyomatosis (Fig C 51-7)	Multiple thin-walled cysts, varying in size from a few millimeters to 5 cm, that progress to become almost uniformly distributed throughout the lungs.	Rare disease of women of childbearing age that is characterized by disordered proliferation within the pulmonary interstitium of benign-appearing smooth muscle. Patients typically present with progressive dyspnea or hemoptysis (or both), with either recurrent pneumothoraces (caused by rupture of peripheral dilated air spaces secondary to air trapping from obstructed airways) or chylous effusion (secondary to dilated and obstructed lymphatics).
Pneumocystis carinii pneumonia (Fig C 51-8)	Predictable evolution of CT pattern that begins as small, thin-walled cysts localized to focal areas of pulmonary consolidation. The cysts may coalesce to more multiseptated, bizarre thick-walled cysts that frequently abut the pleural space.	Even after the underlying infection has been adequately treated, residual cysts may still be seen long after all evidence of parenchymal consolidation has disappeared. In time, most of these cysts will regress, although underlying parenchymal damage may remain.
Tuberculosis (Fig C 51-9)	Mostly thick-walled cavities, although thin-walled lesions are frequently seen in patients undergoing treatment.	Extensive pleural abnormalities are usually also present. There is no correlation between the CT (or radiographic) appearance of tuberculous cavities and disease activity.

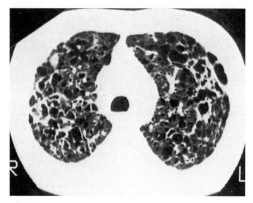

Fig C 51-6
Pulmonary Langerhans cell histiocytosis.
Innumerable thick-walled cysts of various sizes, many with bizarre, branching configurations.[98]

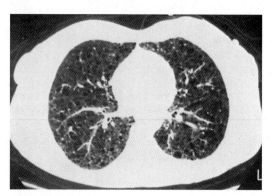

Fig C 51-7
Lymphangioleiomyomatosis. Innumerable thin-walled cysts of approximately equal size that are uniformly distributed throughout both lungs.[98]

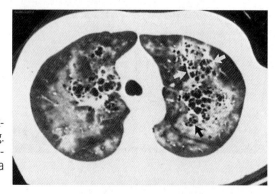

Fig C 51-8
***Pneumocystis carinii* pneumonia.** Discrete thin- and thick-walled cysts occurring in association with consolidated lung. Coalescence of cysts results in the formation of a few bizarre-shaped cysts (arrows). Note that the intervening parenchyma appears grossly normal.[98]

Condition	Imaging Findings	Comments
Septic emboli (Fig C 51-10)	Peripheral nodules in varying stages of cavitation, presumably caused by showers of infected material reaching the lungs at various times.	When seen in cross section, a characteristic "feeding" vessel can often be identified.
Metastases (Fig C 51-11)	Single or multiple cavitary lesions that often are associated with an adjacent feeding pulmonary artery.	Cavitary metastases are rare, occurring in less than 5% of cases. They most often result from primary squamous cell carcinomas (especially from the head and neck, cervix, and bladder). Less frequent causes are primary adenocarcinomas, especially those arising in the gastrointestinal tract, and primary extrathoracic sarcomas.
Sarcoidosis (Fig C 51-12)	Cystic changes in a distinctive subpleural and especially peribronchovascular distribution.	Cystic changes in sarcoidosis are usually attributed to interstitial fibrosis, leading to honeycombing, bronchiectasis, and emphysema with resultant bullae and blebs. These "pseudocavities" are lined with dense fibrous tissue, not granulomas. Indeed, true cavitation of sarcoid nodules due to necrosis is extremely rare.

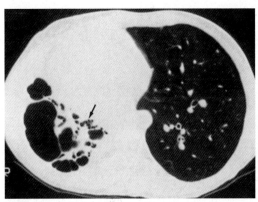

Fig C 51-9
Tuberculosis. Essentially complete replacement of the right lower lobe by cavities and bronchiectasis (arrow). Note that dilated bronchi appear to extend into some of these cavities.[98]

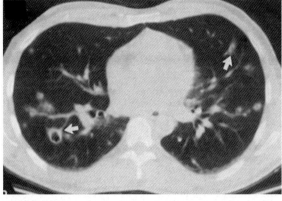

Fig C 51-10
Septic emboli. Scattered nodules in varying stages of cavitation in a patient with staphylococcal endocarditis. Many of the cavities are clearly related to adjacent vessels (arrows).[98]

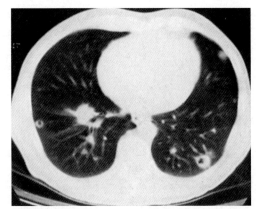

Fig C 51-11
Metastases. In this patient with colon cancer, there are scattered cavitary nodules bilaterally. As in Fig C 43-10, many of the cavities are clearly related to adjacent vessels.[98]

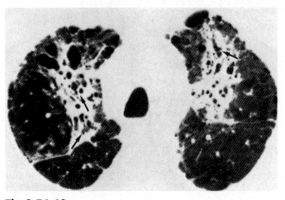

Fig C 51-12
Sarcoidosis. Characteristic pattern of bullae associated with central scarring and bronchiectasis. Note the scattered, poorly marginated nodules, some of which appear to have a perivascular distribution.[98]

Mosaic Pattern on Chest Computed Tomography*

Condition	Imaging Findings	Comments
Primary small airway disease (Fig C 52-1)	Decreased size and number of vessels in lucent lung compared with higher attenuation lung. Air trapping as evidenced by no increase in attenuation or decrease in volume of the lucent lung on expiratory scans.	Small airway diseases that result in focal or poor ventilation of lung parenchyma are the most common causes of the mosaic pattern. Areas of poorly ventilated lung are poorly perfused because of reflex vasoconstriction or because of a permanent reduction in the pulmonary capillary bed. The inciting pathologic processes can be permanent (eg, obliterative bronchiolitis) or reversible (eg, asthma).
Pulmonary vascular disease (Fig C 52-2)	Decreased size and number of vessels in lucent lung compared with higher attenuation lung. No air trapping on expiratory scans.	Can reflect pulmonary thromboembolic disease or pulmonary arterial hypertension. Regions of hyperemic (higher attenuation) lung mimic ground-glass infiltrates when seen adjacent to oligemic (lower attenuation) regions of lung.

A   B

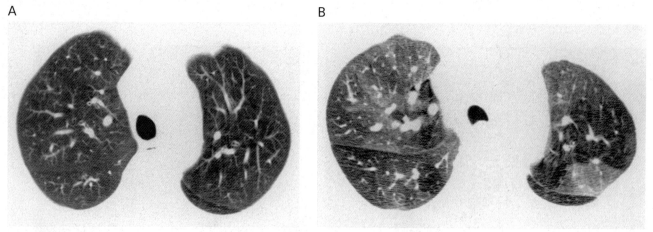

Fig C 52-1
Asthma. (A) CT scan obtained at suspended full inspiration shows normal findings, including a normal gradient of attenuation. (B) Repeat study obtained at suspended full expiration shows patchy diffuse air trapping with typical mosaic pattern of lung attenuation.[99]

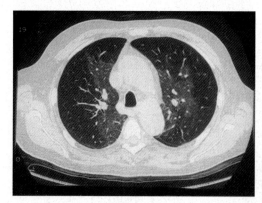

Fig C 52-2
Chronic pulmonary emboli and resulting pulmonary artery hypertension. Mosaic pattern of lung attenuation with perihilar ground-glass attenuation and oligemic peripheral lung. Note that the caliber of vessels in regions of higher attenuation is greater than that in lower attenuation oligemic lung.[99]

*Regional differences in lung perfusion that result in variable lung attenuation in a lobular or multilobular distribution. Vessels in the lucent regions of the lung typically appear smaller than those in denser areas.

Condition	Imaging Findings	Comments
Primary parenchymal disease (Fig C 52-3)	Similar size and number of vessels in both regions of the lung. No air trapping on expiratory scans.	Infiltrative processes with the interstitium of the lung or partial filling of the air spaces by fluid, cells, or fibrosis results in an increase in the CT attenuation of the affected lung compared with that of the normal parenchyma. Diseases that can produce the mosaic pattern include *Pneumocystis carinii* pneumonia, chronic eosinophilic pneumonia, hypersensitivity pneumonia, bronchiolitis obliterans organizing pneumonia, and pyogenic pneumonia.

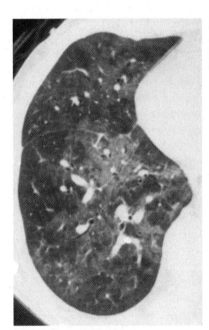

Fig C 52-3
***Pneumocystis carinii* pneumonia in AIDS.** Mosaic pattern is produced by ground-glass infiltrate that spares single lobular and multilobular regions.[99]

Crazy-Paving Pattern on Computed Tomography*

Condition	Comments
Pneumocystis carinii pneumonia (Fig C 53-1)	Common pulmonary infection in the severely immunocompromised patient. Symptoms include dry cough, dyspnea, and low-grade fever. Plain radiographs show bilateral, perihilar reticular opacifications that often progress to alveolar consolidation within a few days.
Bronchioloalveolar (alveolar cell) carcinoma (Fig C 53-2)	The tumor typically spreads through the airways and air spaces with preservation of the lung architecture. A characteristic, though infrequent, clinical feature is bronchorrhea, the expectoration of large quantities of sputum.
Alveolar proteinosis (Fig C 53-3)	Filling of the alveoli by a proteinaceous material that is positive at periodic acid-Schiff staining, associated with an inflammatory response in the adjacent interstitium. Most common between ages 20–50, it typically produces bilateral, symmetric alveolar consolidation, particularly in a perihilar or hilar distribution resembling pulmonary edema.

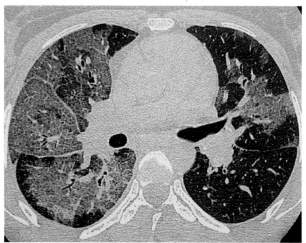

Fig C 53-1
***Pneumocystis carinii* pneumonia.** Ground-glass attenuation with intralobular lines in a young man with acquired immunodeficiency syndrome.[100]

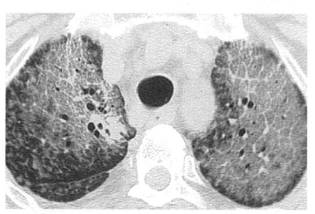

Fig C 53-2
Bronchioloalveolar carcinoma. Bilateral crazy-paving pattern and centrilobular nodules.[100]

Fig C 53-3
Alveolar proteinosis. Diffuse geographic ground-glass attenuation with superimposed intra- and interlobular septal thickening (arrowhead). Note the polygonal appearance, which represents the secondary pulmonary lobule.[100]

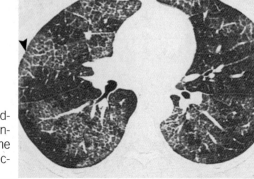

*Scattered or diffuse ground-glass attenuation with superimposed interlobular septal thickening and interlobular lines.

Condition	Comments
Sarcoidosis (Fig C 53-4)	Systemic disorder characterized by the development of noncaseating granulomatous inflammation. More common findings include irregular thickening of the bronchovascular bundles and small nodules along vessels, as well as the typical bilateral hilar and mediastinal lymphadenopathy.
Nonspecific interstitial pneumonia (Fig C 53-5)	Clinical presentation similar to interstitial pulmonary fibrosis, but associated with a much better prognosis. Involvement is usually bilateral and symmetric, predominantly affecting the basal and subpleural regions.
Organizing pneumonia	Also known as cryptogenic organizing pneumonia, this chronic inflammatory process is characterized by focal plugs of granulation tissue in distal small airways and responds well to steroid therapy. Although most cases are idiopathic, there is an association with collagen vascular disease, drug toxicity, and infection.
Lipoid pneumonia (Fig C 53-6)	Pulmonary disorder resulting from chronic aspiration or inhalation of animal, vegetable, or petroleum-based oils or fats. Imaging findings include bilateral lower lobe air-space consolidation, mixed alveolar and interstitial opacities, and even poorly defined mass-like lesions mimicking pulmonary neoplasms. On CT, the lesion typically has low attenuation, indicating the presence of lipid deposition.

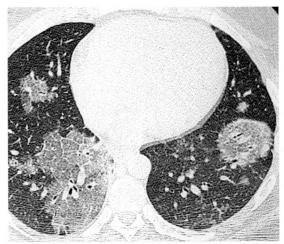

Fig C 53-4
Sarcoidosis. Scattered bilateral areas of ground-glass attenuation associated with inter- and intralobular lines in a young asymptomatic man.[101]

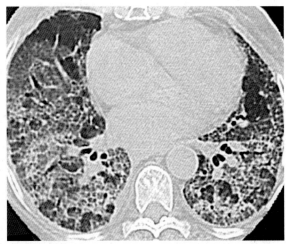

Fig C 53-5
Nonspecific interstitial pneumonia. Bilateral diffuse ground-glass attenuation and inter- and intralobular lines in a patient on Amiodarone therapy. Note the traction bronchiectasis.[100]

Condition	Comments
Adult respiratory distress syndrome (ARDS) (Figs C 53-7 and C 53-8)	Form of pulmonary edema characterized by refractory hypoxemia and respiratory distress. Underlying causes include shock, contusion, infection, sepsis, aspiration, drug abuse, and the inhalation of noxious substances. Chest radiographs typically show bilateral homogeneous pulmonary opacities.
Pulmonary hemorrhage (Fig C 53-9)	Causes include idiopathic pulmonary hemosiderosis, Goodpasture syndrome, collagen vascular disease, drug-induced coagulopathy, and hemorrhage associated with malignancy.

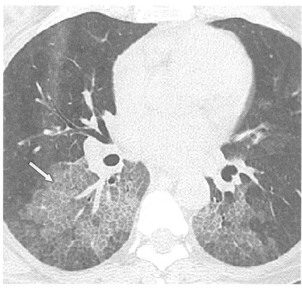

Fig C 53-6
Lipoid pneumonia. Geographic ground-glass attenuation associated with interlobular thickening and inralobular lines (arrow).[100]

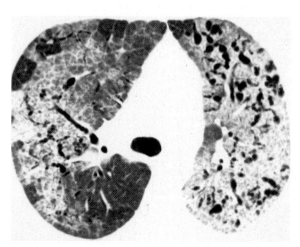

Fig C 53-7
Acute respiratory distress syndrome. Scattered ground-glass attenuation and thickening of the intra- and interlobular septa. In this young man who developed barotraumas, note the air within the areas of interlobular thickening, a finding indicative of pulmonary interstitial emphysema.[102]

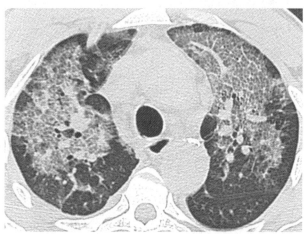

Fig C 53-8
Cocaine abuse. Diffuse bilateral reticular opacities with superimposed thickening of inter- and intralobular interstitium.[11]

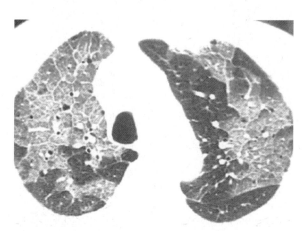

Fig C 53-9
Diffuse pulmonary hemorrhage. In this patient with systemic lupus erythematosus and massive hemoptysis, there are geographic areas of ground-glass attenuation with interlobular septal thickening.[101]

Condition	Comments
Severe acute respiratory syndrome (SARS) (Fig C 53-10)	Atypical pneumonia of unknown etiology, possibly due to a coronavirus. Beginning in Hong Kong, where it initially affected mainly medical personnel, the disease rapidly spread to nearby countries, Europe, North America, and Australia.

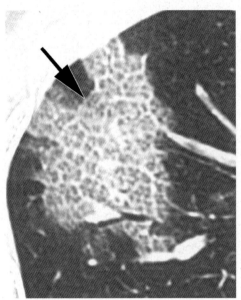

Fig C 53-10
SARS. Ground-glass opacification and thickened interlobular septa (arrow) and intralobular interstitium produce the crazy-paving pattern.[103]

Upper Zone–Predominant Disease

Condition	Comments
Postprimary tuberculosis (Fig C 54-1)	Cavitary disease with patchy areas of consolidation and bronchial wall thickening that primarily involves the apical posterior segment of the upper lobes.
Sarcoidosis (Fig C 54-2)	Predominantly interstitial abnormality that has a bronchovascular distribution on CT. Adenopathy is common, though it usually regresses as the interstitial lung disease worsens.
Pulmonary Langerhans cell histiocytosis (Fig C 54-3)	Nodules evolving into bizarre-shaped cysts that are seen almost exclusively in young smokers and probably represent an allergic reaction to some component of cigarette smoke.
Silicosis/coal-workers' pneumoconiosis (Fig C 54-4)	Nodular interstitial thickening that may progress to pulmonary massive fibrosis (PMF) resulting from long-term exposure to occupational dusts.
Centrilobular emphysema (Fig C 54-5)	Destruction of lung parenchyma, classically near the central arteriole and bronchiole of the secondary pulmonary lobule, with well-defined margins between normal and abnormal lung.

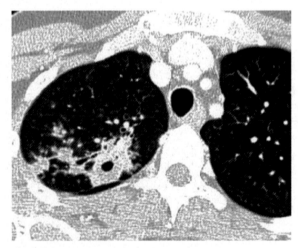

Fig C 54-1
Postprimary tuberculosis. Large cavitary lesion with surrounding consolidation involves the apical posterior segment of the right upper lobe. (Courtesy of Diana Litmanovich, M.D., Boston)

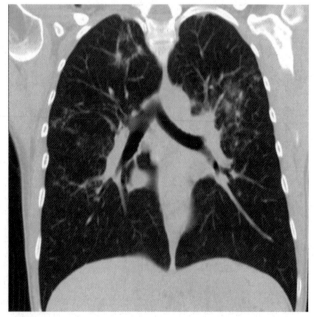

Fig C 54-2
Sarcoidosis. Coronal projection shows that the interstitial abnormalities in a bronchovascular distribution primarily involve the upper lung zones. (Courtesy of Diana Litmanovich, M.D., Boston)

Condition	Comments
Chronic eosinophilic pneumonia (Fig C 54-6)	Peripheral lung consolidation that produces the "photographic negative" of the central "bat-wing" pattern of cardiogenic pulmonary edema. Rapid response to steroid therapy.
Chronic hypersensitivity pneumonitis	Group of allergic lung diseases with various patterns caused by the inhalation of a variety of organic and chemical antigens. The most common types are farmer's lung and bird fancier's lung.

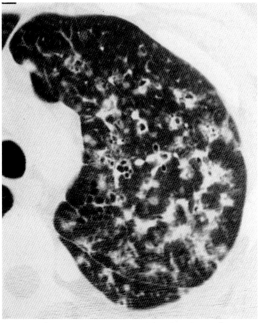

Fig C 54-3
Pulmonary Langerhans cell histiocytosis. Irregular nodules and thick-walled cysts in the upper lung. Lower sections (not shown) showed relative sparing of the lung bases.[104]

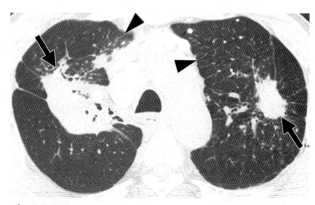

Fig C 54-4
Silicosis. Scan obtained at the level of the aortic arch shows large symmetric bilateral opacities with irregular margins (arrows) indicative of progressive massive fibrosis, as well as numerous small nodules and septal thickening (arrowheads).[105]

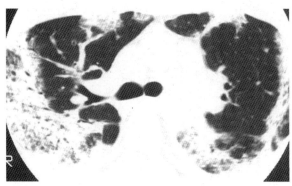

Fig C 54-6
Chronic eosinophilic pneumonia. Air-space consolidation primarily involves the peripheral lung.[106]

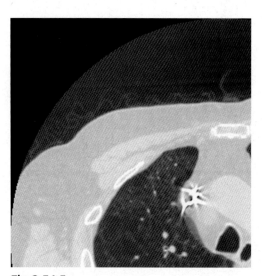

Fig C 54-5
Centrilobular emphysema. Section through the upper lobes shows subtle areas of lung destruction limited to individual secondary pulmonary lobules. The structure of these lobules, including the central core structures, is intact. Such subtle emphysema will often remain undetected on chest radiography. (Courtesy of Diana Litmanovich, MD, Boston)

Condition	Comments
Cystic fibrosis (Fig C 54-7)	Bronchiectasis that is more severe in the upper lobes, especially the right. Autosomal recessive gene disorder that produces thick viscous secretions
Allergic bronchopulmonary aspergillosis (Fig C 54-8)	Central bronchiectasis with peripheral sparing, typically developing as a hypersensitivity reaction in patients with a history of asthma. The condition also occurs as a complication of cystic fibrosis.
Neurogenic pulmonary edema (Fig C 54-9)	Edema due to hydrostatic changes and capillary leak that develops within minutes to hours of any central nervous system insult that acutely raises intracranial pressure.

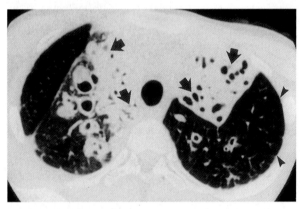

Fig C 54-7
Cystic fibrosis. Scan obtained at the level of the upper lobes demonstrates severe signs of bronchiectasis partly filled with mucus, moderate signs of bronchial wall thickening, multiple areas of consolidation (arrows) with air bronchograms, and emphysema (arrowheads).[107]

A   B

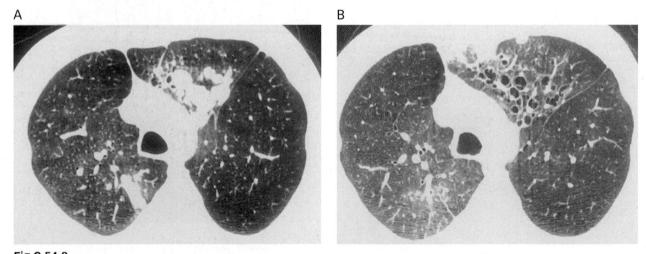

Fig C 54-8
Allergic bronchopulmonary aspergillosis. (A) Initial scan shows multiple tubular areas of increased attenuation in the left upper lobe. (B) Repeat study 2 months later shows cystic bronchiectasis in the region.[46]

Condition	Comments
Smoke inhalation	Noxious gases are concentrated in the upper lung zones, which have a high ventilation/perfusion ratio.
Metastatic pulmonary calcification	The upper lung zones have a high pH and calcium is less soluble in this alkaline environment. May result from deposition of calcium in otherwise normal tissue or in patients with hypercalcemic states, especially renal failure.
Ankylosing spondylitis (Fig C 54-10)	Fibrocystic changes in the upper lobes. Unusual manifestation, seen in fewer than 2% of patients with this disorder.

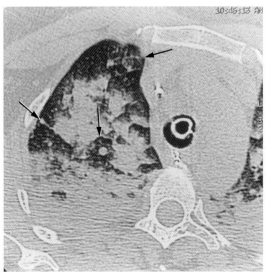

Fig C 54-9
Neurogenic pulmonary edema. Confluent alveolar consolidations in the central portions of the upper lungs. A few thickened interlobular septa are also seen (arrows).[108]

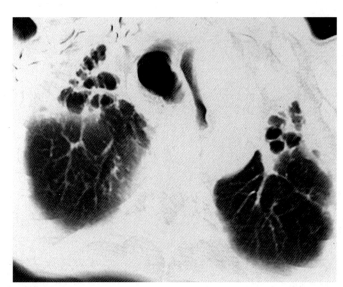

Fig C 54-10
Ankylosing spondylitis. Severe volume loss of the lung apices with traction cystic bronchiectasis.[109]

Basilar-Predominant Disease

Condition	Comments
Usual interstitial pneumonia (UIP) (Fig C 55-1)	Fine or coarse reticular opacities in the subpleural regions of the lung base. Most commonly seen in patients with idiopathic pulmonary fibrosis.
Asbestosis (Fig C 55-2)	Interstitial abnormalities that typically have a subpleural distribution, often with characteristic pleural calcification.
Scleroderma (Fig C 55-3)	Diffuse basilar reticulonodular pattern, often associated with a dilated, air-filled esophagus.
Rheumatoid arthritis (Fig C 55-4)	Diffuse interstitial thickening, at times with superimposed consolidation and nodules. May be associated erosions of the distal clavicles and characteristic changes in the hands, wrists, and other joints.
Sjögren syndrome (Fig C 55-5)	Reticulonodular pattern that primarily involves the lower lung zones. There may be ground-glass attenuation with scattered thin-walled cysts. Clinical triad of dry eyes (keratoconjunctivitis sicca), dry mouth (xerostomia), and arthritis that affects about 0.1% of the general population and 3% of older adults

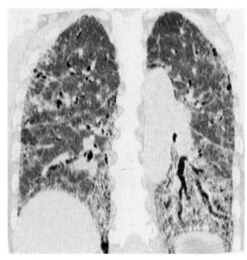

Fig C 55-1
Idiopathic pulmonary fibrosis. Coronal CT clearly shows an apicobasal gradient of fibrotic involvement with areas of honeycombing and traction bronchiectasis.[110]

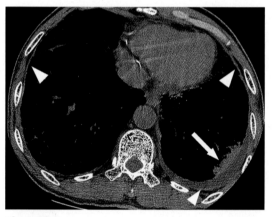

Fig C 55-2
Asbestosis. Scan obtained with mediastinal window settings shows subpleural consolidation (arrow), pleural thickening (arrowheads), and effusion.[105]

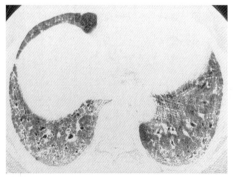

Fig C 55-3
Scleroderma. Scan obtained at the level of the liver dome shows patchy areas of ground-glass attenuation, irregular linear hyperattenuating areas, and traction bronchiectasis.[111]

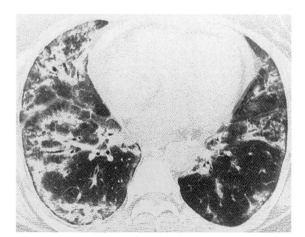

Fig C 55-4
Rheumatoid arthritis. Scan obtained at the level of the inferior pulmonary vein shows patchy areas of ground-glass attenuation and consolidation with a subpleural or peribronchovascular distribution in both lungs.[111]

Condition	Comments
Cryptogenic organizing pneumonia (COP) (Fig C 55-6)	Patchy areas of consolidation, often with nodules and reticular pattern, that may be idiopathic or a reaction to toxic inhaled gases.
Bleomycin drug toxicity (Fig C 55-7)	Often nodular pattern that may mimic hematogenous metastases.
Hematogenous metastases (Fig C 55-8)	Multiple sharply defined pulmonary nodules of varying size that primarily occur within 2 cm of a pleural surface.
Adult respiratory distress syndrome (ARDS)	Pattern varying from diffuse ground-glass opacities to dense consolidation in the dependent lung, related to a wide range of medical and surgical conditions.

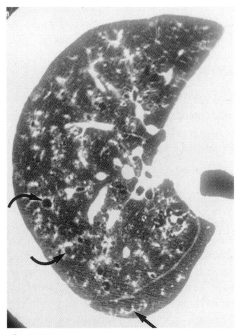

Fig C 55-5
Sjögren syndrome. Centrilobular nodules and branching linear structures (straight arrow) with many thin-walled cysts (curved arrows).[111]

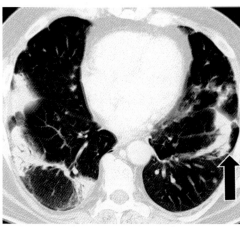

Fig C 55-6
Cryptogenic organizing pneumonia. Peripherally located consolidation with air-bronchograms. In this patient, there is sparing of the subpleural space.[110]

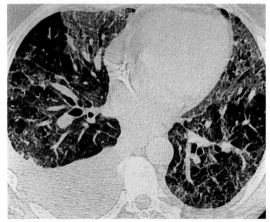

Fig C 55-7
Bleomycin toxicity. Scattered areas of ground-glass opacity and thickening of interlobular septa in the lower lungs with a right pleural effusion. There is architectural distortion and traction bronchiectasis secondary to fibrosis.[112]

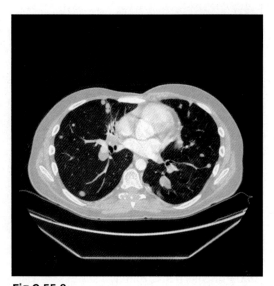

Fig C 55-8
Metastases. Multiple nodules of different size involve both lungs.

Fat-Containing Lesions of the Chest

Condition	Comments
Endobronchial lesions	Chest radiographs are usually normal or demonstrate postobstructive changes such as atelectasis or pneumonia. CT can demonstrate a low-attenuation lesion within the bronchial tree. Common symptoms include a persistent cough, recurrent fever and pneumonia, and wheezing.
Hamartoma (Fig C 56-1)	About 10% to 20% of pulmonary hamartomas arise in an endobronchial location. Frequent inflammation of the lesion can result in non-specific bronchoscopic findings similar to those of bronchogenic carcinoma.
Lipoma	Rare location for this well-circumscribed mesenchymal tumor, which has a predilection for the mainstem bronchi. Hemoptysis is uncommon, due to the avascular nature of lipomas.
Parenchymal lesions Hamartoma (Fig C 56-2)	Most common benign pulmonary neoplasm, which typically presents as a solitary nodule in the periphery of the lung. On plain chest radiographs, the nodule is sharply marginated and may contain popcorn calcifications. On CT, fat is identified in up to half the cases and may be localized or generalized within the nodule. The demonstration of intranodular fat is considered a reliable indicator of hamartoma and may preclude the need for needle aspiration biopsy.

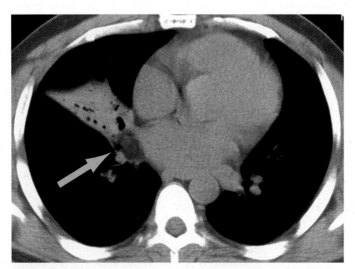

Fig C 56-1
Endobronchial hamartoma. CT scan shows a fat-containing lesion in the right middle lobe bronchus with postobstructive atelectasis. (Case courtesy of H. Page McAdams, M.D., Duke University Medical Center, Durham, N.C.).[59]

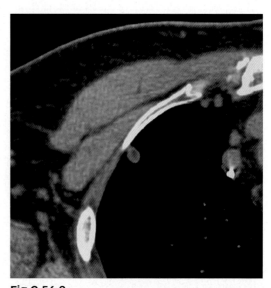

Fig C 56-2
Parenchymal hamartoma. CT scan demonstrates a solitary pulmonary nodule containing a focus of low attenuation.[59]

Condition	Comments
Lipoma (Fig C 56-3)	Although the most common benign neoplasm, involvement of the lung parenchyma is rare. Lipoma is typically detected as an incidental finding on plain chest radiographs as a solitary pulmonary nodule in the periphery surrounded by normal lung tissue. CT shows homogeneous fat attenuation.
Lipoid pneumonia (Fig C 56-4)	Uncommon condition resulting from chronic aspiration of animal, vegetable, or mineral oil into the lung. Plain chest radiographs can show air-space consolidation, an irregular mass-like lesion, or a reticulonodular pattern that most often involves the dependent portions of the lung. The characteristic CT finding is lung consolidation with fat attenuation.
Mediastinal lesions Lipoma/lipomatosis (Fig C 56-5)	Lipomas are well-circumscribed mesenchymal tumors that grow slowly and typically are detected incidentally on routine chest radiographs. They may produce symptoms due to the mass compressing of the primary bronchi, esophagus, veins, or phrenic or vagus nerves. CT and MRI can show the extent and fatty nature of the lesion. Mediastinal lipomatosis is diffuse, unencapsulated infiltrative deposition of fat that is commonly associated with obesity or steroid therapy.
Thymolipoma	Rare, slow-growing, benign tumor of the anterior-superior mediastinum that contains a mixture of thymic parenchyma and mature adipose tissue. The demonstration of a connection between the tumor and the superior mediastinum strongly suggests this diagnosis.

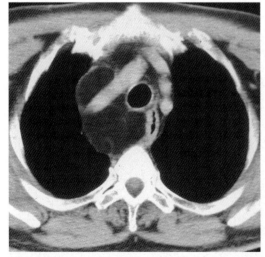

Fig C 56-3
Lipoma. CT scan shows a well-demarcated fatty mass surrounding the right brachiocephalic artery.[59]

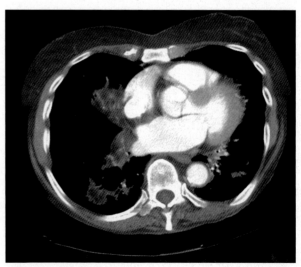

Fig C 56-4
Lipoid pneumonia. CT scan shows bilateral consolidation with low attenuation (arrows).[59]

Condition	Comments
Teratoma/teratocarcinoma (Fig C 56-6)	Teratomas are germ cell neoplasms that typically occur in young patients and appear as spherical, lobulated, encapsulated multicystic masses that predominantly involve the anterior mediastinum. On CT, the lesion appears as a heterogeneous mass containing varying amounts of soft tissue, fluid, fat, and calcification. Fat-suppressed MR imaging sequences can confirm the fat content of the mass. Malignant teratomas are usually more nodular or poorly defined, contain fat less often, and may have a thick capsule that demonstrates contrast enhancement.
Cardiac lesions Lipoma (Fig C 56-7)	Representing about 10% of all primary tumors of the heart and pericardium, a lipoma typically appears on CT as an oval, nonpedunculated mass with fat attenuation.

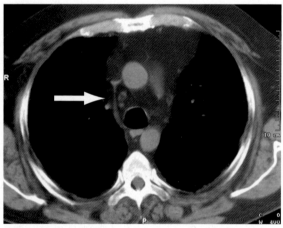

Fig C 56-5
Lipomatosis. CT demonstrates a fatty lesion with mass effect on the superior vena cava and azygos vein. Initial chest radiographs demonstrated upper mediastinal widening with soft-tissue opacity at the level of the aorticopulmonary window.[59]

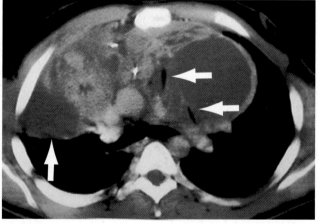

Fig C 56-6
Teratoma. CT scan shows a cystic mass with soft tissue, fluid (arrow), fat (arrowheads), and calcium attenuation.[59]

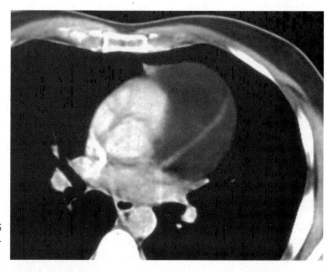

Fig C 56-7
Lipoma. Large, fat-attenuation lesion that surrounds and elevates the left anterior descending artery, a finding consistent with a subpericardial lipoma.[59]

Condition	Comments
Liposarcoma (Fig C 56-8)	Primary cardiac liposarcomas, which usually originate from the right side of the heart, are very rare. They may invade locally, infiltrate the heart, or metastasize to the lungs. MRI can best demonstrate the extent and fatty nature of the lesion.
Lipomatous hypertrophy of the interatrial septum (Fig C 56-9)	Benign accumulation of fat linked to increasing patient age and obesity. On CT, this process appears as a smooth, nonenhancing, well-marginated, fat-containing lesion in the interatrial septum that characteristically has a dumbbell shape with relative sparing of the oval fossa.
Pleural and extrapleural lesions Lipoma (Fig C 56-10)	Soft, encapsulated fatty tumor that demonstrates slow growth and may become extremely large. On CT, it appears as a homogeneous mass with fat attenuation. Extrapleural fat may produce a soft-tissue shadow that can be confused with pleural thickening on plain chest radiographs. Unlike pleural plaques, extrapleural fat is typically bilateral and symmetric and does not calcify. The demonstration of low attenuation on CT confirms the diagnosis.
Diaphragmatic hernias (Figs C 56-11 to C 56-13)	Fat within herniated abdominal contents can be found in hiatal and paraesophageal hernias, as well as hernias through the foramina of Morgagni (anterior) and Bochdalek (posterior).

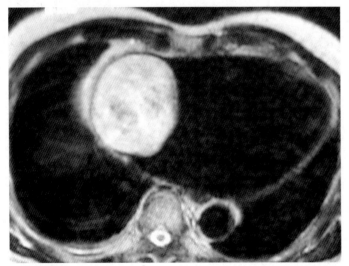

Fig C 56-8
Liposarcoma. Axial T1-weighted MR image shows a lobulated high-signal-intensity mass along the right border of the heart. (Case courtesy of Mark J. Kransdorf, MD, Mayo Clinic, Jacksonville, Fla.).[59]

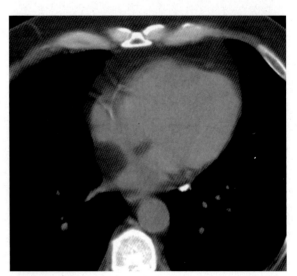

Fig C 56-9
Lipomatous hypertrophy of the interatrial septum. CT scan shows the smooth, well-marginated fat-containing lesion.[59]

A

B

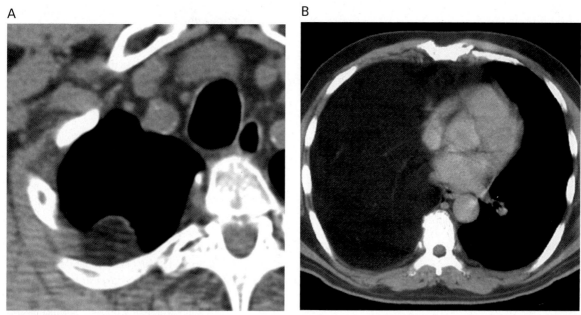

Fig C 56-10
Pleural lipoma. (A) CT scan with mediastinal windowing shows a smoothly marginated mass with fat attenuation in the apex of the right lung. (B) In another patient, there is an extensive mass of low attenuation in the right lung. (B, courtesy of James Pike, MD, Metholdist Hospital, Indianapolis, IN).[59]

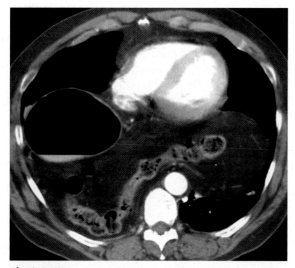

Fig C 56-11
Hiatal hernia. CT scan shows herniation of the stomach and bowel posterior to the heart.[59]

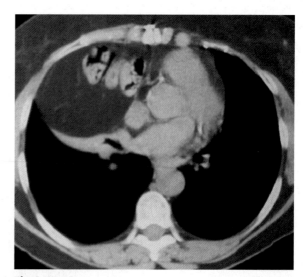

Fig C 56-12
Morgagni hernia. CT scan shows a retrosternal hernia that includes the omentum and colon.[59]

Condition	Comments
Juxtacaval fat (Fig C 56-14)	A focal collection of fat can often be observed medially, adjacent to the lumen of the inferior vena cava (IVC) near the hepatic venous confluence. It is essential to differentiate juxtacaval fat from an intracaval thrombus or tumor. Reformatted sagittal or coronal CT images may be necessary to show the true relationship between the fat collection and the lumen of the IVC.

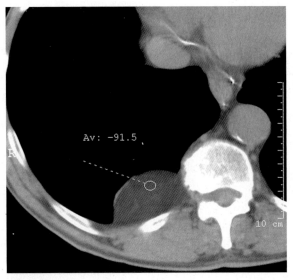

Fig C 56-13
Bochdalek hernia. CT scan shows a posterior paraspinal fat-containing lesion.[59]

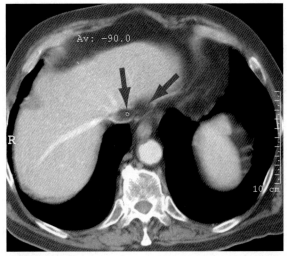

Fig C 56-14
Juxtacaval fat. CT scan shows a fat-containing lesion that appears to be within the lumen of the IVC near the hepatic vein confluence. Continuity between the juxta-caval fat (arrowhead) and paraesophageal fat (arrow) can often be seen.[59]

Filling Defect in Pulmonary Artery on Computed Tomography

Condition	Comments
Acute pulmonary embolism (Fig C 57-1)	Intraluminal clot related to an acute embolism is by far the most common cause of a filling defect within an opacified pulmonary artery on CT. Peripheral filling defects due to acute pulmonary embolism typically form acute angles with the arterial wall. A large occluding embolus prevents any enhancement of the lumen of the artery, which may be enlarged when compared with adjacent patent vessels.
Chronic pulmonary embolism (Figs C 57-2 and C 57-3)	One manifestation is a peripheral, crescent-shaped intraluminal defect that forms obtuse angles with the vessel wall. Other signs include complete occlusion of a vessel that is smaller than adjacent patent vessels, a web or flap within a contrast-filled artery, and extensive bronchial or other systemic collateral vessels. The main pulmonary artery is typically enlarged, reflecting the presence of associated pulmonary arterial hypertension. Chronic pulmonary emboli may show contrast enhancement.
Technical or patient-related artifact (Fig C 57-4)	Among the numerous CT artifacts that can be misinterpreted as pulmonary embolus are respiratory-motion, flow-related, streak, lung-algorithm, and partial-volume artifacts, image noise in large patients, vascular bifurcations, and misidentification of pulmonary veins.

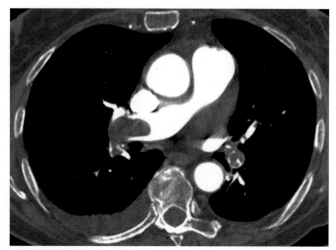

Fig C 57-1
Acute pulmonary embolus. CT pulmonary angiogram demonstrates a large filling defect within the right main and left interlobar pulmonary arteries.[113]

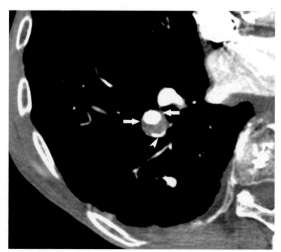

Fig C 57-2
Chronic pulmonary embolus. An eccentrically located thrombus forms obtuse angles with the vessel wall (arrows). Note the dilated collateral bronchial artery (arrowhead).[113]

Condition	Comments
Mucous plug artifact (Fig C 57-5)	A mucous plug within a bronchus, which may also demonstrate peripheral wall enhancement related to inflammation, can mimic acute pulmonary embolism. Detection of an accompanying pulmonary artery that shows normal filling with contrast material should provide a clue to the presence of this artifact. Its true nature can also be understood by viewing the bronchus on contiguous images.

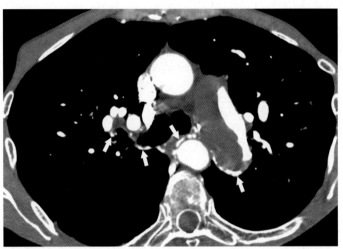

Fig C 57-3
Chronic pulmonary embolus. Extensive collateral bronchial arteries (arrows) associated with the large embolus in the main and left pulmonary arteries (arrowhead).[113]

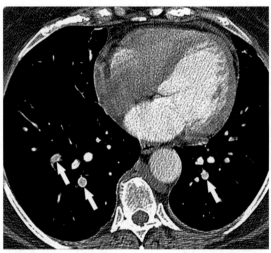

Fig C 57-4
Lung algorithm artifact mimicking pulmonary embolus. Bright rings around normal pulmonary arteries (arrows) produce an appearance mimicking multiple pulmonary emboli.[113]

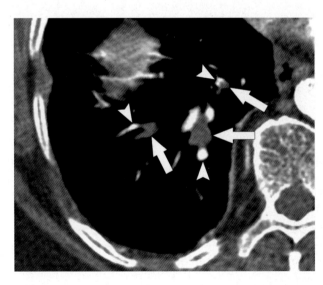

Fig C 57-5
Mucous plugs. Filling defects (arrows) that mimic acute pulmonary emboli. The posterobasal segment of the right lower lobe bronchus is dilated as well as filled with mucus. Identification of the normal accompanying pulmonary arteries (arrowheads) allows the correct interpretation of this finding.[133]

Condition	Comments
Pulmonary artery stump in situ thrombosis (Fig C 57-6)	Thrombus formation can be secondary to vessel injury, disturbance of blood flow, and hypercoagulability, all of which are present in patients who have undergone resection for lung cancer. Intraluminal thrombosis can occasionally be identified in a pulmonary artery stump. The proper diagnosis can be made if thrombus is only seen at the surgical site and all other remote pulmonary vessels are clear.
Primary sarcoma of the pulmonary artery (Fig C 57-7 and C 57-8)	Rare cause, which appears on CT as a unilateral, lobulated, heterogeneously enhancing mass. Unlike acute pulmonary embolism, pulmonary artery sarcoma shows contrast enhancement. Chronic pulmonary embolism also can enhance, but it forms obtuse angles with the vessel wall unlike pulmonary artery sarcoma, which is lobulated and forms acute angles with the wall of the artery.
Tumor emboli (Fig C 57-9)	Large emboli in the main, lobar, and segmental pulmonary arteries can cause intravascular filling defects that mimic acute pulmonary embolism. A rare cause of this appearance, these tumor emboli result from direct invasion of the inferior vena cava or its major branches by various primary neoplasms.

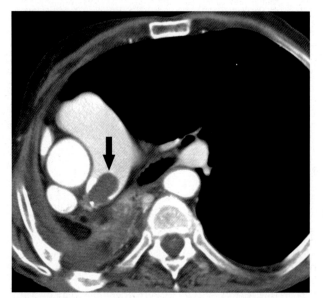

Fig C 57-6
Pulmonary artery stump. In situ thrombosis in the right pulmonary artery stump of an elderly man who had undergone a previous right pneumonectomy for lung cancer.[113]

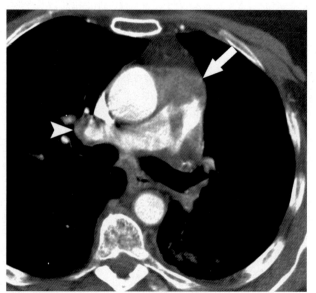

Fig C 57-7
Pulmonary artery sarcoma. Contrast scan shows a heterogeneously enhancing, lobulated mass within the main pulmonary artery (arrow). A metastatic deposit is noted within the right pulmonary artery (arrowhead).[113]

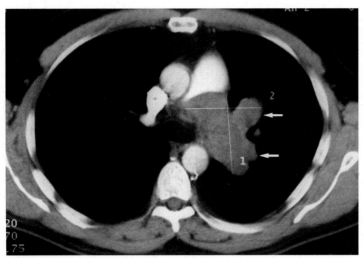

Fig C 57-8
Pulmonary artery leiomyosarcoma. Contrast scan shows a homogeneous mass that fills the left main pulmonary artery and extends into the left upper and lower lobe pulmonary arteries (arrows).[114]

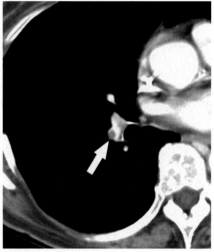

Fig C 57-9
Tumor embolus. Large tumor embolus within the right lower lobe pulmonary artery (artery) from a primary endometrial stromal sarcoma that had invaded the inferior vena cava.[113]

Computed Tomography of Blunt Chest Trauma

Condition	Imaging Findings	Comments
Aortic injury Acute aortic injury (Fig C 58-1)	Blood within the mediastinum, deformity of the aortic contour, intimal flap, thrombosis of debris protruding into the aortic lumen, or abrupt tapering of the diameter of the descending aorta compared with the ascending aorta ("pseudocoarctation").	A normal chest radiograph has a 98% negative predictive value for aortic injury, but an abnormal film has a low positive predictive value. Only 10% to 15% of aortograms obtained to evaluate patients with abnormal radiographic findings demonstrate an aortic tear. Approximately 90% of all injuries visible at CT occur at or just above the level of the ligamentum arteriosum. CT may demonstrate that mediastinal widening seen at chest radiography results not from an aortic injury, but rather from either a hematoma secondary to sternal or vertebral body fracture or such causes as mediastinal lipomatosis, tortuous vessels, vascular anomalies, lymphadenopathy, or pleural fluid.
Chronic pseudoaneurysm (Fig C 58-2)	Frequently calcified mass, typically located at the ligamentum arteriosum.	Only 2% of patients with untreated traumatic aortic injury survive long enough to develop a chronic pseudoaneurysm.
Pulmonary and bronchial injury Pneumothorax (see Fig C 58-6)	Extrapulmonary, intrathoracic collection of air that typically collects in the nondependent portion of the chest.	Pneumothorax occurs in 30% to 40% of cases of blunt chest trauma. CT is far more sensitive than plain chest radiography for detecting pneumothorax, especially in the supine trauma patient.

A

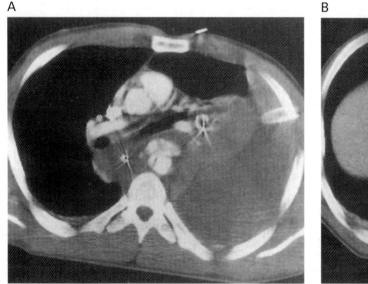

B

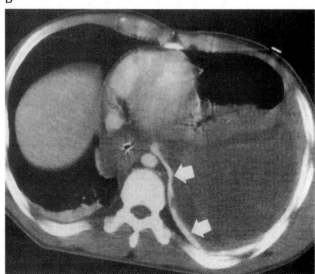

Fig C 58-1
Aortic rupture with active hemorrhage. (A) Gross disruption of the proximal descending aorta with periaortic hematoma. Note the large hemothorax. (B) Scan obtained 7 cm caudad demonstrates active bleeding with extravasation of contrast material into the left pleural space (arrows).[115]

Condition	Imaging Findings	Comments
Pulmonary parenchymal injury		Focal parenchymal injury consisting of edema and interstitial and alveolar hemorrhage, seen in approximately 30% to 70% of patients with blunt chest trauma.
Contusion (see Fig C 58-3)	Poorly defined local area of consolidation, usually in the lung periphery adjacent to the area of trauma.	Traumatic disruption of alveolar spaces with formation of a cavity filled with blood or air. Small lacerations are visible on CT in the majority of patients in whom only contusion is evident at chest radiography.
Laceration (Fig C 58-3)	Localized air collection in an area of consolidation. May be single or multiple, unilateral or bilateral.	Traumatic blood-filled lung cyst. Can persist and result in a traumatic pneumatocele as the hemorrhage resolves.

A

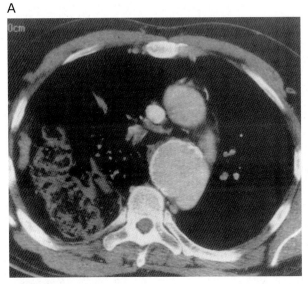

B

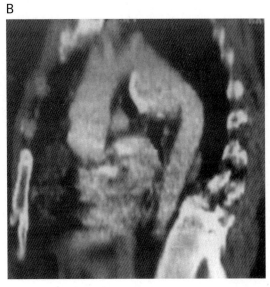

Fig C 58-2
Chronic pseudoaneurysm. The patient had been involved in a motor vehicle accident 32 years earlier. (A) Axial scan shows a large calcified pseudoaneurysm of the proximal descending aorta. Note also the ruptured right hemidiaphragm with herniation of large bowel into the chest. (B) Sagittal reformatted image shows the calcified pseudoaneurysm in the characteristic location just distal to the left subclavian artery.[115]

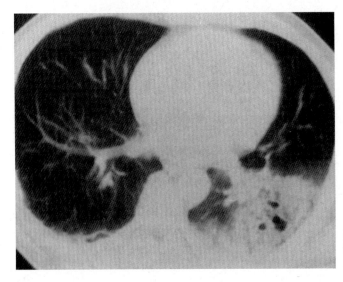

Fig C 58-3
Pulmonary laceration. Multiple small cavities within an area of pulmonary contusion.[115]

Condition	Imaging Findings	Comments
Hematoma (Fig C 58-4)	Well-circumscribed, round area of increased attenuation.	A major clue to tracheal tears on both radiographs and CT is abnormality in the appearance or position of the endotracheal tube. This includes overdistention of the cuff of the tube, protrusion of the tube wall beyond the expected margins of the tracheal lumen, and extraluminal position of the tip of the tube.
Tracheal tear (Fig C 58-5)	Tracheal transactions in the cervical region produce extensive subcutaneous air, and elevation of the hyoid bone (above the level of the C3 vertebral body) or the greater cornu (<2 cm from the angle of the mandible).	Uncommon injury that tends to occur within 2.5 cm of the carina, most often on the right. Associated fractures of the upper thorax, including the first three ribs, clavicle, sternum, and scapula, are seen in about 40% of patients with tracheobronchial injuries. Fallen lung sign is thought to be caused by disruption of the normal hilar attachments of the lung, which leads the collapsed lung to droop peripherally rather than centrally adjacent to the spine.

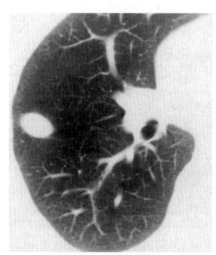

Fig C 58-4
Pulmonary hematoma. Focal, well-circumscribed nodular opacity in the right upper lobe.[115]

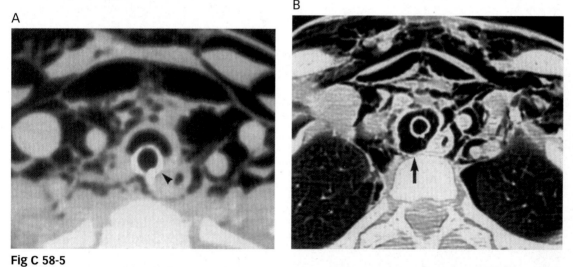

Fig C 58-5
Tracheal tear. (A, B) Eccentric placement of an endotracheal tube with respect to the tracheal ring (arrowhead in A) and disruption of the posterior wall of the trachea (arrow in B). There is extensive subcutaneous air in A, and a small left pneumothorax in B. At surgery, there were three ruptured cartilage rings and a long tear in the posterior tracheal wall.[116]

Condition	Imaging Findings	Comments
Bronchial tear (Fig C 58-6)	Persistent pneumothorax despite adequate placement of one or more chest tubes, massive and increasing subcutaneous emphysema and pneumomediastinum, focal peribronchial collections of air, discontinuity of the bronchial wall, and the "fallen lung" sign (collapsed lung or lobe falling away from the hilum).	Disruption of the diaphragm occurs in 1% to 8% of patients who survive major blunt injury to the chest or abdomen. Chest radiographic findings are abnormal in more than 75%, but are so nonspecific that the diagnosis is initially missed in the majority of cases. The mortality rate in unrecognized cases is 30%, with death occurring from delayed herniation of abdominal viscera and bowel strangulation. Sagittal and coronal reformatted images are superior to axial scans for detecting a diaphragmatic tear and herniation of abdominal contents into the thorax.
Diaphragmatic tear (Figs C 58-7 through C 58-9)	Focal discontinuity of the diaphragm (usually posterolateral, with 75–90% on the left); herniation of peritoneal fat, bowel, or abdominal organs into the chest; focal constriction of bowel or stomach as it projects through the diaphragm ("collar sign"); inability to visualize the diaphragm ("absent diaphragm sign").	More than 80% occur in the cervical and upper thoracic esophagus, most likely secondary to compression of the esophagus between the sternum and spinal column. Distal esophageal tears generally occur just above the gastroesophageal junction along the posterolateral wall on the left, with a mechanism probably similar to that in spontaneous rupture (Boerhaave syndrome) when esophageal pressures rise against a closed glottis. High mortality rate due to rapidly developing mediastinitis, unless the esophageal injury is recognized and treated within 24 hours.

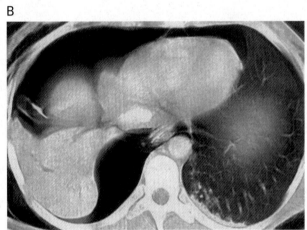

Fig C 58-6
Bronchial tear. (A) Extensive right lung contusion and a large pneumothorax despite multiple chest tubes. The tip of the right chest tube is intraparenchymal. Abnormal focal air collections are noted around the bronchus intermedius, and the wall of the bronchus is disrupted (arrow). (B) Scan obtained at a lower level demonstrates the fallen lung sign. The large right pneumothorax and small left pneumothorax are seen.[116]

Condition	Imaging Findings	Comments
Esophageal rupture	Focal extraluminal air at the site of the tear and hematoma in the mediastinum or in the esophageal wall.	Also plain chest radiographic findings of large left pneumothorax, extensive pneumomediastinum, subcutaneous emphysema, left pleural effusion and lower lobe atelectasis, and the "V sign" of Naclerio (extrapleural air within the lower mediastinum and between the parietal pleura and the diaphragm, which forms a V shape, usually on the left).
Fracture Rib (Fig C 58-10)	Best seen on bone window settings and images reformatted with an edge-enhancing algorithm. Often, associated hemothorax, pneumothorax, subcutaneous emphysema, pulmonary contusion, and soft-tissue hematomas (indicating an underlying rib injury).	Occur in approximately 60% of victims of blunt chest trauma, though only about 20% are detected on portable chest films. A fracture of the first rib indicates severe blunt chest trauma and may be associated with an aortic or bronchial tear and injury to the subclavian vessels. Fractures of five or more ribs in a row or three or more segmental rib fractures (ie, two fractures in one rib) is defined as a flail chest, which must be recognized promptly as respiratory failure may develop because of paradoxical movement of the flail segment.

A

B

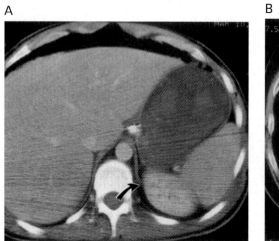
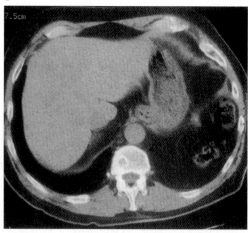

Fig C 58-7
Diaphragmatic tear. (A) Abrupt discontinuity of the left hemidiaphragm (arrow). (B) Absence of the left hemidiaphragm.[115]

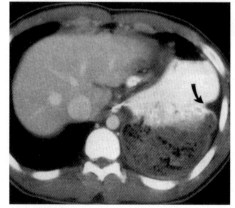

Fig C 58-8
Diaphragmatic tear (collar sign). Focal indentation of the greater curvature of the stomach (arrow).[115]

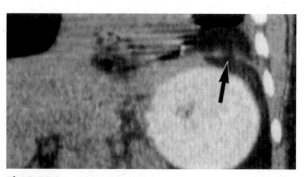

Fig C 58-9
Diaphragmatic tear. Coronal reformatted image demonstrates omental fat herniated through a diaphragmatic defect (arrow).[115]

Condition	Imaging Findings	Comments
Sternum (Fig C 58-11)	Fracture is often associated with a retrosternal mediastinal hematoma with preservation of the fat plane between the hematoma and the aorta (implying that it is not aortic in origin).	Most fractures occur within 2 cm of the manubrial-sternal junction. The fracture usually is not evident on AP portable chest radiographs but obvious at CT.
Thoracic spine (Fig C 58-12)	Paraspinal hematoma associated with disruption or fracture of the vertebral body, pedicle, or spinous process. Mediastinal hematoma confined to the posterior mediastinum is a valuable clue.	Most vulnerable portion is at the thoracoabdominal junction (T9-T11 vertebral bodies). An anterior wedge compression is usually stable, whereas a burst fracture is not. A high percentage of patients with thoracic spine fractures have spinal cord injuries, and many have associated sternal fractures. Only half of thoracic spine fractures are identified on the initial chest radiographs. Compression fractures may be easily overlooked on axial CT scans unless they are displayed with bone windows; sagittal and reformatted images can confirm a simple compression.

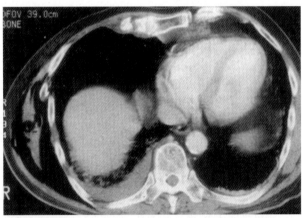

Fig C 58-10
Rib fracture. Displaced fracture with extensive subcutaneous emphysema. There is also a sternal fracture with associated retrosternal hematoma.[115]

Fig C 58-11
Sternal fracture. Midline sternal fracture with an adjacent anterior mediastinal hematoma. Note the preserved fat plane between the hematoma and the great vessels.[115]

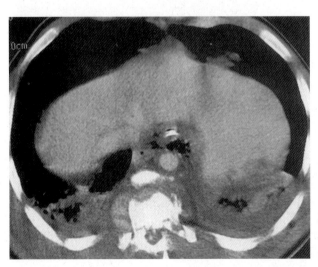

Fig C 58-12
Thoracic spine fracture. Burst fracture of T10 with obliteration of the spinal canal by bone fragments. Note the associated pneumomediastinum and bilateral pleural effusions.[116]

Abnormality of the Cardiophrenic Space on Computed Tomography or Magnetic Resonance Imaging

Condition	Comments
Normal variant Cardiac fat pad (Fig C 59-1)	Large collection of pericardial fat can simulate a neoplastic mass. Recent studies have related the volume of pericardial fat to a possible increase in the risk of cardiovascular disease. The absence of soft-tissue components aids in differentiating prominent fat from benign or malignant fat-containing tumors.
Congenital absence of the pericardium	Infrequent, asymptomatic condition that can be associated with congenital heart disease. When there is associated agenesis of the sternopericardial ligament, the space between the heart and the chest wall can be larger than normal.
Fat-containing lesions Diaphragmatic hernia (Fig C 59-2)	Related to a traumatic, postoperative, or congenital (the most common) origin, herniated fat and other abdominal structures can simulate a tumor in the cardipphrenic space. The presence of air within herniated intestinal loops is pathognomonic. If only omental fat has herniated, it may be difficult to differentiate from lipoma or liposarcoma. The detection of linear opacities corresponding to omental vessels favors the diagnosis of diaphragmatic hernia.

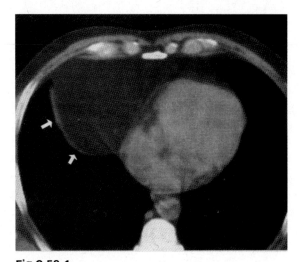

Fig C 59-1
Pericardial fat pad. CT scan shows a large pericardial fat pad (arrows) that simulated a cardiophrenic mass on plain radiographs.[117]

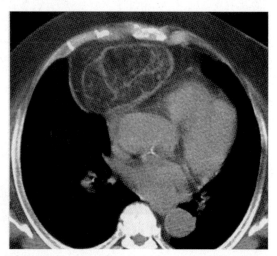

Fig C 59-2
Morgagni hernia. CT scan shows a well-defined fatty mass with numerous omental vessels and fatty infiltration.[117]

Condition	Comments
Pericardial fat necrosis (Fig C 59-3)	Uncommon benign condition that manifests as acute pleuritic chest pain in a previously healthy person. On CT, it appears as an encapsulated fatty lesion with inflammatory changes such as dense strands and thickening of the adjacent pericardium. Follow-up studies show spontaneous improvement or resolution of the findings. Like the pathologically similar fat necrosis in epiploic appendagitis, conservative treatment is indicated for this benign, self-limiting process.
Tumor (Fig C 59-4)	Lipoma and liposarcoma are uncommon tumors in this region and tend to simulate Morgagni hernia. At times, these entities can only be differentiated by demonstrating the diaphragmatic defect associated with the hernia. Thymolipoma may occasionally descend along the mediastinum and occupy the cardiophrenic space. The demonstration of an anatomic connection to the thymic bed may be required to differentiate this from a teratoma.
Cystic lesions Pericardial cyst (Fig C 59-5)	Fluid-filled lesion with well-defined borders, smooth walls, and no contrast enhancement. This asymptomatic and benign condition is usually detected as an incidental finding on plain chest radiographs.
Thymic tumor	Although usually a solid lesion, it infrequently has predominantly cystic contents.
Hydatid cyst (Fig C 59-6)	An echinococcal cyst of the liver can rarely herniate through the foramen of Morgagni.

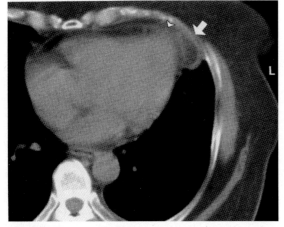

Fig C 59-3
Pericardial fat necrosis. CT scan shows an encapsulated fatty lesion with mild stranding in the left cardiophrenic space (arrow). Arrowhead = associated local pericardial thickening.[117]

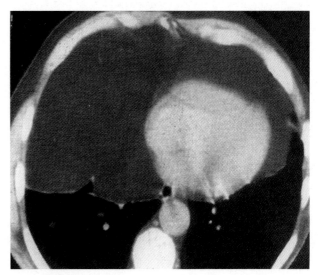

Fig C 59-4
Thymolipoma. CT scan shows a large fatty mass that wraps around the heart.[117]

Condition	Comments
Solid lesions	
Lymphoma (Fig C 59-7)	Most frequent cause of lympadenopathy in this location, which is often overlooked on chest radiographs. The peridiaphragmatic region has a rich lymphatic drainage system, and small (<8 mm) physiologic lymph nodes can normally be visualized in the cardiophrenic space.
Lymphatic metastases (Figs C 59-8 and C 59-9)	In most cases, lymphadenopathy is a sign of distant dissemination from primary tumors located either above or below the diaphragm. Involvement of lymph nodes in the internal mammary chain suggests a metastatic origin regardless of the size. Lung cancer and pleural mesothelioma are the chest tumors that most commonly affect the cardiophrenic space by lymphatic dissemination.

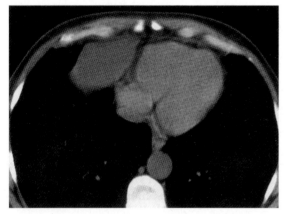

Fig C 59-5
Pleuropericardial cyst. Thin-walled, sharply defined, oval, homogeneous mass with attenuation near that of water.[117]

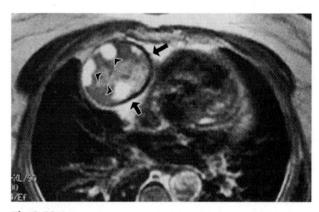

Fig C 59-6
Herniated hydatid cyst. T2-weighted MR image shows a well-defined lesion with a partially calcified wall (arrows) and small cystic lesions within it (arrowhead).[117]

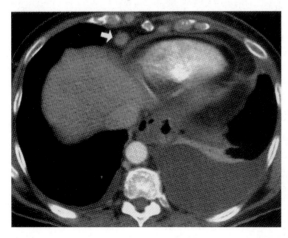

Fig C 59-7
Lymphoma. Lymph node (arrow) in the right cardiophrenic space. Note the associated pericardial and pleural effusions.[117]

Condition	Comments
Thymoma (Fig C 59-10)	Both benign and malignant thymic tumors can be located at the base of the heart and appear as solid or mixed lesions in the cardiophrenic space. The demonstration of a connection between the lesion and the superior mediastinum strongly suggests this diagnosis.
Miscellaneous lesions Abscess	In addition to herniated intestinal loops, the presence of gas within a lesion in the cardiophrenic space may be a manifestation of an abscess caused by a gas-producing microorganism.
Esophageal surgery (Fig C 59-11)	Colonic interposition for esophageal cancer may appear as a gas-containing structure at the base of the anterior mediastinum.

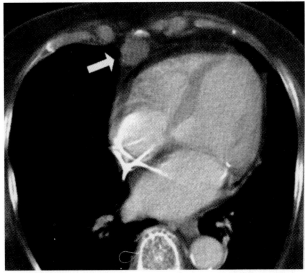

Fig C 59-8
Lymphatic metastases. Lymph node in the right cardiophrenic space from a primary ovarian carcinoma.[117]

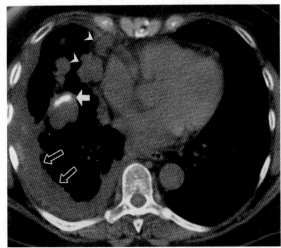

Fig C 59-9
Lymphatic metastases. Multiple nodes in the cardiophrenic space (arrowheads) secondary to metastases from pleural mesothelioma. Note the pleural thickening (open arrows). The pleural calcifications in the right major fissure (solid arrow) are due to previous asbestos exposure.[117]

Condition	Comments
Vascular disorder (Fig C 59-12)	In patients with portal hypertension, collateral circulation may result in cardiophrenic space varices that appear as tortuous tubular structures. Normal vessels in this region may also become substantially dilated secondary to occlusion of the superior vena cava and azygos vein.

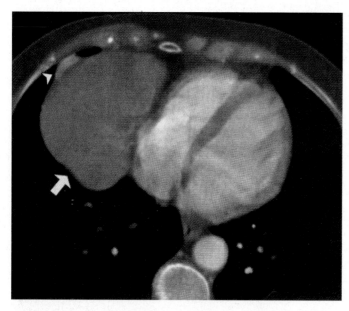

Fig C 59-10
Thymoma. Well-defined mass of soft-tissue attenuation (arrow) in the anterior mediastinum. Note the adjacent compressed lung (arrowhead).[117]

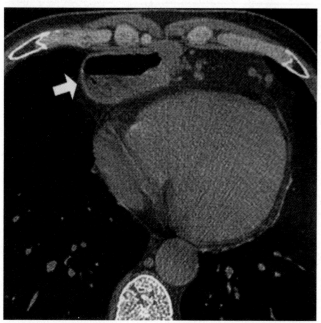

Fig C 59-11
Colonic interposition. The interposed colon (arrow) in the right cardiophrenic space represents a postoperative appearance following surgery for esophageal cancer.[117]

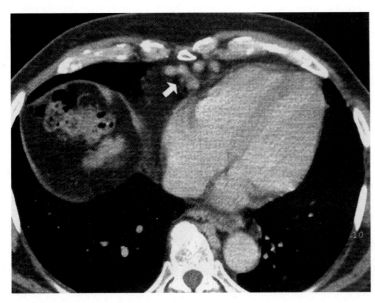

Fig C 59-12
Varices. In this patient with cirrhosis and portal hypertension, varices (arrow) in the right cardiophrenic space simulate lymph nodes.[117]

Axillary Masses on Computed Tomography

Condition	Comments
Breast cancer (Fig C 60-1)	Almost half of the women with breast cancer have axillary metastases when first seen. After primary therapy, up to 20% have local recurrence involving the chest wall; about 5% develop axillary recurrences.
Lymphoma (Fig C 60-2)	Axillary lymph node involvement has been reported in almost half of patients with non-Hodgkin's lymphoma and one-quarter of those with Hodgkin's disease. Even after apparently complete clinical remission, CT may show residual disease, especially in the apex of the axilla.
Metastases (Fig C 60-3)	Primary tumors of the head and neck, lung, and kidney may metastasize to axillary lymph nodes and simulate primary tumors or lymphoma.
Primary malignancy (Fig C 60-4)	Although rare, primary malignant neoplasms of fibrous tissue, muscle, or fat do occur in the axilla. These tumors characteristically do not respect soft tissue or muscle planes and may extend to the apex (producing symptoms of brachial plexus involvement) or spread along the chest wall.
Sarcoidosis (Fig C 60-5)	Unusual manifestation that, when combined with hilar and mediastinal adenopathy, can mimic lymphoma.

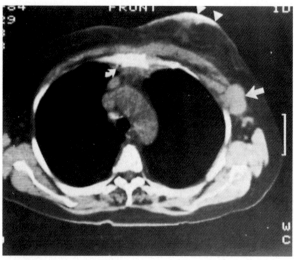

Fig C 60-1
Breast cancer. Left axillary nodes (arrow) and bilateral internal mammary nodes (curved arrows) are seen in this woman with an extensive malignancy of the left breast and involvement of the skin surface (arrowheads).[118]

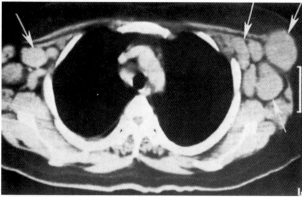

Fig C 60-2
Lymphoma. Extensive bilateral axillary adenopathy with enlarged nodes (arrows) surrounding the neurovascular bundles, but not invading them.[118]

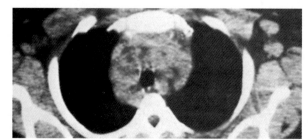

Fig C 60-3
Metastases. Extensive involvement of the left axillary nodes in a young man with neuroblastoma. Note the extension of adenopathy high into the apex of the axilla beneath the pectoralis minor muscle medially.[118]

Condition	Comments
Toxoplasmosis (Fig C 60-6)	Lymphadenopathy is the most common clinical manifestation in acute acquired disease. Although usually affecting cervical nodes, axillary lymph nodes also may be involved.
Cystic hygroma (cystic lymphangioma) (Fig C 60-7)	Congenital anomaly that most likely results from sequestration of primitive embryonic lymph sacs that fail to establish normal communication with the lymphatic system. Although most common in the neck, a hygroma can appear as a smooth, homogeneous axillary mass that displaces but does not invade adjacent muscular structures. It typically has a low attenuation value (10–30 H) that is less than that of soft tissue but much higher than that of fat.
Lipoma (Fig C 60-8)	Well-defined, homogeneous, benign fatty tumor with characteristic low attenuation value (290–2120 H) that is usually less than or equal to that of normal subcutaneous fat. CT can permit differentiation of a lipoma from a liposarcoma, which is a heterogeneous infiltrative lesion with poorly defined margins that shows contrast enhancement.
Desmoid tumor (Fig C 60-9)	Mass of benign but invasive fibrous tissue (considered a low-grade fibrosarcoma by some) that may be either diffusely infiltrative or relatively well defined with a pseudocapsule. After surgery, local recurrence is common.

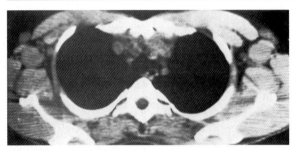

Fig C 60-4
Primary anaplastic carcinoma of the axilla. Peripherally enhancing mass in the right axilla that has infiltrated the neurovascular bundle, resulting in atrophy of the muscles of the right shoulder.[118]

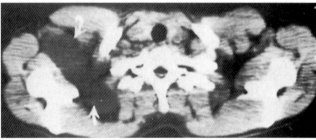

Fig C 60-5
Sarcoidosis. Bilateral axillary and mediastinal adenopathy in a young woman presenting a pattern indistinguishable from that of lymphoma.[118]

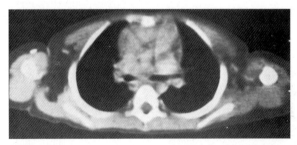

Fig C 60-6
Toxoplasmosis. Bilateral axillary adenopathy in a homosexual man.[118]

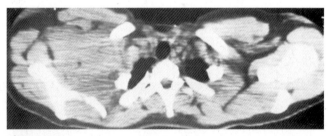

Fig C 60-7
Cystic hygroma. Diffuse mass with low attenuation value that is homogeneous and displaces rather than invades muscle planes.[118]

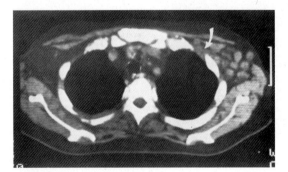

Fig C 60-8
Lipoma. Diffuse mass infiltrating the right axilla that has a characteristic attenuation value of fat.[118]

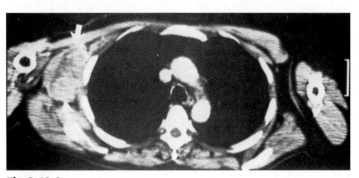

Fig C 60-9
Desmoid tumor. Large mass extensively infiltrating the right axilla (arrows), especially around the level of the neurovascular bundle.[118]

Chest Wall Lesions on Computed Tomography and Magnetic Resonance Imaging

Condition	Imaging Findings	Comments
Benign lesions		
Vascular		
Hemangioma (Fig C 61-1)	On CT, a soft-tissue mass with heterogeneous low levels of attenuation due to the fatty, fibrous, and vascular tissue elements of the mass. Characteristic phleboliths seen in about 30% of cases. On MRI, heterogeneous signal intensity with areas of high signal intensity on both T1-and T2-weighted images. Signal voids may result from rapidly flowing blood.	Cutaneous mass of dilated, tortuous, thin-walled vessels that tend to be large, poorly circumscribed, and can be locally destructive. Typically occurring in infancy or early adulthood, they rarely produce pressure erosion on adjacent bone.
Glomus tumor	CT scans (and chest radiographs) may show a soft-tissue mass with erosion of adjacent bone. On MRI, the well-defined tumor displaces major vessels and is encircled by tortuous vessels branching from a vascular pedicle. The mass usually has heterogeneous signal intensity and demonstrates marked contrast enhancement.	Rare lesion of adulthood that consists of neoplastic cells that closely resemble the smooth muscle cells of the normal glomus body. Most lesions are solitary and painful; multiple tumors are uncommon and usually asymptomatic.
Peripheral nerve		
Schwannoma	Well-circumscribed homogeneous mass similar to muscle on CT and T1-weighted MRI. High signal intensity on T2-weighted images. After contrast administration, there is strong enhancement in small lesions and often non-enhancing central areas of cystic or necrotic change in large lesions.	Common encapsulated, typically slow-growing lesion in an adult that originates in the nerve sheath. Chest wall tumors arise from spinal nerve roots and intercostal nerves. The characteristic finding of bone erosion without destruction, most often of a rib, indicates the benign nature and slow growth of the mass.

A   B

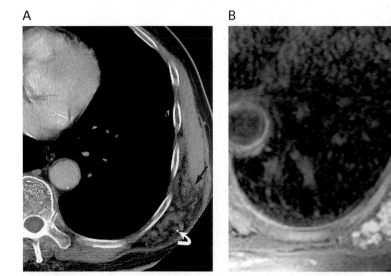

Fig C 61-1
Hemangioma. (A) Contrast CT scan demonstrates a mass (arrow) deep to the left serratus muscles and superficial to the intercostal muscles. The lesion largely has the attenuation of fat and contains multiple discrete nodular areas of soft-tissue attenuation and a small round calcification (curved arrow) that represents a small phlebolith. The lack of enhancement of the mass is related to the timing of the bolus. (B) Axial T2-weighted MR image with frequency-selective fat saturation shows a predominantly hyperintense lobulated mass (arrow) with interspersed areas of low signal intensity that represent fibrofatty septa.[119]

Condition	Imaging Findings	Comments
Neurofibroma (Fig C 61-2)	CT may show rib erosion, calcification, and heterogenous contrast enhancement. On MRI, a well-defined mass with low signal intensity on T1-weighted images and high signal intensity on T2 sequences. T2 often shows a target appearance, with a rim of increased signal surrounding the lower signal central part of the tumor. On contrast studies, the central part of the lesion markedly enhances.	Slow-growing neoplasm that usually develops in early adulthood. About 60% to 90% of affected patients have either type 1 neurofibromatosis or multiple plexiform neurofibromas. The target appearance reflects the histologic feature in many neurofibromas of a central zone composed of highly cellular material and a peripheral zone containing abundant stromal elements.
Osseous and cartilaginous Osteochondroma (Fig C 61-3)	Pedunculated osseous protuberance arising from the surface of the parent bone with a cartilaginous cap that is often calcified on CT and has high signal intensity on T2-weighted MR images.	In the ribs, this common skeletal tumor especially involves the costochondral, junction. Complications include deformity and pathologic fracture. Pain, bone erosion, and irregular calcification raise the possibility of malignant transformation.
Enchondroma (Fig C 61-4)	Expansile mass with calcified cartilaginous matrix.	About 3% of enchondromas occur in the rib and sternum, and they may predispose the patient to pathologic fracture.

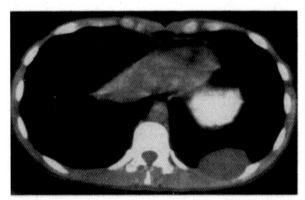

Fig C 61-2
Intercostal neurofibroma. Axial CT scan shows rib erosion caused by pressure from the large posterior mass.[120]

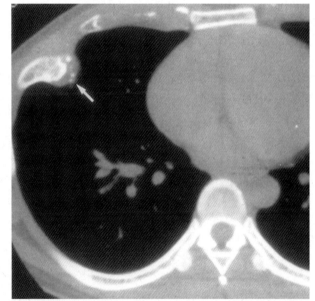

Fig C 61-3
Osteochondroma. CT scan shows a sessile mass with cortical and medullary continuity projecting into the lung. Note the calcification is the cartilaginous cap of the mass.[121]

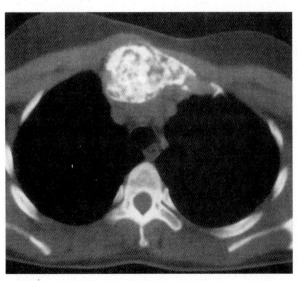

Fig C 61-4
Enchondroma. CT scan demonstrates a central expansile lesion in the upper manubrium with characteristic calcification of cartilaginous matrix.[16]

Condition	Imaging Findings	Comments
Giant cell tumor	Eccentric osteolytic lesion that produces cortical thinning and expansion. Both CT and MRI are valuable in showing the extent of the tumor and its relationship to surrounding structures.	Thoracic tumors often arise in subchondral regions of the flat and tubular bones of the chest wall, including the sternum, clavicle, and ribs. This relatively common benign lesion usually becomes evident in early to middle adulthood, after closing of the epiphyses, and may show a fluid-fluid level on MR (less common than in aneurysmal bone cyst).
Aneurysmal bone cyst	Expansile lesion with cortical thinning. On MR, a lobulated or separated mass with a thin, well-defined rim of low signal intensity. Fluid-fluid level within the tumor suggests the hemorrhagic nature of the cyst contents, but is not pathognomonic.	Network of multiple blood-filled cysts. Soft-tissue extension may make it difficult to distinguish this process from sarcoma. In the chest wall, the lesion most commonly involves the posterior elements of the spine (articular process, lamina, and spinous process).
Fibrous dysplasia (Fig C 61-5)	Fusiform enlargement and deformity of one or more ribs that is often associated with amorphous or irregular calcification on CT. MR is of value in accurately defining the full extent of the lesion.	Developmental anomaly that is monostotic in about 70% to 80% of cases. Complications include pathologic fracture and deformity.

Fatty

Lipoma (Fig C 61-6)	Well-circumscribed, internally homogeneous mass of fat attenuation/signal that shows no contrast enhancement.	Common lesion in adults, especially those who are obese. Septa within the lesion may show slight enhancement.

Non-neoplastic processes

Costochondritis (Fig C 61-7)	CT may show bone destruction and fragmentation of cartilage with soft-tissue swelling. Foci of low attenuation within cartilage may be seen in cases of infection.	Infectious costochondritis, related to various bacterial and fungal organisms, occurs with increased prevalence in intravenous drug abusers
Infection (Figs C 61-8 and C 61-9)	Rib destruction is more accurately detected by CT. Soft-tissue involvement and inflammation of the chest wall are better visualized with MR imaging.	Infections of the chest wall are uncommon but potentially life-threatening. Causative organisms include pyogenic bacteria, tuberculosis, and fungi. Immune compromise, diabetes mellitus, and previous trauma or surgery increase the risk of chest wall infection.

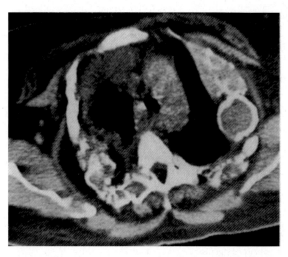

Fig C 61-5
Fibrous dysplasia. CT scan shows fusiform expansion of multiple ribs.[120]

A

B

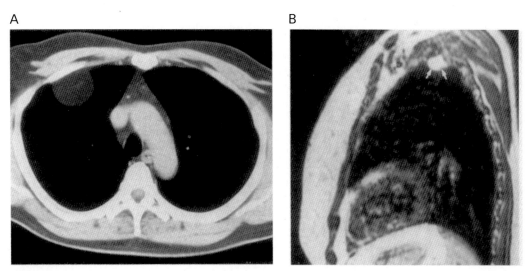

Fig C 61-6
Lipoma. (A) CT scan demonstrates extension of a chest wall lipoma into the intrathoracic extrapleural space. (B) Sagittal T1-weighted MR image in another patient shows a small apical extrapleural lipoma (arrows).[120]

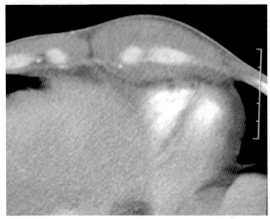

Fig C 61-7
Costochondritis. Soft-tissue mass centered around one of the lower left costochondral junctions (arrows) in an intravenous drug abuser.[10]

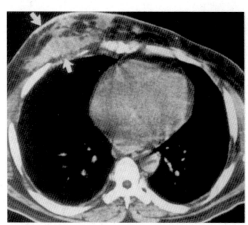

Fig C 61-8
Actinomycosis. CT scan shows extensive chest wall infection.[119]

A

B

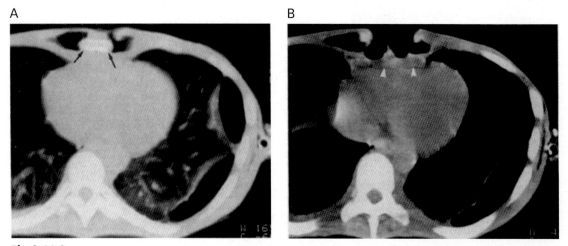

Fig C 61-9
Necrotizing infection in AIDS. CT scans obtained with lung (A) and mediastinal (B) windows show that the infection has eaten through the chest wall and extended around the sternum (arrows in A) and down to the pericardium (arrowheads in B). A pneumothorax and chest tube are present on the left.[120]

Condition	Imaging Findings	Comments
Sternoclavicular septic arthritis (Fig C 61-10)	CT and MRI show destructive changes as well as abscess formation, which is a complication in about 20% of cases.	Insertion of contaminated needles into and around the internal jugular vein may account for the increased frequency of sternoclavicular septic arthritis in intravenous drug abusers.
Paget's disease (Fig C 61-11)	Cortical thickening and bone enlargement are distinctive features, as in other bones.	Relatively uncommon in the ribs and usually an incidental finding noted during the chronic sclerotic phase of the disease.
Hematoma (Fig C 61-12)	Extrapleural mass with a CT attenuation greater than that of soft-tissue, compatible with the presence of blood.	Perivascular hematomas may develop about the subclavian artery or vein. Trauma may result in chest wall hematomas of considerable size.

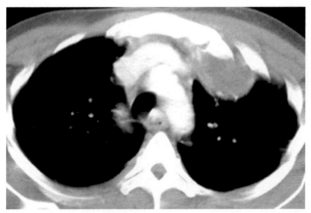

Fig C 61-10
Sternoclavicular septic arthritis. CT shows a low-attenuation collection deep to the left sternoclavicular joint (arrow), which represents an abscess extending from infection of the joint in an intravenous drug abuser.[10]

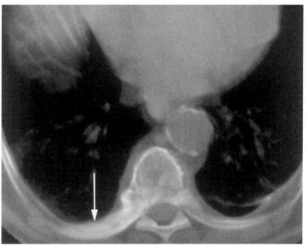

Fig C 61-11
Paget's disease. Bone enlargement with cortical thickening (arrow) involving the right posterior eighth rib.[121]

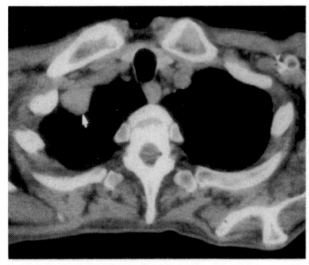

Fig C 61-12
Hematoma. Extrapleural mass (arrow) with attenuation greater than soft tissue, a finding compatible with the presence of blood.[120]

Condition	Imaging Findings	Comments
Lymphangioma (Fig C 61-13)	On CT, a well-defined cystic mass of homogeneous near-water attenuation. The fluid content appears as low signal intensity on T1-weighted MR images and high signal intensity on T2-weighted studies.	Congenital malformation representing sequestered lymphatic sacs that are isolated from the rest of the lymphatic drainage system. Most frequently seen as neck masses, they may extend to involve the mediastinum, chest wall, and axilla.
Malignant *Muscular* Leiomyosarcoma	Large spindle-shaped mass that frequently contains areas of necrosis or cystic change causing a pattern of peripheral contrast enhancement. Often displaces or distorts adjacent vessels.	Frequently painful and typically occurring in adulthood, it is usually a solitary lesion (multiplicity suggests metastases from another site).
Rhabdomyosarcoma	On MR, areas of necrosis with low signal intensity that do show contrast enhancement alternate with ring-like areas of high signal intensity and marked enhancement.	High-grade malignancy that generally affects patients younger than 45 years of age. This rapidly growing lesion causes bone invasion in more than 20% of cases.
Vascular Angiosarcoma	On MR, a large, ill-defined heterogenous mass with strong contrast enhancement. Feeding vessels are often seen in the periphery of the tumor.	In the chest wall, angiosarcomas primarily occur in the breast, most often in association with lymphedema or radiation therapy of breast cancer.
Fibrous Aggressive fibromatosis	Ill-defined mass with signal intensity similar to muscle or lower on T1-weighted images and heterogeneous enhancement.	Most commonly affecting adolescents and young adults, a common neoplastic disease accounting for more than half of low-grade sarcomas of the chest wall. Shoulder involvement is the most common complication.
Malignant fibrous histiocytoma (Fig C 61-14)	Large extraparenchymal mass that usually arises from the musculature of the chest wall. On MRI, heterogeneous signal intensity and marked enhancement are characteristic features.	Most common soft-tissue sarcoma in adults, although a thoracic origin is infrequent. The tumor can be associated with previous bone lesions, including Paget's disease and bone infarcts, and it is the most common sarcoma to develop after irradiation. Its origin within the musculature helps distinguish this tumor from osteosarcoma or chondrosarcoma.

A
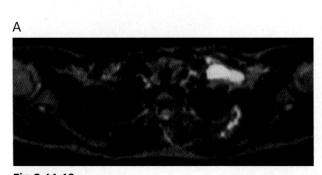

B
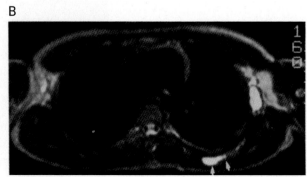

Fig C 61-13
Lymphangioma. Axial T1-weighted MR images, with (A) obtained at a higher level than (B), shows a mass that has high signal intensity because of its high water content. The mass can be traced from the neck into the axilla, where it insinuates between the muscles of the posterior chest wall (arrows in B).[120]

Condition	Imaging Findings	Comments
Peripheral nerves (Fig C 61-15)	Heterogeneous mass with ill-defined contours and heterogeneous contrast enhancement related to areas of necrosis. Primitive neuroectodermal tumors can be associated with adjacent rib destruction, pleural thickening or effusion, and focal invasion of the lung.	Neuroblastoma, ganglioneuroblastoma, malignant peripheral nerve sheath tumor. They usually arise in preexisting neurofibromas of the intercostals nerves or spinal nerve roots or in the brachial plexus.

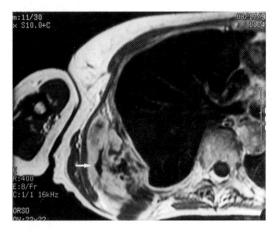

Fig C 61-14
Malignant fibrous histiocytoma. Axial T1-weighted contrast image shows a large extraparenchymal mass in the right upper hemithorax with marked enhancement. Focal areas of low signal intensity (arrow) are consistent with necrosis and fluid. The origin of the lesion within the chest wall musculature helps distinguish this tumor from osteosarcoma or chondrosarcoma.[134]

A

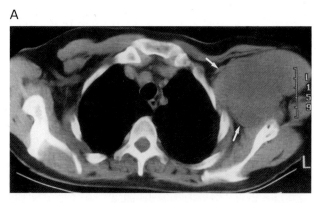

B   C

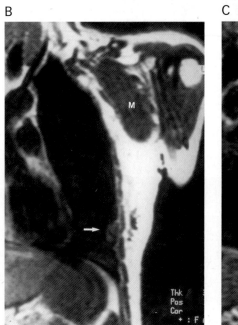

Fig C 61-15
Neurofibrosarcoma. (A) Unenhanced CT scan shows a large, homogeneous mass in the left axilla (arrows). Note the absence of rib destruction. On coronal MR images, the mass (M) is well-circumscribed and demonstrates low signal intensity on a T1-weighted image (B) and high signal intensity on a T2-weighted sequence (C). Note the small neurofibroma with similar signal intensity in the lower lateral aspect of the left hemithorax (arrow).[134]

Condition	Imaging Findings	Comments
Osseous and cartilaginous Chondrosacroma (Figs C 61-16 and C 61-17)	Large well-defined or irregular mass that often demonstrates ring, arc, stippled, or dense calcification in the chondroid matrix on CT. Variable signal intensity on MRI with heterogeneous enhancement.	Most common malignant primary tumor of the chest wall, usually arising anteriorly in an upper rib adjacent to the costal cartilage or in the sternum.

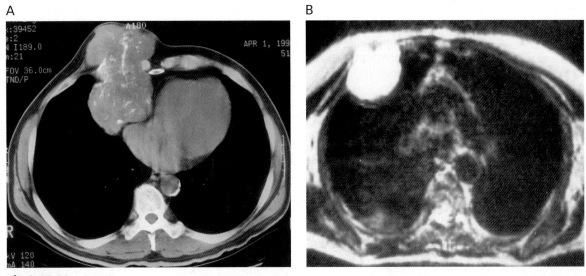

Fig C 61-16
Chondrosarcoma. (A) Unenhanced CT scan shows a large mass that arises from the costochondral junction. The mass extends into the subcutaneous tissue and compresses and displaces the heart. Note the focal punctuate and linear calcifications. The anterior location, origin from the costochondral arches, and chondroid calcification are characteristic of chondrosarcoma of the chest wall.[6]
(B) In another patient, a T2-weighted MR image shows nonspecific areas of high signal intensity within a well-defined extrapleural mass at the costochondral junction of the second rib.[16]

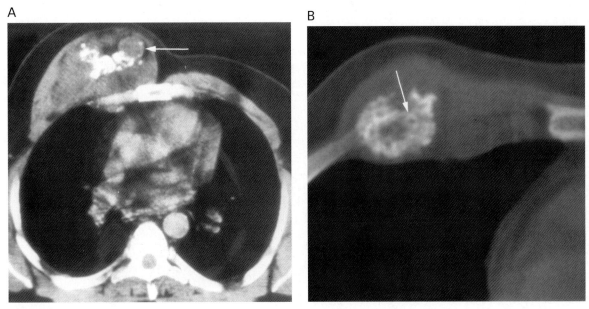

Fig C 61-17
Chondrosarcoma. (A) CT scan shows a large chest wall mass containing nodular and ring calcifications typical of chondroid matrix (arrow). (B) In another patient, a coned view of a smaller chondrosarcoma arising at the costochondral junction shows the characteristic nodular and ring calcifications (arrow).[121]

Condition	Imaging Findings	Comments
Osteosarcoma (Figs C 61-18 and C 61-19)	Large, ill-defined mass that is typically heterogeneous due to necrosis, hemorrhage, and ossification of the tumor matrix.	Rare involvement of the ribs, scapula, or clavicle. It is typically seen in a young adult and associated with an extrapleural mass. Chest wall lesions have a higher incidence of local recurrence and metastatic spread to the lungs and lymph nodes than do tumors of the extremities.
Ewing's sarcoma (Fig C 61-20)	On CT, usually a homogeneous mass when small and heterogeneous when large. On MRI, focal areas of high signal intensity and heterogeneous contrast enhancement are consistent with necrosis and hemorrhage. Extensive bone destruction is common.	About 15% of Ewing's sarcomas arise primarily in the chest wall, usually from a rib or, less frequently, the scapula. They typically occur in children or young adults, and most patients present with a painful chest wall mass. Fever and malaise are common associated systemic manifestations.

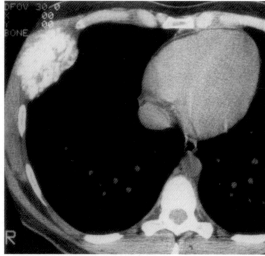

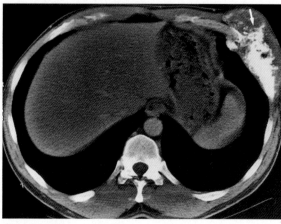

Fig C 61-19
Osteosarcoma. Contrast CT scan shows a left chest wall mass with a characteristic osteoid matrix.[134]

Fig C 61-18
Osteosarcoma. Unenhanced CT scan shows a densely calcified mass destroying the right anterior sixth rib. Although the location of the mass is typical for the more common chondroid tumors, cloudlike osteoid matrix calcification is present.[120]

B

A

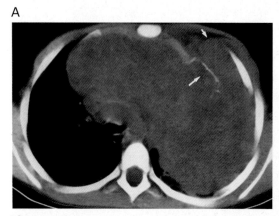

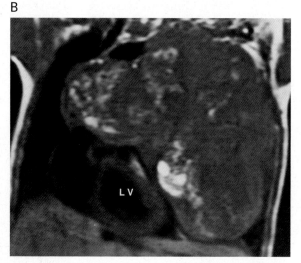

Fig C 61-20
Ewing's sarcoma. (A) Unenhanced CT scan shows a huge heterogeneous mass within the left hemithorax. There is destruction and inward displacement of a left rib (long arrow). Note the local invasion into the subcutaneous tissues (short arrow). (B) Coronal contrast T1-weighted MR image shows heterogeneous enhancement consistent with necrosis and hemorrhage. Note the marked displacement of mediastinal structures into the right hemithorax. LV = left ventricle.[134]

Condition	Imaging Findings	Comments
Liposarcoma (Fig C 61-21)	On CT, the attenuation is slightly higher than normal fat because the tumor contains both fat and soft tissue. Areas of calcification and ossification may be seen within the mass. Various patterns on MRI depending on the histology.	About 10% of these malignant tumors arise in relation to the chest wall.
Hematologic Lymphoma (Figs C 61-22 and C 61-23)	Infiltrating mass (especially along neurovascular bundles) with variable enhancement.	Primary chest wall involvement is infrequent. There is an increased incidence in patients with AIDS and those on immunosuppressive therapy, as well as in patients who have metallic orthopedic implants.

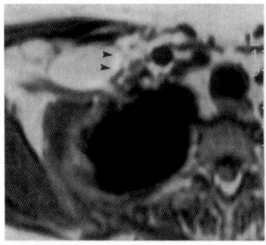

Fig C 61-21
Liposarcoma. Axial T1-weighted MR image shows a mass with high signal intensity equal to that of subcutaneous fat. The arrows point to a chemical shift artifact. The subclavian vessels are patent but displaced posteriorly.[120]

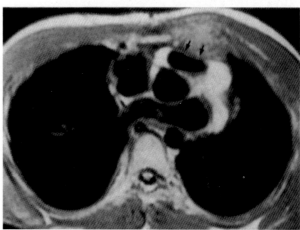

Fig C 61-22
Lymphoma. Axial T1-weighted MR image shows a parasternal mass involving the chest wall and left internal mammary node. The pericardial black line (arrows) is compressed and then obliterated, indicating invasion of this structure.[119]

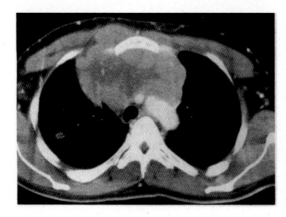

Fig C 61-23
AIDS-related lymphoma. CT scan shows a large mediastinal mass growing through the anterior chest wall in a parasternal location.[120]

Condition	Imaging Findings	Comments
Myeloma	Single or multiple osteolytic lesions with discrete margins in the vertebral column, ribs, or clavicles.	Sclerosis may develop in an osteolytic lesion after pathologic fracture, irradiation, or chemotherapy. Contrast-enhanced MRI can monitor the response to therapy.
Metastases (Fig C 61-24 to C 61-26)	Various patterns of destructive lytic and sclerotic lesions	Hematogenous spread or direct extension of an adjacent primary malignancy.
Bursa and tendon sheath Synovial sarcoma (Fig C 61-27)	Heterogeneous mass, reflecting hemorrhage and necrosis, that occasionally contains calcium.	Because they arise from bursae and tendon sheaths, they most commonly appear as masses in the soft tissues in a juxta-articular location. Although primary thoracic lesions typically occur as chest wall masses, they can rarely arise in the lung and pleura.

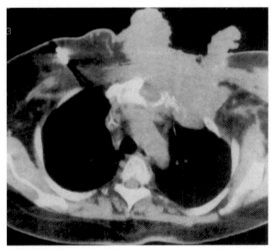

Fig C 61-24
Metastasis (breast cancer). CT scan shows a large ulcerating mass invading the upper chest wall. The sternum is eroded, and the tumor has grown into the suprasternal notch.[120]

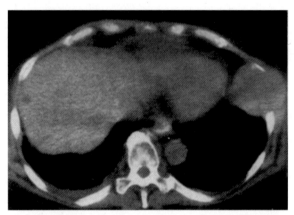

Fig C 61-25
Metastasis (hepatoma). CT scan shows a lytic rib lesion with large soft-tissue component.[120]

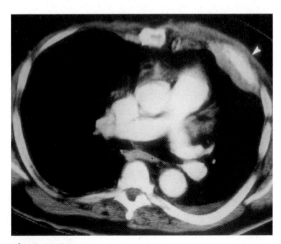

Fig C 61-26
Metastasis (prostate cancer). CT scan demonstrates a mass that arises from the anterior fourth rib and has extensive underlying bone sclerosis.[121]

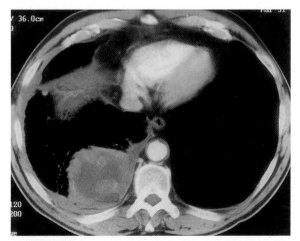

Fig C 61-27
Synovial sarcoma. Contrast CT scan shows a heterogeneous posterior chest wall mass containing areas of low attenuation consistent with extensive necrosis. There is an associated small right pleural effusion.[134]

Condition	Imaging Findings	Comments
Lung apex and pleura		
Pancoast tumor (Fig C 61-28)	Coronal and sagittal MR imaging is more accurate than CT in demonstrating chest wall invasion and involvement of the brachial plexus and adjacent blood vessels.	Superior sulcus tumor, most commonly a primary lung cancer, which invades through the apical fat to involve the brachial plexus and sympathetic stellate ganglion of the upper mediastinum and lower neck. The Pancoast syndrome consists of the clinical triad of ipsilateral arm pain, wasting of the muscles of the hand, and Horner syndrome
Mesothelioma (Fig C 61-29)	Coronal and sagittal MR imaging can directly evaluate the longitudinal extent of the tumor, as well as the degree of chest wall invasion and involvement of the diaphragm.	Typically related to asbestos exposure and often associated with a large pleural effusion that may obscure the underlying neoplasm on chest radiographs.

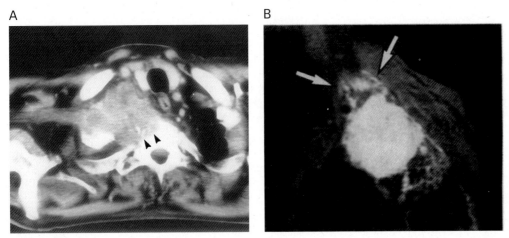

Fig C 61-28
Pancoast tumor. (A) CT scan shows a mass in the apex of the right lung that destroys the first rib and invades the adjacent T2 vertebral body (arrows).[2] (B) In another patient, a sagittal T2-weighted MR image shows a large mass arising in the apex of the right lung that has abnormal high signal intensity and infiltrates the supraclavicular fossa and surrounding brachial plexus.[120]

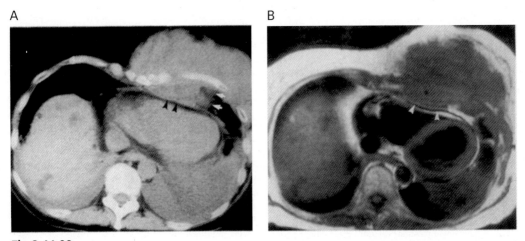

Fig C 61-29
Mesothelioma. (A) CT scan shows a huge mass involving the anterior chest and abdominal wall with growth of tumor (arrows) beneath the xiphoid process and lower ribs. The tumor appears to be contiguous to the pericardium (arrowheads) and it is difficult to determine whether this structure has been invaded. (B) Corresponding axial T1-weighted MR image shows the intact black line of the pericardium (arrowheads), indicating no invasion.[120]

Sources

1. Reprinted with permission from "Spherical Pneumonias in Children Simulating Pulmonary and Mediastinal Masses" by RW Rose and BH Ward, *Radiology* (1973;106:179–182), Copyright ©1973, Radiological Society of North America Inc.

2. Reprinted with permission from "Gram-negative Pneumonia" by JD Unger, HD Rose, and GF Unger, *Radiology* (1973;107:283–291), Copyright ©1973, Radiological Society of North America Inc.

3. Reprinted with permission from "Experience with *Hemophilus influenzae* Pneumonia" by M Vinick, DH Altman, and RE Parks, *Radiology* (1966;86:701–706), Copyright ©1966, Radiological Society of North America Inc.

4. Reprinted with permission from "Pulmonary Blastomycosis" by RA Halvorson et al, *Radiology* (1984;150:1–5), Copyright ©1984, Radiological Society of North America Inc.

5. Reprinted with permission from "The Melting Sign in Resolving Transient Pulmonary Infarction" by ME Woesner, I Sanders, and GW White, *American Journal of Roentgenology* (1971;111:782–790), Copyright ©1971, American Roentgen Ray Society.

6. Restrepo CS, Martinez S, Lemos JA. Imaging Manifestations of Kaposi Sarcoma. *RadioGraphics* 2006;26:1169–1185.

7. Reprinted from *Diagnosis of Diseases of the Chest* by RG Fraser and JAP Pare with permission of WB Saunders Company, ©1979.

8. Reprinted with permission from "The FBI Sign" by WW Wenzel, *Colorado Medicine*, formerly *Rocky Mountain Medical Journal* (1972; 69:71–72), Copyright ©1979.

9. Reprinted with permission from "Amniotic Pulmonary Embolism" by HR Arnold, JE Gardner, and PH Goodman, *Radiology* (1961;77:629–634), Copyright ©1961, Radiological Society of North America Inc.

10. Gotway MB, Marder SR, Hanks DK, et al. Thoracic complications of illicit drug use: an organ system approach. *RadioGraphics* 2002;22: S119–S135.

11. Restrepo CS, Carrillo JA, Martinez S, et al. Pulmonary complications from cocaine and cocaine-based substances: imaging manifstations. *RadioGraphics* 2007;27:941–956.

12. Reprinted with permission from "An Exercise in Radiologic-Pathologic Correlation" by EG Theros, MM Reeder, and JF Eckert, *Radiology* (1968;90:784–791), Copyright ©1968, Radiological Society of North America Inc.

13. Reprinted with permission from "Unilateral Pulmonary Edema" by L Calenoff, GD Kruglik, and A Woodruff, *Radiology* (1978;126:19–24), Copyright ©1978, Radiological Society of North America Inc.

14. Reprinted with permission from "Pulmonary Complications of Drug Therapy" by A Brettner, RE Heitzman, and WG Woodin, *Radiology* (1970;96:31–38), Copyright ©1970, Radiological Society of North America Inc.

15. Leatherwood DL, Heitkamp DE, Emerson RE. Pulmonary langerhans cell histiocytosis. *RadioGraphics* 2007;27:265–268.

16. Meyer CA, White CS. Cartilaginous disorders of the chest. *RadioGraphics* 1998;18:1109–1125.

17. Chong S, Lee KS, Chung MJ, et al. Neuroendocrine tumors of the lung: clinical, pathologic, and imaging findings. *RadioGraphics* 2006;26:21–58.

18. Reprinted with permission from "Bilateral Pulmonary Sequestration: CT Appearance" by KJ Wimbish, FP Agha, and TM Brady, *American Journal of Roentgenology* (1983;140:689–690), Copyright ©1983, American Roentgen Ray Society.

19. Cole TJ, Henry DA, Jolles H, et al. Normal and abnormal vascular structures that simulate neoplasms on chest radiographs: clues to the diagnosis. *RadioGraphics* 1995;15:867–891.

20. Wagner AL, Szabunio M, Hazlett KS, Wagner SG. Radiologic manifestations of round pneumonia in adults. *AJR Am J Roentgenol* 1998;170:723.

21. Seo JB, Im J-G, Goo JM, et al. Atypical pulmonary metastases: spectrum of radiologic findings. *RadioGraphics* 2001;21:403–417.

22. Erasmus JJ, Connolly JE, McAdams HP, Roggli VL. Solitary pulmonary nodules: Part 1. Morphologic evaluation for differentiation of benign and malignant lesions. *RadioGraphics* 2000;20:43–58.

23. Fang W, Washington L, Kumar. Imaging manifestations of blastomycosis: a pulmonary infection with potential dissemination. *RadioGraphics* 2007;27:641–655.

24. Jeung M-Y, Gasser B, Gangi A, et al. Bronchial carcinoid tumor of the thorax: spectrum of radiologic findings. *RadioGraphics* 2002; 22:351–365.

25. Gimenez A, Franquet T, Prats R, et al. Unusual primary lung tumors: a radiologic-pathologic overview. *RadioGraphics* 2002; 22:601–619.

26. Oh YW, Effman EL, Godwin JD. Pulmonary infections in immuno-compromised hosts: the importance of correlating the conventional radiologic appearance with the clinical setting. *Radiology* 2000; 217:647–658.

27. Reprinted from *Radiology of the Heart and Great Vessels* by RN Cooley and MH Schreiber, Williams & Wilkins Company, ©1978, with permission of JH Harris Jr.

28. Reprinted with permission from "The Ruptured Pulmonary Hydatid Cyst" by RFC Kagel and A Fatemi, *Radiology* (1961;76:60–64), Copyright ©1961, Radiological Society of North America Inc.

29. Klein JS, Carter JM. Abnormal intrathoracic gas collections: atypical appearances. *The Radiologist* 1994;1:85–94.

30. Han D, Lee KS, Franquet T, et al. Thrombotic and nonthrombotic pulmonary arterial embolism: spectrum of imaging findings. *RadioGraphics* 2003;23:1521–1539.

31. Reprinted with permission from "Eisenmenger's Syndrome" by HB Spitz, *Seminars in Roentgenology* (1968;3:373–376), Copyright ©1968, Grune & Stratton Inc.

32. Reprinted with permission from "Mediastinal Lymphadenopathy in Bubonic Plague" by VR Sites and JD Poland, *American Journal of Roentgenology* (1970;116:567–570), Copyright ©1970, American Roentgen Ray Society.

33. Reprinted with permission from "Antenatal Ultrasound Findings in Cystic Adenomatoid Malformation" by SM Donn, JN Martin, and SJ White, *Pediatric Radiology* (1981;10:180–182), Copyright ©1981, Springer-Verlag.

34. Reprinted with permission from "Bulging (Sagging) Fissure Sign in *Hemophilus influenzae* Lobar Pneumonia" by JB Francis and PB Francis, *Southern Medical Journal* (1978;71:1452–1453), Copyright ©1978, Southern Medical Association.

35. Reprinted from *Chest Roentgenology* by B Felson with permission of WB Saunders Company, ©1973.

36. Reprinted with permission from "Calcified Pulmonary Lesions: An Overview" by HT Winer-Muram and JI Sebes, *Postgraduate Radiology* (1991;11:3–21), Copyright ©1991.

37. Reprinted with permission from "Diagnosis of Chemotherapy of Lung" by HD Sostman, CE Putnam, and G Gamsu, *American Journal of Roentgenology* (1981;136:33–41), Copyright ©1981, American Roentgen Ray Society.

38. Reprinted from *Clinical Radiology in the Tropics* by WP Cockshott and H Middlemiss with permission of Churchill Livingstone Inc, ©1979.

39. Reprinted with permission from *British Journal of Radiology* (1963;36:889–901), Copyright ©1963, British Institute of Radiology.

40. Reprinted with permission from "Creeping Eruption with Transient Pulmonary Infiltration" by EH Kalmon, *Radiology* (1954;62:222–226), Copyright ©1954, Radiological Society of North America Inc.

41. Franquet T, Muller NL, Gimenez A, et al. Spectrum of pulmonary aspergillosis: histologic, clinical, and radiologic findings. *Radio Graphics* 2001;21:825.

42. Courtesy of the Armed Forces Institute of Pathology.

43. Reprinted with permission from "Computed Tomography in the Evaluation of Mediastinal Widening" by RL Baron et al, *Radiology* (1981;138:107–114), Copyright ©1981, Radiological Society of North America Inc.

44. Glazer HS, Wick MR, Anderson DJ, et al. CT of fatty thoracic masses. *AJR Am J Roentgenol* 1992;159:1181–1187.

45. Nishino M, Ashiku SK, Kocher ON, et al. The Thymus: A Comprehensive Review. *RadioGraphics* 2006;26:335–348.

46. Reprinted from *Computed Body Tomography* by JKT Lee, SS Sagel, and RJ Stanley (Eds) with permission of Raven Press, New York, ©1983.

47. Whitten CR, Khan S, Munneke GJ, Grubnic S. A diagnostic approach to mediastinal abnormalities. *RadioGraphics* 2007;27:657–671.

48. Reprinted with permission from "Parathyroid Scanning by Computed Tomography" by DD Stark et al, *Radiology* (1983;148:297–303), Copyright ©1983, Radiological Society of North America Inc.

49. Ueno T, Tanaka YO, Nagata M, et al. Spectrum of germ cell tumors: From Head to Toe. *RadioGraphics* 2004;24:387–404.

50. Rossi SE, McAdams HP, Rosado-de-Christenson ML, et al. Fibrosing Mediastinits. *RadioGraphics* 2001;21:737–757.

51. Reprinted with permission from "Laceration of the Thoracic Aorta and Brachiocephalic Arteries by Blunt Trauma" by RG Fisher, FP Hadlock, and Y Ben-Menachem, *Radiologic Clinics of North America* (1981;19:91–112), Copyright ©1981, WB Saunders Company.

52. Reprinted with permission from "The 'V' Sign in the Diagnosis of Spontaneous Rupture of the Esophagus" by NA Naclerio, *American Journal of Surgery* (1957;93:291–298), Copyright ©1957, Yorke Medical Group.

53. Reprinted with permission from "The Multiple Roentgen Manifestations of Sclerosing Mediastinitis" by DS Feigin, JC Eggleston, and FS Siegelman, *Johns Hopkins Medical Journal* (1979;144:1–8), Copyright ©1979, Johns Hopkins University Press.

54. Gaerte SC, Meyer CA, Winer-Muram, et al. Fat-containing lesions of the chest. *RadioGraphics* 2002;22:S62–S78.

55. Jeung M-Y, Gasser B, Gangi A, et al. Imaging of cystic masses of the mediastinum. *RadioGraphics* 2002;22:S79–S93.

56. Reprinted from *Computed Tomography of the Body* by AA Moss, G Gamsu, and HK Genant (Eds) with permission of WB Saunders Company, ©1983.

57. Gibbs JM, Chandrasekhar CA, Ferguson EC, Oldham SAA. Lines and Stripes: Where Did They Go? – From Conventional Radiography to CT. *RadioGraphics* 2007;27:33–48.

58. Koyama T, Ueda H, Togashi, et al. Radiologic manifestations of sarcoidosis in various organs. *RadioGraphics* 2004;24:87–104.

59. Reprinted with permission from "CT of Posterior Mediastinal Masses" by A Kawashima, EK Fishman et al, *RadioGraphics* (1991;11:1045–1067), Copyright ©1991, Radiological Society of America Inc.

60. Reprinted with permission from "Abnormalities of the Azygoesophageal Recess at Computed Tomography" by G Lund and HH Lien, *Acta Radiologica: Diagnosis* (1983;24:3–10), Copyright ©1983, Acta Radiologica.

61. Reprinted with permission from "The Lateral Decubitus Film: An Aid in Determining Air-Trapping in Children" by MA Capitanio and JA Kirkpatrick, *Radiology* (1972;103:460–461), Copyright ©1972, Radiological Society of North America Inc.

62. Reprinted with permission from "The Continuous Diaphragm Sign: A Newly Recognized Sign of Pneumomediastinum" by B Levin, *Clinical Radiology* (1973;24:337–338), Copyright ©1973, Royal College of Radiologists.

63. Reprinted with permission from "Mesotheliomas and Secondary Tumors of the Pleura" by K Ellis and M Wolff, *Seminars in*

Roentgenology (1977;12:303–311), Copyright ©1977, Grune & Stratton Inc.

64. Dynes MC, White EM, Fry WA, et al. Imaging manifestations of pleural tumors. *RadioGraphics* 1992;12:1191–1201.

65. Reprinted with permission from "Roentgen Manifestations of Pleural Disease" by VA Vix, *Seminars in Roentgenology* (1977;12:277–286), Copyright ©1977, Grune & Stratton Inc.

66. Reprinted with permission from "Pleural Plaques: A Signpost of Asbestos Dust Inhalation" by EN Sargent, G Jacobson, and JS Gordonson, *Seminars in Roentgenology* (1977;12:287–297), Copyright ©1977, Grune & Stratton Inc.

67. Reprinted with permission from "Radiologic Appearance of Compromised Thoracic Catheters, Tubes, and Wires" by RD Dunbar, *Radiologic Clinics of North America* (1984;22:699–722), Copyright ©1984, WB Saunders Company.

68. Reprinted with permission from "Pneumothorax as a Complication of Feeding Tube Placement" by GL Balogh et al, *American Journal of Roentgenology* (1983;141:1275–1277), Copyright ©1983, American Roentgen Ray Society.

69. Reprinted with permission from "Distribution of Pneumothorax in the Supine and Semirecumbent Critically Ill Adult" by IM Tocino, MH Miller, and WR Fairfax, *American Journal of Roentgenology* (1985;144:901–905), Copyright ©1985, American Roentgen Ray Society.

70. Reprinted with permission from "Plasmacytoma of the Head and Neck" by RC Gromer and AJ Duvall, *Journal of Laryngology and Otology* (1973;87:861–872), Copyright ©1973, Headley Brothers, Ltd.

71. Marom EM, Goodman PC, McAdams HP. Focal abnormalities of the trachea and main bronchi. *AJR* 2001;176:707–711.

72. Prince JS, Duhamel DR, Levin DL, et al. Nonneoplastic lesions of the Tracheobronchial Wall: Radiologic Findings with Bronchoscopic Correlation. *RadioGraphics* 2002;22:S215–S230.

73. Reprinted with permission from "Tracheal Stenosis: An Analysis of 151 Cases" by AL Weber and HC Grillo, *Radiologic Clinics of North America* (1978;16:291–308), Copyright ©1978, WB Saunders Company.

74. Reprinted with permission from "Diffuse Lesions of the Trachea" by RH Choplin, WD Wehunt, and EG Theros, *Seminars in Roentgenology* (1983;18:38–50), Copyright ©1983, Grune & Stratton Inc.

75. Reprinted with permission from "'Saber Sheath' Trachea: A Clinical and Functional Study of Marked Coronal Narrowing of Intrathoracic Trachea" by R Greene and GL Lechner, *Radiology* (1975;15:255–268), Copyright ©1975, Radiological Society of North America Inc.

76. Marom EM, Goodman PC, McAdams HP. Focal abnormalities of the trachea and main bronchi. *AJR* 2001;176:707–711.

77. Marom EM, Goodman PC, McAdams HP. Diffuse abnormalities of the trachea and main bronchi. *AJR* 2001;176:713–717.

78. Chong S, Lee KS, Chung MJ, et al. Neuroendocrine tumors of the lung: Clinical, pathologic, and imaging findings. *RadioGraphics* 2006;26:41–58.

79. Seo JB, Song K-S, Lee JS, et al. Broncholithiasis: Review of the causes with radiologic-pathologic correlation. *RadioGraphics* 2002;22:S199–S213.

80. Seo JB, Lee JW, Ha SY, et al. Primary endobronchial actinomycosis associated with broncholithiasis. *Respiration* 2003;70:110–113.

81. Kim HY, Im JG, Song KS, et al. Localized amyloidosis of the respiratory system: CT features. *J Comput Assist Tomogr* 1999;23:627–631.

82. Song JW, Im JG, Shim YS, et al. Hypertrophied bronchial artery at thin-section CT in patients with bronchiectasis: correlation with CT angiographic findings. *Radiology* 1998;208:187–191.

83. Franquet T, Erasmus JJ, Gimenez A, etal. The retrotracheal space: normal anatomic and pathologic appearances. *RadioGraphics* 2002;22:S231–S246.

84. Reprinted with permission from "The 'Thumb Sign' and 'Little Finger Sign' in Acute Epiglottitis" by JK Podgore and JW Bass,

Journal of Pediatrics (1976;88:154–155), Copyright ©1976, The CV Mosby Company, St. Louis.

85. John SD, Swischuk LE. Stridor and upper airway obstruction in infants and children. *RadioGraphics* 1992;12:625–643.

86. Reprinted with permission from "The Right Paratracheal Stripe in Blunt Chest Trauma" by JH Woodring, CM Pulmano, and RK Stevens, *Radiology* (1982;143:605–608), Copyright ©1982, Radiological Society of North America Inc.

87. Reprinted with permission from "Differential Diagnosis of Chronic Diffuse Infiltrative Lung Disease on High-Resolution Computed Tomography" by NL Müller, *Seminars in Roentgenology* (1991; 26:132–142), Copyright ©1991, WB Saunders Company.

88. Reprinted with permission from Webb WR, Muller NL, Naidich DP: *High-Resolution CT of the Lung* (3rd ed.). Philadelphia, Lippincott Williams & Wilkins, 2001 (pages 259–353).

89. Reprinted with permission from "High-Resolution Computed Tomography of Asbestos-Related Diseases" by DR Aberle, *Seminars in Roentgenology* (1991;26:118–131), Copyright ©1991, WB Saunders Company.

90. Swensen SJ, Aughenbaugh GL, Douglas WW, et al. High-resolution CT of the lungs: findings in various pulmonary diseases. *AJR Am J Roentgenol* 1992;158:971–979.

91. Rossi SE, Franquet T, Valpacchio M, et al. Tree-in-Bud Pattern at Thin-Section CT of the Lungs: Radiologic-Pathologic Overview. *RadioGraphics* 2005;25:789–801.

92. Collins J, Stern EJ. Normal anatomy of the chest. In: Collins J, Stern EJ, eds. *Chest Radiology: The Essentials*. Philadelphia: Lippincott Williams & Wilkins, 1999.

93. Collins J, Blankenbaker D, Stern EJ. CT patterns of bronchiolar disease: what is "tree-in-bud"? *AJR Am J Roentgenol* 1998;171:365.

94. Reprinted with permission from "Computed Tomography of Air-Space Diseases" by SH Hommeyer et al, *Radiologic Clinics of North America* (1991;29:1065–1083), Copyright ©1991, WB Saunders Company.

95. Gervais DA, Whitman GJ, Chew FS. *Pneumocystis carinii* pneumonia. *AJR Am J Roentgenol* 1995;164:1098.

96. Reprinted with permission from "High-Resolution Computed Tomography of Focal Lung Disease" by PA Templeton and EA Zerhouni, *Seminars in Roentgenology* (1991;26:143–150), Copyright ©1991, WB Saunders Company.

97. Reprinted with permission from "Pulmonary Alveolar Proteinosis: CT Findings" by JD Godwin et al, *Radiology* (1988;169:609–613), Copyright ©1988, Radiological Society of North America.

98. Reprinted with permission from "High-Resolution Computed Tomography of Cystic Lung Disease" by DP Naidich, *Seminars in Roentgenology* (1991;26:151–174), Copyright ©1991, WB Saunders Company.

99. Reprinted from Stern EJ, Swensen SJ, Hartman TE, Frank MS. CT mosaic pattern of lung attenuation: distinguishing different causes. *AJR Am J Roentgenol* 1995;165:813.

100. Rossi SE, Erasmus JJ, Volpacchio M, et al. "Crazy-Paving" Pattern at Thin-Section CT of the Lungs: Radiologic-Pathologic Overview. *RadioGraphics* 2003;23:1509–1519.

101. Collins J, Stern EJ. Ground-glass opacity at CT: the ABCs. *AJR* 1997;169:355–367.

102. Stern EJ, Swensen SJ, Collins J, et al. *High-Resolution CT of the Chest*, 2nd ed. Philadelphia: Lippincott Williams & Wilkins, 2000, p. 33.

103. Wong KT, Antonio GE, Hui DSC, et al. Thin-section CT of severe acute respiratory syndrome: evaluation of 73 patients exposed to or with the disease. *Radiology* 2003;228:395–400.

104. Abbott GF, Rosado-de-Christenson ML, Franks TJ, et al. Pulmonary Langerhans cell histiocytosis. *RadioGraphics* 2004;24:821–841.

105. Chong S, Lee KS, Chung MJ, et al. Pneumoconiosis: comparison of imaging and pathologic findings. *RadioGraphics* 2006;26:59–77.

106. Jeong YJ, Kim K-I, Seo IJ, et al. Eosinophilic lung diseases: a clinical, radiological, and pathological overview. *RadioGraphics* 2007;27:617–637.

107. Helbich TH, Heinz-Peer G, Eichler I, et al. Cystic fibrosis: CT assessment of lung involvement in children and adults. *Radiology* 1999;213:537.

108. Gluecker T, Capasso P, Schnyder P, et al. Clinical and radiological features of pulmonary edema. *RadioGraphics* 1999;19:1507–1531.

109. Mayberry JP, Primack SL, Müller NL. Thoracic manifestations of systemic autoimmune diseases: radiographic and high-resolution CT findings. *RadioGraphics* 2000;20:1623–1635.

110. Mueller-Mang C, Grosse C, Schmid K, et al. What every radiologist should know about idiopathic interstitial pneumonias. *RadioGraphics* 2007;27:595–615.

111. Kim EA, Lee KS, Johkoh T, et al. Interstitial lung diseases associated with collagen vascular diseases: radiologic and histopathologic findings. *RadioGraphics* 2002;22:S151–S165.

112. Rossi SE, Erasmus JJ, McAdams HP, et al. Pulmonary drug toxicity: radiologic and pathologic manifestations. *Radiographics* 2000;20:1245–1259.

113. Wittram C, Maher MM, Yoo AJ. CT angiography of pulmonary embolism: diagnostic criteria and causes of misdiagnosis. *RadioGraphics* 2004;24:1219–1238.

114. Gladdish GW, Sabloff BM, Munden RF, et al. Primary thoracic sarcomas. *RadioGraphics* 2002;22:621–637.

115. Reprinted from Van Hise ML, Primack SL, Israel RS, Muller NL. CT in blunt chest trauma: indications and limitations. *RadioGraphics* 1998;18:1071.

116. Reprinted from Kuhlman JE, Pozniak MA, Collins J, Knisely BL. Radiographic and CT findings of blunt chest trauma: aortic injuries and looking beyond them. *RadioGraphics* 1998;18:1085.

117. Pineda V, Andreu J, Caceres J, et al. Lesions of the cardiophrenic space: findings at cross-sectional imaging. *RadioGraphics* 207;27:19–32.

118. Reprinted with permission from "CT of the Axilla: Normal Anatomy and Pathology" by EK Fishman et al, RadioGraphics (1986;6:475–502), Copyright ©1986, Radiological Society of North America Inc.

119. Ly JQ, Sanders TG. Case 65: Hemangioma of the Chest Wall. *Radiology* 2003;229:726–729.

120. Kuhlman JE, Bouchandy L, Fishman EK, Zerhouni EA. CT and MR imaging evaluation of chest wall disorders. *RadioGraphics* 1994;14:571–595.

121. Guttentag AR, Salwen JK. Keep your eyes on the ribs: the spectrum of normal variants and diseases that involve the ribs. *Radio Graphics* 1999;19:1125–1142.

122. Weisbrod GL, Towers MJ, Chamberlain DW, et al. Thin-walled cystic lesions in bronchioalveolar carcinoma. *Radiology* 1992;185:401.

123. Haramati LB, Schulman LL, Austin JH. Lung nodules and masses after cardiac transplantation. *Radiology* 1993;188:491.

124. Remy-Jardin M, Remy J, Cortet B, et al. Lung changes in rheumatoid arthritis: CT findings. *Radiology* 1994;193:375–382.

125. Nishimura K, Itoh H, Kitaichi M, et al. Pulmonary sarcoidosis: correlation of CT and histopathologic findings. *Radiology* 1993;189:105–109.

126. Kim KI, Kim CW, Lee MK, et al. Imaging of occupational lung disease. *RadioGraphics* 2001;21:1371–1391.

2 Cardiovascular Patterns

Right Atrial Enlargement

Condition	Imaging Findings	Comments
Left-to-right shunt	Enlarged right atrium if this chamber is the end point of a shunt.	Atrial septal defect; endocardial cushion defect; anomalous pulmonary venous return; ruptured sinus of Valsalva aneurysm into the right atrium; left ventricular–right atrial shunt.
Right ventricular enlargement/failure	Various patterns, depending on the underlying cause.	Cor pulmonale; chronic left heart failure; mitral stenosis; tetralogy of Fallot.
Tricuspid valve disease (Fig CA 1-1)	Right atrial enlargement (may be extreme); often dilatation of the superior vena cava; right ventricular enlargement in tricuspid insufficiency.	Most commonly the result of rheumatic heart disease. Rarely an isolated lesion and generally associated with mitral or aortic valve disease. Tricuspid insufficiency is usually functional and secondary to marked dilatation of the failing right ventricle. Rare causes of isolated tricuspid valve disease include carcinoid syndrome, endomyocardial fibrosis, and right atrial myxoma.
Pulmonary stenosis or atresia (Fig CA 1-2)	Enlargement of the right atrium and right ventricle; decreased pulmonary vascularity.	Right atrial enlargement secondary to enlargement of the right ventricle.
Hypoplastic left heart syndrome (Fig CA 1-3)	Enlargement of the right atrium and right ventricle produces progressive globular cardiomegaly. Severe pulmonary venous congestion.	Consists of several conditions in which underdevelopment of left side of the heart is related to an obstructive lesion (stenosis or atresia of the mitral valve, aortic valve, or aortic arch). Causes heart failure in the first week of life.

A   B

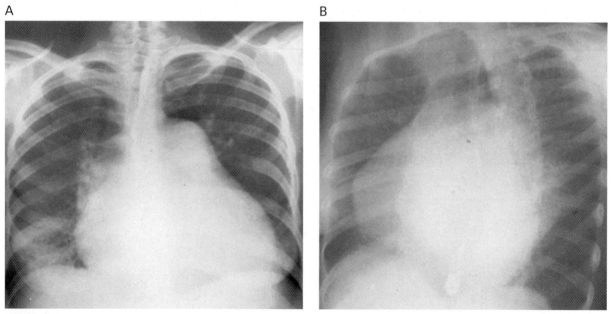

Fig CA 1-1
Tricuspid insufficiency. (A) Frontal and (B) left anterior oblique projections show striking right atrial enlargement.[1]

Condition	Imaging Findings	Comments
Tricuspid atresia	Enlargement of the right atrium and left ventricle; small right ventricle; decreased pulmonary vascularity (usually some degree of pulmonary stenosis).	Right-to-left shunt at the atrial level (patent foramen ovale or true atrial septal defect). Usually a ventricular septal defect or patent ductus arteriosus. Hypoplasia of the right ventricle and the pulmonary outflow tract. The smaller the shunt, the more marked the elevation of right atrial pressure and more striking the enlargement of this chamber.
Ebstein's anomaly (see Fig CA 6-5)	Enlargement of the right atrium causes a characteristic squared or boxed appearance of the heart. Decreased pulmonary vascularity; flat or concave pulmonary outflow tract; narrow vascular pedicle and small aortic arch.	Downward displacement of an incompetent tricuspid valve into the right ventricle so that the upper portion of the right ventricle is effectively incorporated into the right atrium. Functional obstruction to right atrial emptying produces increased pressure and a right-to-left atrial shunt (usually through a patent foramen ovale).
Uhl's disease	Radiographic pattern identical to that in Ebstein's anomaly.	Focal or complete absence of the right ventricular myocardium (the right ventricle becomes a thin-walled fibroelastic bag that contracts poorly and cannot effectively empty blood from the right side of the heart).

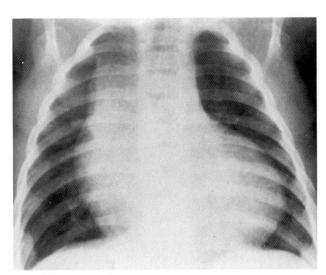

Fig CA 1-2
Pulmonary atresia. Marked right atrial enlargement associated with decreased pulmonary vascularity.

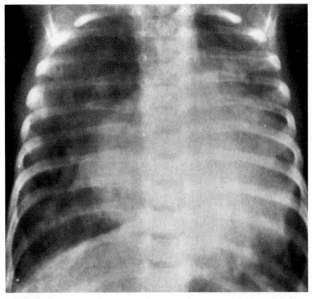

Fig CA 1-3
Hypoplastic left heart syndrome. Globular cardiomegaly with severe pulmonary venous congestion.

Right Ventricular Enlargement

Condition	Imaging Findings	Comments
Tetralogy of Fallot (Fig CA 2-1)	Enlargement of the right ventricle (though overall cardiac size is often normal); decreased pulmonary vascularity; flat or concave pulmonary outflow tract; right aortic arch in approximately 25% of patients.	Consists of (1) high ventricular septal defect, (2) obstruction to right ventricular outflow (usually infundibular pulmonary stenosis), (3) overriding of the aortic orifice above the ventricular defect, and (4) right ventricular hypertrophy. Most common cause of cyanotic congenital heart disease beyond the immediate neonatal period. If there is severe pulmonary stenosis, blood flow from both ventricles is effectively forced into the aorta, causing pronounced bulging of the ascending aorta and prominence of the aortic knob.
Pulmonary stenosis (Fig CA 2-2)	Initially normal heart size; right ventricular enlargement if severe stenosis causes systolic overloading of this chamber; poststenotic dilatation of the pulmonary artery.	Common anomaly found in isolated form or in combination with other abnormalities. The stenosis is most common at the level of the pulmonary valve (supravalvular or infundibular stenosis can occur).
Mitral stenosis (Fig CA 2-3)	Enlargement of the right ventricle (also the pulmonary outflow tract and central pulmonary arteries) reflects pulmonary arterial hypertension from transmitted increased pressure in the left atrium and the pulmonary veins.	Most common rheumatic valvular lesion (results from diffuse thickening of the valve by fibrous tissue or calcific deposits). Decreased left ventricular output causes a small aortic knob. Calcification of the mitral valve (best demonstrated by fluoroscopy) and pulmonary hemosiderosis may develop.

A   B

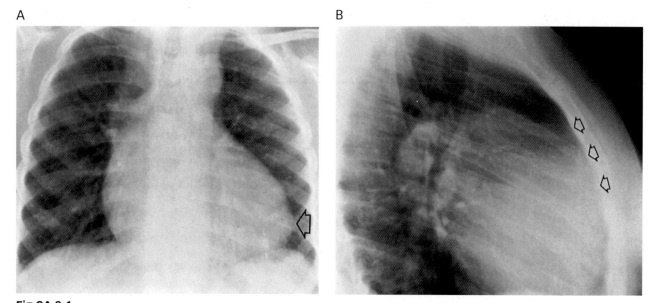

Fig CA 2-1
Tetralogy of Fallot. (A) Frontal view shows right ventricular enlargement as a lateral and upward displacement of the radiographic cardiac apex (arrow). (B) On the lateral view, the enlarged right ventricle fills most of the retrosternal space (arrows).

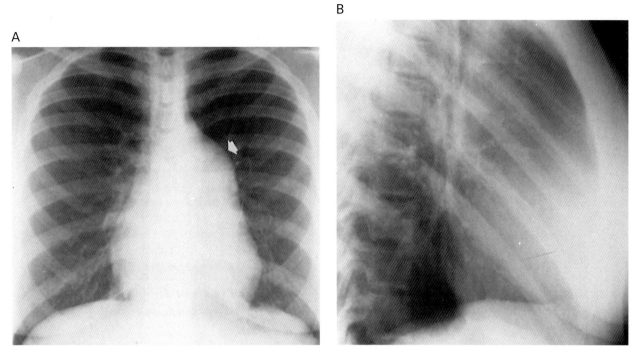

Fig CA 2-2
Pulmonary stenosis. (A) Frontal and (B) lateral views show striking poststenotic dilatation of the pulmonary artery (arrow) in addition to filling of the retrosternal air space, indicating right ventricular enlargement.

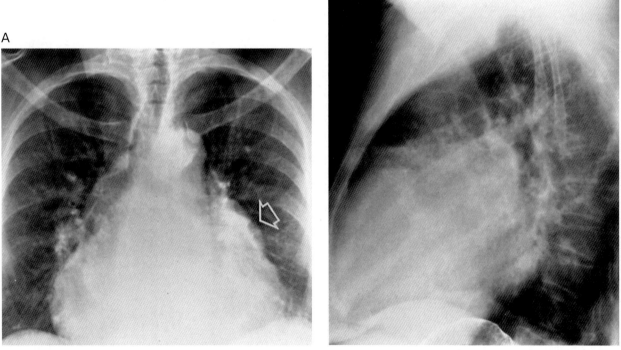

Fig CA 2-3
Mitral stenosis. (A) Frontal and (B) lateral views of the chest demonstrate cardiomegaly with enlargement of the right ventricle and left atrium. The right ventricular enlargement causes obliteration of the retrosternal air space, whereas left atrial enlargement produces a convexity of the upper left border of the heart (arrow, A).

Condition	Imaging Findings	Comments
Cor pulmonale (Fig CA 2-4)	Right ventricular enlargement associated with enlarged central pulmonary vessels, rapid tapering, and small peripheral vessels.	Primary or secondary to such conditions as chronic obstructive emphysema, diffuse interstitial fibrosis, widespread peripheral pulmonary emboli, and Eisenmenger physiology (reversed left-to-right shunt). Rare causes include metastases from trophoblastic neoplasms, immunologic disease, schistosomiasis, multiple pulmonary artery stenoses or coarctations, and vasoconstrictive diseases.
Chronic left heart failure	Enlarged right ventricle associated with left ventricular enlargement and pulmonary venous congestion.	May reflect a myocardiopathy or mitral insufficiency. The transmission of increased pressure from the left side of the heart eventually leads to the development of pulmonary arterial hypertension and enlargement of the right side of the heart.
Left-to-right shunts (see Fig CA 7-1)	Enlarged right ventricle and pulmonary outflow tract with increased pulmonary vascularity. The size of other structures varies depending on the specific underlying lesion.	Most commonly atrial septal defect, ventricular septal defect, or patent ductus arteriosus.
Tricuspid insufficiency	Right ventricular enlargement that may be obscured by the often extreme enlargement of the right atrium.	Usually functional and secondary to marked dilatation of the failing right ventricle.

A   B

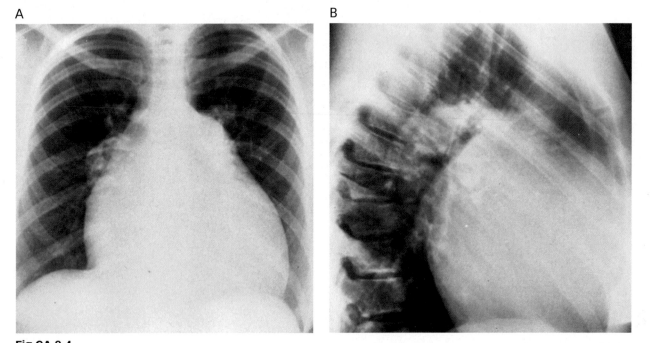

Fig CA 2-4
Cor pulmonale. (A) Frontal and (B) lateral views of the chest in a patient with primary pulmonary hypertension show marked globular cardiomegaly with prominence of the pulmonary trunk and central pulmonary arteries. The peripheral pulmonary vascularity is strikingly reduced. Right ventricular enlargement has obliterated the retrosternal air space on the lateral view.

Condition	Imaging Findings	Comments
Right-to-left shunts and admixture lesions	Various patterns, depending on the underlying cardiac anomaly.	Transposition of great vessels, trilogy of Fallot, Ebstein's anomaly, Uhl's anomaly, persistent truncus arteriosus.
Pseudotruncus arteriosus	Enlargement of the right ventricle; decreased pulmonary vascularity; flat or concave pulmonary outflow tract; right aortic arch in approximately 40% of patients.	Single vessel arising from the heart that is accompanied by a remnant of the atretic pulmonary artery (essentially the same as tetralogy of Fallot with pulmonary atresia).
Hypoplastic left heart syndrome	Right ventricular and right atrial enlargement causes progressive globular cardiomegaly. Severe pulmonary venous congestion.	Consists of several conditions in which underdevelopment of the left side of the heart is related to an obstructive lesion (stenosis or atresia of the mitral valve, aortic valve, or aortic arch). Causes heart failure in the first week of life.
Malformations obstructing pulmonary venous flow	Right ventricular enlargement associated with severe pulmonary venous congestion (increased pressure transmitted to the right side of the heart).	Congenital mitral stenosis; cor triatriatum (incomplete fibromuscular diaphragm dividing the left atrium); congenital pulmonary vein stenosis or atresia.
Pulmonary atresia (with tricuspid insufficiency)	Right ventricular enlargement associated with decreased pulmonary vascularity and a shallow or concave pulmonary artery segment.	May be an isolated anomaly or associated with transposition, atrial septal defect, or common ventricle.

Left Atrial Enlargement

Condition	Imaging Findings	Comments
Mitral stenosis (Figs CA 3-1 and CA 3-2)	Left atrial enlargement; pulmonary venous congestion; enlargement of the right ventricle, pulmonary outflow tract, and central pulmonary arteries; normal-sized left ventricle; small aortic knob (decreased left ventricular output).	Most common rheumatic valvular lesion (results from diffuse thickening of the valve by fibrous tissue or calcific deposits). Obstruction of blood flow from the left atrium into the left ventricle during diastole causes increased left atrial pressure that is transmitted to the pulmonary veins and eventually to the pulmonary arteries and the right side of the heart. Calcification of the mitral valve (best demonstrated by fluoroscopy) and pulmonary hemosiderosis may develop.

A
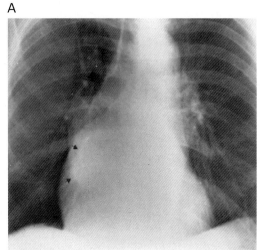

B
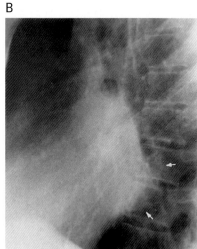

Fig CA 3-1
Mitral stenosis. (A) Frontal chest radiograph demonstrates a double contour (arrows) representing the increased density of the enlarged left atrium. (B) Lateral view confirms the left atrial enlargement (arrows) in this patient with rheumatic heart disease.

A
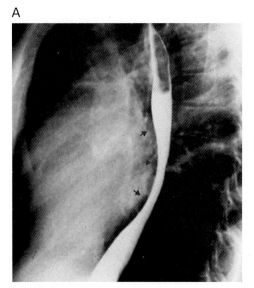

B
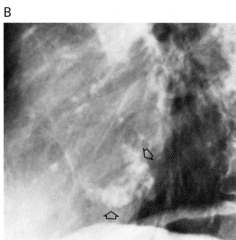

Fig CA 3-2
Mitral stenosis. (A) On a lateral view, the enlarged chamber produces a discrete posterior indentation (arrows) on the barium-filled esophagus. (B) In another patient, there is associated calcification of the mitral valve annulus (arrows).

Condition	Imaging Findings	Comments
Mitral insufficiency (Fig CA 3-3)	Left atrial enlargement (sometimes enormous); enlargement of the left ventricle; normal-sized aortic knob.	Most often caused by rheumatic heart disease. Also rupture of chordae tendineae, papillary muscle dysfunction, or severe left ventricular dilatation that distorts the mitral annulus (congestive heart failure, aortic valve disease, coarctation of the aorta). In mitral insufficiency, the left atrium is usually considerably larger than in mitral stenosis, and pulmonary venous congestion is less frequent and less prominent.
Left-to-right shunts (see Fig CA 7-3)	Left atrial enlargement, increased pulmonary vascularity, and pulmonary outflow tract. The appearance of the right atrium, right ventricle, and aorta depends on the specific lesion.	Ventricular septal defect, patent ductus arteriosus, and aorticopulmonary window are the most common causes. Also coronary artery fistula, persistent truncus arteriosus, and atrial septal defect with reversal of the shunt.
Myxoma of left atrium	Normal heart size and pulmonary vascularity until the tumor causes dysfunction of the mitral valve (radiographic pattern of mitral stenosis). Pathognomonic calcification is seen on fluoroscopy in approximately 10% of cases.	Most common primary cardiac tumor. Almost all arise in an atrium (particularly the left). The tumor is usually pedunculated and causes intermittent obstruction or traumatic injury to the mitral (or tricuspid) valve. A similar ball-valve mechanism may be produced by a left atrial thrombus. Fragmentation of the tumor may produce showers of systemic or pulmonary emboli.
Right-to-left shunts and admixture lesions	Various patterns, depending on the precise intracardiac anomaly. Left atrial enlargement may develop, though other radiographic changes are more diagnostic.	Tricuspid atresia, trilogy of Fallot, transposition of great vessels.
Endocardial fibroelastosis	Striking globular enlargement of the heart. There may be dramatic left atrial enlargement due to often-associated mitral insufficiency. Small aortic knob (decreased left ventricular output). Normal pulmonary vascularity until congestive heart failure supervenes.	Common cause of cardiac failure during the first year of life. Characterized by diffuse thickening of the left ventricular endocardium with collagen and elastic tissue.

A
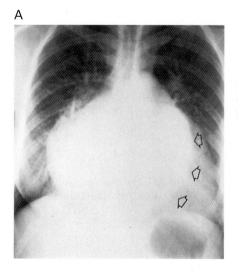

B
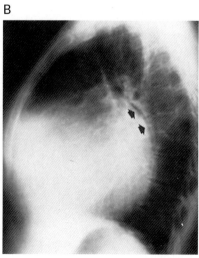

Fig CA 3-3
Mitral insufficiency. (A) Frontal and (B) lateral views of the chest demonstrate gross cardiomegaly with enlargement of the left atrium and left ventricle. Note the striking double-contour configuration (open arrows, A) and elevation of the left main bronchus (closed arrows, B), characteristic signs of left atrial enlargement. The aortic knob is normal in size, and there is no evidence of pulmonary venous congestion.

Left Ventricular Enlargement

Condition	Imaging Findings	Comments
Congestive heart failure	Left ventricular enlargement with pulmonary venous congestion. Pleural effusion is common (bilateral or right sided; unilateral left-sided effusion is rare and suggests another cause).	Precise type and degree of cardiac enlargement depend on the underlying heart disease
High-output heart disease (see figures in Section CA 17)	Left ventricular enlargement associated with prominent pulmonary vascularity (both arteries and veins) and dilatation of the main pulmonary artery.	Causes include anemia, thyrotoxicosis, beriberi, hypervolemia, arteriovenous fistulas, Paget's disease, Pickwickian obesity, polycythemia vera, and pregnancy.
Arteriosclerotic heart disease (myocardial ischemia) (Fig CA 4-1)	Plain chest radiograph is often normal. Left ventricular enlargement is a nonspecific finding that usually reflects the presence of a large quantity of infarcted myocardium.	Coronary artery calcification (see Fig CA 19-5) strongly suggests hemodynamically significant disease. The calcification primarily involves the circumflex and anterior descending branches of the left coronary artery. Best seen with cardiac fluoroscopy (infrequently visualized on routine chest radiographs).
Acute myocardial infarction (Fig CA 4-2)	Generally normal appearance. Left ventricular dilatation is usually related to superimposed pulmonary venous congestion.	Weakening of the myocardial wall at the site of an infarct may permit the development of a ventricular aneurysm, which causes focal bulging or diffuse prominence along the lower left border of the heart near the apex (located anteriorly on lateral view). Characteristic curvilinear calcification in the aneurysm wall and paradoxical or extremely limited pulsation on fluoroscopy.
Hypertension (see figures in Section CA 18)	Initially, increased workload causes left ventricular hypertrophy that produces no radiographic change or only rounding of the left heart border. Eventually, continued strain leads to dilatation and enlargement of the left ventricle. Aortic tortuosity with prominence of the ascending portion often occurs.	Widened superior mediastinum (increased fat deposition) and vertebral compression suggest Cushing's syndrome; figure-3 sign and rib notching indicate coarctation; paravertebral mass suggests pheochromocytoma; erosion of the distal clavicle suggests secondary hyperparathyroidism (renal disease).

A

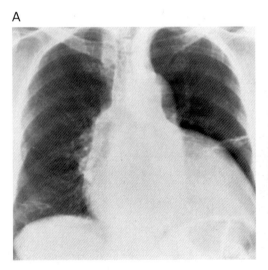

B

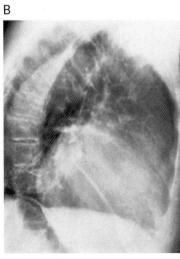

Fig CA 4-1
Arteriosclerotic heart disease. (A) Frontal and (B) lateral views of the chest show marked enlargement of the left ventricle. There is also tortuosity of the aorta and bilateral streaks of fibrosis.

Condition	Imaging Findings	Comments
Aortic insufficiency (Fig CA 4-3)	Left ventricular enlargement (dilatation and hypertrophy). Dilatation of the ascending aorta and aortic knob. As the left ventricle fails, pulmonary venous congestion develops along with left atrial enlargement (due to relative mitral insufficiency).	Most commonly caused by rheumatic heart disease; also caused by infective endocarditis, syphilis, dissecting aneurysm, and Marfan's syndrome. Congenital aortic insufficiency is usually due to a bicuspid valve.
Aortic stenosis (Fig CA 4-4)	Initially, concentric left ventricular hypertrophy produces only some rounding of the cardiac apex (overall heart size is normal). Left ventricular failure and dilatation develop late and are often accompanied by left atrial enlargement, pulmonary venous congestion, and prominence of the right ventricle and pulmonary artery. Poststenotic dilatation of the ascending aorta occurs with valvular stenosis.	May be due to rheumatic heart disease or a congenital valvular deformity (especially a bicuspid valve), or may represent a degenerative process of aging (idiopathic calcific stenosis). An aortic valve disorder due to rheumatic heart disease is rarely isolated and is most commonly associated with a significant lesion of the mitral valve. Aortic valve calcification (best seen with fluoroscopy) is common and indicates severe aortic stenosis.

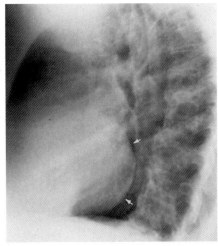

Fig CA 4-2
Acute myocardial infarction. Lateral view of the chest shows marked prominence of the left ventricle (arrows).

A
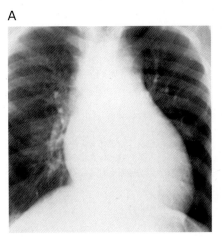

B
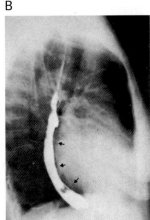

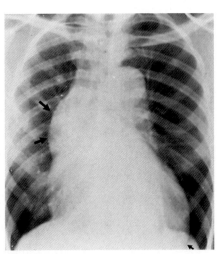

Fig CA 4-3
Aortic insufficiency. Frontal chest radiograph shows left ventricular enlargement with downward and lateral displacement of the cardiac apex. Note that the cardiac shadow extends below the dome of the left hemidiaphragm. The ascending aorta is strikingly dilated (arrows), suggesting some underlying aortic stenosis.

Fig CA 4-4
Aortic stenosis. (A) Frontal view shows downward displacement of the cardiac apex. (B) On a lateral view, the bulging of the lower half of the posterior cardiac silhouette causes a broad indentation on the barium-filled esophagus (arrows).

Condition	Imaging Findings	Comments
Coarctation of aorta (see Fig CA 8-1)	Enlargement of the left ventricle with a characteristic double bulge in the region of the aortic knob (figure-3 sign on plain chest radiographs and reverse figure-3, or figure-E, sign on the barium-filled esophagus). There may be rib notching (usually involving the posterior fourth to eighth ribs) but rarely developing before the age of 6 years.	In the more common "adult" type, aortic narrowing occurs at or just distal to the level of the ductus arteriosus (double bulge represents prestenotic and poststenotic dilatation). In the "infantile" variety, there is a long segment of narrowing lying proximal to the ductus (obligatory right-to-left shunt and early congestive heart failure). There is a relatively high incidence of coarctation in women with Turner's syndrome.
Mitral insufficiency (Fig CA 4-5)	Enlargement (sometimes enormous) of the left ventricle and left atrium. Small or normal aortic knob. Generally normal pulmonary vascularity (there may be pulmonary venous congestion, but it is less frequent and less prominent than in mitral stenosis).	Most often caused by rheumatic heart disease; also may be due to rupture of chordae tendineae, papillary muscle dysfunction, or severe left ventricular dilatation (aortic valve disease, congestive heart failure) distorting the mitral annulus. Coexistent mitral stenosis may produce a bizarre pattern.
Myocardiopathy (Figs CA 4-6 and CA 4-7)	Generalized cardiac enlargement, often with left ventricular predominance. May mimic pericardial effusion. The development of left ventricular failure produces pulmonary venous congestion.	Causes include inflammation (rheumatic, septic, viral, toxoplasmic); infiltration (amyloidosis, glycogen storage disease, leukemia); endocrine imbalance (thyrotoxicosis, myxedema, acromegaly); ischemia; nutritional deficiency (beriberi, alcoholism, potassium or magnesium depletion); toxicity (drugs, chemicals, cobalt); collagen diseases; and postpartum heart disease.

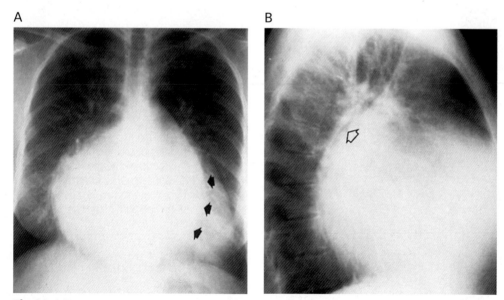

A   B

Fig CA 4-5
Mitral insufficiency. (A) Frontal and (B) lateral views of the chest demonstrate cardiomegaly with enlargement of the left ventricle and left atrium. Note the striking double-contour configuration (closed arrows) and elevation of the left main-stem bronchus (open arrow), characteristic signs of left atrial enlargement.

Condition	Imaging Findings	Comments
Left-to-right shunt (see Figs CA 7-3 and CA 7-5)	Various patterns of abnormal heart size with increased pulmonary vascularity.	Ventricular septal defect (not atrial septal defect), patent ductus arteriosus, endocardial cushion defect, aorticopulmonary window, and, infrequently, persistent truncus arteriosus.
Right-to-left shunt or admixture lesion	Various patterns of abnormal heart size and pulmonary vascularity.	Transposition of great vessels; tricuspid atresia; pulmonary stenosis with intact ventricular septum.
Endocardial fibroelastosis (Fig CA 4-8)	Generalized cardiac enlargement with hypertrophy and dilatation of the left ventricle and often dramatic left atrial enlargement (due to associated mitral insufficiency).	Diffuse thickening of the left ventricular endocardium with collagen and elastic tissue. A common cause of cardiac failure in the first year of life.

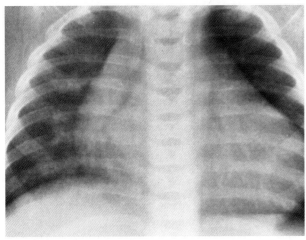

Fig CA 4-6
Glycogen storage disease. Generalized globular cardiac enlargement with a left ventricular prominence.

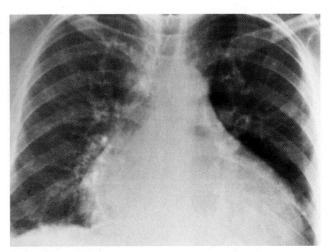

Fig CA 4-7
Alcoholic cardiomyopathy. Generalized cardiac enlargement that involves all chambers but has a left ventricular predominance. There is pulmonary vascular congestion and a right pleural effusion.

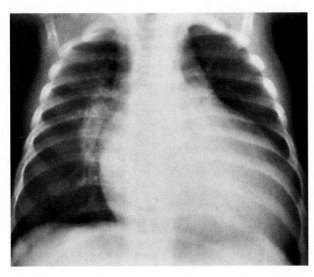

Fig CA 4-8
Endocardial fibroelastosis. Generalized cardiomegaly with prominence of the left ventricle.

Cyanotic Congenital Heart Disease with Increased Pulmonary Vascularity

Condition	Imaging Findings	Comments
Persistent truncus arteriosus (types I, II, and III) (Fig CA 5-1)	Increased pulmonary vascularity; concave pulmonary outflow tract; striking enlargement of the right ventricle, and eventual enlargement of the left atrium and left ventricle.	Failure of the common truncus arteriosus to divide normally into the aorta and the pulmonary artery. Results in a single large arterial trunk that receives the outflow of blood from both ventricles. Variable degree of cyanosis (more profound cyanosis if low pulmonary blood flow).
Transposition of great arteries (Figs CA 5-2 and CA 5-3)	Increased pulmonary vascularity (unless prominent pulmonary stenosis). Various patterns depending on the precise intracardiac anomalies (generally biventricular enlargement with an oval or egg-shaped configuration).	Reversal of the normal relation of the aorta and the pulmonary artery (the aorta arises anteriorly from the right ventricle, whereas the pulmonary artery originates posteriorly from the left ventricle). An intracardiac or extracardiac shunt (atrial and ventricular septal defects, patent ductus arteriosus) must be present to connect the two separate circulations. The shunts are bidirectional and permit mixing of oxygenated and unoxygenated blood (leading to cyanosis).
Taussig-Bing anomaly (Fig CA 5-4)	Increased pulmonary vascularity; generalized cardiomegaly.	Aorta arises from the right ventricle, whereas the pulmonary artery overrides the ventricular septum and receives blood from both ventricles. The pulmonary artery lies to the left of and slightly posterior to the aorta. Also a high ventricular septal defect.
Double-outlet right ventricle (Figs CA 5-5 and CA 5-6)	Increased pulmonary vascularity; generalized cardiomegaly; cardiac waist wider than in other types of transpositions (the aorta and pulmonary artery have a more side-to-side configuration).	Both the aorta and the pulmonary artery arise from the right ventricle. A left-to-right ventricular septal defect permits oxygenated blood from the left ventricle to pass to the right ventricle and then on to the systemic circulation.

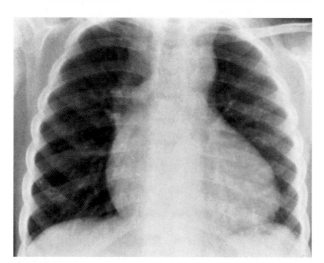

Fig CA 5-1
Persistent truncus arteriosus. Increased pulmonary vascularity, yet typical concave appearance of the pulmonary outflow tract.

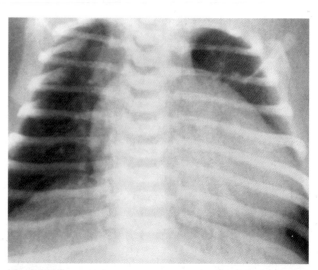

Fig CA 5-2
Transposition of the great arteries. Biventricular enlargement produces a typical oval or egg-shaped heart. Note the narrowing of the vascular pedicle due to superimposition of the abnormally positioned aorta and pulmonary artery.

Condition	Imaging Findings	Comments
Common ventricle (Fig CA 5-7)	Increased or decreased pulmonary vascularity (depending on the presence and degree of associated pulmonary stenosis); marked nonspecific globular enlargement of the heart.	Extremely large septal defect produces a functional "single ventricle." If there is associated severe pulmonary stenosis, the blood flow through the lungs is scanty, and the patient develops profound cyanosis.
Complete endocardial cushion defect (Fig CA 5-8)	Increased pulmonary vascularity; nonspecific globular enlargement of the heart (enlargement of all cardiac chambers).	Low atrial septal defect combined with a large ventricular septal defect plus a contiguous cleft in both the mitral and the tricuspid valves (common atrioventricular canal). Bidirectional shunting with right-to-left components is responsible for producing the cyanosis.

A

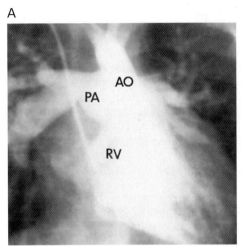

B

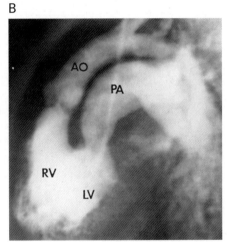

Fig CA 5-3
Transposition of the great arteries. (A) Frontal and (B) lateral views from an angiocardiogram demonstrate contrast material in the right ventricle (RV), which is situated anteriorly and to the right. It communicates through a large ventricular septal defect with the left ventricle (LV), which is located posteriorly and to the left. The transposed aorta (AO) originates from the right ventricular infundibulum directly in front of the pulmonary artery (PA), which arises from the left ventricle.[2]

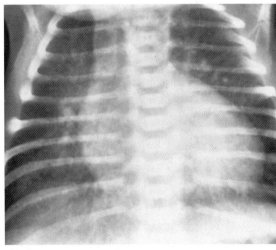

Fig CA 5-4
Taussig-Bing anomaly. Engorged pulmonary vasculature, oval cardiomegaly, and a laterally pointing apex.

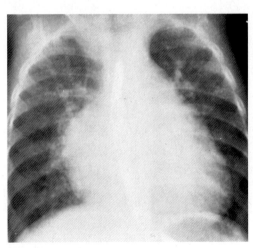

Fig CA 5-5
Double-outlet right ventricle. Generalized cardiomegaly with increased pulmonary vascularity. Because the aorta and the pulmonary artery have a more side-to-side configuration, the cardiac waist is relatively wider than in other types of transpositions.

Condition	Imaging Findings	Comments
Total anomalous pulmonary venous return (Fig CA 5-9)	Increased pulmonary vascularity; "snowman" or figure-8 configuration in types I and II; characteristic indentation on the lower esophagus by the anomalous vein as it descends through the diaphragm in type III.	Pulmonary veins connect to the right atrium directly or to the systemic veins or their tributaries. Because all the pulmonary venous blood returns to the right atrium, a right-to-left shunt through an interatrial communication is necessary for blood to reach the left side of the heart and the systemic circulation (producing cyanosis).
Reversal of left-to-right shunt (Eisenmenger physiology) (Fig CA 5-10)	Increased fullness of the central pulmonary arteries with abrupt narrowing and pruning of peripheral vessels.	Development of pulmonary hypertension causes reversal of the shunt leading to unoxygenated blood entering the systemic circulation (cyanosis). Most commonly develops with atrial and ventricular septal defects and patent ductus arteriosus.

A
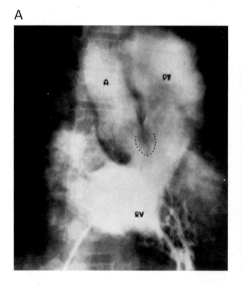

B
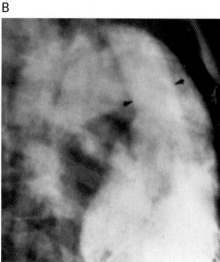

Fig CA 5-6
Double-outlet right ventricle. (A) Frontal view from a selective right ventriculogram shows simultaneous and equal opacification of both great vessels from the right ventricle (RV). The ventricular septal defect was immediately beneath the crista supraventricularis (dotted line). (B) A lateral view shows the aorta (arrows) superimposed over the posterior two-thirds of the pulmonary trunk. (A, aorta; PT, pulmonary trunk.)[3]

A
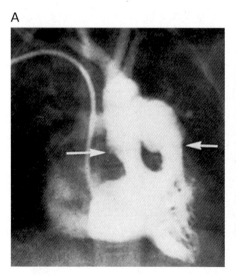

B
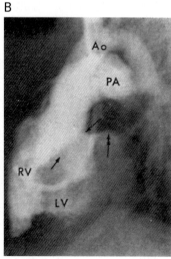

Fig CA 5-7
Single ventricle. (A) Frontal view from a right ventriculogram shows muscular tracts leading from the right ventricle to both great arteries, the valves of which (arrows) are at the same horizontal level. (B) A lateral view shows the anteriorly situated right ventricle (RV) communicating with the left ventricle (LV) via a ventricular septal defect (single arrows). (PA, pulmonary artery; Ao, aorta.)[4]

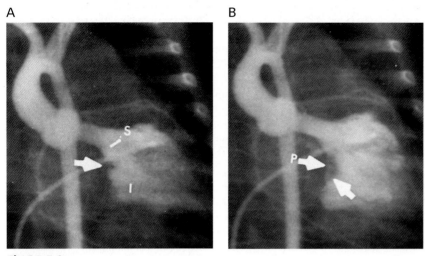

Fig CA 5-8
Common atrioventricular canal. (A) Left ventricular angiogram (frontal view) in early systole shows the cleft (arrow) between the superior (S) and inferior (I) segments of the anterior mitral leaflet located along the right contour of the ventricle. There is no evidence of mitral insufficiency or an interventricular shunt. (B) In diastole, the ventricular outflow tract is narrowed and lies in a more horizontal position than normal. The right border of the ventricle can be followed directly into the scooped-out margin (arrows) of the interventricular septum. The attachment of the posterior mitral leaflet (P) is also visible because of a thin layer of contrast material trapped between the leaflet and the posterior ventricular wall.[5]

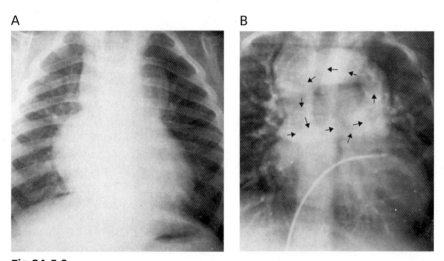

Fig CA 5-9
Total anomalous pulmonary venous return (type I). (A) Frontal chest radiograph demonstrates a snowman, or figure-8, heart with right atrial and right ventricular enlargement. The widening of the superior mediastinum is due to the large, anomalous inverted-U–shaped vein. The pulmonary vascularity is greatly increased. The large pulmonary artery is hidden in the superior mediastinal silhouette. (B) Angiocardiogram demonstrates that all the pulmonary veins drain into the inverted-U–shaped vessel that eventually empties into the superior vena cava (arrows). The widening of the mediastinum produced by this vessel causes the snowman heart.[6]

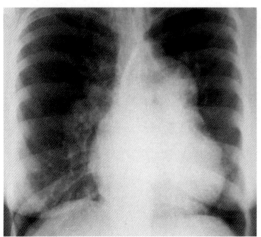

Fig CA 5-10
Eisenmenger physiology in patent ductus arteriosus. There is an increased fullness of the central pulmonary arteries with an abrupt narrowing and paucity of peripheral vessels.

Cyanotic Congenital Heart Disease with Decreased Pulmonary Vascularity

Condition	Imaging Findings	Comments
Tetralogy of Fallot (Fig CA 6-1)	Decreased pulmonary vascularity; flat or concave pulmonary outflow tract; enlargement of the right ventricle; right aortic arch in approximately 25% of cases.	Most common cause of cyanotic congenital heart disease beyond the immediate neonatal period includes (1) high ventricular septal defect, (2) obstruction to right ventricular outflow (usually infundibular stenosis), (3) overriding of the aortic orifice above the ventricular defect, and (4) right ventricular hypertrophy.
Pseudotruncus arteriosus (truncus arteriosus type IV) (Fig CA 6-2)	Decreased pulmonary vascularity; flat or concave pulmonary outflow tract; enlargement of the right ventricle; right aortic arch in approximately 40% of cases.	Single large arterial trunk receives the outflow of blood from both ventricles. The pulmonary arteries are absent, so the pulmonary circulation is supplied by bronchial or other collateral vessels.
Trilogy of Fallot (Fig CA 6-3)	Decreased pulmonary vascularity; poststenotic dilatation of pulmonary artery; heart size often normal (usually some evidence of right ventricular hypertrophy).	Combination of pulmonary valvular stenosis with an intact ventricular septum and an interatrial shunt (patent foramen ovale or true atrial septal defect). Increased pressure on the right side of the heart due to pulmonary stenosis causes the interatrial shunt to be right to left.
Tricuspid atresia/stenosis (Fig CA 6-4)	Decreased pulmonary vascularity (usually some degree of pulmonary stenosis); striking enlargement of the right atrium if small atrial shunt; large left ventricle; small right ventricle.	Right-to-left shunt at the atrial level (patent foramen ovale or true atrial septal defect). Usually there is also a ventricular septal defect or a patent ductus arteriosus. Hypoplasia of the right ventricle and pulmonary outflow tract is evident. The smaller the shunt, the more marked the elevation of right atrial pressure and more striking the enlargement of this chamber. Tricuspid atresia without pulmonary stenosis produces marked cardiomegaly and increased pulmonary vascularity.

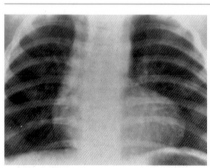

Fig CA 6-1
Tetralogy of Fallot. Plain chest radiograph demonstrates decreased pulmonary vascularity and a flat pulmonary outflow tract. Note the characteristic lateral displacement and upward tilting of the prominent left cardiac apex (*coeur en sabot* appearance).

A
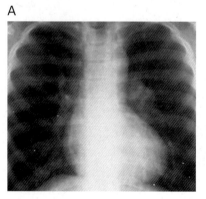

B
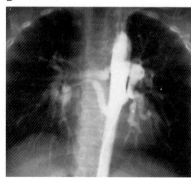

Fig CA 6-2
Pseudotruncus arteriosus. (A) Plain chest radiograph shows the pulmonary vascularity to be strikingly diminished. (B) Angiogram shows that most of the blood supply to the lungs originates from two large arteries arising from the descending aorta.[1]

Condition	Imaging Findings	Comments
Ebstein's anomaly (Fig CA 6-5)	Decreased pulmonary vascularity; flat or concave pulmonary outflow tract; characteristic squared or boxed appearance of the heart (bulging of the right heart border by the enlarged right atrium); narrow vascular pedicle; and small aortic arch.	Downward displacement of an incompetent tricuspid valve into the right ventricle so that the upper portion of the right ventricle is effectively incorporated into the right atrium. The functional obstruction to right atrial emptying produces increased pressure and a right-to-left atrial shunt (usually through a patent foramen ovale).
Uhl's disease	Radiographic pattern identical to that in Ebstein's anomaly.	Focal or complete absence of the right ventricular myocardium (the right ventricle becomes a thin-walled fibroelastic bag that contracts poorly and cannot effectively empty blood from the right side of the heart).
Pulmonary atresia or severe pulmonary stenosis (Fig CA 6-6)	Decreased pulmonary vascularity; shallow or concave pulmonary artery segment; variable cardiomegaly.	May be an isolated anomaly or associated with transposition, atrial septal defect, or common ventricle.

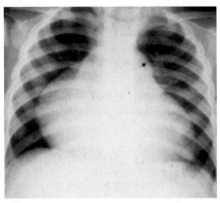

Fig CA 6-3
Trilogy of Fallot. Decreased pulmonary vascularity with prominent poststenotic dilatation (arrow) of the pulmonary artery. There is enormous right atrial and moderate right ventricular enlargement.[6]

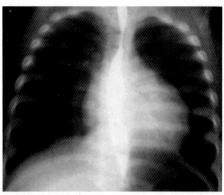

Fig CA 6-4
Tricuspid atresia. Decreased pulmonary vascularity with elongation and rounding of the left border of the heart.

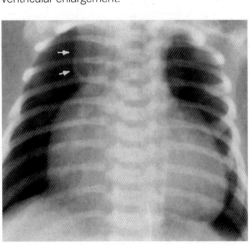

Fig CA 6-5
Ebstein's anomaly. In addition to decreased pulmonary vascularity, there is enlargement of the right atrium, causing upward and outward bulging of the right border of the heart (squared appearance). Widening of the right side of the superior portion of the mediastinum (arrows) reflects marked dilatation of the superior vena cava due to right ventricular failure.

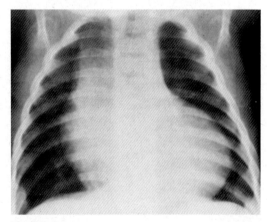

Fig CA 6-6
Pulmonary atresia. Decreased pulmonary vascularity with a concave outflow tract and moderate cardiomegaly.

Acyanotic Congenital Heart Disease with Increased Pulmonary Blood Flow

Condition	Imaging Findings	Comments
Atrial septal defect (Fig CA 7-1)	Increased pulmonary vascularity; enlarged right atrium, right ventricle, and pulmonary outflow tract; normal left atrium and left ventricle; small aorta.	Most common congenital cardiac lesion. The magnitude of the shunt depends on the size of the defect, the relative compliance of the ventricles, and the difference in atrial pressure. May be combined with mitral stenosis (Lutembacher's syndrome) and cause a substantial increase in the workload of the right ventricle.
Ventricular septal defect (Fig CA 7-2)	Increased pulmonary vascularity; enlarged right ventricle, pulmonary outflow tract, left atrium, and sometimes left ventricle (may be normal); normal right atrium; normal or small aorta.	Common congenital cardiac anomaly. The magnitude of the shunt depends on the size of the defect and the difference in ventricular pressure. There may also be a shunt from the left ventricle to the right atrium.
Patent ductus arteriosus (Fig CA 7-3)	Increased pulmonary vascularity; enlargement of the left atrium, left ventricle, aorta, and pulmonary outflow tract; normal right atrium; enlarged or normal right ventricle.	Ductus extends from the bifurcation of the pulmonary artery to join the aorta just distal to the left subclavian artery (shunts blood from the pulmonary artery into the systemic circulation during intrauterine life). The aortic end of the ductus (infundibulum) is often dilated to produce a convex bulge on the left border of the aorta just below the knob.
Endocardial cushion defect (Fig CA 7-4)	Increased pulmonary vascularity; nonspecific globular enlargement of the heart (enlargement of all cardiac chambers).	Low atrial septal defect combined with a high ventricular septal defect. Most often occurs in children with Down's syndrome.

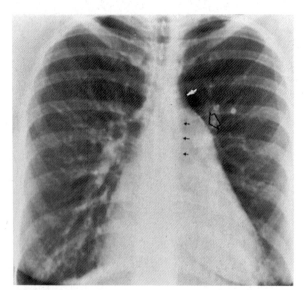

Fig CA 7-1
Atrial septal defect. Frontal view of the chest demonstrates cardiomegaly along with an increase in pulmonary vascularity reflecting the left-to-right shunt. Filling of the retrosternal space indicates enlargement of the right ventricle. The small aortic knob (white arrow) and descending aorta (small black arrows) are dwarfed by the enlarged pulmonary outflow tract (large open arrow).

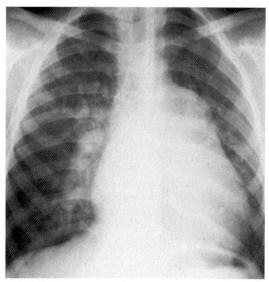

Fig CA 7-2
Ventricular septal defect. The heart is enlarged and somewhat triangular, and there is an increase in pulmonary vascular volume. The pulmonary trunk is very large and over-shadows the normal-sized aorta, which seems small by comparison.[1]

Condition	Imaging Findings	Comments
Aorticopulmonary window (Fig CA 7-5)	Increased pulmonary vascularity; enlargement of the left ventricle, left atrium, and pulmonary outflow tract (similar to patent ductus arteriosus but usually a less prominent aortic knob).	Uncommon anomaly in which a communication between the pulmonary artery and the aorta (just above their valves) is caused by a failure of the primitive truncus arteriosus to separate completely.
Ruptured sinus of Valsalva aneurysm (Fig CA 7-6)	Rapid increase in pulmonary vascularity and enlargement of the right ventricle and the pulmonary outflow tract.	Rupture usually occurs into the right ventricle (occasionally the right atrium). Causes a sudden large left-to-right shunt with the acute onset of chest pain, shortness of breath, and a cardiac murmur.
Coronary artery fistula (Fig CA 7-7)	Increased pulmonary vascularity; enlargement of the pulmonary outflow tract; enlargement of the right ventricle or both the right atrium and the right ventricle (depending on the site of the fistula).	Unusual anomaly in which there is a communication between a coronary artery and a cardiac chamber or the pulmonary artery. The right coronary artery most often communicates with, in order of frequency, the right ventricle, right atrium, coronary sinus, or pulmonary artery.

A

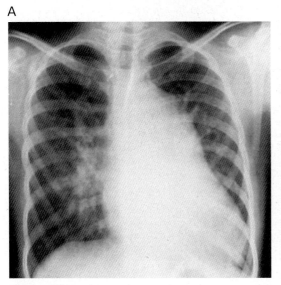

B

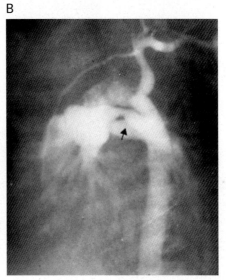

Fig CA 7-3
Patent ductus arteriosus. (A) Preoperative frontal chest film demonstrates cardiomegaly with enlargement of the left atrium, left ventricle, and central pulmonary arteries. There is a diffuse increase in pulmonary vascularity. (B) In another patient, an aortogram shows persistent patency of the ductus arteriosus (arrow).[1]

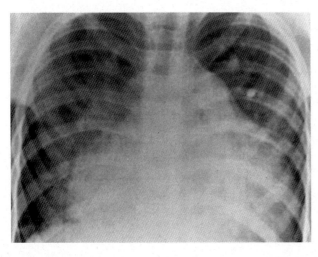

Fig CA 7-4
Endocardial cushion defect. Globular enlargement of the heart with increased pulmonary vascularity.

Condition	Imaging Findings	Comments
Partial anomalous pulmonary venous return (Fig CA 7-8)	Increased pulmonary vascularity; enlarged right atrium, right ventricle, and pulmonary outflow tract; normal left atrium and left ventricle; small aorta.	One (or more) of the pulmonary veins is connected to the right atrium or its tributaries. Virtually indistinguishable from an atrial septal defect radiographically. A "scimitar sign" (crescent-like anomalous venous channel) on the right if associated with hypoplasia of the right lung.

A

B

D

C

E

Fig CA 7-5
Aorticopulmonary window. (A) Plain chest radiograph demonstrates enlargement of the left ventricle, a low position of the apex, and an increase in pulmonary vascularity. (B and C) Contrast material injected into the ascending aorta shows rapid shunting into the pulmonary arteries (arrows). (D and E) Contrast material injected into the descending aorta does not show a shunt, confirming that the shunt is in the ascending aorta.[1]

A

B

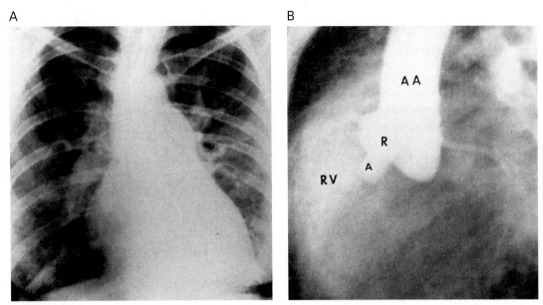

Fig CA 7-6
Ruptured sinus of Valsalva aneurysm. (A) Frontal chest radiograph demonstrates cardiomegaly and increased pulmonary vascularity. (B) Lateral projection from a selective thoracic aortogram shows an aneurysm (A) of the right aortic sinus (R) projecting into the outflow tract of the right ventricle (RV). The contrast material has opacified the right ventricle through the aneurysm. (AA, ascending aorta.)[7]

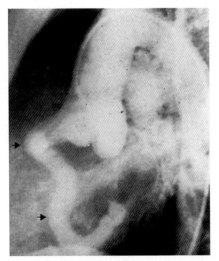

Fig CA 7-7
Coronary artery fistula. Lateral view from an angiocardiogram shows a huge right coronary artery (arrows) draining into the right ventricle.[8]

A

B

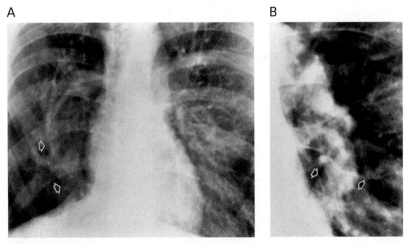

Fig CA 7-8
Partial anomalous pulmonary venous return. Two examples of curvilinear venous pathways (arrows) resembling a Turkish scimitar.

Acyanotic Congenital Heart Disease with Normal Pulmonary Blood Flow

Condition	Imaging Findings	Comments
Coarctation of aorta (Fig CA 8-1)	Characteristic double bulge in the region of the aortic knob (figure-3 sign on plain chest radiographs and reverse figure-3, or figure-E, sign on the barium-filled esophagus). There may be rib notching (usually involving the posterior fourth to eighth ribs) but rarely developing before the age of 6 years.	In the more common "adult" type, the aortic narrowing occurs at or just distal to the level of the ductus arteriosus (double bulge represents prestenotic and poststenotic dilatation). In the "infantile" variety, there is a long segment of narrowing proximal to the ductus (obligatory right-to-left shunt and early congestive heart failure). There is a relatively high incidence of coarctation in women with Turner's syndrome.
Aortic stenosis (Fig CA 8-2)	Increased convexity or prominence of the left heart border (overall heart size often normal). Substantial cardiomegaly reflects left ventricular failure and dilatation.	Valvular, subvalvular, and supravalvular types. Bulging of the right superior mediastinal silhouette (poststenotic dilatation of the ascending aorta) is often seen with valvular stenosis.

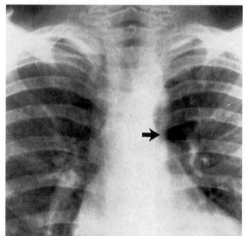

Fig CA 8-1
Coarctation of the aorta. Plain chest radiograph demonstrates the figure-3 sign (arrow points to the center of the 3).

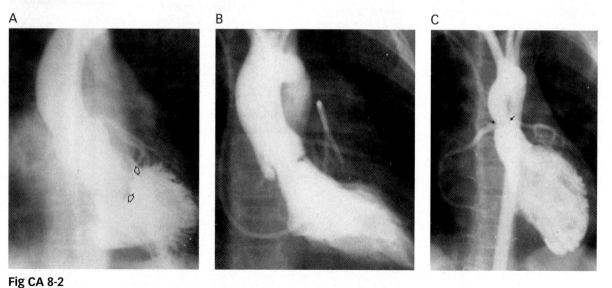

Fig CA 8-2
(A) Subvalvular aortic stenosis. Note the muscular ridge protruding from the upper portion of the ventricular septum (arrows). The ridge is about 2 cm below the aortic valve and encroaches on the outflow tract of the left ventricle. (B) Valvular aortic stenosis. Irregular thickening of aortic valve leaflets and relative rigidity of the left coronary cusp. (C) Supravalvular aortic stenosis. Narrowed segment (arrows) located just above the coronary ostia.[9]

Condition	Imaging Findings	Comments
Pulmonary valvular stenosis (see Fig CA 13-6)	Poststenotic dilatation of the pulmonary artery, often associated with dilatation of the left main pulmonary artery. The heart size is initially normal (right ventricular hypertrophy and dilatation if severe pulmonary stenosis causes systolic overloading of the right ventricle).	Common anomaly found in isolated form or in combination with other abnormalities. The stenosis is most common at the level of the pulmonary valve (supravalvular or infundibular stenosis can occur). Must be differentiated from normal idiopathic poststenotic dilatation of the pulmonary artery in adolescents and young adults, especially women.
Endocardial fibroelastosis (Fig CA 8-3)	Striking globular cardiac enlargement (often with left-sided prominence); small aortic knob.	Diffuse thickening of the left ventricular endocardium with collagen and elastic tissue. A common cause of cardiac failure during the first year of life. The pulmonary vascularity remains normal until congestive heart failure supervenes.
Miscellaneous lesions with normal vascularity (until left-sided failure develops in infancy) (Fig CA 8-4)	Various patterns.	Includes hypoplastic left heart syndrome, mitral stenosis and insufficiency, aortic insufficiency, cor triatriatum, aberrant pulmonary origin of left coronary artery, and cardiomyopathy.

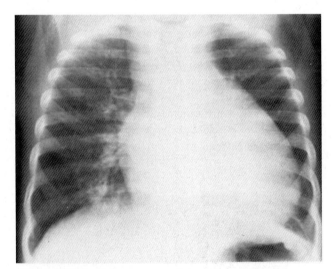

Fig CA 8-3
Endocardial fibroelastosis. Globular enlargement of the heart.

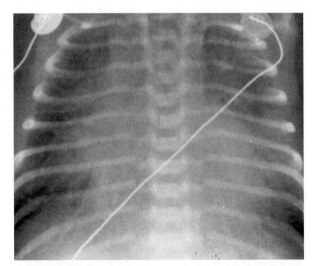

Fig CA 8-4
Hypoplastic left heart syndrome. Globular cardiomegaly with pronounced congestive failure.

Prominent Ascending Aorta or Aortic Arch

Condition	Imaging Findings	Comments
Hypertensive heart disease (see Figs CA 9-1 and CA 18-1)	Aortic tortuosity with prominence of the ascending portion.	Increased workload of the left ventricle causes concentric hypertrophy (rounding of the left heart border). Continued strain eventually leads to dilatation and enlargement of the left ventricle.
Atherosclerosis (Fig CA 9-2)	Generalized tortuosity, elongation, and moderate dilatation of the aorta. Often linear plaques of intimal calcification (especially in the aortic knob and the transverse arch).	Generally considered to be a degenerative condition of old age. However, intimal thickening, plaque formation, and vascular narrowing can develop in younger patients, especially those with diabetes mellitus, hypertension, or familial disorders of lipid metabolism.
Aortic aneurysm (see Fig CA 19-2)	Sharply marginated, saccular, or fusiform mass of homogeneous density (there may be generalized aortic dilatation). Curvilinear calcification may occur in the outer wall.	Causes include atherosclerosis, cystic medial necrosis (there may be associated Marfan's syndrome), syphilis, mycotic infection, and trauma.
Dissecting aneurysm	Progressive widening of the aortic shadow, which may have an irregular or wavy outer border. Separation (more than 4 mm) between the intimal calcification and the outer border of the aortic shadow indicates widening of the aortic wall.	Predisposing factors include atherosclerosis, hypertension, cystic medial necrosis (eg, Marfan's syndrome), trauma, aortic stenosis, coarctation of the aorta, Ehlers-Danlos syndrome, and the intramural injection of contrast material. Most dissections begin as intimal tears immediately above the aortic valve. In two-thirds (type I), the dissection continues into the descending aorta. In the remainder (type II), the dissection is limited to the ascending aorta and stops at the origin of the brachiocephalic vessels. In type III, the dissection begins in the thoracic aorta distal to the subclavian artery and extends proximal and distal to the original site.

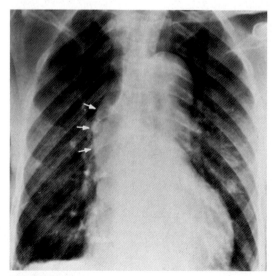

Fig CA 9-1
Hypertensive heart disease. Marked dilatation (arrows) of the ascending aorta caused by increased aortic pressure.

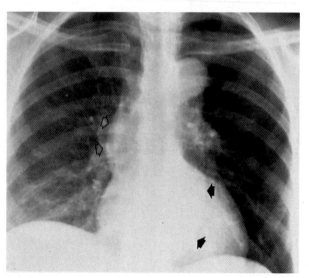

Fig CA 9-2
Atherosclerosis. Generalized tortuosity and elongation of the ascending aorta (open arrows) and descending aorta (closed arrows).

Condition	Imaging Findings	Comments
Aortic valvular stenosis (Fig CA 9-3)	Bulging of the ascending aorta (poststenotic dilatation). Aortic valve calcification (best seen on fluoroscopy) is common and indicates severe stenosis.	May be congenital (usually bicuspid valve) or acquired (generally on a rheumatic basis). Increased prominence of the left heart border (overall heart size is often normal). Substantial cardiomegaly reflects left ventricular failure and dilatation.
Aortic insufficiency (Fig CA 9-4)	Moderate dilatation of the ascending aorta and aortic knob (marked dilatation, especially of the ascending aorta, suggests underlying aortic stenosis). Enlargement of the left ventricle.	Most commonly due to rheumatic heart disease. Other causes include syphilis, infective endocarditis, dissecting aneurysm, and Marfan's syndrome. Left ventricular failure leads to pulmonary venous congestion and left atrial enlargement (relative mitral insufficiency).
Syphilitic aortitis (Fig CA 9-5)	Dilatation of the ascending aorta, frequently with mural calcification.	May cause inflammation of the aortic valvular ring that results in aortic insufficiency. Approximately one-third of patients develop narrowing of the coronary ostia that may lead to symptoms of ischemic heart disease.
Takayasu's disease ("pulseless" disease)	Widening and contour irregularity of the aorta (especially the arch). May also involve major aortic branches. Linear calcifications frequently occur.	Nonspecific obstructive arteritis, primarily affecting young women, in which granulation tissue destroys the media of large vessels. The resulting mural scarring causes luminal narrowing and occlusion. There is usually fever and constitutional symptoms. Characteristic smooth and tapering arterial narrowing on angiography.

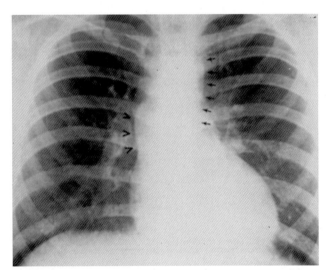

Fig CA 9-3
Aortic valvular stenosis. There is prominence of the left ventricle with poststenotic dilatation of the ascending aorta (arrowheads). The aortic knob and descending aorta (arrows) are normal.[10]

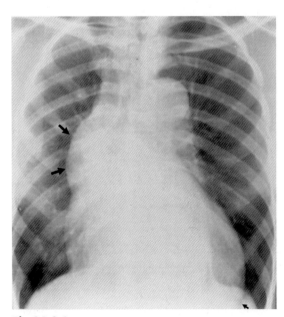

Fig CA 9-4
Aortic insufficiency. Marked dilatation of the ascending aorta (arrows), suggesting some underlying aortic stenosis. The left ventricle is enlarged with downward and lateral displacement of the cardiac apex. Note that the cardiac shadow extends below the dome of the left hemidiaphragm (small arrow).

Condition	Imaging Findings	Comments
Coarctation of aorta (see Fig CA 8-1)	Prominence of the ascending aorta. Characteristic double bulge in the region of the aortic knob (figure-3 sign on plain chest radiographs and reverse figure-3, or figure-E, sign on the barium-filled esophagus). There may be rib notching (usually involving the posterior fourth to eighth ribs but rarely developing before the age of 6 years) and dilated internal mammary arteries (soft-tissue density on lateral films).	In the more common "adult" type, the aortic narrowing occurs at or just distal to the level of the ductus arteriosus. The double bulge represents prestenotic and poststenotic dilatation.
Pseudocoarctation of aorta (Fig CA 9-6)	Two bulges in the region of the aortic knob mimic true coarctation. No rib notching or internal mammary collaterals (as no obstruction or hemodynamic abnormality).	Buckling or kinking of the aortic arch in the region of the ligamentum arteriosum. The bulges represent dilated portions of the aorta just proximal and distal to the kink. The upper bulge is usually higher than the normal aortic knob and can simulate a left superior mediastinal tumor.
Patent ductus arteriosus (Fig CA 9-7)	Prominent aortic knob; increased pulmonary vascularity; enlargement of the left atrium, left ventricle, and pulmonary outflow tract. The aortic end of the ductus (infundibulum) is often dilated to produce a convex bulge on the left border of the aorta just below the knob.	Ductus extends from the bifurcation of the pulmonary artery to join the aorta just distal to the left subclavian artery (shunts blood from the pulmonary artery into the systemic circulation during intrauterine life). Aortic prominence is a differential point from other major left-to-right shunts (atrial and ventricular septal defects).

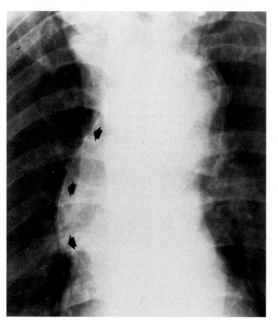

Fig CA 9-5
Syphilitic aortitis. Aneurysmal dilatation of the ascending aorta with extensive linear calcification of the wall (arrows). Some calcification is also seen in the distal aortic arch.

Condition	Imaging Findings	Comments
Tetralogy of Fallot with severe pulmonary stenosis	Pronounced bulging of the ascending aorta and prominence of the aortic knob.	Severe pulmonary stenosis effectively forces the aorta to drain both ventricles. A similar appearance occurs in pseudotruncus arteriosus (essentially tetralogy of Fallot with pulmonary atresia).
Aneurysm of sinus of Valsalva (see Fig CA 7-6)	Large aneurysm produces a smooth local bulge in the right anterolateral cardiac contour (a small aneurysm is undetectable). Curvilinear calcification often occurs in the aneurysm wall.	Primarily involves the sinus above the right cusp of the aortic valve. An acute rupture (usually into the right ventricle) causes a sudden large left-to-right shunt.
Corrected transposition (Fig CA 9-8)	Smooth bulging of the upper left border of the heart replaces the normal double bulge of the aortic knob and the pulmonary artery segment.	Combination of transposition of the origins of the aorta and the pulmonary artery and inversion of the ventricles and their accompanying atrioventricular valves. A single bulge represents the displaced ascending aorta and right ventricular outflow tract.

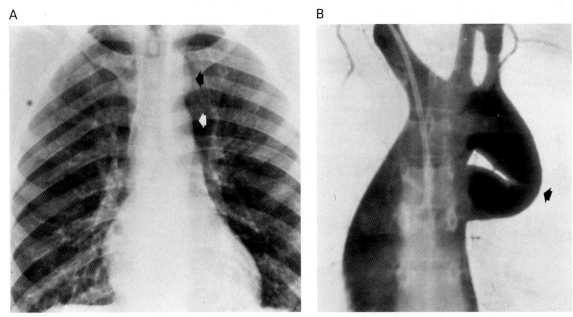

A

B

Fig CA 9-6
Pseudocoarctation of the aorta. (A) Frontal view of the chest demonstrates two bulges (arrows) producing a well-demarcated figure-3 sign in the region of the aortic knob. The upper bulge (black arrow) is higher than the normal aortic knob and simulates a mediastinal mass. Because there is no hemodynamic abnormality, the heart is normal in size, and there is no rib notching. (B) In another patient, an aortogram demonstrates extreme kinking of the descending aorta (arrow) without an area of true coarctation.

Condition	Imaging Findings	Comments
Persistent truncus arteriosus	Bulge in the region of the ascending aorta (represents the large single arterial trunk).	Failure of the common truncus arteriosus to divide normally into the aorta and the pulmonary artery, resulting in a single large arterial trunk that receives the outflow of blood from both ventricles.
Connective tissue disorders (Fig CA 9-9)	Generalized dilatation of the aorta. Increased incidence of aneurysm and dissection.	Conditions include Ehlers-Danlos syndrome, Marfan's syndrome, osteogenesis imperfecta, and pseudoxanthoma elasticum.

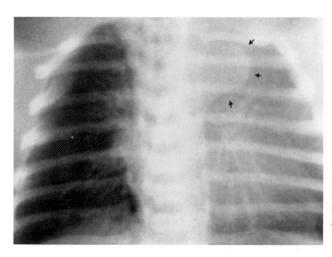

Fig CA 9-7
Patent ductus arteriosus. A convex bulge (arrows) on the left side of the superior mediastinum represents dilatation of the aortic end of the ductus ("ductus bump").

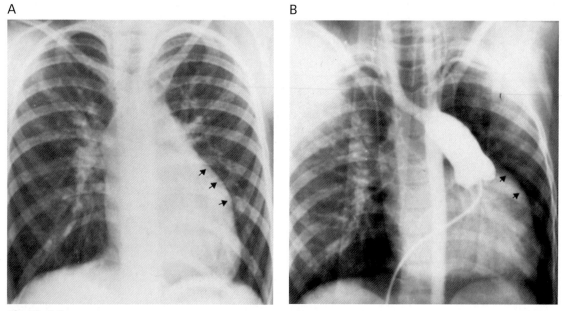

Fig CA 9-8
Corrected transposition with ventricular septal defect. (A) There is fullness of the upper left border of the heart (arrows). Because of the left-to-right ventricular shunt, the pulmonary vasculature is engorged. (B) A film from an angiocardiogram demonstrates the inverted aorta and right ventricular outflow tract (arrows).[6]

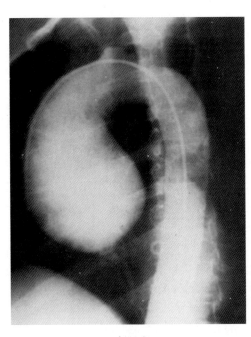

Fig CA 9-9
Marfan's syndrome. Arteriogram shows enormous dilatation of the aneurysmal ascending aorta.

Small Ascending Aorta or Aortic Arch

Condition	Imaging Findings	Comments
Atrial septal defect (see Fig CA 7-1)	Small aorta; increased pulmonary vascularity; enlarged right atrium, right ventricle, and pulmonary outflow tract.	Shunting of blood away from the left side of the heart into the pulmonary circulation causes decreased flow through the aorta.
Ventricular septal defect (see Fig CA 7-2)	Small (or normal) aorta; increased pulmonary vascularity; enlarged right ventricle, pulmonary outflow tract, and left atrium.	Shunting of blood away from the left side of the heart into the pulmonary circulation causes decreased flow through the aorta.
Infantile type of coarctation of aorta	Small (or normal) aorta; pulmonary venous congestion; cardiomegaly (biventricular but more prominent on the right).	Narrowing of a long segment of aorta proximal to the ductus arteriosus. Always a patent ductus arteriosus and often a ventricular septal defect to deliver blood from the pulmonary artery to the descending aorta and the systemic circulation. No rib notching, internal mammary collaterals, or figure-3 or figure-E signs.
Mitral stenosis	Small aorta; enlarged left atrium and increased pulmonary venous congestion; eventual enlargement of the right ventricle, pulmonary outflow tract, and central pulmonary arteries.	Decreased left ventricular output causes diminished aortic blood flow.
Decreased cardiac output	Small aorta; various patterns of heart size; usually pulmonary venous congestion, pleural effusion, and prominence of the superior vena cava.	Gross cardiomegaly in endocardial fibroelastosis and the cardiomyopathies. Normal-sized or small heart with characteristic calcification in chronic constrictive pericarditis.
Endocardial cushion defect	Nonspecific globular enlargement of the heart with increased pulmonary vascularity.	Atrial and ventricular septal defects cause shunting of blood away from the left side of the heart into the pulmonary circulation and thus decreased flow through the aorta.
Hypoplastic left heart syndrome	Small aorta; globular cardiomegaly with severe pulmonary venous congestion.	Underdevelopment of the left side of the heart is related to an obstructive lesion that causes decreased aortic blood flow.
Supravalvular aortic stenosis (Fig CA 10-1)	Aortic knob is often small.	Underdevelopment and stenosis of the supravalvular portion of the aorta. Different from the poststenotic aortic dilation that occurs with valvular aortic stenosis.
Transposition of great vessels (Fig CA 10-2)	Narrowing of the vascular pedicle on frontal projection.	Caused by superimposition of the abnormally positioned aorta and pulmonary artery combined with absence of the normal thymic tissue because of stress atrophy. Widening of the vascular pedicle on lateral projection (due to the anterior position of the aorta with reference to the pulmonary artery).

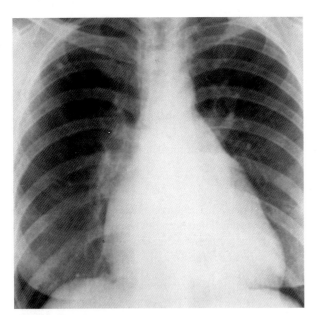

Fig CA 10-1
Congenital aortic stenosis. Small aortic arch with moderate enlargement of the left ventricle.[9]

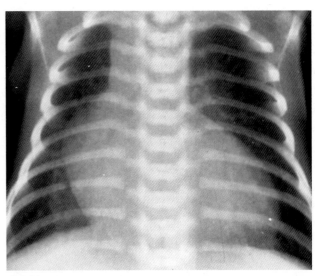

Fig CA 10-2
Transposition of great vessels. Typical oval or egg-shaped heart with a small aortic arch due to narrowing of the vascular pedicle resulting from superimposition of the abnormally positioned aorta and pulmonary artery.

Major Anomalies of the Aortic Arch and Pulmonary Artery

Condition	Imaging Findings	Comments
Right aortic arch Mirror-image pattern (see Fig CA 12-1)	No indentation on the barium-filled esophagus on lateral projection.	No vessel crosses the mediastinum posterior to the esophagus. Frequently associated with congenital heart disease (tetralogy of Fallot, truncus and pseudotruncus, tricuspid atresia, and transposition).
Aberrant left subclavian artery (Fig CA 11-1)	Characteristic oblique posterior indentation on the barium-filled esophagus.	Left subclavian artery arises as the most distal branch of the aorta and courses across the mediastinum posterior to the esophagus to reach the left upper extremity. No associated congenital heart disease.
Isolated left subclavian artery	No esophageal impression.	Left subclavian artery is atretic at its base (totally isolated from the aorta) and receives its blood supply from the left pulmonary artery or via the ipsilateral vertebral artery (congenital subclavian steal syndrome).
Right aortic arch with left descending aorta	Prominent indentation on the posterior wall of the barium-filled esophagus.	Transverse portion of the aorta must cross the mediastinum (posterior to the esophagus) so that the aorta descends on the left.
Cervical aortic arch (Fig CA 11-2)	Posterior impression on the esophagus (caused by the distal arch or the proximal descending aorta).	Ascending aorta extends higher than usual so that the aortic arch is in the neck. Pulsatile mass above the clavicle simulates an aneurysm. No associated congenital heart disease.

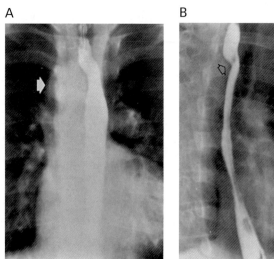
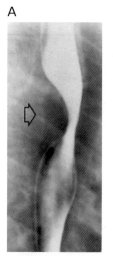
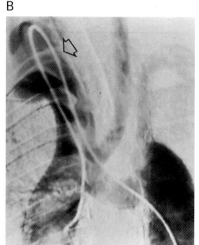

Fig CA 11-1
Right aortic arch with aberrant left subclavian artery.
(A) Frontal view from an esophagram demonstrates the right aortic arch (arrow). (B) Oblique posterior impression on the esophagus (arrow) represents the aberrant left subclavian artery as it courses to reach the left upper extremity.

Fig CA 11-2
Cervical aortic arch. (A) Posterior esophageal impression (arrow) is caused by the retroesophageal course of the distal arch or the proximal descending aorta. (B) Subtraction film from an aortogram demonstrates the aortic arch extending into the neck (arrow).

Condition	Imaging Findings	Comments
Double aortic arch (Fig CA 11-3)	Bulges on both sides of the superior mediastinum (the right is usually larger and higher than the left). Reverse S-shaped indentation on the barium-filled esophagus.	In most patients, the aorta ascends on the right, branches, and finally reunites on the left. The two limbs of the aorta completely encircle the trachea and the esophagus, forming a ring.
Aberrant right subclavian artery (Fig CA 11-4)	Posterior esophageal indentation on lateral views. On frontal views, characteristic impression running obliquely upward and to the right.	Arises as the last major vessel of the aortic arch (just distal to the left subclavian) and must course across the mediastinum behind the esophagus to reach the right upper extremity. No associated congenital heart disease.
Aberrant left pulmonary artery (pulmonary sling) (Fig CA 11-5)	Typical impression on the posterior aspect of the trachea just above the carina and a corresponding indentation on the anterior wall of the barium-filled esophagus.	Aberrant left pulmonary artery arises from the right pulmonary artery and must cross the mediastinum (between the trachea and the esophagus) to reach the left lung.

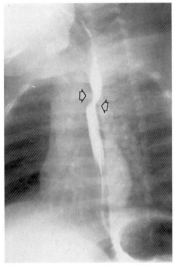

Fig CA 11-3
Double aortic arch. Characteristic reverse S-shaped indentation on the esophagus (arrows). As usual, the right (posterior) arch is higher and larger than the left (anterior) arch.[6]

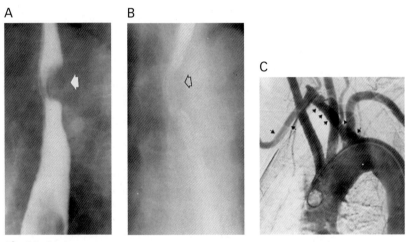

Fig CA 11-4
Aberrant right subclavian artery. (A) Lateral view from an esophagram demonstrates a posterior esophageal impression (arrow). (B) On a frontal view, the esophageal impression (arrow) runs obliquely upward and to the right. (C) Subtraction film from an arteriogram shows the aberrant vessel (arrows) arising distal to the left subclavian artery.

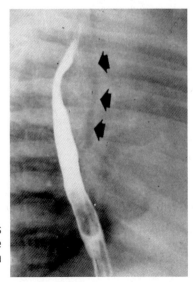

Fig CA 11-5
Aberrant left pulmonary artery. Lateral esophagram demonstrates the characteristic indentation of the anterior wall of the esophagus. Note the posterior impression and anterior displacement of the trachea (arrows) caused by the aberrant artery.[11]

Congenital Heart Disease Associated with the Right Aortic Arch (Mirror-Image Branching)

Condition	Imaging Findings	Comments
Pseudotruncus arteriosus	Decreased pulmonary vascularity; flat or concave pulmonary outflow tract; enlargement of the right ventricle.	Right aortic arch in approximately 40% of cases. Single vessel arising from the heart is accompanied by a remnant of the atretic pulmonary artery (essentially the same as tetralogy of Fallot with pulmonary atresia).
Tetralogy of Fallot	Decreased pulmonary vascularity; flat or concave pulmonary outflow tract; enlargement of the right ventricle.	Right aortic arch in approximately 25% of cases. Consists of (1) high ventricular septal defect, (2) obstruction to right ventricular outflow (usually infundibular pulmonary stenosis), (3) overriding of the aortic orifice above the ventricular defect, and (4) right ventricular hypertrophy.
Persistent truncus arteriosus (Fig CA 12-1)	Increased pulmonary vascularity; concave pulmonary outflow tract; striking enlargement of the right ventricle and eventual enlargement of the left atrium and left ventricle.	Right aortic arch in approximately 25% of cases. Failure of the common truncus arteriosus to divide normally into the aorta and the pulmonary artery results in a single large arterial trunk that receives the outflow from both ventricles.
Tricuspid atresia	Decreased pulmonary vascularity; striking enlargement of the right atrium if small atrial shunt; large left ventricle; small right ventricle.	Right aortic arch in approximately 5% of cases. An obligatory right-to-left shunt at the atrial level (there may also be a ventricular septal defect or patent ductus arteriosus). Hypoplasia of the right ventricle and pulmonary outflow tract.
Transposition of great vessels	Increased pulmonary vascularity; generally biventricular enlargement (oval or egg-shaped configuration); narrowed vascular pedicle.	Right aortic arch in approximately 5% of cases. Reverse of the normal relation of the aorta and the pulmonary artery (the aorta arises anteriorly from the right ventricle and the pulmonary artery originates posteriorly from the left ventricle).

A   B

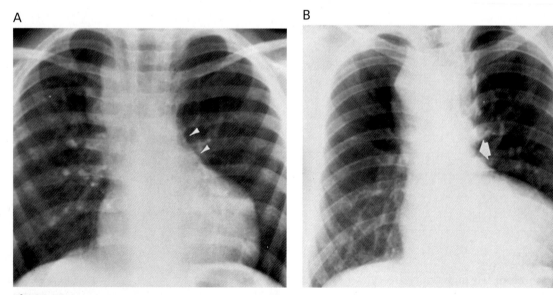

Fig CA 12-1
Persistent truncus arteriosus. Two patients with the characteristic concave appearance of the pulmonary outflow tract (arrowheads, arrow) associated with a right aortic arch.

Dilatation of the Main Pulmonary Artery

Condition	Imaging Findings	Comments
Normal variant (Fig CA 13-1)	Isolated prominence of pulmonary artery segment; normal pulmonary vascularity; no associated cardiac abnormality.	Common appearance in adolescents and adults younger than 30 years of age (especially women).
Congestive heart failure	Cardiomegaly with evidence of pulmonary venous congestion. Often pleural effusion and Kerley's lines.	Failure of the left side of the heart leads to increased blood volume in the pulmonary circulation.
High-output heart disease (Fig CA 13-2)	Cardiomegaly with prominent pulmonary vascularity (both arteries and veins).	Anemia; thyrotoxicosis; beriberi; hypovolemia (fluid overload, overtransfusion); peripheral arteriovenous fistulas; Paget's disease; Pickwickian obesity; polycythemia vera; pregnancy.
Cor pulmonale (Figs CA 13-3 and CA 13-4)	Enlargement of the main and hilar pulmonary arteries with rapid tapering and small peripheral vessels. Initially normal heart size, then right ventricular enlargement, and eventually distention of the superior vena cava.	Caused by diffuse lung disease (obstructive emphysema, interstitial fibrosis); diffuse pulmonary arterial disease (thromboembolism, arteritis, primary pulmonary hypertension); chronic heart disease (reversed left-to-right shunt, left ventricular failure, mitral valve disease); and chronic hypoxia (chest deformity, neuromuscular disease, Pickwickian obesity, high-altitude dwelling).

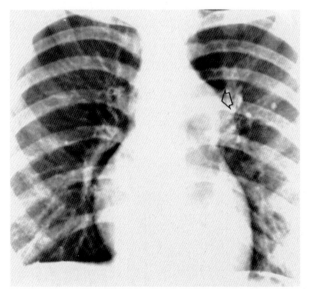

Fig CA 13-1
Idiopathic dilatation of the pulmonary artery. Plain chest radiograph in a normal young woman demonstrates prominence of the pulmonary artery (arrow) that simulates the poststenotic dilatation associated with pulmonary valvular stenosis.

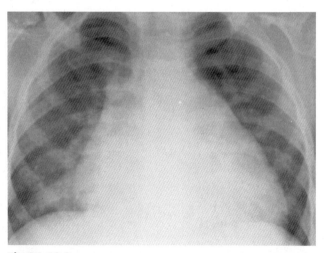

Fig CA 13-2
Thyrotoxicosis. Generalized cardiomegaly with increased pulmonary vascularity.

A

B

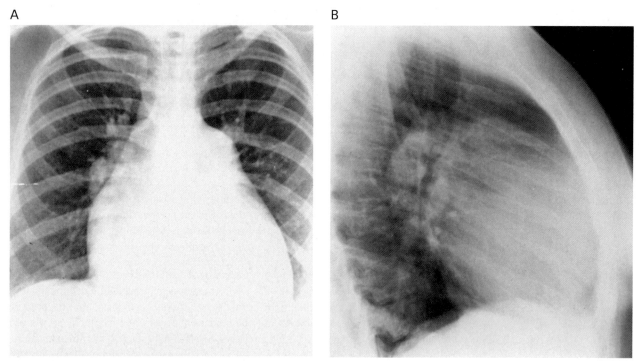

Fig CA 13-3
Cor pulmonale (primary pulmonary hypertension). (A) Frontal and (B) lateral views of the chest show prominence of the pulmonary outflow tract and markedly dilated central pulmonary vessels. The lateral displacement of the cardiac apex and filling of the retrosternal air space indicate right ventricular enlargement.

A

B

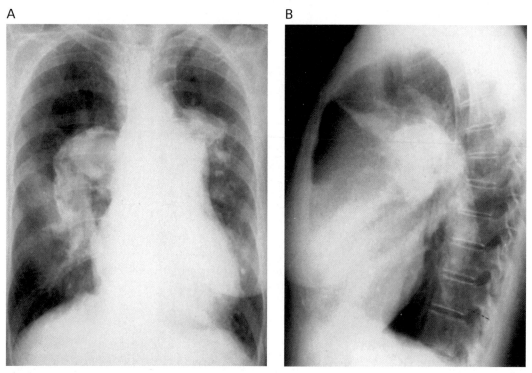

Fig CA 13-4
Eisenmenger syndrome in atrial septal defect. (A) Frontal and (B) lateral films demonstrate slight but definite cardiomegaly and a great increase in the size of the pulmonary trunk. The right and left pulmonary artery branches are huge, but the peripheral pulmonary vasculature is relatively sparse. Long-standing pulmonary hypertension has produced degenerative intimal changes in the pulmonary arteries, which have become densely calcified.[1]

Condition	Imaging Findings	Comments
Left-to-right shunt (Fig CA 13-5)	Various patterns, depending on the level and extent of the shunt.	Most commonly atrial septal defect, ventricular septal defect, or patent ductus arteriosus.
Pulmonary thromboembolic disease (see Fig C 10-4)	Enlargement of the main pulmonary artery segment.	Caused by pulmonary hypertension or distention of the vessel by bulk thrombus. This sign is primarily of value when serial radiographs demonstrate progressive enlargement.
Pulmonary valvular stenosis (Fig CA 13-6)	Prominence of the main pulmonary artery segment.	Common anomaly with poststenotic dilatation of the left pulmonary artery (central dilatation of the right pulmonary artery, but the dilated segment is hidden in the mediastinum).
Mitral stenosis or insufficiency	Enlargement of the left atrium and right ventricle; normal-sized left ventricle and small aortic arch; pulmonary vascular congestion.	Obstruction of flow from the left atrium to the left ventricle during diastole results in increased pressure and enlargement of the left atrium. The increased pressure is transmitted to the pulmonary veins and eventually to the pulmonary arteries and the right side of the heart. Usually caused by rheumatic valvular lesion; also by congenital mitral stenosis and the parachute deformity (all chordae tendineae originating from a single papillary muscle). There is a similar mechanism in the hypoplastic left heart syndrome and a large left atrial myxoma.

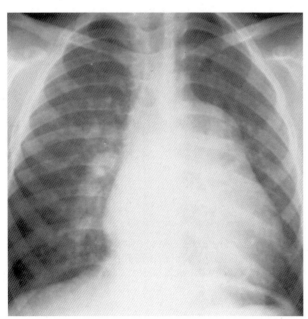

Fig CA 13-5
Ventricular septal defect. The pulmonary trunk is very large and overshadows the normal-sized aorta, which seems small by comparison. The pulmonary artery branches in the hilum and in the periphery of the lung are enlarged, and the pulmonary vascular volume is increased. The heart is enlarged and somewhat triangular.[1]

Condition	Imaging Findings	Comments
Partial anomalous pulmonary venous return (see Fig CA 7-8)	Increased pulmonary vascularity; enlarged right atrium, right ventricle, and main pulmonary artery segment; normal left atrium and left ventricle; small aorta.	One or more pulmonary veins connected to the right atrium or its tributaries. Virtually indistinguishable from an atrial septal defect radiographically. Scimitar sign (crescent-shaped anomalous venous channel) on the right if associated with hypoplasia of the right lung.
Trilogy of Fallot (Fig CA 13-7)	Poststenotic dilatation of the pulmonary artery; decreased pulmonary vascularity; heart size often normal (usually some evidence of right ventricular hypertrophy).	Combination of pulmonary valvular stenosis with an intact ventricular septum and an interatrial shunt (patent foramen ovale or true atrial septal defect). Increased pressure on the right side of the heart due to pulmonary stenosis causes the interatrial shunt to be right to left (patient is cyanotic).
Tricuspid atresia without pulmonary stenosis	Marked cardiomegaly and increased pulmonary vascularity.	May be associated with transposition of the great vessels.
Total anomalous pulmonary venous return (see Fig CA 5-9)	Increased pulmonary vascularity and enlarged main pulmonary artery segment; various patterns and characteristic "snowman," or figure-8, sign.	All pulmonary veins connect to the right atrium directly or to the systemic veins or their tributaries. Because all pulmonary venous blood returns to the right atrium, a right-to-left shunt through an interatrial communication is necessary for blood to reach the left side of the heart and the systemic circulation.

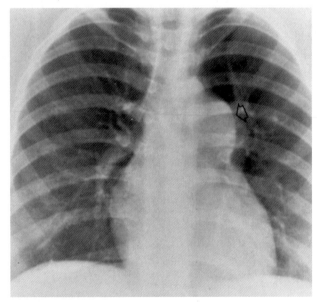

Fig CA 13-6
Pulmonary valvular stenosis. Severe poststenotic dilatation of the pulmonary outflow tract (arrow). The heart size and pulmonary vascularity remain within normal limits.

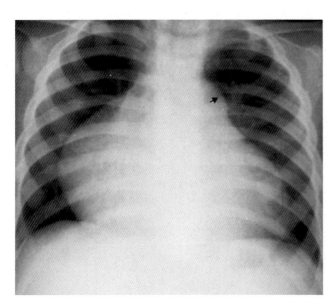

Fig CA 13-7
Trilogy of Fallot. Marked poststenotic dilatation (arrow) of the pulmonary artery with decrease in overall pulmonary vascularity. There is enormous right atrial and moderate right ventricular enlargement.[6]

Dilatation of the Superior Vena Cava*

Condition	Comments
Increased central venous pressure (Fig CA 14-1)	In the great majority of cases, this pattern is caused by congestive heart failure or by cardiac tamponade due to pericardial effusion or constrictive pericarditis.
Intrathoracic neoplasm (Figs CA 14-2 to CA 14-4)	There is often an associated soft-tissue mass. Primarily bronchogenic carcinoma (especially oat cell carcinoma), but also tumors of the esophagus and the mediastinum.

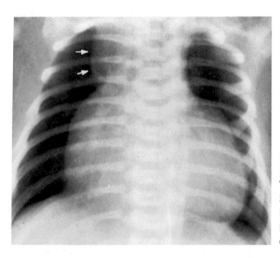

Fig CA 14-1
Right ventricular failure. Plain chest radiograph in a patient with Ebstein's anomaly shows widening of the right side of the superior portion of the mediastinum (arrows), reflecting marked dilatation of the superior vena cava. There is enlargement of the right atrium, causing upward and outward bulging of the right border of the heart (squared appearance).

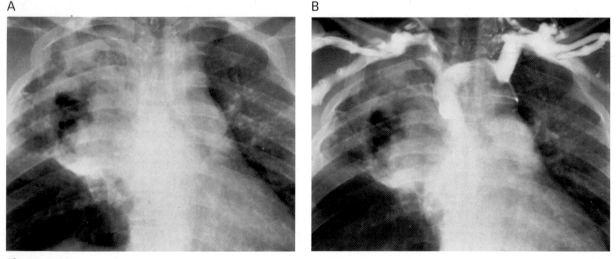

Fig CA 14-2
Bronchogenic carcinoma. (A) Frontal view of the chest shows a bulky, irregular mass filling much of the right upper lobe. (B) Bilateral upper extremity venograms show almost complete occlusion of the superior vena cava by the large malignant neoplasm.

*Pattern: Smooth, well-defined widening of the right side of the upper half of the mediastinum.

Condition	Comments
Mediastinal fibrosis	Idiopathic or secondary to chronic histoplasmosis, irradiation, or methylsergide ingestion.
Lymphadenopathy	Most commonly histoplasmosis or bronchogenic carcinoma.
Aneurysm of aorta or great vessels	Associated with a large soft-tissue mass representing the aneurysm. Usually due to atherosclerotic or dissecting aneurysms (syphilitic aneurysms were formerly more common but are now rare).
Severe mediastinal emphysema	Striking increase in mediastinal pressure causes venous compression.
Thrombosis of superior vena cava	Reported after surgery for repair of tetralogy of Fallot and in patients with ventriculoatrial shunts for hydrocephalus.

A

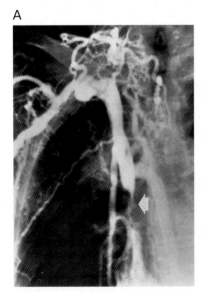

B

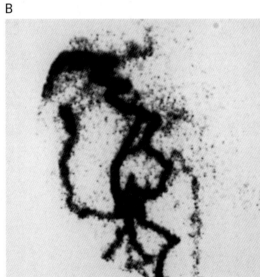

Fig CA 14-3
Bronchogenic carcinoma. (A) Right upper extremity venogram shows extensive venous collaterals bypassing an obstruction of the superior vena cava (arrow). (B) Radionuclide scan in another patient shows extensive venous collaterals bypassing an obstruction of the superior vena cava.

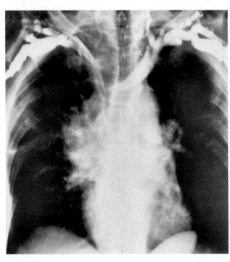

Fig CA 14-4
Bronchogenic carcinoma. Bilateral upper extremity venogram shows virtual occlusion of the superior vena cava by a large oat cell tumor in the right hilar and perihilar region.

Dilatation of the Azygos Vein*

Condition	Comments
Increased central venous pressure (Fig CA 15-1)	Underlying causes include congestive heart failure, pericardial tamponade due to pericardial effusion, constrictive pericarditis, and tricuspid valvular lesions. Dilatation of the azygos vein may be obscured by a dilated superior vena cava. A dilated azygos vein may be differentiated from an enlarged azygos lymph node by demonstrating a marked increase in the diameter of the shadow in the supine position.
Portal hypertension	Intrahepatic or extrahepatic portal vein obstruction (tumor thrombus). Enlarged azygos and hemiazygos veins may produce widening and irregularity of the right and left paraspinal lines, respectively (this appearance also occurs with superior vena caval obstruction and congenital infrahepatic interruption of the inferior vena cava).
Occlusion of superior vena cava	Smooth, well-defined widening of the right side of the upper half of the mediastinum may obscure or obliterate the shadow of the enlarged azygos vein.
Azygos continuation of inferior vena cava	Congenital infrahepatic interruption of the inferior vena cava. Often associated with a congenital cardiac malformation, error in abdominal situs, asplenia, or polysplenia. Characteristic absence of the shadow of the inferior vena cava at the posterior border of the heart on a lateral chest radiograph.
Pregnancy	Dilatation of the azygos vein is probably secondary to generalized hypervolemia and disappears after delivery.
Traumatic aneurysm/ arteriovenous fistula	Extremely rare occurrence.

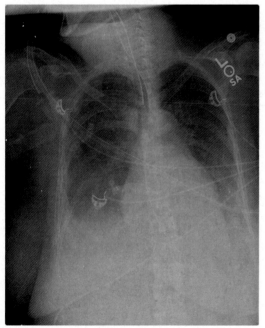

Fig CA 15-1
Increased central venous pressure. Dilatation of the azygos vein is associated with evidence of congestive failure and bilateral pleural effusions.

*Pattern: Round or oval shadow in the right tracheobronchial angle that measures more than 10 mm in diameter on standard upright radiographs. The azygos vein decreases in size with inspiration, upright position, and the Valsalva maneuver.

Congestive Heart Failure in Neonates Less Than 4 Weeks Old

Condition	Imaging Findings	Comments
Hypoplastic left heart syndrome (Fig CA 16-1)	Severe pulmonary venous congestion. Progressive cardiomegaly with a globular or oval heart (combination of right atrial and right ventricular enlargement).	Consists of several conditions in which underdevelopment of the left side of the heart is related to an obstructive lesion (stenosis or atresia of mitral valve, aortic valve, or aortic arch). Causes heart failure in the first week of life.
Coarctation of aorta (Fig CA 16-2)	Pulmonary venous congestion. Cardiomegaly (biventricular but more prominent on the right).	"Infantile" type in which there is narrowing of a long segment of the aorta proximal to the ductus. Always a patent ductus arteriosus and often a ventricular septal defect to deliver blood from the pulmonary artery to the descending aorta and the systemic circulation. Because the shunted blood is unoxygenated, the lower half of the body is cyanotic.
Tetralogy of Fallot	Decreased pulmonary vascularity; flat or concave pulmonary outflow tract; enlargement of the right ventricle; right aortic arch in approximately 25% of cases.	Consists of (1) high ventricular septal defect, (2) obstruction to right ventricular outflow (usually infundibular pulmonary stenosis), (3) overriding of the aortic orifice above the ventricular defect, and (4) right ventricular hypertrophy.
Transposition of great vessels	Pulmonary vascularity and heart size are normal in the newborn. Progressive cardiac enlargement and vascular engorgement occur within a few days.	Reverse of the normal relation of the aorta and the pulmonary artery. A left-to-right shunt is required to connect the two separate circulations. The shunts are bidirectional and permit the mixing of oxygenated and unoxygenated blood.
Pseudotruncus arteriosus	Decreased pulmonary vascularity; flat or concave pulmonary outflow tract; enlargement of right ventricle; right aortic arch in approximately 40% of cases.	Single vessel arising from the heart that is accompanied by a remnant of the atretic pulmonary artery (essentially the same as tetralogy of Fallot with pulmonary atresia).
Large left-to-right shunt (Fig CA 16-3)	Increased pulmonary vascularity; diastolic overloading and enlargement of the left atrium and the left ventricle.	Congestive heart failure may develop early in severe ventricular septal defect, patent ductus arteriosus, or common atrioventricular canal.

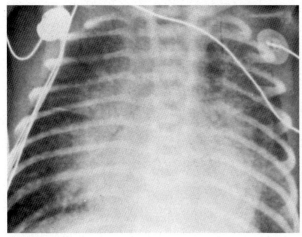

Fig CA 16-1
Hypoplastic left heart syndrome.

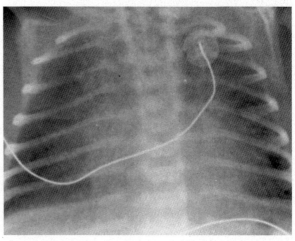

Fig CA 16-2
Coarctation of the aorta.

Condition	Imaging Findings	Comments
Persistent truncus arteriosus	Increased pulmonary vascularity; concave pulmonary outflow tract.	Early congestive heart failure if a severe left-to-right shunt. The development of pulmonary hypertension is a protective factor (reduces the pulmonary flow and the diastolic overloading of the heart).
Tricuspid atresia with transposition and no pulmonary stenosis	Increased pulmonary vascularity; marked cardiomegaly.	Because the pulmonary blood flow is exuberant, there is less cyanosis, but diastolic overloading of the left side of the heart leads to early congestive heart failure.
Pulmonary atresia	Decreased pulmonary vascularity; concave pulmonary artery segment.	If the ventricular septum is intact, blood enters the pulmonary circulation via the ductus arteriosus. Once the ductus closes, the infant's condition deteriorates rapidly.
Ebstein's anomaly	Decreased pulmonary vascularity; flat or consquared or boxed appearance of the heart.	Downward displacement of an incompetent tricuspid valve into the right ventricle so that the upper portion of the right ventricle is effectively incorporated into the right atrium. A right-to-left atrial shunt causes cyanosis.
Uhl's disease	Radiographic pattern identical to that of Ebstein's anomaly.	Focal or complete absence of the right ventricular myocardium (the right ventricle becomes a thin-walled fibroelastic bag that contracts poorly and cannot effectively empty blood from the right side of the heart).
Common ventricle	Increased pulmonary vascularity; marked nonspecific globular enlargement of the heart.	Extremely large septal defect produces a functional "single ventricle." If there is no pulmonary stenosis, there is marked diastolic overloading of the ventricular chamber and early congestive heart failure.
Premature (prenatal) closure of foramen ovale (Fig CA 16-4)	Appearance identical to that of hypoplastic left heart syndrome.	Premature closure of the foramen ovale in the fetus leads to severe left-sided hypoplasia with marked elevation of pulmonary venous pressure (no possibility for left-to-right shunting).

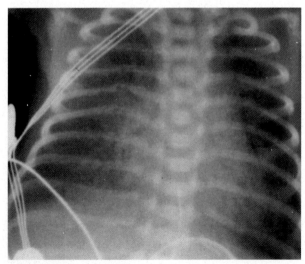

Fig CA 16-3
Patent ductus arteriosus.

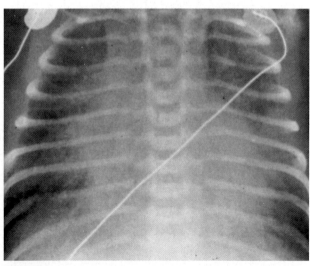

Fig CA 16-4
Premature closure of the foramen ovale.

Condition	Imaging Findings	Comments
Malformations obstructing pulmonary venous flow	Severe pulmonary venous congestion; left atrial enlargement in some conditions.	Congenital mitral stenosis; cor triatriatum (incomplete fibromuscular diaphragm dividing the left atrium); congenital pulmonary vein stenosis or atresia; total anomalous pulmonary venous return with high-grade pulmonary venous obstruction.
Myocardiopathy	Pulmonary venous congestion with striking cardiomegaly.	Endocardial fibroelastosis; glycogen storage disease (Pompe's); myocarditis (toxoplasmosis, rubella, coxsackievirus); myocardial ischemia (neonatal hypoxia; infantile coronary arteriosclerosis); anomalous left coronary artery arising from the pulmonary artery.
Arteriovenous fistula or hemangioma	High-output congestive failure.	Vein of Galen aneurysm; peripheral or pulmonary arteriovenous fistula; cutaneous or hepatic cavernous hemangioma.
Intracranial disease with increased intracranial pressure	Pulmonary venous congestion.	Cerebral birth injury.
Conduction and rhythm abnormalities	Pulmonary vascular congestion.	Tachycardia (>200 beats per minute); complete heart block; arrhythmia.
Iatrogenic	Pulmonary venous congestion.	Fluid overload; sodium chloride poisoning.
Polycythemia	Pulmonary venous congestion.	Maternal-fetal hemorrhage; placental and twin-to-twin transfusion.
Maternal diabetes/neonatal hypoglycemia	Pulmonary venous congestion.	
High-output states	High-output congestive failure.	Severe anemia (eg, erythroblastosis); neonatal hyperthyroidism.
Asplenia or polysplenia syndrome	Pulmonary venous congestion. There may be a symmetric midline liver or a small midline stomach.	High incidence of complex congenital cardiac anomalies that may produce a bizarre configuration of the heart. The spleen may be absent or there may be multiple accessory spleens on radionuclide studies.

High-Output Heart Disease

Condition	Comments
Anemia (Fig CA 17-1)	Hemolytic anemia (eg, sickle celldisease, thalassemia) with characteristic marrow hyperplasia (widening of the medullary spaces with thinning of the cortices and coarsening of the trabecular pattern). May also occur in severe chronic blood-loss anemia. May interfere with myocardial function by producing myocardial anoxia.
Thyrotoxicosis (Fig CA 17-2)	Direct impairment of myocardial metabolism in a patient with the characteristic clinical features of hyperthyroidism.
Beriberi (Fig CA 17-3)	Thiamine (vitamin B_1) deficiency causes direct impairment of myocardial metabolism. The diagnosis requires a good dietary history and observation of the response to treatment.

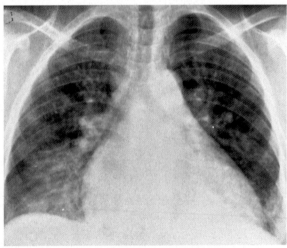

Fig CA 17-1
Sickle cell anemia. Marked cardiomegaly with a generalized increase in pulmonary vascular markings.

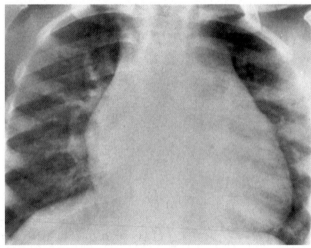

Fig CA 17-2
Thyrotoxicosis. Generalized enlargement of the heart and engorged pulmonary vascularity.

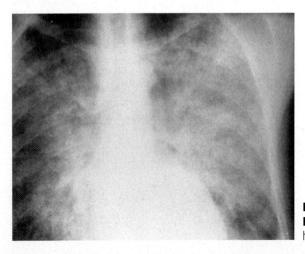

Fig CA 17-3
Beriberi. Diffuse pulmonary edema due to severe high-output failure.

Condition	Comments
Hypervolemia	Fluid overload; overtransfusion.
Arteriovenous fistulas	Rapid shunting of blood from the arterial to the venous system. The fistulas may be peripheral, abdominal, or cerebral.
Paget's disease	Caused by multiple microscopic arteriovenous malformations in pagetoid bone. Characteristic destructive changes are followed by an extensive reparative phase.
Polycythemia vera	Hematologic disorder characterized by hyperplasia of the bone marrow resulting in an increased production of erythrocytes, granulocytes, and platelets. The increased blood volume and viscosity cause prominence of the pulmonary vascularity, simulating congenital heart disease. Usually there is massive splenomegaly and an increased incidence of peptic ulcer disease and urate stones (secondary gout).
Pickwickian obesity (Fig CA 17-4)	Extreme obesity causes profound hypoventilation (diffuse elevation of the diaphragm and bibasilar atelectatic changes) that results in hypoxia and secondary polycythemia.
Pregnancy	Increased blood volume and flow.

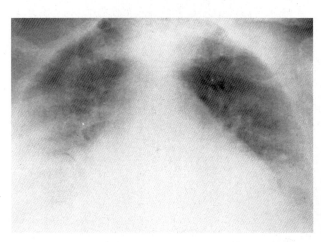

Fig CA 17-4
Pickwickian syndrome. Profound obesity has led to severe hypoventilation and secondary polycythemia, causing marked cardiomegaly and engorgement of the pulmonary vessels.

Hypertensive Cardiovascular Disease*

Condition	Comments
Essential (idiopathic) hypertension (Fig CA 18-1)	Represents the vast majority of patients with elevated blood pressure.
Renovascular disease	Suggestive findings on rapid-sequence excretory urography include (1) unilateral delayed appearance and excretion of contrast material, (2) difference in kidney size greater than 1.5 cm, (3) irregular contour of the renal silhouette (suggesting segmental infarction or atrophy), (4) indentations on the ureter or renal pelvis due to dilated, tortuous ureteral arterial collaterals, and (5) hyperconcentration of contrast material in the collecting system of the smaller kidney on delayed films. Approximately 25% of patients with renovascular hypertension have a normal rapid-sequence excretory urogram (though this modality is also of value in detecting other causes of hypertension, such as tumor, pyelonephritis, polycystic kidneys, or renal infarction).

A   B

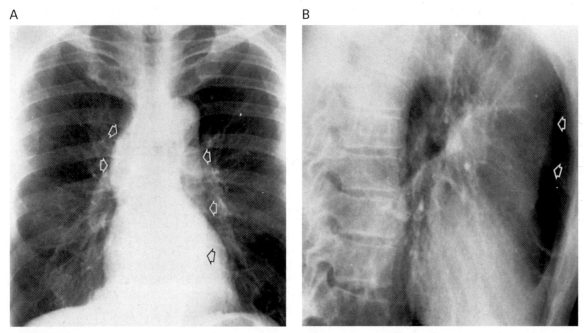

Fig CA 18-1
Essential (idiopathic) hypertension. (A) Frontal and (B) lateral views of the chest demonstrate characteristic tortuosity of the aorta (arrows), especially the ascending portion. Because the elevated blood pressure has caused left ventricular hypertrophy without dilatation, the radiographic appearance of the cardiac silhouette remains normal.

---

*Pattern: The increased workload of the left ventricle due to chronic hypertension initially causes concentric hypertrophy, which produces little if any change in the radiographic appearance of the cardiac silhouette. Eventually, the continued strain leads to dilatation and enlargement of the left ventricle along with downward displacement of the cardiac apex, which often projects below the left hemidiaphragm. Aortic tortuosity with prominence of the ascending portion commonly occurs.

Condition	Comments
Renal artery stenosis (Fig CA 18-2)	Most commonly due to arteriosclerotic narrowing that tends to occur in the proximal portion of the vessel close to its origin from the aorta. Poststenotic dilatation is common. Bilateral renal artery stenoses are noted in up to one-third of the patients. At times, renal artery stenosis may be detected only on oblique projections that demonstrate the vessel origins in profile.
Fibromuscular hyperplasia (Fig CA 18-3)	Characteristic "string-of-beads" pattern, in which there are alternating areas of narrowing and dilatation (representing microaneurysms). Smooth, concentric stenoses occur less frequently. Most commonly affects young women and is often bilateral.
Perirenal hematoma (Page kidney)	Dense fibrous encasement of the kidney after healing of a subcapsular or perirenal hematoma compresses the renal parenchyma and causes an alteration of the intrarenal hemodynamics that produces ischemia and hypertension. The kidney is often enlarged and demonstrates a mass effect with distortion of the collecting system. Arteriography reveals splaying and stretching of the intrarenal arteries and often irregular staining in the healing portion of the hematoma. Removal of the kidney or evacuation of the offending mass may result in clearing of the hypertension.
Renal parenchymal disease	Causes include glomerulonephritis, chronic pyelonephritis, polycystic kidney, renal tumor, and renal agenesis or hypoplasia.

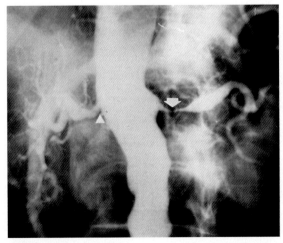

Fig CA 18-2
Renovascular hypertension. Bilateral arteriosclerotic renal artery stenoses (arrowhead, arrow).

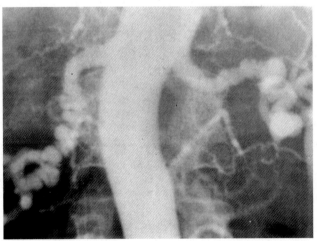

Fig CA 18-3
Renovascular hypertension. String-of-beads pattern of fibromuscular dysplasia bilaterally.

Condition	Comments
Coarctation of aorta (see Fig CA 8-1)	Suggestive radiographic findings include inordinate dilatation of the ascending aorta, widening of the left superior mediastinum, the figure-E or figure-3 sign, and rib notching.
Adrenal disease	Causes include Cushing's syndrome (suggested by widening of the superior mediastinum due to increased fat deposition associated with osteoporosis and compression changes in the dorsal vertebrae), pheochromocytoma (may produce a paravertebral mass), adrenocortical adenoma, carcinoma, primary aldosteronism, and the adrenogenital syndrome.
Other endocrine disorders	Hyperthyroidism, acromegaly, and the use of estrogen-containing oral contraceptives (this may be the most common form of secondary hypertension).
Collagen disease	Systemic lupus erythematosus; polyarteritis nodosa.
Neurogenic	Dysautonomia (familial autonomic dysfunction; Riley-Day syndrome); psychogenic.

Cardiovascular Calcification

Condition	Comments
Aortic wall Arteriosclerosis (Fig CA 19-1)	Elongation and tortuosity of the aorta with linear plaques of calcification that most commonly occur in the aortic knob and transverse arch. In severe disease, the entire aorta may be outlined by extensive calcification in its wall.
Aneurysm	An increased diameter of the aorta indicates an aneurysm, whereas an increased distance between intimal calcification and the outer wall of the aorta suggests a dissection.
Aortitis (Fig CA 19-2)	Dilatation and prominence of the ascending aorta with thin, curvilinear streaks of calcification (often extensive) is characteristic of syphilitic aortitis; linear calcification also frequently occurs in patients with Takayasu's aortitis ("pulseless" disease), a nonspecific obstructive arteritis that primarily affects young women.
Valvular/annulus Aortic annulus or valve (Fig CA 19-3)	Calcification of the annulus tends to be heavy and distinct, unlike valvular calcification, which is usually stippled and often not detected on plain radiographs (best demonstrated on fluoroscopic examination). Causes include arteriosclerosis, rheumatic aortic valve disease, infective endocarditis, and a congenital defect of the aortic valve.

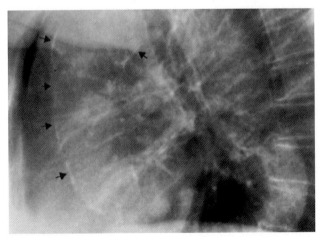

Fig CA 19-1
Arteriosclerosis. Lateral view of the chest demonstrates calcification of the anterior and posterior walls of the ascending aorta (arrows). The descending thoracic aorta is tortuous.

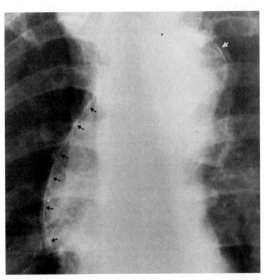

Fig CA 19-2
Syphilitic aortitis. Aneurysmal dilatation of the ascending aorta with extensive linear calcification of the wall (black arrows). Some calcification is also seen in the distal aortic arch (white arrow).

Condition	Comments
Mitral valve	Develops in patients with long-standing severe mitral stenosis and is often indistinct and easily missed on plain radiographs (best demonstrated by fluoroscopy). The amount of calcification does not reflect the degree of functional disturbance. Multiple calcific or ossific nodules throughout the lower portions of the lungs may develop in areas of chronic interstitial edema.
Mitral annulus (Fig CA 19-4)	Dense curved or annular calcified band around the mitral valve that usually reflects underlying arteriosclerosis. Although usually insignificant, a rigid annulus may cause functional insufficiency of the mitral valve.

A

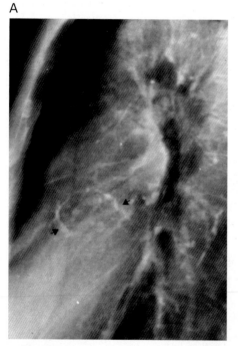

B

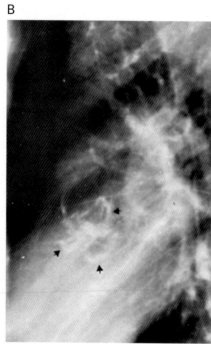

Fig CA 19-3
Aortic stenosis. Calcification in (A) the aortic annulus (arrows) and (B) the three leaflets of the aortic valve (arrows).

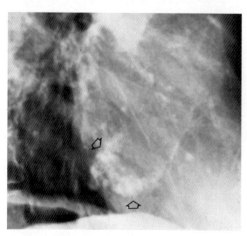

Fig CA 19-4
Mitral annulus calcification (arrows) in mitral stenosis.

Condition	Comments
Coronary artery (Fig CA 19-5)	Punctate, patchy, or tubular densities that primarily involve the circumflex and anterior descending branches of the left coronary artery and are most commonly seen along the left margin of the heart below the pulmonary artery segment. Although infrequently visualized on routine chest radiographs, calcification of a coronary artery strongly suggests the presence of hemodynamically significant arteriosclerotic coronary artery disease. Cardiac fluoroscopy is far more sensitive than plain chest radiography in demonstrating coronary artery calcification, though there is controversy about the prognostic significance of fluoroscopically identified coronary artery calcification in patients with ischemic heart disease. In patients younger than 50 years of age, coronary artery calcification is a strong predictor of major narrowing in women and a moderate predictor in men. In older patients, calcification has less predictive value.
Sinus of Valsalva	Calcification primarily involves the wall of an aortic sinus aneurysm and is usually best seen on the lateral view.
Left atrium (Figs CA 19-6 and CA 19-7)	Calcification of the left atrial wall usually reflects long-standing severe mitral stenosis and appears as a thin curvilinear rim. Atrial myxomas calcify in approximately 10% of cases and are best seen by fluoroscopy (may present the pathognomonic appearance of a calcified mass prolapsing into the ventricle during systole). Calcification in the left atrial appendage represents a calcified thrombus.
Ventricular aneurysm (Fig CA 19-8)	Complication of myocardial infarction in which weakening of the myocardial wall permits the development of a local bulge at the site of the infarct. Curvilinear calcification in the wall of an aneurysm is an infrequent but important finding.

A B

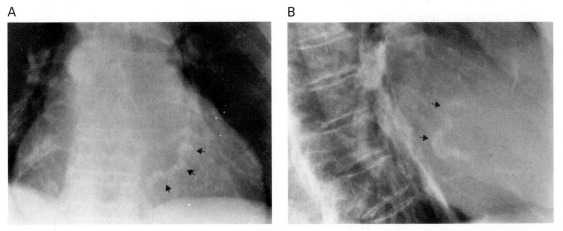

Fig CA 19-5
Coronary artery calcification (arrows) in ischemic heart disease. (A) Frontal and (B) lateral views of the chest.

Condition	Comments
Myocardium	Most commonly a manifestation of an old myocardial infarct. Rare causes include myocardial damage (trauma, myocarditis, and rheumatic fever), hyperparathyroidism, and vitamin D toxicity.
Pericardium (Fig CA 19-9)	Calcific plaques in a thickened pericardium are present in approximately half of patients with constrictive pericarditis. Though the heaviest deposits of calcium are located anteriorly, posterior calcification and calcification of the pericardium adjacent to the diaphragm can often be seen. At times, the heart appears to be encased in a virtually pathognomonic calcific shell.
Ductus arteriosus (Fig CA 19-10)	Calcification mimicking involvement of the aortic wall may rarely occur in patients with a patent or a closed ductus arteriosus.

A

B

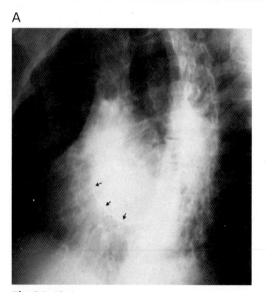
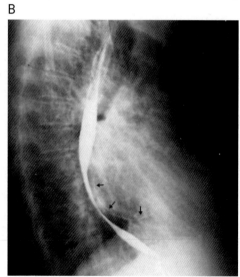

Fig CA 19-6
Left atrial calcification. (A) Overpenetrated film in the left anterior oblique position and (B) lateral view with barium in the esophagus show enlargement of the left atrium and calcification of the wall of this chamber (arrows) in a patient with mitral stenosis.[12]

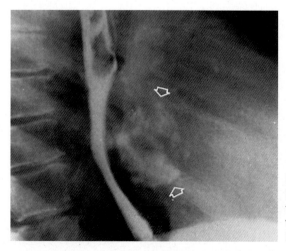

Fig CA 19-7
Left atrial myxoma. The arrows point to calcification in the tumor. The myxoma has led to destruction of the mitral valve with resulting left atrial enlargement that causes an impression on the barium-filled esophagus.

A

B

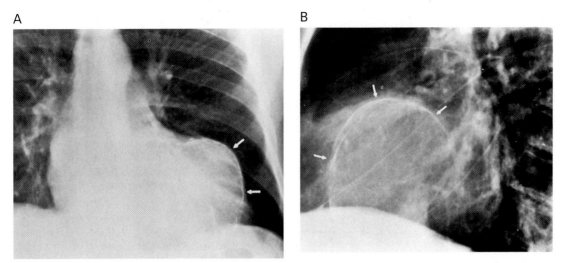

Fig CA 19-8
Ventricular aneurysm. (A) Frontal and (B) lateral views of the chest demonstrate bulging and curvilinear peripheral calcification (arrows) along the lower left border of the heart near the apex. Note the relatively anterior position of the aneurysm on the lateral view.

A

B

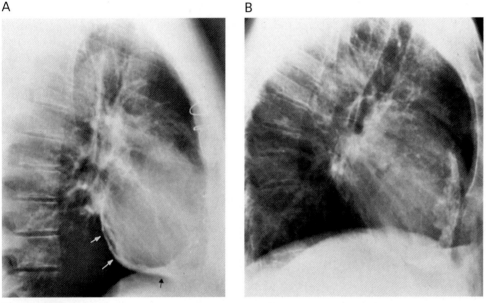

Fig CA 19-9
Pericardial calcification (A and B). Lateral views of the chest demonstrate dense plaques of pericardial calcification (arrows) in two patients with chronic constrictive pericarditis due to tuberculosis.

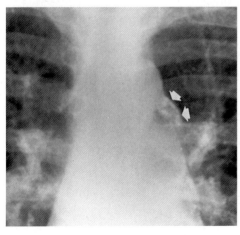

Fig CA 19-10
Ductus arteriosus calcification (arrows).

Pericardial Effusion

Condition	Comments
Congestive heart failure	Evidence of pulmonary venous congestion. An associated pleural effusion is common (frequently unilateral on the right, rarely on the left; may be bilateral).
Collagen disease (see Fig CA 34-9)	Systemic lupus erythematosus; scleroderma; polyarteritis nodosa; rheumatoid disease. There may be unilateral or bilateral pleural effusion (especially in lupus). Generalized reticulonodular disease (more prominent in the lung bases) may occur.
Infectious pericarditis (Fig CA 20-1)	Most commonly coxsackievirus. Also other infections (eg, bacterial, tuberculous, histoplasmic, amebic, toxoplasmic).
Postcardiac surgery	Accumulation of fluid after pericardiotomy. Evidence of surgical clips and sutures.
Postmyocardial infarction syndrome (Dressler's syndrome) (Fig CA 20-2)	Autoimmune phenomenon characterized by fever and pleuropericardial chest pain beginning 1 to 6 weeks after an acute myocardial infarction. Other manifestations include pleural effusion that is bilateral in 50% of patients (usually greater on the left) and an ill-defined pneumonia (often with atelectatic streaks) that may be bilateral or involve only the left base.

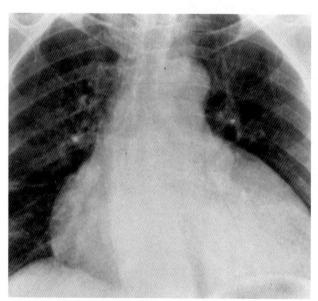

Fig CA 20-1
Infectious pericarditis. Globular enlargement of the cardiac silhouette reflects a combination of pericarditis and pericardial effusion in a patient with coxsackievirus infection. There are small pleural effusions bilaterally.

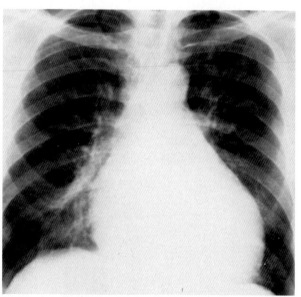

Fig CA 20-2
Dressler's syndrome. Chest film obtained 3 weeks after an acute myocardial infarction demonstrates a large pericardial effusion appearing as a rapid increase in heart size in comparison with an essentially normal-sized heart 1 week earlier.

Condition	Comments
Trauma	Rapid development of a pericardial effusion may produce severe alteration of cardiac function with minimal change in the radiographic cardiac silhouette.
Tumor of pericardium or heart	Direct invasion from carcinoma of the lung or mediastinal lymphoma, or metastases from melanoma or tumors of the lung or breast. Radiation therapy may produce complete (but usually temporary) resolution of the fluid.
Uremia (Fig CA 20-3)	Develops in approximately 15% of patients on prolonged hemodialysis. May collect rapidly and be life threatening.

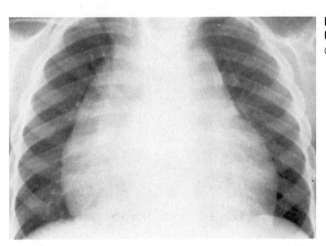

Fig CA 20-3
Uremia. Globular enlargement of the cardiac silhouette in a child on prolonged hemodialysis.

A

B

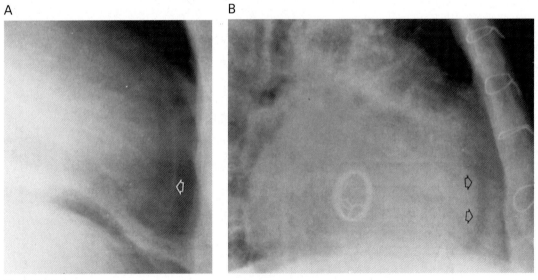

Fig CA 20-4
Epicardial fat pad sign in pericardial effusion. (A) In a normal person, a thin, relatively dense line (arrow) representing the normal pericardium lies between the anterior mediastinal and subepicardial fat. (B) Lateral chest radiograph demonstrates a wide soft-tissue density separating the subepicardial fat stripe (arrows) from the anterior mediastinal fat. This is a virtually pathognomonic sign of pericardial effusion or thickening.

Condition	Comments
Radiation therapy	May follow the use of moderately high doses (4000 rads in 4 to 5 weeks, as in the treatment of Hodgkin's disease or breast carcinoma).
Myxedema	May cause massive chronic pericardial effusion (rarely tamponade).
Bleeding diathesis	Severe chronic anemia; erythroblastosis fetalis; excessive anticoagulant therapy.
Idiopathic	Diagnosis of exclusion for acute pericardial effusion.

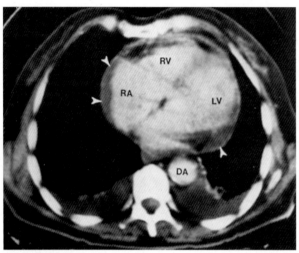

Fig CA 20-5
Pericardial effusion. CT scan made after the injection of intravenous contrast material shows the pericardial effusion as a low-density area (arrowheads) that is clearly demarcated from the contrast-enhanced blood in the intracardiac chambers and descending aorta. Note the bilateral pleural effusions posteriorly. (DA, descending aorta; LV, left ventricle; RA, right atrium; RV, right ventricle.)[13]

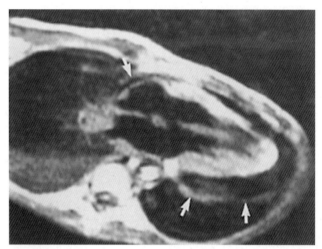

Fig CA 20-6
Pericardial effusion. MRI scan shows the pericardium (arrows) to be displaced away from the heart by a huge pericardial effusion that has very little signal intensity. The effect of gravity is seen in the posterior location of both the pericardial and the right pleural effusions.[14]

Constrictive Pericarditis

Condition	Comments
Tuberculosis (Figs CA 21-1 and CA 21-2)	Etiologic agent in up to one-third of older series. Now an infrequent cause.
Other infections	Pyogenic (especially staphylococcal or pneumococcal); histoplasmosis; viral (especially coxsackie B).
Radiation therapy	May follow the use of moderately high doses (4000 rads in 4 to 5 weeks, as for the treatment of Hodgkin's disease or carcinoma of the breast).
Uremia	Relatively high incidence in patients on prolonged hemodialysis.
Trauma	Hemopericardium leading to dense fibrosis.
Idiopathic	Underlying cause of pericardial disease is often undetermined. Probably represents an asymptomatic or forgotten bout of acute pericarditis.

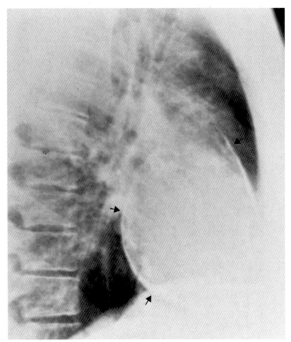

Fig CA 21-1
Chronic constrictive pericarditis. Dense calcification in the pericardium (arrows) completely surrounding a normal-sized heart.

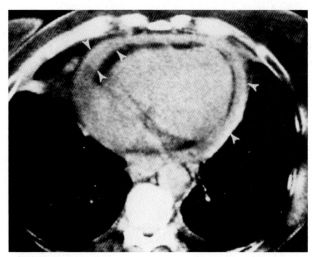

Fig CA 21-2
Chronic constrictive pericarditis. CT scan performed during an infusion of contrast material shows enhancement of the soft-tissue-density pericardium (arrowheads), which is up to 6 mm thick.[13]

Pericardial Disease on Computed Tomography and Magnetic Resonance Imaging

Condition	Imaging Findings	Comments
Pericardial effusion (Figs CA 22-1 to CA 22-4)	On CT, a simple pericardial effusion has attenuation close to that of water. A higher attenuation suggests malignancy, hemopericardium, purulent exudates, or an effusion associated with hypothyroidism. Low attenuation effusions have been reported with chylopericardium. On MRI, the intensity of nonhemorrhagic pericardial effusion is low on T1-weighted images and high on GRE images. The appearance is reversed with hemorrhagic pericardial effusions, which have high signal intensity of T1-weighted images and low intensity on GRE images. Malignant effusions may be associated with an irregularly thickened pericardium of pericardial nodularity.	Develops from obstruction of the venous or lymphatic drainage of the heart secondary to heart failure, renal insufficiency, infection (bacterial, viral, or tuberculosis), neoplasm (carcinoma of lung or breast, or lymphoma), or injury (trauma or myocardial infarction). Although echocardiography is considered the primary imaging modality, both CT and MRI can help characterize the underlying abnormality as well as provide a wider field of view that enables detection of associated abnormalities in the mediastinum and lungs.

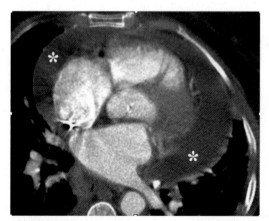

Fig CA 22-1
Pericardial effusion (simple). Contrast CT scan shows an effusion (*) with the same attenuation as water.[15]

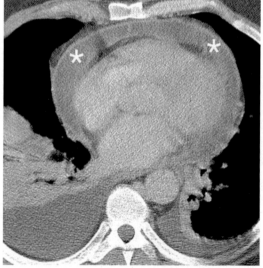

Fig CA 22-2
Pericardial effusion (serosanguinous). Contrast CT scan shows a moderate-sized enhancing effusion (*).[15]

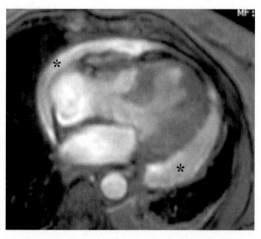

Fig CA 22-3
Pericardial effusion (nonhemorrhagic). Cine GRE image shows a high-signal-intensity effusion (*), consistent with nonhemorrhagic fluid.[15]

Condition	Imaging Findings	Comments
Constrictive pericarditis (Figs CA 22-5 to CA 22-7)	Pericardial thickness of 4 mm or more is abnormal and, when accompanied by clinical findings of heart failure, is highly suggestive of constrictive pericarditis. CT is exquisitely sensitive for detecting pericardial calcification, which is also associated with constrictive pericarditis.	Most frequent causes are cardiac surgery and radiation therapy. Less common etiologies include infection (viral or tuberculous), connective tissue disease, uremia, and neoplasm. The demonstration of pericardial thickening on CT and MRI can aid in making the critical distinction between constrictive pericarditis and restrictive cardiomyopathy, which have similar clinical manifestations and findings on cardiac catheterization and echocardiography.

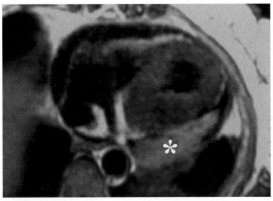

Fig CA 22-4
Pericardial effusion (hemorrhagic). Axial T1-weighted MR image shows an effusion with high signal intensity (*), suggestive of hemorrhage.[15]

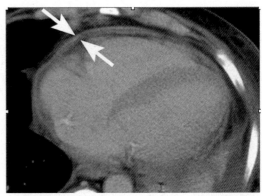

Fig CA 22-5
Constrictive pericarditis. Contrast CT scan shows pericardial thickening (arrows) in this patient, who presented with symptoms of heart failure after mediastinal irradiation for Hodgkin's lymphoma.[15]

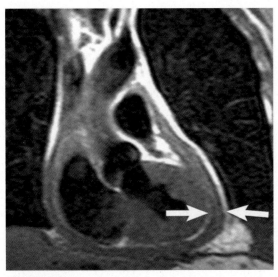

Fig CA 22-6
Constrictive pericarditis. Coronal T1-weighted MR image shows abnormally thickened pericardium (arrows) outlined by epicardial and mediastinal fat.[15]

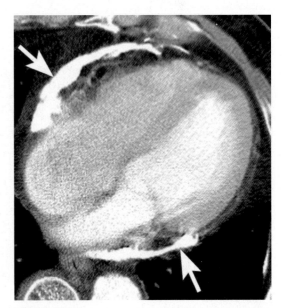

Fig CA 22-7
Constrictive pericarditis. Contrast CT shows dense pericardial calcification (arrows) in a patient with a history of hemopericardium.[15]

Condition	Imaging Findings	Comments
Pericarditis without constriction (Figs CA 22-8 and CA 22-9)	Enhancement of the thickened pericardium on CT indicates inflammation. On MRI, the normal pericardium (composed primarily of fibrous tissue), as well as the purely fibrous or calcified pericardium in chronic pericardial disease, has a low signal intensity on both T1- and T2-weighted images. Thickened pericardium with moderate-to-high signal is seen in subacute pericarditis, and contrast enhancement also is a sign of pericardial inflammation.	Pericardial thickening without clinical symptoms of constrictive pericarditis can be caused by inflammation secondary to acute pericarditis, uremia, rheumatic heart disease, rheumatoid arthritis, sarcoidoisis, and mediastinal irradiation.

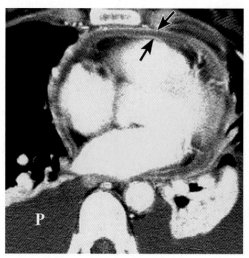

Fig CA 22-8
Infectious pericarditis. Contrast CT scan shows enhancement of the pericardium (arrows), indicative of inflammation. Note the associated small pericardial effusion and large bilateral pleural effusions (P).[15]

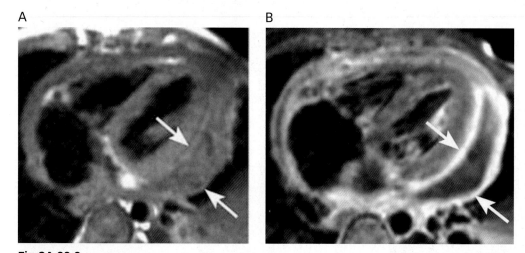

Fig CA 22-9
Infectious pericarditis. (A) T1-weighted MR image shows a crescent-shaped area of intermediate signal intensity (arrows) surrounding the ventricles, which indicates either pericardial thickening or effusion. (B) Contrast T1-weighted image with fat saturation shows marked thickening and enhancement of the pericardium (arrows), findings consistent with inflammation. There is also a moderate-sized pericardial effusion.[15]

Condition	Imaging Findings	Comments
Pericardial masses		Although pericardial masses are often detected initially with echocardiography, CT attenuation or MR signal intensity characteristics, the degree of contrast enhancement, and the presence or absence of blood flow on cine MR images can help differentiate among them.
Cysts (Figs CA 22-10 and CA 22-11)	Thin-walled structure without internal septa that typically has the attenuation and signal intensity of pure water. Occasionally, a cyst may contain highly proteinaceous fluid that produces high signal intensity on T1-weighted MR images.	Congenital pericardial cysts are formed when a portion of the pericardium is pinched off during early development. Generally found in the right cardiophrenic angle, they may occur anywhere in the mediastinum. In unusual sites, they may be indistinguishable from brochogenic or thymic cysts.

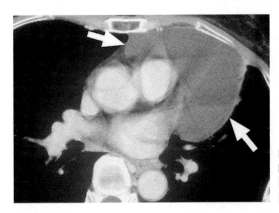

Fig CA 22-10
Pericardial cyst. Contrast CT scan shows a nonenhancing homogeneous mass (arrows) with the attenuation of water, located adjacent to the pulmonary artery.[15]

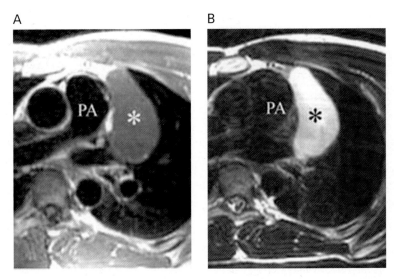

Fig CA 22-11
Pericardial cyst. (A) T1-weighted contrast MR image shows a nonenhancing mass (*) of intermediate signal intensity adjacent to the main pulmonary artery. (B) On a T2-weighted image, the mass (*) has homogeneous high signal intensity.[15]

Condition	Imaging Findings	Comments
Hematomas (Figs CA 22-12 and CA 22-13)	Acute hematomas have homogeneous high signal intensity on T1 and T2 images. Subacute hematomas (1 to 4 weeks old) typically show heterogeneous signal, with areas of hyperintensity on both these sequences. On T1-weighted and GRE images, chronic organized hematomas may show a dark peripheral rim and low-signal-intensity internal foci that may represent calcification, fibrosis, or hemosiderin deposition. High-signal areas on T1- and T2-weighted images often correspond to hemorrhagic fluid.	Coronary or ventricular pseudoaneurysms or neoplaasms may resemble hematomas on MR images. However, these entities demonstrate contrast enhancement, which is not seen with hematomas. The detection of internal flow in a pseudoaneurysm on velocity-encoded cine MR imaging also can differentiate this condition from a hematoma.

A
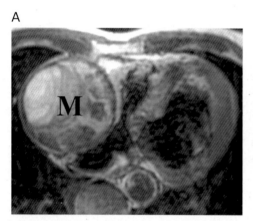
B
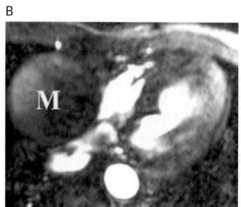

Fig CA 22-12
Pericardial hematoma. (A) T1-weighted contrast image shows a nonenhancing mass of heterogeneous signal intensity (M) in the right atrioventricular groove. (B) Phase velocity-encoded cine image shows no blood blow in the mass (M), a finding indicative of hematoma rather than pseudoaneurysm.[15]

A
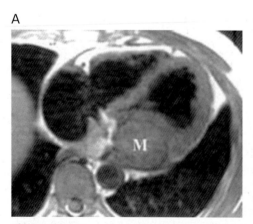
B
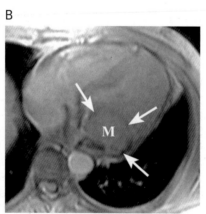

Fig CA 22-13
Pericardial hematoma (chronic, organized). (A) T1-weighted MR image in a patient who had sustained blunt chest trauma 8 years previously shows a well-circumscribed mass (M) with intermediate signal intensity in the left atrioventricular groove that compresses the left atrium and ventricle. (B) Cine GRE image shows a mass (M) with low-signal-intensity foci and a low-signal-intensity rim (arrows), which are indicative of central and peripheral calcifications.[15]

Condition	Imaging Findings	Comments
Neoplasms Metastases (Fig CA 22-14)	On CT, metastatic involvement is suggested by an irregularly thickened pericardium or pericardial mass associated with an effusion. On MRI, tumor invasion of the pericardium causes focal obliteration of the pericardial line, which remains intact if an adjacent tumor extends only up to it. Hemorrhagic pericardial effusions secondary to metastases usually have high signal intensity on all SE images. The signal intensity of most neoplasms is low on T1 and high on T2. An exception is metastatic melanoma, which may have high signal intensity on T1-weighted images because of the paramagnetic metals bound by melanin. Most metastases show significant contrast enhancement.	Pericardial metastases are much more common than primary pericardial tumors. They may seed the pericardium via the blood stream or lymphatics, or directly invade from the lung or mediastinum. Cancers of the breast and lung are the most common sources of metastases to the pericardium, followed by lymphoma and melanoma.
Primary neoplasms (Figs CA 22-15 and CA 22-16)	Lipoma typically has low attenuation on CT images and high signal intensity on T1-weighted MR images. The CT demonstration of calcium or fat in a pericardial mass suggests a teratoma. Fibroma generally has low signal intensity on T2-weighted images and shows poor or no enhancement due to poor vascularization. Mesotheliomas occasionally demonstrate pericardial nodules or plaques in addition to a pericardial effusion. Lymphoma, sarcoma, and liposarcoma typically appear as large heterogeneous masses, frequently associated with a serosanguineous effusion.	Primary pericardial neoplasms are rare. Benign tumors include lipoma, teratoma, fibroma, and hemangioma; malignant primary tumors include mesothelioma, lymphoma, sarcoma, and liposarcoma.

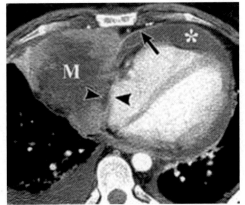

Fig CA 22-14
Metastatic lymphoma. Contrast CT scan shows a large heterogeneous anterior mediastinal mass (M) with central necrosis, which has invaded the pericardium (arrowheads). Note the moderate pericardial effusion (*) and associated enhancement of the pericardium.[15]

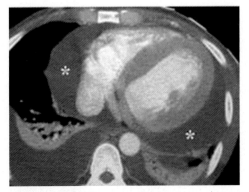

Fig CA 22-15
Primary pericardial mesothelioma. Contrast CT scan shows a large pericardial effusion (*) and no pericardial nodules (which occur in this disease but are rare).[15]

Condition	Imaging Findings	Comments
Congenital absence of the pericardium (Fig CA 22-17)	Interposition of lung tissue between the aorta and the main segment of the pulmonary artery with rotation of the heart toward the left (normally, the aorticopulmonary window is covered by pericardium and contains some fat). At times, the left atrial appendage bulges through the defect.	Congenital absence of the pericardium is rare. Most pericardial defects are partial and occur on the left.

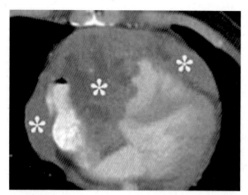

Fig CA 22-16
Primary pericardial lymphoma. Contrast CT scan shows an irregular, enhancing soft-tissue mass (*), which has infiltrated the entire pericardium.[15]

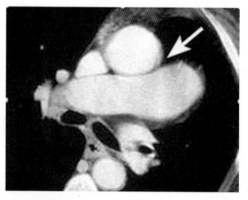

Fig CA 22-17
Congenital absence of the pericardium. Contrast CT scan shows interposition of lung tissue between the aorta and the main segment of the pulmonary artery (arrow), indicating the absence of the pericardium in this area. Note the rotation of the heart toward the left.[15]

Sources

1. Reprinted from *Radiology of the Heart and Great Vessels* by RN Cooley and MH Schreiber, Williams & Wilkins Company, ©1978, with permission of JH Harris Jr.

2. Reprinted with permission from "Transposition of the Great Arteries" by A Barcia et al, *American Journal of Roentgenology* (1967;100:249–261), Copyright ©1967, American Roentgen Ray Society.

3. Reprinted with permission from "Roentgenographic Features in a Case with Origin of Both Great Vessels from the Right Ventricle without Pulmonary Stenosis" by LS Carey and JE Edwards, *American Journal of Roentgenology* (1965;93:268–287), Copyright ©1965, American Roentgen Ray Society.

4. Reprinted with permission from "Angiocardiographic and Anatomic Findings in Origin of Both Great Arteries from the Right Ventricle" by FJ Hallerman et al, *American Journal of Roentgenology* (1970;109:51–66), Copyright ©1970, American Roentgen Ray Society.

5. Reprinted with permission from "Endocardial Cushion Defects" by MG Baron, *Radiologic Clinics of North America* (1968;6:43–52), Copyright ©1968, WB Saunders Company.

6. Reprinted from *Plain Film Interpretation in Congenital Heart Disease* by LE Swischuk with permission of Williams & Wilkins Company, ©1979.

7. Reprinted with permission from "Other Forms of Left-to-Right Shunt" by LP Elliott, *Seminars in Roentgenology* (1966;1:120–136); Copyright ©1966, Grune & Stratton Inc.

8. Reprinted with permission from "Coronary Arteriovenous Fistula" by I Steinberg and GR Holswade, *American Journal of Roentgenology* (1972;116:82–90), Copyright ©1972, American Roentgen Ray Society.

9. Reprinted with permission from "Congenital Aortic Stenosis" by FB Takekawa et al, *American Journal of Roentgenology* (1966;98:800–821), Copyright ©1966, American Roentgen Ray Society.

10. Reprinted from *Diagnostic Imaging in Internal Medicine* by RL Eisenberg with permission of McGraw-Hill Book Company, ©1985. Courtesy of Marvin Belasco, MD.

11. Reprinted with permission from "Anomalous Origin of the Left Pulmonary Artery from the Right Pulmonary Artery" by KL Jue et al, *American Journal of Roentgenology* (1965;95:598–610), Copyright ©1965, American Roentgen Ray Society.

12. Reprinted with permission from "Left Atrial Calcification" by SCW Vickers et al, *Radiology* (1959;72:569–575), Copyright ©1959, Radiological Society of North America Inc.

13. Reprinted from *Computed Body Tomography* by JKT Lee, SS Sagel, and RJ Stanley (Eds) with permission of Raven Press, New York, ©1989.

14. Reprinted with permission from "Cardiac Magnetic Resonance Imaging" by SW Miller et al, *Radiological Clinics of North America* (1985;23:745–764), Copyright ©1985, WB Saunders Company.

15. Wang ZJ, Reddy GP, Gotway MB, et al. CT and MR Imaging of Pericardial Disease. *RadioGraphics* 2003;23:S167–S180.

3

Gastrointestinal Patterns

Esophageal Motility Disorders

Condition	Imaging Findings	Comments
Cricopharyngeal achalasia (Fig GI 1-1)	Hemispherical or horizontal, shelf-like protrusion on the posterior aspect of the esophagus at approximately the C5-C6 level.	Failure of the upper esophageal sphincter to relax. Can result in dysphagia by obstructing the passage of a swallowed bolus. In severe disease, can cause aspiration and pneumonia.
Total laryngectomy (pseudodefect)	Appearance identical to that of cricopharyngeal achalasia.	Clinically, the patient complains of dysphagia on the way down and dysphonia with esophageal speech on the way up.
Scleroderma (Fig GI 1-2)	Dilated, atonic esophagus involving only the smooth muscle portion (from the aortic arch down). Normal stripping wave in the upper third of the esophagus (which is composed primarily of striated muscle). Patulous lower esophageal sphincter with gastroesophageal reflux. In the upright position, barium flows rapidly into the stomach.	Atrophy of smooth muscle with replacement by fibrosis. Often asymptomatic, though the patient may be required to eat or drink in a sitting or an erect position. High incidence of gastroesophageal reflux leading to peptic esophagitis and stricture formation.

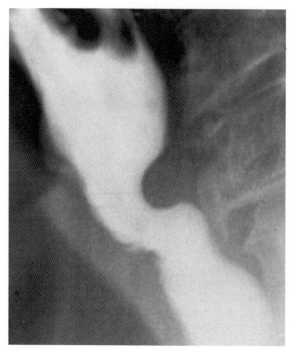

Fig GI 1-1
Cricopharyngeal achalasia.

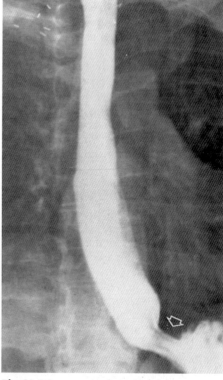

Fig GI 1-2
Scleroderma. Note the patulous esophagogastric junction (arrow).

Condition	Imaging Findings	Comments
Achalasia (Figs GI 1-3 to GI 1-5)	Dilatation and tortuosity of the esophagus that can produce a widened mediastinum (often with an air-fluid level) primarily on the right side adjacent to the cardiac shadow. Multiple uncoordinated tertiary contractions. Smoothly tapered, conical narrowing of the distal esophagus (beak sign). In the erect position, small spurts of barium enter the stomach (jet effect). Length of narrowed segment (<3.5 cm) and degree of proximal dilatation (>4 cm) suggests primary achalasia.	Incomplete relaxation of the lower esophageal sphincter related to a paucity or absence of ganglion cells in the myenteric plexuses (Auerbach's) of the distal esophageal wall. Denervation hypersensitivity response to Mecholyl (synthetic acetylcholine). A similar appearance may be produced by any generalized or localized interruption of the reflex arc controlling normal esophageal motility (eg, diseases of the medullary nuclei, abnormality of the vagus nerve, destruction of myenteric ganglion cells by inflammatory disease, or carcinoma of the distal esophagus or the gastric cardia).

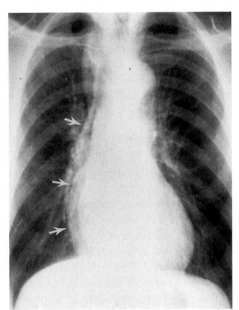

Fig GI 1-3
Achalasia. The margin of the dilated, tortuous esophagus (arrows) parallels the right border of the heart.

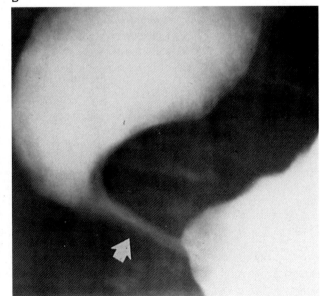

B

A

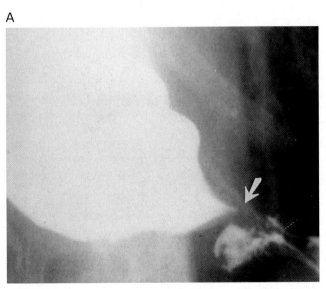

Fig GI 1-4
Achalasia. (A) Beak sign (arrow). (B) Jet effect (arrow).

Condition	Imaging Findings	Comments
Chagas' disease	Pattern identical to that of achalasia.	Destruction of the myenteric plexuses by the protozoan *Trypanosoma cruzi*, which also causes megacolon with chronic constipation, ureteral dilatation, and myocarditis.
Diffuse esophageal spasm (Fig GI 1-6)	Tertiary contractions of abnormally high amplitude that can obliterate the lumen. Corkscrew pattern of transient sacculations or pseudodiverticular (rosary bead esophagus).	Classic clinical triad of massive uncoordinated esophageal contractions, chest pain, and increased intramural pressure. Symptoms are frequently caused or aggravated by eating, but can occur spontaneously and even awaken the patient at night.
Presbyesophagus	Nonpropulsive tertiary contractions that are usually occasional and mild but may become frequent and strong.	Condition of aging that may be the result of a minor cerebrovascular accident affecting the central nuclei. Usually asymptomatic but can cause moderate dysphagia.
Esophagitis (Fig GI 1-7)	Initially, repetitive nonperistaltic tertiary contractions that occur distal to the point of disruption of the primary wave. If severe, can result in complete aperistalsis.	Disordered esophageal motility is the earliest and most frequent radiographic abnormality in esophageal inflammation, whether secondary to reflux, corrosive agents, infection, amyloidosis, or radiation injury.
Primary muscle disorders (Fig GI 1-8)	Disordered peristalsis involving the upper third of the esophagus (containing striated muscle). In myasthenia gravis, the initial swallow is often normal, but peristalsis weakens on repeated swallows. In myotonic dystrophy, there is reflux across the cricopharyngeus muscle (continuous column of barium extending from the hypopharynx to the cervical esophagus even when the patient is not swallowing).	Patient unable to develop a good pharyngeal peristaltic wave. In myasthenia gravis, muscular fatigue results from failure of neural transmission between the motor end plate and the muscle fiber. In myotonic dystrophy, an anatomic abnormality of the motor end plate leads to atrophy and an inability of the contracted muscle to relax. Other primary muscle disorders include polymyositis, dermatomyositis, amyotrophic lateral sclerosis, myopathies secondary to steroids and abnormal thyroid function, and oculopharyngeal myopathy.
Primary neural disorders	Various patterns of abnormal motility, including profound motor incoordination of the pharynx and the upper esophageal sphincter, diffuse tertiary contractions, and an achalasia pattern.	Causes include peripheral or central cranial nerve palsy, cerebrovascular occlusive disease affecting the brainstem, high unilateral cervical vagotomy, bulbar poliomyelitis, syringomyelia, multiple sclerosis, and familial dysautonomia (Riley-Day syndrome).
Diabetes mellitus	Various patterns of abnormal motility, including tertiary contractions and esophageal dilatation with a substantial delay in esophageal emptying when the patient is recumbent.	Markedly decreased amplitude of pharyngeal and peristaltic contractions. Primarily involves diabetics with a neuropathy of long duration.
Alcoholism	Diminished peristalsis, most pronounced in the distal portion.	Probably reflects a combination of alcoholic myopathy and neuropathy.
Drugs	Aperistalsis and dilatation of the esophagus (mimics scleroderma).	Anticholinergic agents (atropine, Pro-Banthine).
Obstructive lesions	Initially, tertiary contractions are produced in an attempt to pass the obstruction. Eventually, there may be a dilated and virtually aperistaltic esophagus.	Lesions that may cause esophageal obstruction include tumors, foreign bodies, webs, strictures, and Schatzki's rings.

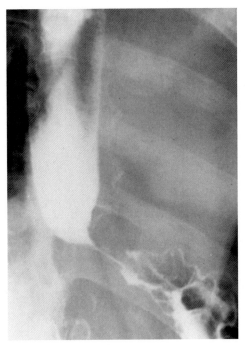

Fig GI 1-5
Achalasia pattern caused by the proximal extension of carcinoma of the fundus of the stomach.

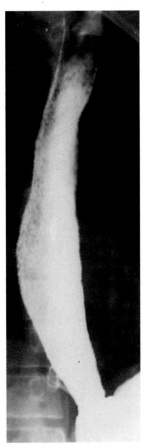

Fig GI 1-6
Diffuse esophageal spasm.

Fig GI 1-7
Candidiasis. Aperistalsis and esophageal dilatation are associated with diffuse ulceration.

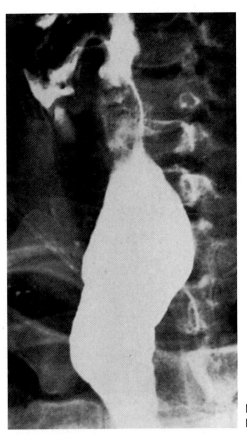

Fig GI 1-8
Myotonic dystrophy.[1]

Extrinsic Impressions on the Cervical Esophagus

Condition	Imaging Findings	Comments
Cricopharyngeus muscle (Fig GI 2-1)	Relatively constant posterior impression on the esophagus at approximately the C5-C6 level.	Caused by failure of the cricopharyngeus muscle to relax. A similar posterior impression can often be observed after total laryngectomy.
Pharyngeal venous plexus (Fig GI 2-1)	Anterior impression on the esophagus at about the C6 level. Appearance varies from swallow to swallow.	Caused by prolapse of lax mucosal folds over the rich central submucosal pharyngeal venous plexus. Occurs in 70% to 90% of adults and is thus considered a normal finding.
Esophageal web (Figs GI 2-1 through GI 2-3)	Smooth, thin lucent band (occasionally multiple) arising from the anterior wall of the esophagus near the pharyngoesophageal junction.	Usually an incidental finding of no clinical importance, but can be associated with epidermolysis bullosa, benign mucous membrane pemphigus, or the "Plummer-Vinson syndrome."
Anterior marginal osteophyte (Fig GI 2-4)	Smooth, regular indentation on the posterior wall of the esophagus at the level of an intervertebral disk space.	Usually asymptomatic but may produce pain or difficulty in swallowing (especially with profuse osteophytosis and diffuse idiopathic skeletal hyperostosis).
Thyroid enlargement or mass (Fig GI 2-5)	Smooth impression on and displacement of the lateral wall of the esophagus, usually with parallel displacement of the trachea.	Caused by localized or generalized hypertrophy of the gland, inflammatory disease, or thyroid malignancy.
Parathyroid mass	Impression on and displacement of the lateral wall of the esophagus.	Can aid in determining the site of the lesion in a patient with symptoms of hyperparathyroidism due to a functioning parathyroid tumor.
Lymphadenopathy	Smooth impression on and displacement of the esophagus.	May be calcified.
Soft-tissue abscess or hematoma	Impression on and displacement of the esophagus.	Abscess may contain gas.
Spinal neoplasm or inflammation	Posterior impression on the esophagus (may be irregular).	Suggested if there is associated destruction of a vertebral body.
Ectopic gastric mucosal rest (Fig GI 2-6)	Persistent ring-like narrowing of the upper esophagus.	Congenital condition that is almost always asymptomatic but rarely can produce dysphagia.
Narrow thoracic inlet	Extrinsic compression of esophagus at the cervicodorsal junction.	Rare anatomic variant. CT is required to exclude a mass and permit measurement of the thoracic inlet.

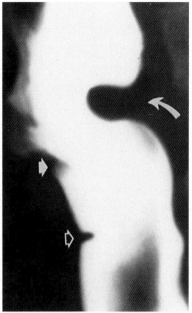

Fig GI 2-1
Three impressions on the cervical esophagus: **cricopharyngeal impression** (curved arrow), **pharyngeal venous plexus** (short closed arrow), and **esophageal web** (short open arrow).[2]

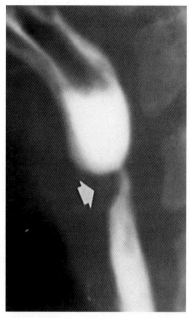

Fig GI 2-2
Epidermolysis bullosa. A stenotic web (arrow) results from the healing of subepidermal blisters involving the mucous membranes.

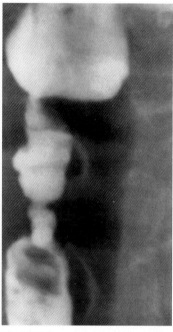

Fig GI 2-3
Benign mucous membrane pemphigus. Postinflammatory scarring causes a long, irregular area of narrowing suggestive of a malignant process.

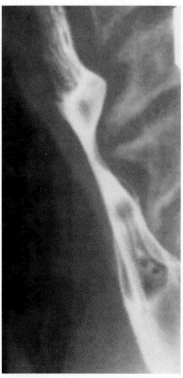

Fig GI 2-4
Anterior marginal osteophytes.

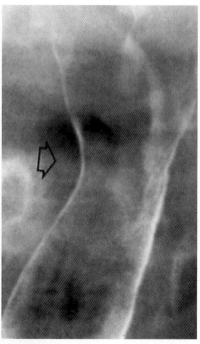

Fig GI 2-5
Enlargement of the thyroid gland. Smooth impression in the cervical esophagus (arrow).

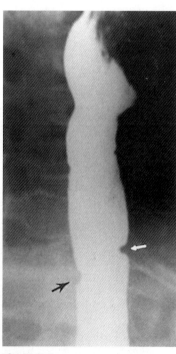

Fig GI 2-6
Ectopic gastric mucosa. Persistent ring-like narrowing (arrows) in the upper esophagus at the level of the thoracic inlet.[3]

Extrinsic Impressions on the Thoracic Esophagus

Condition	Imaging Findings	Comments
Normal structures		
Aortic knob (Fig GI 3-1)	Broad impression on the esophagus at the level of the transverse arch.	More prominent as the aorta becomes increasingly dilated and tortuous with age.
Left main-stem bronchus (Fig GI 3-1)	Narrower impression on the esophagus at the level of the carina.	
Left inferior pulmonary vein/confluence of left pulmonary veins	Impression on the anterior aspect of the left wall of the esophagus 4 to 5 cm below the carina.	Seen in approximately 10% of patients (especially in a steep left posterior oblique [LPO] projection). The vascular nature of the indentation can be confirmed by the Valsalva and Mueller maneuvers (the impression becomes smaller and more prominent, respectively).
Right inferior supra-azygous recess	Smooth extrinsic impression on the right posterolateral wall of the upper thoracic esophagus between the thoracic inlet and the aortic arch.	Seen in approximately 10% of individuals, this impression should not be mistaken for lymphadenopathy or other mediastinal mass.
Vascular abnormalities		
Right aortic arch (Fig GI 3-2)	Impression on the right lateral wall of the esophagus at a level slightly higher than the normal left aortic knob. Deviation of the trachea to the left.	If no posterior esophageal impression (mirror-image pattern), congenital heart disease (especially tetralogy of Fallot) is frequently associated. If there is an oblique posterior indentation on the esophagus (aberrant left subclavian artery), congenital heart disease is rarely associated.
Cervical aortic arch (see Fig CA 11-2)	Pulsatile mass causing a posterior impression on the esophagus above the clavicle.	Caused by the retroesophageal course of the distal arch or the proximal descending aorta. No coexistent intracardiac congenital heart disease.

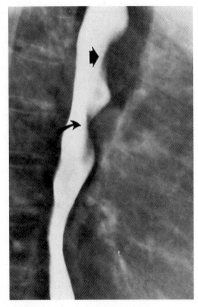

Fig GI 3-1
Normal esophageal impressions caused by the aorta (short arrow) and left main-stem bronchus (long arrow).

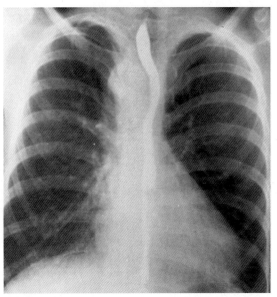

Fig GI 3-2
Right aortic arch.

Condition	Imaging Findings	Comments
Double aortic arch (see Fig CA 11-3)	Reverse S-shaped impression on the esophagus. Right (posterior) arch is generally higher and larger than the left (anterior) arch. Infrequently, the two esophageal impressions are directly across from each other.	Aorta generally ascends on the right, branches, and finally reunites on the left. The two limbs of the aorta encircle the trachea and esophagus, forming a ring.
Coarctation of aorta (see Fig CA 8-1)	Characteristic figure-3 sign on plain chest radiographs. Reverse figure-3, or figure-E, impression on the barium-filled esophagus.	Usually occurs at or just distal to the level of the ductus arteriosus. Much less frequently, the area of narrowing is more proximal. The more cephalad bulge represents prestenotic dilatation, whereas the lower bulge reflects poststenotic dilatation. Relative obstruction of aortic blood flow leads to left ventricular hypertrophy and rib notching (collateral circulation).
Aortic aneurysm or tortuosity (Fig GI 3-3)	Sickle-like deformity that typically displaces the esophagus anteriorly and to the left.	May cause esophageal symptoms ("dysphagia aortica").
Aberrant right subclavian artery (see Fig CA 11-4)	Posterior impression on the esophagus that runs obliquely upward and to the right on the frontal view.	Usually asymptomatic and not associated with congenital heart disease. The aberrant artery arises as the last major vessel of the aortic arch and courses across the mediastinum behind the esophagus.
Aberrant left pulmonary artery (Fig GI 3-4)	Characteristic figure-3 sign on plain chest radiographs. Reverse figure-3, or figure-E, impression on the barium-filled esophagus.	Aberrant artery crosses the mediastinum between the trachea and the esophagus.
Anomalous pulmonary venous return (type III)	Anterior impression on the lower portion of the esophagus, just above the diaphragm but slightly below the expected site of the left atrial indentation.	Anomalous pulmonary vein travels with the esophagus through the diaphragm to insert into the portal vein or a systemic vein.
Persistent truncus arteriosus	Discrete impression (often multiple) on the posterior wall of the esophagus that is located somewhat lower than the usual position of an aberrant left subclavian artery.	Caused by dilated bronchial artery collaterals that develop because of the absence of the pulmonary artery.

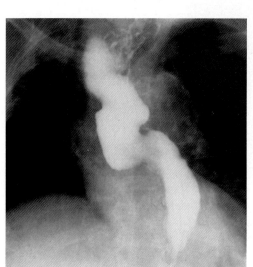

Fig GI 3-3
Dysphagia aortica. Tortuosity of the descending thoracic aorta produces characteristic displacement of the esophagus to the left. Note the retraction of the upper esophagus to the right, caused by chronic inflammatory disease, which simulates an extrinsic mass arising from the opposite side.

Condition	Imaging Findings	Comments
Left atrial enlargement (see Figs in Section CA 3)	Anterior impression on and posterior displacement of the esophagus beginning approximately 2 cm below the carina.	Associated signs include posterior displacement of the left main-stem bronchus, widening of the carina, bulging of the left atrial appendage, and a "double-density" sign on frontal views.
Left ventricular enlargement (see Figs in Section CA 4)	Anterior impression on and posterior displacement of the esophagus at a level somewhat inferior to an enlarged left atrium.	Most often caused by aortic valvular disease or cardiac failure.
Mediastinal or pulmonary masses (Figs GI 3-5 through GI 3-7)	Focal or broad impression on and displacement of the esophagus. The appearance depends on the size and the position of the mass.	Most common causes are inflammatory and metastatic lesions involving lymph nodes in the carinal and subcarinal regions. Also tumors and cysts of the mediastinum, lung, and trachea.
Thoracic osteophyte (Fig GI 3-8)	Posterior impression on the thoracic esophagus.	Infrequent cause of dysphagia that usually occurs in association with diffuse idiopathic skeletal hyperostosis (DISH). Anterior marginal osteophytes much more commonly cause posterior compression of the esophagus in the cervical region.
Paraesophageal hernia (Fig GI 3-9)	Usually displaces the distal esophagus posteriorly and to the right.	Extent of the impression depends on the amount of herniated stomach. The esophagogastric junction remains in its normal position below the diaphragm.
Pericardial lesions	Localized or broad impression on the anterior wall of the esophagus.	Tumors and cysts usually cause localized impressions, whereas effusions are generally broader.
Apical pleuropulmonary fibrosis (pseudo-impression)	Retraction of the upper thoracic esophagus toward the side of the pulmonary lesion.	Simulates the appearance of an extrinsic mass arising from the opposite side. Usually a complication of chronic inflammatory disease, especially tuberculosis.

A

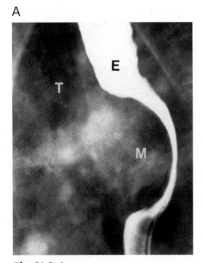

B

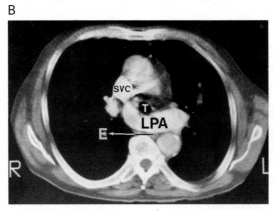

Fig GI 3-4
Aberrant left pulmonary artery. (A) Lateral esophagram shows a smooth, ovoid soft-tissue mass (M) lying between the distal trachea (T) and mid-esophagus (E) and causing marked esophageal narrowing. (B) Dynamic CT scan of the thorax shows that the mass is actually the proximal portion of a dilated left pulmonary artery (LPA), which has an anomalous origin from the right pulmonary artery and courses between the trachea (T) and the esophagus (E) toward the left hilum. (SVC, superior vena cava.)[4]

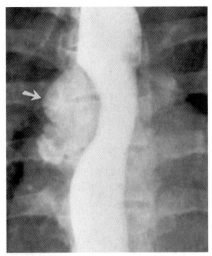

Fig GI 3-5
Calcified mediastinal lymph nodes at the carinal level (arrow) cause a focal impression on and displacement of the esophagus.

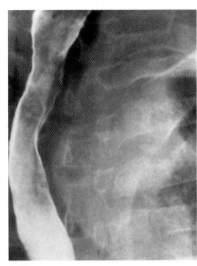

Fig GI 3-6
Squamous cell carcinoma of the lung produces a broad impression on the upper thoracic esophagus.

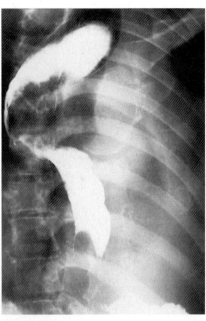

Fig GI 3-7
Squamous cell carcinoma of the lung impressing and invading the mid-thoracic esophagus.

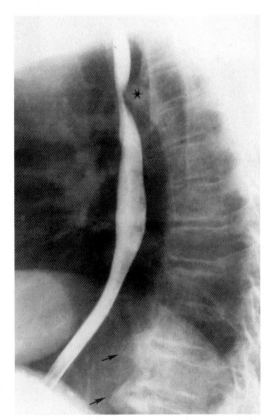

Fig GI 3-8
Thoracic osteophyte. Posterior extrinsic defect on the esophagus anterior to the T4 vertebral body. The osteophyte (*) was better shown on CT. Note the osteophytes and the flowing ossification anterior to the lower thoracic vertebral bodies (arrows) with preservation of the disk spaces.[5]

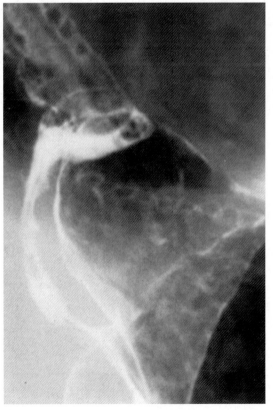

Fig GI 3-9
Paraesophageal hernia impressing the distal esophagus.

Esophageal Ulceration

Condition	Imaging Findings	Comments
Reflux esophagitis (Figs GI 4-1 through GI 4-3)	Initially, superficial ulcerations or erosions appear as streaks or dots of barium superimposed on the flat mucosa of the distal esophagus. Ulcers may be linear and associated with radiating folds and slight retraction of the esophageal wall. In advanced disease, there may be deep erosions or penetrating ulcers with nodular thickening of folds.	Increased incidence with hiatal hernia, repeated vomiting, prolonged nasogastric intubation, scleroderma, and late pregnancy. Also occurs after surgical procedures in the region of the gastroesophageal junction that impair the normal function of the lower esophageal sphincter (eg, Heller procedure for achalasia). May be associated with a disorder of esophageal motility and fine transverse folds (feline esophagus).

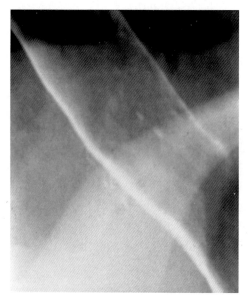

Fig GI 4-1
Reflux esophagitis. Superficial ulcerations appear as streaks of contrast material superimposed on the flat mucosa of the distal esophagus.

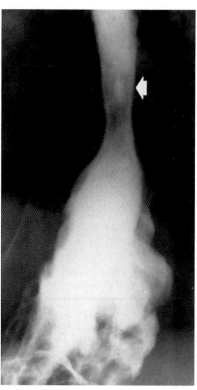

Fig GI 4-2
Reflux esophagitis. Large penetrating ulcer (arrow).

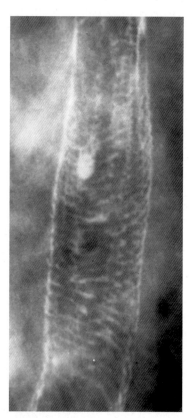

Fig GI 4-3
Feline esophagus.[6]

Condition	Imaging Findings	Comments
Barrett esophagus (Fig GI 4-4)	Ulceration can occur anywhere along the columnar epithelium and tends to be deep and penetrating like peptic gastric ulcers. Postinflammatory stricture of the esophagus often develops.	Often associated with hiatal hernia and reflux, though the ulcer is generally separated from the hernia by a variable length of normal-appearing esophagus. High propensity for developing adenocarcinoma in the columnar-lined portion of the esophagus.
Infectious esophagitis *Candida* (Fig GI 4-5)	Multiple ulcerations of various sizes that can involve the entire thoracic esophagus. Irregular nodular mucosal pattern with marginal serrations. May be a single large ulcer in patients with AIDS.	Most frequently develops in patients with chronic debilitating diseases or undergoing immunosuppressive therapy. Disordered esophageal motility (dilated, atonic esophagus) is often an early finding.
Herpetic (Fig GI 4-6)	Similar to candidiasis, though the background mucosa is often otherwise normal.	Self-limited viral inflammation that predominantly affects patients with disseminated malignancy or abnormal immune systems.

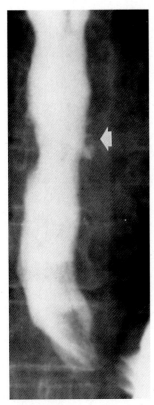

Fig GI 4-4
Barrett esophagus. Ulcerations (arrow) have developed at a distance from the esophagogastric junction.

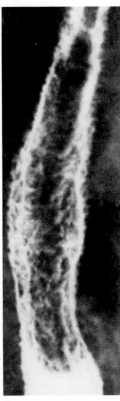

Fig GI 4-5
***Candida* esophagitis.** Multiple ulcers and nodular plaques produce the grossly irregular contour of a shaggy esophagus. This manifestation of far-advanced candidiasis is now infrequent because of earlier and better treatment of the disease.[7]

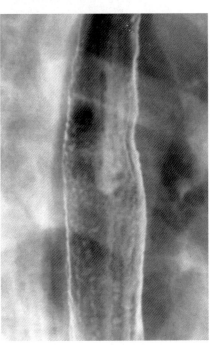

Fig GI 4-6
Herpes simplex esophagitis. Innumerable punctate and linear areas of ulceration.[8]

Condition	Imaging Findings	Comments
Cytomegalovirus (Fig GI 4-7)	Diffuse or segmental ulcerating colitis, primarily affecting the distal half of the esophagus with extension into the gastric fundus. Often solitary, large, relatively flat ulcer.	Most frequently develops in patients with AIDS or other cause of compromised immune system. Widely distributed organism that usually causes only a subclinical infection in a normal adult host.
Tuberculous (Fig GI 4-8)	Single or multiple ulcers that may mimic malignancy. Sinuses and fistulous tracts are common.	Intense fibrotic response often narrows the esophageal lumen. Numerous miliary granulomas can produce multiple nodules.
Human immunodeficiency virus (Fig GI 4-9)	Giant, relatively flat, ovoid or irregular lesions that typically involve the middle third of the esophagus.	Causes odynophagia in patients with acute or chronic HIV infection who have no evidence of the usual opportunistic fungal or viral organisms. Ulcers heal spontaneously or respond to oral steroids (thus must be distinguished from giant ulcers of cytomegalovirus, which require treatment with potentially toxic antiviral agents).

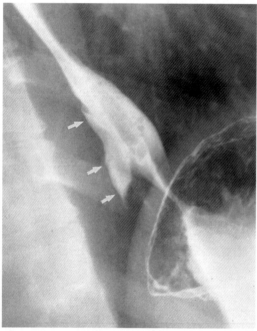

Fig GI 4-7
Cytomegalovirus. Deep focal ulcer in the distal esophagus (arrows).[9]

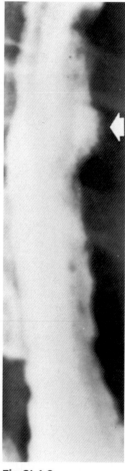

Fig GI 4-8
Tuberculosis. Diffuse mucosal irregularity of the esophagus associated with sinus tracts extending anteriorly into the mediastinum (arrow).[10]

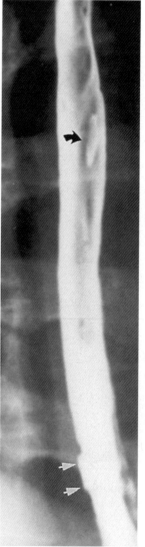

Fig GI 4-9
Human immunodeficiency virus. Long, ovoid lesion seen en face in the upper esophagus (black arrow). Note the more distal lesion (white arrows) seen in profile.

Condition	Imaging Findings	Comments
Other organisms	Various patterns of ulceration, nodularity, and fistulous tracts.	Rare manifestation of syphilis and histoplasmosis.
Carcinoma of the esophagus (Figs GI 4-10 and GI 4-11)	Ulcer crater (often irregular) surrounded by an unchanging bulging mass projecting into the esophageal lumen.	In the relatively uncommon primary ulcerative esophageal carcinoma, virtually all of an eccentric, flat mass is ulcerated. Ulceration is an infrequent manifestation of esophageal lymphoma.
Corrosive esophagitis (Fig GI 4-12)	Diffuse superficial or deep ulceration involves a long portion of the esophagus.	Most severe corrosive injuries are caused by alkali. Fibrous healing results in gradual esophageal narrowing.
Radiation injury	Multiple ulcerations of various sizes that can involve the entire thoracic esophagus. Irregular nodular mucosal pattern with marginal serrations.	Appearance indistinguishable from that of *Candida* esophagitis (which is far more common in patients undergoing chemotherapy or radiation therapy for malignant disease). Develops after relatively low radiation doses in patients who simultaneously or sequentially receive Adriamycin or actinomycin D.
Crohn's disease/ eosinophilic esophagitis (Fig GI 4-13)	Various patterns of ulceration, nodularity, and fistulous tracts.	Infrequent esophageal involvement.

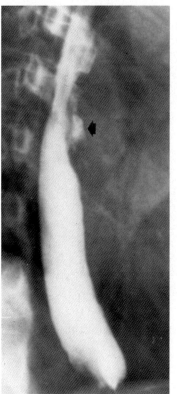

Fig GI 4-10
Squamous carcinoma of the esophagus. On a profile view, the lesion appears as an ulcer crater (arrow) surrounded by a bulging mass projecting into the esophageal lumen.

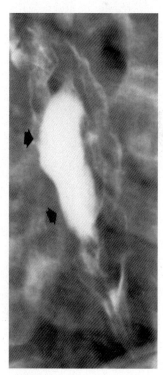

Fig GI 4-11
Primary ulcerative carcinoma. Characteristic meniscoid ulceration (arrows) surrounded by a tumor mass.

Condition	Imaging Findings	Comments
Drug-induced esophagitis (Fig GI 4-14)	Various patterns of superficial or deep esophageal ulcerations.	Primarily occurs in patients who have delayed esophageal transit time (abnormal peristalsis, hiatal hernia with reflux, or relative obstruction). Most commonly associated with potassium chloride tablets; other causes include tetracycline, emperonium bromide, quinidine, and ascorbic acid.
Sclerotherapy of esophageal varices (Fig GI 4-15)	Focal or diffuse ulceration that varies in size, shape, and depth.	Most frequent cause of rebleeding. The degree of ulceration is directly related to the amount of sclerosant solution used, the number of injections, and the number of columns of varices injected.
Intramural esophageal pseudodiverticulosis (Fig GI 4-16)	Multiple, small (1–3 mm), ulcer-like projections arising from the esophageal wall. There is frequently an associated smooth stricture in the upper esophagus.	Rare disorder in which the pseudodiverticula represent the dilated ducts of submucosal glands. *Candida albicans* can be cultured from approximately half the patients, though there is no evidence suggesting the fungus as a causative agent.

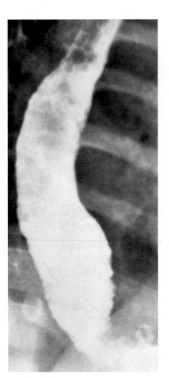
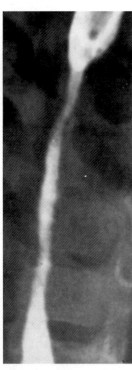

Fig GI 4-12
Corrosive esophagitis. (A) Dilated, boggy esophagus with ulceration 8 days after the ingestion of a caustic agent. (B) Stricture formation is evident on an esophagram obtained 3 months after the caustic injury.

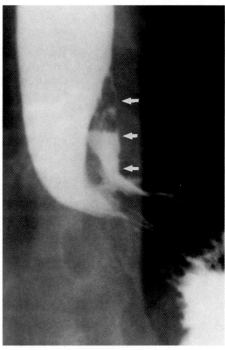

Fig GI 4-13
Crohn's esophagitis. Long intramural sinus tract (arrows).[11]

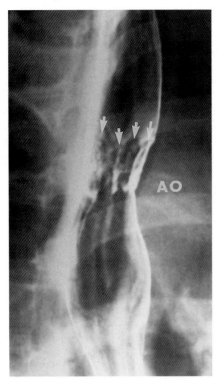

Fig GI 4-14
Drug-induced esophagitis. Several focal and linear ulcers (arrows) coalescing in the proximal thoracic esophagus at the level of the aortic arch (AO), related to the ingestion of penicillin tablets for pharyngitis.[12]

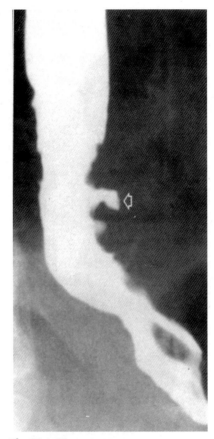

Fig GI 4-15
Variceal sclerotherapy. Barium esophagram performed 2 weeks after two courses of endoscopic injection sclerotherapy shows diffuse ulceration in the distal third of the esophagus and one intramural sinus tract (arrow).[13]

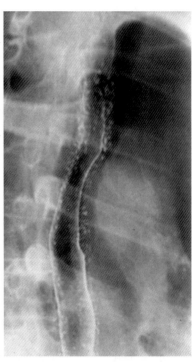

Fig GI 4-16
Intramural pseudodiverticulosis.

Esophageal Narrowing

Condition	Imaging Findings	Comments
Esophageal web (Fig GI 5-1)	Smooth, thin lucent band arising from the anterior wall of the esophagus near the pharyngo-esophageal junction. Rarely distal or multiple.	Usually an incidental finding of no clinical importance, but can be associated with epidermolysis bullosa, benign mucous membrane pemphigus, chronic graft-versus-host disease, or the Plummer-Vinson syndrome. Fluoroscopically guided balloon dilatation has been reported as an easy and highly effective technique for treating symptomatic webs.
Lower esophageal ring (Schatzki's ring) (Fig GI 5-2)	Smooth, concentric narrowing of the esophagus arising several centimeters above the diaphragm.	Can cause dysphagia if the width of the lumen is less than 12 mm.
Carcinoma of esophagus (Fig GI 5-3)	Initially, a flat plaque-like lesion on one wall of the esophagus. Later, an encircling mass with irregular luminal narrowing and overhanging margins.	Major cause of dysphagia in patients older than 40. Close association with drinking and smoking and with head and neck carcinomas. Spreads rapidly and often ulcerates.
Malignancy of fundus of the stomach (Fig GI 5-4)	Irregular narrowing and nodularity of the distal esophagus.	Develops in 10% to 15% of adenocarcinomas and in 2% to 10% of lymphomas arising in the cardia.

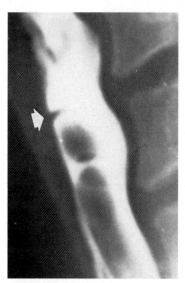

Fig GI 5-1
Esophageal web (arrow).

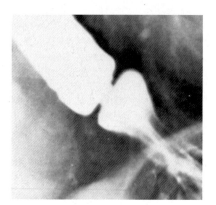

Fig GI 5-2
Lower esophageal ring.

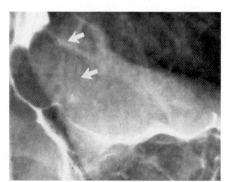

Fig GI 5-4
Adenocarcinoma of the fundus involving the esophagus. An irregular tumor of the superior aspect of the fundus extends proximally as a large mass (arrows) that almost obstructs the distal esophagus.

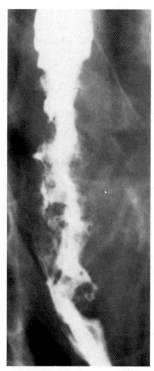

Fig GI 5-3
Esophageal carcinoma. Irregular narrowing of an extensive segment of the thoracic portion of the esophagus.

Condition	Imaging Findings	Comments
Reflux esophagitis (Figs GI 5-5 and GI 5-6)	Asymmetric, often irregular, stricture of the esophagus that usually extends to the cardio-esophageal junction.	Often, but not always, associated with a hiatal hernia.
Barrett esophagus (Fig GI 5-7)	Smooth stricture that generally involves the midportion of the thoracic esophagus.	Usually a variable length of normal-appearing esophagus separates the stricture from the cardio esophageal junction. A technetium scan can demonstrate the columnar tissue in the lower esophagus.

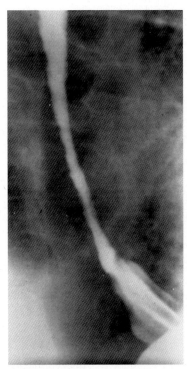

Fig GI 5-5
Reflux esophagitis. The long esophageal stricture is associated with a hiatal hernia.

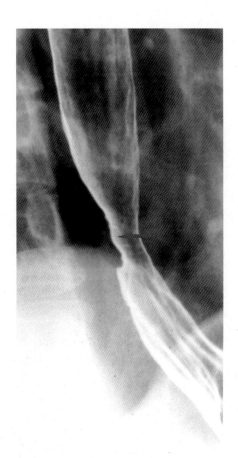

Fig GI 5-6
Reflux esophagitis. Eccentric area of narrowing in the distal esophagus (arrow), which resulted from asymmetric scarring.[14]

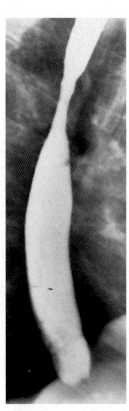

Fig GI 5-7
Barrett esophagus. Smooth stricture in the upper thoracic esophagus.

Condition	Imaging Findings	Comments
Corrosive esophagitis (Fig GI 5-8)	Long stricture that involves a large portion of the esophagus down to the cardioesophageal junction.	Most severe injuries are caused by the ingestion of alkali.
Drug ingestion (Fig GI 5-9)	Segmental area of concentric narrowing.	Drugs such as quinidine, potassium chloride, alendronate, and aspirin or other nonsteroidal anti-inflammatory agents may cause severe esophagitis with large areas of ulceration and the development of strictures. The esophagitis typically results from prolonged irritation of that mucosa caused by pills that lodge in the esophagus at sites of extrinsic compression by adjacent structures, such as the aortic arch, left main bronchus, or enlarged left chambers of the heart.
Prolonged nasogastric intubation (Fig GI 5-10)	Smooth narrowing of the distal esophagus.	Caused by reflux esophagitis (tube prevents hiatal closure) or mucosal ischemia (compression effect of the tube).

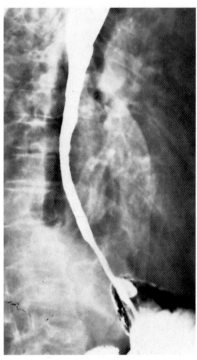

Fig GI 5-8
Extensive caustic stricture due to lye ingestion that involves almost the entire thoracic esophagus.

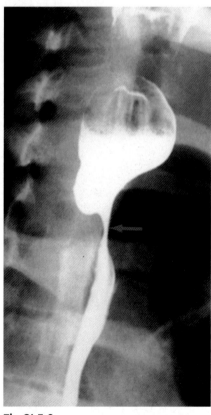

Fig GI 5-9
Drug-induced stricture. Slightly asymmetric focal area of narrowing in the upper thoracic esophagus (arrow) above the level of the aortic arch in a patient who developed dysphagia 6 months after taking potassium chloride for hypokalemia.[14]

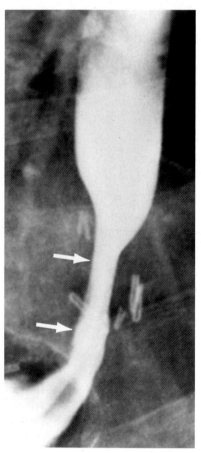

Fig GI 5-10
Nasogastric intubation stricture. Relatively long segment of narrowing in the distal esophagus (arrows), which developed 5 months after prolonged nasogastric intubation.[14]

Condition	Imaging Findings	Comments
Radiation (Fig GI 5-11)	Relatively long segment of smooth, concentric, tapered narrowing within a pre-existing radiation portal	This appearance can usually be distinguished from the more irregular narrowing, asymmetric mass effect, and ulceration associated with recurrent tumor in the mediastinum.
Infectious or granulomatous disorders (Fig GI 5-12)	Various patterns of esophageal narrowing.	Tuberculosis; histoplasmosis; syphilis; herpes simplex; Crohn's disease; eosinophilic esophagitis.
Motility disorders (see Fig GI 1-4)	Various patterns of esophageal narrowing.	Achalasia (failure of the lower esophageal sphincter to relax, beak sign); diffuse esophageal spasm (prolonged strong contractions).

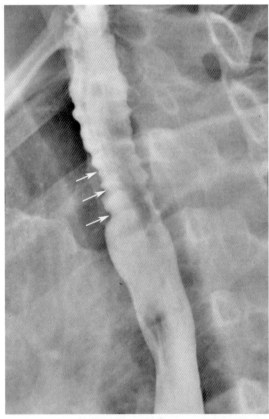

Fig GI 5-11
Radiation-induced stricture. Long segment of smooth tapered narrowing (arrows) in the upper esophagus in a patient who had undergone medistinal irradiation.[15]

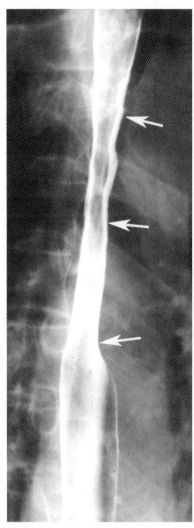

Fig GI 5-12
Eosinophilic esophagitis. Moderately long stricture in the upper thoracic esophagus. Note the multiple distinctive ring-like indentations (arrows) in the region of the stricture that are frequently seen in this condition.[16]

Condition	Imaging Findings	Comments
Intramural esophageal pseudodiverticulosis (Fig GI 5-13)	Smooth stricture in the upper third of the esophagus associated with multiple small ulcer-like projections arising from the esophageal wall.	Dilatation of the stricture generally ameliorates the symptoms of dysphagia.
Skin disease (Fig GI 5-14)	Concentric or asymmetric narrowing in the upper or mid-esophagus, sometimes with associated webs.	Epidermolysis bullosa dystrophica and benign mucous membrane pemphigoid.
Congenital esophageal stenosis (Fig GI 5-15)	Focal stricture containing ring-like indentations in the mid-esophagus.	A severe form that occurs in newborns or infants and usually requires surgery. However, a milder form is occasionally seen in young or even middle-aged adults with a lifelong history of mild, "compensated" dysphagia and recurrent food impactions.
Miscellaneous causes (Figs GI 5-16 to GI 5-17)	Various patterns of esophageal narrowing.	Endoscopic sclerotheraphy of esophageal varices, glutaraldehyde contamination at endoscopy, graft-versus-host disease, and Behcet disease.

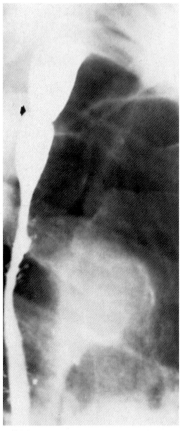

Fig GI 5-13
Intramural esophageal pseudo-diverticulosis. The arrow points to the upper esophageal stricture.

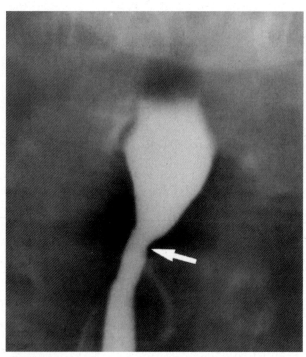

Fig GI 5-14
Benign mucous membrane pemphigoid. Focal stricture in the upper esophagus (arrow) near the thoracic inlet.[14]

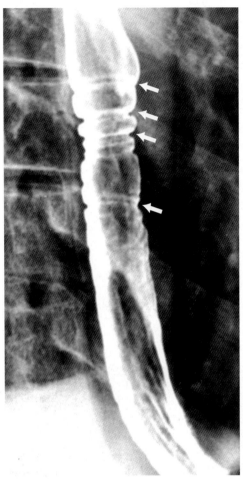

Fig GI 5-15
Congenital esophageal stenosis. Mild narrowing in the mid-esophagus with ring-like indentations (arrows) in the region of the stricture.[14]

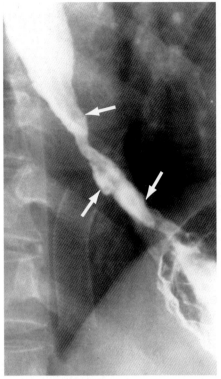

Fig GI 5-16
Endoscopic sclerotherapy. Long, irregular stricture in the distal esophagus (straight white arrows) that resulted from scarring caused by prior endoscopic sclerotherapy for esophageal varices. Note also the flat ulcer in the region of the stricture (white arrow). Black arrows indicate a transjugular intrahepatic portosystemic shunt.[14]

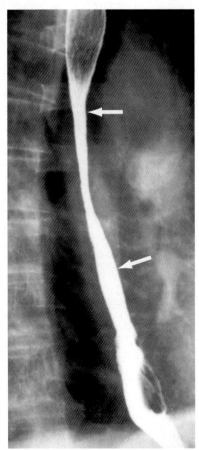

Fig GI 5-17
Glutaraldehyde-induced stricture. Long stricture involving the middle and distal esophagus (arrows). In the absence of any other predisposing factors, this stricture was presumed to be caused by toxicity from residual glutaraldehyde contamination at endoscopy.[14]

Esophageal Filling Defects

Condition	Imaging Findings	Comments
Benign tumors		
Spindle cell tumor (Fig GI 6-1)	Smooth, rounded intramural defect that is sharply demarcated from the adjacent esophageal wall. No infiltration, ulceration, or overhanging margins.	Most commonly leiomyoma, which is usually asymptomatic and rarely ulcerates, bleeds, or undergoes malignant transformation. Occasionally contains pathognomonic amorphous calcification.
Fibrovascular polyp (Fig GI 6-2)	Large, oval or elongated, sausage-like intraluminal mass.	Though rare, the second most common type of benign esophageal tumor. Large polyps can locally widen the esophagus, but do not cause complete obstruction or wall rigidity as with carcinoma.
Inflammatory esophagogastric polyp (Fig GI 6-3)	Filling defect in the region of the esophagogastric junction that is usually in continuity with a markedly thickened gastric fold.	Probably represents a stage in the evolution of chronic esophagitis (polyp reflects thickening of the proximal aspect of an inflamed gastric fold).
Villous adenoma	Filling defect with typical barium filling of the frond-like interstices.	Tumor of intermediate malignant potential.

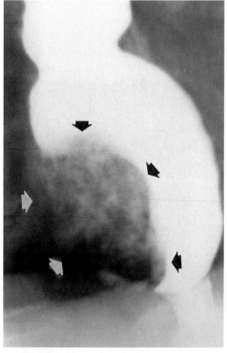

Fig GI 6-1
Leiomyoma. Note the amorphous calcifications in this smoothly lobulated intramural tumor (arrows).[17]

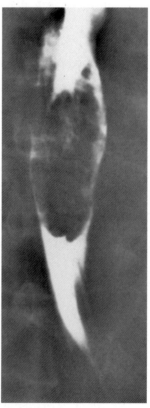

Fig GI 6-2
Fibrovascular polyp.

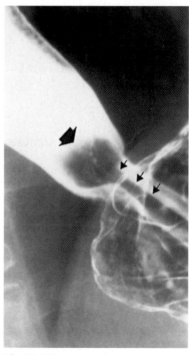

Fig GI 6-3
Inflammatory esophagogastric polyp. Distal esophageal filling defect (large arrow) in continuity with a thickened gastric fold (small arrows).

Condition	Imaging Findings	Comments
Malignant tumors		
Carcinoma of esophagus (Fig GI 6-4)	Irregular circumferential lesion with destruction of mucosal folds, overhanging margins, and abrupt transition to adjacent normal tissue.	Less frequently, carcinoma can present as a localized polypoid mass, often with deep ulceration and a fungating appearance.
Carcinoma or lymphoma of fundus of stomach (see Fig GI 5-4)	Irregular filling defect of the lower esophagus.	Continuous with malignancy of the gastric cardia.
Sarcoma (Fig GI 6-5)	Bulky mass that may ulcerate.	Rare lesions. Leiomyosarcoma; carcinosarcoma (nests of squamous epithelium surrounded by interlacing bundles of spindle-shaped cells with numerous mitoses); pseudosarcoma (low-grade nonsquamous malignancy often associated with adjacent squamous cell carcinoma).
Other malignancies (Fig GI 6-6)	Variable appearance.	Rare cases of melanoma, lymphoma, metastases, or verrucous carcinoma (exophytic, papillary, or warty tumor that rarely metastasizes and has a much better prognosis than typical squamous cell carcinoma).

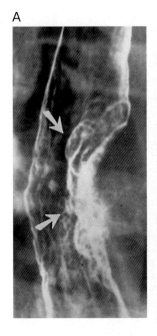

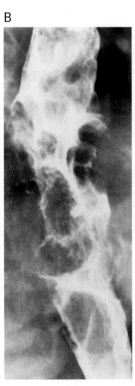

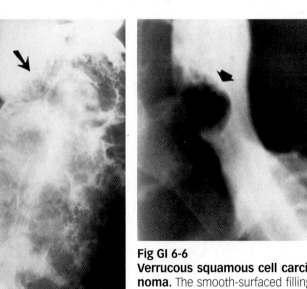

Fig GI 6-6
Verrucous squamous cell carcinoma. The smooth-surfaced filling defect in the distal esophagus (arrow) has a benign appearance.

Fig GI 6-4
Carcinoma of the esophagus. (A) Localized polypoid mass with ulceration (arrows). (B) Bulky irregular filling defect with destruction of mucosal folds.

Fig GI 6-5
Carcinosarcoma. Bulky, intraluminal, polypoid mass (arrows).

Condition	Imaging Findings	Comments
Lymph node enlargement (see Fig GI 3-5)	Extrinsic impression simulating an intramural esophageal lesion.	Usually caused by metastases or a granulomatous process (especially tuberculosis). Occasionally due to syphilis, sarcoidosis, histoplasmosis, or Crohn's disease.
Infectious esophagitis (Fig GI 6-7)	Diffuse pattern of multiple round and oval nodular defects.	Most commonly candidiasis, which is usually associated with ulceration and a shaggy contour of the esophageal wall. Rarely, herpetic esophagitis.
Esophageal varices (Fig GI 6-8)	Diffuse, round and oval filling defects reflecting serpiginous thickening of folds.	Dilated venous structures of varices change size and appearance with variations in intrathoracic pressure. Distal esophagus involved in portal hypertension. "Downhill" varices in the upper esophagus are due to superior vena cava obstruction.
Duplication cyst (Fig GI 6-9)	Eccentric impression simulating an intramural mass.	Alimentary tract duplications occur least commonly in the esophagus. They rarely communicate with the esophageal lumen.

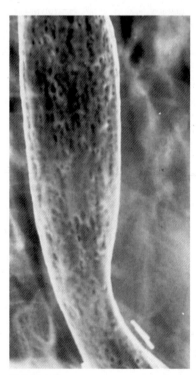

Fig GI 6-7
***Candida* esophagitis.** Numerous plaque-like defects in the middle and distal esophagus. Note that the plaques have discrete margins and a predominantly longitudinal orientation.

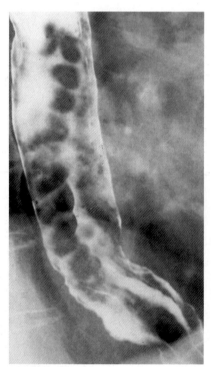

Fig GI 6-8
Esophageal varices.

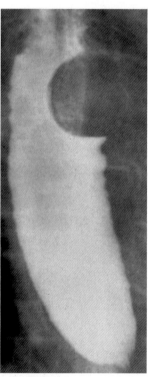

Fig GI 6-9
Duplication cyst. Eccentric impression on the barium-filled esophagus simulates an intramural mass.

Condition	Imaging Findings	Comments
Foreign bodies (Fig GI 6-10)	Various patterns depending on the material swallowed.	Usually impacted in the distal esophagus just above the level of the diaphragm. Often a distal stricture, especially if the impaction is in the cervical portion of the esophagus. Irregular margins may mimic an obstructing carcinoma.
Intramural hematoma	Soft, elongated filling defect with smooth borders.	Submucosal bleeding with intramural dissection of the esophageal wall has been described as resulting from emetics, after endoscopic instrumentation, and in patients having impaired hemostasis (hemophilia, thrombocytopenia) or receiving anticoagulant therapy.
Hirsute esophagus	Single or multiple filling defects representing a mass of hair or multiple hair follicles, respectively.	Complication of reconstructive surgery of the pharynx and esophagus in which skin flaps are mobilized and rotated to reconstruct a "skin tube esophagus" to restore anatomic continuity of the gastrointestinal tract.
Prolapsed gastric folds	Irregular filling defect in the distal esophagus.	Serial radiographs demonstrate reduction of the prolapse, return of the gastric folds below the diaphragm, and a normal distal esophagus.

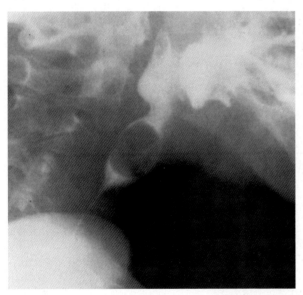

Fig GI 6-10
Foreign body. Cherry pit impacted in the cervical esophagus proximal to a caustic stricture.

Esophageal Diverticula

Condition	Imaging Findings	Comments
Zenker's diverticulum (Figs GI 7-1 and GI 7-2)	Arises from the upper esophagus with its neck lying in the midline of the posterior wall at the pharyngoesophageal junction (approximately the C5–C6 level).	Pulsion diverticulum that is apparently related to premature contraction or other motor incoordination of the cricopharyngeus muscle. May cause dysphagia or even esophageal obstruction.
Cervical traction diverticulum (Fig GI 7-3)	Variable appearance. Arises from any portion of the esophageal wall.	Rare condition resulting from fibrous healing of an inflammatory process in the neck or secondary to postsurgical changes (eg, laryngectomy).
Lateral diverticulum	Arises in a lateral or anterolateral direction at the level of the pharyngoesophageal junction (just below the transverse portion of the cricopharyngeus muscle).	Also known as Killian-Jamieson diverticula, they are considerably smaller than Zenker's diverticula and are much less likely to be associated with overflow aspiration and consequent pneumonia (because the diverticulum lies below the cricopharyngeus and allows the muscle to close above it).
Thoracic diverticulum (Fig GI 7-4)	Arises in the middle third of the thoracic esophagus opposite the bifurcation of the trachea in the region of the hilum of the lung.	Traction diverticulum that develops in response to the pull of fibrous adhesions after mediastinal lymph node infection. There are often adjacent calcified mediastinal lymph nodes from healed granulomatous disease.

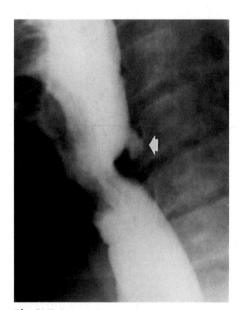

Fig GI 7-1
Small Zenker's diverticulum (arrow).

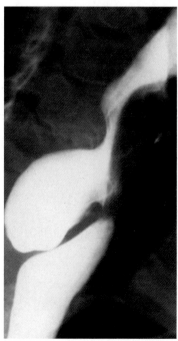

Fig GI 7-2
Large Zenker's diverticulum almost occluding the esophageal lumen.

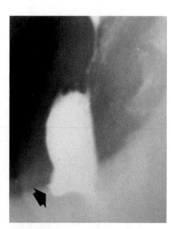

Fig GI 7-3
Cervical traction diverticulum (arrow) caused by postoperative scarring after total laryngectomy.

Condition	Imaging Findings	Comments
Epiphrenic diverticulum (Fig GI 7-5)	Occurs in the distal 10 cm of the esophagus and tends to have a broad, short neck.	Pulsion diverticulum that is probably related to incoordination of esophageal peristalsis and relaxation of the lower sphincter. If small, can simulate an esophageal ulcer (though the mucosal pattern of the adjacent esophagus is normal).
Intramural esophageal pseudodiverticulosis (Fig GI 7-6)	Multiple small (1–3 mm), ulcer-like projections arising from the esophageal wall. There is frequently an associated smooth stricture in the upper esophagus. Approximately half of the patients have diffused disease, whereas the rest have segmental disease (typically with evidence of chronic esophagitis or distal esophageal strictures).	Rare disorder with pseudodiverticula (mimicking Rokitansky-Aschoff sinuses of the gallbladder) representing dilated ducts of submucosal glands. *Candida albicans* can be cultured from approximately half the patients, though there is no evidence suggesting that the fungus is a causative agent. Intramural tracks bridging two or more pseudodiverticula and running parallel to the lumen may mimic ulceration or frank perforation.
Intraluminal diverticulum (Fig GI 7-7)	Thin radiolucent line separates the barium-filled pouch of mucosal membrane that is open proximally and closed distally.	Rare entity that usually is related to mucosal damage secondary to increased intraluminal pressure in an esophagus that has been constricted by an inflammatory process.

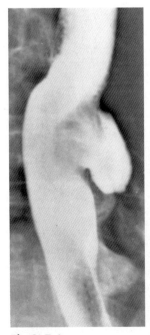

Fig GI 7-4
Thoracic diverticulum.

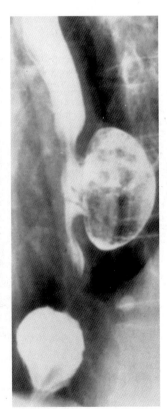

Fig GI 7-5
Epiphrenic diverticulum.

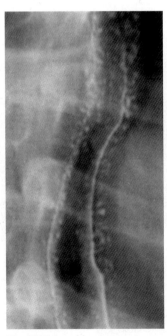

Fig GI 7-6
Intramural esophageal pseudodiverticulosis.

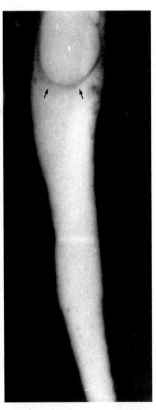

Fig GI 7-7
Intraluminal esophageal diverticulum.
The wall of the diverticulum appears as a thin radiolucent line (arrows). Note the moderate irregular stenosis of the distal esophagus secondary to the acid ingestion that resulted in the formation of the intraluminal diverticulum.[18]

Gastric Ulceration

Condition	Imaging Findings	Comments
Peptic ulcer disease (Fig GI 8-1)	Classic signs of benignancy include penetration, Hampton line, ulcer collar, ulcer mound, and radiation of smooth, slender mucosal folds to the edge of the crater.	If the ulcer crater is very shallow, a thin layer of barium coating results in a ring shadow. Irregular folds merging into a mound of polypoid tissue around the crater suggest a malignancy. Fundal ulcers above the level of the cardia are usually malignant.
Gastritis (Fig GI 8-2)	Ulcers vary from superficial erosions to deep niches.	Superficial erosions occur with gastritis due to alcohol, anti-inflammatory agents, or Crohn's disease. Frank ulcerations develop in patients with corrosive gastritis or granulomatous infiltration.
Benign tumor	Central ulceration in a mass.	Predominantly spindle cell tumors, especially leiomyoma.
Radiation injury	Discrete ulcerations identical to peptic disease.	Pain is unrelenting and has no relation to meals. High incidence of perforation and hemorrhage. Healing is minimal even with intensive medical therapy.
MALT lymphoma (Fig GI 8-3)	Discrete ulcer surrounded by a mass and associated with regional or generalized enlargement of rugal folds.	Previously termed *pseudolymphoma*, mucosa-associated lymphoid tissue lymphoma has a much more favorable prognosis than high-grade lymphoma; early diagnosis and prompt treatment may lead to cure.

A

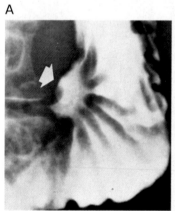

B

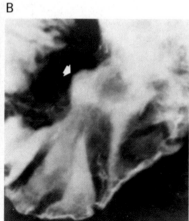

Fig GI 8-1
Fold patterns in gastric ulcers (arrow). (A) Small, slender folds radiating to the edge of a benign ulcer. (B) Thick folds radiating to an irregular mound of tissue surrounding a malignant gastric ulcer (arrow).

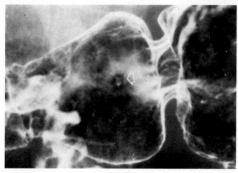

Fig GI 8-2
Gastritis. Superficial gastric erosions (arrow). Tiny flecks of barium, representing erosions, are surrounded by radiolucent halos, representing mounds of edematous mucosa.

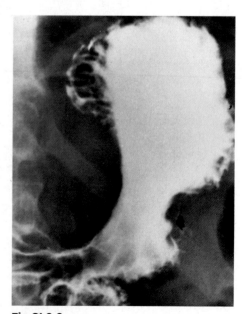

Fig GI 8-3
MALT lymphoma. Greater curvature ulcer (arrow) surrounded by a soft-tissue mass and associated with regional enlargement of rugal folds.

Condition	Imaging Findings	Comments
Carcinoma (Fig GI 8-4)	Ulcers vary from shallow erosions in superficial mucosal lesions to huge excavations in fungating polypoid masses.	Signs of malignant ulcer include Carman's meniscus sign (and Kirklin complex) and abrupt transition between normal mucosa and abnormal, usually nodular, tissue surrounding the ulcer. The ulcer does not penetrate beyond the normal gastric lumen.
Lymphoma (Fig GI 8-5)	Irregular ulcer that often is larger than the adjacent gastric lumen. Combination of a large ulcer and an extraluminal mass may suggest extravasation of barium.	May be indistinguishable from carcinoma. Findings suggestive of lymphoma include splenomegaly and extrinsic impressions on the barium-filled stomach (due to retrogastric and other regional lymph nodes).
Sarcoma (Fig GI 8-6)	Large central ulceration in a mass that often has a prominent exophytic component.	Primarily leiomyosarcoma, which often is radiographically indistinguishable from its benign spindle cell counterpart.
Metastases (Fig GI 8-7)	Single or multiple bull's-eye lesions.	Most commonly caused by malignant melanoma. An identical appearance can be due to metastases from carcinoma of the breast or lung.

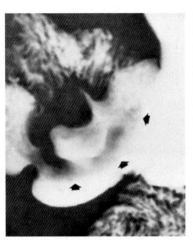

Fig GI 8-4
Carcinoma of the stomach. Carman's meniscus sign in malignant gastric ulcer. The huge ulcer has a semicircular configuration with its inner margin convex toward the lumen. The ulcer is surrounded by the radiolucent shadow of an elevated ridge of neoplastic tissue (arrows).

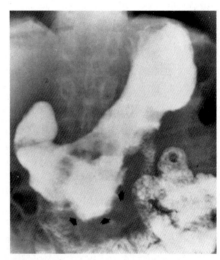

Fig GI 8-5
Gastric lymphoma. Huge, irregular ulcer (arrows) in a neoplastic gastric mass.

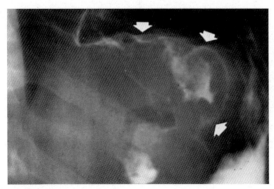

Fig GI 8-6
Leiomyosarcoma of the stomach. The large fundal mass (arrows) shows exophytic extension and ulceration.

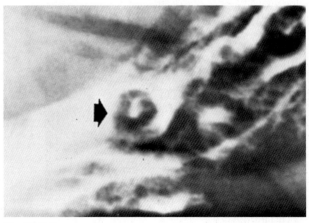

Fig GI 8-7
Gastric metastases from melanoma (arrow).

Narrowing of the Stomach

Condition	Imaging Findings	Comments
Carcinoma (Figs GI 9-1 and GI 9-2)	Thickening and fixation of the stomach wall, usually beginning near the pylorus and progressing upward.	By far the most common cause of the linitis plastica pattern. Tumor invasion of the gastric wall stimulates a strong desmoplastic response. Gastric carcinoma can also cause segmental narrowing.
Lymphoma	Luminal narrowing that primarily involves the antral region, mimicking scirrhous carcinoma.	Unlike the rigidity and fixation of scirrhous carcinoma, residual peristalsis and flexibility of the stomach wall are often preserved in Hodgkin's disease.
Metastases (Fig GI 9-3)	Circumferential narrowing of the stomach, usually with more segmental involvement than in a primary gastric malignancy.	Direct extension from carcinoma of the pancreas or transverse colon or desmoplastic hematogenous metastases (eg, carcinoma of the breast).
Peptic ulcer disease (Fig GI 9-4)	Antral narrowing and rigidity due to intense spasm.	Acute ulcer may not be seen because of the lack of antral distensibility. Peptic ulcer–induced rigidity usually heals with adequate antacid therapy. Midgastric ulcer in an elderly patient may heal with an hour-glass deformity.
Crohn's disease (Fig GI 9-5)	Smooth, tubular antrum flaring into a normal gastric body and fundus (ram's horn sign).	Often cobblestoning of antral folds with fissures and ulceration. Concomitant involvement of the adjacent duodenal bulb and proximal sweep produces the pseudo–Billroth-I pattern.
Other infiltrative disorders (Fig GI 9-6)	Mural thickening and luminal narrowing predominantly involve the antrum.	Sarcoidosis; syphilis; tuberculosis; strongyloidiasis; cytomegalovirus; toxoplasmosis; eosinophilic gastritis; polyarteritis nodosa.

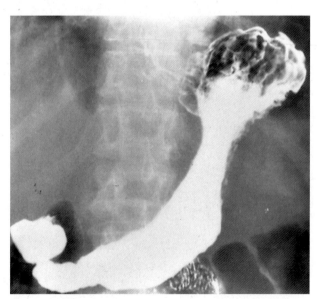

Fig GI 9-1
Scirrhous carcinoma of the stomach producing a linitis plastica pattern.

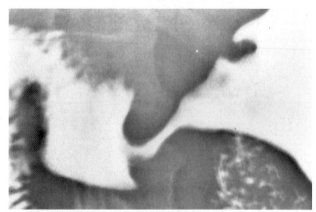

Fig GI 9-2
Adenocarcinoma of the stomach causing segmental constriction of the antrum.

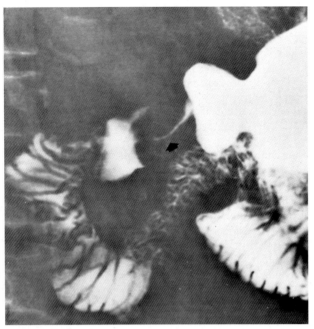

Fig GI 9-3
Metastatic pancreatic carcinoma. Circumferential narrowing of the distal stomach (arrow) secondary to enlarged perigastric lymph nodes.

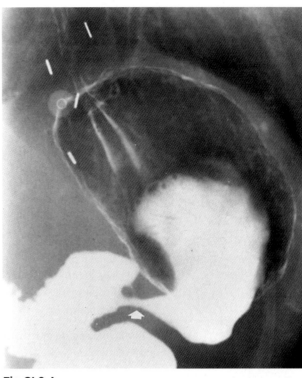

Fig GI 9-4
Peptic ulcer disease causing antral narrowing and rigidity (arrow). Note the metallic clips from a previous vagotomy.

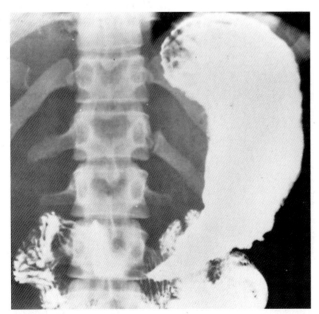

Fig GI 9-5
Crohn's disease of the stomach (ram's horn sign).[19]

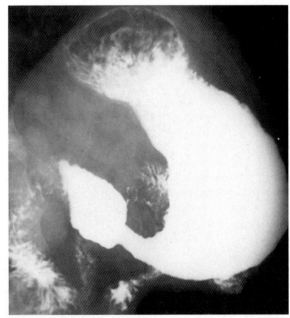

Fig GI 9-6
Tuberculosis of the stomach. Fibrotic healing narrows and stiffens the distal antrum.

Condition	Imaging Findings	Comments
Phlegmonous gastritis (Fig GI 9-7)	Diffuse irregular narrowing mimicking infiltrating carcinoma.	Extremely rare. Bacterial invasion thickens the gastric wall. The development of intramural gas bubbles is an ominous finding.
Corrosive gastritis (Fig GI 9-8)	Stricturing of the antrum (within several weeks of the injury).	Acute inflammatory reaction (most severe with ingested acids) that heals by fibrosis and scarring.
Gastric irradiation or freezing (Fig GI 9-9)	Various degrees of fixed luminal narrowing and mural rigidity.	Represents fibrotic healing of an acute injury. Irradiation and freezing were once used to treat intractable peptic ulcer disease.
Iron intoxication	Antral stricture (within 6 weeks of ingestion).	Ingestion of ferrous sulfate causes intense corrosion, which is often fatal.
Hepatic arterial infusion chemotherapy	Narrowing and rigidity of the gastric antrum and body. Return to normal appearance after chemotherapy is discontinued.	Complications of gastroduodenal ulceration and narrowing that are probably related to leakage of the chemotherapeutic agent directly into the blood supply of nonhepatic organs.
Amyloidosis	Narrowing and rigidity that primarily involve the antrum.	Deposition of eosinophilic, extracellular protein–polysaccharide complex in the gastric wall.
MALT lymphoma	Narrowing that usually involves a large segment of the body or antrum of the stomach.	Almost invariably associated with a large gastric ulcer crater. Benign condition mimicking lymphoma clinically and histologically.
Exogastric mass (Fig GI 9-10)	Luminal narrowing due to extrinsic pressure on the stomach.	Most commonly caused by severe hepatomegaly. Also occurs with pancreatic pseudocysts or enlargement of other upper abdominal organs.

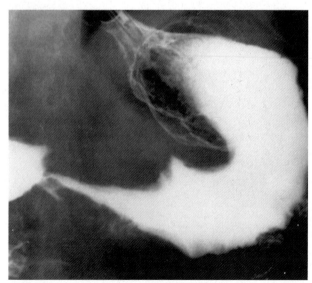

Fig GI 9-7
Phlegmonous gastritis. Irregular narrowing of the antrum and distal body of the stomach with effacement of mucosal folds along the lesser curvature and marked thickening of folds along the greater curvature.[20]

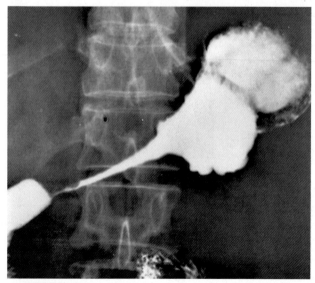

Fig GI 9-8
Corrosive stricture of the antrum after the ingestion of hydrochloric acid.

Condition	Imaging Findings	Comments
Gastroplasty	Narrowing at the operative site.	Clinical history of weight-reduction surgery and evidence of metallic suture material.
Hypertrophic pyloric stenosis (see Fig GI 12-9)	Elongation and narrowing of the pyloric canal. Symmetric concave, crescentic indentation on the base of the duodenal bulb (partial invagination of the hypertrophied muscle mass into the bulb).	Histologic, anatomic, and radiographic abnormalities in adult hypertrophic pyloric stenosis are indistinguishable from those in the infantile form (may be the same entity but milder and later in its clinical appearance).

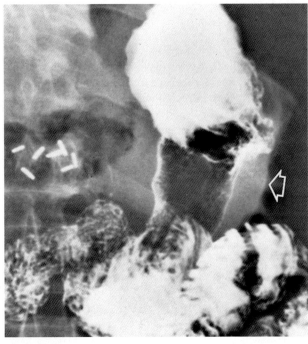

Fig GI 9-9
Radiation therapy. Luminal narrowing and severe thickening of the wall of the stomach (arrow).

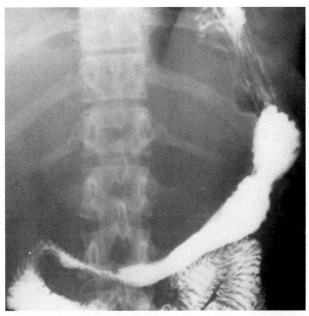

Fig GI 9-10
Echinococcal cystic disease. Narrowing of the lumen of the stomach secondary to extrinsic impression by a huge liver.

Filling Defects in the Stomach

Condition	Imaging Findings	Comments
Areae gastricae	Fine reticular pattern surrounded by barium-filled grooves, simulating multiple filling defects.	Represents a normal anatomic feature seen on double-contrast studies. Most commonly identified in the antrum. Prominent areae gastricae (état mamelonné) may represent nonspecific inflammation.
Benign tumors/tumor-like conditions		
Hyperplastic polyp (Fig GI 10-1)	Small (1 cm), often multiple, sharply defined mass.	Most common cause of a discrete gastric filling defect. Represents excessive regenerative hyperplasia in an area of chronic gastritis rather than a true neoplasm.
Adenomatous polyp (Fig GI 10-2)	Large (2 cm or more), usually single and sessile lesion with an irregular surface.	As with hyperplastic polyps, adenomatous polyps tend to develop in patients with chronic atrophic gastritis (associated with a high incidence of carcinoma). Increased incidence of gastric polyps in familial polyposis of the colon and the Cronkhite-Canada syndrome.

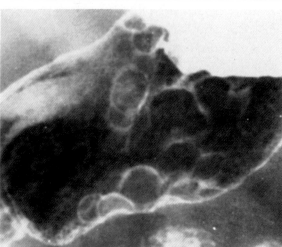

Fig GI 10-1
Hyperplastic polyps. Multiple smooth filling defects of similar sizes.

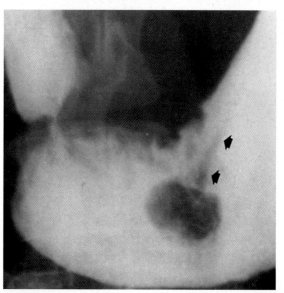

Fig GI 10-2
Adenomatous polyp. A long, thin pedicle (arrows) extends from the head of the polyp to the stomach wall.

Condition	Imaging Findings	Comments
Hamartoma	Multiple filling defects.	No malignant potential. Occurs in Peutz-Jeghers syndrome and Cowden's disease.
Spindle cell tumor (Fig GI 10-3)	Single intramural mass, often with central ulceration.	Most commonly, leiomyoma. A large lesion may have an intraluminal component or produce an extensive exogastric mass mimicking extrinsic gastric compression.
Malignant tumors Polypoid carcinoma (Fig GI 10-4)	Sessile mass that is usually relatively large, irregular, and ulcerated.	Increased incidence in patients with atrophic gastritis and pernicious anemia. May be difficult to distinguish from a benign gastric polyp.
Lymphoma (Fig GI 10-5)	Large, bulky polypoid lesion that is usually irregular and ulcerated.	Factors favoring lymphoma rather than carcinoma include multiple ulcerating polypoid tumors and adjacent thickening of folds (rather than the atrophic mucosal pattern often seen in carcinoma).

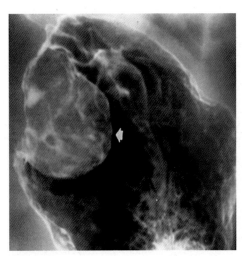

Fig GI 10-3
Leiomyoma of the fundus (arrow).

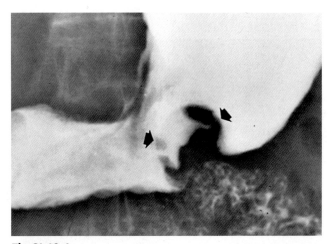

Fig GI 10-4
Carcinoma of the stomach. A huge ulcer is evident in the smooth, fungating polypoid mass (arrows).

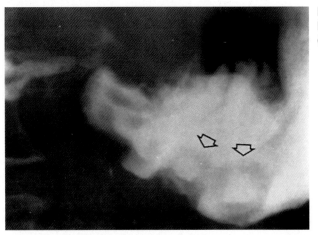

Fig GI 10-5
Lymphoma. Multiple ulcerated, polypoid gastric masses (arrows).

Condition	Imaging Findings	Comments
Metastases (see Fig GI 8-7)	Usually multiple, often ulcerated (bull's-eye appearance).	Most commonly due to malignant melanoma. Also caused by carcinomas of the breast and lung.
Sarcoma (Fig GI 10-6)	Large, bulky mass that is often ulcerated.	Most are leiomyosarcomas, which are difficult to differentiate from their benign spindle cell counterparts (large exogastric mass suggests malignancy).
Villous adenoma	Characteristic barium filling of the interstices of the tumor. Often multiple.	Rare lesion with a substantial incidence of malignancy.
Carcinoid	Broad-based mass that is often ulcerated.	Slow-growing lesion with long survivals (even in the presence of regional or hepatic dissemination).
Ectopic pancreas (Fig GI 10-7)	Smooth submucosal mass with central umbilication.	Most commonly found on the greater curvature of the distal antrum close to the pylorus. Central umbilication represents the orifice of an aberrant pancreatic duct rather than ulceration.
Enlarged gastric folds (Fig GI 10-8)	Multiple nodular filling defects (if viewed end-on).	Ménétrier's disease; gastric varices; Crohn's disease; sarcoidosis; tuberculosis; eosinophilic gastritis.

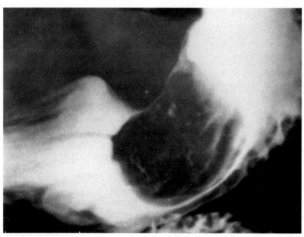

Fig GI 10-6
Leiomyosarcoma. There is scattered ulceration in this bulky tumor.

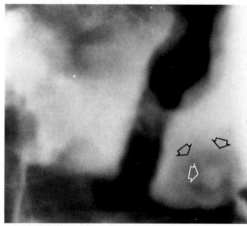

Fig GI 10-7
Ectopic pancreas. Central opacification (white arrow) of a rudimentary pancreatic duct in a soft-tissue mass (black arrows) in the distal antrum.

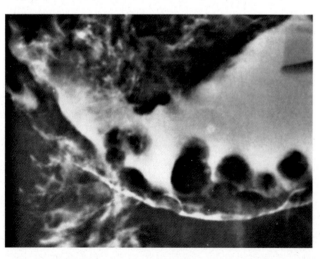

Fig GI 10-8
Alcoholic gastritis. Multiple nodular filling defects (suggesting polyps) are due to enlarged gastric folds viewed on end.

Condition	Imaging Findings	Comments
Bezoar (Fig GI 10-9)	Large mass that may fill the entire stomach. Occasionally completely smooth (simulating an enormous gas bubble).	Contrast material coating the mass and infiltrating the interstices may produce a characteristic mottled or streaked appearance. Phytobezoars (undigested vegetable material) and trichobezoars (hairballs).
Foreign body/blood clot	Single or multiple filling defects.	Variety of ingested substances and any cause of esophageal or gastric bleeding.
Peptic ulcer disease (Figs GI 10-10 and GI 10-11)	Various appearances (with or without ulceration).	Can represent a large mound of edema surrounding an acute ulcer, an incisura on the wall opposite an ulcer crater, or a double pylorus.
Langerhans cell histiocytosis (inflammatory fibroid polyp)	Sharply defined, smooth, round or oval mass (usually in the antrum).	Nonspecific inflammatory infiltrate that is usually asymptomatic (no food allergy or peripheral eosinophilia as in eosinophilic gastritis).
Duplication cyst	Filling defect or extrinsic mass impression.	Very rare. Tends to be asymptomatic, to involve the greater curvature, and to not communicate with the gastric lumen.
Fundoplication (Fig GI 10-12)	Prominent filling defect at the esophagogastric junction. The mass is generally smoothly marginated and symmetric on both sides of the distal esophagus.	Fundal pseudotumor secondary to a surgical procedure for hiatal hernia repair. In a Nissen fundoplication, the gastric fundus is wrapped around the lower esophagus to create an intra-abdominal esophageal segment with a natural valve mechanism at the esophagogastric junction.

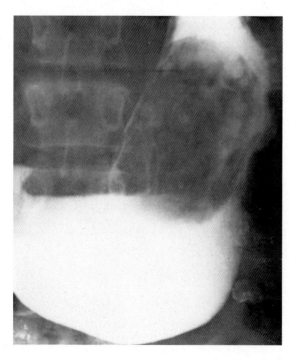

Fig GI 10-9
Glue bezoar in a young model-airplane builder. The smooth mass simulates an enormous air bubble.

Condition	Imaging Findings	Comments
MALT lymphoma	Multiple, rounded, often confluent nodules of varying size (<1 cm) that primarily involve the body and antrum of the stomach.	Appearance may mimic enlarged areae gastricae. Larger single masses are often ulcerated.

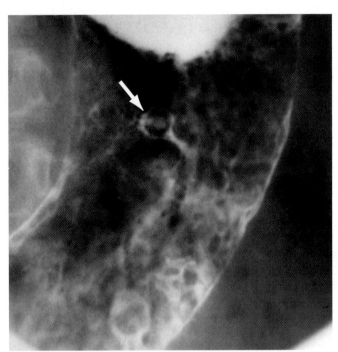

Fig GI 10-10.
Peptic ulcer disease. There are innumerable small mucosal and submucosal polypoid masses, several of which contain ulcer craters (arrow).[21]

A

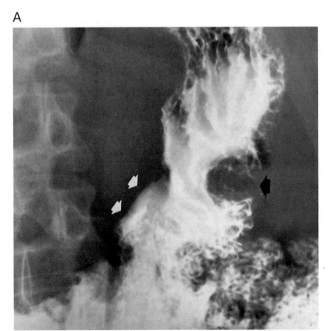

B

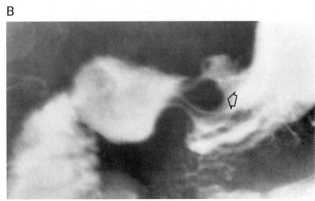

Fig GI 10-11
Peptic ulcer disease. (A) Large incisura (black arrow) simulating a filling defect on the greater curvature. The incisura is incited by a long ulcer (white arrows) on the lesser curvature. (B) Double pylorus. The true pylorus and the accessory channel along the lesser curvature are separated by a bridge, or septum, that produces the appearance of a discrete lucent filling defect (arrow).

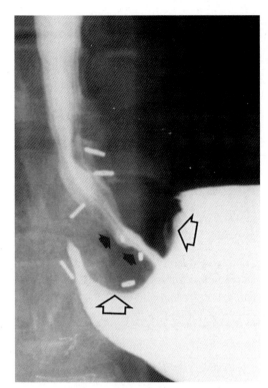

Fig GI 10-12
Normal Nissen fundoplication. The distal esophagus with normal mucosal pattern (closed arrows) passes through the fundal pseudotumor (open arrows).[22]

Thickening of Gastric Folds

Condition	Imaging Findings	Comments
Normal variant	Apparent thickening of folds in the fundus and along the greater curvature.	Folds in the fundus and proximal body tend to be thicker and more tortuous than those in the distal stomach, especially if the stomach is partially empty or contracted.
Alcoholic gastritis (Fig GI 11-1)	Generalized thickening of folds that usually subsides after withdrawing of alcohol.	Bizarre thickening may mimic malignant disease. There is a relative absence of folds in chronic alcoholic gastritis.
Hypertrophic gastritis (Fig GI 11-2)	Generalized thickening of folds, more prominent proximally.	Probably reflects a hypersecretory state and is often associated with peptic ulcer disease.
Antral gastritis (Fig GI 11-3)	Fold thickening localized to the antrum.	Controversial entity that most likely reflects one end of the spectrum of peptic ulcer disease. Isolated antral gastritis appears without fold thickening or acute ulceration in the duodenal bulb.

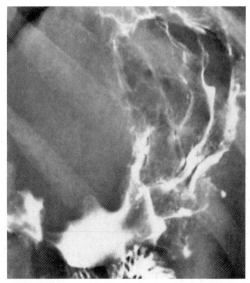

Fig GI 11-1
Alcoholic gastritis with bizarre, large folds simulating a malignant process.

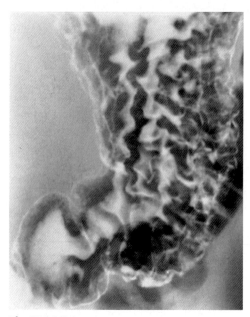

Fig GI 11-2
Hypertrophic gastritis in a patient with high acid output and peptic ulcer disease.

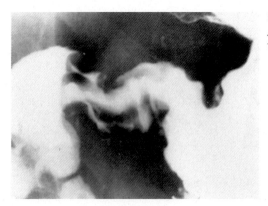

Fig GI 11-3
Antral gastritis. Thickening of gastric rugal folds is confined to the antrum.

Condition	Imaging Findings	Comments
Corrosive gastritis	Predominantly distal involvement with associated ulcers, atony, and rigidity.	Ingested acids cause the most severe injury. The pylorus is usually fixed and open. Gas in the wall of the stomach is an ominous sign.
Infectious gastritis	Fold thickening may be localized or diffuse.	Due to bacterial invasion of the stomach wall or bacterial toxins (eg, botulism, diphtheria, dysentery, typhoid fever). Gas-forming organisms can produce gas in the stomach wall.
Gastric irradiation or freezing	Generalized fold thickening.	Previous therapy for intractable gastric ulcer disease.
Peptic ulcer disease (Fig GI 11-4)	Fold thickening diffusely involves the body and fundus.	Represents hypersecretion of acid and may be associated with large amounts of retained gastric fluid. Localized fold thickening with radiation of folds toward the crater is a traditional sign of gastric ulcer.
Ménétrier's disease (Fig GI 11-5)	Massive enlargement of rugal folds. Classically described as a lesion of the fundus and body, but may involve the entire stomach.	Usually hyposecretion of acid, excessive secretion of gastric mucus, and protein loss into the gastric lumen. The lesser curvature of the body of the stomach is infrequently involved (different from lymphoma).

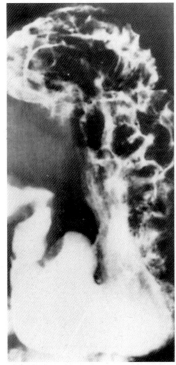

Fig GI 11-4
Zollinger-Ellison syndrome. Diffuse thickening of gastric folds is associated with hypersecretion of acid and peptic ulcer disease.

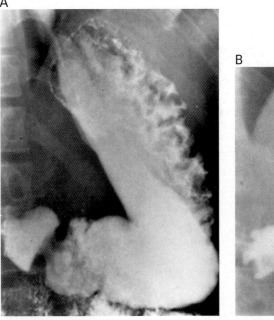

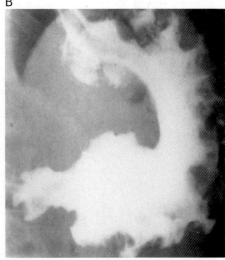

Fig GI 11-5
Ménétrier's disease. (A) Fold thickening involves the greater curvature of the fundus and body and spares the lesser curvature and antrum. (B) Generalized rugal fold thickening involves the entire stomach.

Condition	Imaging Findings	Comments
Lymphoma (Fig GI 11-6)	Generalized or localized thickening, distortion, and nodularity of folds.	May mimic Ménétrier's disease, though more commonly also involves the distal stomach and lesser curvature. Splenomegaly or an extrinsic impression by enlarged nodes suggests lymphoma; lack of ulceration and rigidity or the presence of excess mucus suggests Ménétrier's disease.
MALT lymphoma	Thickened, lobulated folds, often associated with a large gastric ulcer.	Previously termed *pseudolymphoma*, this condition has a much more favorable prognosis than high-grade lymphoma; early diagnosis and prompt treatment may lead to cure.
Carcinoma (Fig GI 11-7)	Enlarged, tortuous, coarse gastric folds.	Carcinoma rarely produces this pattern (simulating lymphoma). Associated punctate calcification is virtually diagnostic of colloid carcinoma or mucinous adenocarcinoma of the stomach.
Gastric varices (Figs GI 11-8 and GI 11-9)	Fundal varices appear as multiple smooth, lobulated filling defects. Occasionally a single varix. Nonfundal gastric varices occasionally occur.	Usually associated with esophageal varices. Isolated gastric varices suggest splenic vein occlusion. Unlike malignancy, varices are changeable in size and shape.
Infiltrative processes (Fig GI 11-10)	Diffuse thickening of rugal folds, especially in the distal half of the stomach.	Causes include eosinophilic gastritis, Crohn's disease, sarcoidosis, tuberculosis, syphilis, and amyloidosis.

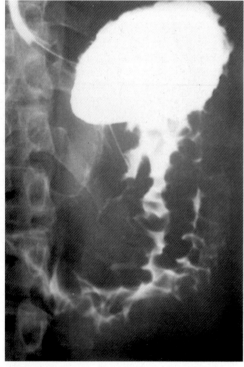

Fig GI 11-6
Lymphoma. Diffuse thickening, distortion, and nodularity of gastric folds.

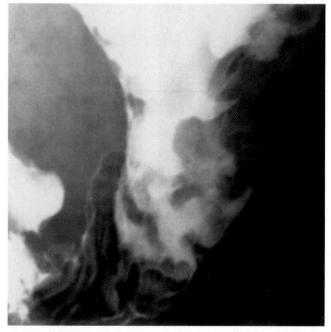

Fig GI 11-7
Carcinoma of the stomach. Enlarged, tortuous, coarse rugal folds simulate lymphoma.

Condition	Imaging Findings	Comments
Adjacent pancreatic disease (Fig GI 11-11)	Fold thickening primarily involves the posterior wall and the lesser curvature.	Most commonly reflects severe acute pancreatitis.

A

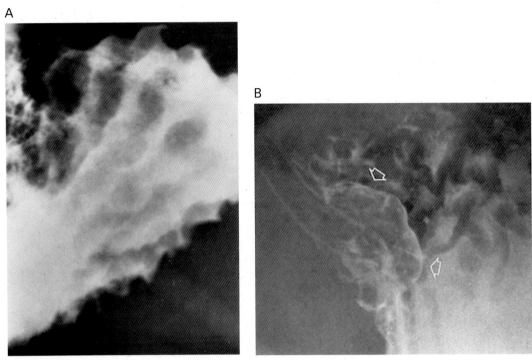

B

Fig GI 11-8
Fundal gastric varices. (A) Multiple smooth, lobulated filling defects representing the dilated venous structures. (B) Single large gastric varix (arrows).

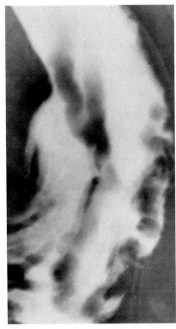

Fig GI 11-9
Nonfundal gastric varices.[23]

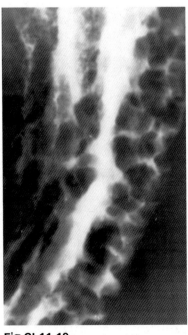

Fig GI 11-10
Amyloidosis. Huge, nodular folds caused by diffuse infiltration of the stomach by amyloid.

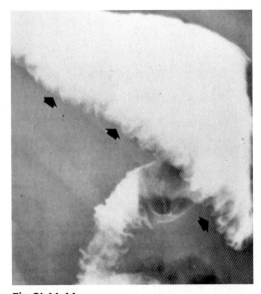

Fig GI 11-11
Acute pancreatitis. Prominence of mucosal folds on the posterior wall of the stomach (arrows) and a large retrogastric mass.

Gastric Outlet Obstruction

Condition	Imaging Findings	Comments
Peptic ulcer disease (Fig GI 12-1)	Severe luminal narrowing resulting from spasm, acute inflammation and edema, muscular hypertrophy, or contraction of scar tissue. The obstructing lesion is usually in the duodenum, occasionally in the pyloric channel or prepyloric gastric antrum, and rarely in the body of the stomach.	By far the most common cause of gastric outlet obstruction in adults (60% to 65% of cases). Distortion and scarring of the duodenal bulb make peptic ulcer disease the most likely cause of obstruction, whereas a radiographically normal bulb increases the likelihood of underlying malignant disease.
Malignant tumor (Fig GI 12-2)	Luminal narrowing due to an annular constricting lesion or diffuse mural infiltration by tumor.	Second leading cause of gastric outlet obstruction (30% to 35% of cases). Unlike patients with underlying peptic disease, who typically have a long history of ulcer pain, approximately one-third of patients with obstruction due to malignancy have no pain, and most of the others have a history of pain of less than 1 year's duration.

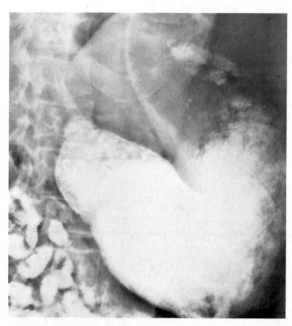

Fig GI 12-1
Peptic ulcer disease. The mottled density of nonopaque material represents excessive overnight gastric residue.

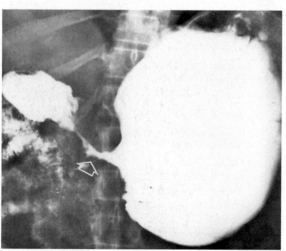

Fig GI 12-2
Annular constricting carcinoma of the stomach (arrow).

Condition	Imaging Findings	Comments
Inflammatory disorder (Figs GI 12-3 through GI 12-5)	Spasm, mural infiltration, or stricture formation causing severe luminal narrowing.	Causes include Crohn's disease, pancreatitis, cholecystitis, corrosive stricture, sarcoidosis, syphilis, tuberculosis, and amyloidosis.

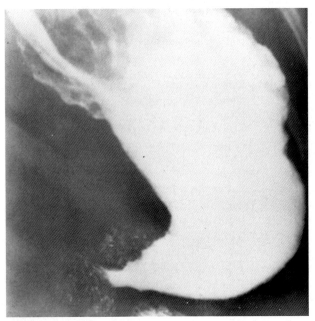

Fig GI 12-3
Crohn's disease.

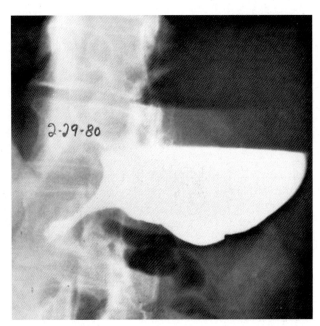

Fig GI 12-4
Corrosive gastritis.

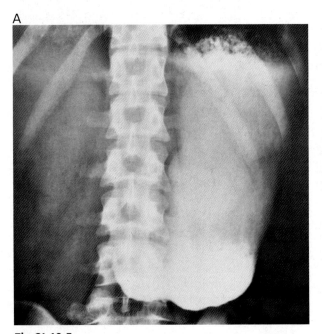

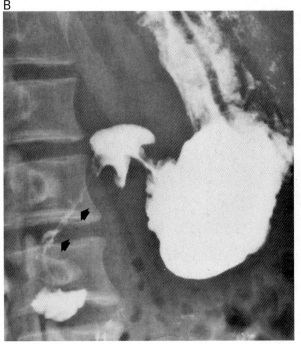

Fig GI 12-5
Acute pancreatitis. (A) Complete gastric outlet obstruction. (B) As the acute inflammatory process subsides, some barium passes through the severely spastic and narrowed second portion of the duodenum (arrows).

Condition	Imaging Findings	Comments
Congenital disorders		
Antral mucosal diaphragm (Fig GI 12-6)	Persistent, sharply defined, band-like defect, 2 to 3 cm wide, in the barium column that arises at a right angle to the gastric wall. Best seen when the stomach proximal and distal to the defect is distended. The portion of the antrum proximal to the pylorus and distal to the mucosal diaphragm can mimic a second duodenal bulb.	Thin membranous septum is usually situated within 3 cm of the pyloric canal and runs perpendicular to the long axis of the stomach. Probably a congenital anomaly resulting from failure of the embryonic foregut to recanalize. Symptoms of gastric outlet obstruction do not occur if the diameter of the diaphragm exceeds 1 cm.
Gastric duplication (Fig GI 12-7)	Extrinsic narrowing and deformity of the antrum.	Rare manifestation (usually causes only an indentation on the stomach).
Annular pancreas	Extrinsic narrowing and deformity of the descending duodenum.	Rare manifestation (more commonly produces an extrinsic impression on the lateral aspect of the descending duodenum).
Gastric volvulus (Fig GI 12-8)	Double air-fluid level on upright films, inversion of the stomach with the greater curvature above the level of the lesser curvature, positioning of the cardia and pylorus at the same level, and downward pointing of the pylorus and duodenum. Usually occurs in conjunction with a large esophageal or paraesophageal hernia that permits part or all of the stomach to assume an intrathoracic position.	Uncommon acquired twist of the stomach on itself that can lead to gastric outlet obstruction. *Organoaxial volvulus* refers to rotation of the stomach upward around its long axis so that the antrum moves from an inferior to a superior position. In the mesenteroaxial type of gastric volvulus, the stomach rotates from right to left or left to right about the long axis of the gastrohepatic omentum (line connecting the middle of the lesser curvature with the middle of the greater curvature).

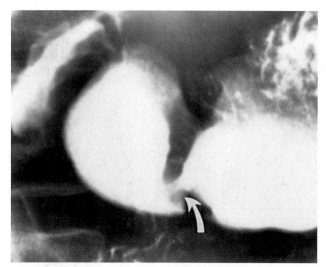

Fig GI 12-6
Antral mucosal diaphragm (arrow).

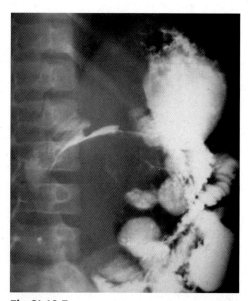

Fig GI 12-7
Duodenal duplication. Extrinsic mass indenting and partially obstructing the gastric antrum, pylorus, and duodenum. This 5-year-old boy was asymptomatic but had a palpable epigastric mass.[24]

Condition	Imaging Findings	Comments
Hypertrophic pyloric stenosis (Fig GI 12-9)	Elongation and narrowing of the pyloric canal with a characteristic symmetric, concave, crescentic indentation on the base of the duodenal bulb (presumably due to partial invagination of the hypertrophied muscle mass into the bulb).	The histologic, anatomic, and radiographic abnormalities in adult hypertrophic pyloric stenosis are indistinguishable from those in the infantile form (the disease in adults may be the same entity observed in infants and children but milder and later in clinical appearance).
Bezoar	Gastric outlet obstruction.	Masses of foreign material in the stomach are rarely of sufficient size to cause obstruction.
Prolapsed antral mucosa/ antral polyp	Intermittent pyloric obstruction.	Rare causes of intermittent gastric outlet obstruction. Prolapsed mucosa can undergo erosion or ulceration, leading to gastrointestinal bleeding and iron deficiency anemia.

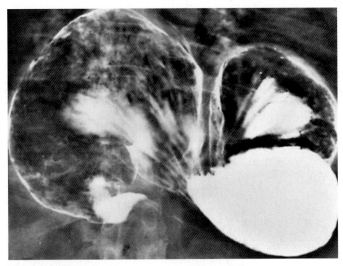

Fig GI 12-8
Organoaxial volvulus.

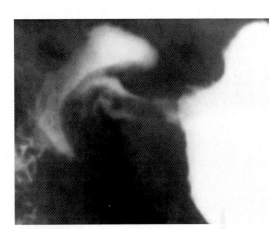

Fig GI 12-9
Adult hypertrophic pyloric stenosis.

Gastric Dilatation without Outlet Obstruction

Condition	Comments
Acute gastric dilatation	
Abdominal surgery (Fig GI 13-1)	The incidence of this postoperative complication has dramatically decreased with the advent of nasogastric suction, improved anesthetics, close monitoring of acid-base and electrolyte balance, and meticulous care in the handling of tissues at surgery.
Abdominal trauma (especially involving the back) (Fig GI 13-2)	Probably caused by a reflex paralysis of the gastric motor mechanism that permits the stomach to distend abnormally as fluid and air accumulate in it.
Severe pain/abdominal inflammation	Reflex neurologic pathway causes acute gastric dilatation in patients with severe renal colic, biliary colic, migraine headaches, and infectious and inflammatory conditions (peritonitis, pancreatitis, appendicitis, subphrenic abscess, and septicemia).
Immobilization	Patients who are immobilized (body plaster cast, paraplegia) may develop acute gastric dilatation because of difficulty in belching or because of compression of the transverse portion of the duodenum.

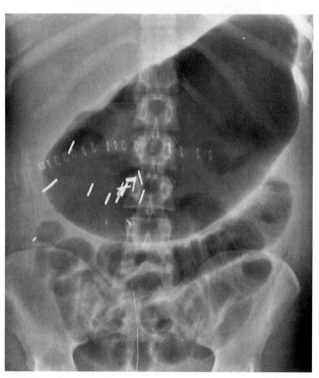

Fig GI 13-1
Acute gastric dilatation after abdominal surgery.

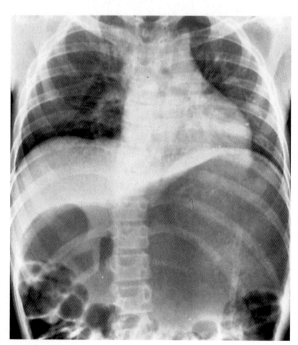

Fig GI 13-2
Acute gastric dilatation after abdominal trauma.

Condition	Comments
Chronic gastric dilatation	
Diabetes mellitus (gastric paresis) (Fig GI 13-3)	Gastric motor abnormalities occur in up to 30% of diabetics, primarily those who have long-term disease under relatively inadequate control and evidence of peripheral neuropathy or other complications.
Neuromuscular abnormalities (Fig GI 13-4)	Decreased peristalsis and visceral dilatation (more commonly involving the esophagus) may develop in patients with brain tumor, bulbar poliomyelitis, tabes dorsalis, scleroderma, or muscular dystrophy.
Vagotomy	Surgical or chemical (atropine or drugs with an atropine-like action).
Electrolyte or acid-base imbalance	Dilatation of abdominal viscera (most likely the colon) presumably develops because of alteration in muscle tone in patients with diabetic ketoacidosis, hypercalcemia, hypocalcemia, hypokalemia, hepatic coma, uremia, or myxedema.
Lead poisoning/porphyria	Gastric distention reflects an alteration in muscle tone.
Emotional distress	Gastric dilatation can be due to a reflex neurologic abnormality or to hyperventilation associated with the excessive swallowing of air.

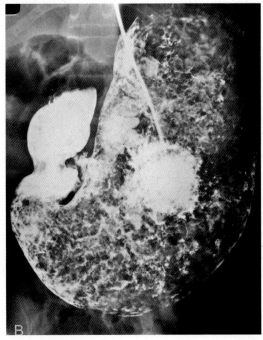

Fig GI 13-3
Gastric dilatation due to chronic diabetic neuropathy. Tremendous amount of particulate material in the massively distended stomach.

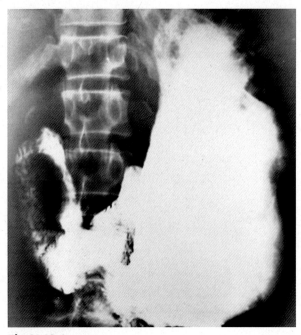

Fig GI 13-4
Gastric dilatation without obstruction in a patient with scleroderma.

Widening of the Retrogastric Space

Condition	Imaging Findings	Comments
Obesity/ascites/previous surgery/gross hepatomegaly (especially of caudate lobe)	Generalized widening without a discrete mass.	Anterior displacement of the stomach with no discrete posterior impression.
Pancreatic mass (Fig GI 14-1)	Extrinsic impression on the antrum (head of the pancreas) or the body and fundus (body and tail of the pancreas).	Most common cause of a discrete lesion widening the retrogastric space. Causes include pancreatitis, pseudocyst, cystadenoma, and carcinoma. Findings suggest invasive carcinoma including fixation of the gastric wall, mucosal destruction or ulceration, and a high-grade gastric outlet obstruction.
Retroperitoneal mass (Fig GI 14-2)	Single or lobulated impression on the posterior wall of the stomach.	Causes include benign and malignant neoplasms, enlargement of retroperitoneal lymph nodes (lymphoma, tuberculosis), cysts, abscesses, and hematomas.
Tumor arising from posterior wall of stomach	Usually an intraluminal component in addition to the posterior impression and the widened retrogastric space.	Most commonly occurs in gastric tumors with large exogastric components (leiomyoma, leiomyosarcoma).
Aortic aneurysm/ choledochal cyst	Discrete retrogastric mass.	Diagnosis can be made by ultrasound or CT.

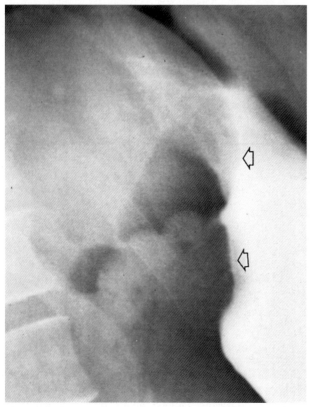

Fig GI 14-1
Pancreatic pseudocyst. Widening of the retrogastric space with a lobulated impression (arrows) on the posterior wall of the stomach.

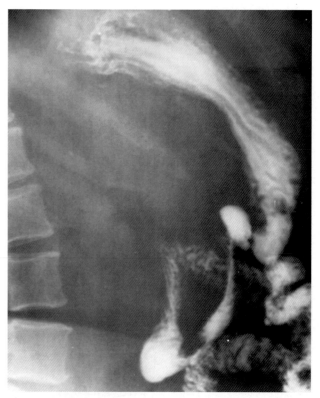

Fig GI 14-2
Retroperitoneal sarcoma. Pronounced anterior displacement of the stomach and duodenum.

Filling Defects in the Gastric Remnant

Condition	Imaging Findings	Comments
Surgical deformity	Various patterns depending on the type of surgical procedure.	Because the appearance may closely simulate a neoplastic process, a baseline upper gastrointestinal series is often obtained soon after partial gastric resection.
Suture granuloma (Fig GI 15-1)	Well-defined, rounded mass at the level of the surgical anastomosis.	Can mimic a gastric neoplasm and lead to an unnecessary reoperation. Occurs only with nonabsorbable suture material.
Bezoar (Fig GI 15-2)	Mottled filling defect simulating a mass of retained food.	Usually consists of the fibrous, pithy component of fruits (especially citrus) and vegetables. Can cause gastric outlet obstruction or pass into and obstruct the small bowel.

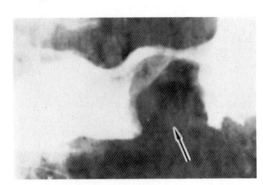

Fig GI 15-1
Suture granuloma. Large mass at the greater curvature side of the antrum (arrow) projects as a smooth tumor into the gastric lumen.[21]

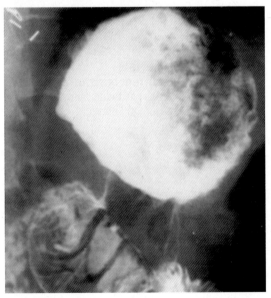

Fig GI 15-2
Bezoar. The mass of retained food particles produces a mottled appearance.

Condition	Imaging Findings	Comments
Gastric stump carcinoma (Fig GI 15-3)	Irregular polypoid mass that may be ulcerated. Uniform infiltration by the tumor can narrow the gastric remnant.	Refers to a malignancy occurring in the gastric remnant after resection for peptic ulcer or other benign disease. Tends to occur 10 to 20 years after the initial surgery (after a long period of relatively good health). Must be differentiated from benign marginal ulceration, which occurs on the jejunal side of the anastomosis within 2 years of surgery (ulcer on the gastric side must be considered malignant).
Recurrent carcinoma (Fig GI 15-4)	Narrowing of the stoma with local mucosal destruction or a discrete filling defect.	May be difficult to distinguish from a second primary if it occurs less than 10 years after the initial resection for malignant disease.
Bile (alkaline) reflux gastritis (Fig GI 15-5)	Thickened folds, often with ulceration, on the gastric side of the anastomosis.	Reactive response of the stomach to reflux of bile and pancreatic juices from the jejunum (normally prevented by the intact pylorus).

A

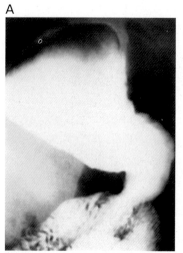

B

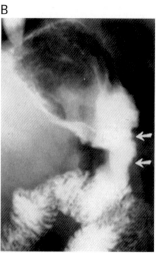

Fig GI 15-3
Gastric stump carcinoma. (A) Normal gastric remnant and Billroth-II anastomosis after surgery for peptic disease. (B) Irregular narrowing of the perianastomotic region (arrows) several years later represents a gastric stump carcinoma.

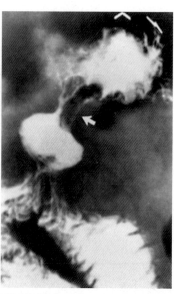

Fig GI 15-4
Recurrent gastric carcinoma. Tumor infiltration narrows the gastric lumen (arrow).

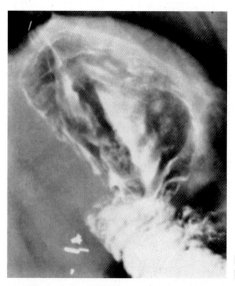

Fig GI 15-5
Bile reflux gastritis.

Condition	Imaging Findings	Comments
Hyperplastic polyps	Discrete polypoid masses.	Masses developing within a few years of surgery are more likely to be hyperplastic polyps than carcinoma (but endoscopy and biopsy are essential for confirmation).
Jejunogastric intussusception (Fig GI 15-6)	Spherical or ovoid intraluminal filling defect. Contrast material may outline the stretched jejunal folds.	Rare, but potentially lethal, complication of partial gastrectomy with Billroth-II anastomosis. The efferent loop alone is included in 75% of cases; the afferent loop or the afferent in combination with the efferent intussuscepts in the remaining cases. Acute intussusception is a surgical emergency.
Gastrojejunal mucosal prolapse (Fig GI 15-7)	Smooth, sharply marginated intraluminal mass in the efferent or afferent loop.	Antegrade prolapse occurs much more frequently than retrograde jejunogastric intussusception. Can cause partial obstruction if the anastomotic stoma is small.

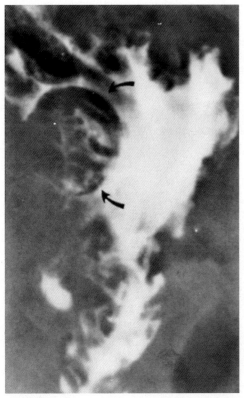

Fig GI 15-6
Jejunogastric intussusception (afferent loop) producing a large, sharply defined filling defect (arrows).

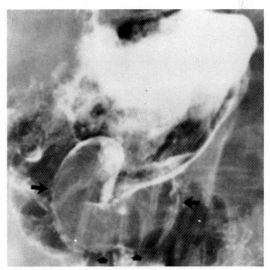

Fig GI 15-7
Gastrojejunal mucosal prolapse producing a large, partially obstructing mass in the efferent loop (arrows).

Simultaneous Involvement of the Gastric Antrum and Duodenal Bulb

Condition	Imaging Findings	Comments
Lymphoma (Fig GI 16-1)	Contour deformities, polypoid filling defects, and ulceration.	Transpyloric extension of tumor seen in up to 33% of patients.
Carcinoma (Fig GI 16-2)	Narrowing and irregularity, polypoid filling defects, and ulceration.	Radiographically detectable invasion of the duodenum in 5% of patients with antral carcinoma. Because carcinoma of the stomach is 50 times more frequent than gastric lymphoma, transpyloric extension of tumor in an individual patient makes carcinoma the more likely diagnosis.
Peptic ulcer disease	Mucosal thickening or ulceration of both areas.	Fibrotic healing can produce narrowing and deformity involving both the antrum and the bulb.
Crohn's disease (Fig GI 16-3)	Blending of the antrum, pylorus, and duodenal bulb into a single tubular or funnel-shaped structure.	Pylorus and duodenal bulb lose their identity as anatomic features between the antrum and the second portion of the duodenum. Simulates the radiographic appearance after a Billroth-I anastomosis.
Tuberculosis	Mural nodularity and ulceration of the pyloroduodenal area.	Rare. Duodenal involvement occurs in 10% of patients with gastric tuberculosis and in half of those in whom the pylorus is involved.
Strongyloidiasis	Nodular intramural defects, ulceration, and luminal narrowing.	Rare appearance seen only in advanced cases.
Eosinophilic gastroenteritis (Fig GI 16-4)	Mural narrowing and mucosal fold thickening.	Associated with specific food allergies and peripheral eosinophilia.

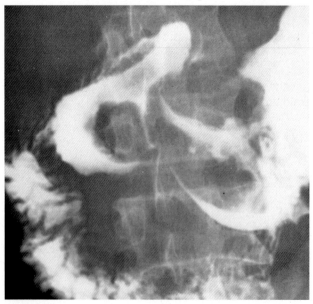

Fig GI 16-1
Gastric lymphoma. There are large lymphomatous masses in the distal stomach and duodenal bulb with irregular ulceration.

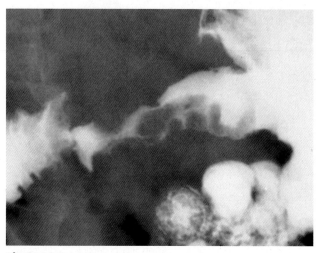

Fig GI 16-2
Gastric carcinoma. Rigid, abnormal folds in the distal stomach extend to involve the base of the duodenal bulb.

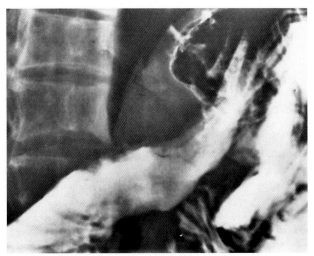

Fig GI 16-3
Crohn's disease (pseudo–Billroth-I pattern). There are no recognizable anatomic landmarks between the antrum and the second portion of the duodenum.

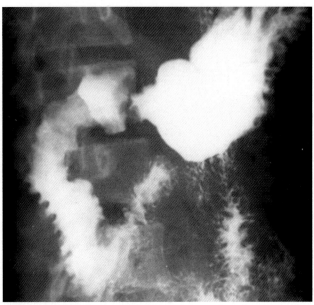

Fig GI 16-4
Eosinophilic gastroenteritis. Irregular fold thickening involves the antrum and proximal duodenum.

Duodenal Filling Defects

Condition	Imaging Findings	Comments
Pseudotumors (Figs GI 17-1 and GI 17-2)	Intraluminal filling defects or extrinsic impressions.	Prominent gallbladder; severe edema surrounding a small ulcer crater; retained blood clot; ingested foreign body; gallstone; prolapsed gastrostomy tube; stitch abscess; pylorus seen on end; gas-filled duodenal diverticulum.
Flexure defect	Pseudodefect on the inner margin of the junction between the first and second portions.	Acute change in the axis of the duodenum at this point causes heaping up of redundant loose mucosa and an apparent filling defect.
Ectopic pancreas (see Fig GI 10-7)	Smooth, round or oval, well-demarcated filling defect.	Usually asymptomatic. Typically contains a central collection of barium representing filling of ductal structures (mimics an ulcerated mass).
Prolapsed antral mucosa	Mushroom-, umbrella-, or cauliflower-shaped mass at the base of the duodenal bulb.	Active peristalsis causes prolapse of redundant antral folds through the pylorus. As the wave relaxes, the mucosal folds tend to return into the antrum, and the defect at the base of the bulb diminishes or disappears.
Brunner's gland hyperplasia (Fig GI 17-3)	Multiple nodular filling defects, primarily in the bulb and the proximal half of the second portion.	Probably represents a response of the duodenal mucosa to peptic ulcer disease. May present as a large discrete filling defect (Brunner's gland "adenoma").
Benign lymphoid hyperplasia (Fig GI 17-4)	Innumerable tiny nodular defects evenly scattered throughout the duodenum.	No clinical significance. Unlike Brunner's gland hyperplasia associated with peptic disease, there is normal distensibility of the duodenal bulb.
Heterotopic gastric mucosa (Fig GI 17-5)	Multiple, abruptly marginated, angular filling defects scattered over the surface of the duodenal bulb.	Smaller and less uniform than Brunner's gland hyperplasia. Unlike benign lymphoid hyperplasia, heterotopic gastric mucosa is more irregular and involves only the duodenal bulb.

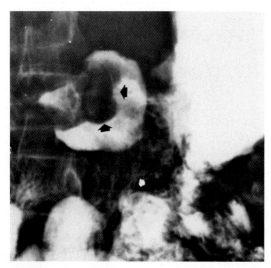

Fig GI 17-1
Large blood clot (arrows) in a giant ulcer of the duodenal bulb.

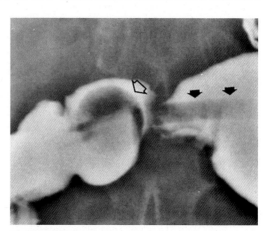

Fig GI 17-2
Feeding gastrostomy tube (open arrow) prolapsed into the duodenal bulb. The tube could be mistaken for a polyp on a large stalk (solid arrows).

Condition	Imaging Findings	Comments
Nonerosive duodenitis	Nodular pattern or thickened folds.	Most cases are not accompanied by discrete ulceration.
Papilla of Vater (Fig GI 17-6)	Normal "filling defect" on the medial wall of the midportion of the descending duodenum.	Situated on or immediately below the promontory, just above the straight segment. For the differential diagnosis of enlargement of the papilla (>1.5 cm), see GI-18.
Choledochocele (Fig GI 17-7)	Well-defined, smooth filling defect on the medial wall of the descending duodenum.	Cystic dilatation of the intraduodenal portion of the common bile duct in the region of the ampulla of Vater. This bulbous terminal portion of the common bile duct fills at cholangiography.

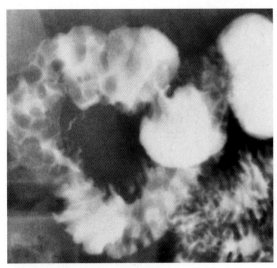

Fig GI 17-3
Brunner's gland hyperplasia.

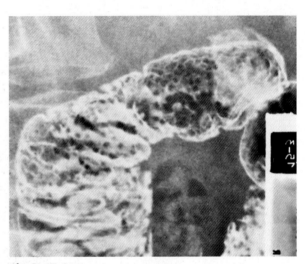

Fig GI 17-4
Benign lymphoid hyperplasia.[25]

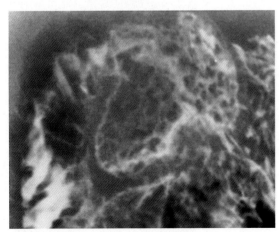

Fig GI 17-5
Heterotopic gastric mucosa.

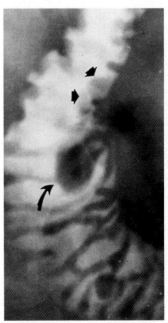

Fig GI 17-6
Papilla of Vater (straight arrows). Note the large benign polyp (curved arrow) that is clearly separate from the papilla.

Condition	Imaging Findings	Comments
Duplication cyst	Sharply defined intramural defect (usually in the concavity of the first and second portions of the duodenum).	Because the cyst is fluid-filled, it may change shape with compression and on serial films. Communicates with the duodenal lumen in 10% to 20% of cases.
Pancreatic pseudocyst (Fig GI 17-8)	Intramural duodenal filling defect.	Pseudocyst may rarely extend into the duodenal wall and even cause various degrees of duodenal obstruction.
Duodenal varices or mesenteric arterial collaterals (Fig GI 17-9)	Solitary or, more commonly, diffuse serpiginous thickening of duodenal folds.	Duodenal varices are almost always associated with esophageal varices and are often complicated by gastrointestinal bleeding. Enlarged mesenteric arterial collaterals develop secondary to occlusion of the celiac trunk or the superior mesenteric artery.

A

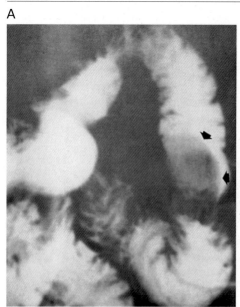

B

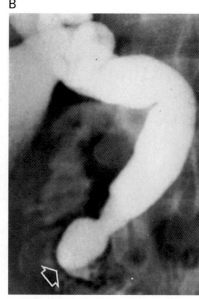

Fig GI 17-7
Choledochocele (arrows). (A) Barium study. (B) Cholangiogram.

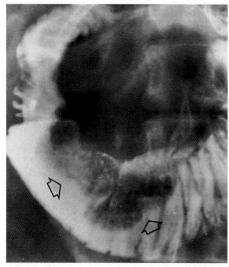

Fig GI 17-8
Pancreatic pseudocyst extending into the wall of the duodenum and producing a large intramural filling defect (arrows).

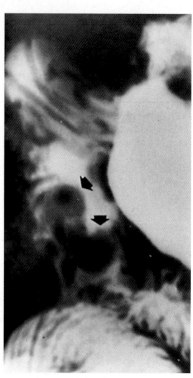

Fig GI 17-9
Duodenal varices (arrows).

Condition	Imaging Findings	Comments
Intramural hematoma (Fig GI 17-10)	Sharply defined intramural mass that usually causes stenosis or even complete obstruction of the duodenum.	Develops in patients receiving anticoagulant therapy or with congenital bleeding diatheses, or after blunt abdominal trauma (the retroperitoneal portion of the duodenum is the most fixed part of the small bowel).
Benign tumors	Single or multiple filling defects that may ulcerate.	Adenoma; leiomyoma; lipoma; hamartoma; cavernous lymphangioma; prolapsed antral polyp. Approximately 90% of bulb tumors are benign, whereas most tumors in the fourth portion of the duodenum are malignant. Equal frequency of benign and malignant tumors in the second and third portions.
Villous adenoma (Fig GI 17-11)	Often-irregular filling defect with barium coating the interstices between the frond-like projections of the tumor.	Variable malignant potential. No definite radiographic criteria to differentiate benign from early malignant lesions.
Carcinoid tumor	Solitary (occasionally multiple) submucosal filling defect, usually arising proximal to the papilla.	High endocrine activity (serotonin, insulin, gastrin). May be associated with multiple endocrine adenomatosis. There is usually progressive and intractable peptic ulceration or severe diarrhea. Low-grade malignancy that may eventually metastasize to adjacent structures or the liver.
Malignant tumors	Various appearances (annular constricting lesion with mucosal destruction; ulcerating intraluminal polypoid mass).	Approximately 80% to 90% are adenocarcinomas, most of which occur at or distal to the papilla. Sarcomas (mainly leiomyosarcomas) and primary lymphoma are rare. Metastases involve the duodenum by direct invasion (gastric carcinoma or lymphoma; carcinoma of the pancreas, gallbladder, colon, or kidney). Hematogenous metastases (primarily melanoma) are rare.

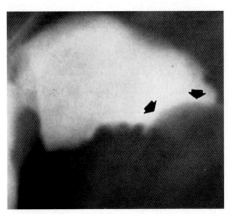

Fig GI 17-10
Intramural duodenal hematoma. The sharply defined intramural mass (arrows) obstructs the lumen in the immediate post-bulbar area.

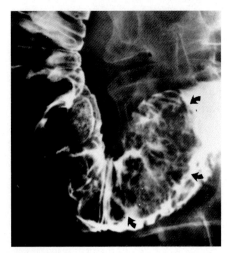

Fig GI 17-11
Villous adenoma. Large mass at the junction of the second and third portions of the duodenum. The irregular surface of the mass (arrows), with its crevices filled with barium, is characteristic of a villous tumor.[26]

Enlargement of the Papilla of Vater (>1.5 centimeters)

Condition	Imaging Findings	Comments
Normal variant (Fig GI 18-1)	Smooth enlargement.	Found in 1% of normal examinations and is a diagnosis of exclusion (if all other causes ruled out).
Impacted stone in distal common bile duct	Papillary edema (smooth enlargement).	Typical symptoms of acute biliary colic. The papilla may rarely be irregular and mimic a peri-Vaterian neoplasm.
Acute pancreatitis (Fig GI 18-2)	Papillary edema (smooth enlargement).	Very early sign (Poppel's) that is usually present before pancreatic enlargement can be detected. There may be pancreatic calcification if the acute process represents a subacute exacerbation of disease.

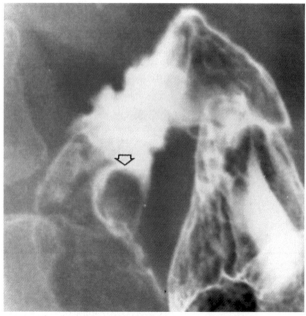

Fig GI 18-1
Normal variant.

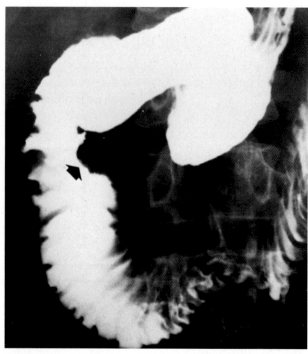

Fig GI 18-2
Acute pancreatitis.

Condition	Imaging Findings	Comments
Acute duodenal ulcer disease (Fig GI 18-3)	Papillary edema (smooth enlargement).	Papillary fold participates in the generalized duodenal edema. There is almost invariably diffuse enlargement of folds and an acute ulcer crater in the duodenal bulb.
Periampullary neoplasm (Fig GI 18-4)	Irregular enlargement, often with ulceration.	Collective term for malignancies arising in the duodenum, head of the pancreas, distal common bile duct, and ampulla of Vater. There is usually a history of progressive jaundice and no thickening of the surrounding duodenal folds.
Papillitis	Polypoid enlargement.	Periductal inflammatory reaction rather than a true neoplasm. Exuberant fibrosis may eventually produce sphincter stenosis.
Iatrogenic	Papillary edema.	Following surgery or instrumentation of the distal biliary tree.
Lesions simulating enlarged papilla	Variable appearance.	Benign spindle cell tumor or ectopic pancreatic tissue on the inner aspect of the second portion of the duodenum can mimic papillary enlargement unless the papilla itself is clearly demonstrated. Central barium collection (ulcer or rudimentary duct) in an apparently enlarged papilla suggests a spindle cell tumor (especially leiomyoma) or ectopic pancreas.

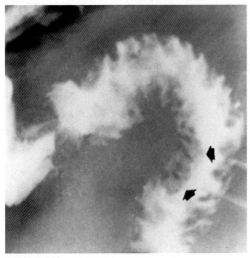

Fig GI 18-3
Diffuse peptic ulcer disease.

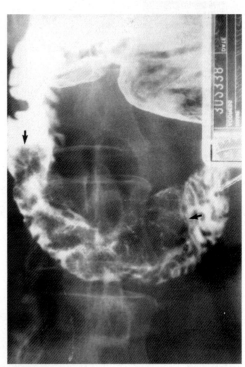

Fig GI 18-4
Ampullary carcinoma. Large, smooth filling defect (arrows) in the medial portion of the duodenum representing a well-differentiated malignant neoplasm.[26]

Condition	Imaging Findings	Comments
Congenital anomalies		
Duodenal atresia (Fig GI 19-1)	Double bubble sign. Absence of gas in the small and large bowel.	Complete obliteration of the duodenal lumen is the most common cause of congenital duodenal obstruction. Relatively high incidence in infants with Down's syndrome.
Duodenal stenosis (Fig GI 19-2)	Double bubble sign. Some gas in the bowel distal to the obstruction.	High-grade but incomplete congenital stenosis of the duodenum.
Annular pancreas	In infants, double bubble sign with some gas in the distal bowel. In adults, a notch-like defect on the lateral wall of the duodenum causing eccentric luminal narrowing.	Incomplete obstruction with gas in the bowel distal to the level of the high-grade duodenal stenosis. Relatively high incidence in infants with Down's syndrome.
Duodenal diaphragm (web) (Fig GI 19-3)	Thin lucent line across the lumen, often with proximal duodenal dilatation.	Usually involves the second part of the duodenum. May balloon out distally, producing a rounded, barium-filled, comma-shaped sac (intraluminal diverticulum).

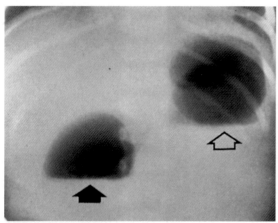

Fig GI 19-1
Duodenal atresia with double-bubble sign. The left bubble (open arrow) represents air in the stomach; the right bubble (solid arrow) reflects duodenal gas. There is no gas in the small or large bowel distal to the level of the complete obstruction.

Fig GI 19-2
Congenital duodenal stenosis. The presence of small amounts of gas distal to the obstruction indicates that the stenosis is incomplete.

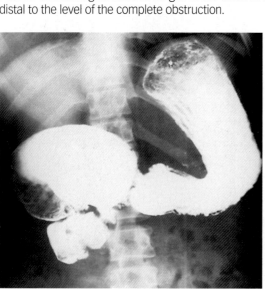

Fig GI 19-3
Duodenal diaphragm. The presence of gas in the bowel distal to the diaphragm indicates that the high-grade obstruction is not complete.

Condition	Imaging Findings	Comments
Midgut volvulus	High-grade duodenal obstruction. Spiral course of bowel loops on the right side of the abdomen.	Occurs with incomplete rotation of the bowel. The duodenojejunal junction (ligament of Treitz) is located inferiorly and to the right of its expected position.
Congenital peritoneal (Ladd's) bands (Fig GI 19-4)	Intermittent partial duodenal obstruction. Symptoms often increase with standing (bands tighten) and decrease when lying down (bands relax).	Dense fibrous bands extending from an abnormally placed, malrotated cecum or hepatic flexure over the anterior surface of the second or third portion of the duodenum to the right gutter and the inferior surface of the liver.
Duodenal duplication cyst	Intramural or extrinsic duodenal mass.	Usually asymptomatic. Rarely causes high-grade stenosis or complete obstruction.
Postbulbar ulcer (Fig GI 19-5)	Eccentric duodenal narrowing (spasm or fibrosis) or a ring stricture.	Incisura represents indrawing of the lateral wall of the duodenum. Often appears similar to annular pancreas, though granular mucosa in the narrowed segment suggests healed ulceration.
Crohn's disease (Fig GI 19-6)	Fusiform and concentric narrowing of the duodenum.	Usually evidence of Crohn's disease elsewhere. Crohn's disease of the duodenal bulb and antrum produces tubular narrowing (pseudo–Billroth-I appearance).

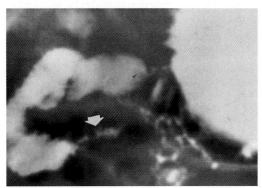

Fig GI 19-4
Ladd's bands. Obstruction of the third portion of the duodenum (arrow) in a newborn infant, due to dense fibrous bands.

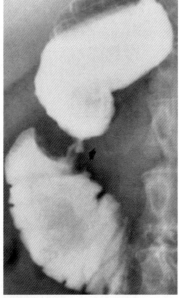

Fig GI 19-5
Postbulbar ulcer. The deep incisura associated with the medial wall postbulbar ulcer (arrow) causes severe narrowing of the second portion of the duodenum.

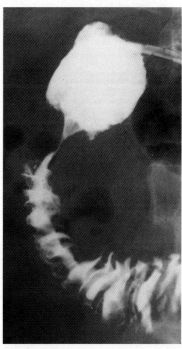

Fig GI 19-6
Crohn's disease. Severe postbulbar narrowing with distal fold thickening.

Condition	Imaging Findings	Comments
Tuberculosis	Appearance indistinguishable from that of Crohn's disease.	Extremely rare. Almost always associated with antropyloric disease. There may be fistulas and sinus tracts.
Strongyloidiasis/sprue	Single or multiple areas of stenosis of the duodenum.	Strongyloidiasis is indistinguishable from Crohn's disease. In long-standing nontropical sprue, narrowing represents healing of ulceration.
Pancreatitis/cholecystitis (Fig GI 19-7)	Narrowing and deformity of the duodenum with fold thickening and spiculation.	May represent irritability and spasm due to severe acute inflammation or postinflammatory fibrotic healing.
Pancreatic pseudocyst (Fig GI 19-8)	Extrinsic compression of the duodenal sweep.	Mucosal folds of the duodenum may be thickened, splayed, and distorted, but are not destroyed as with pancreatic cancer.
Pancreatic carcinoma (Fig GI 19-9)	Extrinsic impression and double-contour effect. Often associated with ulceration and mucosal destruction.	May be difficult to distinguish from pancreatitis. Duodenal mucosal destruction suggests malignancy, though some pancreatic tumors can infiltrate the submucosa and produce stenosis without mucosal destruction.
Duodenal carcinoma	Annular constricting lesion with overhanging edges, nodular mucosal destruction, and ulceration.	Approximately 90% are adenocarcinomas, which usually arise at or distal to the ampulla of Vater. May be impossible to differentiate from secondary neoplastic invasion of the duodenum due to extension of tumors of the pancreas, gallbladder, or colon.

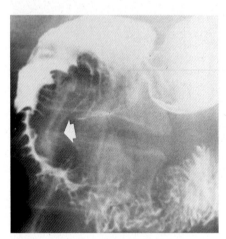

Fig GI 19-7
Chronic pancreatitis with acute exacerbation. The inflammatory mass narrows the second portion of the duodenum and causes marked mucosal edema and spiculation (arrow).

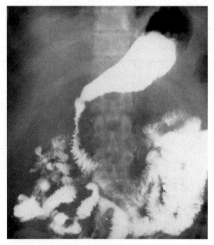

Fig GI 19-8
Pancreatic pseudocyst. Although there is narrowing of the second portion of the duodenum with widening of the duodenal sweep, the mucosal folds are intact.

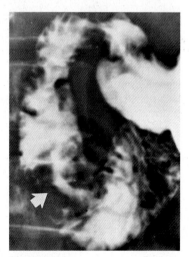

Fig GI 19-9
Carcinoma of the pancreas producing an annular constricting lesion (arrow). The radiographic appearance is indistinguishable from that of primary duodenal carcinoma.

Condition	Imaging Findings	Comments
Metastatic malignancy	Irregular narrowing of the duodenum associated with mass effect and ulceration.	Primarily metastases to lymph nodes (peripancreatic, celiac, para-aortic) along the second and third portions of the duodenum.
Intramural duodenal hematoma (Fig GI 19-10)	Tumor-like intramural mass causing narrowing of the duodenal lumen.	Secondary to anticoagulant therapy, abnormal bleeding diathesis, or blunt trauma (the duodenum is the most fixed portion of the small bowel).
Aorticoduodenal fistula	Extrinsic mass compressing and displacing the third portion of the duodenum.	Often fatal complication of an abdominal aortic aneurysm or the placement of a prosthetic graft.
Radiation injury	Smooth stricture, primarily involving the second portion of the duodenum.	Infrequent complication after radiation therapy to the upper abdomen.
Superior mesenteric artery syndrome (Fig GI 19-11)	Narrowing or obstruction of the third portion of the duodenum with proximal dilatation.	Controversial entity referring to compression of the transverse duodenum between the aorta and the superior mesenteric artery due to any process that decreases duodenal peristalsis or thickens the bowel wall or the root of the mesentery.

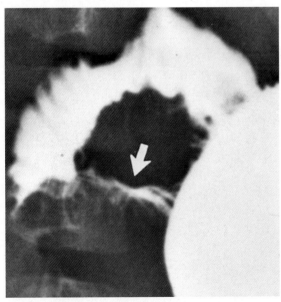

Fig GI 19-10
Intramural duodenal hematoma. High-grade stenotic lesion (arrow) that developed in a young child, who had been kicked in the abdomen.

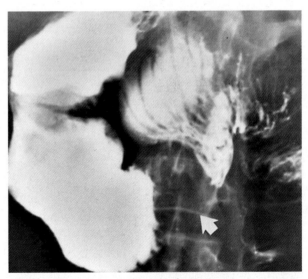

Fig GI 19-11
Superior mesenteric artery syndrome in scleroderma. There is severe atony and dilatation of the duodenum proximal to the aorticomesenteric angle (arrow).

Thickening of Duodenal Folds

Condition	Imaging Findings	Comments
Peptic ulcer disease (see Fig GI 17-3)	Diffuse fold thickening, primarily involving the bulb and proximal sweep.	Most common cause. Nodular, cobblestone appearance suggests Brunner's gland hyperplasia (response of the duodenal mucosa to an ulcer diathesis).
Zollinger-Ellison syndrome (Fig GI 20-1)	Diffuse fold thickening.	Associated findings include ulceration in atypical positions (third and fourth portions of the duodenum, proximal jejunum) and chemical enteritis of the proximal jejunum.
Pancreatitis (Fig GI 20-2)	Thickened folds in the second portion.	Associated findings include mass impression and elevated serum amylase.
Uremia (chronic dialysis)	Nodular fold thickening, primarily involving the bulb and second portion.	Simulates the appearance of pancreatitis, which frequently complicates prolonged uremia and may be responsible for producing the radiographic pattern.
Crohn's disease/ tuberculosis (Fig GI 20-3)	Diffuse fold thickening, often with ulceration and luminal narrowing.	In Crohn's disease, usually involvement of the terminal ileum. In tuberculosis, the antrum and pylorus are generally affected.
Infectious disorders (see Fig GI 26-6)	Nodular fold thickening.	Giardiasis (increased secretions causing a blurred appearance), strongyloidiasis (ulcerations and luminal stenosis), and cryptosporidiosis, cytomegalovirus, and *Mycobacterium avium-intracellulare* (in patients with AIDS).

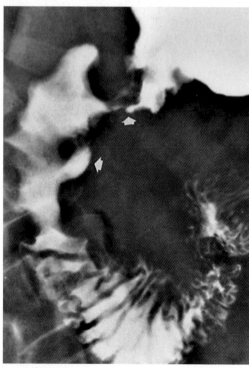

Fig GI 20-1
Zollinger-Ellison syndrome. Diffuse thickening of folds in the proximal duodenal sweep is associated with bulbar and postbulbar ulceration (arrows).

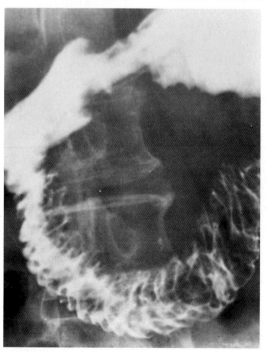

Fig GI 20-2
Acute pancreatitis. Note the widening of the duodenal sweep, double-contour effect, and sharp spiculations.

Condition	Imaging Findings	Comments
Nontropical sprue	Bizarre nodular thickening of folds.	Early manifestation of the disease.
Neoplastic disorders (Fig GI 20-4)	Various patterns of fold thickening.	Lymphoma (coarse, nodular, irregular folds) and metastases to peripancreatic lymph nodes (localized duodenal impressions simulating thickened folds).
Infiltrative disorders	Diffuse fold thickening (usually generalized involvement of the small bowel).	Whipple's disease; amyloidosis; mastocytosis; eosinophilic enteritis; intestinal lymphangiectasia.
Duodenal varices (Fig GI 20-5)	Nodular or serpiginous fold thickening.	Esophageal varices are almost always also present.
Mesenteric arterial collaterals	Serpiginous, nodular filling defects simulating thickened folds.	Collateral vessels of the pancreaticoduodenal arcade due to occlusion of the celiac axis or the superior mesenteric artery.
Cystic fibrosis (Fig GI 20-6)	Coarse, thickening of folds.	Probably related to the lack of pancreatic bicarbonate, which results in inadequate buffering of normal amounts of gastric acid.

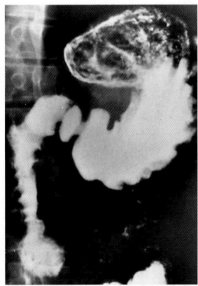

Fig GI 20-3
Tuberculosis. Diffuse fold thickening, spasm, and ulceration of the proximal duodenum.

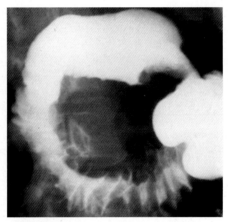

Fig GI 20-4
Metastases to peripancreatic lymph nodes cause localized impressions on the duodenum simulating thickened folds.

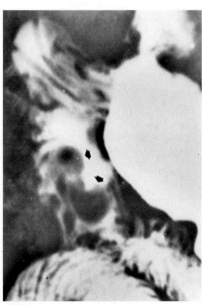

Fig GI 20-5
Duodenal varices (arrows).

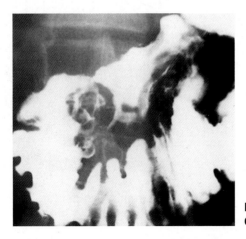

Fig GI 20-6
Cystic fibrosis.

Widening of the Duodenal Sweep

Condition	Imaging Findings	Comments
Normal variant	Illusion of generalized widening.	Especially in an obese patient with a high transverse stomach and a long vertical course of the descending duodenum.
Acute pancreatitis (Fig GI 21-1)	Generalized widening with mucosal ulcerations, fold thickening, and mass effect.	Associated radiographic findings include elevation of a hemidiaphragm, basilar atelectasis, pleural effusion (left side), colon cutoff sign, and sentinel loop.
Chronic pancreatitis	Generalized widening with fold effacement and spiculation. Pancreatic calcification is often visible radiographically.	History of alcoholism in more than half the patients. Biliary tract disease (usually with gallstones) in approximately one-third.
Pancreatic pseudocyst (Fig GI 21-2)	Generalized widening and compression of the duodenal sweep.	Common complication of pancreatitis. May also develop after pancreatic injury.
Pancreatic malignancy (Fig GI 21-3)	Diffuse widening with mass impression, spiculation, and double-contour effect.	Often difficult to distinguish radiographically from benign pancreatic disease. A similar pattern may be produced by cystadenocarcinoma and metastatic lesions.
Lymph node enlargement	Generalized widening.	Lymphadenopathy due to lymphoma, metastases to lymph nodes, or inflammatory disease.
Cystic lymphangioma of mesentery (Fig GI 21-4)	Generalized widening.	Benign cystic structure containing serous or chylous fluid resulting from the congenital obliteration of draining lymphatics or an acquired lymphatic obstruction.

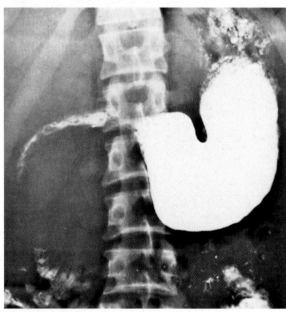

Fig GI 21-1
Acute pancreatitis. Severe inflammation causes widening of the sweep and a high-grade duodenal obstruction.

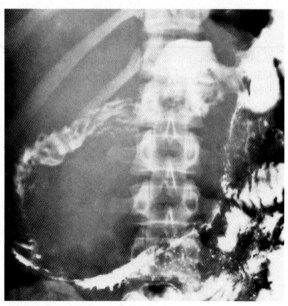

Fig GI 21-2
Pancreatic pseudocyst.

Condition	Imaging Findings	Comments
Retroperitoneal mass	Generalized widening.	Primary or metastatic neoplasm; cyst.
Aortic aneurysm	Downward displacement of the third portion of the duodenum.	Definitive diagnosis made on ultrasound or CT.
Choledochal cyst	Generalized widening of the duodenal sweep or a localized impression near the papilla.	Definitive diagnosis made on ultrasound or CT.

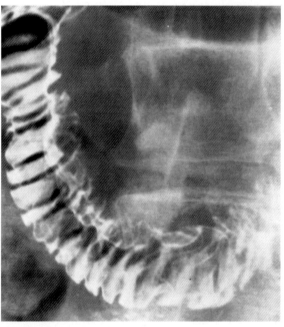

Fig GI 21-3
Carcinoma of the pancreas. Note the double-contour effect along the medial aspect of the duodenal sweep.

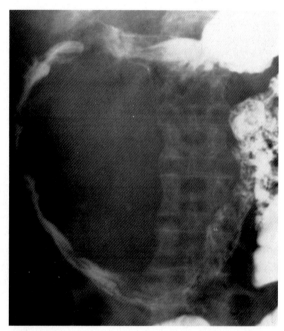

Fig GI 21-4
Cystic lymphangioma of the mesentery. Scattered clumps of calcification are present in the lesion.

Adynamic Ileus*

Condition	Imaging Findings	Comments
Surgical procedure	Generalized ileus.	Usually resolves spontaneously or clears with the aid of intubation and suction. If progressive, can cause intestinal rupture and pneumoperitoneum.
Peritonitis	Generalized ileus, often with blurring of the mucosal pattern and intestinal edema.	Suggestive findings include free peritoneal fluid, restricted diaphragmatic movement, and pleural effusion. Gastroenteritis or enterocolitis without peritonitis can also present as generalized adynamic ileus.
Medication	Generalized ileus.	Drugs with atropine-like effects (morphine, Lomotil, L-dopa, barbiturates, and other sympathomimetic agents).
Electrolyte imbalance/ metabolic disorder	Generalized ileus.	Most commonly hypokalemia, but also occurs with hypochloremia, calcium or magnesium abnormalities, and hormonal deficits (hypothyroidism, hypoparathyroidism).
Other abdominal or chest conditions	Generalized ileus.	Abdominal trauma; retroperitoneal hemorrhage; spinal or pelvic fractures; generalized gram-negative sepsis; shock; acute pulmonary disease; mesenteric vascular occlusion.
Sentinel loop (Fig GI 22-2)	Localized distended loop of small or large bowel (associated with an adjacent acute inflammatory process).	Portion of bowel involved can suggest the underlying disease (jejunum or transverse colon in acute pancreatitis, hepatic flexure in acute cholecystitis, terminal ileum in acute appendicitis, descending colon in acute diverticulitis).
Colonic ileus (Fig GI 22-3)	Disproportionate gaseous distention of the large bowel without organic obstruction. Massive distention of the cecum (often horizontally oriented).	Usually related to abdominal surgery or acute inflammation. The clinical presentation simulates mechanical obstruction.
Chronic idiopathic intestinal pseudo-obstruction (Fig GI 22-4)	Distention of the small bowel mimicking intestinal obstruction, but without any demonstrable obstructive lesion.	Episodic symptoms of intestinal obstruction. Recognition of the true nature of this nonobstructive condition is essential to prevent the patient from undergoing unnecessary laparotomies.
Pelvic surgery	Mimics small bowel obstruction.	Develops between the second and fifth postoperative days, especially if there was manipulation of the small bowel. Self-limited and rarely requires surgery.
Urinary retention	Mimics small bowel obstruction.	Symptoms often completely disappear after emptying of the distended bladder.

*Pattern: The entire small and large bowel appears almost uniformly dilated with no demonstrable point of obstruction (Fig GI 22-1).

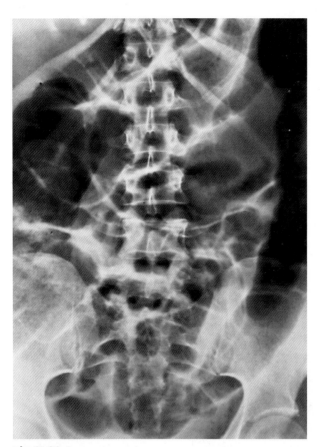

Fig GI 22-1
Adynamic ileus pattern.

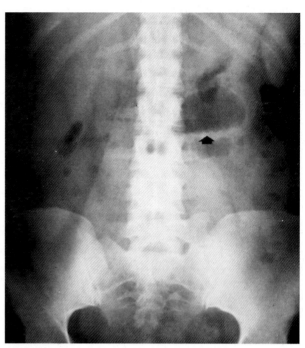

Fig GI 22-2
Sentinel loop (arrow) in a patient with acute pancreatitis.

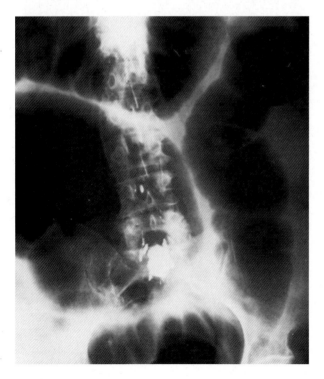

Fig GI 22-3
Colonic ileus in a patient with severe diabetes and hypokalemia.

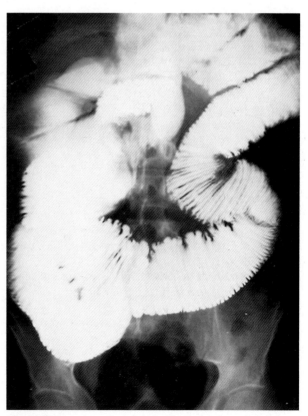

Fig GI 22-4
Chronic idiopathic intestinal pseudo-obstruction. The diffuse small bowel dilatation simulates mechanical obstruction.[27]

Condition	Imaging Findings	Comments
Acute intermittent porphyria (Fig GI 22-5)	Mimics small bowel obstruction.	Familial metabolic disease. The diagnosis is suggested by the characteristic neurologic symptoms or the urine becoming dark on exposure to light.
Ceroidosis	Mimics small bowel obstruction.	Diffuse accumulation of a brown lipofuscin pigment in the muscularis due to long-standing malabsorption and prolonged depletion of vitamin E. May lead to unnecessary bowel resection for nonexistent obstruction.
Neonatal adynamic ileus	Mimics small bowel obstruction.	Causes include septicemia, hormonal or chemical deficits, hypoxia-induced vasculitis, respiratory distress syndrome, intestinal infection, peritonitis, and mesenteric thrombosis.

A   B

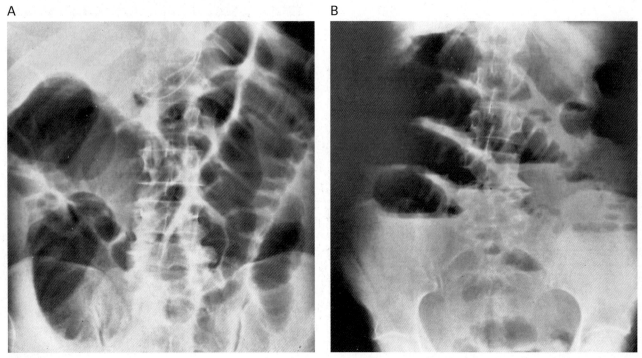

Fig GI 22-5
Acute intermittent porphyria. Adynamic ileus simulating mechanical obstruction on (A) supine and (B) upright views.

Small Bowel Obstruction

Condition	Imaging Findings	Comments
Fibrous adhesions (Fig GI 23-1)	Most frequently involves the ileum (site of most abdominal inflammatory processes and operative procedures).	Fibrous adhesions caused by previous surgery or peritonitis account for almost 75% of all small bowel obstructions.
External hernias	May have gas or excessive soft-tissue density on the affected side.	External hernias (inguinal, femoral, umbilical, and incisional) are the second most frequent cause of small bowel obstruction.
Internal hernias	Various patterns.	Results from congenital abnormalities or surgical defects in the mesentery. More than half are paraduodenal (mostly on the left).
Volvulus/congenital bands	Duodenal obstruction.	Usually associated with malrotation anomalies.
Neoplasms (Fig GI 23-2)	Luminal occlusion or extrinsic impression.	Can be caused by benign or malignant neoplasms and involve any level of the small bowel.
Gallstone ileus (Fig GI 23-3)	Classic triad of jejunal or ileal filling defect, gas or barium in the biliary tree, and small bowel obstruction.	Caused by a large gallstone entering the small bowel via a fistula from the gallbladder or the common bile duct to the duodenum. Usually occurs in elderly women.
Bezoar (Fig GI 23-4)	Filling defect on barium studies.	Primarily seen in patients who are mentally retarded or edentulous or who have undergone partial gastric resection.

A   B

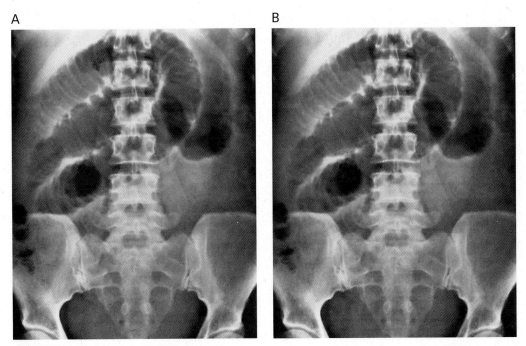

Fig GI 23-1
Typical small bowel obstruction on (A) supine and (B) upright projections.

Condition	Imaging Findings	Comments
Intussusception (Fig GI 23-5)	May produce the classic coiled-spring appearance (barium trapped between the intussusceptum and the surrounding portions of bowel).	A major cause of small bowel obstruction in children (much less common in adults). The leading edge of an intussusception (usually a pedunculated polypoid tumor) can be demonstrated in 80% of adults. In children, there is infrequently any apparent anatomic etiology.

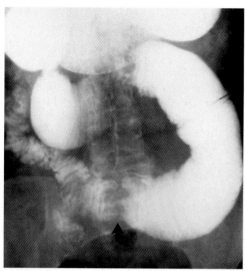

Fig GI 23-2
Carcinoma of the jejunum causing small bowel obstruction. There is pronounced dilatation of the duodenum and proximal jejunum to the level of the annular constricting tumor (arrow).

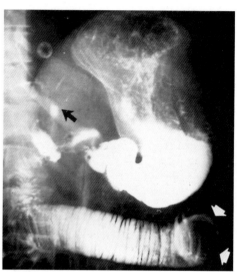

Fig GI 23-3
Gallstone ileus. Upper gastrointestinal series demonstrates the obstructing stone (white arrows) and barium in the biliary tree (black arrow).

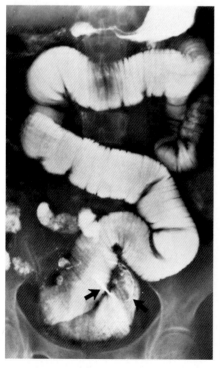

Fig GI 23-4
Impacted bezoar (arrows) causing small bowel obstruction.

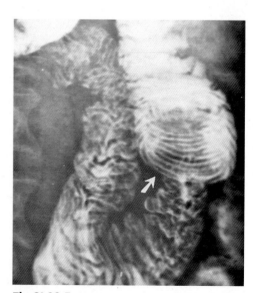

Fig GI 23-5
Intussusception. Coiled-spring appearance (arrow) in jejuno-jejunal intussusception.

Condition	Imaging Findings	Comments
Meconium ileus (Fig GI 23-6)	Infant with a bubbly or frothy pattern superimposed on dilated loops of small bowel.	Caused by thick and sticky meconium due to the absence of normal pancreatic and intestinal gland secretions during fetal life. Often occurs with cystic fibrosis. A microcolon is seen on barium enema examination.
Congenital intestinal atresia or stenosis (Fig GI 23-7)	Double bubble (duodenal atresia) or triple bubble (proximal jejunal atresia) signs, or a typical obstructive pattern.	Barium enema may be required to distinguish small from large bowel in a low ileal obstruction. Microcolon in ileal atresia; normal-caliber colon in duodenal atresia. Meconium peritonitis (often calcified) is a complication of small bowel atresia.
Stricture of bowel wall	May involve any level of the small bowel.	Causes include neoplasm, inflammation (Crohn's disease, tuberculosis, and parasitic infections), chemical irritation (medicines such as enteric-coated potassium chloride tablets), radiation therapy, massive deposition of amyloid, and intestinal ischemia (arterial or venous occlusion).

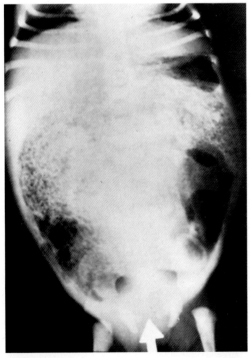

Fig GI 23-6
Meconium ileus. Massive small bowel distention with a profound soap-bubble effect of gas mixed with meconium.[28]

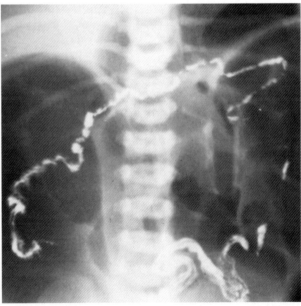

Fig GI 23-7
Ileal atresia with microcolon. Barium enema examination shows the colon to be thin and ribbon-like. Note the markedly distended loops of small bowel extending to the point of obstruction in the lower ileum.

Small Bowel Dilatation

Condition	Imaging Findings	Comments
Mechanical obstruction (see Figs in Section GI 23)	Dilatation proximal to the level of the obstruction.	Distinct difference in caliber between loops proximal and distal to the point of the obstruction. Generally a paucity of colonic gas.
Adynamic ileus (see Figs in Section GI 22)	Generalized dilatation of the small (and large) bowel.	No point at which the caliber of the bowel dramatically changes.
Vagotomy (surgical or chemical) (Fig GI 24-1)	Generalized dilatation of the small bowel.	Vagotomy clips or a history of previous ulcer surgery; atropine-like medications (morphine, L-dopa, Lomotil, barbiturates).
Sprue (Fig GI 24-2)	Generalized dilatation, but often most marked in the mid and distal jejunum. Excessive amount of fluid in the bowel lumen (coarse, granular appearance of the barium). Moulage sign and frequent transient intussusception.	Classic disease of malabsorption that includes idiopathic (nontropical) sprue, tropical sprue, and celiac disease of children. Diagnosis is made by jejunal biopsy (flattening or atrophy of intestinal villi). Nontropical sprue is treated with a gluten-free diet, tropical sprue with antibiotics or folic acid.
Lymphoma	Occasionally has an appearance indistinguishable from that of sprue.	Rare manifestation of intestinal lymphoma. More commonly, thickening of the bowel wall, displacement of intestinal loops, and extraluminal masses.

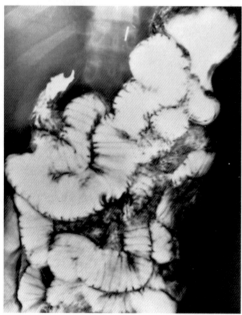

Fig GI 24-1
Surgical vagotomy with partial gastrectomy and Billroth-II anastomosis.

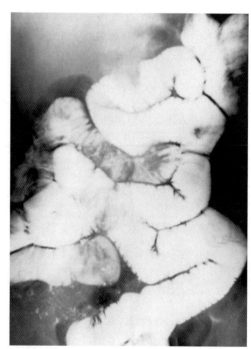

Fig GI 24-2
Idiopathic (nontropical) sprue. Note the pronounced hypersecretion.

Condition	Imaging Findings	Comments
Scleroderma (Fig GI 24-3)	Dilatation that is usually most marked in the duodenum proximal to the aorticomesenteric angle. The entire small bowel can be diffusely involved.	"Hidebound" sign of folds abnormally packed together despite bowel dilatation. Hypomotility of the small bowel with extremely prolonged transit time. There may be pseudosacculations simulating small bowel diverticula. Similar findings occasionally occur with dermatomyositis.
Lactase deficiency (Fig GI 24-4)	Generalized dilatation with dilution of barium, rapid transit time, and reproduction of symptoms after the administration of lactose.	Most common of the disaccharidase-deficiency syndromes; especially frequent in North American blacks, Mexicans, and Chinese. Patients experience abdominal discomfort, cramps, and watery diarrhea 30 minutes to several hours after ingesting milk or milk products.

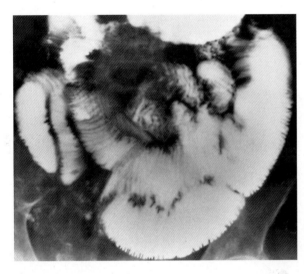

Fig GI 24-3
Scleroderma. For the degree of dilatation, the small bowel folds are packed remarkably close together (hidebound pattern).

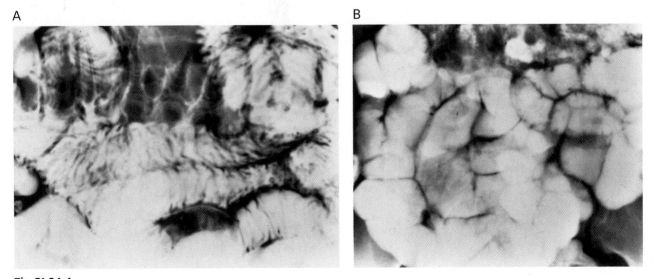

Fig GI 24-4
Lactase deficiency. (A) Normal conventional small bowel examination. (B) After the addition of 50 g of lactose to the barium mixture, there is marked dilatation of the small bowel with dilution of barium, rapid transit, and reproduction of symptoms.

Condition	Imaging Findings	Comments
Diabetes with hypokalemia	Generalized dilatation of the small bowel.	Small bowel is usually normal in patients with diabetes mellitus unless complicated by hypokalemia (probably represents a visceral neuropathy).
Vascular insufficiency/ vasculitis (Figs GI 24-5 and GI 24-6)	Generalized dilatation of the small bowel.	Occasional manifestation of mesenteric ischemia (if a disturbance of intestinal motility, rather than intramural bleeding, is the major abnormality). Also occurs with the vasculitis due to systemic lupus erythematosus or massive amyloid deposition.
Chronic idiopathic intestinal pseudo-obstruction (see Fig GI 22-4)	Small bowel obstruction pattern.	Episodic signs and symptoms of mechanical obstruction without any organic lesion. Recognition of this condition may prevent unnecessary laparotomies.
Chagas' disease	Generalized dilatation of the small bowel.	Trypanosomes extensively invade the smooth muscle and destroy intrinsic neurons and ganglion cells in the bowel wall.

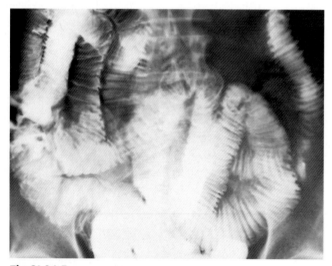

Fig GI 24-5
Systemic lupus erythematosus.

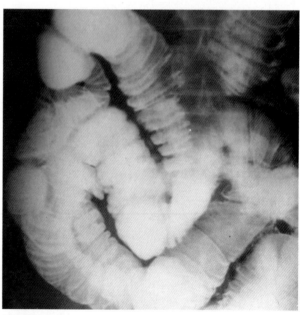

Fig GI 24-6
Amyloidosis.

Regular Thickening of Small Bowel Folds

Condition	Comments
Hemorrhage into bowel wall (Fig GI 25-1)	Usually segmental involvement of the small bowel (especially the jejunum) with scalloping and thumbprinting. Concomitant bleeding into the mesentery often results in separation of bowel loops and even an eccentric mass simulating malignancy. Causes include anticoagulant therapy, ischemic bowel disease, vasculitis (connective tissue diseases, Buerger's disease, Henoch-Schönlein purpura), hemophilia, idiopathic thrombocytopenic purpura, trauma, and coagulation defects secondary to other diseases (hypoprothrombinemia, leukemia, multiple myeloma, lymphoma, metastatic carcinoma, disorders of the fibrinogen system).
Intestinal edema (Fig GI 25-2)	Generalized involvement of the small bowel. Causes include hypoproteinemia (cirrhosis, nephrotic syndrome, protein-losing enteropathies), lymphatic blockage (especially tumor infiltration), and angioneurotic edema (tends to be episodic and more localized).
Intestinal lymphangiectasia	Generalized small bowel involvement. Occurs in primary and secondary forms. Regular thickening represents a combination of intestinal edema (lymphatic obstruction or severe protein loss) and lymphatic dilatation.
Abetalipoproteinemia	Generalized small bowel involvement. Extremely rare disease manifested clinically by malabsorption of fat, progressive neurologic deterioration, and retinitis pigmentosa. Acanthocytosis (thorny appearance of red blood cells) is a characteristic finding. The small bowel folds may also be irregular or nodular.
Eosinophilic enteritis/ amyloidosis	Generalized regular thickening of small bowel folds may occur at an early stage before the development of the more characteristic irregular thickening of folds.

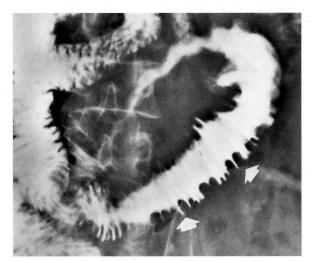

Fig GI 25-1
Small bowel ischemia producing a segmental picket-fence pattern of regular thickening of small bowel folds (arrows).

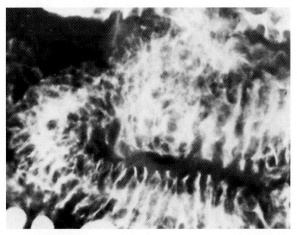

Fig GI 25-2
Hypoproteinemia causing regular thickening of small bowel folds in a patient with cirrhosis.

Generalized, Irregular, Distorted Small Bowel Folds

Condition	Imaging Findings	Comments
Whipple's disease (Fig GI 26-1)	Most frequently involves the duodenum and proximal jejunum. Small bowel appearance may revert to normal after antibiotic therapy.	Infiltration of the lamina propria by large macrophages containing multiple glycoprotein granules that react positively to the periodic acid-Schiff (PAS) stain. Clinically, malabsorption syndrome and often extraintestinal symptoms (arthritis, fever, lymphadenopathy). Characteristic low-attenuation lymph nodes on CT.
Giardiasis (Fig GI 26-2)	Primarily involves the duodenum and jejunum. Small bowel pattern returns to normal after treatment with Atabrine or Flagyl.	Usually a history of travel to areas where the parasite is endemic (eg, Leningrad, India, or the Rocky Mountains of Colorado). May complicate an immune deficiency state (especially nodular lymphoid hyperplasia).
Lymphoma (Fig GI 26-3)	Localized, multifocal, or diffuse. Most commonly involves the ileum (site of the greatest amount of lymphoid tissue).	May be primary or secondary (25% of patients with disseminated lymphoma have small bowel involvement at autopsy). Today, a substantial proportion of small bowel lymphomas occur in patients with AIDS or other cause of immune compromise.

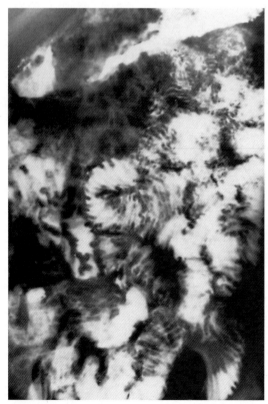

Fig GI 26-1
Whipple's disease.

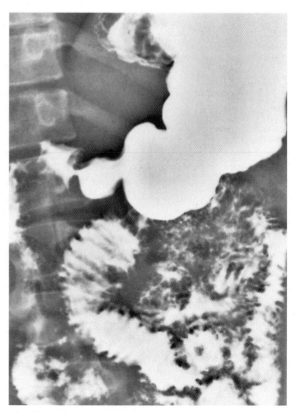

Fig GI 26-2
Giardiasis. Irregular fold thickening is most prominent in the proximal small bowel.

Condition	Imaging Findings	Comments
Amyloidosis (Fig GI 26-4)	Generalized involvement of the small bowel.	Small intestinal involvement occurs in at least 70% of cases of generalized amyloidosis. May be primary or secondary to a chronic inflammatory or necrotizing process (eg, tuberculosis, osteomyelitis, ulcerative colitis, rheumatoid arthritis, and malignant neoplasm), multiple myeloma, or familial Mediterranean fever.
Eosinophilic enteritis (Fig GI 26-5)	Primarily involves the jejunum, though the entire small bowel is sometimes affected.	There is often concomitant eosinophilic infiltration of the stomach. Typical food allergies and peripheral eosinophilia.
Crohn's disease	Most often involves the terminal ileum, but can affect any part of the small bowel.	Characteristic findings include skip lesions, string sign, severe narrowing, separation of bowel loops, and fistula formation.
Tuberculosis	Radiographic pattern indistinguishable from that of Crohn's disease.	Tends to be more localized than Crohn's disease and predominantly affects the ileocecal region.
Histoplasmosis	Generalized involvement of the small bowel.	Fungal disease that rarely affects the gastrointestinal tract. Folds seen end-on may appear as innumerable small filling defects. Focal stenotic lesions may mimic neoplastic disease.

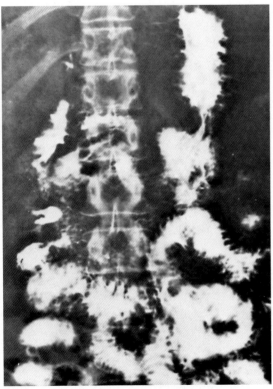

Fig GI 26-3
Lymphoma. In addition to diffuse, irregular thickening of the small bowel folds, there is mesenteric involvement causing separation of bowel loops.

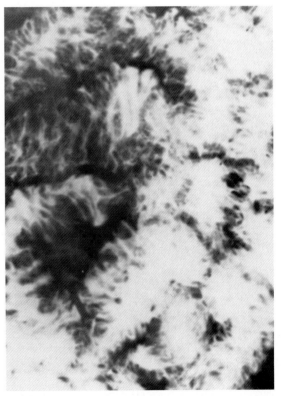

Fig GI 26-4
Amyloidosis.

Condition	Imaging Findings	Comments
Mastocytosis	Generalized involvement of the small bowel.	Systemic mast cell proliferation in the reticuloendothelial system and the skin. Often lymphadenopathy and hepatosplenomegaly and occasionally sclerotic bone lesions. High incidence of peptic ulcers and episodic pruritus, flushing, tachycardia, asthma, and headaches.
Strongyloidiasis (Fig GI 26-6)	Predominantly involves the proximal small bowel (a severe infestation can affect the entire alimentary tract).	Roundworm that lives in warm, moist climates where there is frequent fecal contamination of the soil.
Yersinia enterocolitis (Fig GI 26-7)	Predominantly a focal disease involving short segments of the terminal ileum. Infrequently affects the colon and rectum.	Gram-negative rod that causes acute enteritis with fever and diarrhea in children and an acute terminal ileitis or mesenteric adenitis (simulating appendicitis) in adolescents and adults.
Typhoid fever	Involvement limited to the terminal ileum.	Caused by *Salmonella typhosa*. Mimics Crohn's disease, though in typhoid fever the ileal involvement is symmetric, skip areas and fistulas do not occur, and there is usually evidence of splenomegaly.
Other infections (Fig GI 26-8)	Various patterns.	*Campylobacter, Shigella, Escherichia coli*, anisakiasis. In AIDS and other immunocompromised patients, *Cryptosporidium, Mycobacterium avium-intracellulare*, and *Candida*.

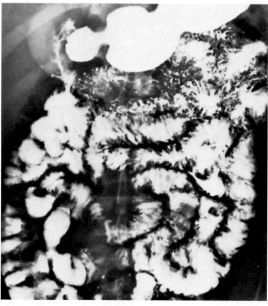

Fig GI 26-5
Eosinophilic enteritis. The irregular thickening of folds primarily involves the jejunum. There is no concomitant involvement of the stomach.

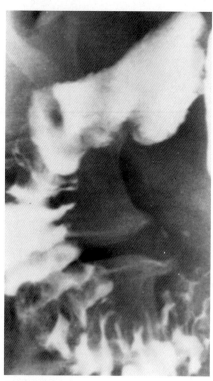

Fig GI 26-6
Strongyloidiasis. Predominant involvement of the duodenal sweep.

Condition	Imaging Findings	Comments
Alpha-chain disease	Generalized involvement of the small bowel.	Disorder of immunoglobulin peptide synthesis that probably permits bacterial overgrowth.
Abetalipoproteinemia	Generalized involvement of the small bowel.	Rare inherited disease manifested clinically by malabsorption of fat, progressive neurologic deterioration, and retinitis pigmentosa. The folds may be regularly thickened.

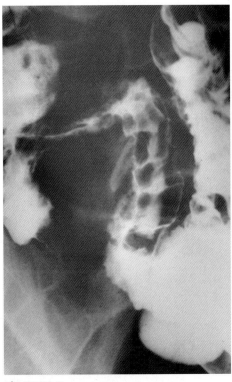

Fig GI 26-7
***Yersinia* enterocolitis.** Nodular pattern of thickened folds in the terminal ileum.[29]

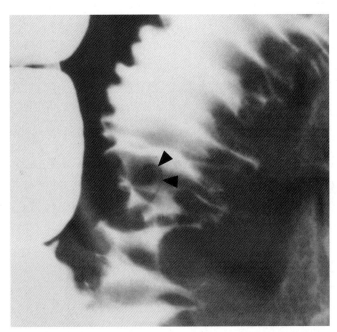

Fig GI 26-8
Anisakiasis. Coned view shows a thread-like filling defect (arrows), representing the worm, surrounded by irregular thickening of folds.[30]

Filling Defects in the Jejunum and Ileum

Condition	Imaging Findings	Comments
Benign spindle cell tumor (Fig GI 27-1)	Usually a single, well-circumscribed filling defect that may ulcerate. Pedunculated tumor may cause intussusception.	Leiomyomas are most common in the jejunum; adenomas most frequently involve the ileum; lipomas primarily affect the distal ileum and the ileocecal valve area.
Hemangioma (Fig GI 27-2)	Usually multiple, but often small and frequently missed on barium studies.	Combination of phleboliths and multiple filling defects in the small bowel is pathognomonic of multiple hemangiomas.
Polyposis syndrome (Fig GI 27-3)	Multiple filling defects, often associated with colonic and even gastric tumors.	In Peutz-Jeghers syndrome, hamartomas are associated with mucocutaneous pigmentation. In Gardner's syndrome, adenomatous polyps are associated with osteomas and soft-tissue tumors.
Adenocarcinoma of small bowel (Fig GI 27-4)	Usually a single broad-based intraluminal mass. Pedunculated polyp is extremely rare.	Most common malignant tumor of the small bowel. The tumor is usually aggressively invasive and causes luminal narrowing that soon produces obstruction.
Lymphoma (Figs GI 27-5 and GI 27-6)	Discrete polypoid mass that is often large and bulky with irregular ulcerations.	Relatively infrequent manifestation of lymphoma. Multiple small or large masses can occur.

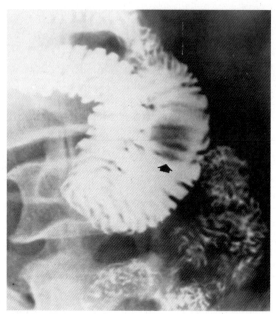

Fig GI 27-1
Leiomyoma of the jejunum (arrow).[31]

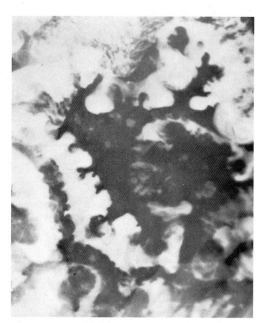

Fig GI 27-2
Hemangiomatosis of the small bowel and mesentery. Characteristic phleboliths are associated with multiple filling defects in the small bowel.

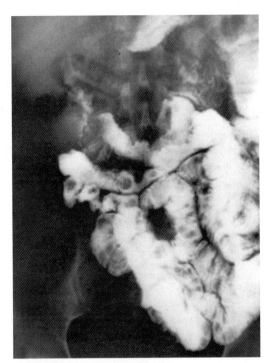

Fig GI 27-3
Peutz-Jeghers syndrome. Multiple small bowel hamartomas are present in a patient with mucocutaneous pigmentation.[32]

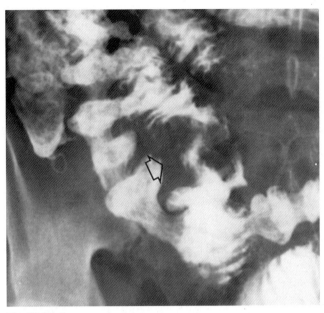

Fig GI 27-4
Primary adenocarcinoma of the ileum (arrow) appearing as an annular constricting lesion.

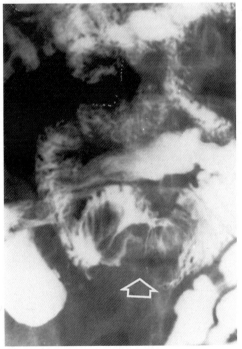

Fig GI 27-5
Lymphoma. Note the large, bulky, irregular lesion (arrow).

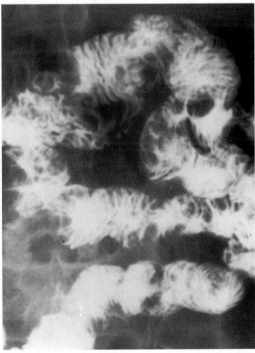

Fig GI 27-6
Lymphoma. Multiple large irregular masses.

Condition	Imaging Findings	Comments
Sarcoma (Fig GI 27-7)	Usually a single, large, bulky, irregular lesion, often with central ulceration.	Most tumors primarily project into the peritoneal cavity so that their major manifestation is displacement of adjacent, uninvolved barium-filled loops of small bowel.
Metastases (Fig GI 27-8)	Usually multiple filling defects, often with central ulceration (bull's-eye appearance).	Most commonly due to melanoma and carcinomas of the breast and lung. Other tumors include Kaposi's sarcoma and primary neoplasms of the ovary, pancreas, kidney, stomach, and uterus.
Carcinoid tumor (Fig GI 27-9)	Initially a small, sharply defined filling defect (often missed radiographically).	Most common primary neoplasm of the small bowel. Rule of one-third (frequency of metastases, second malignancy, and multiplicity). Most often occurs in the ileum. Carcinoid syndrome (liver metastases) is infrequent.
Gallstone ileus (Fig GI 27-10)	Single filling defect (lucent or opaque).	Classic triad of small bowel filling defect, mechanical small bowel obstruction, and gas or barium in the biliary tree.

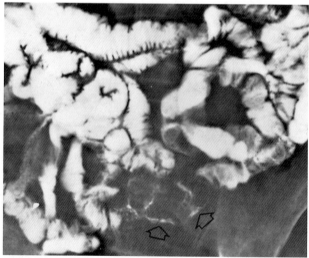

Fig GI 27-7
Leiomyosarcoma. Large, bulky, irregular lesion (arrows).

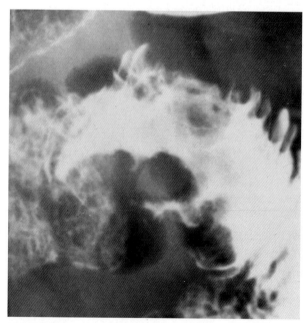

Fig GI 27-8
Metastatic hypernephroma. Multilobulated nodular mass in the proximal jejunum.

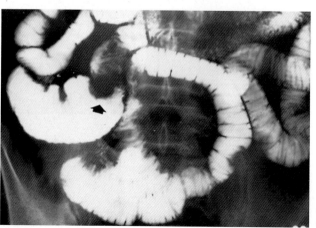

Fig GI 27-9
Carcinoid tumor (arrow).

Condition	Imaging Findings	Comments
Parasites (Fig GI 27-11)	Usually multiple linear intraluminal defects. A clump of coiled worms can produce a single intraluminal filling defect.	Most commonly *Ascaris lumbricoides* (barium can fill the intestinal tract of the worm). Other parasites include *Strongyloides stercoralis*, *Ancylostoma duodenale* (hookworm), and *Taenia solis* (tapeworm).
Endometrioma	Single filling defect.	In premenopausal women with associated pelvic endometriosis.
Duplication cyst	Single filling defect.	Typically, changes contour with external pressure and rarely communicate with the small bowel lumen.
Nodular lymphoid hyperplasia (Fig GI 27-12)	Single filling defect or multiple nodules diffusely scattered through the small bowel.	Larger filling defects may mimic polypoid masses.
Ingested material (Fig GI 27-13)	Single or multiple filling defects.	Food particles, fruit pits, foreign bodies, bezoars, and pills.
Crohn's disease (Fig GI 27-14)	Single or multiple filling defects.	Rare manifestation of the disease.
Amyloidosis (Fig GI 27-15)	Multiple filling defects.	More commonly diffuse thickening of folds.
Varices	Multiple polypoid or serpiginous filling defects.	Dilatation of jejunal veins can occur as part of a syndrome (with multiple phlebectasia involving the oral mucosa, tongue, and scrotum) and should be suspected as a possible cause of gastrointestinal bleeding when mucocutaneous manifestations are present.

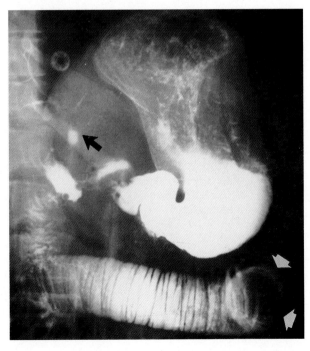

Fig GI 27-10
Gallstone ileus. The obstructing stone (white arrows) in the jejunum is associated with evidence of barium in the biliary tree (black arrow).

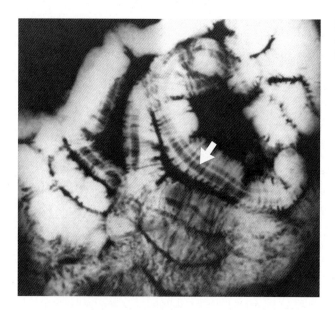

Fig GI 27-11
Ascaris. The linear intestinal tract of the roundworm is filled with barium (arrow).[32]

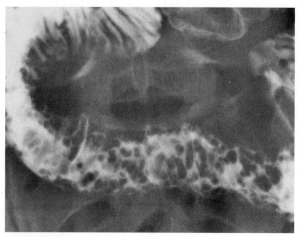

Fig GI 27-12
Nodular lymphoid hyperplasia. Large filling defects suggest multiple polypoid masses.

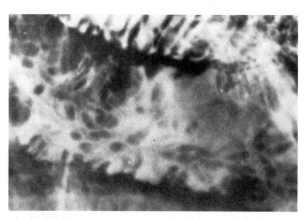

Fig GI 27-14
Crohn's disease. Multiple polypoid lesions in the distal jejunum and proximal ileum show both smooth and lobulated contours.[34]

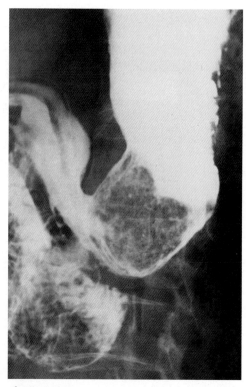

Fig GI 27-13
Phytobezoar. Large, irregular, proximal jejunal filling defect containing barium within the interstices of the lesion. Note the second bezoar in the stomach.[33]

A

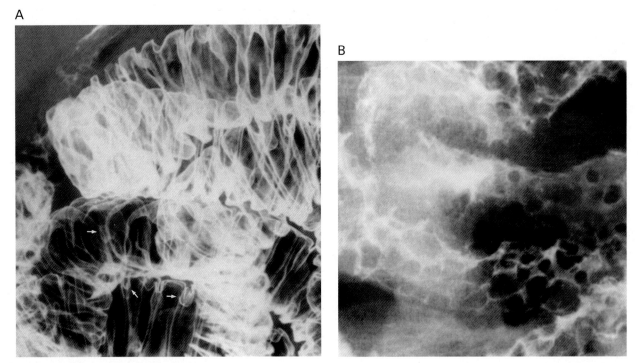

B

Fig GI 27-15
Amyloidosis. (A) Multiple polypoid protrusions (arrows) associated with diffusely thickened jejunal folds. (B) Multiple nodular filling defects in the jejunum of another patient.[35]

Sand-like Lucencies in the Small Bowel

Condition	Imaging Findings	Comments
Macroglobulinemia (Waldenström's disease) (Fig GI 28-1)	Generalized involvement of the small bowel.	Plasma cell dyscrasia with a highly elevated level of immunoglobulin M (IgM) in the serum. Insidious onset in late adult life. Characterized by anemia, bleeding, lymphadenopathy, and hepatosplenomegaly.
Mastocytosis	Generalized involvement of the small bowel.	Sand-like lucencies superimposed on a generally irregular, thickened fold pattern.
Nodular lymphoid hyperplasia (Figs GI 28-2 through GI 28-4)	Primarily involves the jejunum, but can occur throughout the entire small bowel.	In adults, almost invariably associated with late-onset immunoglobulin deficiency. Frequently associated with *Giardia lamblia* infection and irregular thickening of folds. In children, a pattern of multiple small symmetric nodules in the terminal ileum is a normal finding, and there is usually no immune deficiency.
Intestinal lymphangiectasia (Fig GI 28-5)	Generalized involvement of the small bowel.	Usually the early onset of massive edema, hypoproteinemia, and lymphocytopenia.
Whipple's disease	Primarily involves the duodenum and the proximal jejunum.	Extensive infiltration of the lamina propria by large macrophages with a positive periodic acid-Schiff (PAS) reaction.
Yersinia enterocolitis	Primarily involves the ileum.	Healing stage of the disease (follicular ileitis) that can persist for many months.

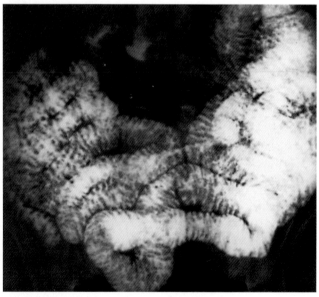

Fig GI 28-1
Waldenström's macroglobulinemia.

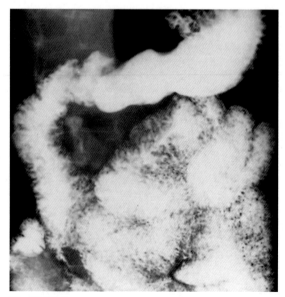

Fig GI 28-2
Nodular lymphoid hyperplasia. Innumerable tiny polypoid masses are uniformly distributed throughout the involved segments of small bowel. The underlying fold pattern is normal. The patient showed no evidence of associated disease.

Condition	Imaging Findings	Comments
Histoplasmosis (Fig GI 28-6)	Generalized involvement of the small bowel.	Rarely involves the gastrointestinal tract. May be superimposed on irregular, distorted folds.
Miscellaneous causes	Generalized involvement of the small bowel.	Sand-like pattern reported in eosinophilic enteritis (often with gastric involvement), Cronkhite-Canada syndrome (associated with colonic polyposis), cystic fibrosis, amyloidosis, radiation enteritis, pancreatic glucagonoma, protein-losing enteropathy, and small bowel ischemia.

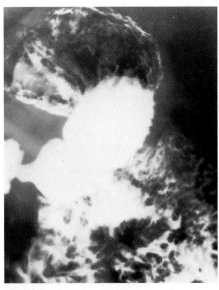

Fig GI 28-3
Nodular lymphoid hyperplasia in a patient with an immune deficiency and *Giardia lamblia* infestation. The relatively larger nodules are superimposed on an irregularly thickened and grossly distorted underlying fold pattern.

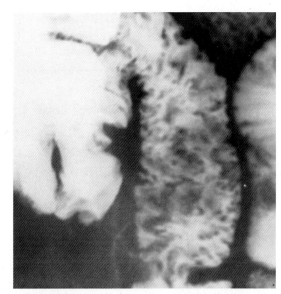

Fig GI 28-4
Normal terminal ileum in an adolescent. The multiple small nodules represent normal prominence of lymphoid follicles.

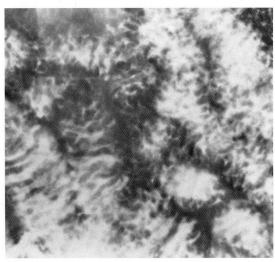

Fig GI 28-5
Intestinal lymphangiectasia.

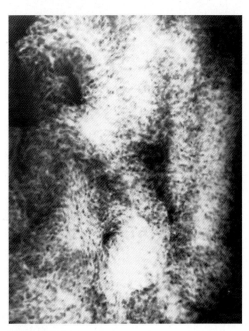

Fig GI 28-6
Histoplasmosis.

Separation of Small Bowel Loops

Condition	Imaging Findings	Comments
Thickening or infiltration of bowel wall or mesentery (Figs GI 29-1 and GI 29-2)	May be associated with extrinsic masses, luminal narrowing, and regular or irregular thickening of folds.	Causes include Crohn's disease, tuberculosis, intestinal hemorrhage or mesenteric vascular occlusion, Whipple's disease, amyloidosis, graft-versus-host disease, and lymphoma.
Radiation injury	May be associated with shallow mucosal ulceration, irregular fold thickening, and nodular filling defects.	Probably secondary to an endarteritis with vascular occlusion and bowel ischemia.
Carcinoid tumor (Figs GI 29-3 and GI 29-4)	Localized or generalized separation of loops.	Severe desmoplastic response typically produces one or several intramural nodules coexisting with a bizarre pattern of severe intestinal kinking and angulation.

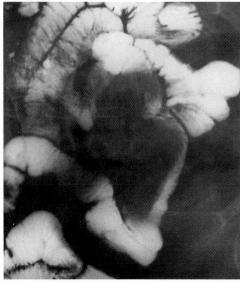

Fig GI 29-1
Crohn's disease. Marked thickening of the mesentery and mesenteric nodes produces a lobulated mass that widely separates small bowel loops.

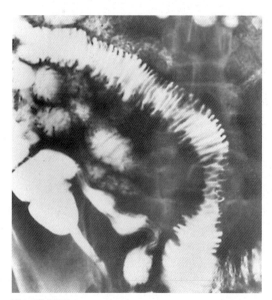

Fig GI 29-2
Intestinal hemorrhage with bleeding into the bowel wall and mesentery.

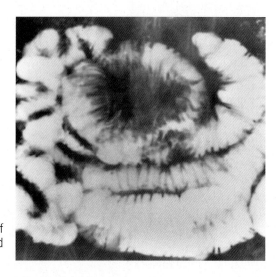

Fig GI 29-3
Carcinoid tumor. Localized separation of bowel loops with luminal narrowing and fibrotic tethering of mucosal folds.

Condition	Imaging Findings	Comments
Ascites	General abdominal haziness (ground-glass appearance).	Causes include hepatic cirrhosis, peritonitis, congestive failure, constrictive pericarditis, peritoneal carcinomatosis, and primary or metastatic disease of the lymphatic system.
Neoplasms	Often single or multiple mass impressions or angulated segments of small bowel.	Causes include metastases (peritoneal carcinomatosis) and primary tumors of the peritoneum and mesentery. Stretching and fixation of mucosal folds transverse to the long axis of the bowel lumen is an important sign.
Intraperitoneal abscess	Soft-tissue mass often associated with extraluminal bowel gas (multiple small lucencies ["soap bubbles"] or linear lucencies following fascial planes).	Localized collection of pus after generalized peritonitis or a more localized intra-abdominal disease process or injury. May have adjacent localized ileus (sentinel loop).
Retractile mesenteritis (Fig GI 29-5)	Bizarre pattern of diffuse separation of loops.	Fibroadipose thickening and sclerosis of the mesentery. If there is prominent fibrosis, the bowel tends to be drawn into a central mass with kinking, angulation, and conglomeration of adherent loops.
Retroperitoneal hernia (Fig GI 29-6)	Separation of normal loops from loops of bowel crowded closely together in the hernia sac.	Occurs in fossae formed by peritoneal folds in paraduodenal, paracecal, or intrasigmoidal locations. The normal small bowel remains free in the peritoneal cavity.

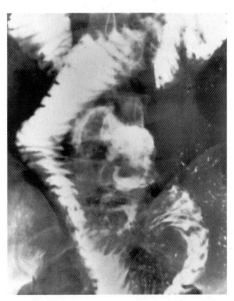

Fig GI 29-4
Carcinoid tumor. An intense desmoplastic reaction incited by the tumor causes kinking and angulation of the bowel and separation of small bowel loops in the mid-abdomen.

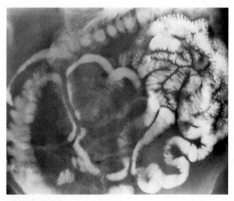

Fig GI 29-5
Retractile mesenteritis.[36]

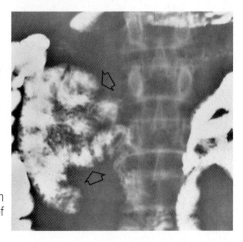

Fig GI 29-6
Right paraduodenal hernia. The loops of bowel crowded together in the hernia sac (arrows) are widely separated from other segments of small bowel that remain free in the peritoneal cavity.

Small Bowel Diverticula and Pseudodiverticula

Condition	Imaging Findings	Comments
Duodenal diverticulum	Smooth, rounded shape with normal mucosal folds. Generally changes configuration during the study. Often multiple.	Incidental finding in 1% to 5% of barium examinations. Most commonly found along the medial border of the descending duodenum in the peri-ampullary region; 30% to 40% arise in the third and fourth portions. Anomalous insertion of the common bile duct and pancreatic duct into a duodenal diverticulum can promote retrograde inflammation.
Giant duodenal ulcer (Fig GI 30-1)	Rigid-walled cavity that lacks a normal mucosal pattern and remains constant in size and shape throughout the study.	Usually there is narrowing of the pylorus proximal to the giant ulcer and of the duodenum distal to the ulcer (may be severe enough to produce gastric outlet obstruction). Great propensity for perforation and massive hemorrhage (high mortality rate) unless there is a prompt diagnosis and the institution of appropriate therapy.
Pseudodiverticulum of duodenal bulb	Deformity representing spasm or fibrosis.	Exaggerated outpouchings of the inferior and superior recesses at the base of the bulb related to duodenal ulcer disease.
Intraluminal duodenal diverticulum (Fig GI 30-2)	Finger-like sac separated from contrast material in the duodenal lumen by a lucent band representing the diverticular wall (halo sign).	Related to forward pressure by food and strong peristaltic activity on a congenital duodenal web originating near the papilla of Vater.
Jejunal diverticulum (Fig GI 30-3)	Usually multiple and with a wider neck than a colonic diverticulum.	May produce the blind loop syndrome with bacterial overgrowth and folic acid deficiency. A major cause of pneumoperitoneum without peritonitis or surgery. Diverticulitis is a rare complication.

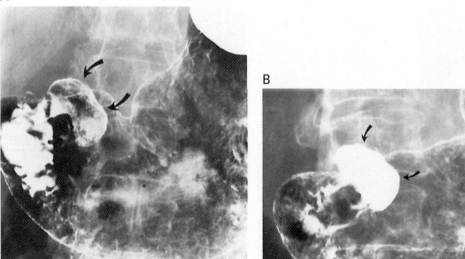

A

B

Fig GI 30-1
Giant duodenal ulcer. There is little change in the appearance of the rigid-walled cavity (arrows) in air-contrast (A) and barium-filled (B) views.[37]

Condition	Imaging Findings	Comments
Pseudodiverticula of jejunum or ileum (Fig GI 30-4)	Simulate intestinal diverticula.	Occur in scleroderma (sacculations resulting from smooth muscle atrophy and fibrosis), Crohn's disease (strictures and characteristic mucosal changes), and lymphoma (fusiform aneurysmal dilatation of the bowel).
Meckel's diverticulum (Fig GI 30-5)	Arises on the antimesenteric side of the ileum within 100 cm of the ileocecal valve.	Most frequent congenital anomaly of the intestinal tract. An outpouching of the rudimentary omphalomesenteric duct (embryonic communication between the gut and yolk sac that is normally obliterated in utero). May be inflamed and simulate acute appendicitis or may contain heterotopic gastric mucosa (see on a technetium scan).

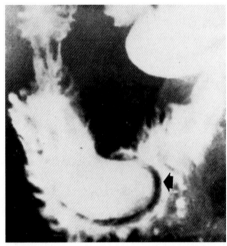

Fig GI 30-2
Halo sign (arrow) of intraluminal duodenal diverticulum.[38]

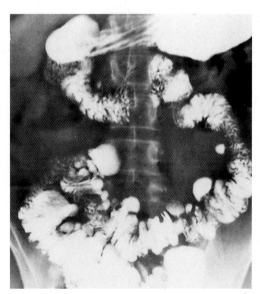

Fig GI 30-3
Jejunal diverticulosis.

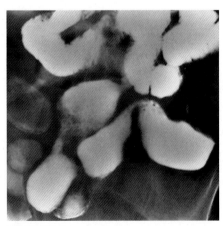

Fig GI 30-4
Pseudodiverticula in Crohn's disease.

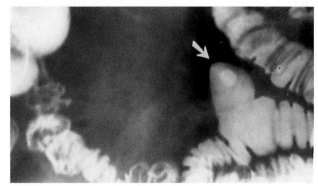

Fig GI 30-5
Meckel's diverticulum (arrow) with a small diverticulum (area of increased density) arising from it.

Condition	Imaging Findings	Comments
Ileal diverticulum (Fig GI 30-6)	Small, often multiple, and situated in the terminal portion near the ileocecal valve.	Least common of the small bowel diverticula. Ileal diverticulitis mimics acute appendicitis.

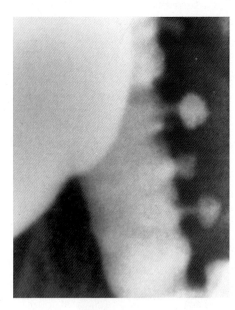

Fig GI 30-6
Ileal diverticula. Note that these diverticula are near the ileocecal valve, unlike Meckel's diverticula, which are situated more proximally.

Simultaneous Fold Thickening of the Stomach and Small Bowel

Condition	Imaging Findings	Comments
Lymphoma (see Figs GI 16-1 and GI 26-3)	Generalized, irregular fold thickening.	May also be a discrete mass or malignant ulceration in the stomach and an ulcerated filling defect, extrinsic impressions, or separation of loops in the small bowel.
Crohn's disease (see Figs GI 16-3 and GI 29-1)	Generalized, irregular fold thickening.	Narrowing and pseudo–Billroth-I deformity in the stomach; strictures, ulceration, cobblestoning, fistulas, and sinus tracts in the small bowel.
Eosinophilic gastroenteritis (see Fig GI 26-5)	Generalized, irregular fold thickening.	Characteristic clinical pattern of food allergies and peripheral eosinophilia.
Zollinger-Ellison syndrome (Fig GI 31-1)	Extreme prominence of gastric rugae, irregular thickening of folds in the proximal small bowel, and often ulcerations in unusual locations in the distal duodenum or jejunum.	Hyperrugosity reflects a hypersecretory state in response to a gastrin-secreting islet cell tumor of the pancreas. An excessive volume of acidic gastric secretions floods the small bowel and produces chemical enteritis.
Ménétrier's disease (see Fig GI 11-5)	Giant hypertrophy of gastric rugae and diffuse regular thickening of small bowel folds.	Protein-losing enteropathy associated with giant gastric folds. Hypoproteinemia results in regular thickening of small bowel folds.
Gastric varices with hypoproteinemia (see Figs GI 11-8 and GI 11-9)	Gastric varices with diffuse regular thickening of small bowel folds.	Gastric varices (prominent rugae or nodular fundal masses) reflect severe liver disease, which causes hypoproteinemia that results in regular thickening of small bowel folds.
Amyloidosis/Whipple's disease (Fig GI 31-2)	Generalized, irregular fold thickening.	Both conditions can also infiltrate the wall of the distal stomach and narrow the antrum.

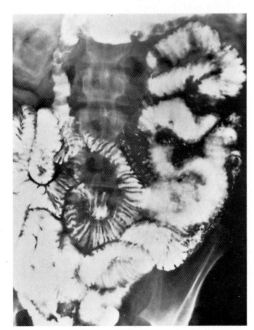

Fig GI 31-1
Zollinger-Ellison syndrome. In addition to prominent thickening of gastric and duodenal folds, there is dilatation of the small bowel with excessive secretions causing the barium to have a granular, indistinct quality.

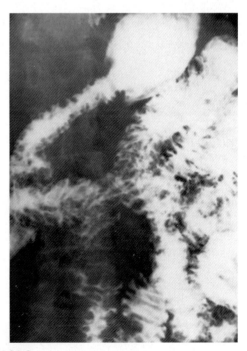

Fig GI 31-2
Amyloidosis. Diffuse thickening of mucosal folds involving the stomach, duodenum, and visualized small bowel. Infiltration of amyloid into the wall of the distal stomach narrows the antrum.

Coned Cecum

Condition	Imaging Findings	Comments
Amebiasis (Fig GI 32-1)	Initially, small shallow ulcers produce a finely granular mucosa and an irregular bowel margin. Eventually, the ileocecal valve is thickened, rigid, and fixed in an open position.	Cone shape represents fibrotic narrowing of the cecum, which is involved in approximately 90% of cases of chronic amebiasis. Terminal ileum is not involved (unlike Crohn's disease or tuberculosis). Rapid return to normal appearance after antiamebic therapy.
Crohn's disease (Fig GI 32-2)	Narrowing and rigidity of the cecum.	Terminal ileum almost invariably involved, often with a thin, linear collection of barium (string sign) representing incomplete filling due to the irritability and spasm accompanying the severe ulceration. CT may demonstrate a target appearance of the thickened cecal wall.

A

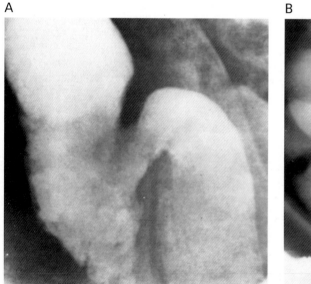

B

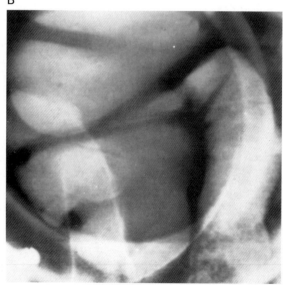

Fig GI 32-1
Amebiasis. (A) The small, shallow ulcers produce an irregular bowel margin and finely granular mucosa. The terminal ileum is not involved. (B) After a course of antiamebic therapy, the cecum returns to a normal appearance.

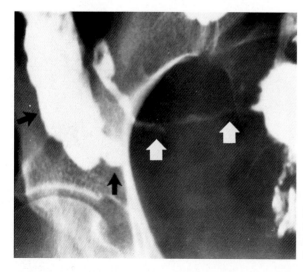

Fig GI 32-2
Crohn's disease. In addition to rigid narrowing of the cecum (black arrows), there is incomplete filling of the terminal ileum (string sign; white arrows).

Condition	Imaging Findings	Comments
Tuberculosis (Fig GI 32-3)	Shortening and narrowing of the purse-shaped cecum.	Usually there is involvement of the terminal ileum, which may appear to empty directly into the stenotic ascending colon with nonopacification of the fibrotic, contracted cecum (Stierlin's sign).
Ulcerative colitis (Fig GI 32-4)	Cecal narrowing usually limited to a short segment.	Terminal ileum involvement (backwash ileitis) in 10% to 25% of cases. Gaping ileocecal valve.
Appendicitis (see Fig GI 33-1)	Eccentric defect at the base of the cecum, most commonly on its medial aspect.	Appendiceal abscess can impress the cecum and produce a cone-shaped appearance.
Carcinoma of cecum (Fig GI 32-5)	Stiffness and rigidity of the cecal wall.	Cecum may be narrowed because of either the tumor itself or an inflammatory reaction from necrosis and perforation of the tumor. Perforated cecal carcinoma should be included in the differential diagnosis of right lower quadrant pain in patients more than 50 years old. A confident CT diagnosis can be made in the presence of contiguous organ invasion, malignant peritoneal implants, and distant metastases.

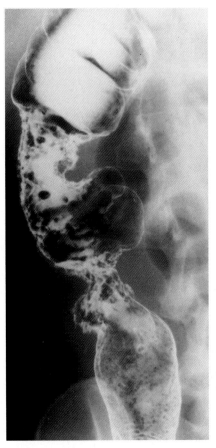

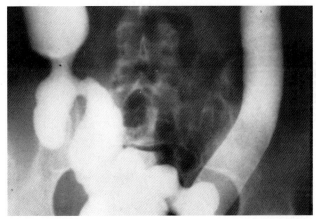

Fig GI 32-4
Ulcerative colitis. Concentric narrowing of the cecum with a gaping ileocecal valve.

Fig GI 32-3
Tuberculosis. The cecum is fibrotic and contracted, the ileocecal valve is irregular, gaping, and incompetent, and the terminal ileum appears to empty directly into the ascending colon (Stierlin's sign). Note the diffuse ulcerations in the ascending colon and the lymphoid follicles in the terminal ileum.[39]

Condition	Imaging Findings	Comments
Perforated cecal diverticulum (Fig GI 32-6)	Extrinsic impression narrowing the cecum.	Walled-off pericecal abscess (mimicking acute appendicitis) from a perforated cecal diverticulum (which is uncommon, frequently solitary, and usually situated within 2 cm of the ileocecal valve). CT demonstrates mild asymmetric thickening of the cecal wall and focal pericolic inflammation; the presence of diverticula supports the diagnosis. Differentiation of cecal diverticulitis from appendicitis or perforated carcinoma may be difficult if the normal appendix is not seen or if a prominent soft-tissue mass component is present, respectively.
Actinomycosis	Inflammatory narrowing of the cecum.	Uncommon infection. The combination of a palpable abdominal mass and an indolent sinus tract draining through the abdominal wall is highly suggestive of this condition.
South American blastomycosis	Narrowing and rigidity of the cecum.	Granulomatous fungal disease caused by *Paracoccidioides brasiliensis* that also usually involves the terminal ileum (mimics Crohn's disease).
Anisakiasis (Fig GI 32-7)	Narrowing and rigidity of the cecum.	Caused by an ascaris-like nematode in patients eating raw fish (especially in Japan, Holland, and Scandinavia). Terminal ileum often involved.
Typhoid fever/ *Yersinia* enterocolitis (Figs GI 32-8 and GI 32-9)	Narrowing and irregularity of the cecum.	Most severe inflammatory changes usually involve the terminal ileum.

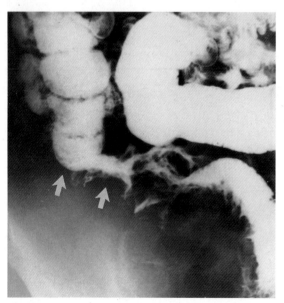

Fig GI 32-5
Carcinoma of the cecum. Severe narrowing and rigidity (arrows) give the radiographic appearance of a coned cecum. Note the extension of the process to involve the terminal ileum.

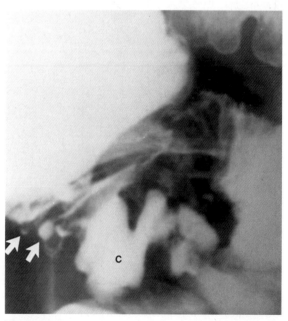

Fig GI 32-6
Cecal diverticulitis. Deformity and contraction of the cecum on a barium enema examination performed approximately 3 weeks after the onset of symptoms in a 27-year-old man. Several diverticula (arrows) are seen along the lateral wall of the cecum (C).[40]

Condition	Imaging Findings	Comments
Cytomegalovirus	Narrowing and rigidity of the cecum.	Opportunistic infections in patients with AIDS or other disorders that compromise the immune system.
Treated leukemia/lymphoma	Irritability and distortion of the cecum.	Rare, but well-recognized, complication (especially in children). Most cases are probably related to progressive ulceration and infection by enteric organisms after potent antimetabolite therapy.

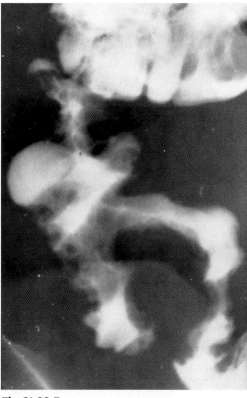

Fig GI 32-7
Anisakiasis. Severe inflammatory changes in the cecum, ascending colon, and ileocecal valve in a patient who developed severe abdominal pain after eating raw fish.

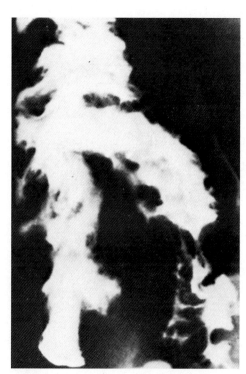

Fig GI 32-8
Typhoid fever. Nodularity and irregularity of the terminal ileum with deformity of the cecum. There was a rapid return to a normal appearance after appropriate therapy.[41]

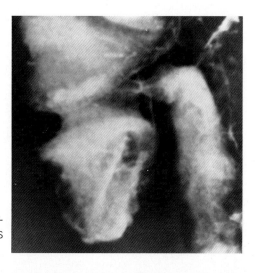

Fig GI 32-9
***Yersinia* enterocolitis.** Conical narrowing and irregular margins of the cecum are present with mild inflammatory changes in the terminal ileum.

Filling Defects in the Cecum

Condition	Imaging Findings	Comments
Appendicitis/appendiceal abscess (Figs GI 33-1 and GI 33-2)	Irregular extrinsic impression at the base of the cecum associated with the failure of barium to enter the appendix. If the appendix is retrocecal, the cecal impression is more proximal and is usually on its lateral aspect.	Appendicolith is virtually diagnostic and is associated with a high incidence of complications (especially perforation and abscess formation). Failure of barium to fill the appendix is not a reliable sign of appendicitis (occurs in 20% of normal patients).
Crohn's disease	Large extrinsic mass impinging on the cecal tip and the medial cecal wall.	Crohn's disease is rarely limited to the appendix with no evidence of terminal ileal involvement.
Inverted appendiceal stump (Fig GI 33-3)	Smooth filling defect at the base of the cecum in the expected site of the appendix.	Often very prominent for several weeks after surgery until the postoperative edema and inflammation subside. May be indistinguishable from a neoplasm, especially if lobulated or irregular.

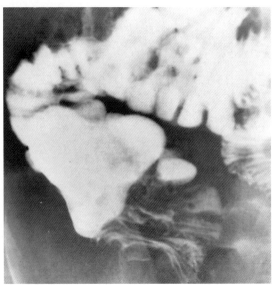

Fig GI 33-1
Periappendiceal abscess. There is fixation and a mass effect at the base of the cecum with no filling of the appendix.

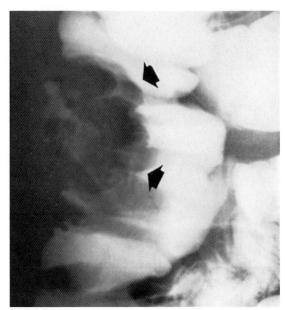

Fig GI 33-2
Periappendiceal abscess. Severe inflammatory mucosal changes and a mass effect on the lateral aspect of the ascending colon (arrows) in a patient with a ruptured retrocecal appendix.

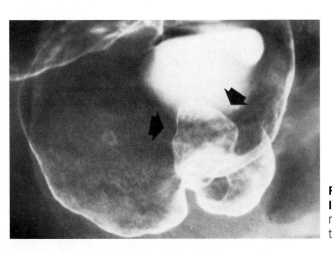

Fig GI 33-3
Inverted appendiceal stump. In this example, the mass (arrows) is large and irregular, simulating a neoplasm at the base of the cecum.

Condition	Imaging Findings	Comments
Mucocele of appendix (Fig GI 33-4)	Sharply outlined, smooth-walled, broad-based filling defect indenting the lower part of the cecum. Usually on the medial side and associated with nonfilling of the appendix.	May result from proximal luminal obstruction or represent a mucinous cystadenoma. May have a mottled or rimlike calcification around the periphery. Rupture of a mucocele of the appendix (or ovary) can lead to the development of pseudomyxoma peritonei.
Myxoglobulosis	Smooth extramucosal mass impressing the cecum that is associated with the failure of barium to enter the appendix.	Rare type of mucocele composed of multiple round or oval translucent globules mixed with mucus. Characteristic finding is a calcified rim about the periphery of individual globules.
Intussusception of appendix (Fig GI 33-5)	Oval, round, or finger-like filling defect projecting into the medial wall of the cecum. Appendix is not visible.	Invagination of the appendix into the cecum that simulates a cecal tumor. Can present as an acute surgical emergency or as a subacute recurring condition.
Benign neoplasm of appendix	Small filling defect (rarely diagnosed radiographically).	Approximately 90% are carcinoids (almost always benign; rarely metastasize or cause the carcinoid syndrome). Others are spindle cell tumors.
Malignant neoplasm of appendix (Fig GI 33-6)	Extrinsic mass deforming and displacing the cecum.	Most appendiceal malignancies are adenocarcinomas. Extensive tumor may form an acute angle between the mass and the adjacent cecal wall and mimic an intramural or even an intraluminal cecal mass.
Metastases (Fig GI 33-7)	Localized defect on the medial aspect of the cecum below the ileocecal valve.	Primary pancreatic carcinoma typically spreads along the mesentery to this region. Intraperitoneal seeding from carcinoma of the ovary, colon, or stomach can cause an extrinsic impression in the region of the ileocecal junction or on the lateral and posterior aspects of the cecum.

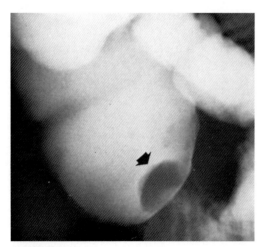

Fig GI 33-4
Mucocele of the appendix. Smooth, broad-based filling defect (arrow) indents the lower medial part of the cecum. There is no filling of the appendix with barium.

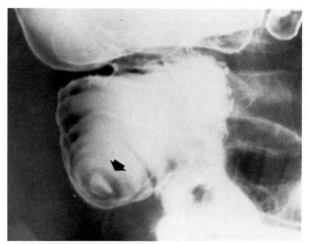

Fig GI 33-5
Intussusception of the appendix (arrow). After reduction, the cecum and appendix appeared normal on another barium enema examination.

Condition	Imaging Findings	Comments
General colonic lesions	Various patterns of filling defects.	Inflammatory masses (especially ameboma), benign and malignant primary cecal neoplasms, and ileocecal intussusception.
Ileocecal diverticulitis (see Fig GI 32-4)	Smooth eccentric mass that is sharply demarcated from the adjacent colonic wall.	Localized mural abscess in the wall of the colon that often occurs in young patients (unlike colonic diverticulitis) and mimics acute appendicitis. There may be extraluminal barium in a fistula or abscess cavity.
Solitary benign cecal ulcer (Fig GI 33-8)	Filling defect simulating a discrete tumor mass.	Mass represents granulation tissue caused by the healing of a solitary benign ulcer of the cecum (the ulcer itself is infrequently detected).

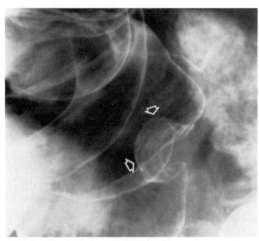

Fig GI 33-6
Adenocarcinoma of the appendix. The extensive tumor produces a large mass (arrows) that mimics an intraluminal cecal neoplasm.

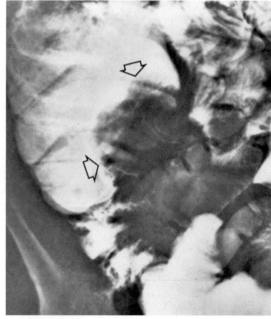

Fig GI 33-7
Carcinoma of the pancreas metastatic to the cecum. There is a localized extrinsic pressure defect (arrows) on the medial and inferior aspects of the cecum and no filling of the appendix.

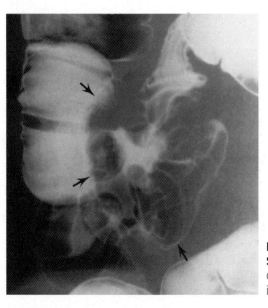

Fig GI 33-8
Solitary benign ulcer of the cecum. Lobular soft-tissue mass centered at the ileocecal valve (arrows) with a central irregular barium collection representing ulceration.[42]

Condition	Imaging Findings	Comments
Adherent fecalith (Fig GI 33-9)	Persistent tumorlike mass in the cecum.	Sticky fecal material that is most commonly found in patients with cystic fibrosis and simulates a colonic neoplasm.
Endometriosis	Intramural, extramucosal lesion with a smooth surface and sharp margins.	Rarely associated with the fibrotic compression and kinking of the colon that are characteristic of the disease in the sigmoid region.
Burkitt's lymphoma (Fig GI 33-10)	Large mass in the ileocecal area.	Childhood tumor of the reticuloendothelial system that may cause intussusception or obstruction (primarily reported in the North American variety).

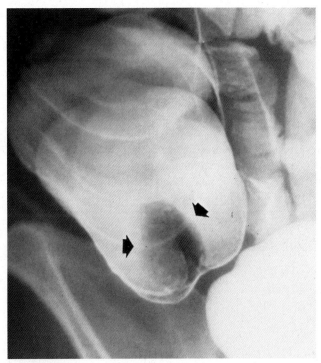

Fig GI 33-9
Adherent fecalith (arrows) in cystic fibrosis.

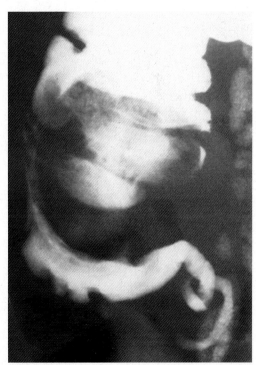

Fig GI 33-10
Burkitt's lymphoma. A huge mass fills essentially the entire cecum.[10]

Ulcerative Lesions of the Colon

Condition	Imaging Findings	Comments
Ulcerative colitis (Fig GI 34-1)	Initially, fine mucosal granularity. Later, discrete ulcers of various sizes symmetrically distributed around the bowel wall.	Primarily involves the rectosigmoid, though pancolitis can occur. Mild involvement of the terminal ileum (backwash ileitis) in 10% to 25% of cases. Complications include colon carcinoma, stricture formation, perforation, and toxic megacolon.
Crohn's colitis (Fig GI 34-2)	Initially, aphthous ulcers on a background of normal mucosa. Later, random and asymmetric distribution of deep, irregular ulcers.	Primarily affects the proximal colon. Terminal ileal involvement in approximately 80% of cases. Non-continuous skip lesions are common (never occur in ulcerative colitis) and fistulas and sinus tracts are characteristic.
Ischemic colitis (Fig GI 34-3)	Initially, fine superficial ulceration. Later, deep penetrating ulcers may occur.	Characteristic clinical presentation (abrupt onset of lower abdominal pain and rectal bleeding). Most patients are older than age 50 (except women taking birth control pills). Usually involves a relatively short segment (pancolitis can occur) and returns to a normal appearance (postischemic strictures can develop).
Infectious colitides Amebiasis (Fig GI 34-4)	Initially, superficial ulcerations especially involving the cecum. Later, deep penetrating ulcers may produce a bizarre appearance.	May present as a segmental process with skip lesions (simulating Crohn's disease) or as a diffuse colitis mimicking ulcerative colitis. The terminal ileum is virtually never involved.

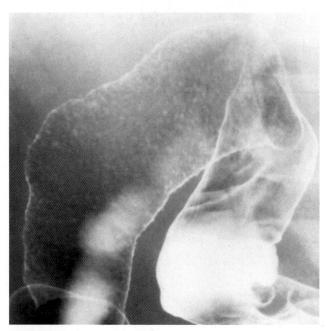

Fig GI 34-1
Early ulcerative colitis. Fine granularity of the mucosa reflects the hyperemia and edema that are seen endoscopically.

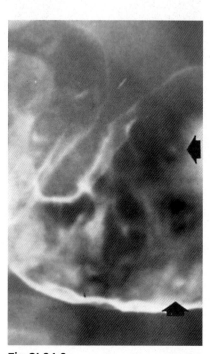

Fig GI 34-2
Aphthoid ulcers of early Crohn's colitis. Punctate collections of barium are surrounded by lucent halos of edema (arrows).

Condition	Imaging Findings	Comments
Schistosomiasis	Diffuse granular pattern of tiny ulcerations simulating ulcerative colitis.	Primarily involves the descending and sigmoid colon (adult worms have a predilection for invading the inferior mesenteric vein). Multiple, small filling defects constitute a more characteristic appearance.
Shigellosis/salmonellosis (Fig GI 34-5)	Initially, diffuse fine ulcerations. Later, deep ulceration.	Frequently, it is impossible to distinguish the colonic involvement of shigellosis (bacillary dysentery) from salmonellosis (food poisoning, typhoid fever). Involvement of the terminal ileum strongly suggests salmonellosis.

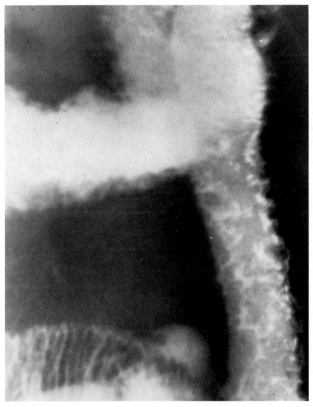

Fig GI 34-3
Ischemic colitis. Superficial ulcers and inflammatory edema produce a serrated outer margin of the barium-filled colon simulating ulcerative colitis.

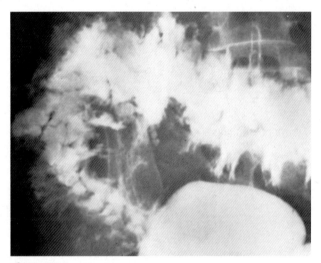

Fig GI 34-4
Amebic colitis. Deep, penetrating ulcers produce a bizarre appearance.

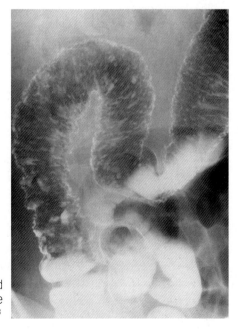

Fig GI 34-5
***Salmonella* colitis.** Multiple small ulcers and a stippled appearance representing fine ulcerations or erosions are diffusely visible in the ascending and transverse colon.[43]

Condition	Imaging Findings	Comments
Tuberculous colitis	Appearance virtually indistinguishable from that of Crohn's disease.	Predominantly involves the cecum with concomitant disease in the distal ileum. May extend to affect the ascending and transverse colon. There is rarely segmental involvement in the sigmoid region.
Gonorrheal proctitis	Rectal ulceration and mucosal edema.	Barium enema examination is usually normal.
Staphylococcal colitis	Generalized ulcerating colitis.	Cause of postantibiotic diarrhea after orally administered broad-spectrum antibiotics (usually tetracycline).
Yersinia colitis (see Fig GI 32-7)	Multiple small colonic ulcerations.	Primarily involves the terminal ileum and cecum (often indistinguishable from Crohn's colitis).
Campylobacter fetus colitis	Ulcerative colitis pattern.	Most common cause of specific infectious colitis. Usually self-limited and probably responsible for most single episodes of alleged ulcerative colitis.
Fungal infections	Mucosal ulcerations are occasionally identified.	Histoplasmosis, mucormycosis, actinomycosis, and candidiasis. More typical appearance is irritable bowel with irregularly thickened mucosal folds.
Lymphogranuloma venereum	Multiple shaggy ulcers primarily involving the rectum.	Venereal disease (especially common in the tropics). A rectal stricture typically develops, and fistulas and sinus tracts often occur.
Herpes zoster	Segmental ulcerating colitis.	Typical clinical history and skin lesions.
Cytomegalovirus	Ulceration primarily involves the cecum.	Major cause of severe lower gastrointestinal bleeding in patients with AIDS and in renal transplant recipients undergoing immunosuppressive therapy.
Strongyloidiasis	Diffuse ulcerating colitis.	Unusual manifestation due to larval invasion of the colon wall.
Pseudomembranous colitis (Fig GI 34-6)	Diffuse irregular ulceration associated with multiple, flat, raised lesions.	Follows drug administration (tetracycline, penicillin, ampicillin, clindamycin, and lincomycin). May reflect infection by a resistant strain of *Clostridium difficile*. The clinical hallmark is a severe debilitating diarrhea.
Radiation injury (see Fig GI 35-6)	Fine superficial (occasionally deep) ulceration, primarily involving the rectosigmoid region.	Usually follows pelvic irradiation for carcinoma of the cervix, endometrium, ovary, bladder, or prostate. Strictures and fistulas often develop.
Caustic colitis (see Fig GI 35-8)	Severe ulcerating process after an irritating enema (soapsuds, detergents).	Irritant enema tends to produce spasm of the rectosigmoid, resulting in rapid expulsion of the solution from this segment. Because the fluid trapped in the proximal colon is not promptly expelled, corrosive damage is most severe in this region.
Pancreatitis (Fig GI 34-7)	Pattern of ulcerating colitis involving the superior margin of the transverse colon and the splenic flexure.	Close anatomic relation between the pancreas and transverse colon provides a pathway for the dissemination of pancreatic inflammatory products.

Condition	Imaging Findings	Comments
Adenocarcinoma of colon (Fig GI 34-8)	Various patterns of ulceration.	May present as an excavation in a large fungating mass or as mucosal destruction in an annular apple-core tumor.

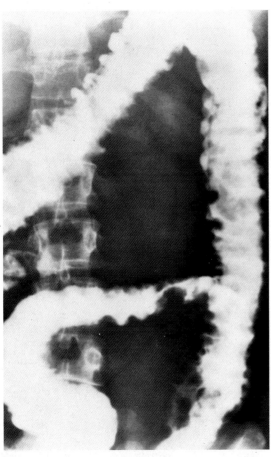

Fig GI 34-6
Pseudomembranous colitis. The shaggy and irregular margins reflect the pseudomembrane and superficial necrosis with mucosal ulceration.

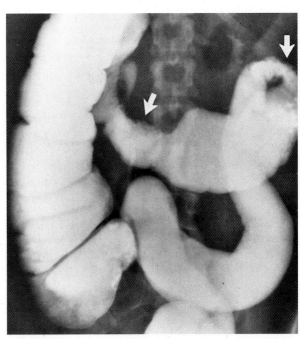

Fig GI 34-7
Pancreatitis. Spiculation of the proximal transverse colon and splenic flexure (arrows) simulates an ulcerating colitis.

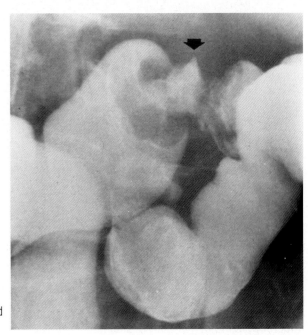

Fig GI 34-8
Ulcerated primary carcinoma of the sigmoid colon (arrow).

Condition	Imaging Findings	Comments
Metastases (Figs GI 34-9 and GI 34-10)	Various patterns of ulceration.	May produce marginal and deep ulcerations associated with nodular masses and multiple eccentric strictures.
Behçet's syndrome	Various patterns of ulceration (segmental involvement by multiple discrete ulcers; diffuse ulceration).	Uncommon multiple-system disease characterized by ulceration of the buccal and genital mucosa, ocular inflammation, and a variety of skin lesions. Colitis often leads to perforation or hemorrhage.
Solitary rectal ulcer syndrome	Usually a single ulceration within 15 cm of the anal verge.	Primarily occurs in young patients complaining of rectal bleeding and may lead to stricturing. Often difficult to distinguish from inflammatory bowel disease or malignancy.
Nonspecific benign ulceration of colon (Fig GI 34-11)	Usually single (20% are multiple) ulcer primarily involving the cecum and ascending colon in the region of the ileocecal valve.	Associated intense inflammatory reaction produces a mass-like effect simulating carcinoma. Suggested causes include peptic ulceration, solitary diverticulitis, mucosal trauma, infection, and vascular disease.
Amyloidosis	Nonspecific ulcerating colitis.	Histologic material and special amyloid stains (Congo red) required for diagnosis.
Inorganic mercury poisoning	Nonspecific ulcerating colitis.	Clinical history and concomitant renal involvement are usually diagnostic.

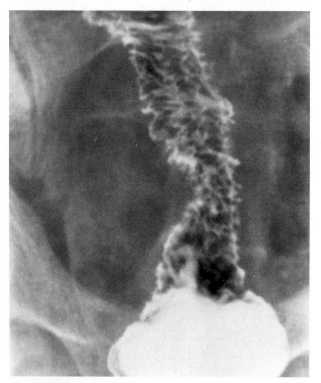

Fig GI 34-9
Carcinoma of the prostate metastatic to the rectum and rectosigmoid. The diffuse circumferential ulceration mimics ulcerative colitis.

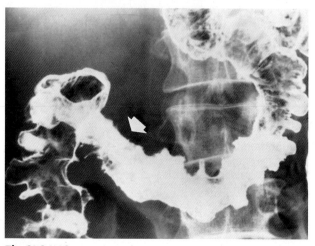

Fig GI 34-10
Carcinoma of the stomach metastatic to the transverse colon. Localized right-sided ulceration and narrowing (arrow) simulate Crohn's colitis.

Condition	Imaging Findings	Comments
Drug-induced colitis	Nonspecific ulcerating colitis.	Cancer chemotherapeutic agents, methyldopa, nonsteroidal anti-inflammatory agents, cimetidine, the antifungal agent flucytosine, and elemental gold.
Collagenous colitis	Fine mucosal granularity that predominantly involves the rectosigmoid region.	Chronic or intermittent watery diarrhea, often with colicky abdominal pain, that usually occurs in middle-aged or older women.
Diversion colitis	Nonspecific ulcerating colitis.	Inflammation in a segment of colon that has been surgically isolated from the fecal stream by placement of a proximal colostomy or ileostomy.
Postrectal biopsy	Shallow, ring-like ulcer surrounded by a radiolucent elevation.	May be seen on barium enema examinations performed within several days following rectal biopsy or polypectomy.

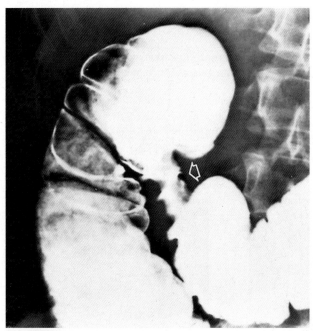

Fig GI 34-11
Nonspecific benign ulcer of the colon. Area of narrowing in the proximal transverse colon with ulceration along its inferior aspect and marginal spiculation (arrow).[44]

Narrowing of the Colon

Condition	Imaging Findings	Comments
Ulcerative colitis (Figs GI 35-1 and GI 35-2)	Rigidity and narrowing of the bowel lumen ("lead pipe" colon) with foreshortening.	Colonic strictures with smooth contours and pliable, tapering margins occur in up to 10% of patients. Carcinoma in these patients can have an indistinguishable appearance.
Crohn's colitis (Fig GI 35-3)	Narrowing and stricture formation.	May appear identical to ulcerative colitis, though there are usually characteristic features of Crohn's disease elsewhere (deep ulcerations, pseudopolyposis, skip lesions, sinus tracts, fistulas).
Infectious colitides Ischemic colitis (Fig GI 35-4)	Short segment of tubular narrowing.	Rectum is rarely involved because of its excellent collateral blood supply. May produce an annular constricting lesion simulating malignancy.
Amebiasis (Fig GI 35-5)	Annular constriction (ameboma) simulating malignancy.	Localized granulomatous mass. Factors favoring ameboma rather than malignancy include multiplicity, longer length and pliability of the lesion, and rapid improvement on antiamebic therapy.
Schistosomiasis	Segmental narrowing, primarily involving the sigmoid colon.	Stenosing granulomatous process simulating Crohn's disease or colonic malignancy.
Bacillary dysentery	Segmental rigidity and tubular narrowing.	Repeated episodes can produce a pattern simulating chronic ulcerative colitis.

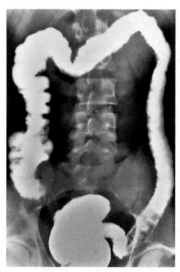

Fig GI 35-1
Chronic ulcerative colitis. Fibrosis and muscular spasm cause shortening and rigidity of the colon and a loss of haustral markings.

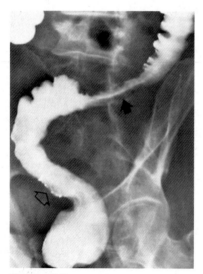

Fig GI 35-2
Benign stricture in chronic ulcerative colitis. In addition to the severe narrowing in the sigmoid colon (closed arrow), there are ulcerative changes in the upper rectum and proximal sigmoid colon (open arrow).

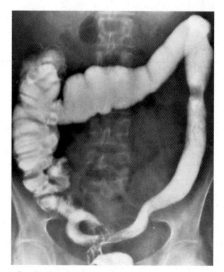

Fig GI 35-3
Chronic Crohn's colitis. Foreshortening and loss of haustra involving the colon distal to the hepatic flexure simulate the appearance of chronic ulcerative colitis.

Condition	Imaging Findings	Comments
Tuberculosis	Segmental narrowing and rigidity.	May produce an annular ulcerating lesion mimicking carcinoma.
Lymphogranuloma venereum (see Fig GI 39-2)	Rectal stricture beginning just above the anus.	Varies from a short isolated narrowing to a long stenotic segment with multiple deep ulcers. There are often associated fistulas and sinus tracts.
Other infectious causes	Various patterns of narrowing.	Herpes zoster; cytomegalovirus (in renal transplant patients undergoing immunosuppressive therapy or in those with AIDS); strongyloidiasis; fungal infestations.
Radiation injury (Fig GI 35-6)	Long smooth stricture of the rectum and sigmoid colon.	Develops 6 to 24 months after irradiation. Probably related to chronic ischemia caused by an obliterative arteritis in the bowel wall. A short, irregular, radiation-induced stricture can mimic malignancy.

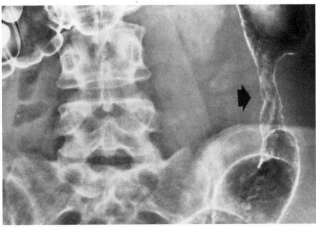

Fig GI 35-4
Ischemic colitis. A stricture in the descending colon (arrow) followed healing of the ischemic episode.[45]

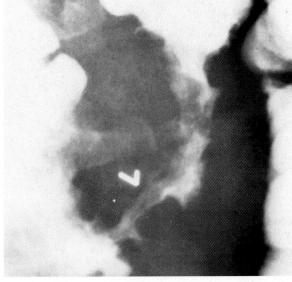

Fig GI 35-5
Amebiasis. Irregular constricting lesion in the transverse colon. The relatively long area of involvement tends to favor an inflammatory etiology.

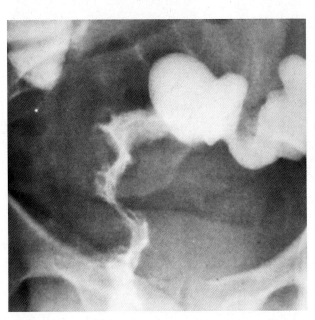

Fig GI 35-6
Radiation injury. Smooth stricture of the rectosigmoid developed 18 months after irradiation.

Condition	Imaging Findings	Comments
Cathartic colon (Fig GI 35-7)	Bizarre contractions and inconstant areas of narrowing, primarily involving the right colon.	Due to the prolonged use of stimulant and irritant cathartics, especially in women of middle age. May mimic "burned-out" chronic ulcerative colitis.
Caustic colitis (Fig GI 35-8)	Stricture formation primarily involving the transverse and descending colon.	Fibrosis with luminal narrowing is a late complication.
Solitary rectal ulcer syndrome	Rectal stricture.	Without previous evidence of mucosal nodularity or ulceration, it may be impossible to differentiate this condition from inflammatory bowel disease, lymphogranuloma venereum, or rectal malignancy.
Nonspecific benign ulcer of colon (see Fig GI 34-10)	Smooth or irregular area of narrowing, most frequently involving the cecum.	May be radiographically indistinguishable from carcinoma. Perforation and hemorrhage are complications.
Colonic "sphincters"	Transient areas of narrowing, primarily in the transverse, descending, and sigmoid portions.	Areas of spasm that probably reflect localized nerve and muscle imbalance. Unlike annular carcinoma, colonic sphincters change on sequential films, have tapering margins and intact mucosa, and usually can be relieved by intravenous glucagon.
Annular carcinoma of colon (Fig GI 35-9)	Short segment of luminal narrowing with an abrupt change from tumor to normal bowel (overhanging margins).	Initially produces a flat plaque of tumor (saddle lesion) involving only a portion of the circumference of the colon wall. In the sigmoid, an apple-core lesion may be difficult to distinguish from diverticulitis (annular carcinoma tends to be shorter with more sharply defined margins and mucosal destruction).

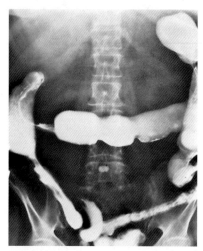

Fig GI 35-7
Cathartic colon. Bizarre contractions with irregular areas of narrowing primarily involve the right colon. Although the ileocecal valve is gaping, simulating ulcerative colitis, no ulcerations are identified.

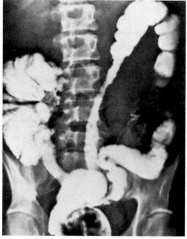

Fig GI 35-8
Caustic colitis. Narrowing of the midtransverse colon 2 months after a detergent enema.[46]

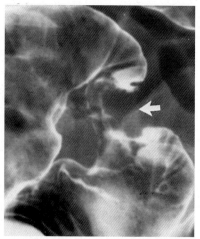

Fig GI 35-9
Annular carcinoma of the sigmoid colon. The relatively short lesion (arrow) has sharply defined proximal and distal margins.

Condition	Imaging Findings	Comments
Scirrhous carcinoma of colon (Fig GI 35-10)	Long segment (up to 12 cm) of luminal narrowing due to intense desmoplastic reaction infiltrating the bowel wall.	Rare variant of annular carcinoma with a very poor prognosis. Unlike the more common annular form, the mucosa in scirrhous carcinoma is often partially preserved and the margins of the lesion tend to taper.
Metastases (Figs GI 35-11 and GI 35-12)	Various patterns of narrowing. May be associated with ulceration, extrinsic masses, and a "striped colon" (transverse folds that do not completely traverse the colonic lumen).	Metastases to the colon can arise from direct invasion (prostate, ovary, uterus; stomach and pancreas via mesenteric reflections), intraperitoneal seeding (especially involving the pouch of Douglas, inferomedial border of the cecum, right paracolic gutter, and sigmoid mesocolon), hematogenous spread (especially breast carcinoma; infrequently lung and melanoma), or lymphangitic spread.

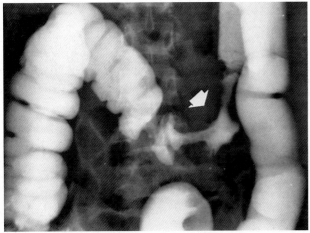

Fig GI 35-10
Scirrhous carcinoma of the colon. The long, circumferentially narrowed area (arrow) simulates segmental colonic encasement due to metastatic disease.

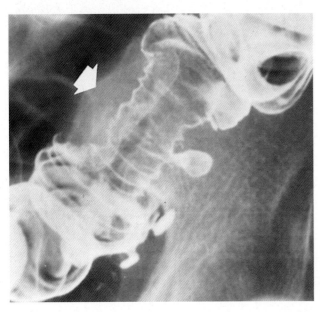

Fig GI 35-11
Intraperitoneal metastases from carcinoma of the pancreas. The nodular mass in the region of the pouch of Douglas (arrows) was clinically palpable (Blumer's shelf).

Fig GI 35-12
Intraperitoneal seeding of undifferentiated carcinoma involving the sigmoid mesocolon. There is a mass effect and tethering localized to the superior border of the sigmoid colon (arrow).

Condition	Imaging Findings	Comments
Carcinoma complicating other conditions (Fig GI 35-13)	Various patterns of narrowing.	Ulcerative colitis (filiform stricture); Crohn's colitis (fungating mass); ureterosigmoidostomy (adjacent to the urine-diverting stoma).
Carcinoid tumor	Infiltrating, constricting lesion.	Infrequent presentation (usually produces a polypoid mass).
Lymphoma	Localized annular narrowing.	Rare presentation (more commonly a polypoid mass or diffuse infiltration).
Diverticulitis (Fig GI 35-14)	Eccentric narrowing or severe spasm. Definitive diagnosis requires evidence of diverticular perforation (extravasation or a pericolic mass due to a localized abscess).	May be indistinguishable from carcinoma (diverticulitis is usually longer with intact, though often distorted, mucosa and tapering margins).
Pancreatitis	Narrowing primarily involving the distal transverse colon and splenic flexure.	Reflects the spread of liberated digestive enzymes along the mesenteric attachments joining the pancreas and transverse colon. May simulate pancreatic or colon carcinoma.
Amyloidosis	Narrowing and rigidity, primarily in the rectum and sigmoid.	Thickening of the bowel wall due to direct mural deposition of amyloid or secondary to ischemic colitis. May mimic chronic ulcerative colitis.
Endometriosis	Smooth constriction, usually involving the rectosigmoid.	Occurs in women of childbearing age. May simulate malignancy but is usually longer with more tapering margins and an intact mucosa.

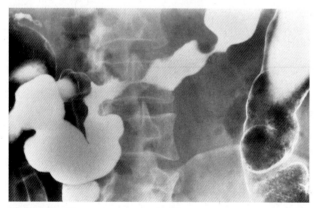

Fig GI 35-13
Carcinoma of the colon developing in a patient with long-standing chronic ulcerative colitis. There is a long, irregular lesion with a bizarre pattern in the transverse colon. Note the pseudopolyps in the visualized portion of the descending colon.

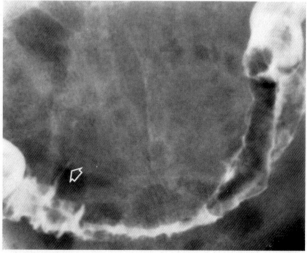

Fig GI 35-14
Acute sigmoid diverticulitis. Severe spasm of the sigmoid colon due to the intense adjacent inflammation. Note the thin projection of contrast material (arrow) representing extravasation from the colonic lumen.

Condition	Imaging Findings	Comments
Pelvic lipomatosis	Vertical elongation of the sigmoid colon with narrowing of the rectosigmoid. Increased pelvic lucency on plain films.	Benign increased deposition of normal, mature adipose tissue in the pelvis. Almost all cases occur in men. Teardrop bladder. The major complication is urinary tract obstruction.
Retractile mesenteritis (see Fig GI 29-5)	Narrowing of the rectosigmoid simulating pelvic carcinomatosis.	Rare condition in which fibroadipose proliferation causes thickening and retraction of the mesentery. Usually involves the small bowel rather than the colon.
Adhesive bands	Short, smooth areas of circumferential narrowing with normal mucosal contours.	Most bands are due to previous abdominal or pelvic surgery, though some are secondary to development of the mesentery or to inflammatory disease of the appendices epiploicae.
Site of surgical anastomosis	Smooth segmental narrowing.	Distensibility of the narrowed area and a history of previous surgery permit distinction from a malignant process.
Rectal suppository (Fig GI 35-15)	Smooth or irregular rectal narrowing.	Can develop after prolonged use of suppositories containing various analgesics.

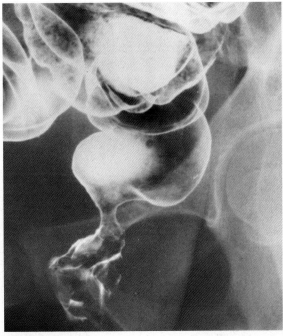

Fig GI 35-15
Rectal stenosis due to suppositories of Veganine.[47]

Filling Defects in the Colon

Condition	Imaging Findings	Comments
Hyperplastic polyp	Smooth, sessile mucosal elevation less than 5 mm in size.	Constitutes more than 90% of all colonic polyps. No malignant potential.
Adenomatous polyp (Fig GI 36-1)	Sessile, protuberant, or pedunculated appearance; often multiple. An increasing incidence with advancing age.	Premalignant condition. Adenomas measuring 5 to 9 mm have a 1% probability of containing invasive malignancy. Polyps measuring 1 to 2 cm have a 4% to 10% incidence of malignancy. Polyps more than 2 cm in diameter have a 20% to 40% incidence of malignancy.
Carcinoma (Fig GI 36-2)	Various appearances (saddle lesion, discrete intraluminal polyp, annular constriction). Often ulcerated. There is a 1% risk of multiple synchronous colon cancers and a 3% risk of metachronous cancers.	Signs of malignancy include large size; irregular or lobulated surface; retraction (puckering) of the colon wall on profile view; interval growth or change in shape; and short, thick, irregular stalk (if pedunculated).
Villous adenoma (Fig GI 36-3)	Bulky mass with barium filling the interstices of the tumor. Usually solitary.	Some 40% have infiltrating carcinoma (usually at the base). There may be mucous diarrhea causing severe fluid, protein, and electrolyte (especially potassium) depletion.
Lipoma (Fig GI 36-4)	Smooth submucosal filling defect that is usually single and most often involves the right colon.	Second most common benign colonic tumor. Fatty consistency makes the tumor changeable in size and shape with palpation. Other spindle cell tumors are rare.

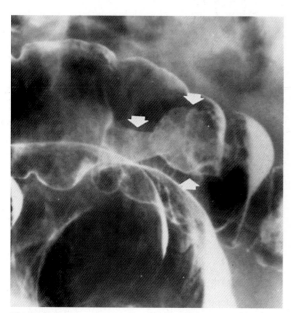

Fig GI 36-1
Pedunculated colonic polyp (arrows).

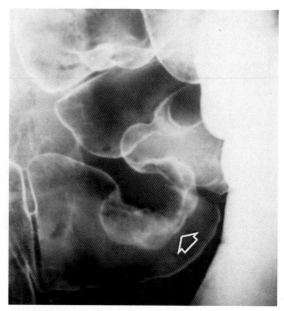

Fig GI 36-2
Saddle cancer of the colon. The tumor (arrow) appears to sit on the upper margin of the distal transverse colon like a saddle on a horse.

Condition	Imaging Findings	Comments
Carcinoid tumor (Fig GI 36-5)	Small (<1 cm), solitary, polypoid filling defect in the rectum.	Metastases develop in approximately 10% of patients (primarily when lesions are larger than 2 cm). Most are asymptomatic and found incidentally (rarely cause the carcinoid syndrome).

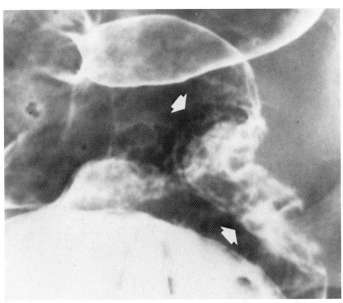

Fig GI 36-3
Benign villous adenoma of the rectum (arrows). Barium is seen filling the deep clefts between the multiple fronds.

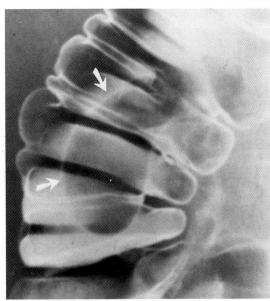

Fig GI 36-4
Lipoma. Ascending colon mass that is extremely lucent and has smooth margins and a teardrop shape (arrows).

A   B

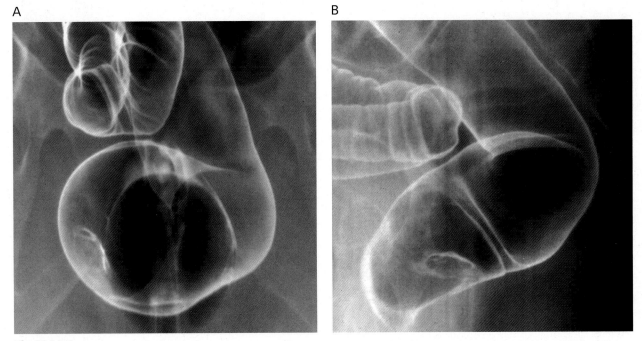

Fig GI 36-5
Rectal carcinoid. (A) Anteroposterior and (B) lateral spot radiographs show a smoothly marginated sessile polyp (arrow) on the right lateral wall of the rectum.[48]

Condition	Imaging Findings	Comments
Metastases (Figs GI 36-6 and GI 36-7)	Filling defects that are most commonly multiple.	Major primary sites include the breast, lung, stomach, ovary, pancreas, and uterus. Also melanoma.
Lymphoma (Fig GI 36-8)	Single (rarely multiple) bulky polypoid mass.	Unlike carcinoma, lymphoma often produces a large mass or extensively infiltrates a longer segment of the colon.

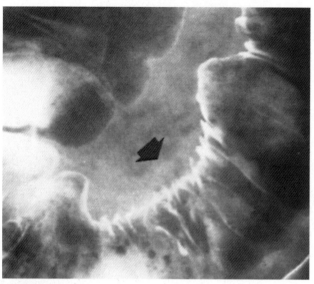

Fig GI 36-6
Carcinoma of the pancreas metastatic to the transverse colon. Shallow extrinsic pressure defect with multiple spiculations (arrow).

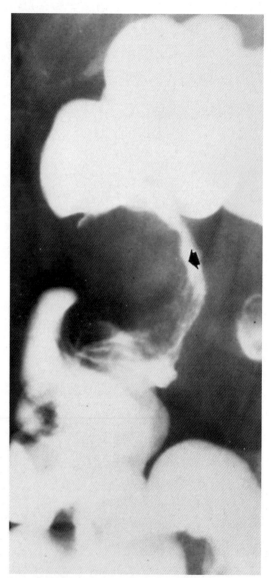

Fig GI 36-7
Carcinoma of the ovary metastatic to the ascending colon (arrow). Large mass mimicking an intramural, extramucosal tumor.

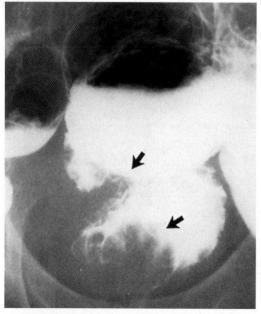

Fig GI 36-8
Lymphoma. Bulky, irregular, ulcerated mass involving much of the rectum (arrows).

Condition	Imaging Findings	Comments
Polyposis syndromes Familial polyposis (Figs GI 36-9 and GI 36-10)	Multiple adenomatous polyps.	Inherited disorder (autosomal dominant) with a 100% risk of developing colorectal cancer.
Gardner's syndrome (Fig GI 36-11)	Multiple adenomatous polyps.	Inherited disorder (autosomal dominant) with a 100% risk of developing colorectal cancer. There are often sinus osteomas and soft-tissue tumors.
Peutz-Jeghers syndrome	Multiple hamartomatous polyps (primarily involving the small bowel).	Inherited disorder (autosomal dominant) with no malignant potential (2% of patients develop gastrointestinal carcinoma elsewhere; 5% of women have ovarian cysts or tumors). Characteristic abnormal mucocutaneous pigmentation (especially affecting the lips and buccal mucosa).
Turcot syndrome	Multiple adenomatous polyps.	Extremely rare. Polyps are associated with brain tumors (usually supratentorial glioblastoma).

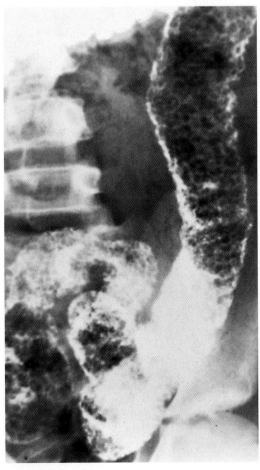

Fig GI 36-9
Familial polyposis.

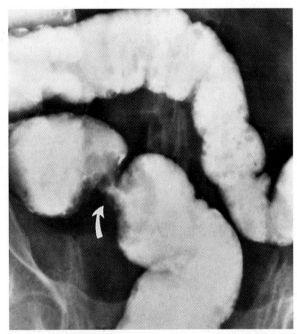

Fig GI 36-10
Carcinoma of the sigmoid (arrow) developing in a patient with long-standing familial polyposis.

Condition	Imaging Findings	Comments
Cronkhite-Canada syndrome	Multiple hamartomatous juvenile polyps.	No malignant potential. Presents later in life with malabsorption and severe diarrhea. Associate hyperpigmentation, alopecia, and atrophy of the fingernails and toenails.
Multiple juvenile polyps	Multiple hamartomatous polyps.	Childhood disorder with no malignant potential (polyps tend to autoamputate or regress). Surgery is indicated only if there are significant or repeated episodes of rectal bleeding or intussusception.
Cowden's disease	Multiple hamartomatous polyps.	Rare hereditary disorder associated with multiple malformations and tumors of various organs. Typically, there is circumoral papillomatosis and nodular gingival hyperplasia.
Neurocrest and colonic tumors	Multiple adenomatous polyps.	Associated with malignant tumors of neurocrest origin (pheochromocytoma; carcinoid; multiple endocrine neoplasia syndrome type II B with malignant medullary thyroid carcinoma).
Ruvalcaba-Myhre-Smith syndrome	Multiple hamartomatous polyps.	Rare inherited disorder (autosomal dominant) with macrocephaly and pigmented genital lesions.
Inflammatory pseudopolyposis (Fig GI 36-12)	Islands of hyperplastic, inflamed mucosa (between areas of ulceration) mimicking multiple filling defects. Occasionally a large single inflammatory pseudopolyp.	Most commonly a manifestation of ulcerative colitis and Crohn's colitis. Usually there is other radiographic evidence of the inflammatory process (ulceration, absence or irregularity of haustral folds, luminal narrowing) and a history of chronic diarrhea. A similar pattern may develop in infectious colitis (amebiasis, schistosomiasis, strongyloidiasis, and trichuriasis).
Ameboma	Single or multiple polypoid filling defects.	Focal hyperplastic granuloma (secondary bacterial infection of an amebic abscess in the bowel wall). Usually produces an annular, nondistensible lesion with irregular mucosa simulating colonic carcinoma.

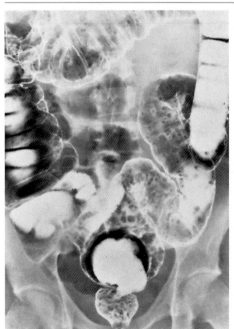

Fig GI 36-11
Gardner's syndrome. Innumerable adenomatous polyps throughout the colon present a radiographic appearance indistinguishable from that of familial polyposis.

Condition	Imaging Findings	Comments
Fecal material (Fig GI 36-13)	Innumerable filling defects or a single large, irregular intraluminal mass (impaction).	Usually freely movable (occasionally tightly adherent and resembling a polyp). Plain radiographs are usually diagnostic of fecal impaction (soft-tissue density in the rectum containing multiple small, irregular lucent areas reflecting pockets of gas in the fecal mass).
Other artifacts; foreign bodies	Bizarre array of multiple filling defects.	Air bubbles; mucous strands (long and slender); ingested foreign bodies.
Endometriosis (Fig GI 36-14)	Single or multiple intramural defects involving the sigmoid colon.	Extrauterine foci of endometrium in women of childbearing age. May cause pleating of the adjacent mucosa (secondary fibrosis) or present as a constricting lesion simulating annular carcinoma.
Intussusception (Fig GI 36-15)	Mass causing obstruction to the retrograde flow of barium. Often the characteristic coiled-spring appearance.	Most occur in children (younger than age 2) and are ileocolic without a specific leading point. Frequently can be reduced by the increased hydrostatic pressure of a carefully performed barium enema examination.
Gallstone (see Fig GI 53-2)	Filling defect in the rectum or distal sigmoid. May contain laminated calcification.	Rare. The gallstone enters the bowel via a cholecystoduodenal fistula (passing through the terminal ileum) or a direct cholecystocolic fistula.
Internal hemorrhoids (Fig GI 36-16)	Multiple rectal filling defects simulating polyps.	Usually associated with linear shadows of the veins from which they arise.

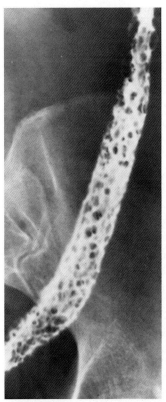

Fig GI 36-12
Inflammatory pseudopolyposis in Crohn's colitis.

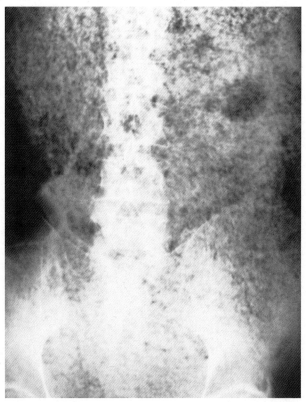

Fig GI 36-13
Fecal impaction.

Condition	Imaging Findings	Comments
Diverticulum	Barium-coated, air-filled diverticulum may mimic a filling defect.	Ring of barium coating a diverticulum has a smooth, well-defined outer border and a blurred, irregular inner border (opposite of a polyp). "Filling defects" can be projected clear of the colonic lumen on oblique views.
Pneumatosis intestinalis (see Fig GI 37-4)	Intramural collections of gas simulating multiple colonic polyps.	"Filling defects" are extremely lucent and change shape when the abdomen is palpated.
Colitis cystica profunda	Multiple, irregular filling defects in the rectosigmoid. Single rectal mass may mimic a sessile polyp.	Large submucosal, mucous epithelium–lined cysts involving a short segment of the bowel. Benign condition with no malignant potential.
Nodular lymphoid hyperplasia (Fig GI 36-17)	Multiple tiny nodular filling defects evenly distributed throughout the involved bowel.	Aggregates of lymphoid tissue that can simulate familial polyposis, pseudopolyposis of inflammatory bowel disease, or nodular lymphoma. Characteristic fleck of barium in the center of each "polyp" (umbilication at the apices of the lymphoid nodules).
Lymphoid follicular pattern (Fig GI 36-18)	Multiple tiny nodular filling defects evenly distributed throughout the involved bowel.	Normal finding in children. Also occurs in 10% to 15% of adults on double-contrast examination. No flecks of barium in the centers of the "polyps."
Cystic fibrosis	Multiple poorly defined filling defects simulating polyposis.	Adherent collections of viscid mucus that can rarely be adequately cleansed before a barium enema examination.
Submucosal edema pattern (Fig GI 36-19)	Large, round or polygonal, raised plaques in grossly dilated bowel.	Initially described as "colonic urticaria" (hypersensitivity reaction predominantly involving the right colon). Can also occur secondary to obstructing carcinoma, cecal volvulus, ischemia, colonic ileus, benign colonic obstruction, and herpes zoster infection.

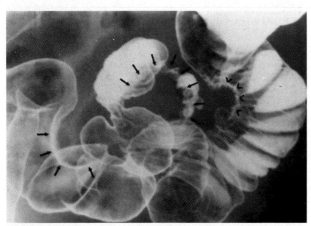

Fig GI 36-14
Endometriosis. Three separate endometrial implants (arrows and arrowheads) in the sigmoid colon. The most distal lesion has a smooth interface with the bowel wall, indicating no intramural invasion. The two more proximal lesions demonstrate crenulations indicating intramural or submucosal invasion.[49]

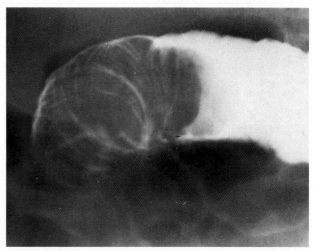

Fig GI 36-15
Intussusception. Obstruction of the colon at the hepatic flexure. Note the characteristic coiled-spring appearance.

Condition	Imaging Findings	Comments
Ulcerative pseudopolyps proximal to an obstruction	Prominent nodularity with pseudopolyp formation (simulates ulcerating colitis).	Probably caused by ischemia (due to distention of the bowel with decreased bowel flow). Bowel distal to the point of obstruction appears normal.
Amyloidosis	Single or multiple discrete filling defects.	Single collection of amyloid usually involves the rectum and simulates a neoplasm.
Other conditions	Various patterns.	Colonic varices, hypertrophied anal papilla, and extramedullary plasmacytoma.

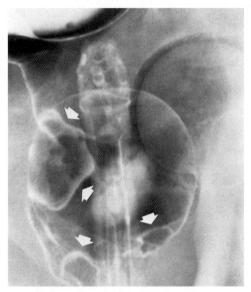

Fig GI 36-16
Internal hemorrhoids. Multiple rectal filling defects (arrows) simulate polyps.

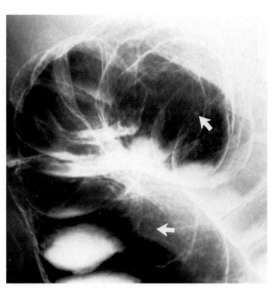

Fig GI 36-17
Nodular lymphoid hyperplasia. The arrows point to characteristic flecks of barium in the centers of several of the lymphoid masses.

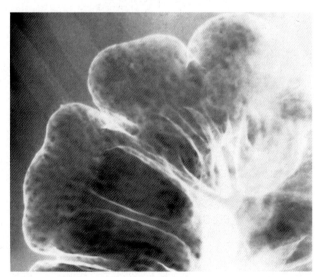

Fig GI 36-18
Lymphoid follicular pattern in an adult.[50]

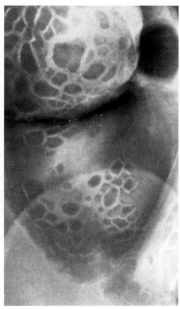

Fig GI 36-19
Colonic urticaria. Large polygonal, raised plaques in a dilated cecum and ascending colon.

Thumbprinting of the Colon*

Condition	Comments
Ischemic colitis (Fig GI 37-1)	Segmental involvement resulting from occlusive vascular disease or intramural hemorrhage (anticoagulant overdose, bleeding diathesis). Usually reverts to a normal radiographic appearance if good collateral circulation is established. May heal by stricture formation.
Ulcerative colitis and Crohn's colitis	Multiple symmetric contour defects simulating thumbprinting. Usually involves the rectum in ulcerative colitis (rectal involvement is infrequent in ischemic colitis). Transverse linear ulcers, skip areas, and terminal ileal disease suggest Crohn's colitis.
Infectious colitis	Rare manifestation of amebiasis, schistosomiasis, strongyloidiasis, salmonellosis, anisakiasis, and cytomegalovirus.
Pseudomembranous colitis (Fig GI 37-2)	Generalized thumbprinting involving the entire colon, unlike the segmental pattern in ischemic disease. Develops after a course of antibiotic therapy, with the thumbprinting reflecting marked thickening of the bowel wall.
Malignant lesion (Fig GI 37-3)	Often asymmetric or irregular pattern of thumbprinting that is caused by submucosal cellular infiltrate in lymphoma and hematogenous metastases. Insidious onset, unlike the acute presentation of ischemic colitis.

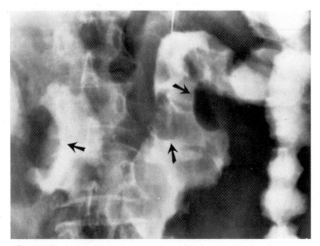

Fig GI 37-1
Ischemic colitis. Multiple filling defects (arrows) indent the margins of the transverse and descending portions of the colon.

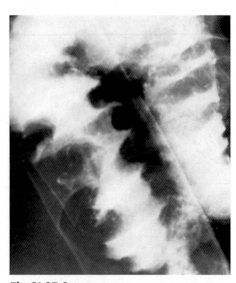

Fig GI 37-2
Pseudomembranous colitis. Wide transverse bands of mural thickening.[51]

*Pattern: Sharply defined, finger-like marginal indentations along the wall of the colon.

Condition	Comments
Endometriosis	Multiple intramural filling defects simulating thumbprinting that develop in women of childbearing age.
Amyloidosis	Deposition of amyloid in the submucosal layer of the colon.
Pneumatosis intestinalis (Fig GI 37-4)	The polypoid masses indenting the barium column are composed of air rather than soft-tissue density.
Diverticulosis	Accordion-like effect simulating thumbprinting that reflects accentuated haustral markings due to extensive muscular hypertrophy of the bowel wall. There are usually multiple diverticula and evidence of muscular thickening and spasm.
Hereditary angioneurotic edema	Thumbprinting pattern develops during acute attacks and reverts to a normal radiographic appearance once the acute episode subsides.

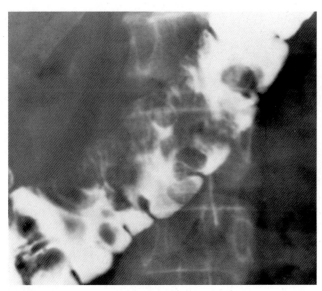

Fig GI 37-3
Lymphoma. Submucosal cellular infiltrate produces the radiographic pattern of thumbprinting.

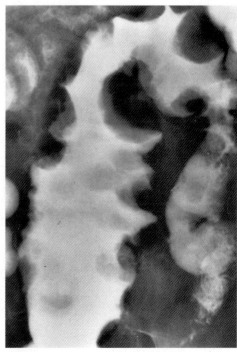

Fig GI 37-4
Pneumatosis intestinalis. Polypoid masses indenting the barium column are composed of air rather than soft-tissue density.

Double Tracking in the Colon

Condition	Comments
Diverticulitis (Figs GI 38-1 and GI 38-2)	Primarily involves the sigmoid region. Represents a dissecting sinus tract that probably resulted from multiple fistulous communications with a paracolic diverticular abscess.
Crohn's disease (Fig GI 38-3)	Long extraluminal sinus tract that may be indistinguishable from diverticulitis both clinically and radiographically. Ulceration, edematous and distorted folds, and other sites of colon involvement suggest Crohn's disease.
Carcinoma of colon (Fig GI 38-4)	Primarily involves the sigmoid colon. Caused by transmural ulceration leading to perforation with abscess formation in the pericolic fat. Difficult to distinguish from diverticulitis unless there is clear radiographic evidence of bowel inflammation.

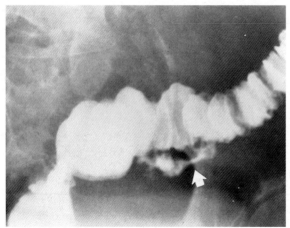

Fig GI 38-1
Dissecting peridiverticulitis. There is a short extraluminal track (arrow) along the antimesocolic border of the sigmoid colon. Note the apparent absence of other demonstrable diverticula.

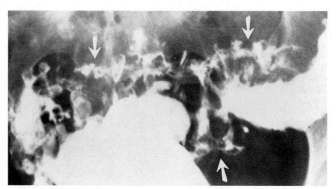

Fig GI 38-2
Dissecting peridiverticulitis. There is diffuse sigmoid involvement with extraluminal tracks extending along both the mesocolic (upper arrows) and antimesocolic (lower arrow) borders.

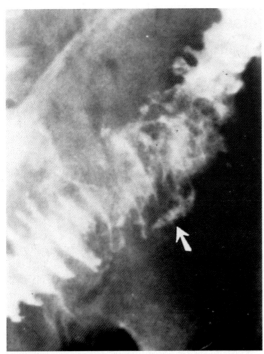

Fig GI 38-3
Crohn's colitis grafted on diverticulosis. A 1.5-cm
track of barium (arrow) is visible along the antimesocolic border of the sigmoid. The mucosal fold pattern
appears granular and ulcerated and multiple diverticula are apparent.[52]

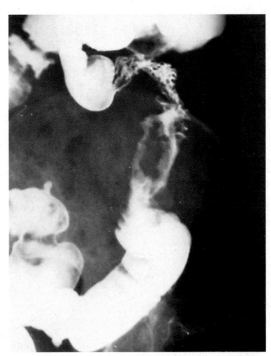

Fig GI 38-4
Primary carcinoma of the distal descending colon
producing a double-track appearance due to transmural perforation.[52]

Enlargement of the Retrorectal Space

Condition	Imaging Findings	Comments
Normal variant (Fig GI 39-1)	Widening of the retrorectal space with no evidence of an abnormality of the rectum, sacrum, or presacral soft tissues.	More than one-third of individuals have an "enlarged" retrorectal space (>1.5 cm) with no underlying abnormality. Most are large or obese.
Inflammatory bowel disease (Fig GI 39-2)	Rectal involvement (ulceration, narrowing).	Most commonly due to ulcerative colitis. Other causes include Crohn's disease and, infrequently, tuberculosis, amebiasis, lymphogranuloma venereum, radiation, or ischemia. Rarely, retrorectal abscess from diverticulitis, perforated appendix, malignant perforation, or infected developmental cyst.
Benign retrorectal tumor	Smooth, extrinsic impression on the posterior wall. Overlying rectal mucosa remains intact.	Most commonly due to a developmental cyst (especially dermoid cyst). Rare causes include lipomas and hemangioendotheliomas.
Primary or metastatic malignancy (Fig GI 39-3)	Irregular narrowing of the rectum. There may be mucosal destruction and shelf formation (even with metastases).	Almost all primary tumors are adenocarcinomas (rare lymphomas, sarcomas, cloacogenic carcinomas). Metastases include carcinomas of the prostate, bladder, cervix, and ovary. It may be difficult to distinguish a widened retrorectal space caused by radiation effects from that due to recurrent tumor.
Neurogenic tumor	Anterior displacement of the rectum without bowel wall invasion.	Chordomas often cause expansion and destruction of the sacrum (50% show amorphous calcifications). A neurofibroma arising in a sacral foramen can enlarge and distort it.

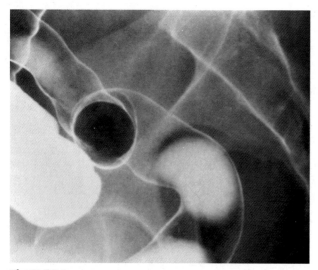

Fig GI 39-1
Normal variant. Although the retrorectal space measured 2 cm, the patient had no abnormality by clinical history, digital rectal examination, or proctoscopy.

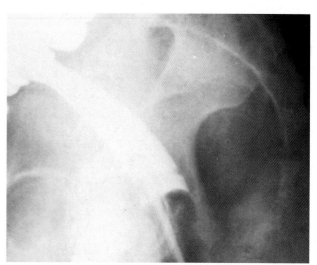

Fig GI 39-2
Lymphogranuloma venereum. Characteristic smooth narrowing of the rectum with widening of the retrorectal space.

Condition	Imaging Findings	Comments
Sacral tumor	Various abnormalities involving the sacrum.	Primary and secondary malignancies cause bone destruction; an anterior sacral meningocele is associated with an anomalous sacrum; and sacrococcygeal teratomas frequently contain calcification.
Pelvic lipomatosis/ Cushing's disease	Narrowed rectum with an excessively lucent retrorectal space.	Massive deposition of fat in the pelvis.
Previous sacral fracture	Evidence of an old sacral fracture.	Bleeding into the presacral soft tissues causes a widened retrorectal space.
Colitis cystica profunda	Multiple intraluminal filling defects in the rectum.	Filling defects represent cystic dilatation of colonic mucous glands.
Partial sigmoid resection (Fig GI 39-4)	Shortening of the rectosigmoid colon.	Operative trauma alters the normal anatomic relations in the pelvis.

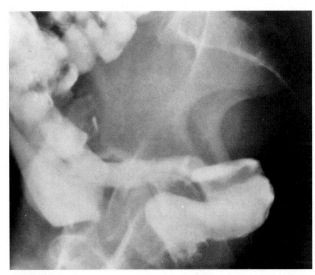

Fig GI 39-3
Lymphoma. Marked widening of the retrorectal space with narrowing of a long segment of the rectosigmoid.

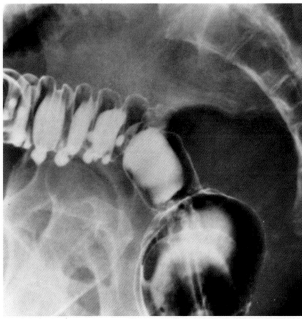

Fig GI 39-4
Sigmoid resection for carcinoma. Widening of the retrorectal space is due to operative trauma altering the normal anatomic relations in the pelvis.

Alterations in Gallbladder Size

Condition	Imaging Findings	Comments
Courvoisier phenomenon (Fig GI 40-1)	Enlarged gallbladder.	Caused by extrahepatic neoplastic disease (arising in the head of the pancreas, duodenal papilla, ampulla of Vater, or lower common bile duct). Usually produces jaundice and a nontender, palpable gallbladder.
Hydrops/empyema	Enlarged gallbladder.	Complications of acute cholecystitis. No jaundice.
Vagotomy	Enlarged gallbladder.	No evidence of biliary tract obstruction. Size of the gallbladder in the resting state is approximately twice normal after a truncal vagotomy.
Diabetes mellitus	Enlarged gallbladder.	Seen in 20% of patients with diabetes and probably reflects an autonomic neuropathy. Increased incidence of gallstones.
Chronic cholecystitis (Fig GI 40-2)	Small, shrunken gallbladder.	Thickening and fibrous contraction of the gallbladder wall.
Cystic fibrosis	Small, contracted gallbladder.	In 30% to 50% of patients with cystic fibrosis, the gallbladder has multiple web-like trabeculations, and is filled with thick, tenacious, colorless bile and mucus. Increased incidence of gallstones.
Congenital multiseptate gallbladder	Small gallbladder with honeycomb pattern.	Multiple intercommunicating septa divide the lumen of the gallbladder. Increased incidence of infection and gallstone formation.
Hypoplasia of gallbladder	Very small gallbladder.	Gallbladder is merely a small, rudimentary pouch at the end of the cystic duct.

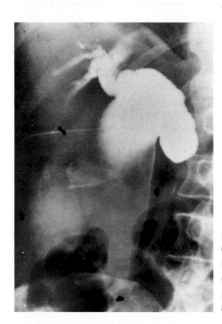

Fig GI 40-1
Courvoisier phenomenon. Huge gallbladder (arrows) injected by error at percutaneous hepatic cholangiography. The patient had carcinoma of the pancreas and presented with painless jaundice.

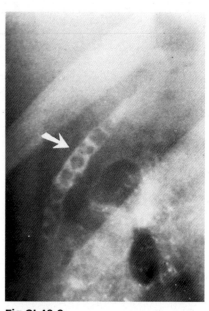

Fig GI 40-2
Chronic cholecystitis. Multiple radiolucent stones (arrow) fill the small, shrunken gallbladder.

Filling Defects in an Opacified Gallbladder

Condition	Imaging Findings	Comments
Gallstones (Figs GI 41-1 through GI 41-3)	Variable size, shape, number, and degree of calcifications. They are usually freely movable and settle in the dependent portion of the gallbladder (the level depends on the relation of the specific gravity of the stone to that of the surrounding bile).	Approximately 80% are lucent cholesterol stones, whereas 20% contain sufficient calcium to be radiographically detectable. The incidence of gallstones increases in several disease states (hemolytic anemias, cirrhosis, diabetes, Crohn's disease, hyperparathyroidism, pancreatic disease) and various metabolic disorders. Infrequently, a gallstone coated by tenacious mucus adheres to the gallbladder wall.

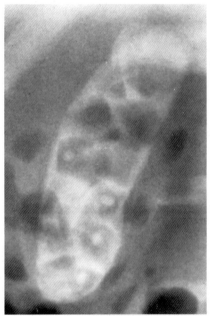

Fig GI 41-1
Multiple radiolucent gallstones, many of which contain a central nidus of calcification.

A   B

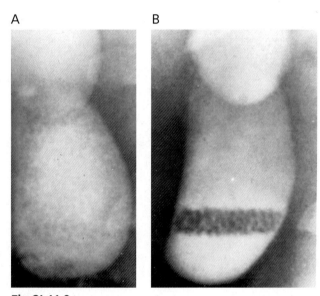

Fig GI 41-2
Layering of gallstones. (A) With the patient supine, the stones are poorly defined and have a gravel-like consistency. (B) On an erect film taken with a horizontal beam, the innumerable gallstones layer out and are easily seen.

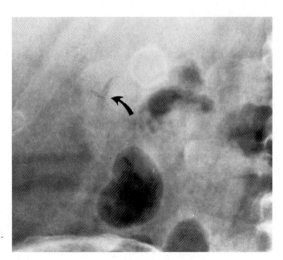

Fig GI 41-3
Fissuring in a gallstone. Mercedes-Benz sign (arrow). Note the adjacent gallstone with a radiopaque rim.

Condition	Imaging Findings	Comments
Cholesterolosis (strawberry gallbladder) (Fig GI 41-4)	Single or multiple, small polypoid filling defects (best seen after a fatty meal).	Abnormal deposits of cholesterol esters in fat-laden macrophages in the lamina propria of the gallbladder wall. No malignant potential.
Adenomyoma (Figs GI 41-5 and GI 41-6)	Single filling defect situated at the tip of the fundus.	In adenomyomatosis, single or multiple oval collections of contrast material (Rokitansky-Aschoff sinuses) are projected just outside the lumen of the gallbladder.
Benign tumor	Fixed filling defect.	Rare. Mainly adenomatous polyps and papillary adenomas (papilloma, villous adenoma).
Carcinoma of gallbladder (Fig GI 41-7)	Solitary fixed polyp or irregular mural filling defect.	Rare manifestation (the gallbladder is usually not visualized in the presence of a carcinoma). Primarily affects elderly women and is usually associated with cholelithiasis.
Metastases	Single or multiple fixed filling defects.	Most commonly, melanoma (occurs in approximately 15% of patients with the disease but is rarely detectable radiographically).
Parasitic granuloma	Single or multiple fixed nodules.	Eggs of *Ascaris lumbricoides* or *Paragonimus westermani* deposited in the gallbladder wall incite an intense inflammatory cell infiltration.
Metachromatic leukodystrophy	Single or multiple filling defects.	Very rare condition in which there is deposition of metachromatic sulfatides due to an enzyme deficiency.

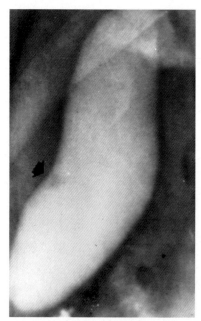

Fig GI 41-4
Cholesterol polyp (arrow).

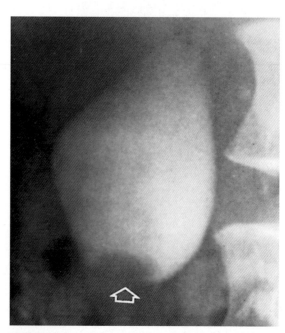

Fig GI 41-5
Solitary adenomyoma. A broad mass (arrow) is evident at the tip of the fundus of the gallbladder.

Condition	Imaging Findings	Comments
Pseudopolyp	Fixed filling defect that may simulate a true tumor.	Congenital fold or septum (eg, Phrygian cap); heterotopic gastric or pancreatic tissue; projectional artifacts (folding or coiling of the junction between the neck of the gallbladder and the cystic duct or a lucent cystic duct superimposed on the opaque neck of the gallbladder).

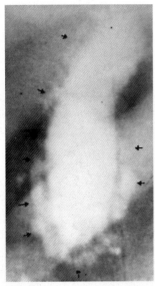

Fig GI 41-6
Adenomyomatosis. Rokitansky-Aschoff sinuses are scattered diffusely throughout the gallbladder. The collections of intramural contrast material appear to parallel the opacified gallbladder lumen (arrows), from which they are separated by a lucent space representing the thickness of the mucosa and muscularis.

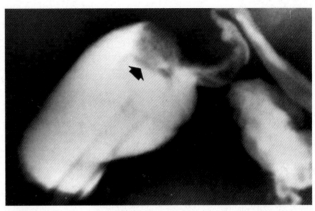

Fig GI 41-7
Carcinoma of the gallbladder. Irregular mural mass (arrow) with tumor growth extending into the cystic duct.

Filling Defects in the Bile Ducts

Condition	Imaging Findings	Comments
Biliary calculi (Figs GI 42-1 and GI 42-2)	Single or multiple filling defects that move freely and change location with alterations in patient position.	Usually arise in the gallbladder and reach the bile duct either by passage through the cystic duct or by fistulous erosion through the gallbladder wall. May impact in the distal common duct and cause obstruction (smooth, sharply defined meniscus).
Pseudocalculus (Fig GI 42-3)	Smooth, arcuate filling defect simulating an impacted gallstone. Serial radiographs show the pseudocalculus disappearing as the sphincter relaxes.	Cyclic contraction of the sphincter of Oddi that occurs after surgical manipulation or instrumentation of the common bile duct. Never completely obstructs the bile duct (some contrast material flows into the duodenum).

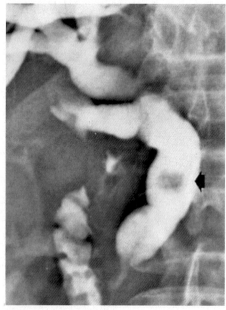

Fig GI 42-1
Common bile duct stone (arrow).

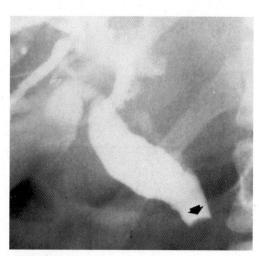

Fig GI 42-2
Impacted common bile duct stone (arrow). Characteristic smooth, concave intraluminal filling defect.

A

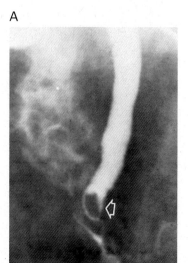

B

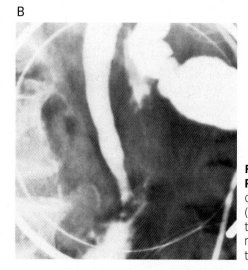

Fig GI 42-3
Pseudocalculus. (A) Contrast material encircles the stone-like filling defect (arrow). (B) After relaxation of the sphincter of Oddi, the distal common bile duct appears normal and contrast material flows freely into the duodenum.

Condition	Imaging Findings	Comments
Air bubbles	Smooth, round, generally multiple filling defects.	Vexing artifacts on T-tube cholangiography. If the patient is raised toward the upright position, the air bubbles rise (lighter than contrast-laden bile), while true calculi remain in a stationary position or fall with gravity.
Malignant tumors (Fig GI 42-4)	Single or multiple filling defects.	Rare manifestation of cholangiocarcinoma, ampullary carcinoma, hepatoma, or villous tumors.
Benign tumors (Figs GI 42-5 and GI 42-6)	Small polypoid filling defects.	Very rare. Mostly adenomas and papillomas.

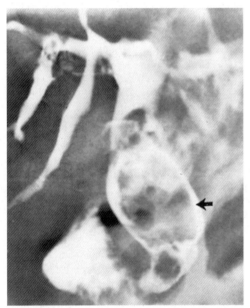

Fig GI 42-4
Cholangiocarcinoma presenting as a large filling defect (arrow) in the common bile duct.

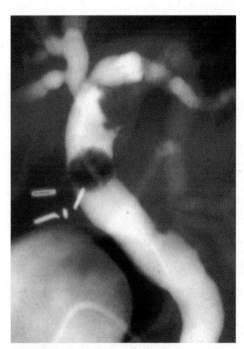

Fig GI 42-5
Adenoma. Lobulated sessile mass in the common hepatic duct.[53]

Condition	Imaging Findings	Comments
Ascaris lumbricoides	Long, linear filling defects.	Coiling of worms can rarely produce a discrete mass.
Liver flukes (Fig GI 42-7)	Smooth filling defects simulating calculi (when viewed en face). Typical linear filling defects when the worms are seen in profile.	*Clonorchis sinensis* (in raw or partially cooked fish) and *Fasciola hepatica* (in pond water or watercress in sheep-growing areas).
Hydatid cyst (*Echinococcus*) (Fig GI 42-8)	Round or irregular filling defect in a bile duct or a cyst cavity.	If a liver cyst communicates with the biliary tree, the periodic discharge of cyst membranes, daughter cysts, or scolices causes recurrent episodes of biliary colic.
Other causes	Various patterns.	Blood clot; right hepatic artery (extrinsic impression); bile duct varices following extrahepatic obstruction of the portal vein.

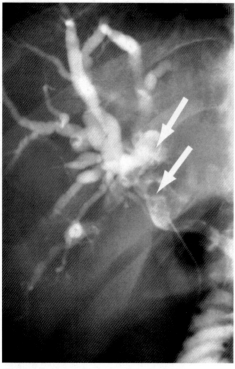

Fig GI 42-6
Biliary papillomatosis. Multiple polypoid filling defects in dilated intra- and extrahepatic bile ducts (straight arrows). The filling defect in the left hepatic duct (curved arrow) prevents contrast material filing of the left intrahepatic ducts.[53]

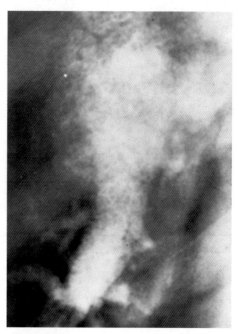

Fig GI 42-7
Liver flukes *(Clonorchis sinensis)* causing multiple filling defects in the biliary system. Many of the filling defects represent co-existing calculi, which are often seen in this condition.

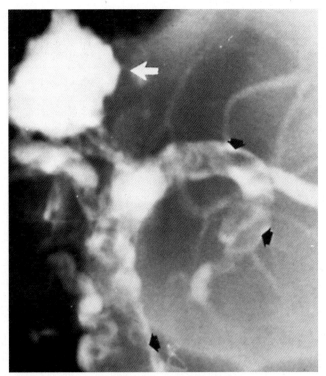

Fig GI 42-8
Hydatid disease of the liver and biliary tree. Multiple cysts present as filling defects in the bile ducts (black arrows). Note contrast material filling a large communicating cystic cavity in the liver parenchyma (white arrow).

Bile Duct Narrowing or Obstruction

Condition	Imaging Findings	Comments
Cholangiocarcinoma (Figs GI 43-1 and GI 43-2)	Short, well-demarcated, segmental narrowing of the bile duct. There may be diffuse ductal narrowing (extensive desmoplastic response). Rarely multicentric (mimicking sclerosing cholangitis).	Most commonly affects the retroduodenal or supraduodenal segments of the common bile duct. Lesions are usually far advanced at the time of diagnosis (extend along the bile duct and spread to regional lymph nodes). Klatskin tumors arising at the junction of the right and left hepatic ducts tend to grow slowly and metastasize late.
Ampullary carcinoma (Fig GI 43-3)	Obstruction of the distal end of the bile duct.	Small neoplasm that can appear as a polypoid mass or merely obstruct the bile duct without a demonstrable tumor mass.
Adjacent malignancy (Figs GI 43-4 and GI 43-5)	Asymmetric narrowing or obstruction of the bile duct.	Primary carcinoma of the pancreas or the duodenum; metastases (usually from a gastrointestinal tract primary); lymphoma (nodes in the porta hepatis).
Benign tumor (Fig GI 43-6)	Polypoid filling defect with some degree of obstruction.	Extremely rare. Usually occurs in the distal bile duct and simulates a biliary stone.

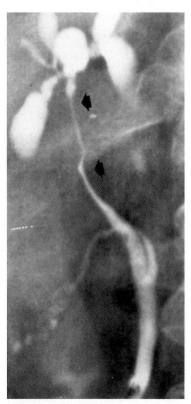

Fig GI 43-1
Cholangiocarcinoma causing severe narrowing of a long segment of the common hepatic duct (arrows).

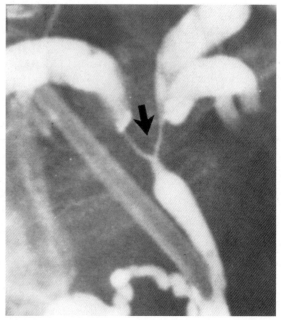

Fig GI 43-2
Klatskin tumor. Sclerosing cholangiocarcinomas arising at the junction of the right and left hepatic ducts (arrow).

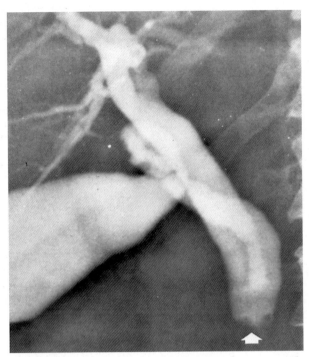

Fig GI 43-3
Ampullary carcinoma. Abrupt occlusion (arrow) of the distal common bile duct.

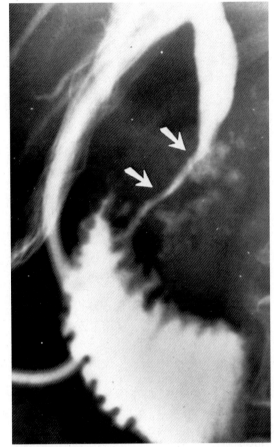

Fig GI 43-4
Carcinoma of the head of the pancreas. Irregular narrowing of the common bile duct (arrows). The calcifications reflect underlying chronic pancreatitis.

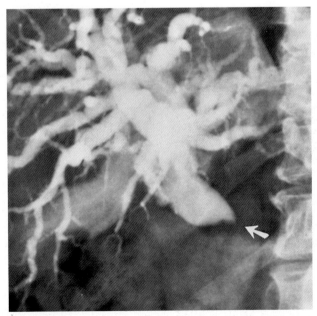

Fig GI 43-5
Extrinsic obstruction of the common bile duct (arrow) due to nodal metastases from carcinoma of the colon.

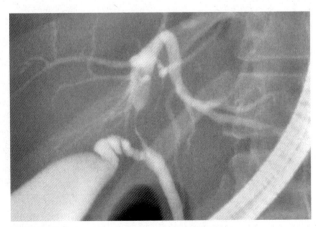

Fig GI 43-6
Granular cell tumor. Focal stricture in the distal common hepatic duct (arrow).[53]

Condition	Imaging Findings	Comments
Cholangitis (Fig GI 43-7)	Multiple biliary strictures of various lengths with beading of the duct between narrowed segments. Almost always involves the extrahepatic ducts; there may be progressive involvement of the intrahepatic ducts.	Most commonly an inflammatory disorder secondary to long-standing partial obstruction. Primary sclerosing cholangitis is a rare condition that tends to occur in patients with inflammatory bowel disease.
Cholangiolitic hepatitis (Fig GI 43-8)	Diffuse or focal ductal narrowing with diminished branching of the intrahepatic biliary ductal system.	Rare, chronic, slowly progressive intrahepatic disease of unknown etiology. Extrahepatic ducts are not involved (unlike sclerosing cholangitis).
Chronic pancreatitis (Fig GI 43-9)	Smooth, concentric inflammatory stricture with gradual tapering.	Involves the intrapancreatic portion of the common bile duct. Often associated with pancreatic calcifications.
Acute pancreatitis	Circumferential narrowing of the common bile duct.	Usually reversible when the acute inflammatory process subsides.
Papillary stenosis	Smooth narrowing of the terminal portion of the bile duct.	Controversial entity that is associated with chronic inflammatory disease of the biliary tract and pancreas. May be the cause of postcholecystectomy symptoms resembling biliary colic. Successfully treated by surgical relief of the obstruction at the choledochoduodenal junction.
Parasitic infestation	Relative obstruction usually due to an inflammatory stricture and stone formation.	*Clonorchis sinensis, Fasciola hepatica, Ascaris lumbricoides.* Conglomeration of worms can cause an obstructive mass. In *Echinococcus* infestation, daughter cysts shed into the bile ducts can cause obstruction at the ampullary level.

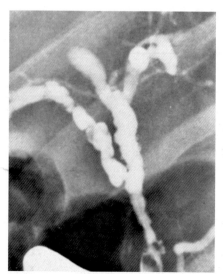

Fig GI 43-7
Primary sclerosing cholangitis in a patient with chronic ulcerative colitis.

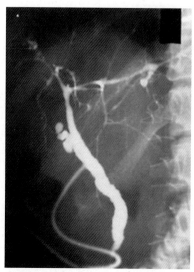

Fig GI 43-8
Cholangiolitic hepatitis. Decreased branching of the intrahepatic ducts with associated diffuse and focal narrowing. The extrahepatic bile ducts are normal.[54]

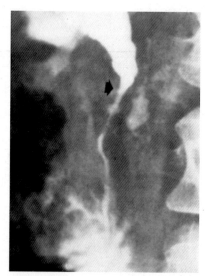

Fig GI 43-9
Chronic pancreatitis. Note the abrupt transition between the encased pipe stem segment and the dilated suprapancreatic portion of the common bile duct (arrow). Calcification suggestive of chronic pancreatitis can also be seen.

Condition	Imaging Findings	Comments
Granulomatous disease	Compression and narrowing of the bile duct, primarily in the region of the porta hepatis.	Periductal lymph node involvement in tuberculosis, sarcoidosis, and other chronic granulomatous diseases.
Impacted biliary calculus (see Fig GI 42-2)	Smooth, concave intraluminal filling defect.	Impacted ampullary stone and papillary edema secondary to a recently passed stone are common causes of bile duct obstruction. Calculi enter the common bile duct via the cystic duct or by erosion.
Surgical or traumatic stricture (Fig GI 43-10)	Smooth, concentric narrowing of the bile duct. If the bile duct is obstructed, it appears convex (unlike the concave margin of an obstructing stone).	Most are related to previous biliary tract surgery. Infrequently, blunt abdominal trauma causes torsion injury to the common bile duct. Unlike malignant lesions, benign strictures usually involve long segments and have a gradual transition without complete obstruction.
Biliary atresia	Obliteration of the ductal lumen (often segmental and irregular in distribution).	Most common cause of persistent neonatal jaundice. Rather than a congenital defect, it probably develops postpartum as a complication of a chronic inflammatory process.
Membranous diaphragm (Fig GI 43-11)	Luminal web in the common bile duct.	Extremely rare. Chronic partial biliary obstruction results in bile stasis, stone formation, and recurring cholangitis.
Duodenal diverticulum	Distal obstruction of the common bile duct.	Common duct that empties directly into a duodenal diverticulum may be obstructed by anatomic distortion, diverticulitis, or an enterolith in the sac.
Cirrhosis	Irregular, tortuous or corkscrew appearance of the intrahepatic bile ducts.	Distortion of the hepatic parenchyma by fatty infiltration and subsequent regenerating nodules and fibrosis.

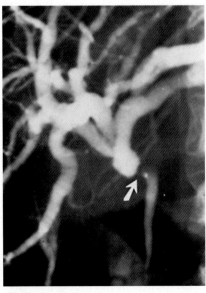

Fig GI 43-10
Benign stricture of the common bile duct (arrow) related to previous biliary tract surgery.

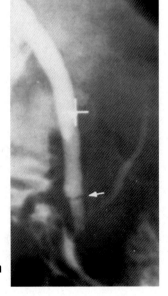

Fig GI 43-11
Congenital membranous diaphragm (web) of the common bile duct (arrow).

Cystic Dilatation of the Bile Ducts

Condition	Imaging Findings	Comments
Choledochal cyst (Fig GI 44-1)	Cystic or fusiform dilatation that primarily affects the common bile duct and adjacent portions of the common hepatic and cystic ducts. There can also be dilatation of intrahepatic bile ducts.	Typically associated with a localized constriction of the distal common bile duct. Classic clinical triad of upper abdominal pain, mass, and jaundice.
Choledochocele (Fig GI 44-2)	Cystic dilatation of the intraduodenal portion of the common bile duct.	Well-defined, smooth duodenal filling defect on an upper gastrointestinal series. On cholangiography, it mimics the urographic appearance of ureterocele.
Caroli's disease (Fig GI 44-3)	Segmental saccular dilatation of intrahepatic bile ducts throughout the liver.	Rare condition in which the dilated cystic segments contain bile and communicate freely with the biliary tree and each other. Approximately 80% of patients have associated medullary sponge kidney.
Congenital hepatic fibrosis (Fig GI 44-4)	Large or small cystic spaces communicating with intrahepatic bile ducts (lollipop-tree appearance).	Rare condition that radiographically simulates Caroli's disease but is far more serious. Massive periportal fibrosis leads to fatal liver failure and portal hypertension at an early age.
Papillomatosis of intrahepatic biliary ducts	Intrahepatic or extrahepatic bile duct dilatation proximal to multiple filling defects.	Rare condition in which biliary obstruction is caused by thick mucous material produced by the villous tumors, fragmentation of the papillary fronds, or amputation of entire polyps into the biliary tract. High incidence of carcinoma.

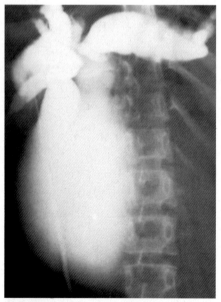

Fig GI 44-1
Choledochal cyst. Cholangiographic contrast material fills the huge fusiform dilatation of the common bile duct and the markedly dilated intrahepatic ducts.

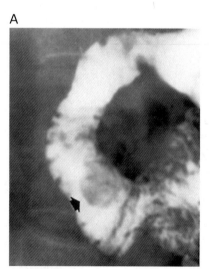 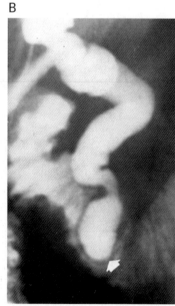

Fig GI 44-2
Choledochocele. (A) A well-defined, smooth filling defect (arrow) projects into the duodenal lumen on an upper gastrointestinal series. (B) At cholangiography, the bulbous terminal portion of the common bile duct fills with contrast material and projects into the duodenal lumen (arrow). It is separated from contrast material in the duodenum by a radiolucent membrane.

Condition	Imaging Findings	Comments
Choledocholithiasis (Oriental)	Ductal dilatation proximal to obstructing calculi or masses of worms.	In Asian countries, intrahepatic lithiasis and cystic dilatation of bile ducts are frequent complications of parasitic infestation (*Ascaris lumbricoides, Clonorchis sinensis*).
Cholangitis (Fig GI 44-5)	Areas of cystic dilatation combined with strictures of various lengths.	Caused by diffuse periductal inflammatory fibrosis. Cystic dilatation can also be due to communicating hepatic abscesses.
Cholangiohepatitis (recurrent pyogenic hepatitis) (Fig GI 44-6)	Segmental dilatation of bile ducts with areas of rapid peripheral tapering (arrowhead sign).	Major cause of acute abdomen in the Far East. Frequently leads to stone formation, biliary obstruction, and portal septicemia.

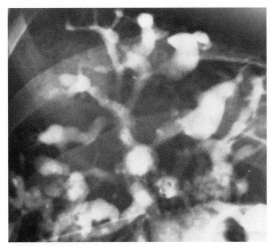

Fig GI 44-3
Caroli's disease.

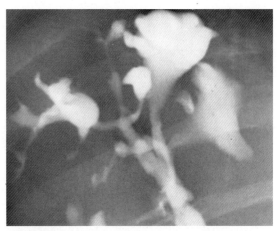

Fig GI 44-4
Congenital hepatic fibrosis.[55]

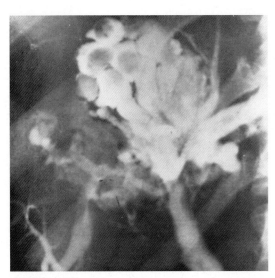

Fig GI 44-5
Cholangitis. Communicating hepatic abscess simulating localized cystic dilatation of an intrahepatic bile duct.

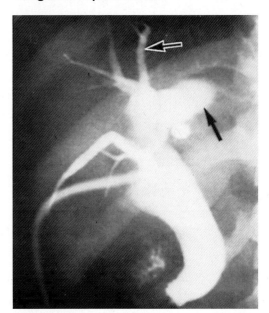

Fig GI 44-6
Cholangiohepatitis. A T-tube cholangiogram demonstrates that the common bile duct and intrahepatic duct (lower arrow) are dilated. The upper arrow shows a moderately dilated bile duct with short branches arising at right angles to the duct.[56]

Pneumoperitoneum

Condition	Comments
Pneumoperitoneum with peritonitis	
Perforated viscus (Figs GI 45-1 and GI 45-2)	The most frequent cause is perforated ulcer (gastric or duodenal). In 30% of perforated peptic ulcers, no free intraperitoneal gas can be detected. The absence of stomach gas with gas present distally suggests gastric perforation, whereas the absence of colonic gas in the presence of a gastric gas-fluid level and small bowel distention suggests colonic perforation. Colonic perforation can be due to obstructing malignancy, severe ulcerating colitis (toxic megacolon), and, rarely, diverticulitis or appendicitis. A precise diagnosis of the site of perforation often requires a barium study.
Ulcerative bowel disease	Tuberculosis; typhoid fever; ulcerated Meckel's diverticulum; ulcerative colitis (toxic megacolon); lymphogranuloma venereum. There is often evidence of bowel inflammation on the plain abdominal radiograph.
Infection/trauma	Infection of the peritoneal cavity by a gas-forming organism; blunt or penetrating trauma causing rupture of a hollow viscus.
Delayed complication of renal transplantation	Spontaneous perforation of the colon may develop in a patient on long-term immunosuppressive therapy. High mortality rate.
Pneumoperitoneum without peritonitis	
Iatrogenic causes	Abdominal surgery; endoscopy; diagnostic pneumoperitoneum.
Abdominal causes	Pneumatosis intestinalis (rupture of mural gas-filled cysts); forme fruste of perforation; jejunal diverticulosis.
Gynecologic causes	Rubin test for tubal patency; vaginal douching; postpartum exercises or examination; orogenital intercourse (ascent of air through the normal female genital tract into the peritoneal cavity).
Intrathoracic causes	Pneumomediastinum; ruptured emphysematous bulla (dissection of gas downward into the extraperitoneal tissues followed by perforation into the peritoneal cavity).

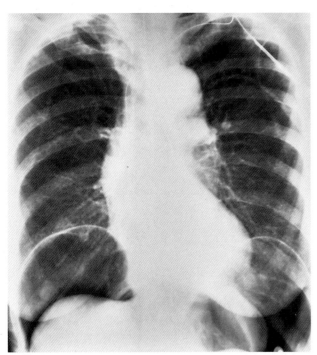

Fig GI 45-1
Extensive pneumoperitoneum after colonic perforation.

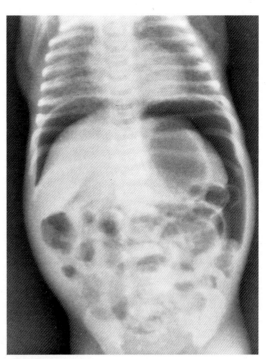

Fig GI 45-2
Pneumoperitoneum after perforation of an ulcerated Meckel's diverticulum in a child.

Gas in the Bowel Wall (Pneumatosis Intestinalis)

Condition	Imaging Findings	Comments
Primary (idiopathic) pneumatosis intestinalis (Fig GI 46-1)	Radiolucent clusters of cysts along the contours of the bowel that are compressible on palpation and can simulate polyps, thumbprinting, or even an annular constriction.	Benign condition with multiple thin-walled, noncommunicating, gas-filled cysts in the bowel wall. Primarily involves the colon (especially the left side). No associated gastrointestinal or respiratory abnormalities, but may cause asymptomatic pneumoperitoneum.
Necrotizing enterocolitis (Fig GI 46-2)	Frothy or bubbly appearance of gas in the wall of diseased bowel loops. Often resembles fecal material in the right colon (normal in adults, but abnormal in premature infants).	Primarily occurs in premature or debilitated infants and has a low survival rate. Most commonly affects the ileum and right colon. Pneumoperitoneum and portal vein gas are ominous signs.

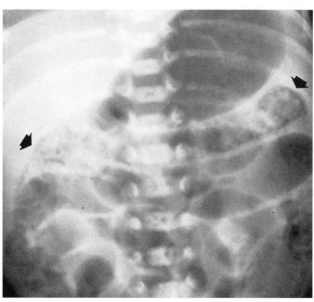

Fig GI 46-2
Pneumatosis intestinalis in a premature infant with necrotizing **enterocolitis.** The bubbly appearance of gas in the wall of the diseased colon represents fecal material (arrows).

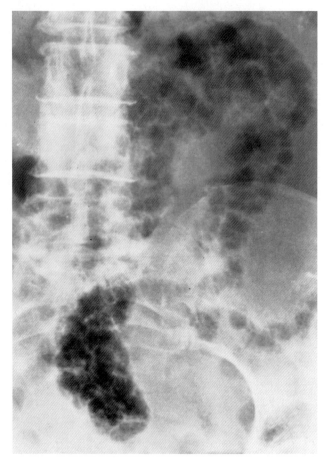

Fig GI 46-1
Primary pneumatosis intestinalis in an asymptomatic man.

Condition	Imaging Findings	Comments
Mesenteric vascular disease (Fig GI 46-3)	Crescentic linear gas collections in the walls of ischemic bowel loops.	Due to loss of mucosal integrity or increased intraluminal pressure in the bowel (ischemic necrosis; intestinal obstruction, especially if strangulation; corrosive ingestion; primary infection of the bowel wall). Portal vein gas indicates irreversible intestinal necrosis.
Gastrointestinal tract lesion without necrosis of bowel wall (Fig GI 46-4)	Short, sharply defined intramural gas collections parallel to the bowel wall.	May develop in conditions resulting in mucosal ulceration or intestinal obstruction (obstructive pyloroduodenal peptic ulcer disease, inflammatory bowel disease, connective tissue disease, jejunoileal bypass surgery, obstructive colonic lesions in children, steroid therapy, and complication of gastrointestinal endoscopy or colonoscopy).
Obstructive pulmonary disease	Segmental intramural gas collections parallel to the bowel wall.	Partial bronchial obstruction and coughing presumably cause alveolar rupture with gas dissecting along peribronchial and perivascular tissue planes into the mediastinum and passing through various diaphragmatic openings to reach the retroperitoneal arch. Gas then dissects between the leaves of the mesentery to reach the bowel wall.

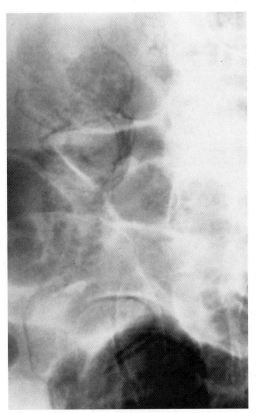

Fig GI 46-3
Pneumatosis intestinalis due to mesenteric arterial thrombosis.

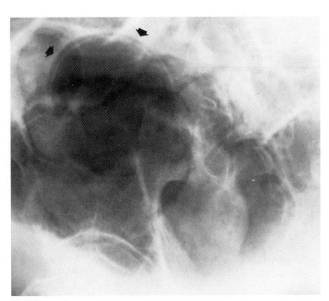

Fig GI 46-4
Pneumatosis intestinalis involving the colon (arrows) in a patient with severe pyloric stenosis.

Extraluminal Gas in the Upper Quadrants

Condition	Imaging Findings	Comments
Pneumoperitoneum (Fig GI 47-1)	Best seen on upright or decubitus views with a horizontal beam. Double-wall, inverted-V, and urachal signs on supine views. Falciform ligament and football signs in children.	Secondary to visceral perforation, surgery, or a variety of nonemergent abdominal, gynecologic, and intrathoracic causes.
Retroperitoneal gas (Fig GI 47-2)	Outlines the kidney and, on the right, the undersurface of the liver. Does not move freely when the patient changes position (unlike intraperitoneal gas).	Most common cause is perforation of the duodenum or rectum due to trauma, diverticulitis, or ulcerative disease. Can be a complication of an endoscopic procedure.
Subhepatic gas	Triangular or crescent-shaped gas collection overlying the right kidney inferior to the liver edge. Subhepatic abscess has a round or oval configuration and often contains a gas-fluid level.	Most common cause is perforation of a duodenal ulcer. Less frequently, perforation of the appendix or a sigmoid diverticulum or leakage of a gastro-enteric or ileotransverse colon anastomosis. Sub-hepatic abscess may complicate enteric perforation or pelvic inflammation.
Subphrenic abscess (Fig GI 47-3)	Mottled radiolucent appearance, often with a gas-fluid level. Unlike bowel gas, gas in an abscess is constant in multiple projections and on serial films.	Primarily a complication of intra-abdominal surgery and associated with a high mortality rate. Usually there is elevation and restricted motion of the ipsilateral hemidiaphragm and often a nonpurulent (sympathetic) pleural effusion.

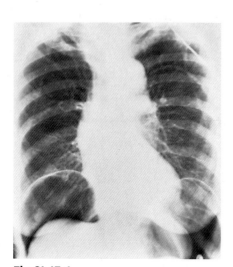

Fig GI 47-1
Pneumoperitoneum.

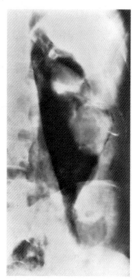

Fig GI 47-2
Retroperitoneal gas surrounding the left kidney after colonoscopy.

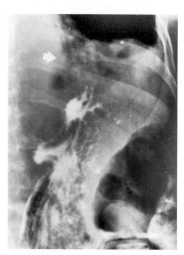

Fig GI 47-3
Left subphrenic abscess. Characteristic mottled radiolucent appearance of the abscess (arrow), which is located above the fundus of the stomach, is due to gas bubbles intermixed with necrotic material and pus.

Condition	Imaging Findings	Comments
Renal or perirenal abscess (Fig GI 47-4)	Gas within and surrounding the kidney.	Caused by antecedent urinary tract disease (infection, obstruction, trauma, instrumentation) or direct or hematogenous spread of an extraurinary infection.
Liver abscess	Bubbly gas collection overlying the liver.	Caused by pyogenic organisms (especially *Klebsiella*) or amebic infestation.
Pancreatic abscess (Fig GI 47-5)	Mottled lucent pattern in the mid-abdomen.	Complication of acute pancreatitis that is associated with a high mortality rate.
Lesser sac abscess (Fig GI 47-6)	Mottled collection in the left upper abdomen, often with a gas-fluid level.	Displaces the stomach anteriorly and the colon inferiorly. May extend slightly over the midline but does not reach the diaphragm.
Gas in bowel wall (pneumatosis intestinalis) (Fig GI 47-7)	Multiple gas-filled mural cysts (primary) or crescentic linear gas collections (secondary).	Benign primary condition or secondary to necrotizing enterocolitis, mesenteric vascular disease, and a variety of gastrointestinal and obstructive pulmonary conditions.

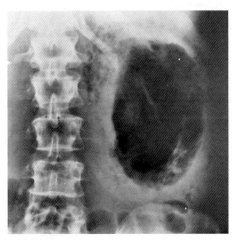

Fig GI 47-4
Renal and perirenal abscess.

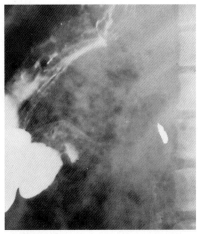

Fig GI 47-5
Pancreatic abscess.

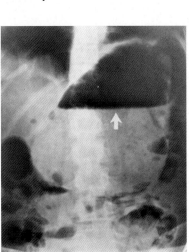

Fig GI 47-6
Lesser sac abscess with a prominent gas-fluid level (arrow).

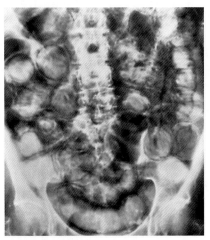

Fig GI 47-7
Pneumatosis intestinalis secondary to primary amyloidosis of the small bowel.

Condition	Imaging Findings	Comments
Gas in biliary system (Fig GI 47-8)	Gas in larger, more centrally situated bile ducts.	Caused by inflammatory fistulization between the gallbladder or bile duct and the stomach or duodenum, or due to previous surgery (sphincterotomy), cholecystitis, severe peptic ulcer disease, trauma, or a tumor.
Emphysematous cholecystitis (Fig GI 47-9)	Gas in the lumen or the wall of the gallbladder or in pericholecystic tissues.	Caused by gas-forming organisms and usually occurs in patients with poorly controlled diabetes mellitus, most of whom have cystic duct obstruction by stones.
Gas in portal venous system (Fig GI 47-10)	Radiating tubular lucencies branching from the porta hepatis to the periphery of the liver.	Usually an ominous prognostic sign in children with necrotizing enterocolitis or adults with mesenteric ischemia and bowel necrosis. A benign form in children is related to the placement of an umbilical venous catheter.

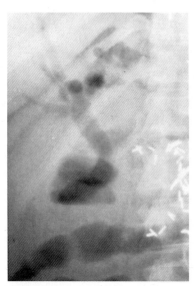

Fig GI 47-8
Gas in the biliary tree in a patient who had undergone a surgical procedure to relieve biliary obstruction.

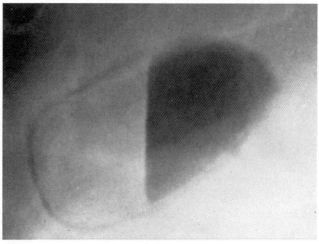

Fig GI 47-9
Emphysematous cholecystitis. There is gas in the gallbladder lumen and wall.

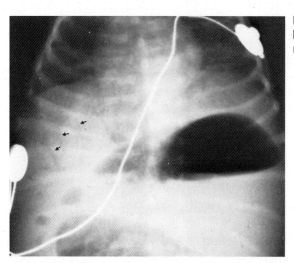

Fig GI 47-10
Portal vein gas (arrows) in an infant with necrotizing enterocolitis.

Condition	Imaging Findings	Comments
Chilaiditi's syndrome (Fig GI 47-11)	Gas in the hepatic flexture of the colon interposed between the liver and the diaphragm.	No clinical significance. Primarily seen in mentally retarded or psychotic patients with chronic colonic enlargement. Must not be confused with pneumoperitoneum.
Perforation due to foreign body	Offending foreign body seen if opaque.	Most ingested foreign bodies pass through the gastrointestinal tract without incident. Sharp or elongated foreign bodies may cause perforation and localized abscess formation (which may be associated with signs of peritonitis, mechanical bowel obstruction, or pneumoperitoneum).
Abdominal wall gas/abscess (Fig GI 47-12)	Gas in the region of the abdominal wall musculature.	May be a normal finding after surgery or reflect postoperative wound infection or localized abscess formation.

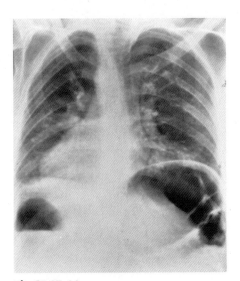

Fig GI 47-11
Chilaiditi's syndrome.

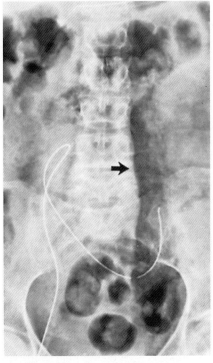

Fig GI 47-12
Gas in a wound infection in the rectus sheath (arrow) after abdominal surgery.

Bull's-Eye Lesions of the Gastrointestinal Tract

Condition	Comments
Melanoma (Fig GI 48-1)	Multiple ulcerated lesions frequently involve the small bowel and stomach.
Primary neoplasms (Fig GI 48-2)	Single ulcerated lesion that is most commonly due to a spindle cell tumor (especially leiomyoma). Infrequent manifestation of lymphoma, carcinoma, or carcinoid.
Hematogenous metastases (Fig GI 48-3)	Multiple ulcerating lesions most commonly due to carcinomas of the breast or lung (especially in the stomach and duodenum).

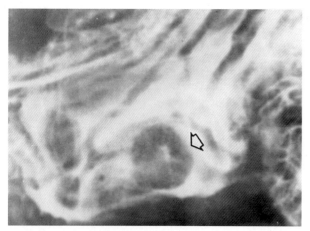

Fig GI 48-1
Metastatic melanoma. Large, ulcerated filling defect (arrow) in the stomach.

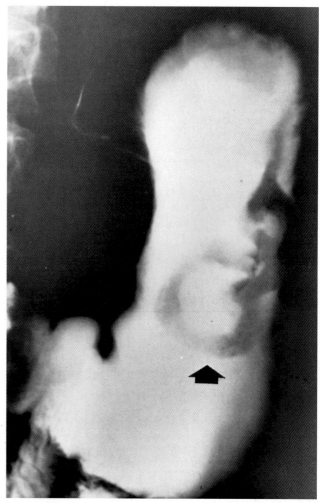

Fig GI 48-3
Carcinoma of the breast metastatic to the stomach.
There is a huge, centrally ulcerated lesion (arrow).

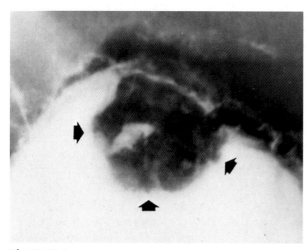

Fig GI 48-2
Ulcerated leiomyoma of the fundus of the stomach (arrows).

Condition	Comments
Kaposi's sarcoma	Multiple ulcerating lesions that primarily involve the small bowel. Associated with characteristic ulcerated hemorrhagic dermatitis in patients with AIDS and other immune deficiency disorders.
Langerhans cell histiocytosis	Single ulcerated polypoid mass that most frequently involves the stomach, but can occur in the small bowel, colon, or rectum. Unlike eosinophilic gastroenteritis, the inflammatory mass of Langerhans cell histiocytosisis not associated with specific food intolerance or peripheral blood eosinophilia.
Ectopic pancreas (Fig GI 48-4)	Single "ulcerated" polypoid mass in the stomach or duodenum. The central barium collection represents umbilication of a rudimentary pancreatic duct rather than necrotic ulceration.
Mastocytosis	Multiple nodules with central barium collections have been reported in one case of this rare disorder characterized by mast cell proliferation in the skin, bones, lymph nodes, and parenchymal organs.
Behçet's syndrome	Central ring-like collections of barium in multiple, large, discrete nodular lesions in the terminal ileum have been reported as a specific gastrointestinal manifestation.

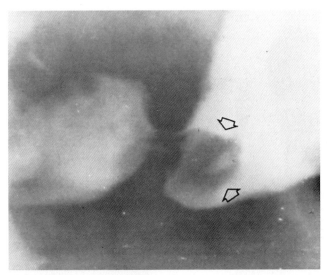

Fig GI 48-4
Ectopic pancreas. Central collection of barium in a rudimentary duct in a filling defect in the gastric antrum (arrows).

Abdominal Hernias

Condition	Comments
Paraduodenal (duodenojejunal flexure) (Figs GI 49-1 to GI 49-4)	Result from failure of the mesentery to fuse with the parietal peritoneum at the ligament of Treitz. May be left (75% to 80%) or right, depending on the position of the duodenum and the orientation of the opening of the paraduodenal fossa.

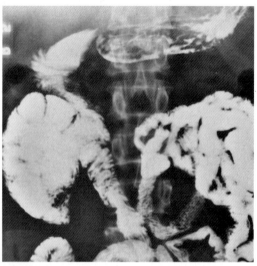

Fig GI 49-1
Right paraduodenal hernia. The jejunal loops are bunched together on the right side of the abdomen, and the junction of the duodenum and jejunum has a low right paramedian position.

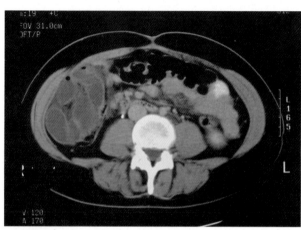

Fig GI 49-2
Right paraduodenal hernia. Contrast CT scan shows a sac-like mass of fluid-filled bowel loops, most of which were jejunal and proximal ileal loops.[57]

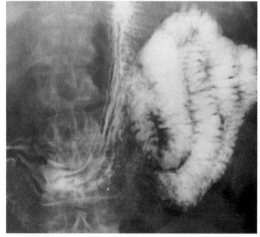

Fig GI 49-3
Left paraduodenal hernia. Small bowel loops are clustered in the left upper quadrant lateral to the fourth portion of the duodenum and stomach.

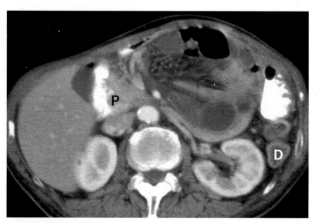

Fig GI 49-4
Left paraduodenal hernia. Contrast CT scan shows a sac-like mass of dilated jejunal loops between the pancreatic head (P) and stomach. The descending mesocolon (D) and stomach are displaced laterally. The dilated inferior mesenteric vein is located at the anterior border of the encapsulated loops.[57]

Condition	Comments
Lesser sac (Figs GI 49-5 to GI 49-7)	Herniation into the lesser peritoneal sac through the foramen of Winslow is a rare condition that typically presents as an acute abdominal emergency that may lead to intestinal strangulation and death if not promptly relieved by surgery. May contain small bowel, colon, gallbladder, or merely omentum.
Inguinal (Fig GI 49-8)	Classified as indirect or direct, depending on their relation to the inferior epigastric vessels.
Indirect (Fig GI 49-9)	Occurs predominantly in males, in whom the peritoneal sac passes down the course of the inguinal canal, anterior to the spermatic cord, and lateral to the inferior epigastric vessels. In females, the hernia sac follows the course of the round ligament into the labium. Indirect inguinal hernias account for 15% of intestinal obstructions (only neoplasms and adhesions are more common causes).

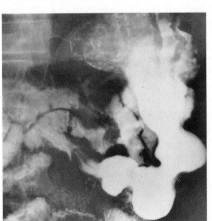

Fig GI 49-5
Cecal herniation through the foramen of Winslow. Loops of bowel are seen in an abnormal position along the lesser curvature medial and posterior to the stomach.

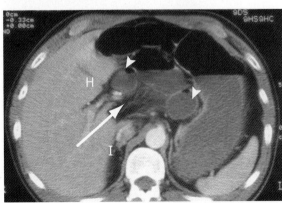

Fig GI 49-7
Lesser sac hernia. CT scan shows a cluster of dilated small bowel loops (arrowheads) in the lesser sac. There are stretched and converging mesenteric vessels (arrow) between the portal vein in the hepatoduodenal ligament (H) and the inferior vena cava (I).[57]

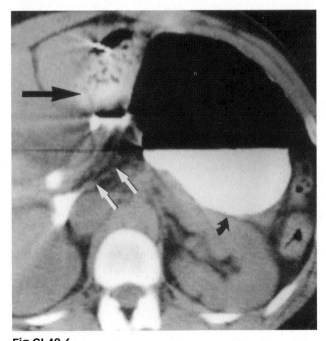

Fig GI 49-6
Cecal herniation into the lesser sac. CT scan shows air and contrast material in a dilated cecum (curved arrow) posterior to the stomach (large black arrow). Note the beak-like contour of herniated bowel and stretched mesenteric vessels (small white arrows) at the foramen of Winslow.[58]

Condition	Comments
Direct (Figs GI 49-10 and GI 49-11)	Visceral protrusion directly through the lower abdominal wall in a weak area medial to the inferior epigastric vessels (also primarily occurs in males). It generally does not traverse the inguinal canal. Because of its short and blunt aperture, a direct hernia seldom becomes incarcerated.

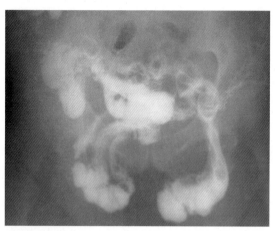

Fig GI 49-8
Inguinal hernia. Barium-filled loops of small bowel in bilateral hernias.

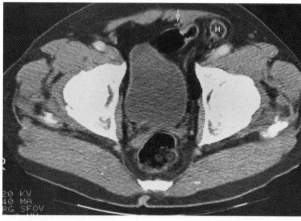

Fig GI 49-9
Indirect inguinal hernia. The neck of the hernia (H) is situated just lateral to the inferior epigastric vessels (arrow).[59]

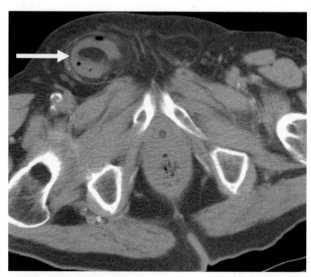

Fig GI 49-10
Direct inguinal hernia. The hernia (arrow) is situated medial to the inferior epigastric vessels of the right side of the groin. Note the presence of bowel loops in the hernia sac.[2]

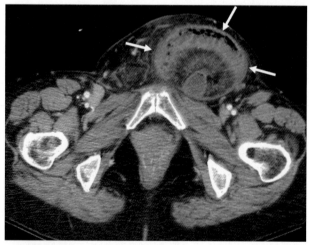

Fig GI 49-11
Strangulated inguinal hernia. C-shaped configuration (arrows) of bowel wall thickening, severe fat stranding, mesenteric engorgement, and extraluminal fluid that is confined to the hernia sac. These findings suggest strangulation.[2]

Condition	Comments
Femoral (Figs GI 49-12 and GI 49-13)	More common in women, the hernia protrudes through the femoral ring and appears at the saphenous opening. It can displace or narrow the femoral vein and descend along the saphenous vein. Although less frequent than inguinal hernias, femoral hernias are more prone to incarceration and strangulation because of the firm and unyielding margins of the femoral ring. On CT, hernia emerging from the femoral canal lies below and lateral to the pubic tubercle, in contrast to an inguinal hernia that lies above and medial to the tubercle.
Obturator (Fig GI 49-14)	Rare lesion that is most frequent in thin, older women and typically occurs on the right side. May contain any or all of the internal female genital organs, urinary bladder, variable segments of small and large bowel, appendix, and omentum. A highly suggestive (though not always present) indication of obturator hernia is the Howship-Romberg sign, which consists of pain along the inner aspect of the thigh to the knee or below that is due to compression of the obturator nerve by the hernial contents.

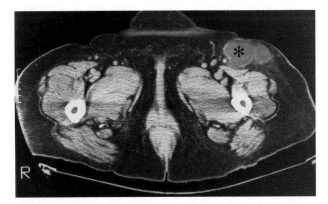

Fig GI 49-12
Femoral hernia. Fluid-filled loops of bowel (asterisk) lie along the course of the saphenous vein.[54]

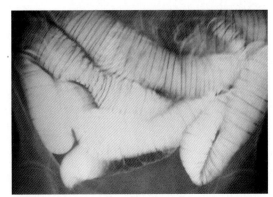

Fig GI 49-13
Femoral hernia causing strangulating obstruction. Dilated loops of barium-filled small bowel are seen proximal to the point of obstruction.

Condition	Comments
Sciatic (Fig GI 49-15)	Rare lesion that passes from the pelvis through the sciatic foramen into the buttocks. May involve the ureter, bowel, bladder, or ovary.
Perineal (Fig GI 49-16)	Rare protrusion through a defect in the pelvic floor musculature. Herniated loops of bowel may be seen adjacent to the distal rectum and anal canal or extending to one of the buttocks.

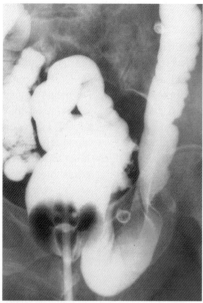

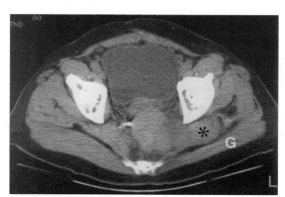

Fig GI 49-15
Sciatic hernia. Recurrent rectal carcinoma (asterisk) herniating through the sciatic foramen lies behind the ischial spine deep to the gluteus maximus muscle (G).[54]

Fig GI 49-14
Obturator hernia containing sigmoid colon.

A

B

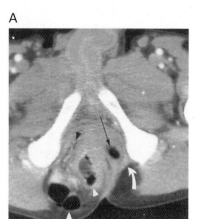

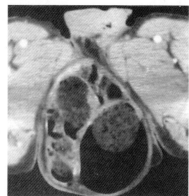

Fig GI 49-16
Perineal hernia. (A) Herniated loops of sigmoid colon (white arrowheads) are situated in the right ischiorectal fossa. Note the vessels coursing in the sigmoid mesocolon (black arrowhead). The rectum (black arrow) is deviated to the left. The levator ani muscle (white arrow) is seen on the left but not on the right. (B) Scan 2 cm inferior shows multiple loops of sigmoid colon filling the entire clinically evident mass.[55]

Condition	Comments
Umbilical (Figs GI 49-17 to GI 49-19)	Much more common in women. Risk factors include multiple pregnancies, liver failure, ascites, obesity, and large intraabdominal masses. Because bowel loops herniated into an anterior abdominal wall sac are superimposed on normal intraperitoneal loops on an anteroposterior view, oblique or lateral radiographs are required for optimal evaluation.
Epigastric (Fig GI 49-20)	Type of ventral hernia that arises in the linea alba above the umbilicus.

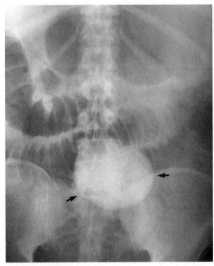

Fig GI 49-17
Strangulated umbilical hernia. Large soft-tissue mass (arrows) in the mid-abdomen and lower pelvis. The loops of the small bowel proximal to the point of obstruction are dilated.

Fig GI 49-18
Umbilical hernia. Contrast CT scan obtained during a Valsalva maneuver shows small bowel loops (arrows) within the hernia. The initial study demonstrated herniation of only omental fat.[60]

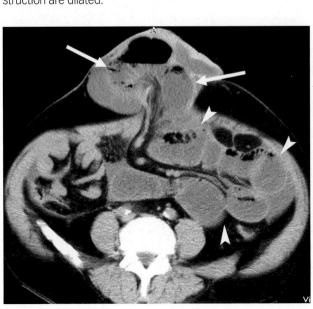

Fig GI 49-19
Strangulated umbilical hernia. The strangulated hernia (arrows) causes small bowel obstruction (arrowheads). The herniated bowel loop has a C-shaped configuration and there is discrete mesenteric engorgement as well as ascitic fluid with the hernia sac.[60]

Condition	Comments
Incisional (Fig GI 49-21)	Common complication of abdominal surgery. Best appreciated on CT, as they may be impossible to palpate due to the patient's obesity or abdominal pain or distention and be undetectable on abdominal radiographs due to their intermittency and easy reducibility.
Omphalocele (Fig GI 49-22)	Protrusion of the abdominal viscera into the base of the umbilical cord (with an associated defect in the abdominal wall). It represents persistence of normal fetal herniation with failure of complete withdrawal of the midgut from the umbilical cord during the 10th fetal week.

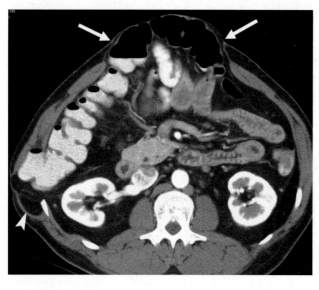

Fig GI 49-20
Epigastric hernia. The hernia (arrows) contains the transverse colon and small bowel loops. Note also the interparietal hernia through the right lateral aspect of the abdominal wall (arrowhead) containing the hepatic flexure of the colon.[60]

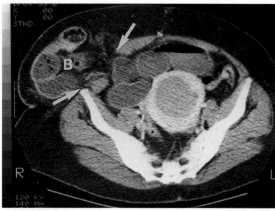

Fig GI 49-21
Obstructed incisional hernia. Dilated loops of bowel (B) extend into the abdominal wall through a defect in the region of the linea semilunaris (arrows). This was the site of a previous surgical incision.[59]

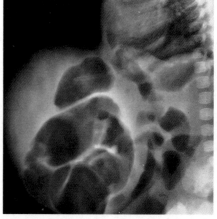

Fig GI 49-22
Omphalocele. Loops of gas-filled small bowel can be seen within the lesion.

Condition	Comments
Spigelian (Figs GI 49-23 and GI 49-24)	Lateral herniation through a spontaneous defect of the abdominal wall that arises along the linea semilunaris (where the sheaths of the lateral abdominal muscles fuse to form the lateral rectus sheath). Almost always found just above the point where the inferior epigastric vessels pierce the posterior wall of the rectus sheath. Although rare, spigelian hernias frequently incarcerate.
Lumbar (Figs GI 49-25 to GI 49-27)	Occur through two areas of relative weakness in the flank: the superior lumbar triangle, which is bounded by the 12th rib superiorly, the internal oblique muscle anteriorly, and the erector spinae muscle posteriorly; and the inferior lumbar triangle, which is bordered inferiorly by the iliac crest, anteriorly by the external oblique muscle, and posteriorly by the latissimus dorsi muscle. They occur most commonly on the left side and in middle-aged men.
Transmesenteric (Figs GI 49-28 and GI 49-29)	About one-third occur during the pediatric period and are most likely caused by a congenital mechanism. In adults, most mesenteric defects are probably the result of surgery, trauma, or inflammation.
Transomental (Fig GI 49-30)	Herniation may occur through a free greater omentum with no sac (more common) or into the lesser sac through the gastrocolic ligament (rare).

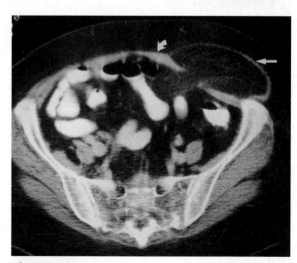

Fig GI 49-24
Spigelian hernia. Herniation of fat through a defect in the aponeurosis between the left rectus abdominis (curved arrow) and the aponeurosis of the left transversus abdominis and internal oblique muscles. The lateral margin of the hernia sac is the external oblique muscle and fascia (straight arrow).[61]

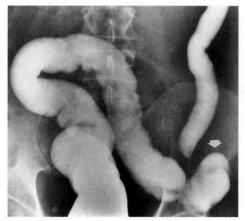

Fig GI 49-23
Spigelian hernia. Small bowel is trapped in the hernia sac (arrow), which arises along the left semilunar line.

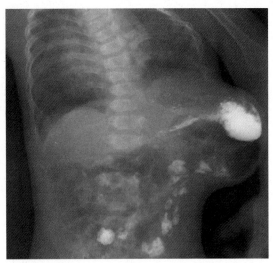

Fig GI 49-25
Lumbar hernia through the superior triangle.
Note the multiple bony anomalies.

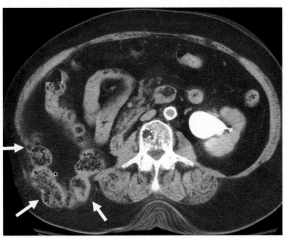

Fig GI 49-26
Superior lumbar hernia. The incisional type of hernia (arrows) developed following right nephrectomy for renal cell carcinoma. Note the protrusion of the ascending colon in the subcutaneous tissue. The extrarenal pelvis on the left was an incidental finding.[60]

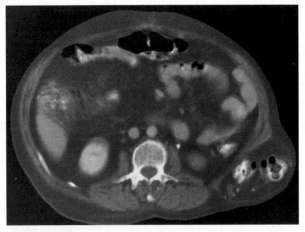

Fig GI 49-27
Lumbar hernia through the inferior triangle.

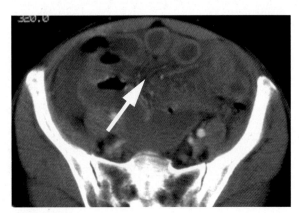

Fig GI 49-28
Transmesenteric hernia. Crowding of bowel loops and converging vessels (arrow) are seen at the orifice of the hernia.[57]

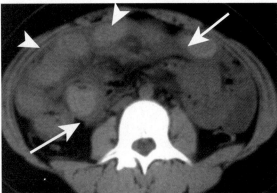

Fig GI 49-29
Transmesenteric hernia with gangrene. Unenhanced CT scan in a young girl shows diffuse mesenteric fluid and haziness (arrows) and mildly dilated small bowel loops. The attenuation of the intraluminal fluid is increased (arrowheads) because red blood cells may have been released in the lumen.[57]

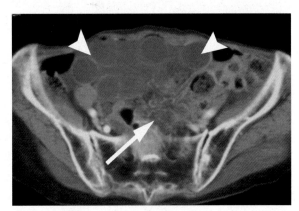

Fig GI 49-30
Transomental hernia. Contrast CT of the pelvis shows a cluster of fluid-filled small bowel loops (arrowheads) with poor or absent enhancement of bowel walls adjacent to the mid-abdominal wall. The mesenteric vascular pedicle (arrow), which is crowded and engorged with vessels, is seen at the orifice of the hernia.[57]

Condition	Comments
Pericecal (Fig GI 49-31)	Herniation through any of the four different pericecal recesses formed by folds of the peritoneum.
Sigmoid mesocolon (Fig GI 49-32)	Herniation through the peritoneal fold that attaches the sigmoid colon to the pelvic wall.
Broad ligament (Fig GI 49-33)	This type of herniation typically occurs in middle-aged women who have been pregnant and have no history of abdominal surgery
Perirectal fossa (Fig GI 49-34)	Extremely rare type of hernia.

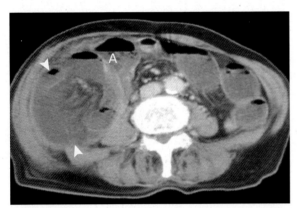

Fig GI 49-31
Pericecal hernia. Contrast CT scan shows a cluster of encapsulated small bowel loops (arrowheads) in the lateral aspect of the right paracolic gutter and behind the ascending colon (A). Dilated and stretched mesenteric vessels are seen within the cluster.[57]

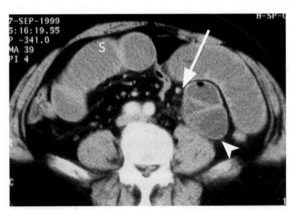

Fig GI 49-32
Sigmoid mesocolon hernia. Contrast CT shows multiple dilated small bowel loops (S). A dilated inferior mesenteric vein (arrow) appears as a landmark at the edge of the inferior mesentery. A sac-like mass of incarcerated jejunal loops (arrowhead) is located anterior to the left psoas muscle.[57]

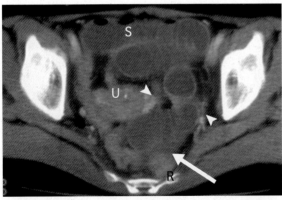

Fig GI 49-33
Broad ligament hernia. Contrast CT shows dilated small bowel loops (S) and a cluster of small bowel loops with air-fluid levels (arrow) between the uterus (U) and rectum (R). Stenosis of an incarcerated bowel loop (arrowheads) can be seen because of the fat layer around the uterus. The C-shaped configuration of the bowel loop suggests a closed-loop obstruction.[57]

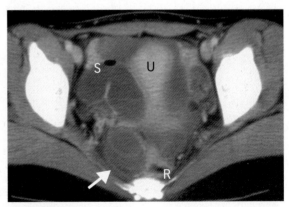

Fig GI 49-34
Perirectal hernia. Contrast CT scan shows dilated and fluid-filled small bowel loops (S). A cluster of dilated bowel loops (arrow) is located to the right of the rectum (R) and behind the uterine cervix (U).[57]

Liver Calcification

Condition	Imaging Findings	Comments
Tuberculosis/histoplasmosis (Fig GI 50-1)	Small (1–3 cm), multiple, dense, discrete calcifications scattered throughout the liver.	Healed foci of granulomatous disease are the most common intrahepatic calcifications. Usually there are also calcifications in the lung and spleen.
Echinococcus granulosus (Fig GI 50-2)	Complete oval or circular calcification at the periphery of a mother cyst. There may be multiple daughter cysts with arc-like calcifications.	Hydatid cyst calcification generally develops 5 to 10 years after liver infection. Extensive dense calcifications suggest an inactive cyst, whereas segmental calcifications suggest cystic activity and are often considered an indication for surgery.
Echinococcus multilocularis (Fig GI 50-3)	Multiple small lucencies surrounded by rings of calcification which, in turn, lie within large areas of amorphous calcification.	Calcification occurs in approximately 70% of patients with this rarer and more malignant form ("alveolar type") of hydatid disease.

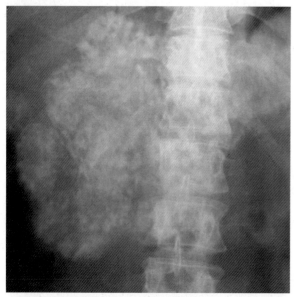

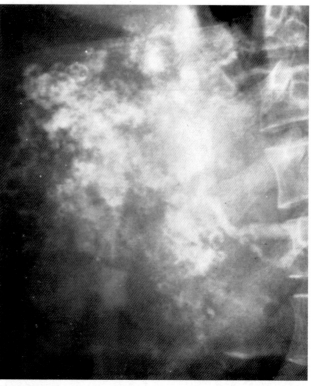

Fig GI 50-1
Hepatobiliary tuberculosis. Multiple, confluent coarse or chalky calcifications.[62]

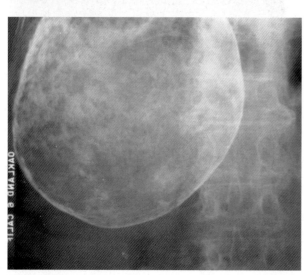

Fig GI 50-2
Hydatid liver cyst. Extensive calcification of a huge right upper quadrant mass.

Fig GI 50-3
Alveolar hydatic disease (*Echinococcus multilocularis*).[63]

Condition	Imaging Findings	Comments
Amebic or pyogenic abscess (Fig GI 50-4)	Dense, mottled calcifications that are usually solitary but are occasionally multiple.	Patient is usually asymptomatic when the hepatic calcification is detected.
Brucellosis (see Fig GI 51-1)	Snowflake appearance of fluffy calcifications.	Usually there are similar calcifications in the spleen.
Other parasitic infestations (Fig GI 50-5)	Various patterns of calcification.	*Armillifer armillatus* (tongue worm); guinea worm; filariasis; toxoplasmosis; cysticercosis; schistosomiasis.
Cavernous hemangioma	Sunburst pattern of spicules of calcification (radiating from the central area toward the periphery of the lesion).	Appearance similar to that of hemangiomas in flat bones (eg, skull and sternum). Most hemangiomas are not calcified. Rarely associated with calcified phleboliths (unlike hemangiomas elsewhere).
Primary carcinoma of liver	Various patterns of calcification (small irregular flecks to discrete spherical calculi).	Tumors most often calcify in children as a result of dystrophic calcification of necrotic tissue.
Metastases to liver (Fig GI 50-6)	Diffuse, finely granular calcifications.	Calcification most commonly occurs in metastatic colloid carcinoma of the colon or rectum. Less frequently, carcinomas of the breast, stomach, and ovary. Metastases from other primary tumors are usually larger and denser. Calcification within liver metastases may also develop as a result of radiation treatment or systemic chemotherapy.
Portal vein thrombus (Fig GI 50-7)	Linear opacity crossing the vertebral column.	Usually associated with cirrhosis and portal hypertension.
Hepatic artery aneurysm	Circular, cracked-eggshell pattern.	Most hepatic artery aneurysms do not calcify.
Calcification of liver capsule (Fig GI 50-8)	Opaque shell around part or all of the liver.	May reflect alcoholic cirrhosis, pyogenic infection, meconium peritonitis, pseudomyxoma peritonei, or lipoid granulomatosis after the intraperitoneal instillation of mineral oil. A similar pattern can follow the inadvertent introduction of barium into the peritoneal cavity through a colonic perforation.

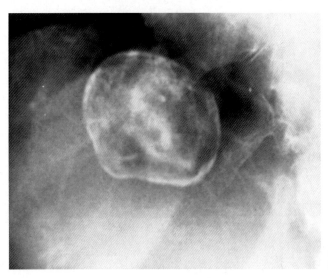
Fig GI 50-4
Calcified pyogenic liver abscess.

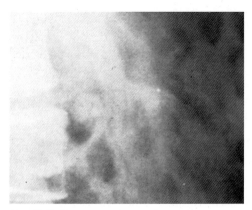

Fig GI 50-5
Calcified guinea worm in the right lobe of the
liver.[64]

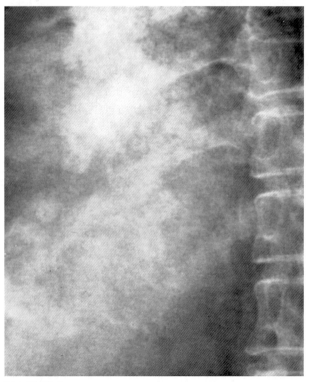

Fig GI 50-6
Calcified liver metastases from colloid carcinoma of the
colon producing a diffuse, finely granular pattern.

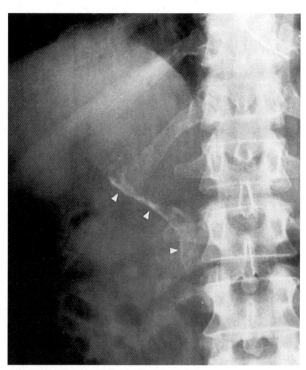

Fig GI 50-7
Portal vein. Track-like calcification with irregular margins
directed along the course of the portal vein (arrows).[65]

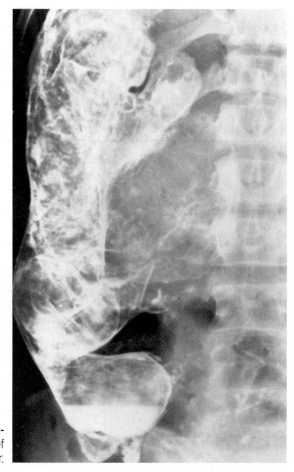

Fig GI 50-8
Appearance simulating intrinsic hepatic calcification due to inadvertent intraperitoneal extravasation of
barium, which produced an opaque shell around the liver.

Condition	Imaging Findings	Comments
Generalized increased liver density (without specific demonstrable calcification) (Figs GI 50-9 and GI 50-10)	Uniform or patchy increased density.	Causes include hemochromatosis, siderosis, cirrhosis (contracted liver), and a previous injection of Thorotrast.

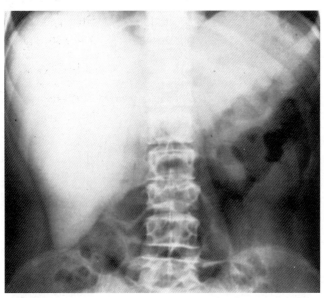

Fig GI 50-9
Hemochromatosis. Extremely dense liver shadow in the right upper quadrant is caused by parenchymal deposition of iron.[66]

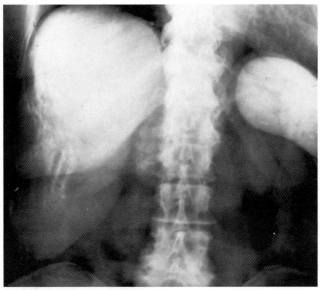

Fig GI 50-10
Prior injection of Thorotrast causing generalized increased density of the liver and spleen.

Spleen Calcification

Condition	Imaging Findings	Comments
Histoplasmosis/tuberculosis (Fig GI 51-1)	Multiple, small, round, or ovoid calcified nodules distributed throughout the spleen.	Healed foci of granulomatous disease are the most common intrasplenic calcifications. There are usually also calcifications in the lung and occasionally in the liver.
Brucellosis (Fig GI 51-2)	Snowflake appearance of fluffy calcifications that are generally larger than those in other granulomatous diseases.	The lesions in chronic brucellosis, unlike those in histoplasmosis and tuberculosis, tend to be active and suppurating even in the presence of calcification.
Phleboliths	Small, round, or ovoid calcified nodules, often with lucent centers.	Usually diffusely distributed in veins throughout the spleen.
Cysts Nonparasitic (Fig GI 51-3)	Thin peripheral calcification.	Infrequent manifestation of congenital or post-traumatic cyst.
Echinococcal (hydatid) (Fig GI 51-4)	Peripheral calcification that is often multiple and tends to be thicker and coarser than nonparasitic cystic calcification.	Echinococcal calcification can reflect a hydatid cyst in the spleen or extension of cysts arising from neighboring organs.

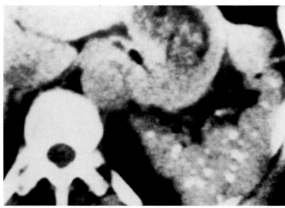

Fig GI 51-1
Histoplasmosis. CT scan shows multiple small calcifications in the spleen.

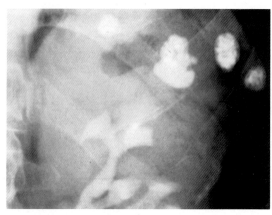

Fig GI 51-2
Brucellosis. Large calcified splenic granulomas.

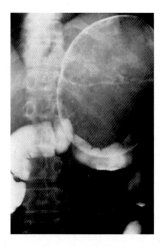

Fig GI 51-3
Huge calcified nonparasitic splenic cyst.

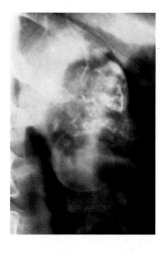

Fig GI 51-4
Calcified hydatid cyst of the spleen (echinococcal disease).

Condition	Imaging Findings	Comments
Calcification of splenic capsule (Fig GI 51-5)	Opaque shell around part or all of the spleen.	May be secondary to a pyogenic or tuberculous abscess, infarct, or hematoma. Although they infrequently calcify, splenic infarcts may have a characteristic triangular or wedge-shaped appearance, with the apex of the calcification appearing to point toward the center of the organ.
Splenic artery (Fig GI 51-6)	Characteristic tortuous, corkscrew appearance.	Extremely common finding. When viewed end-on, splenic artery calcification appears as a thin-walled ring.
Splenic artery aneurysm (Fig GI 51-7)	Circular pattern or bizarre configuration of calcification.	
Generalized increased splenic density (without demonstrable calcification) (Fig GI 51-8)	Uniform or patchy increased density.	Causes include sickle cell anemia, hemochromatosis, Fanconi's anemia, multiple transfusions, and a previous injection of Thorotrast.

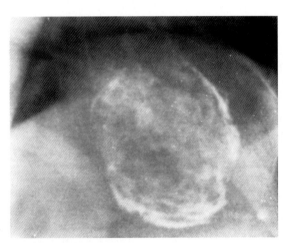

Fig GI 51-5
Calcified splenic hematoma.

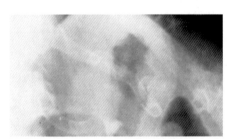

Fig GI 51-6
Calcification of the splenic artery.

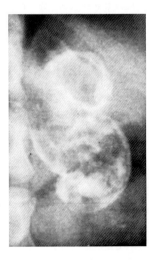

Fig GI 51-7
Splenic artery aneurysm producing bizarre, lobulated calcification.

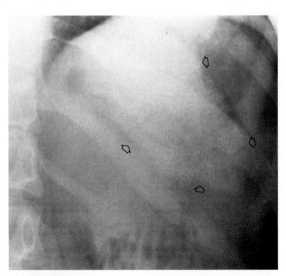

Fig GI 51-8
Sickle cell anemia causing generalized increase in splenic density (arrows).

Alimentary Tract Calcification

Condition	Imaging Findings	Comments
Appendicolith (Fig GI 52-1)	Round or oval, laminated stones of various sizes.	Found in 10% to 15% of cases of acute appendicitis. Suggests a gangrenous appendix that is likely to perforate and is usually an indication for surgery. May be retrocecal (simulating a gallstone) or pelvic (mimicking a ureteral stone).
Other enterolith (Fig GI 52-2)	Faceted, laminated stone in a Meckel's diverticulum, a colonic diverticulum, or the rectum.	Probably results from stasis and is usually found proximal to an area of stricture or within a diverticulum. May cause mucosal ulceration and lower abdominal pain.
Calcified mucocele of appendix	Large crescent-shaped or circular calcification.	Mucocele represents a mucus-containing dilatation of the appendix distal to a fibrotic obstruction of the lumen.
Calcified appendices epiploicae (Fig GI 52-3)	Cyst-like calcifications adjacent to the gas-filled colon (especially the ascending portion).	May become detached from the colon and appear as small, ring-shaped calcifications lying free in the peritoneal cavity (they change position on serial films).

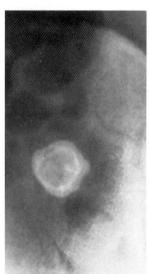

Fig GI 52-1
Appendicolith.

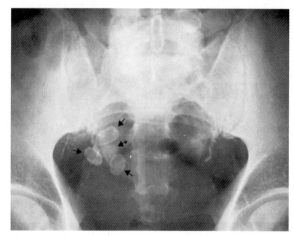

Fig GI 52-2
Faceted stones in a Meckel's diverticulum. Four radiopaque calculi (arrows) are seen in the right side of the pelvis.[67]

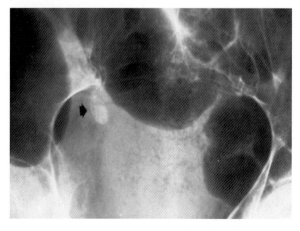

Fig GI 52-3
Calcified appendix epiploica (arrow). The cyst-like calcific density was detached from the colon and changed position on serial films.

Condition	Imaging Findings	Comments
Ingested foreign bodies (Fig GI 52-4)	Various calcific and metallic densities.	Ingested birdshot (metallic) may be trapped in the appendix or colonic diverticula. Trapped seeds and pits may develop ring-like calcium deposits around them.
Mucinous carcinoma of stomach or colon (Fig GI 52-5)	Small mottled or punctate deposits of calcium in the tumor.	Calcification may be limited to the tumor mass or involve regional lymph nodes, adjacent omentum, or metastatic foci in the liver.
Leiomyoma of stomach or esophagus (see Fig GI 16-1)	Stippled or punctate calcification scattered throughout the mass.	Simulates the pattern of calcification in uterine leiomyomas (fibroids).
Mesenteric calcification (Fig GI 52-6)	Various patterns of calcification.	Calcified fat deposits in the omentum; peripheral calcification in mesenteric cysts; rarely, calcified mesenteric lipomas or hydatid cysts in the peritoneal cavity.

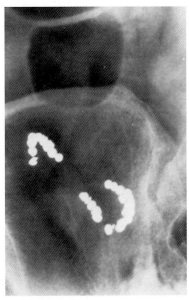

Fig GI 52-4
Metallic foreign bodies in the appendix representing ingested birdshot.

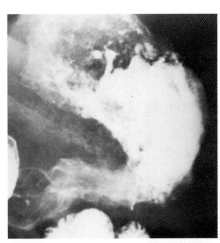

Fig GI 52-5
Calcified mucinous adenocarcinoma of the stomach causing irregular narrowing of the antrum and body.

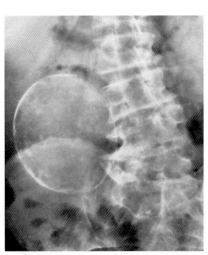

Fig GI 52-6
Calcified mesenteric cyst.

Pancreatic Calcification

Condition	Imaging Findings	Comments
Chronic pancreatitis (Fig GI 53-1)	Multiple irregular, small concretions widely scattered throughout the gland (limited to the head or tail in approximately 25% of cases). Solitary pancreatic calculi are rare.	Primarily alcoholic pancreatitis (calcification in 20% to 40% of patients with chronic alcoholic pancreatitis; 90% of patients with pancreatic calcification have high alcohol intake). Calcification is much less common (2% of cases) in pancreatitis secondary to biliary tract disease.
Pancreatic pseudocyst (Fig GI 53-2)	Typical calcifications of chronic pancreatitis, occasionally with a rim of calcification outlining the wall of the pseudocyst.	Calcification can be detected in approximately 20% of patients who develop a pseudocyst as a complication of chronic pancreatitis.
Hyperparathyroidism	Chronic pancreatitis pattern of calcification.	Pancreatitis occurs in up to 20% of patients with hyperparathyroidism. There is often associated renal calcification (nephrocalcinosis or nephrolithiasis).
Cystadenoma/ cystadenocarcinoma (Fig GI 53-3)	Sunburst pattern of calcification.	Tumor calcification (often nonspecific) in approximately 10% of cases. No calcification in adenocarcinoma of the pancreas (though there may be calcification from associated chronic pancreatitis). Sunburst calcification suggests an insulinoma.

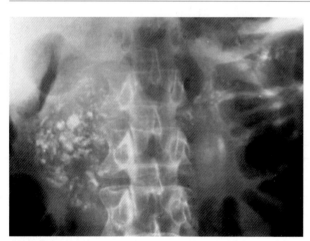

Fig GI 53-1
Chronic alcoholic pancreatitis.

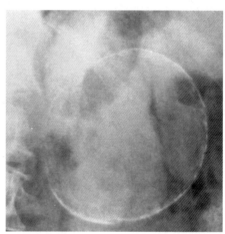

Fig GI 53-2
Pancreatic pseudocyst. A rim of calcification outlines the wall of the pseudocyst.

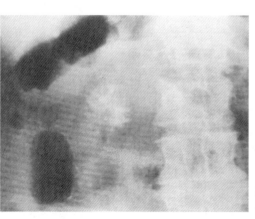

Fig GI 53-3
Pancreatic insulinoma. Sunburst pattern of calcification.[68]

Condition	Imaging Findings	Comments
Cavernous lymphangioma (Fig GI 53-4)	Multiple phleboliths within and adjacent to the pancreas.	Very rare pancreatic tumor.
Hereditary pancreatitis (Fig GI 53-5)	Large, rounded calcification (larger than in cystic fibrosis).	More than 50% of children with this inherited (autosomal dominant) condition have pancreatic calcification. Some 20% die from pancreatic cancer.
Cystic fibrosis (Fig GI 53-6)	Fine granular calcifications (smaller than in hereditary pancreatitis).	In children and young adults, pancreatic calcification usually implies marked fibrosis with diabetes mellitus.
Kwashiorkor (protein malnutrition)	Various patterns of calcification.	Occurs in underdeveloped countries and is often associated with diabetes and steatorrhea.
Intraparenchymal hemorrhage	Calcified pancreatic mass.	Calcified hematoma due to trauma, infarction, or a bleeding intrapancreatic aneurysm.
Idiopathic pancreatitis	Various patterns of calcification.	Calcified hematoma due to trauma, infarction, or a bleeding intrapancreatic aneurysm.

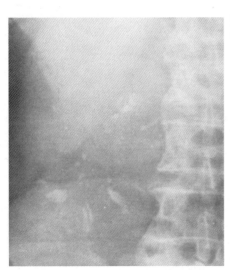

Fig GI 53-4
Cavernous lymphangioma.

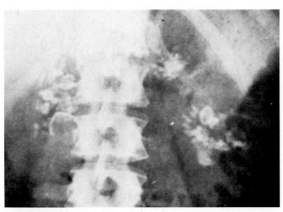

Fig GI 53-5
Hereditary pancreatitis. The calcifications are rounder and larger than those usually found in other pancreatic diseases.[69]

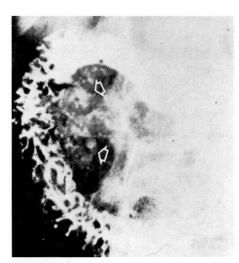

Fig GI 53-6
Cystic fibrosis. Finely granular calcification (arrows) primarily found in the head of the pancreas.[38]

Gallbladder and Bile Duct Calcification

Condition	Imaging Findings	Comments
Gallstone (Figs GI 54-1 and GI 54-2)	Single or multiple, smooth or faceted, and often laminated (alternating opaque and lucent rings).	Approximately 20% of gallstones contain sufficient calcium to be radiopaque. If there is a fistula between the biliary and alimentary tracts, a gallstone can be demonstrated at any point in the duodenum, small bowel, or colon.
Porcelain gallbladder (Fig GI 54-3)	Extensive mural calcification around the perimeter of the gallbladder.	High incidence of carcinoma (up to 60% of cases). Therefore, a prophylactic cholecystectomy is usually performed even if the patient is asymptomatic.

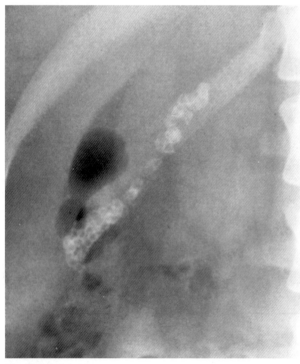

Fig GI 54-1
Multiple faceted gallstones.

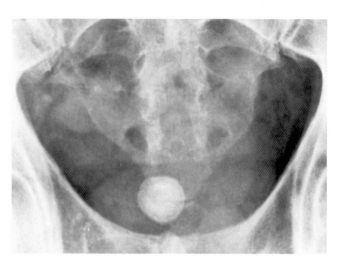

Fig GI 54-2
Calcified gallstone in the rectum.

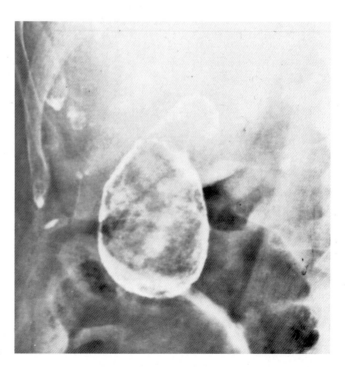

Fig GI 54-3
Porcelain gallbladder.

Condition	Imaging Findings	Comments
Milk of calcium bile (Fig GI 54-4)	Opacification of the entire gallbladder (simulates a normal gallbladder with contrast material).	Gallbladder is filled with bile that appears opaque because of the high concentration of calcium carbonate. Secondary to chronic cholecystitis with a thickened gallbladder wall and an obstructed cystic duct.
Common duct stone	Single or multiple calcified calculi.	Often difficult to diagnose (the stone is situated close to the spine and often overlies a transverse process).
Mucinous adenocarcinoma of gallbladder	Fine, granular, punctate flecks of calcification.	Rare manifestation. Similar to tumors of the same cell type in the stomach and colon.

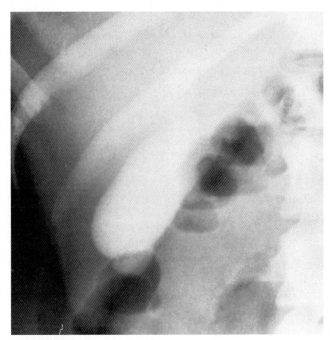

Fig GI 54-4
Milk of calcium bile on a plain abdominal radiograph. The patient had not received any cholecystographic agent.

Adrenal Calcification

Condition	Imaging Findings	Comments
Neonatal adrenal hemorrhage (Fig GI 55-1)	Triangular or circular calcification about the periphery of the gland.	Most common cause of adrenal calcification. Usually occurs in infants born to diabetic mothers or those with an abnormal obstetric history (prematurity, use of forceps, breech delivery).
Tuberculosis (Fig GI 55-2)	Discrete, stippled densities that often outline the entire gland.	Seen in approximately one-fourth of patients with adrenal tuberculosis. Infrequently produces confluent and dense calcific masses.

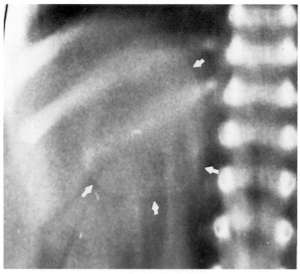

Fig GI 55-1
Neonatal adrenal hemorrhage. Circular calcification about the periphery of the gland (arrows).[70]

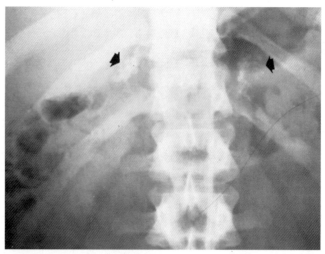

Fig GI 55-2
Adrenocortical insufficiency (Addison's disease). There are bilateral adrenal calcifications (arrows) in this patient with tuberculous adrenal disease.

Condition	Imaging Findings	Comments
Neuroblastoma (Fig GI 55-3)	Multiple finely stippled, punctate, or flocculent calcifications. May be dense and confluent or extend across the midline.	Calcification with areas of hemorrhage and necrosis occurs in approximately 50% of cases. There may be calcification in metastatic foci in regional lymph nodes and the liver.
Adrenal cyst	Thin rim of curvilinear calcification outlining the cyst wall.	May represent serous cyst, pseudocyst (necrosis and resolution of old hemorrhage), parasitic (usually echinococcal) cyst, or cystic adenoma.
Adrenal cortical carcinoma	Scattered calcifications in a mass.	Calcification is fairly common in these tumors.
Pheochromocytoma	Tiny flecks of calcification scattered throughout the tumor.	Approximately 10% are multiple and 10% arise in an extrarenal location (primarily the retroperitoneal ganglia).
Wolman's disease (Fig GI 55-4)	Diffuse punctate calcifications throughout both glands.	Rare familial xanthomatosis that causes death in early infancy. Adrenal glands are enlarged but have a normal shape.

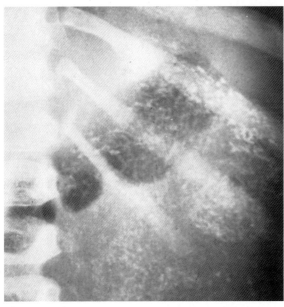

Fig GI 55-3
Neuroblastoma. Diffuse granular calcification in the large left upper quadrant mass.

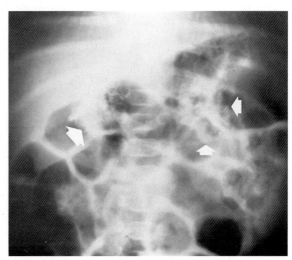

Fig GI 55-4
Wolman's disease. Diffuse punctate calcifications in bilaterally enlarged adrenal glands (arrows).

Renal Calcification

Condition	Imaging Findings	Comments
Calculus (Fig GI 56-1)	Single or multiple stones in the calyces and renal pelvis.	Approximately 80% of renal calculi are opaque. Urinary stasis and infection are important predisposing factors.
Nephrocalcinosis (Fig GI 56-2)	Diffuse calcium deposition in the renal parenchyma (especially the medullary pyramids). Varies from a few scattered punctate densities to very dense and extensive calcifications throughout both kidneys.	Causes include skeletal deossification (hyperparathyroidism, primary and secondary bone malignancy, severe osteoporosis, Cushing's syndrome, and steroid therapy), increased intestinal absorption of calcium (sarcoidosis, milk-alkali syndrome, hypervitaminosis D), renal tubular acidosis, and hyperoxaluria.
Medullary sponge kidney (Fig GI 56-3)	Small, round calculi clustering around the apices of renal pyramids.	Cystic dilatations of the distal collecting ducts.

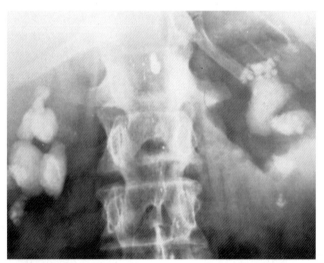

Fig GI 56-1
Bilateral staghorn calculi.

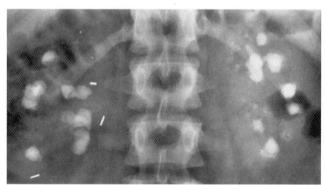

Fig GI 56-2
Milk-alkali syndrome causing nephrocalcinosis.

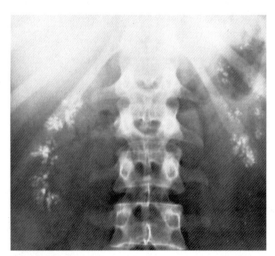

Fig GI 56-3
Medullary sponge kidney.

Condition	Imaging Findings	Comments
Papillary necrosis (Fig GI 56-4)	Triangular lucency surrounded by a dense opaque band (ring shadow) representing calcification of a sloughed papilla.	Infarction of renal papillae resulting in necrosis with sloughing of involved tissue. Causes include analgesic abuse (phenacetin), diabetes mellitus, sickle cell anemia, pyelonephritis, and urinary tract obstruction.
Tuberculosis	Various patterns of calcification.	Flecks of calcification in multiple tuberculous granulomas. Massive amorphous calcification in nonfunctioning renal parenchyma (autonephrectomy).
Cystic disease (Fig GI 56-5)	Thin, curvilinear calcification around the periphery of a renal cyst.	Approximately 3% of simple renal cysts have this pattern (but up to 20% of renal carcinomas have a similar appearance). Peripheral calcification also occurs in polycystic or multicystic disease and in more than half of echinococcal cysts.
Perirenal hematoma/ abscess	Large cyst-like calcification.	Calcification tends to be thicker than in a simple renal cyst.
Renal cell carcinoma (Fig GI 56-6)	Typically nonperipheral, mottled, or punctate calcification in a mass. There may be cyst-like peripheral calcification of the fibrous pseudocapsule.	About 10% contain calcification (primarily in reactive fibrous zones about areas of tissue necrosis). Approximately 90% of masses containing calcium in a nonperipheral location are malignant.
Wilms' tumor	Peripheral cystic calcification in approximately 10% of cases.	Differs from the fine, granular, or stippled calcification that occurs in 50% of neuroblastomas.
Other neoplasms	Various patterns of calcification.	Infrequently reported causes include cortical adenoma, angiomyolipoma, dermoid, fibroma, osteosarcoma, oncocytoma, spindle cell sarcomas, transitional cell carcinoma, and metastases (thyroid, Hodgkin's disease).

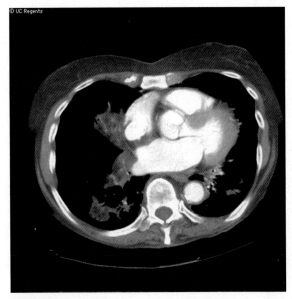

Fig GI 56-4
Lipoid pneumonia. Multifocal areas of consolidation in the right lung containing areas of fat attenuation. (Courtesy of Michael B. Gotway, MD, Scottsdale, AZ.)

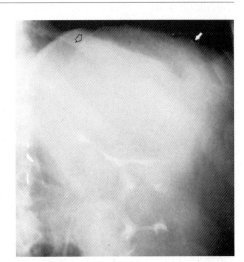

Fig GI 56-5
Simple renal cyst. Curvilinear, peripheral calcification outlines part of the cyst wall (arrows). Smooth splaying of upper pole calyces is demonstrated on this film from an excretory urogram.[71]

Condition	Imaging Findings	Comments
Xanthogranulomatous pyelonephritis (Fig GI 56-7)	Diffuse parenchymal calcification, often with an obstructing pelvocalyceal stone.	Chronic inflammatory disease that predominantly occurs in women with a long history of renal infection and is characterized by multiple inflammatory masses that often simulate renal carcinoma.
Cortical calcification	Punctate or linear (tramline) calcification around the renal margin.	Occurs in acute cortical necrosis (rare form of acute renal failure with sparing of the medulla), chronic glomerulonephritis, and hereditary nephritis, and also occurs in dialysis patients.
Renal artery aneurysm (Fig GI 56-8)	Circular calcification with a cracked-eggshell appearance.	Calcification develops in one-third of these saccular structures situated at the renal hilum.

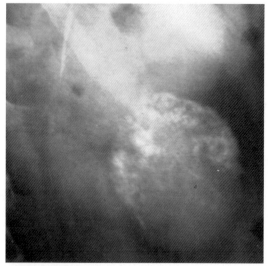

Fig GI 56-6
Calcification in a renal cell carcinoma. If there is no peripheral calcification, mottled or punctuate calcium that appears to be within a mass is highly indicative of a malignant lesion.[72]

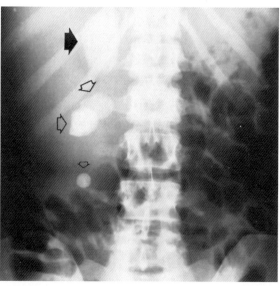

Fig GI 56-7
Xanthogranulomatous pyelonephritis. Several large radioplaque calculi at the ureteropelvic junction and in the proximal ureter on the right (open arrows). The closed arrow points to an opacified gallbladder. At excretory urography, the right kidney showed no function.

A

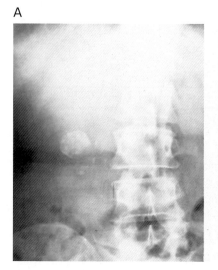

B

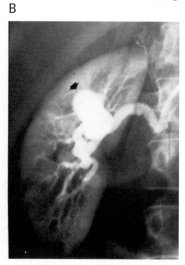

Fig GI 56-8
Calcification in a renal artery aneurysm. (A) Plain abdominal radiograph demonstrates the circular calcification with a cracked-eggshell appearance at the renal hilum. (B) Selective right arteriogram shows contrast material filling the saccular aneurysm (arrow).

Condition	Imaging Findings	Comments
Arteriovenous malformation	Curvilinear calcification.	Congenital malformation that usually presents with hematuria and frequently an abdominal bruit.
Renal milk of calcium (Fig GI 56-9)	Simulates a typical round or oval solid calculus on supine views. Characteristic half-moon contour with the patient in an upright or sitting position (calcific material gravitates to the bottom of the cyst).	Suspension of fine sediment containing calcium that is most commonly found in a cyst or calyceal diverticulum. Usually asymptomatic and an incidental finding. May be related to stasis and infection.
Dysplastic (Fig GI 56-10)	Thin curvilinear calcification outlining cyst walls.	Nonhereditary congenital dysplasia, usually unilateral and asymptomatic, in which the kidney is composed almost entirely of large, thin-walled cysts with only a little solid renal tissue. Absent or severely atretic renal artery and an atretic ureter with a blind proximal end.
Residual Pantopaque in renal cyst	Heavy-metal density simulating a swallowed coin.	Pantopaque instilled after renal cyst puncture takes several years to be absorbed (unlike water-soluble contrast material).

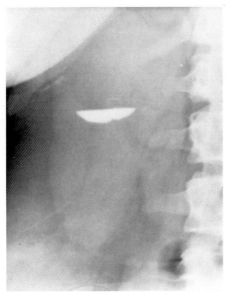

Fig GI 56-9
Renal milk of calcium. On an upright view, the calcium-containing sediment gravitates to the bottom of the renal cyst, resulting in the characteristic half-moon contour.

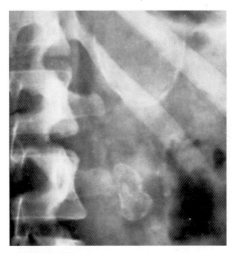

Fig GI 56-10
Congenital unilateral multicystic kidney.
There are three peripherally calcified masses, with no excretion of contrast material on excretory urography.[72]

Ureteral Calcification

Condition	Imaging Findings	Comments
Calculus (Figs GI 57-1 and GI 57-2)	Small, irregular, and poorly calcified. Often oval with its long axis paralleling the course of the ureter.	Most commonly lodges in the lower portion of the ureter (especially at the ureterovesical junction and the pelvic brim). Situated medially above the interspinous line (unlike the far more common phleboliths, which are spherical and located in the lateral portion of the pelvis below a line joining the ischial spines).
Schistosomiasis (see Fig GI 58-1)	Two roughly parallel, dense lines separated by the caliber of the ureter.	Ureteral calcification occurs in approximately 15% of patients. It is heaviest in the pelvic portion and gradually decreases proximally. Diffuse bladder calcification is present almost invariably.
Tuberculosis (Fig GI 57-3)	Linear calcification of the ureteral wall.	Much less frequent than renal calcification in tuberculosis. Calcification of the bladder is relatively rare.

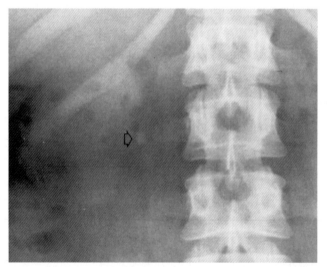

Fig GI 57-1
Ureteral calculus (arrow).

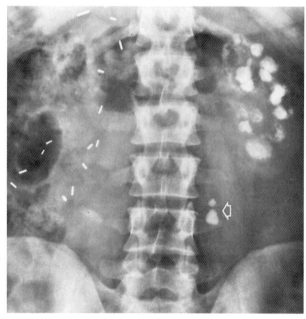

Fig GI 57-2
Ureteral calculi. Two stones (one of which is causing obstruction) in the midportion of the left ureter (arrow) in a patient with renal tubular acidosis causing nephrocalcinosis.

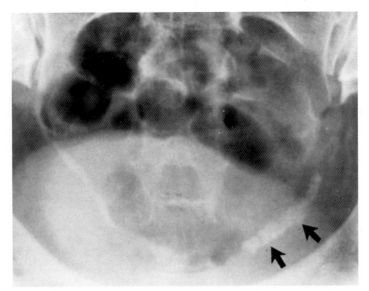

Fig GI 57-3
Tuberculosis. Linear calcification of the distal ureter (arrows).

Bladder Calcification

Condition	Imaging Findings	Comments
Schistosomiasis (Fig GI 58-1)	Linear opaque shadow that initially involves the base of the bladder and eventually encircles the entire bladder.	Worldwide, the most common cause of bladder wall calcification. The bladder often retains relatively normal capacity and distensibility (unlike other inflammatory causes of calcification). Disruption in the continuity of the line of calcification suggests superimposed bladder carcinoma.
Tuberculosis	Faint, irregular rim of calcium outlining the wall of a markedly contracted bladder.	When bladder wall calcification is detectable, extensive tuberculous changes are usually evident in the kidneys and ureters.
Other types of cystitis	Various patterns of amorphous calcification.	Rare manifestation of postirradiation cystitis, bacterial cystitis, and nonspecific infections (encrusted cystitis) with calcium deposited on mucosal erosions.
Bladder calculus (Figs GI 58-2 and GI 58-3)	Single or multiple and varying in size from tiny concretions to an enormous single calculus occupying the entire bladder lumen.	May represent a migrating stone from the upper urinary tract or a de novo bladder stone (predominantly in elderly men with obstruction or infection of the lower urinary tract). The calcification is usually circular or oval, but may be amorphous, laminated, or spiculated.
Bladder neoplasm (Fig GI 58-4)	Punctate, coarse, or linear calcification that is usually encrusted on the tumor surface.	Most common in epithelial lesions (transitional cell and squamous cell carcinomas). Occasionally occurs in mesenchymal tumors (leiomyosarcoma, hemangioma, neuroblastoma, osteogenic sarcoma).

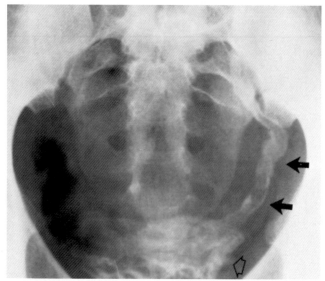

Fig GI 58-1
Schistosomiasis. Calcification of the bladder (open arrow) and distal ureter (solid arrows).

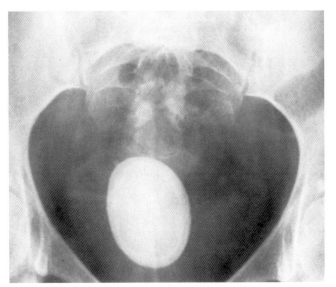

Fig GI 58-2
Bladder calculus. Single, huge, laminated, calcified stone.

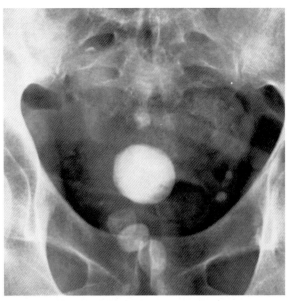

Fig GI 58-3
Multiple bladder stones of various sizes.

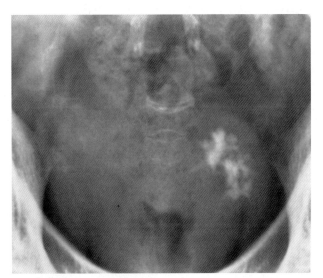

Fig GI 58-4
Calcified transitional cell carcinoma of the bladder. Coarse tumor calcification was associated with an intravesical mass.

Female Genital Tract Calcification

Condition	Imaging Findings	Comments
Uterine fibroid (leiomyoma) (Fig GI 59-1)	Stippled, mottled, or whorled calcification.	Most common calcified lesion of the female genital tract. A huge fibroid may occupy the entire pelvis or even extend beyond it.
Dermoid cyst (Fig GI 59-2)	May contain partially or completely formed teeth. Less frequently, the wall of the cyst is partially calcified.	Approximately half of dermoid cysts contain some calcification. Demonstration of the relatively radiolucent fatty material in the lesion is diagnostic.
Cystadenoma/ cystadenocarcinoma of ovary (Fig GI 59-3)	Scattered, fine amorphous shadows (psammomatous bodies), which are barely denser than normal soft tissue.	Calcification is often found in serosal and omental implants throughout the abdomen.
Gonadoblastoma of ovary (Fig GI 59-4)	Unilateral or bilateral circumscribed, mottled calcifications.	Rare, potentially malignant gonadal neoplasm that is usually hormonally active and is composed of germ cells, cells of sex cord origin, and mesenchymal elements.
Spontaneous amputation of ovary	Small, coarsely stippled, calcified mass that moves on serial films or with changes in patient position.	Probably the result of torsion of the adnexa with subsequent ischemic infarction. Ultrasound or CT shows evidence of a missing ovary on one side.
Pseudomyxoma peritonei (Fig GI 59-5)	Curvilinear calcification at the periphery of the jelly-like masses.	Complication of spontaneous or surgical rupture of pseudomucinous carcinoma of the ovary or mucocele of the appendix.
Tuberculous salpingitis	Bilateral "string-of-pearls" calcification.	Fallopian tubes have an irregular contour, small lumen, and multiple strictures.

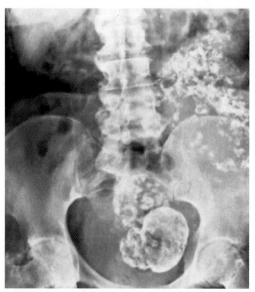

Fig GI 59-1
Calcified uterine fibroid (leiomyoma). The calcified mass extends well beyond the confines of the pelvis.

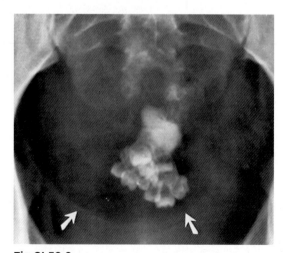

Fig GI 59-2
Dermoid cyst containing multiple well-formed teeth. Note the relative lucency of the mass (arrows), which is composed largely of fatty tissue.

Condition	Imaging Findings	Comments
Placental calcification	Fine lace-like pattern outlining the crescent shape of the placenta.	Physiologic phenomenon associated with involution of the placenta (usually occurs after the 32nd week of fetal life).
Lithopedion (Fig GI 59-6)	Calcification or ossification of fetal skeletal parts.	Rare. May be intrauterine (old missed abortion) or extrauterine (previous ectopic pregnancy).
Complication of parametrial gold therapy	Bilateral laminated calcification closely approximating the lateral pelvic wall.	Complication of parametrial injections of [198]Au colloid (previous therapy for carcinoma of the cervix). Gold seed implants for pelvic malignancy can appear as multiple, short, thin metallic densities.

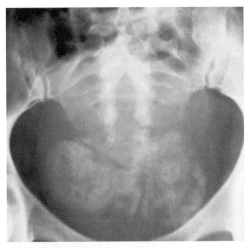

Fig GI 59-3
Calcified cystadenocarcinoma of the ovary. Diffuse, ill-defined collections of granular amorphous calcification.

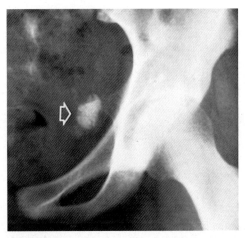

Fig GI 59-4
Calcified gonadoblastoma of the ovary (arrow).[73]

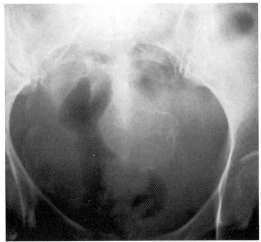

Fig GI 59-5
Pseudomyxoma peritonei. Complication of spontaneous rupture of pseudomucinous carcinoma of the ovary.

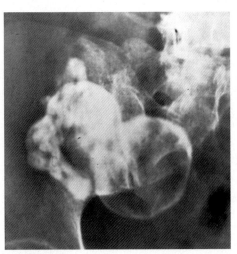

Fig GI 59-6
Lithopedion in a 78-year-old woman.

Male Genital Tract Calcification

Condition	Imaging Findings	Comments
Vas deferens (Fig GI 60-1)	In diabetics, typically bilaterally symmetric, parallel tubular densities that run medially and caudally to enter the medial aspect of the seminal vesicles at the base of the prostate (simulates arteriosclerotic calcification).	Most commonly seen in diabetic males, but also occurs as a degenerative phenomenon. In patients with chronic inflammatory diseases (tuberculosis, syphilis, nonspecific urinary tract infection), vas deferens calcification is largely intraluminal and produces an irregular pattern of calcification.
Seminal vesicle (Fig GI 60-2)	Multiple, small concretions near the proximal end of the vas deferens.	Usually associated with seminal vesiculitis (primarily due to neisserial infections, tuberculosis, or bilharziasis) and can be mistaken clinically and radiographically for ureteral calculi.
Prostate (Fig GI 60-3)	Multiple small calcifications extending to either side of the midline overlying or directly above the level of the symphysis pubis.	Usually represent calculi in older men. Occasionally, tuberculous calcification of the prostate gland can produce a radiographically indistinguishable appearance.

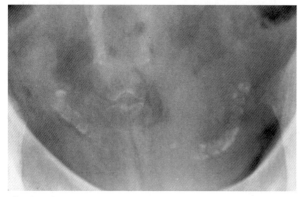

Fig GI 60-1
Vas deferens. Vascular-like calcification in a man with diabetes mellitus.

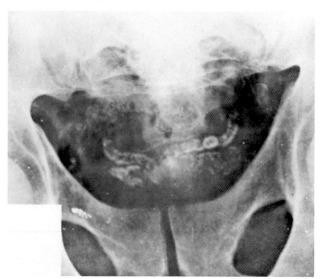

Fig GI 60-2
Seminal vesicles and vas deferens (nondiabetic).[74]

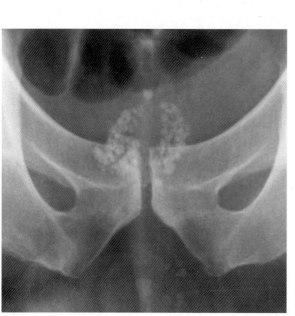

Fig GI 60-3
Prostatic calculi.

Condition	Imaging Findings	Comments
Scrotum (Fig GI 60-4)	Various patterns.	Calcification may occur in the ductus deferens, hydroceles, spermatoceles, and testicular tumors. A dense oval collection of calcification can be due to infection of the testicle or to testicular infarction secondary to torsion.
Penile implant (Fig GI 60-5)	Large pelvic opacification.	

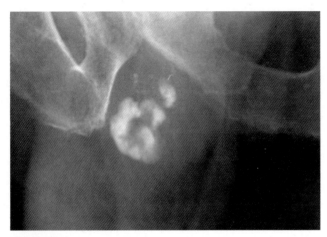

Fig GI 60-4
Testicular calcification. The clumps of amorphous calcification presumably developed after infarction secondary to testicular torsion.[75]

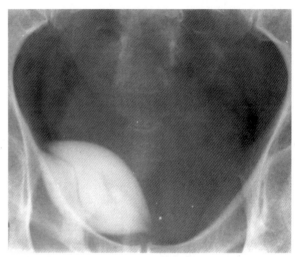

Fig GI 60-5
Penile implant.

Widespread Abdominal Calcification

Condition	Imaging Findings	Comments
Psammomatous calcification (cystadenocarcinoma of ovary) (Fig GI 61-1)	Scattered granular or sand-like shadows that are often barely denser than normal soft tissue.	May be confined to the primary tumor or diffusely involve metastases throughout the abdomen.
Pseudomyxoma peritonei (see Fig GI 59-5)	Widespread abdominal calcifications that are annular and tend to be most numerous in the pelvis.	Caused by rupture of a pseudomucinous cystadenoma of the ovary or a mucocele of the appendix.
Undifferentiated abdominal malignancy (Fig GI 61-2)	Bizarre masses of calcification that do not conform to any organ.	Patients with this condition have large soft-tissue masses with multiple linear or nodular calcific densities that can coalesce to form distinctive conglomerate masses.
Tuberculous peritonitis	Widespread mottled abdominal calcifications.	May simulate residual barium in the gastrointestinal tract.
Meconium peritonitis	Multiple, small calcific deposits scattered widely throughout the abdomen in a newborn.	Chemical inflammation of the peritoneum caused by the escape of sterile meconium into the peritoneal cavity. Meconium peritonitis usually results from perforation in utero secondary to a congenital stenosis or atresia of the bowel or to meconium ileus.

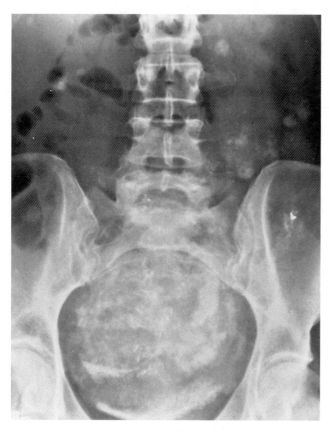

Fig GI 61-1
Psammomatous calcification of ovarian cystadenocarcinoma. The granular, sand-like calcifications represent metastatic spread throughout the abdomen.

Condition	Imaging Findings	Comments
Oil granulomas (Fig GI 61-3)	Widespread annular or plaque-like deposits simulating pseudomyxoma peritonei.	Late effect of the instillation of liquid petrolatum into the peritoneal cavity to prevent adhesions. The calcifications are located in masses of fibrous tissue surrounding the oil droplets. Clinically, oil granulomas can produce hard palpable masses that simulate carcinomatosis or cause intestinal obstruction.

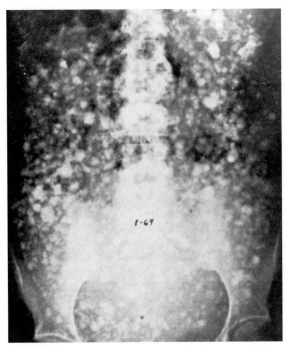

Fig GI 61-2
Undifferentiated abdominal malignancy.[76]

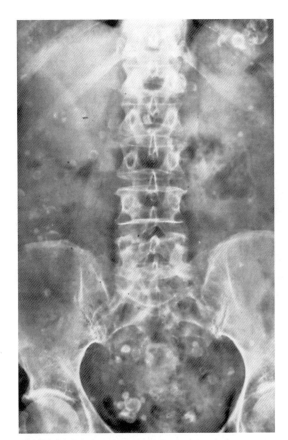

Fig GI 61-3
Intraperitoneal granulomatosis.

Gastric Diseases on Computed Tomography

Condition	Imaging Findings	Comments
Neoplasms Adenocarcinoma (Figs GI 62-1 to GI 62-5)	Variable appearances including a focal area of mural thickening, diffuse infiltration and narrowing (linitis plastica), and a bulky mass that is often ulcerated. Mucinous tumors may show calcification.	Occurring twice as frequently in males as in females, adenocarcinoma is the most common gastric tumor, accounting for approximately 95% of primary neoplasms of the stomach. It remains a deadly disease, with a 5-year survival rate of only 20%, though when detected at an early stage there is a much better prognosis. Predisposing conditions include atrophic gastritis, pernicious anemia, gastric polyps, partial gastrectomy, and Ménétrier's disease.

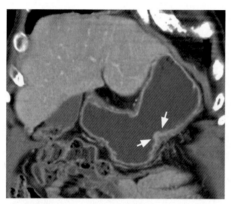

Fig GI 62-1
Early gastric carcinoma. Coronal reformatted image shows an elevated lesion in the greater curvature that protrudes less than 5 mm into the lumen. There is marked focal enhancement of the inner layer of the gastric wall (arrows).[77]

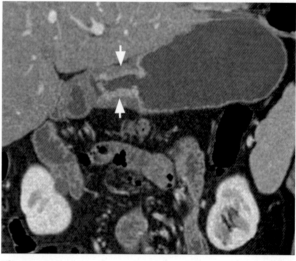

Fig GI 62-2
Antral carcinoma. Coronal reformatted image shows focal wall thickening of the antrum with marked enhancement of the mucosal layer (arrows). The subtle irregularities of the mucosal surface corresponded to ulcers at histology. Note the clear fat plane around the tumor.[77]

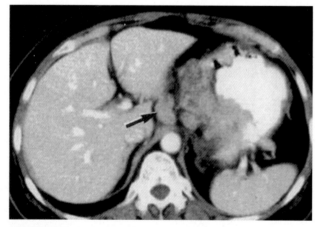

Fig GI 62-3
Advanced gastric carcinoma. Large ulcerating mass with spread of tumor beyond the gastric wall. There is evidence of adenopathy in the celiac nodal chain.[78]

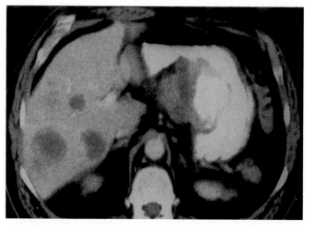

Fig GI 62-4
Advanced gastric carcinoma. Large, ulcerating exophytic mass with liver metastases. The tumor appears to involve the pancreas.[78]

Condition	Imaging Findings	Comments
Lymphoma (Figs GI 62-6 and GI 62-7)	Infiltrative lesions manifest as focal or diffuse enlargement of gastric folds due to submucosal spread of tumor. Localized polypoid tumors often ulcerate.	The stomach is the most frequent site of lymphomatous involvement of the gastrointestinal tract. About 80% of lesions are of the non-Hodgkin's type. The imaging findings may be indistinguishable from adenocarcinoma. However, most patients with lymphoma have adenopathy, and the nodes are usually bulkier than with carcinoma and extend beneath the renal hilum. Moreover, the degree of thickening of the gastric wall tends to be much more prominent than in carcinoma.
Metastasis (Figs GI 62-8 and GI 62-9)	Variable pattern ranging from bull's-eye lesions in melanoma to linitis plastic in breast cancer. At time, the appearance of primary gastric cancer and metastatic disease may be identical.	Metastases to the stomach are infrequent, found in less than 2% of patients who die of cancer. Spread to the stomach may be by hematogenous (breast or lung cancer, malignant melanoma) or lymphatic spread (esophageal or colon cancer), or by direct extension from malignancies arising in neighboring structures (pancreas, liver, gallbladder, colon, kidney).

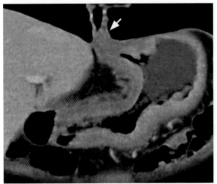

Fig GI 62-5
Linitus plastica. Oblique coronal reformatted image shows circumferential thickening of the wall of the stomach with loss of gastric folds. The tumor extends into the distal esophagus (arrow).[77]

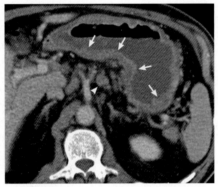

Fig GI 62-6
Lymphoma. Large areas of gastric wall thickening (arrows) with enlarged lymph nodes (arrowhead).[77]

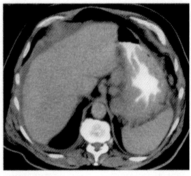

Fig GI 62-7
Lymphoma. Marked thickening of gastric folds with extensive adenopathy and ascites.[78]

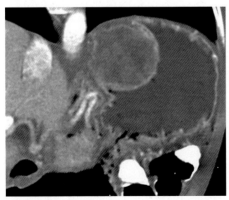

Fig GI 62-8
Metastasis. Submucosal gastric masses from a primary esophageal carcinoma.[77]

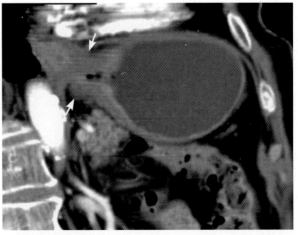

Fig GI 62-9
Metastasis. Direct infiltration of the stomach by an esophageal carcinoma (arrows).[77]

Condition	Imaging Findings	Comments
Gastrointestinal stromal tumors (GIST) (Figs GI 62-10 to GI 61-13)	Submucosal mass. Large tumors have a prominent exogastric component and often show intratumoral necrosis and ulceration.	Now recognized as the most common mesenchymal neoplasm of the gastrointestinal tract. Many, but not all, mesenchymal tumors previously diagnosed as leiomyomas, leiomyoblastomas, leiomyosarcomas, and other lesions are placed in this category. About 60% to 70% of GISTs are found in the stomach. Up to 30% are malignant, and the risk increases with extragastric location, larger diameter (>5 cm), and extension into adjacent organs.
Lipoma	Smooth mass of variable fat attenuation.	Rare tumor that is usually detected as an incidental finding.

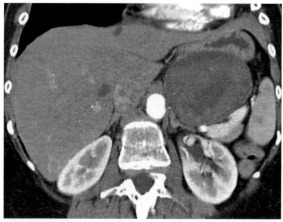

Fig GI 62-10
Gastrointestinal stromal tumor. Oblique coronal reformatted image shows a large, inhomogeneous, round mass that compresses the fundus of the stomach. Note the obtuse angle on the medial side and the rounded angle on the lateral side, which are compatible with the subserosal location seen at histology.[77]

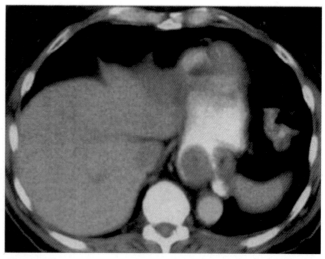

Fig GI 62-11
Leiomyoma. Smooth ulcerating mass in the fundus of the stomach.[78]

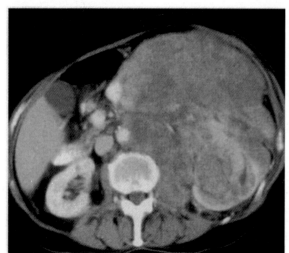

Fig GI 62-12
Leiomyosarcoma. Huge gastric mass that invades the spleen and left kidney. The tumor extends downward to invade the left psoas muscle as well.[78]

Condition	Imaging Findings	Comments
Gastric polyps Hyperplastic (Fig GI 62-14a)	Smooth, sessile, round or oval filling defects, typically 5–10 mm in diameter, that usually occur as multiple lesions of similar size, clustered in the body or fundus of the stomach on the posterior gastric wall.	Accounting for at least 75% of gastric polyps, they are often seen in the setting of chronic gastritis, atrophic gastritis, or bile reflux gastritis. Although they have no malignant potential, patients with hyperplastic polyps are at increased risk for harboring separate, coexisting gastric carcinomas.
Adenomatous (Fig GI 62-14b)	Larger (approximately 2 cm in diameter) and more commonly pedunculated and lobulated than hyperplastic polyps. They are generally solitary and occur adjacent to the antrum.	Larger polyps contain carcinomatous foci in approximately 40% of cases.
Inflammatory disease Gastritis	Thickened gastric folds or wall thickening. The attenuation is generally similar to that of soft tissue, though there may be low attenuation due to edema	Common disease with such predisposing factors as alcohol abuse, aspirin, nonsteroidal and anti-inflammatory drugs. Polypoid and lobulated folds may be difficult to distinguish from gastric cancer and lymphoma, and biopsy is required in questionable cases.

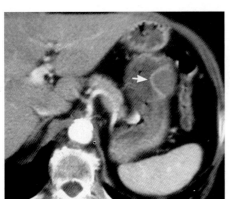

Fig GI 62-13
Schwannoma. A submucosal soft-tissue mass with only minor enhancement but with markedly enhancing intact mucosa. Note that the perigastric fat plane around the tumor is clear.[77]

A

B

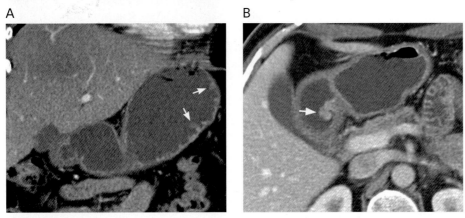

Fig GI 62-14
Gastric polyps. (A) Hypertrophic polyps appear as multiple small nodular masses arising from the gastric wall (arrows). (B) Adenomatous polyp appears as a single larger lesion in the gastric antrum (arrow).[77]

Condition	Imaging Findings	Comments
Helicobacter pylori infection (Fig GI 62-15)	Thickened gastric folds and wall thickening. Infrequently, it can stimulate an infiltrating carcinoma or focal gastric mass.	*H. pylori* bacillus is identified in nearly 80% of patients with gastric ulcers and almost 100% of those with chronic gastritis. However, up to 60% of adults over age 60 are infected with this organism, but are usually asymptomatic. The role of *H. pylori* in gastric cancer is more controversial, though approximately 80% to 90% of patients with this malignancy that arises outside the cardia of the stomach have antibodies to this organism.
Gastric ulcer disease (Fig GI 62-16)	Variable findings including perforating or penetrating ulcer, gastritis with wall thickening, pneumoperitoneum, and extravasation of contrast material.	Most gastric ulcers develop along the lesser curvature or the posterior wall of the antrum or body of the stomach. Fewer than 5% involve the anterior wall.
Radiation gastritis (Fig GI 62-17)	Symmetric thickening of the gastric wall, often with small ulcerations and a "shaggy" appearance of the mucosa.	Although often confused with recurrent or residual tumor, radiation gastritis typically has sharp margins that correspond to the therapy ports.
Eosinophilic gastritis (Fig GI 62-18)	Thickening of the gastric wall, especially affecting the antrum. Concurrent involvement of the small bowel is common.	Uncommon disease of unknown origin in which there is eosinophilic infiltration of the wall of the stomach or small bowel.

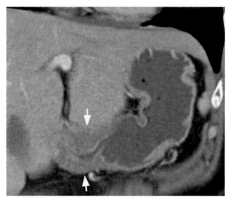

Fig GI 62-15
***Helicobacter pylori*-induced gastritis.**
Focal thickening and enhancement of the gastric wall (arrows). Note the preserved mucosal lining.[77]

A

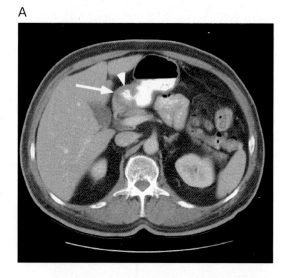

B

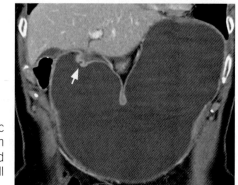

Fig GI 62-16
Gastric ulcer. (A) Axial image shows focal asymmetric thickening (arrow) of the wall of the gastric antrum with barium trapped in the ulcer cavity (arrowhead).[79] (B) Coronal reformatted image in another patient shows mucosal hyperemia and wall thickening in the antrum with a central ulcer (arrow).[77]

Condition	Imaging Findings	Comments
Miscellaneous diseases Ménétrier's disease (Fig GI 62-19)	Grossly thickened, lobulated folds that primarily involve the fundus.	Rare chronic gastric disorder of unknown origin that results in hypertrophy of gastric folds. The enlargement most commonly occurs in the gastric fundus, but any part of the stomach may be involved. The appearance may simulate an infiltrating process such as lymphoma.

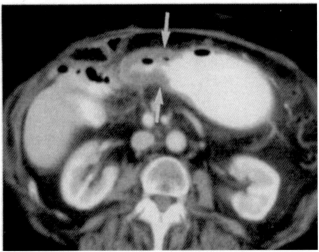

Fig GI 62-17
Radiation gastritis. Thickening and narrowing of the gastric antrum (arrows), which correspond to the postoperative radiation ports in a woman who had undergone a Whipple procedure for pancreatic cancer.[78]

A

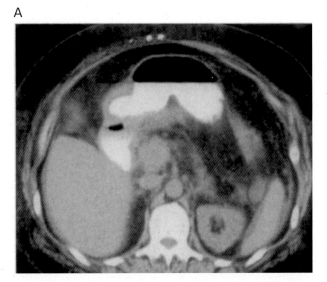

B

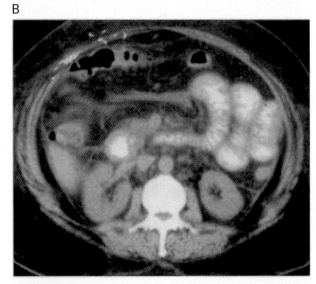

Fig GI 62-18
Eosinophilic gastritis. (A, B) Thickening of the gastric antrum and dilated loops of proximal small bowel. Note the "wet" appearance of the small bowel folds and minimal fluid in the mesentery.[78]

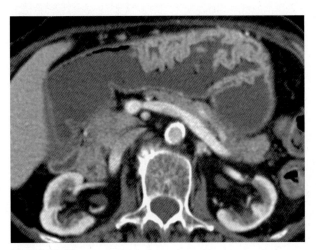

Fig GI 62-19
Ménétrier's disease. Large, lobulated folds with preserved gastric mucosa that primarily involve the fundus.[77]

Condition	Imaging Findings	Comments
Emphysematous gastritis (Fig GI 62-20)	Mottled gas in the wall of the stomach with associated thickening of gastric folds.	Life-threatening condition with a high mortality rate caused by bacterial invasion of the gastric wall with gas production. Emphysematous gastritis can be caused by ingestion of toxic or caustic substances, alcohol abuse, trauma, gastric infarction, and gastroduodenitis. The offending organism is most often *E. coli*.
Gastric emphysema (Fig GI 62-21)	Thin, linear streaks of gas in the gastric wall, which is not thickened.	Benign condition, typically in an asymptomatic patient, which resolves spontaneously without long-term sequelae. It may be related to placement of a nasogastric tube.
Gastric outlet obstruction (Fig GI 62-22)	Severe narrowing of the distal stomach.	In adults, usually caused by peptic ulcer disease in about two-thirds of cases and by an annular constricting carcinoma of the distal antrum or pylorus in most of the remainder. Occasionally, this appearance may result from other infiltrating primary or metastatic tumors, severe inflammatory disease, or extensive fibrous scarring after the ingestion of corrosive substances.
Gastric varices (Fig GI 62-23)	Enhancing tubular structures that are most commonly seen in the fundus of the stomach. Collateral vessels are often apparent in the region of the gastrohepatic ligament, near the lesser omentum, and along the course of the coronary vein.	Commonly associated with splanchnic obstruction or portal hypertension. The presence of gastric varices without esophageal varices is a classic sign of isolated splenic vein occlusion, most commonly secondary to pancreatitis or pancreatic carcinoma. On non-contrast scans, gastric varices can be confused with thickened gastric folds.

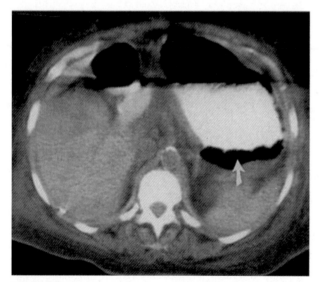

Fig GI 62-20
Emphysematous gastritis. Gas in the gastric wall (arrow) that is best seen posteriorly. Endoscopy demonstrated massive infarction of the entire posterior wall of the stomach.[78]

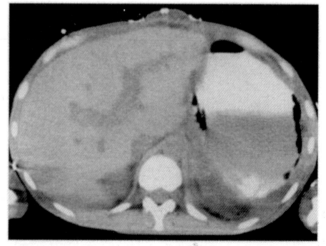

Fig GI 62-21
Gastric emphysema. Gas in the gastric wall without evidence of perforation or extravasation of contrast material. The changes were thought to be due to placement of a gastrotomy tube, and the patient recovered with conservative treatment.[78]

Condition	Imaging Findings	Comments
Hiatal hernia (Fig GI 62-24)	Focal wall thickening or filling defect in the posteromedial wall with no evidence of contrast enhancement.	The appearance is caused by incomplete distension of the hiatal hernia, with prolapse of the hernia into the fundus.
Unusual infiltrative processes (Fig GI 62-25)	Focal or diffuse narrowing of the stomach simulating a gastric neoplasm.	Especially in immune-compromised patients, this pattern may be produced by a variety of infections such as tuberculosis, syphilis, and cytomegalovirus. Sarcoidosis can cause a similar appearance.

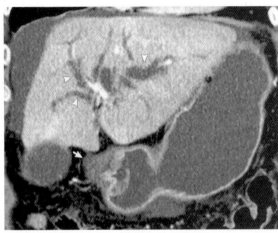

Fig GI 62-22
Gastric outlet obstruction. Coronal reformatted image shows distal stomach obstruction due to infiltration by a cholangiocarcinoma (arrow). Note the dilated intrahepatic bile ducts (arrowheads).[77]

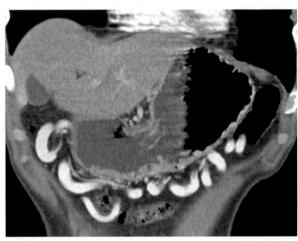

Fig GI 62-23
Gastric varices. Coronal reformatted image shows varices of the small gastric veins in a patient with chronic pancreatitis and obstruction of the splenic vein.

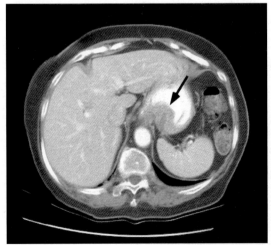

Fig GI 62-24
Hiatal hernia. Focal asymmetric thickening (arrow) of the posteromedial wall of the gastric fundus in the region of the cardia with no evidence of enhancement.[79]

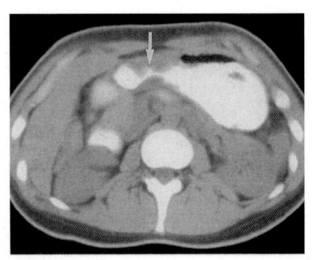

Fig GI 62-25
Cytomegalovirus infection (acquired immunodeficiency syndrome). Ulceration in the gastric antrum with thickened folds suspicious for a neoplasm (arrow).[78]

Duodenal Diseases on Computed Tomography

Condition	Comments
Developmental anomaly	
Diverticulum (Fig GI 63-2)	Most frequently develops in the medial wall of the second and third portions of the duodenum, usually within 2 cm of the ampulla of Vater.
Duplication (Fig GI 63-3)	Well-circumscribed cystic mass with fluid attenuation that most often involves the medial wall of the second and third portions of the duodenum and does not communicate with the lumen.
Annular pancreas (Fig GI 63-4)	Often presenting with duodenal stenosis and vomiting in the first decade of life, in about half of cases the diagnosis is not made until adulthood. Demonstration by CT is often difficult in children due to the paucity of intra-abdominal fat and the narrow width of the pancreatic band.

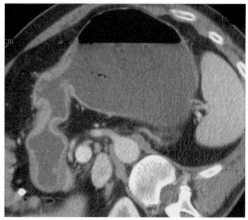

Fig GI 63-1
Normal duodenum. Contrast scan obtained with oral administration of whole milk and the patient in the right posterior oblique position shows the lumen, mural enhancement, and the gastroduodenal artery.[80]

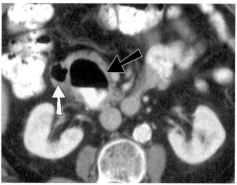

Fig GI 63-2
Diverticulum. Contrast scan shows two "duodenal lumina," with the true lumen lateral to the diverticulum (straight arrow). The diverticulum contains an air-fluid level and causes medial displacement of the pancreatic head (curved arrow).[80]

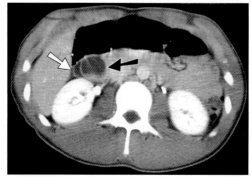

Fig GI 63-3
Duplication. Scan without oral contrast shows two fluid-attenuation structures in the second portion of the duodenum. The duplicated segment (curved arrow) is medial to the true lumen and contains debris. The true lumen is narrowed (straight arrow).[80]

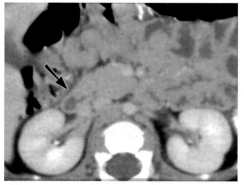

Fig GI 63-4
Annular pancreas. A band of ectopic pancreatic tissue is seen posterior to the second portion of the duodenum (arrow).[80]

Condition	Comments
Trauma (Figs GI 63-5 and GI 63-6)	Penetrating or blunt injury can cause contusion or transection. Findings suggesting duodenal injury include gas or extravasated oral contrast adjacent to the duodenum in the retroperitoneum, retroperitoneal fluid, edema in the duodenal wall, stranding of the peripancreatic fat, and pancreatic transection. Iatrogenic duodenal perforation is a rare complication of endoscopy.
Inflammatory process Pancreatitis (Fig GI 63-7)	Release of exocrine enzymes causes mild to severe duodenal edema and can produce gastric outlet obstruction. In severe disease, enzymatic disruption of the intramural vasculature can cause an intramural duodenal hematoma.
Perforated ulcer (Fig GI 63-8)	Suggestive findings include wall thickening, periduodenal fluid, retroperitoneal gas, free intraperitoneal gas, and the intraperioneal extravasation of oral contrast material.

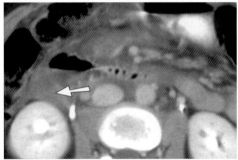

Fig GI 63-5
Ruptured duodenum (motor vehicle accident). There is fluid in the duodenum and leakage of fluid into the right anterior pararenal space (arrow).[80]

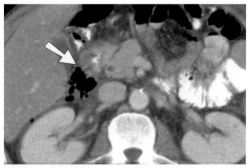

Fig GI 63-6
Duodenal perforation (endoscopy). Thick-walled, contracted duodenum with gas in the adjacent retroperitoneum (arrow).[80]

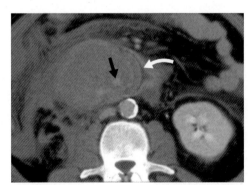

Fig GI 63-7
Pancreatitis. Extensive stranding of the peripancreatic fat indicates pancreatitis. Intramural hemorrhage has caused massive enlargement of the lateral duodenal wall, accompanied by a focal area of increased attenuation at the site of bleeding (black arrow). The duodenal lumen, which contains low-attenuation fluid, is narrowed and displaced medially (white arrow).[80]

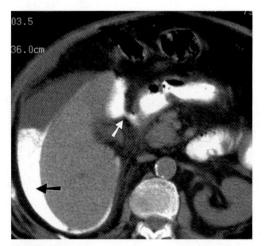

Fig GI 63-8
Perforated ulcer. Intraperitoneal extravasation of oral contrast material from the lateral portion of the duodenum (white arrow) and leakage of contrast around the liver (black arrow).

Condition	Comments
Gastric outlet obstruction (duodenal ulcer) (Fig GI 63-9)	Severe duodenal ulcer disease can result in severe strictures and obstruction of the gastric outlet.
Other inflammatory processes (Fig GI 63-10)	Crohn's disease, duodenitis, inflammation of the duodenal papilla in patients with acquired immunodeficiency syndrome or radiation therapy, and adjacent cholecystitis that can cause erosion of a stone through the gallbladder wall into the duodenum and result in gallstone ileus.
Henoch-Schonlein purpura (Fig GI 63-11)	Systemic hypersensitivity disease of unknown etiology in which the deposition of immune complexes within small vessels throughout the body results in abnormal permeability of small blood vessels. This can result in a purpuric rash, glomerulonephritis, and hemorrhage in the gastrointestinal tract. CT shows multifocal areas of bowel wall thickening and mesenteric edema.
Neoplastic process	The duodenum is the most common site of tumors in the small bowel.
Benign (Figs GI 63-12 to GI 63-14)	Leiomyoma is the most common symptomatic benign neoplasm of the duodenum. On CT, it appears as a heterogeneous mass with moderate enhancement and an annular narrowing of the lumen with abrupt concentric or irregular edges. Lipomas are typically asymptomatic, smooth-marginated lesions of characteristic fat attenuation. Tubular and Brunner gland adenomas are benign; villous adenomas have some malignant potential and are surgically resected. The multiple hamartomatous polyps of Peutz-Jeghers syndrome may affect the duodenum.

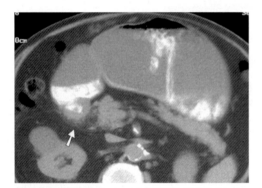

Fig GI 63-9
Gastric outlet obstruction (duodenal ulcer). Dilated stomach and thickened wall of the duodenal bulb, associated with stranding of the periduodenal fat (arrow).[80]

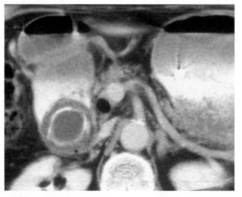

Fig GI 63-10
Gallstone ileus. Gallstone within the duodenum (arrow) with proximal duodenal and gastric dilatation.[80]

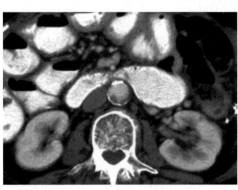

Fig GI 63-11
Henoch-Schonlein purpura. Marked thickening of the second and fourth portions of the duodenal wall (arrows). The lumen was narrowed, but there was no obstruction of the gastric outlet.[80]

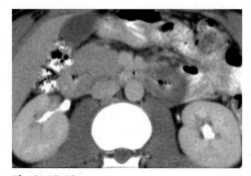

Fig GI 63-12
Lipoma. Low-attenuation lesion with well-circumscribed margins (arrow).[80]

Condition	Comments
Malignant (Figs GI 63-15 to GI 63-17)	Adenocarcinoma is the most common of the rare primary malignant neoplasms of the duodenum. Most patients are at an advanced stage, with signs of bleeding, jaundice, or obstruction. Paragangliomas and lymphoma also occur. Metastases to the duodenum may be from local extension or distant sites.

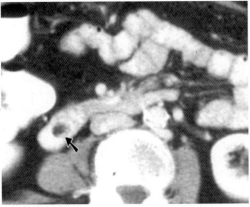

Fig GI 63-13
Villous adenoma. Soft-tissue mass (white arrow) arising from the medial wall of the duodenum. The duodenal lumen is narrowed (black arrow).[80]

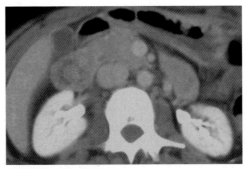

Fig GI 63-14
Peutz-Jeghers syndrome. Soft-tissue filling defect in the duodenal lumen (arrow), outlined by water. There were several polyps in the proximal small bowel.[80]

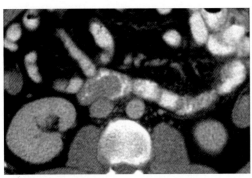

Fig GI 63-15
Adenocarcinoma. A solid intraluminal soft-tissue mass (arrow) without transmural invasion or retroperitoneal adenopathy.[80]

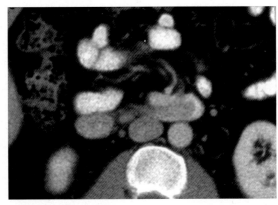

Fig GI 63-16
Paraganglioma. Subtle, smoothly marginated soft-tissue mass (arrows) in the second and third portions of the duodenum.[80]

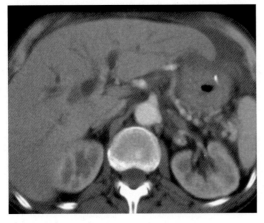

Fig GI 63-17
Metastasis (colon cancer). Mass of soft-tissue attenuation that causes lateral displacement of the duodenum (arrow). The lesion mimics a mass arising in the duodenum or pancreatic head.[80]

Attenuation Patterns in the Abnormal Bowel Wall

Condition	Imaging Findings	Comments
White attenuation (Figs GI 64-1 and GI 64-2)	Avid contrast enhancement that uniformly affects the majority of a thickened bowel wall.	One mechanism is injury to intramural vessels with accompanying interstitial leakage, exemplified by the diffuse ischemia of the small bowel in hypotensive adults who have sustained blunt trauma ("shock bowel"). Hypoperfusion results in increased vascular permeability to macromolecules and albumin, which leads to diffuse bowel wall thickening and increased enhancement on CT because of slowed perfusion and interstitial leakage of molecules of contrast material. Although decreased or absent enhancement may be the most specific sign of bowel ischemia, at times the ischemic segment may also have increased enhancement due to altered vascular permeability and perfusion problems (ie, delayed return of venous blood with subsequent slowing of the arterial supply or arteriospasm). The increased bowel wall enhancement associated with inflammatory bowel disease reflects the hyperemic and hypervascular state of acute inflammation, in which there is also dilatation and tortuosity of mesenteric vessels.
Gray attenuation (Figs GI 64-3 and GI 64-4)	Thickened bowel wall that shows little definite contrast enhancement and has a homogeneous attenuation comparable with that of enhanced muscle.	The least specific of the patterns, it is common in both benign and malignant conditions and additional morphologic criteria must be used. In general, when compared with malignant disorders, benign processes have tapered rather than heaped up edges; uniform, symmetric, and thinner bowel wall thickness; and the presence of valvulae conniventes or haustra.

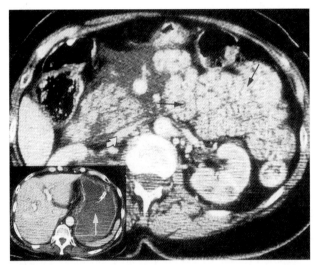

Fig GI 64-1
White attenuation in shock bowel. Increased enhancement in the jejunum (black arrows). Note that the attenuation is greater than that of the inferior vena cava (curved arrow). The enhancement qualities could be mistaken for oral contrast material in the lumen, but none was given. (Straight white arrow = fluid in stomach.)[81]

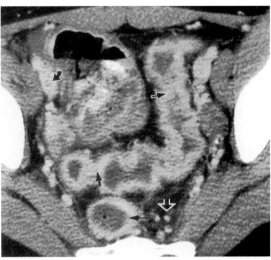

Fig GI 64-2
White attenuation in acute ulcerative colitis. Uniform increased enhancement (straight black arrow) in the thickened wall of the rectosigmoid. The attenuation of this segment of the colon is similar to that of the external iliac vein (curved arrow). The pericolonic vessels are dilated (white arrow).[81]

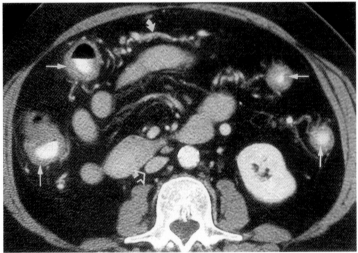

Fig GI 64-3
Gray attenuation in ischemic colitis. The attenuation of the enhancing walls of the colon (solid straight arrows) falls short of that of the superior mesenteric venous branch (curved arrow) and inferior vena cava (open arrow). Therefore, interpretation in this case should be assigned to the gray attenuation pattern.[81]

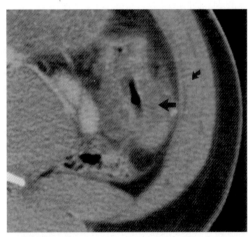

Fig GI 64-4
Gray attenuation in colon carcinoma. The thickened wall of the mid-descending colon (straight arrow) has an attenuation similar to that of the adjacent muscle (curved arrow).[81]

Condition	Comments
Water halo sign (Figs GI 64-5 and GI 64-6)	Stratification with a thickened bowel wall that consists of either two or three continuous, symmetrically thickened layers. When there are two layers (double halo sign), either a higher attenuation outer ring (muscularis propria) surrounds a second, luminally oriented ring of gray attenuation (submucosal edema) or there is a higher attenuation inner layer and an outer ring of gray attenuation. In the three-layer "target" sign, there is an outer high-attenuation muscularis propria, a middle ring of gray attenuation, and a luminally oriented ring of high attenuation. Numerous disorders of the large and small bowel can cause the water halo sign. The most common are idiopathic inflammatory bowel disease, vascular disorders, infectious disease, and radiation damage. The value of the water halo sign is that it is an unequivocal indication of bowel wall injury, usually of an acute nature. Moreover, malignancy rarely produces the classic water halo sign.

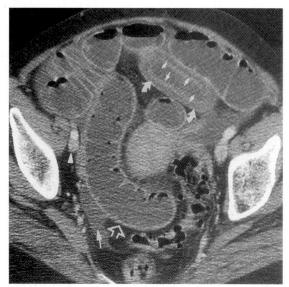

Fig GI 64-5
Water halo sign in bowel obstruction. Inner layer of a strangulated, ischemic segment of small bowel (small straight solid arrows) is surrounded by a lower attenuation layer (curved arrows). Note the brightness of the dilated, obstructed proximal small bowel wall (open arrow), which approximates the attenuation of the external iliac vein (arrowhead). However, since the wall of the dilated bowel is not thickened, it would not be considered abnormal (large straight arrow indicates ascites).[81]

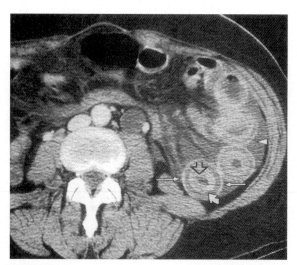

Fig GI 64-6
Target sign in angioedema. Several segments of small bowel demonstrate three uniformly thick layers. The layers grossly correspond to the muscularis propria (straight solid arrows), submucosa (curved arrow), and mucosa (open arrow). Arrowhead indicates ascites.[81]

Condition	Imaging Findings	Comments
Fat halo sign (Figs GI 64-7 and GI 64-8)	Three-layered target sign of thickened bowel in which the middle ("submucosal") layer has a fatty attenuation. The darker attenuation of intramural fat usually can be visually distinguished from the grayer tone of the water halo sign.	In the small bowel, the fat halo sign is virtually diagnostic of Crohn's disease. In the colon, the differential diagnosis includes ulcerative colitis. An unusual cause is chronic radiation enteritis.
Black attenuation (Fig GI 64-9)	The equivalent of pneumatosis.	Other than the rare large cystic collections, pneumatosis should be considered as part of an acute injury to bowel that causes a break in the integrity of the mucosa (ischemia, infection, or trauma). Although usually considered life-threatening, it may be seen as an incidental finding after intestinal anastomotic surgery.

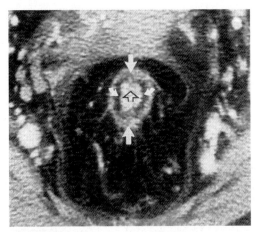

Fig GI 64-7
Fat halo sign in ulcerative colitis. An outer enhanced layer (straight solid arrows) surrounds a fat-attenuation layer (curved arrows). Contrast material is seen within the colonic lumen (open arrow).[81]

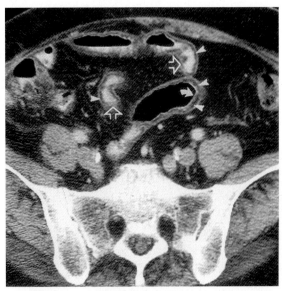

Fig GI 64-8
Fat halo sign in chronic radiation enteritis. Several segments of small bowel have walls thickened by a central band of lower attenuation consistent with fat (arrowheads). The target configuration is evident in one segment that lacks luminal oral contrast material (solid arrow). Other segments with a fatty layer have luminal contrast enhancement, which conceivably could be obscuring a higher attenuation "mucosal" layer (open arrows).[81]

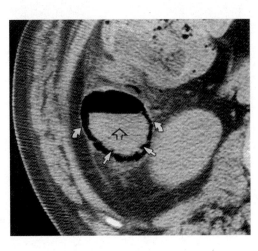

Fig GI 64-9
Black attenuation in cecal pneumatosis. There are rounded collections of mural gas attenuation (straight solid arrows) in this patient with ischemic colitis. Mural gas attenuation is also seen at the outer margin of the colonic wall (curved arrows) and lumen (open arrow).[81]

Ileocecal Diseases on Computed Tomography

Condition	Imaging Findings	Comments
Malignant tumors *Adenocarcinoma* 　Cecum 　(Fig GI 65-1)	Large, polypoid, and bulky mass that may occupy a large proportion of the lumen of the colon but rarely causes obstruction (often asymptomatic for a long period).	Cecal lesions account for about one-fourth of all colonic carcinomas. The distal ileum may be abnormally thickened in up to 10% of patients with cancer of the right colon due to tumor extension or, less commonly, congestion and edema.
Terminal ileum 　(Fig GI 65-2)	Annular and constricting lesion causing eccentric or circumferential wall thickening that involves a short segment of ileum and shows contrast enhancement.	May be difficult to distinguish from Crohn's disease, though this inflammatory process tends to involve longer or multiple segments.
Appendix	Most often detected as a mucocle reflecting their high mucin content.	Although less common than appendiceal carcinoids, they are more likely to be detected due to their larger size and higher complication rate. Soft-tissue thickening and irregularity of the wall of a mucocele and surrounding fat should suggest the possibility of a malignancy, though this nonspecific appearance may also reflect secondary inflammation.

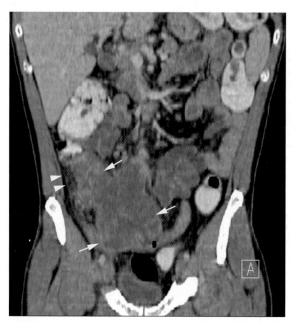

Fig GI 65-1
Adenocarcinoma (colon). Coronal oblique reformatted image shows a bulky, irregular heterogeneous mass (arrows) involving both the cecum and the terminal ileum with abrupt transition in the right colon, mild fat stranding (arrowheads), and small mesenteric lymph nodes.[82]

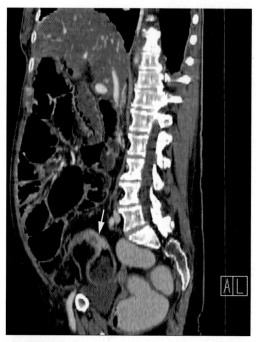

Fig GI 65-2
Adenocarcinoma (terminal ileum). Oblique sagittal reformatted obtained through the ileocecal junction shows obstructive stenosis of the terminal ileum (arrow) in a woman with Crohn's disease who presented with a sudden occlusive syndrome. Surgery revealed a small adenocarcinoma located 2 cm from the ileocecal valve.[82]

Condition	Imaging Findings	Comments
Carcinoid Terminal ileum (Fig GI 65-3)	Hypervascular nodular wall thickening or a small, smooth submucosal mass.	Larger lesions rarely cause narrowing of the lumen due to annular constriction or kinking of the bowel wall. Mesenteric desmoplastic reaction can produce an ill-defined mass (often calcified) with a stellate pattern of mesenteric stranding extending toward surrounding bowel loops.
Appendix	Tumors at the base of the appendix usually appear as appendicitis, though there may be diffuse mural thickening.	Usually less than 1 cm and found in the distal third of the appendix. Most are asymptomatic and only discovered incidentally at surgery or pathologic examination.
Lymphoma (Fig GI 65-4)	Single or multiple areas of marked circumferential thickening with homogeneous attenuation and poor enhancement. It may produce a polypoid lesion of variable size that may act as the lead point of an intussusception.	The ileum and cecum are the most common sites of involvement by primary lymphoma in the small and large bowel, respectively. Characteristic features include excavating masses and the development of fistulous tracts to adjacent bowel.

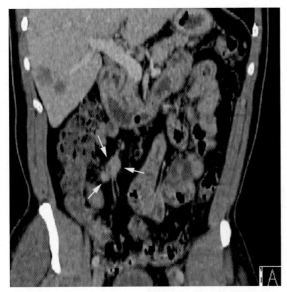

Fig GI 65-3
Carcinoid tumor (terminal ileum). Coronal oblique reformatted image shows an ill-defined, spiculated mesenteric mass (arrows).[82]

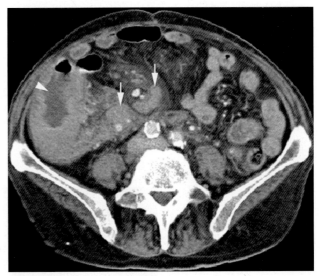

Fig GI 65-4
Non-Hodgkin's lymphoma. Marked homogeneous symmetric thickening of the cecal wall without any stenosis of the lumen (arrowhead). There is large regional and mesenteric lymphadenopathy (arrows). Note the presence of fat stranding, though it is less severe than the wall thickening.[82]

Condition	Imaging Findings	Comments
Metastasis (Fig GI 65-5)	Variable pattern including increased bowel wall thickening, annular stenosis with severe luminal narrowing and angulation, and a polypoid mass that may rarely cavitate.	Neoplastic lesions may spread to the small bowel hematogenously, by direct invasion, and by intraperitoneal seeding (the termination of the small bowel mesentery in the right lower is a predominant site of implantation).
Benign tumors Lipoma (Fig GI 65-6)	Low-attenuation intramural mass that is round or oval and well defined.	The ileum and cecum are common sites of this fatty lesion. A true lipoma must be differentiated from lipomatosis, which appears as symmetric enlargement of the ileocecal valve.
Appendiceal adenoma (Fig GI 65-7)	Round, sharply defined paracecal mass.	Most are mucinous lesions that manifest as mucoceles with homogeneous contents of near-water or soft-tissue attenuation depending on the amount of mucin they contain.
Intussusception (Fig GI 65-8)	Pathognomonic bowel-within-bowel appearance that may contain fat and mesenteric vessels; proximal bowel obstruction; and sometimes a mass corresponding to the lead point.	The lead point of an ileocolic intussusception may be a benign mass (lipoma, ileal polyp, appendiceal mucocele, duplication cyst), a polypoid malignant tumor (lymphoma, carcinoma), or a Meckel's diverticulum.
Inflammatory condition *Noninfectious* Appendicitis (Fig GI 65-9)	Enlargement of the appendix (>6 mm) with thickened enhancing wall, periappendiceal fat stranding, and sometimes focal thickening of the terminal ileum or colon.	Patients with mild isolated appendiceal dilatation (<9 mm) are unlikely to have appendicitis. Less than one-third of patients with an identifiable normal appendix surrounded by inflammatory stranding have appendicitis.

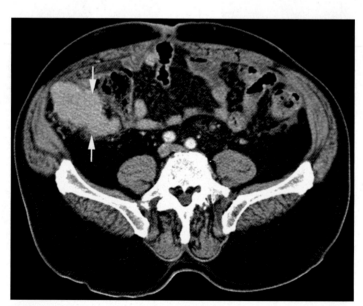

Fig GI 65-5
Metastasis. Large, hyperattenuating subserosal cecal mass (arrows) representing metastasis from hepatocellular carcinoma.[82]

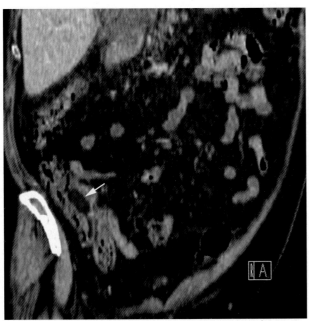

Fig GI 65-6
Lipoma of the ileocecal valve. Sagittal oblique reformatted image shows a small, well-defined fatty mass (arrow) at the level of the ileocecal valve.[82]

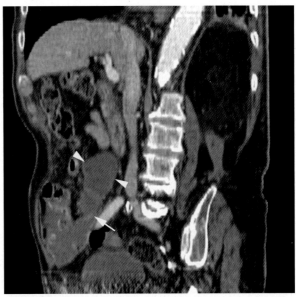

Fig GI 65-7
Mucocele (mucinous appendiceal adenoma). Coronal oblique reformatted image shows a long cystic mass (arrowheads) situated close to the base of the cecum (arrow).[82]

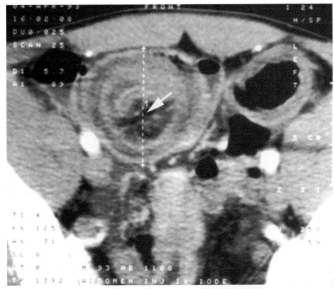

Fig GI 65-8
Ileoileal intussusception (lead point an inverted Meckel's diverticulum). Contrast scan demonstrates a central focus of fat attenuation with concentric rings of alternating fat and soft-tissue attenuation (arrow). These findings represent a core of mesenteric fat surrounded by the wall of the diverticulum and the intestinal wall.[82]

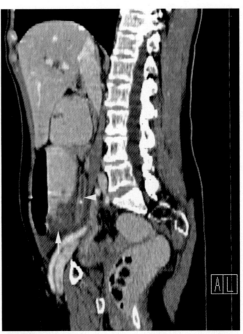

Fig GI 65-9
Appendicitis. Sagittal oblique reformatted image shows the full length of an inflamed appendix (arrowhead) and mild thickening of the base of the cecum (arrow).[82]

Condition	Imaging Findings	Comments
Cecal diverticulitis (Fig GI 65-10)	Asymmetric or circumferential thickening of the cecal wall with focal pericolic inflammation and demonstration of diverticula.	Often mistaken clinically for appendicitis, visualization of a normal appendix or inflammatory changes involving the ascending colon at a level above the ileocecal valve favors the diagnosis of diverticulitis.
Meckel's diverticulitis	Inflammatory process occurring at some distance (60–100 cm) from the ileocecal valve.	The diagnosis requires identification of a blind-ending, tubular, round or oval structure in the right lower quadrant with surrounding inflammation. There may be an enterolith within the inflamed diverticulum.
Epiploic appendagitis (Fig GI 65-11)	Oval paracecal mass (representing the infracted or inflamed appendix epiploica) with a well-circumscribed hyperattenuating rim and sometimes a high-attenuation central dot. There may be reactive thickening in the cecal wall.	Patients present with acute abdominal pain, which can mimic appendicitis that is secondary to spontaneous torsion, ischemia, or inflammation of an epiploic appendage of the colon.
Crohn's disease (Fig GI 65-12)	Segmental thickening of the bowel wall, narrowing of the lumen, mesenteric fat stranding, creeping fat, enlargement of mesenteric lymph nodes, and skip lesions. Layered contrast enhancement of the bowel may be seen in acute disease.	The terminal ileum and cecum are frequently involved in this process. Thickening of a long segment of the terminal ileum, circumferential thickening of the cecum, and inflammation centered away from the appendix, fistulas, sinus tracts, and abscesses make the diagnosis of Crohn's disease much more likely than appendicitis.
Infectious Tuberculosis	Asymmetric thickening of the ileocecal valve and medial wall of the cecum, exophytic extension engulfing the terminal ileum, and massive lymph nodes with central low-attenuation areas.	The ileocecal area is the portion of the gastrointestinal tract that is most commonly affected by tuberculosis.

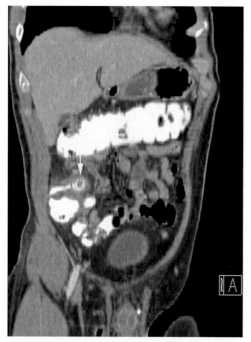

Fig GI 65-10
Cecal diverticulitis. Coronal oblique reformatted image shows mild thickening of the cecal wall, an inflamed enhancing diverticulum with a thickened wall (arrow), and mild stranding of peridiverticular and pericecal fat. The patient had previously undergone an appendectomy.[82]

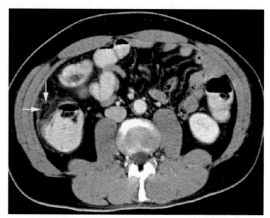

Fig GI 65-11
Epiploic appendagitis. Oval, paracecal fatty mass (arrows) with surrounding fat stranding.[82]

Condition	Imaging Findings	Comments
Infectious terminal ileitis (Fig GI 65-13)	Circumferential wall thickening of the terminal ileum (and often cecum) with enlargement of mesenteric lymph nodes in the right lower quadrant.	The most frequent causative organisms are *Yersinia*, *Campylobacter*, and *Salmonella*. The clinical diagnosis is evident when the patient presents with symptoms of acute diarrhea, and stool cultures are confirmatory.
Typhlitis (neutropenic colitis) (Figs GI 65-14 and GI 65-15)	Segmental bowel wall thickening with pericolic fluid collection or fat stranding. Intramural low-attenuating areas indicate edema or necrosis, and there may be gas in the bowel wall	Inflammatory condition seen in immunocompromised patients that primarily involves the cecum and ascending colon but may also affect the terminal ileum and appendix. Early diagnosis and aggressive treatment are necessary to prevent transmural necrosis and perforation.

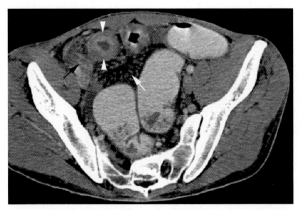

Fig GI 65-12
Crohn's disease. Enlarged appendix (black arrow), stratified symmetric thickening of the terminal ileum (arrowheads), and adjacent creeping fat (white arrow).[82]

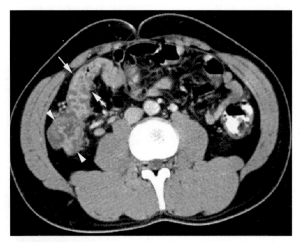

Fig GI 65-13
Terminal ileitis. (A) In a young adult with *Campylobacter* infection, there is marked thickening of the cecum (arrowheads) and terminal ileum (arrows) with preservation of a layered enhancement pattern. Note the small regional lymph nodes and the absence of fat stranding.[82]

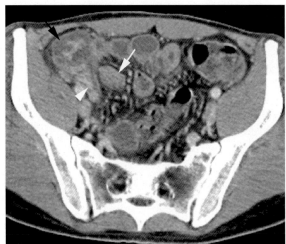

Fig GI 65-14
Typhlitis. Thickened cecum (black arrow), appendix (arrowhead), and terminal ileum (white arrow), associated with marked submucosal edema, in a young man with acute myeloblastic leukemia and sepsis who presented with sudden, violent right lower quadrant pain and fever.[82]

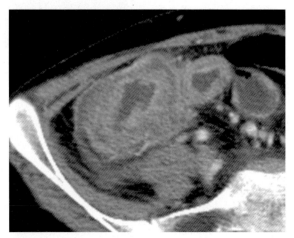

Fig GI 65-15
Typhlitis. Marked thickening and increased enhancement of the fluid-filled cecum and terminal ileum in a young girl several months after bone marrow transplantation for lymphoma.[83]

Condition	Imaging Findings	Comments
Ischemia of the cecum (Fig GI 65-16)	Circumferential thickening of the cecal wall, a mural stratification pattern due to submucosal edema, and mild pericolic stranding. More specific signs are isolated gas in the bowel wall, mesenteric or portal vein gas, and pneumoperitoneum.	Rare, potentially life-threatening condition that may occur spontaneously or be related to chronic heart disease, cardiopulmonary bypass surgery, cholesterol embolization, or aortitis. A normal appendix and absence of diverticula should suggest this diagnosis if the patient is elderly or has predisposing risk factors.
Cecal volvulus	Whorled pattern due to torsion of the afferent and efferent loops around the fixed and twisted mesentery.	The distended cecum is usually located in the left upper quadrant.
Ileocecal enteric duplication cyst	Smooth fluid-filled cyst or tubular structure with thin enhancing walls, located in or adjacent to the bowel wall.	Uncommon congenital anomaly that most often involves the ileum. A cyst near the ileocecal valve can occasionally serve as the lead point for an intussusception.

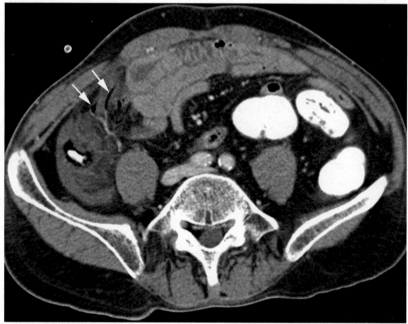

Fig GI 65-16
Ischemic necrosis of the cecum. Prominent thickening of the cecal wall associated with gas (arrows) in the veins that drain the cecum. The patient had a history of cardiac failure with arrhythmia. At surgery, there was necrotic cecal mucosa without perforation.[82]

Mesenteric Lymph Node Enlargement

Condition	Comments
Malignancy	
Lymphoma (Figs GI 66-1 and GI 66-2)	Most common malignancy resulting in mesenteric lymphadenopathy. Enlarged nodes may be seen in the mesenteric root, scattered throughout the peripheral mesentery, or in a mixed root-peripheral pattern. Early during the course of the disease, the lymph nodes may be small and discrete. As the disease progresses, the nodes often coalesce, forming a conglomerate soft-tissue mass. When there is extensive involvement, the softness of the neoplasm can result in the characteristic appearance of tumor growing around and displacing normal anatomic structures in the area of the nodal mass, such as blood vessels or bowel. Although rare prior to treatment, calcification may occur in involved mesenteric nodes following therapy. Lymphomatous mesenteric nodes usually have soft-tissue attenuation and demonstrate homogeneous enhancement. Because mesenteric lymphadenopathy in patients with lymphoma does not necessarily indicate active disease, it may be necessary to perform serial scans to demonstrate interval growth of specific nodes.
Metastasis (Figs GI 66-3 to GI 66-5)	Primary malignancies that most commonly cause metastatic mesenteric lymphadenopathy include carcinomas of the breast, lung, pancreas, and gastrointestinal tract. Carcinoid tumor also can result in mesenteric lymphadenopathy. Somewhat less frequent are melanoma, carcinoma of the bladder, leukemia, and sarcomas arising from the mesentery, gastrointestinal tract, or peritoneum. Metastatic lymph nodes may undergo central necrosis, which produces an area of lower attenuation, and show peripheral contrast enhancement.
Kaposi's sarcoma (Fig GI 66-6)	In patients with AIDS, extensive involvement of nodes in the mesenteric root and throughout the periphery of the mesentery should suggest this diagnosis. The concomitant presence of small bowel nodules may aid in differentiating Kaposi's sarcoma from other causes of conglomerate mesenteric lymphadenopathy.
Inflammation (Figs GI 66-7 to GI 66-11)	Mesenteric lymphadenopathy may be related to a localized inflammatory process (appendicitis, diverticulitis, cholecystitis, pancreatitis, or the inflammatory response following perforation of an abdominal viscus), inflammatory bowel disease (especially Crohn's), connective tissue disease, sarcoidosis, amyloidosis, or mesenteric panniculitis (nonspecific inflammatory and fibrotic process affecting the fatty tissue of the mesentery).

A
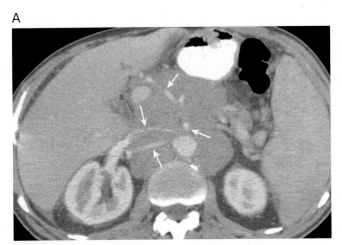
B
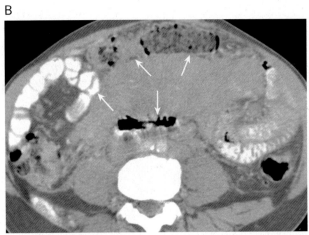

Fig GI 66-1
Lymphoma. (A) Homogeneous conglomerate mass formed by coalescent mesenteric and retroperitoneal adenopathy. The mass surrounds but does not occlude the mesenteric vessels (arrows). (B) On this image, the mass displaces bowel loops but does not occlude them (arrows).[84]

A

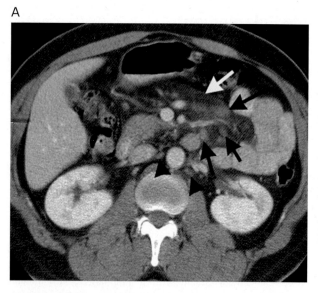

B

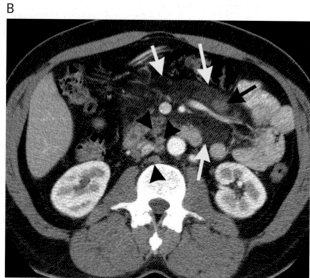

C

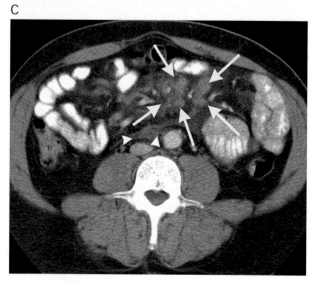

Fig GI 66-2
Lymphoma. (A) There is increased attenuation of the mesentery ("misty mesentery"; white arrow) and soft-tissue nodules (black arrows) along the superior mesenteric vessels. Note the subcentimeter retroperitoneal lymph nodes (arrowheads). (B) The misty mesentery (white arrows) and soft-tissue nodules (black arrows) are seen again. The fat (white arrowheads) immediately adjacent to mesenteric vessels along their long axes is preserved. Note the retroperitoneal lymph nodes (black arrowheads). (C) Prominent nodules (arrows) surround mesenteric vessels. There is soft-tissue stranding (arrowheads) anterior to the inferior vena cava and aorta.[85]

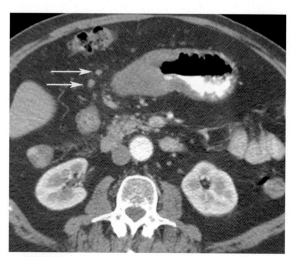

Fig GI 66-3
Metastases (from gastric carcinoma). Small mesenteric lymph nodes (arrows) associated with a concentrically thickened gastric antrum.[84]

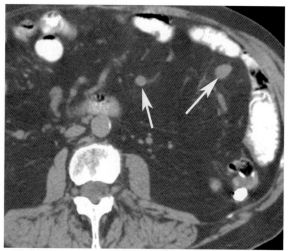

Fig GI 66-4
Metastases (from colon carcinoma). Mesenteric lymphadenopathy (arrows), which is easily seen against the intra-abdominal fat.[84]

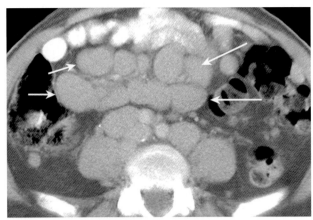

Fig GI 66-5
Leukemia. Extensive bulky lymphadenopathy both at the mesenteric root and throughout the periphery of the mesentery (arrows).[84]

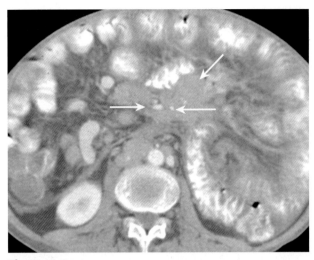

Fig GI 66-6
Kaposi's sarcoma. Homogeneous soft-tissue mass formed by mesenteric lymphadenopathy (top arrow). The mass surrounds the mesenteric vessels (bottom arrows) but does not occlude them.[84]

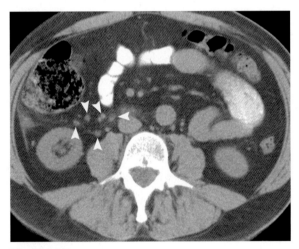

Fig GI 66-7
Appendicitis. Multiple lymph nodes in the mesentery of the right lower quadrant (arrowheads).[84]

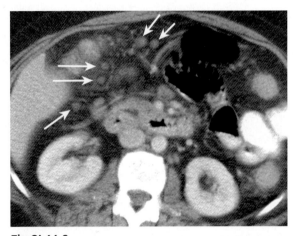

Fig GI 66-8
Crohn's disease. Lmphadenopathy throughout the periphery of the mesentery (arrow) and in the mesentery of the right lower quadrant.[84]

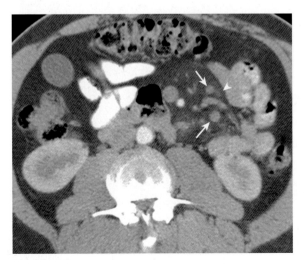

Fig GI 66-9
Mesenteric panniculitis. Multiple enlarged nodes in the mesentery (arrows). Note the inflammatory changes in the surrounding mesentery (arrowhead).[84]

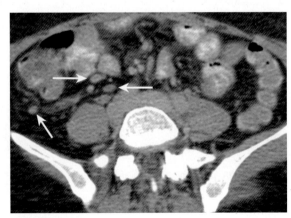

Fig GI 66-10
Systemic lupus erythematosus. Multiple enlarged lymph nodes throughout the mesentery (arrows).[84]

Condition	Comments
Infection Mesenteric adenitis (Fig GI 66-12)	Mesenteric lymphadenopathy associated with abominal pain, malaise, lethargy, and sometimes fever in the absence of an underlying cause.
Yersinia HIV (human immunodeficiency virus) (Fig GI 66-13)	Concomitant bowel wall thickening in the right lower quadrant, mimicking Crohn disease. Although isolated mesenteric lymphadenopathy may result from direct infection by the virus, this appearance is more likely related to an opportunistic infection or even an underlying malignancy. An important secondary cause is *Mycobacterium avium* complex (MAC), which often is associated with massive mesenteric lymphadenopathy forming a conglomerate mass. About 20% of nodes infected with MAC have low central attenuation.

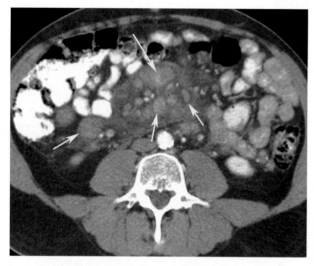

Fig GI 66-11
Amyloidosis. Diffuse mesenteric lymphadenopathy (arrows).

A

B

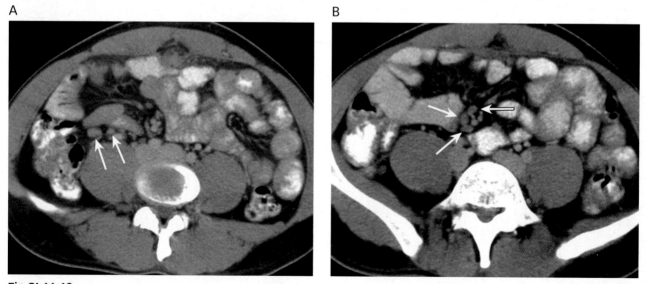

Fig GI 66-12
Mesenteric adenitis. Innumerable lymph nodes in the mesentery of the right lower quadrant (arrows in A) and at the mesenteric root (arrows in B).[84]

Condition	Comments
Tuberculosis	Infected nodes generally have a lower attenuation value (closer to that of fluid or fat) than enlarged inflammatory or malignant nodes. Contrast enhancement is often peripheral in tuberculosis, rather than homogeneous as in other causes of mesenteric lymphadenopathy.
Whipple's disease	Affected nodes have a high fat content responsible for the characteristic low attenuation value. The lymphadenopathy responds to antibiotic therapy.
Cavitating mesenteric lymph node syndrome (Fig GI 66-14)	A manifestation of celiac disease, the low-attenuation mesenteric lymphadenopathy in this condition actually represents cavitating nodes. The presence of fat-fluid levels within nodes permits an imaging-specific diagnosis. These nodes regress when the underlying celiac disease is treated with a gluten-free diet. It is important to distinguish this appearance from the homogeneous lymphadenopathy in lymphoma, which occurs at a higher incidence in patients with celiac disease.
Familial Mediterranean fever	Mesenteric lymphadenopathy has been reported in up to one-third of patients during an acute attack.

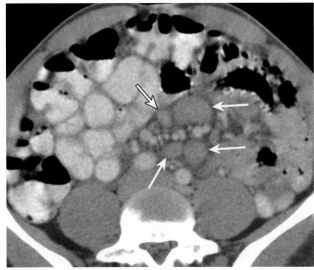

Fig GI 66-13
***Mycobacterium avium* complex (MAC) infection in HIV.**
Extensive mesenteric lymphadenopathy of uniform soft-tissue attenuation (arrows). The lymph nodes are discrete with no formation of a conglomerate mass or displacement of vessels or intestines.[84]

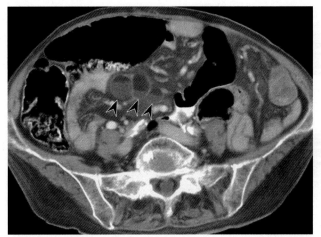

Fig GI 66-14
Cavitating mesenteric lymph node syndrome. Enlarged mesenteric lymph nodes with characteristic fat-fluid levels (arrowheads). (Case courtesy of Denise Reddy, Loyola University Medical Center, Maywood, IL).[86]

Thickened Gallbladder Wall (>3 millimeters)

Condition	Comments
Cholecystitis (Figs GI 67-1 and GI 67-2)	Thickening of the gallbladder wall is frequently observed on sonograms of patients with acute cholecystitis, though it is a nonspecific finding that can be seen in several other conditions. Measurements of gallbladder wall thickness should be made on the anterior surface of the gallbladder where it abuts the liver, as the posterior wall is often more difficult to define because of acoustic enhancement and adjacent bowel. Gallbladder wall thickening may occur in patients with chronic cholecystitis (with or without stones) and has also been described in complications of cholecystitis (eg, empyema of the gallbladder, gangrenous necrosis, and pericholecystic abscess).
Xanthogranulomatous cholecystitis (Fig GI 67-3)	Unusual form of chronic cholecystitis that may simulate malignancy radiologically and pathologically. It is predominantly seen in women between the ages of 60 and 70. Extravastion of bile in the gallbladder wall is thought to have a role, and the infiltrative process may extend into the adjacent soft tissues, liver, colon, or duodenum. Stones are present in the majority of patients.

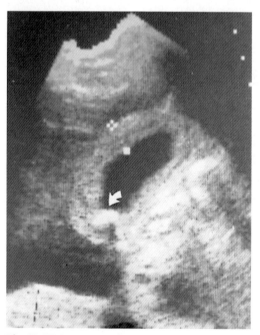

Fig GI 67-1
Acute cholecystitis. Marked thickening of the gallbladder neck (1.1 cm between the cursors). There is a densely echogenic stone (arrow) with posterior acoustic shadowing in the neck of the gallbladder.

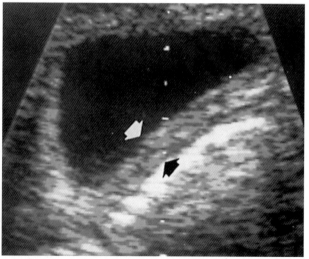

Fig GI 67-2
Acalculous cholecystitis. Enlarged gallbladder with a thickened, edematous wall (arrows). There is no evidence of gallstones or posterior acoustic shadowing.

Condition	Comments
Hypoalbuminemia (Fig GI 67-4)	Thickening of the gallbladder wall may be associated with markedly depressed levels of serum albumin in the absence of any other known etiologic factor. The postulated mechanism for wall thickening in this setting is edema from increased extravascular fluid (due to low plasma oncotic pressure). Hypoalbuminemia may well be the underlying cause for the gallbladder wall thickening seen in patients with ascites, renal disease, and elevated venous pressure secondary to congestive heart disease.
Ascites (Fig GI 67-5)	May reflect an underlying hypoalbuminemic state. The apparent gallbladder wall thickening in this condition may result from improper transducer placement or angulation.

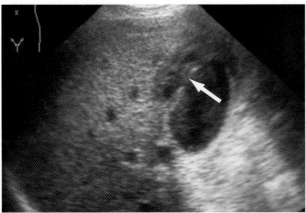

Fig GI 67-3
Xanthogranulomatous cholecystitis. Longitudinal sonogram of the right upper quadrant shows disruption of the mucosal line of the gallbladder (arrow), which contains echogenic material. There is pericholecystic fluid, focal hypoattenuation in the adjacent liver, and loss of the normal plane between the gallbladder and liver.[87]

Fig GI 67-4
Hypoalbuminemia with marked ascites. Thickening of the gallbladder wall (arrow).

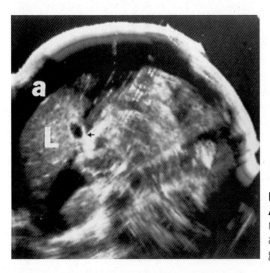

Fig GI 67-5
Ascites. A large amount of sonolucent ascitic fluid (a) separates the liver (L) and other soft-tissue structures from the anterior abdominal wall. Note the relative thickness of the gallbladder wall (arrow).

Condition	Comments
Congestive heart failure (Fig GI 67-6)	Probably reflects edema of the gallbladder wall due to increased systemic and portal venous engorgement.
Hepatitis (Fig GI 67-7)	A postulated mechanism is that the viruses excreted into the biliary system may produce a mild pericholecystic inflammation that is appreciated as wall thickening on ultrasound.
Incomplete fasting	The most common reason for apparent thickening of the gallbladder wall (not related to any pathologic abnormality). Normal patients who have incompletely fasted will often show a contracted gallbladder with a wall thickness of greater than 3 mm, so an accurate history of dietary intake before the examination is essential. Especially common in infants, in whom prolonged fasting before the examination is not possible.
Extrahepatic portal vein obstruction	Variceal collaterals and edema cause thickening of the gallbladder wall. May be secondary to pancreatitis, carcinoma of the pancreas or stomach, or neonatal omphalitis.
Lymphatic obstruction	Nodal enlargement in the porta hepatis causes dilation of lymphatics in the gallbladder wall.
Carcinoma of gallbladder	Diffuse or focal thickening of the gallbladder wall is a relatively unusual manifestation. Metastases may very rarely cause segmental wall thickening.

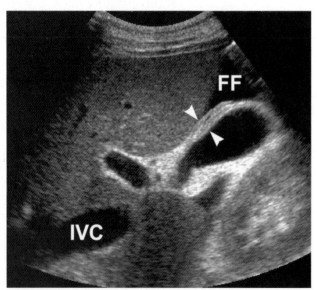

Fig GI 67-6
Congestive heart failure. Sagittal sonogram shows edema of the wall of the gallbladder (arrowheads), pericholecystic fluid (FF), and distension to the inferior vena cava (IVC).[88]

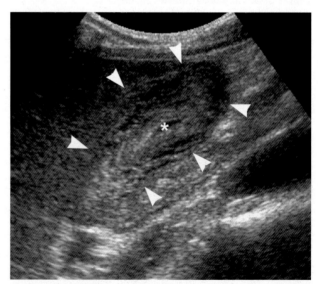

Fig GI 67-7
Acute viral hepatitis. Sagittal sonogram shows a tiny, slit-like gallbladder lumen (*) with massive "onion-peel" edema of the wall (arrowheads).[88]

Condition	Comments
Adenomyomatosis	Diffuse or focal thickening of the muscular layer of the gallbladder. Characteristic glandlike, barium-filled outpouchings projecting just outside the gallbladder lumen on oral cholecystography.
Cirrhosis (Fig GI 67-8)	Secondary gallbladder wall thickening in patients with liver cirrhosis is presumably due to elevated portal venous pressure and decreased intravascular osmotic pressure.

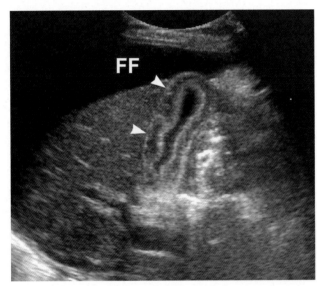

Fig GI 67-8
Cirrhosis. Sagittal sonogram shows a thickened gallbladder wall (arrowheads) and free fluid (FF).[88]

Focal Anechoic (Cystic) Liver Masses

Condition	Comments
Congenital cyst (Fig GI 68-1)	Most common benign cystic lesion of the liver that develops secondary to an excess of intrahepatic ductules that fail to involute. Although generally asymptomatic, hepatic cysts may grow large (even causing obstructive jaundice), become infected, or bleed.
Polycystic disease of liver (Fig GI 68-2)	Minimal to virtually complete replacement of the hepatic parenchyma by cystic lesions occurs in approximately one-third of patients with adult-type polycystic kidney disease.
Caroli's disease (Fig GI 68-3)	Multiple focal cystic collections throughout the liver representing communicating cavernous ectasia of the biliary tree. Although the appearance superficially is that of polycystic disease, careful scanning usually shows that the collections communicate with the biliary tree (unlike the isolated cysts of polycystic disease).

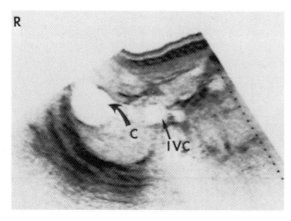

Fig GI 68-1
Simple nonparasitic hepatic cyst. Transverse sonogram of the upper abdomen in a patient with suspected metastatic disease and a defect on a radionuclide scan shows a completely sonolucent mass (C) that meets the criteria for a simple uncomplicated cyst. (IVC, inferior vena cava; R, right.)[89]

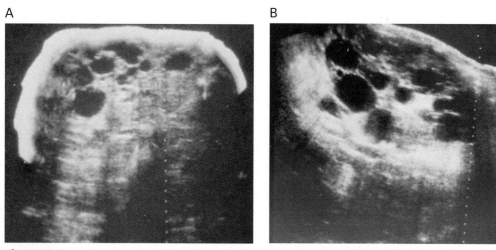

Fig GI 68-2
Polycystic liver disease. (A) Multiple anechoic cysts of various sizes throughout the liver in extensive adult-type polycystic kidney disease. (B) Prone longitudinal sonogram on the same patient shows multiple renal cysts.

Condition	Comments
Acquired cysts	Occasionally develop after an episode of trauma or a localized inflammatory process of the liver. Segmental obstruction of the biliary tree (stricture from previous surgery, infection, or neoplasm) may produce focal anechoic areas that mimic true cysts but generally are not as well defined.
Intrahepatic gallbladder	Most common positional anomaly, which appears as a cystic intrahepatic lesion lying in the main interlobar fissure between the right and left lobes. The diagnosis can usually be made by careful scanning and noting that the gallbladder is not present in its normal location. If unclear on ultrasound, a radionuclide scan can document the biliary origin of the lesion.
Hematoma (Fig GI 68-4)	May appear cystic, but generally not as well defined as a simple cyst. Subcapsular hematomas tend to be elliptical and are located peripherally.
Biloma (Fig GI 68-5)	Round or elliptical, often loculated mass. Radionuclide scanning may show persistent communication between the lesion and the normal biliary tree.
Abscess	Although an early pyogenic abscess tends to be echogenic and poorly demarcated, as it evolves, it tends to become well demarcated and nearly anechoic.
Echinococcal cyst (Fig GI 68-6)	May present as a purely fluid collection in the liver (1 to 20 cm in size) and with localized thickening of the cyst wall. There is often a more complex appearance with multiple septations and daughter cysts or scolices.

A

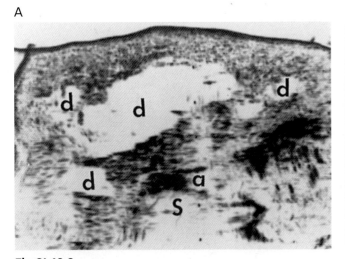

B

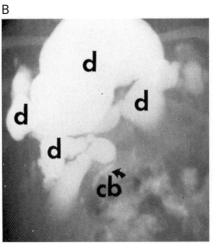

Fig GI 68-3
Caroli's disease. (A) Transverse supine sonogram demonstrates multiple dilated bile ducts (d) as sonolucent spaces in the liver. (S, spine; a, aorta.) (B) Frontal view of a transhepatic cholangiogram in a projection corresponding to that in (A) shows cystic dilatation of the distal intrahepatic ducts (d) with a normal-sized common bile duct (cb).[90]

Condition	Comments
Metastases (Fig GI 68-7)	Usually develop in patients with primary neoplasms that have a cystic component. Also seen in some melanomas, carcinoids, and bronchogenic carcinomas, as well as in metastatic sarcomas that have undergone extensive central necrosis. In most cases, the findings of a thick rim, irregular margins, mural nodules, or a fluid-fluid level should suggest the appropriate diagnosis.

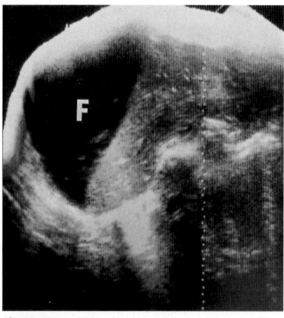

Fig GI 68-4
Traumatic subcapsular hematoma. Transverse scan shows an elliptical fluid collection (F) that developed after blunt trauma to the abdomen.

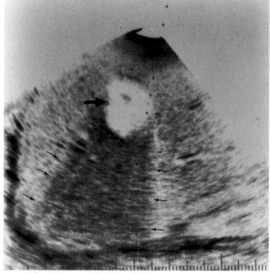

Fig GI 68-5
Biloma. Anechoic mass (large arrow) with a few internal echoes and excellent distal sonic enhancement (small arrows) that developed following a gunshot wound to the liver.[91]

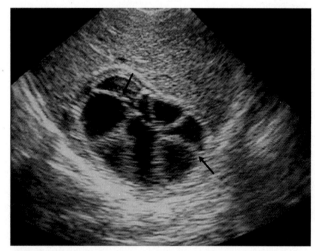

Fig GI 68-6
Echinococcal cyst. Longitudinal sonogram of the liver shows a well-defined multilocular hypoechoic lesion (cursors) with echogenic internal septa (arrows).[92]

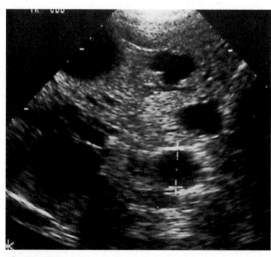

Fig GI 68-7
Metastases. Multiple anechoic defects in the liver. (Courtesy of Carol Krebs, Shreveport, LA.)

Condition	Comments
Biliary cystadenoma (Fig GI 68-8)	Large multicystic mass that tends to occur in middle-aged women and is generally considered to be a premalignant lesion. The presence of mural nodules and irregular thickening of the wall suggests malignancy (but these are not reliable signs).
Choledochal cyst	If there is dilatation of the intrahepatic bile ducts.
Hepatic artery aneurysm (Fig GI 68-9)	Second most common splanchnic aneurysm (after splenic artery). Most are secondary to atherosclerosis, infection (often mycotic), or trauma. On real-time ultrasound, a hepatic artery aneurysm appears as a focal anechoic lesion, often with proximal dilatation of ducts. Duplex and color-flow Doppler clearly demonstrate the characteristic arterial pulsations and waveform.

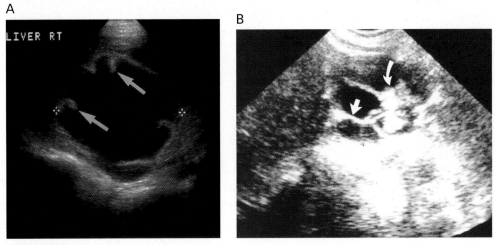

Fig GI 68-8
Biliary cystadenoma. (A) Transverse image shows a well-defined anechoic cyst with enhanced through transmission. There are multiple echogenic tumor excrescences extending into the cyst lumen (arrows). (B) In another patient, the complex anechoic cyst contains echogenic septa (straight arrow) and tumor nodules (curved arrow).[93]

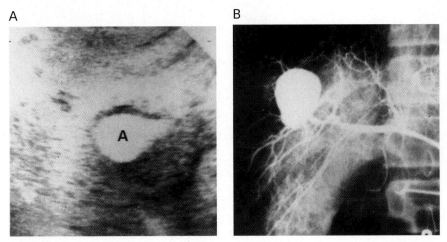

Fig GI 68-9
Hepatic artery aneurysm. (A) Sagittal sonogram shows the well-circumscribed anechoic aneurysm (A), which has good sound transmission. (B) Arteriogram confirms the aneurysm, which arises from the right hepatic artery.[94]

Complex or Solid Liver Masses

Condition	Comments
Hepatocellular carcinoma (hepatoma) (Figs GI 69-1 and GI 69-2)	Because primary hepatic carcinoma usually (but not always) arises on a background of underlying liver disease, such as cirrhosis or parasitic infection, the areas of tumor tend to appear hypoechoic when contrasted with the remainder of the liver. When a hepatoma arises in an otherwise normal liver, it may be echogenic. Because the tumor is often multifocal, the demonstration of multiple lesions cannot differentiate between primary and secondary tumors. Unlike metastases, a hepatoma commonly invades the portal venous system and thus should be strongly suspected if tumor thrombus can be visualized in the portal venous radicles.
Metastases (Figs GI 69-3 through GI 69-5)	Variable pattern (large or small, echogenic or echolucent, partially cystic, focal or diffuse). No correlation between the histology of a metastasis and its sonographic appearance.

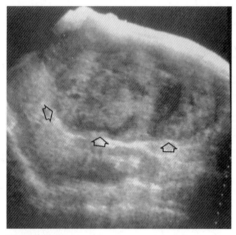

Fig GI 69-1
Hepatoma. Complex mass (arrows) with a large echogenic component.

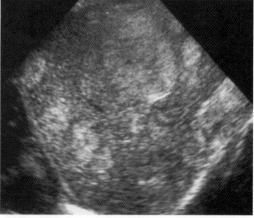

Fig GI 69-2
Multinodular hepatocellular carcinoma mimicking metastatic disease. Sagittal scan demonstrates multiple hyperechoic masses.[95]

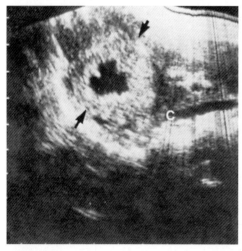

Fig GI 69-3
Metastasis. Sagittal scan shows a large echogenic mass (arrows) with central necrosis. (C, inferior vena cava.)[96]

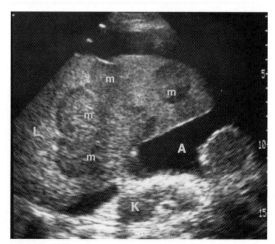

Fig GI 69-4
Multiple metastases. Sagittal scan demonstrates multiple hypoechoic masses (m) in the liver (L). Note the prominent ascitic fluid (A). (K, kidney.)[95]

Condition	Comments
Abscess (Figs GI 69-6 to GI 69-8)	May appear as focal or diffuse areas of increased or decreased parenchymal echoes. In the more chronic stage, an abscess typically appears as a well-defined cavity with various degrees of internal echogenicity and a well-defined, thickened, irregular wall. Microabscesses may appear as "targets" with sonolucent peripheries and echogenic centers. Serial scans may be helpful because echogenic abscesses usually evolve toward a more cystic appearance.

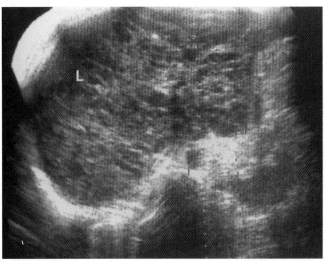

Fig GI 69-5
Diffuse metastases. Transverse scan shows a heterogeneous echo pattern in which areas of hypoechogenicity are mixed with hyperechogenic regions. (L, liver.)[95]

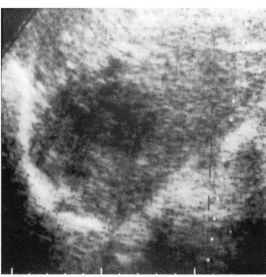

Fig GI 69-6
Pyogenic hepatic abscess. Ill-defined complex mass with irregular margins.

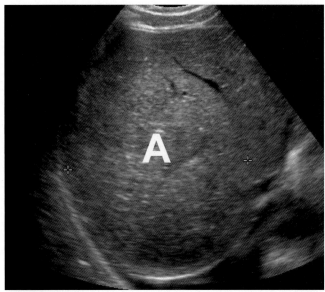

Fig GI 69-7
Hepatic abscess. Large, solid-appearing mass (A) in the right lobe of the liver in a young man with fever and pain in the right upper quadrant.[97]

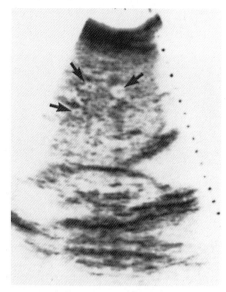

Fig GI 69-8
***Candida albicans* abscesses.** Numerous, rounded, fluid-filled lesions (arrows) with a target appearance.[98]

Condition	Comments
Cavernous hemangioma (Fig GI 69-9)	Virtually pathognomonic appearance of a small (1 to 3 cm), highly echogenic focus superimposed on a background of normal liver parenchyma. The increased echogenicity is due to the interfaces caused by the walls of the cavernous venous sinuses and the blood in these vessels. A slightly more irregular pattern develops as the hemangioma undergoes degeneration and fibrous replacement.
Hydatid disease (Fig GI 69-10)	Variable appearance ranging from purely cystic to solid-appearing pseudotumors. Within the cyst there may be wavy bands of delaminated endocyst (water lily sign). Daughter cysts are frequently seen and may be surrounded by echogenic debris. Peripheral calcification is common, varying from tiny to massive. This severe and common parasitic disease is endemic to the Mediterranean basin and other sheep-rearing areas. Humans become infected by ingestion of eggs of the tapeworm *E. granulosus*, either by eating contaminated food or from contact with dogs. Although the liver filters out most of the resultant embryos, those that are not destroyed become hepatic hydatid cysts.

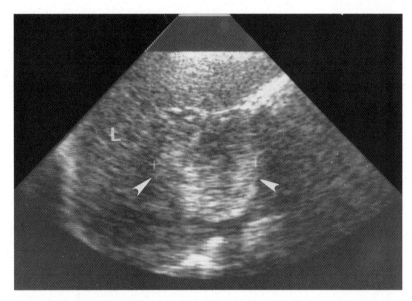

Fig GI 69-9
Hemangioma. Transverse sonogram shows a characteristic hyperechoic mass containing homogeneous echoes. (L, liver.)[95]

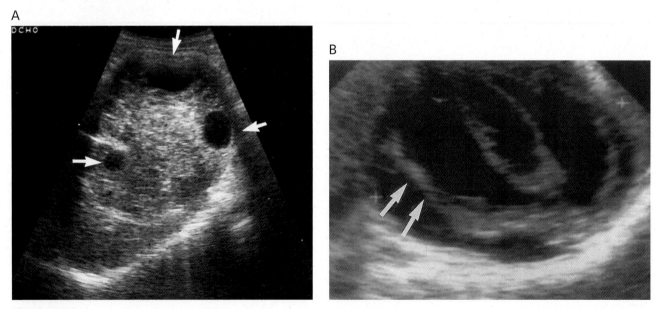

Fig GI 69-10
Echinococcal cyst. (A) Three distinct daughter cysts (arrows) with the typical peripheral location within the mother cyst.[99] Hydatid matrix with a solid appearance is seen filling the rest of the cavity. (B) A hydatid cyst in the right lobe of the liver contains wavy bands of delaminated endocyst (water lily sign) (arrows).[100]

Condition	Comments
Echinococcal multilocularis (Fig GI 69-11)	Rare alveolar form of Echinococcus infection, which produces multilocular cysts that resemble alveoli and grow by exogenous proliferations. More than 90% of infected patients have liver involvement. At ultrasound, these lesions usually manifest with the "hailstorm pattern," which is characterized by multiple echogenic nodules with irregular and indistinct margins. Lesions with liquefactive necrosis appear hypoechoic with some internal echoes and an irregular hyperechoic border.
Schistosomiasis (Fig GI 69-12)	The infectious organisms live in the bowel lumen and lay their eggs in the mesenteric veins. The eggs may then embolize to the portal vein, where they incite an inflammatory reaction with a granulomatous response that eventually leads to fibrosis and presinusoidal hypertension. The eggs themselves do not survive and may subsequently calcify. Chronic infection results in cirrhosis and the risk of developing hepatocellular carcinoma. The typical ultrasound appearance is an irregular mosaic pattern with echogenic septa outlining polygonal areas of relatively normal parenchyma that vary from 15 to 30 mm.

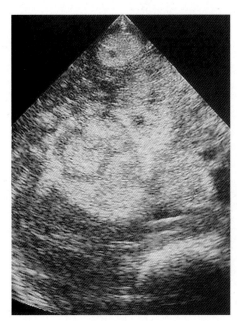

Fig GI 69-11
***Echinococcal multilocularis* cyst.** Transverse sonogram of the liver shows a typical hailstorm pattern, characterized by multiple echogenic nodules with irregular and indistinct margins.[100]

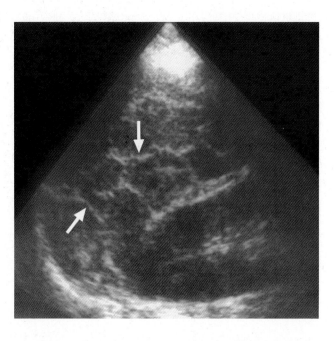

Fig GI 69-12
Schistosomiasis. Longitudinal sonogram through the liver shows the characteristic network pattern, with echogenic septa (arrows) outlining polygonal areas of relatively normal liver parenchyma.[100]

Condition	Comments
Ascariasis (Fig GI 69-13)	Ascariasis infects about 1 billion people worldwide and spreads through fecal contamination. After an egg is swallowed, larvae hatch in the small intestine and invade its mucosa, migrate through the circulatory system to the lungs, invade the alveoli, ascend the tracheobronchial tree, and then are swallowed into the small intestine where they mature into adult worms that may reach 40 cm in length. Migration of worms into the biliary tree may result in biliary colic, cholecystitis, cholangitis, intrahepatic abscesses, or pancreatitis. The worm typically appears as an echogenic structure with a relatively hypoechoic center and a more echogenic wall. Multiple worms may completely fill the bile duct and mimic a neoplasm.
Focal nodular hyperplasia/ liver cell adenoma (Figs GI 69-14 and GI 69-15)	Sonographically indistinguishable lesions that appear as solid masses of increased or decreased echogenicity. Adenomas may contain sonolucent areas (due to necrosis or hemorrhage) and are frequently seen in women taking oral contraceptives and in patients with type 1 glycogen storage disease (von Gierke). Unlike hepatic adenoma, which is composed entirely of hepatocytes without Kupffer's cells, focal nodular hyperplasia contains these technetium-avid cells and thus often appears normal on ^{99m}Tc-sulfur colloid scans.

A
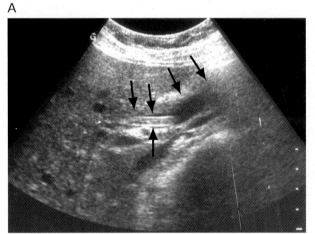

B
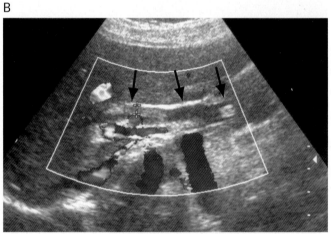

Fig GI 69-13
Ascariasis. (A) Sagittal sonogram of the porta hepatic shows a tubular echogenic region (arrow) within the slightly dilated common bile duct (arrowheads). (B) Oblique sonogram in a slightly different plane shows the echogenic region in lengthwise section (open arrow) in the common hepatic and common bile ducts and in cross section (solid arrow) more distally in the common bile duct. The intraluminal abnormality measured approximately 5 mm. The arrowhead denotes the common bile duct.[101]

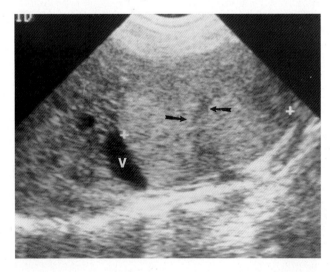

Fig GI 69-14
Focal nodular hyperplasia. The hyperechoic mass (between cursor marks) has a central scar (arrows) and was found in an otherwise normal liver. The middle hepatic vein (v) is displaced.[102]

Condition	Comments
Hemangioendothelioma (Fig GI 69-16)	Most common hepatic lesion producing symptoms during infancy (the vast majority of these tumors present before 6 months of age). Although generally considered benign, there have been rare reports of distant metastases. Extensive arteriovenous shunting in the lesion may lead to high-output congestive heart failure. The tumor has a nonspecific sonographic pattern and may appear as a hypoechoic, complex, or hyperechoic lesion.
Hepatoblastoma (Fig GI 69-17)	Most common primary liver neoplasm in childhood. It usually develops with the first 3 years of life and is very aggressive (often metastasizing to the lung at the time of diagnosis). May show acoustic shadowing secondary to intratumoral calcification. Intense neovascularity of the tumor is associated with high Doppler frequency shifts.

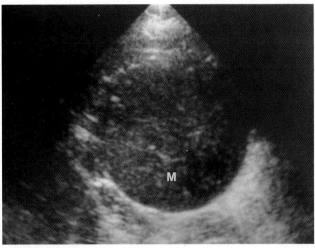

Fig GI 69-15
Hepatic adenoma. Well-defined exophytic right lobe mass (M) containing heterogeneous internal echoes in a young woman taking oral contraceptive pills.[102]

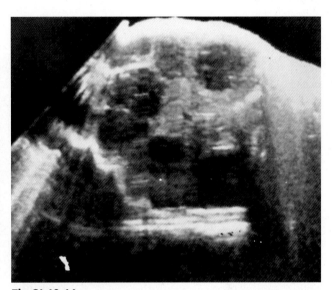

Fig GI 69-16
Hemangioendothelioma. Sagittal sonogram shows multiple, discrete, hypoechoic solid masses.[103]

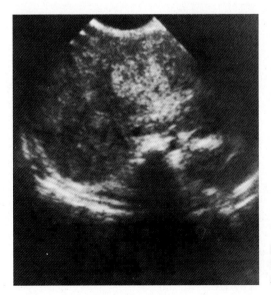

Fig GI 69-17
Hepatoblastoma. Transverse scan demonstrates the echogenic mass.[32]

Condition	Comments
Fibrolamellar carcinoma (Fig GI 69-18)	Slow-growing neoplasm that typically arises in adolescents and adults younger than 40 who do not have cirrhosis or any other predisposing risk factor. Average survival of 4 to 5 years (compared with only 6 months in hepatocellular carcinoma). Typically appears as a large, hyperechoic, homogeneous mass, often containing shadowing calcification.
Undifferentiated (embryonal) sarcoma	Unusual hepatic malignancy found in children and young adults. The sonographic appearance ranges from a multiseptate cystic mass to an inhomogeneous, predominantly echogenic solid lesion.
Cholangiocarcinoma (Fig GI 69-19)	Approximately 10% to 20% are exophytic, intrahepatic masses indistinguishable from other hepatic malignancies.
Biliary cystadenoma/ cystadenocarcinoma (Fig GI 69-20)	Typically produces large, multicystic, septated mass that may have mural nodules.

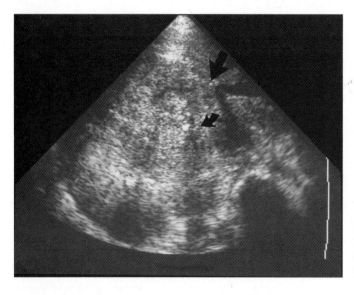

Fig GI 69-18
Fibrolamellar carcinoma. Sonogram shows mixed echogenicity and calcification (curved arrow) within a mass (straight arrow).[104]

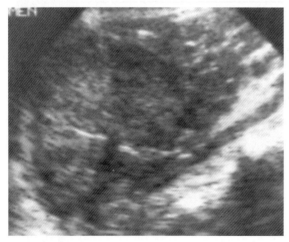

Fig GI 69-19
Intrahepatic cholangiocarcinoma. Sagittal scan shows a large hyperechoic mass in the right lobe of the liver.[105]

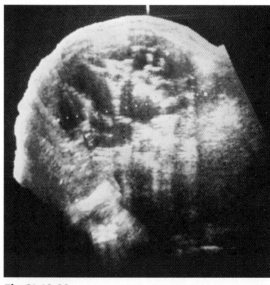

Fig GI 69-20
Biliary cystadenoma. Multiloculated liver mass. Note that the internal septa show nodular thickening and papillary excrescences.[106]

Condition	Comments
Focal fatty infiltration (Figs GI 69-21 and GI 69-22)	Although this condition typically produces a diffuse increase in echogenicity of the liver, at times focal deposits of fat may appear as discrete areas of increased echogenicity on a background of otherwise normal liver parenchyma. Features suggestive of fatty infiltration include the lack of mass effect or displacement of hepatic vessels and the rapid change with time.
Lipoma (Fig GI 69-23)	Extremely uncommon lesion consisting of mature adipose tissue. On ultrasound, it has the characteristic appearance of a well-circumscribed, uniformly hyperechoic lesion.

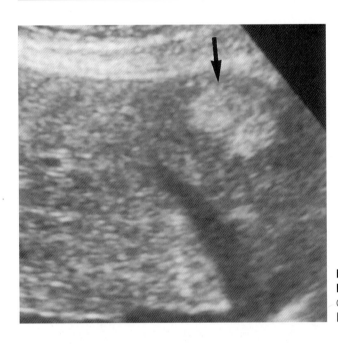

Fig GI 69-21
Focal fatty infiltration. Axial sonogram of the liver shows an ovoid, uniformly hyperechoic focus (arrow) consistent with a localized collection of fat.[107]

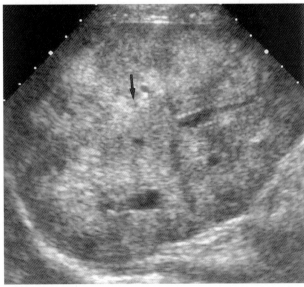

Fig GI 69-22
Multifocal nodular fatty infiltration. Axial sonogram shows a diffuse pattern of patchy hyperechoic foci (arrow) simulating an infiltrative tumor. The combination of in-phase and opposed-phased MR imaging allows this appearance to be reliably differentiated from metastatic disease.[107]

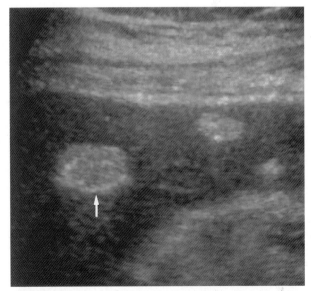

Fig GI 69-23
Lipoma. Axial sonogram shows uniformly hyperechoic lesions (arrow).[107]

Generalized Increased Echogenicity of the Liver

Condition	Comments
Fatty infiltration (Figs GI 70-1 and GI 70-2)	Alcohol abuse is by far the most common cause of fatty liver. Other underlying causes include obesity, diabetes, chemotherapy, parenteral nutrition, protein malnutrition, intestinal bypass operations, steroid therapy, inflammatory bowel disease, severe hepatitis, carbon tetrachloride toxicity, hyperlipidemia, and congestive heart failure. At times, fatty infiltration may involve only portions of the liver, producing discrete areas of increased echogenicity alternating with normal parenchyma (may be confused with metastatic disease). Although the ultrasound pattern is indistinguishable from generalized hepatic fibrosis, the two entities can be clearly separated by the different CT attenuation values of fat and fibrous tissue.
Fibrosis (Figs GI 70-3 through GI 70-5)	Most commonly the result of cirrhosis. Usually due to alcohol abuse, though it may be secondary to chronic viral hepatitis, schistosomiasis, other parasitic diseases, or glycogen storage disease. Cirrhosis should be suspected if the hepatic size is decreased and when there is nodularity of the liver surface, accentuation of fissures, coarsening of hepatic architecture, enlargement of the caudate lobe, regenerating nodules, ascites, or signs of portal hypertension. Careful sagittal scans of the left lobe should be performed to detect the recanalized umbilical vein, an indicator of portal hypertension.

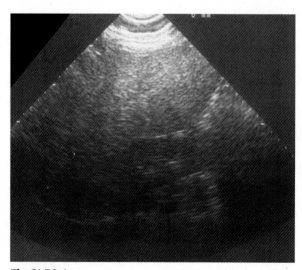

Fig GI 70-1
Fatty infiltration. Sagittal scan demonstrates a diffuse increase in echogenicity of the hepatic parenchyma with marked attenuation of the sound beam.[95]

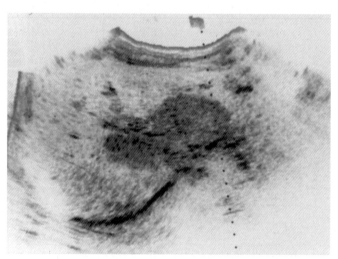

Fig GI 70-2
Focal fatty infiltration. Longitudinal scan shows a well-defined, densely echogenic focus within the liver.[108]

Condition	Comments
Diffuse malignancy	Generalized permeating infiltration of the liver by primary hepatocellular carcinoma, metastases, or lymphoma.
Technical artifact (Fig GI 70-6)	Occurs if scanning is performed with too much overall system gain. In most normal patients, the liver and kidney parenchyma are very similar in their gray-scale texture (echogenicity of the liver may be slightly higher). A definite mismatch of the two tissues is strong evidence for parenchymal disease of the organ showing the greater echogenicity.

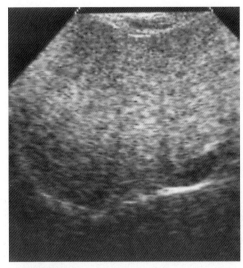

Fig GI 70-3
Fibrosis. Diffuse increased echogenicity of the liver secondary to chronic hepatitis.

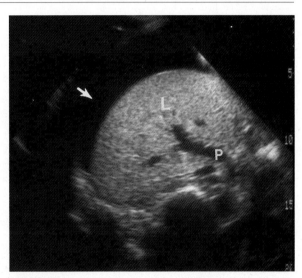

Fig GI 70-4
Cirrhosis. Transverse scan shows a small, contracted liver (L) with increased echogenicity surrounded by ascitic fluid (arrow). (P, portal vein.)[95]

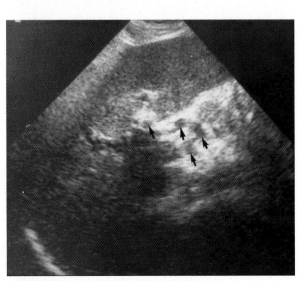

Fig GI 70-5
Cirrhosis with portal hypertension. Transverse scan shows multiple venous collaterals (arrowheads).[95]

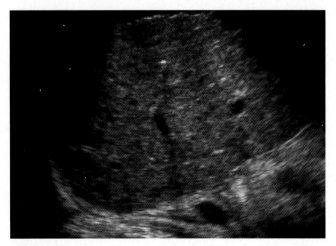

Fig GI 70-6
Kaposi sarcoma. Sagittal sonogram through the right upper quadrant shows abnormal heterogeneous increase in echogenicity of the liver, with multiple hyperechoic lesions throughout the hepatic parenchyma.[109]

Generalized Decreased Echogenicity of the Liver

Condition	Comments
Cellular infiltration	Most commonly due to lymphoma, which may also produce hypoechoic or echogenic focal lesions. Other causes include leukemia and amyloidosis.
Hepatitis (Figs GI 71-1 and GI 71-2)	Although the liver parenchyma appears normal in many cases of acute viral hepatitis, swelling of liver cells may produce an overall decreased echogenicity of the liver associated with accentuated brightness of the portal vein walls. In chronic hepatitis, the parenchymal echo pattern is coarsened because of periportal fibrosis and inflammatory cells.

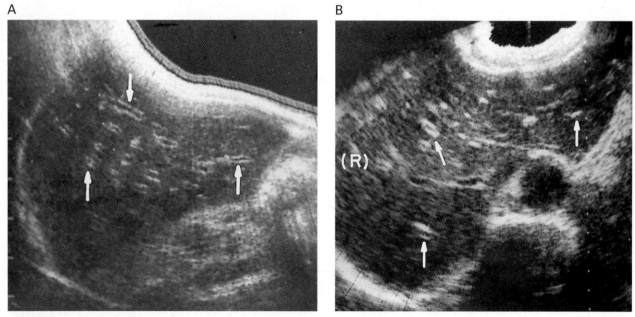

A

B

Fig GI 71-1
Acute hepatitis. (A) Longitudinal and (B) transverse scans of the right lobe in two different patients show an overall decrease in the echo pattern. Note that the portal vein radicle walls (arrows) are brighter than usual.[110]

A

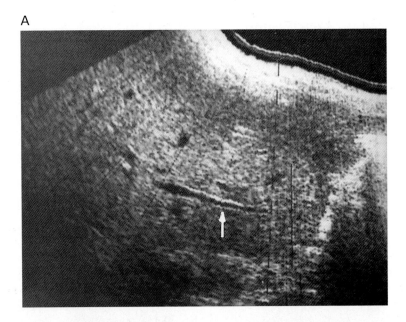

B

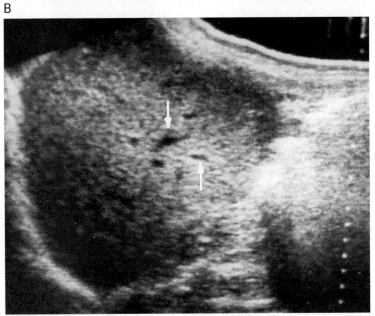

Fig GI 71-2
Chronic hepatitis. (A) Longitudinal scan of the right lobe shows marked coarsening of the liver echoes. Note the decrease in the brightness and number of the portal vein radicle walls (arrow). (B) In another patient, the liver pattern is even more coarsened. Note the increased brightness of the band through the mid-portion of the liver, corresponding to the maximum zone of sensitivity. The portal vein radicle walls seen within this bright zone have no internal echoes (arrows).[110]

Shadowing Lesions in the Liver

Condition	Comments
Calcification (Figs GI 72-1 through GI 72-3)	Usually reflects previous inflammatory disease (granulomatous or parasitic). Also may occur with hepatic metastases (mucinous tumors of the gastrointestinal tract in adults, neuroblastoma in children).

Gas
    Biliary tree
    (Figs GI 72-4 and GI 72-5)
	Most commonly due to a surgical connection between the biliary tree and the alimentary tract. If there is no history of previous surgery, the most common causes are gallstone ileus and penetrating duodenal ulcer disease.

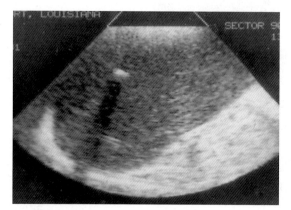

Fig GI 72-1
Calcified granuloma in the liver. Note the posterior shadowing.[111]

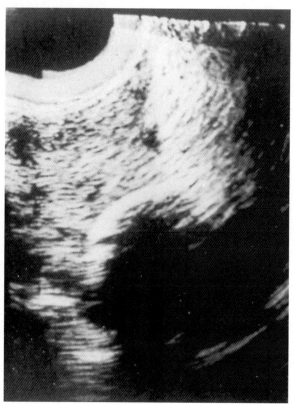

Fig GI 72-2
Calcified hydatid cyst. The calcified wall is sharply delineated and there is posterior acoustic shadowing.[112]

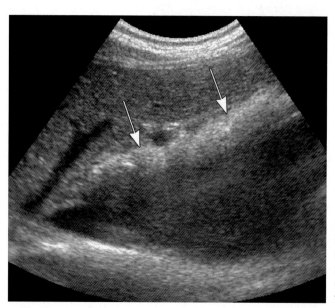

Fig GI 72-3
Recurrent pyogenic cholangiohepatitis. Sagittal sonogram of the right lobe of the liver shows a linear band of shadowing stones (arrows) in the bile ducts. The bile ducts are close to the edge of the liver, an appearance that reflects marked atrophy of the involved hepatic segment.[113]

Condition	Comments
Portal vein	Much less common than biliary gas and generally related to necrotizing enterocolitis, mesenteric arterial occlusion and bowel infarction, or an eroding abscess. Shadowing lesions due to portal vein gas appear in the periphery of the liver, unlike the more central location when the shadowing is secondary to gas in the biliary tree.
Normal shadowing	On sagittal scans near the neck of the gallbladder in normal patients, there is often a discrete shadow projected on the posterior aspect of the liver. This may be secondary to a refractive effect caused by tangential incidence of the ultrasound beam to the interface between the liver and gallbladder or to either thick fibrous tissue surrounding the right portal vein or the spiral valves of Heister in the gallbladder. Decubitus scans are required to search for tiny biliary calculi that may be lodged in the cystic duct and produce a similar appearance.

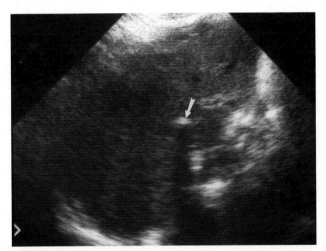

Fig GI 72-4
Gas in the biliary tree. Focal hyperechoic structure with shadowing (arrow).[95]

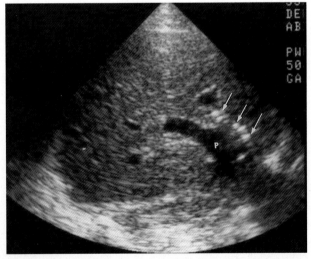

Fig GI 72-5
Gas in the biliary tree. Multiple hyperechoic foci (arrows) anterior to the portal vein (P).[95]

Focal Decreased-Attenuation Masses in the Liver

Condition	Imaging Findings	Comments
Cyst		
Nonparasitic cyst (Fig GI 73-1)	Sharply delineated, round or oval, near–water attenuation lesion with a very thin wall, no internal septations, and no contrast enhancement.	Most commonly congenital, but may be secondary to inflammation or trauma. Although more frequently single, hepatic cysts may be multiple (innumerable multifocal cysts occur in polycystic liver disease). May occasionally be difficult to differentiate from a cystic neoplasm or an old hematoma (on ultrasound, cystic tumors may have internal septations and irregular inner margins, whereas non-neoplastic hepatic cysts have no internal septations and have completely smooth walls).
Echinococcal cyst (Fig GI 73-2)	Sharply defined, rounded, near–water attenuation mass with a thin wall. May appear multilocular with internal septations representing the walls of daughter cysts.	Tissue infection of humans caused by the larval stage of a small tapeworm, for which dogs, sheep, cattle, and camels are the major intermediate hosts. The wall of the cyst may show dense calcification, and gas may form in the cyst because of superimposed infection or communication with the intestinal lumen through the bile duct. The rare finding of a fat-fluid level in an echinococcal cyst has been reported as an indication of communicating rupture into the biliary tree.
Polycystic disease (Fig GI 73-3)	Multiple low-attenuation cysts of various sizes.	Approximately one-third of patients with adult polycystic kidney disease have associated cysts of the liver, which do not interfere with hepatic function.

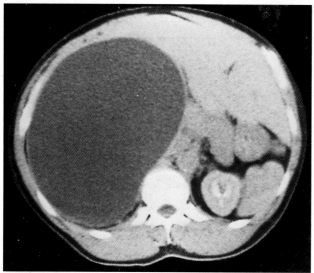

Fig GI 73-1
Simple hepatic cyst. A 20-cm fluid-filled mass in the right lobe of the liver displaces the abdominal contents and compresses the inferior vena cava. After aspiration and the instillation of alcohol, there was virtual ablation of the cyst.[114]

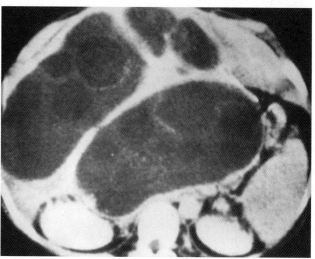

Fig GI 73-2
Echinococcal cyst. Multiple large cysts filling a massively enlarged liver.

Condition	Imaging Findings	Comments
Caroli's disease (Fig GI 73-4)	Multiple low-attenuation cystic masses in the liver.	Rare disorder characterized by segmental saccular dilatation of the intrahepatic bile ducts throughout the liver. The dilated cystic segments contain bile and communicate freely with the biliary tree and with each other, in contrast to polycystic liver disease in which the cysts contain a clear serous fluid and do not communicate with the biliary tree or other cysts. About 80% of patients have associated medullary sponge kidney.

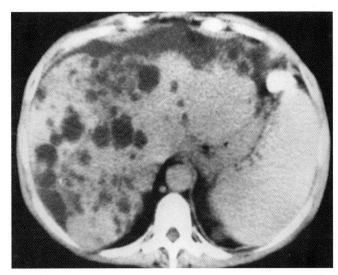

Fig GI 73-3
Polycystic liver disease. Innumerable lucent lesions of various sizes in a markedly enlarged liver. The patient also had severe polycystic kidney disease.

A

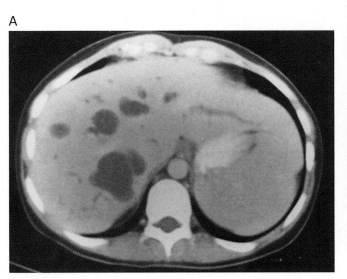

B

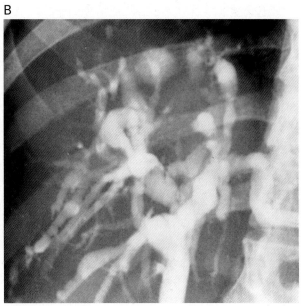

Fig GI 73-4
Caroli's disease. (A) CT scan shows fluid-filled cystic masses in the liver. (B) Cholangiogram shows the characteristic dilatation of intrahepatic ducts.

Condition	Imaging Findings	Comments
Choledochal cyst (Fig GI 73-5)	Cystic or fusiform dilatation of the common bile duct.	Classic clinical triad of upper abdominal pain, mass, and jaundice.
Abscess Pyogenic abscess (Figs GI 73-6 and GI 73-7)	Sharply defined homogeneous area with an attenuation usually greater than that of a benign cyst but lower than that of a solid neoplasm. No enhancement after intravenous injection of contrast material, though a rim of tissue around the cavity may become denser than normal liver (also seen with a necrotic neoplasm).	Results from such diverse causes as ascending biliary tract infection (especially secondary to calculi or carcinoma in the extrahepatic biliary ductal system), hematogenous spread via the portal venous system, generalized septicemia with involvement of the liver by way of the hepatic arterial circulation, direct extension from intraperitoneal infection, and hepatic trauma. May be solitary or multilocular (a single abscess is usually located in the right lobe). The demonstration of gas in a low-density hepatic mass is highly suggestive of an abscess.
Amebic abscess (Fig GI 73-8)	Sharply defined homogeneous area with an attenuation usually greater than that of a benign cyst but lower than that of a solid neoplasm. No enhancement after intravenous injection of contrast material, though a rim of tissue around the cavity may become denser than normal liver (also seen with a necrotic neoplasm).	Most frequent extracolonic complication of amebiasis, occurring in approximately one-third of patients with amebic dysentery. About two-thirds are solitary, with the remainder being multiple and often coalescing into a single large liver abscess. Most often located in the posterior portion of the right lobe of the liver, since this region receives most of the blood draining the right colon (where amebas tend to settle) because of the streaming effect in portal blood flow.

A

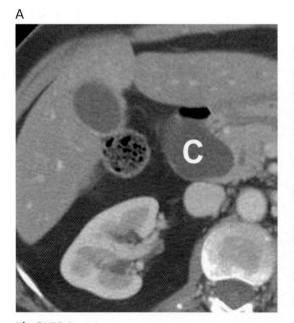

B

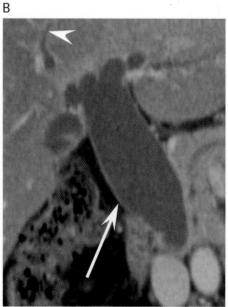

Fig GI 73-5
Choledochal cyst. (A) Contrast CT shows a cystic mass (C) that is well demarcated due to the dilation of the distal portion of the common bile duct. (B) Coronal oblique reformatted image shows fusiform dilatation of the common bile duct (arrow). Note also the dilatation of the intrahepatic biliary tree (arrowhead).[115]

A

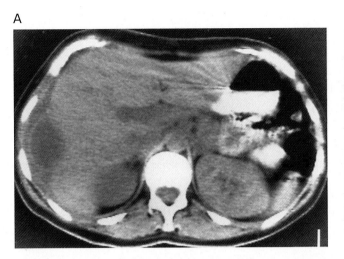

B

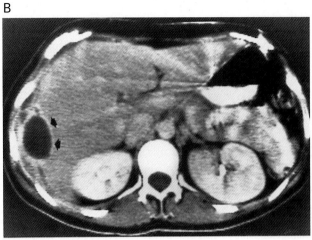

C

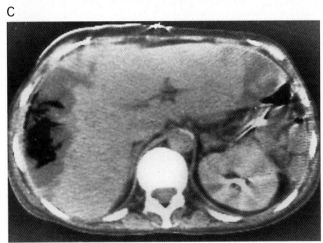

Fig GI 73-6
Hepatic abscess. (A) Unenhanced scan shows a single low-density lesion with poorly defined margins at the periphery of the liver. (B) After infusion of contrast material, there is rim enhancement with the margins of the abscess seen as a white line (arrows) of higher density than the surrounding normal liver. (C) CT scan in another patient shows a large collection of gas in a pyogenic abscess in the lateral aspect of the right lobe of the liver.[116]

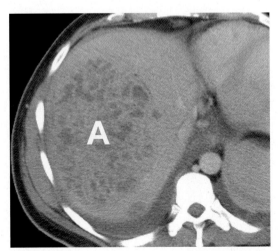

Fig GI 73-7
Pyogenic abscess. Large mass (A) in the right lobe of the liver that contains low-attenuation areas reflecting early liquefaction.[117]

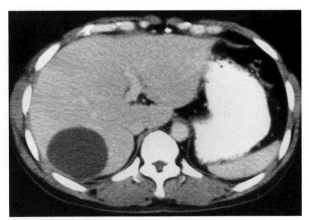

Fig GI 73-8
Amebic abscess. Well-circumscribed, fluid-attenuation mass (consistent with a simple cyst) in the posterior portion of the right lobe of the liver.[102]

Condition	Imaging Findings	Comments
Fungal abscess (Fig GI 73-9)	Multiple, small, rounded low-attenuation lesions, some of which have a central higher density focus producing a target appearance.	Uncommon condition that usually occurs in patients with compromised immune systems (especially acute myelogenous and lymphocytic leukemia). The abscesses are usually scattered rather uniformly throughout the liver, spleen, and even the kidneys.
Hydatid disease (Fig GI 73-10)	Large, well-defined, mass of low attenuation with a distinguishable wall, usually with multiple internal septa. Coarse peripheral calcifications are common, as are multiple daughter cysts.	Echinococcal disease is common in sheep-rearing areas, where humans become infected by ingestion of eggs of the tapeworm *E. granulosus*, either by eating contaminated food or from contact with dogs. Although the liver filters out most of the resultant embryos, those that are not destroyed become hepatic hydatid cysts
Echinococcus multilocularis (Fig GI 73-11)	Multiple, irregular, ill-defined low-attenuation lesions scattered through the liver. Irregular calcifications and central necrosis may be seen.	Rare alveolar form of Echinococcus infection, which produces multilocular cysts that resemble alveoli and grow by exogenous proliferations. More than 90% of infected patients have liver involvement. The appearance may mimic either metastases or pyogenic abscesses, though unlike these conditions in *E. multilocularis* infestation there is little or no contrast enhancement (reflecting the poor vascularization of the parasitic lesion).
Schistosomiasis (Fig GI 73-12)	A pathognomonic pattern is the presence of calcified septa, usually aligned perpendicular to the liver capsule ("tortoise shell" or "turtle back" appearance). Other common findings are capsular calcification, junctional notches or depressions, an irregular hepatic contour, and extension of periportal vein deep into the liver resulting from fibrosis and parenchymal retraction.	An inflammatory reaction to the eggs of this parasite, which embolize from bowel vessels to the portal vein, causes a granulomatous response that eventually leads to fibrosis and presinusoidal hypertension. The eggs themselves do not survive and may subsequently calcify. Chronic infection results in cirrhosis and an increased risk of developing hepatocellular carcinoma.

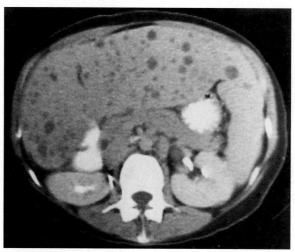

Fig GI 73-9
Fungal abscesses. Numerous low-density lesions in a massively enlarged liver representing multiple abscesses containing *Candida albicans*.[98]

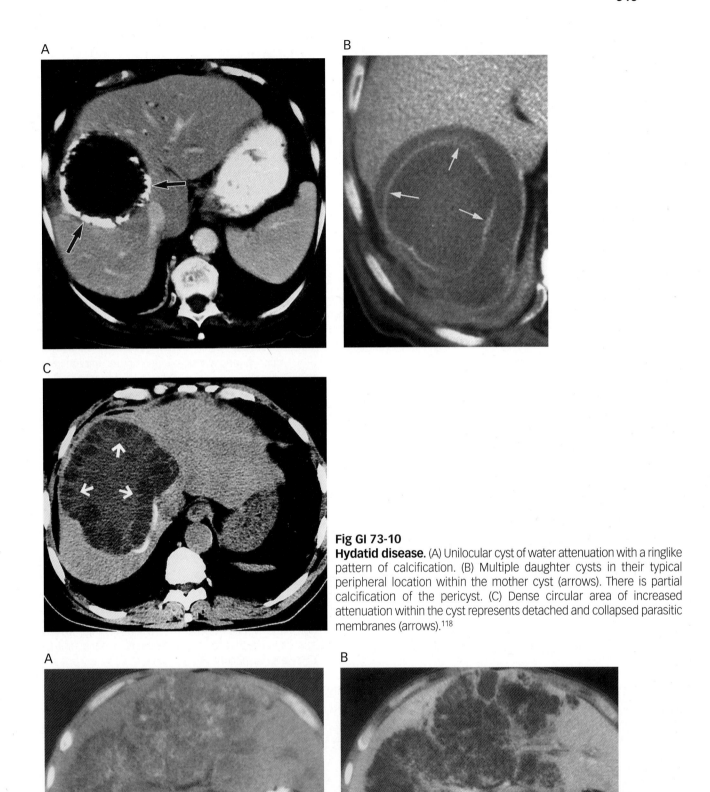

Fig GI 73-10
Hydatid disease. (A) Unilocular cyst of water attenuation with a ringlike pattern of calcification. (B) Multiple daughter cysts in their typical peripheral location within the mother cyst (arrows). There is partial calcification of the pericyst. (C) Dense circular area of increased attenuation within the cyst represents detached and collapsed parasitic membranes (arrows).[118]

Fig GI 73-11
Echinococcal multilocularis. (A) Unenhanced and (B) contrast-enhanced scans demonstrate a large, irregular, hypoattenuating lesion with dense punctuate calcifications, which are more clearly seen on the unenhanced image. Note the poor enhancement of the lesion.[119]

Condition	Imaging Findings	Comments
Tuberculosis (Fig GI 73-13)	Multiple lesions of low attenuation on scans both with and without contrast material.	There are frequently similar masses in the spleen. Miliary tuberculosis of the liver is common, but is usually not detected at imaging.
Fascioliasis (Fig GI 73-14)	Clusters of microabscesses arranged in a characteristic tract-like fashion, usually in the subcapsular region. A large cyst-like necrotic lesion may also occur.	Infestation by the liver fluke that infects cattle and sheep and involves humans as accidental hosts when they ingest water or raw aquatic plants contaminated with metacercariae, which later penetrate the intestinal wall and migrate through the peritoneal cavity to the liver after penetrating Glisson's capsule.
Neoplasm Cavernous hemangioma (Fig GI 73-15)	Well-circumscribed, low-attenuation area. After the bolus injection of contrast material, the periphery of the lesion becomes hyperdense; serial scans show a centripetally advancing border of enhancement as the central area of low density becomes progressively smaller.	Most common benign tumor of the liver. Usually single, small, and asymptomatic and found incidentally at surgery or autopsy or during an unrelated radiographic procedure. Large symptomatic hemangiomas may present as palpable masses, and spontaneous rupture infrequently causes massive intraperitoneal hemorrhage.

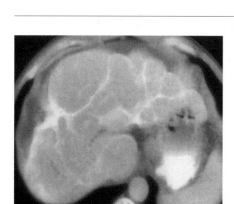

Fig GI 73-12
Schistosomiasis. Characteristic pericapsular and periportal calcifications, which give the liver a tortoise shell appearance.[119]

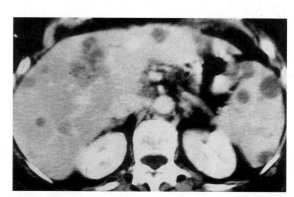

Fig GI 73-13
Tuberculosis. Multiple low-attenuation areas of varying size in the liver and spleen. The imaging findings are not specific, and thus biopsy is required whenever this disease is suspected.[119]

A

B

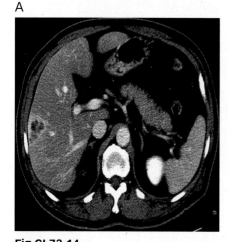
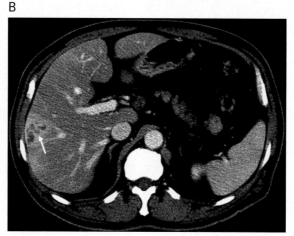

Fig GI 73-14
Fascioliasis. (A, B) Contrast scans show clustered small low-attenuating lesions with peripheral enhancement in the subcapsular area of the right hepatic lobe. Note the characteristic crooked tract-like lesion (burrow tract) in B (arrows).[120]

Condition	Imaging Findings	Comments
Adenoma (Fig GI 73-16)	Low-density or almost isodense mass that demonstrates a variable degree of enhancement. Recent hemorrhage appears as a central area of increased attenuation, while a remote bleeding episode may produce a central area of low attenuation reflecting an evolving hematoma or central cellular necrosis.	Benign lesion that is generally solitary and composed entirely of hepatocytes without Kupffer's cells. The tumor has a strong hormonal association and most often develops in women taking oral contraceptives. When the tumor occurs in men, it may be associated with hormonal therapy of carcinoma of the prostate. Spontaneous hemorrhage, sometimes of life-threatening proportions, is relatively common.

A

B

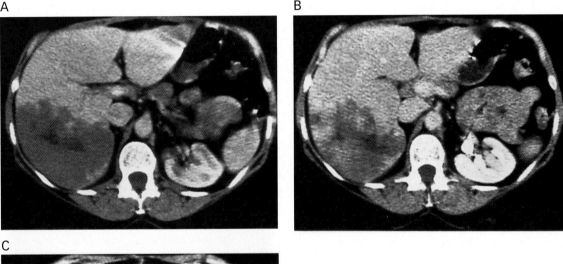

C

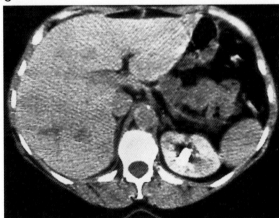

Fig GI 73-15
Cavernous hemangioma. (A) Initial scan after a bolus injection of contrast material demonstrates a large low-density lesion in the posterior segment of the right lobe of the liver.[121](B and C) Delayed scans show progressive enhancement of the lesion until it becomes nearly isodense with normal hepatic parenchyma.

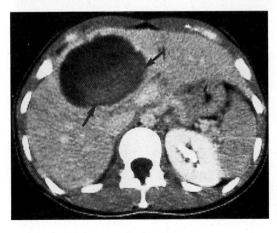

Fig GI 73-16
Adenoma. Large low-density mass in the liver. Note the area of higher density (arrows), which represents a blood clot, along the posterior aspect of the lesion.

Condition	Imaging Findings	Comments
Focal nodular hyperplasia (Fig GI 73-17)	Nonspecific low-attenuation mass that often demonstrates substantial enhancement after intravenous injection of contrast material. Central scar may occasionally be large enough to appear as a relatively low-density stellate area in a generally enhancing mass.	Controversial entity that probably represents an uncommon benign liver tumor composed of normal hepatocytes and Kupffer's cells. The characteristic morphologic feature is a central stellate, fibrous scar with peripherally radiating septa that divide the mass into lobules. Often in a subcapsular location or pedunculated along the inferior margin of the liver (infrequently situated deep in the hepatic parenchyma). The normal uptake of ^{99m}Tc-sulfur colloid virtually excludes other hepatic neoplasms that do not contain Kupffer's cells.
Angiomyolipoma (Fig GI 73-18)	Variable appearance depending on the amount of intratumoral fat.	Benign, unencapsulated mesenchymal tumor composed of varying proportions of smooth muscle cells, thick-walled blood vessels, and mature adipose tissue. Most commonly occurring in the kidneys, angiomyolipoma is rare in the liver.
Hemangioendothelioma (Fig GI 73-19)	Multiple, well-demarcated masses of decreased attenuation. After a bolus injection of contrast material, there is early enhancement of the lesions, which may be isodense with normal liver on delayed scans.	Most common hepatic lesion producing symptoms during infancy (the vast majority of these tumors presents before 6 months of age). Although generally considered benign, there have been rare reports of distant metastases. Extensive arteriovenous shunting in the lesion may lead to high-output congestive heart failure. May rarely occur in adults with long-term exposure to vinyl chloride or who have received Thorotrast.

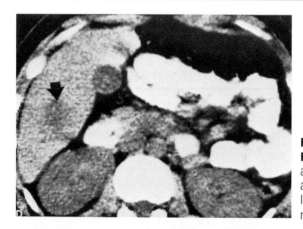

Fig GI 73-17
Focal nodular hyperplasia. Noncontrast scan shows an area of low attenuation (arrow) that is indistinguishable from a primary or secondary hepatic neoplasm. The lesion became isodense after the administration of contrast material.[122]

A   B

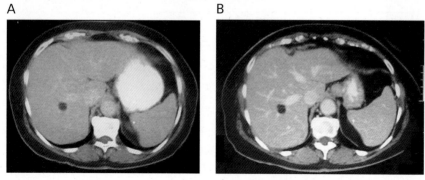

Fig GI 73-18
Angiomyolipoma. Well-defined hepatic mass (arrow) with the attenuation of fat.[123]

Condition	Imaging Findings	Comments
Hamartoma	Variable appearance, ranging from a single large hypoattenuating mass with internal septa to multiple small lesions mimicking metastases.	Benign liver malformation consisting of focal disorderly collections of bile ducts surrounded by abundant fibrous stroma.
Primary hepatocellular carcinoma (Figs GI 73-20 and GI 73-21)	Single or multiple solid masses with low attenuation. Dense, diffuse, nonuniform contrast enhancement.	In the United States, primary liver cell carcinoma most commonly occurs in patients with underlying diffuse hepatocellular disease, especially alcoholic or postnecrotic cirrhosis. Extremely common in Africa and Asia, where this tumor may account for up to one-third of all types of malignancies. Unlike metastases, primary hepatocellular carcinoma tends to be solitary or produce a small number of lesions. The demonstration of one or a few large focal lesions in association with a pattern of generalized cirrhosis strongly suggests this diagnosis. The lung, abdominal lymph nodes, and bone are the most common extrahepatic sites of metastatic hepatocellular carcinoma. Incidental extrahepatic lesions detected on CT in less common sites (brain, gastrointestinal tract) in patients without known metastases are unlikely to represent metastatic disease.
Other primary neoplasms (Figs GI 73-22 through GI 73-25)	Various patterns.	Fibrolamellar carcinoma (characteristic central scar); cholangiocarcinoma (often dense areas of calcification); biliary cystadenoma/cystadenocarcinoma; angiosarcoma (history of Thorotrast exposure); undifferentiated (embryonal) sarcoma.
Metastases (Figs GI 73-26 and GI 73-27)	Single or, more commonly, multiple low-density masses adjacent to normally enhancing hepatic parenchyma after contrast material administration. Metastases may rarely have an attenuation value higher than that of liver parenchyma (due to diffuse calcification, recent hemorrhage, or fatty infiltration of surrounding hepatic tissue).	By far the most common malignant tumor involving the hepatic parenchyma. Cystic metastases (sarcoma, melanoma, ovarian and colon carcinoma) may closely simulate benign cysts, though they often have somewhat shaggy and irregular walls. Amorphous punctate deposits of calcification in an area of diminished density may be seen in metastases from mucin-producing tumors (carcinomas of the gastrointestinal tract).

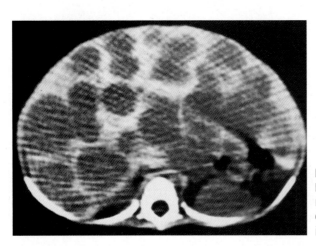

Fig GI 73-19
Infantile hepatic hemangioendothelioma. Multiple, rounded, hypodense masses throughout the liver. On a delayed postcontrast scan, all of the lesions became isodense to the surrounding liver.[124]

A
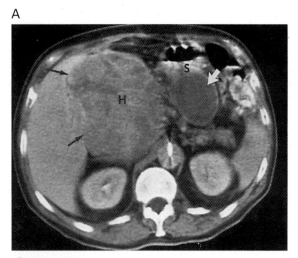
B
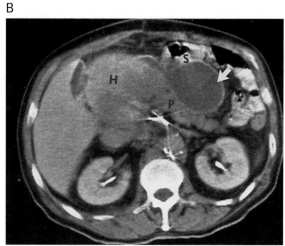

Fig GI 73-20
Primary hepatocellular carcinoma. (A) Huge mass with an attenuation value slightly less than that of normal liver. The black arrows point to the hematoma (H)–normal liver interface. Of incidental note is a pancreatic pseudocyst (white arrow) in the lesser sac between the stomach (S) and the pancreas. (B) On a slightly lower scan, there is absence of the fat plane surrounding the head of the pancreas (P), indicating invasion of the pancreas by the tumor.

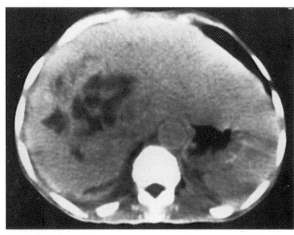

Fig GI 73-21
Primary hepatocellular carcinoma. Multiple low-attenuation masses in the liver.

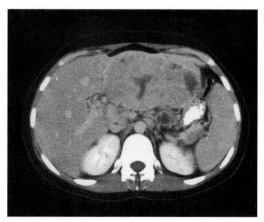

Fig GI 73-22
Fibrolamellar carcinoma. Contrast-enhanced scan shows a solitary lobulated, low-attenuation mass in the lateral segment of the left lobe with punctate calcification and central stellate scar. Note the retroperitoneal metastasis.[104]

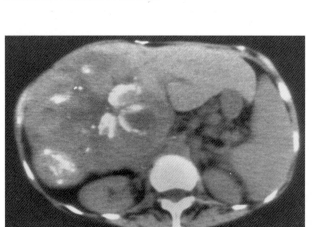

Fig GI 73-23
Cholangiocarcinoma. Large, lobulated mass containing multiple, large, chunky, dense areas of calcification. Note the central areas of decreased attenuation corresponding to fibrosis.[105]

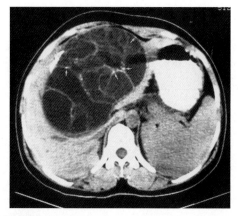

Fig GI 73-24
Biliary cystadenoma. Nonenhanced scan shows a well-defined, ovoid, low-attenuation liver mass with multiple internal septations. Multiple calcifications (arrows) are seen along the wall and internal septa.[96]

Condition	Imaging Findings	Comments
Kaposi's sarcoma (Fig GI 73-28)	Multiple low-attenuation nodules with irregular enlargement of the hilum and peripheral portal branches. Most nodules demonstrate contrast enhancement on delayed scans. Similar findings can be seen in the spleen.	Most common intrahepatic neoplasm in patients with AIDS. Cutaneous manifestations of Kaposi's sarcoma are usually evident and help differentiate the imaging appearance from metastases, fungal microabscesses, or multiple hemangiomas.
Lymphoma (Fig GI 73-29)	Multiple focal masses of diminished attenuation, often associated with lymphadenopathy.	Secondary involvement of the liver is common, though CT is relatively insensitive in detecting the usually small foci. Diffuse lymphomatous infiltration is generally isodense.

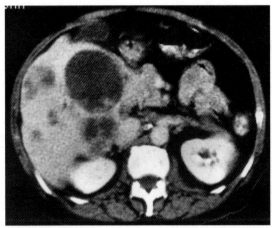

Fig GI 73-25
Angiosarcoma. Contrast-enhanced scan shows multiple low-attenuation lesions in a patient with previous exposure to Thorotrast.[125]

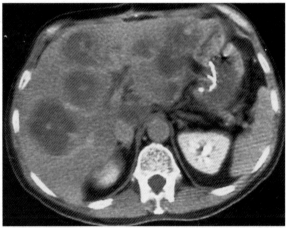

Fig GI 73-26
Metastases. Multiple, low-density metastases with high-density centers.

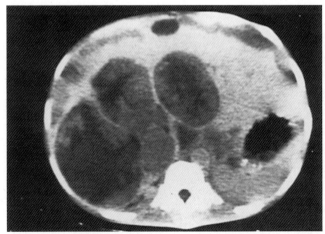

Fig GI 73-27
Metastases. Several large, low-density lesions filling much of the liver. Although these lesions simulate benign cysts, their walls are somewhat shaggy and irregular.

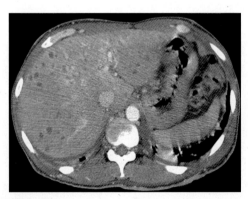

Fig GI 73-28
Kaposi's sarcoma. Multiple, ill-defined peripheral portal liver nodules (arrows) in a patient with disseminated AIDS-related disease. Some of the nodules show hypoattenuation, whereas others show enhancement.[123]

Condition	Imaging Findings	Comments
Trauma		
Subcapsular hematoma (Fig GI 73-30)	Well-marginated, crescentic or lenticular fluid collection located just beneath the hepatic capsule. Variable attenuation depending on its age and composition.	May be the result of blunt or penetrating abdominal trauma or a complication of surgery, percutaneous cholangiography, biopsy, portography, or biliary drainage procedures. Hematomas generally have high attenuation during the first few days, and then diminish gradually over several weeks to become low-density lesions.
Intrahepatic hematoma (Fig GI 73-31)	Round or oval mass of variable attenuation depending on its age and composition.	Hematomas generally have high attenuation during the first few days, then diminish gradually over several weeks to become low-density lesions. Dependent layering of cellular debris may produce a fluid-fluid interface in the mass.

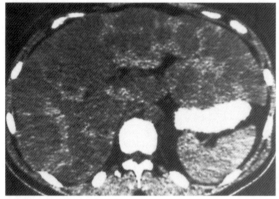

Fig GI 73-29
Lymphoma. Multiple nodules are scattered throughout the liver.[126]

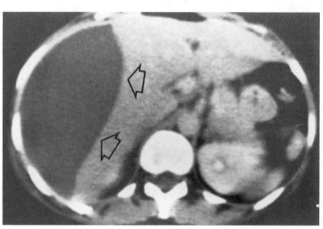

Fig GI 73-30
Subcapsular hematoma. Well-circumscribed elliptical area of low-attenuation density (arrows) in the periphery of the right lobe of the liver. The patient had sustained blunt trauma to the upper abdomen 2 weeks previously.

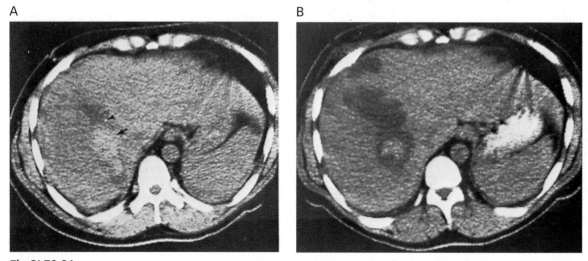

Fig GI 73-31
Intrahepatic hematoma. The patient had sustained a gunshot wound of the liver that was not appreciated at the time of laparotomy. (A) CT scan shows the bullet fragment (arrowhead) in a mixed low- and high-density collection. The high-density area (arrow) represents clotted blood. (B) One week later, the hematoma is larger and of lower density.[89]

Condition	Imaging Findings	Comments
Parenchymal laceration (Fig GI 73-32)	Irregularly shaped cleft or mass of low attenuation that often extends to the periphery of the liver and may have a branching pattern superficially resembling dilated bile ducts.	Small hyperdense foci, representing clotted blood, are frequently detected in the larger low-density site of a lysed clot and damaged parenchyma. Recent hemorrhage and clot have higher density than older hematomas that have matured.
Biloma (Fig GI 73-33)	Low-attenuation mass.	Intrahepatic or extrahepatic collection of bile due to traumatic rupture of the biliary tree.
Intraoperative retraction	Sharply marginated, wedge-shaped hypoattenuation lesion in the lateral segment of the left lobe of the liver.	The location of the lesion corresponds to the site of retractor placement during surgery. The CT appearance is most likely secondary to contusion or focal hepatic necrosis from compression by the surgical retractor.
Radiation injury (Fig GI 73-34)	Sharply defined band of diminished density in the liver corresponding to the radiation port.	Low attenuation in the irradiated area reflects the histologic combination of panlobular congestion, evolving hemorrhage, and fatty change. May become apparent days to months after radiation therapy (>3,500 rads). Usually a transient phenomenon that is not seen on follow-up scans until several months after the initial discovery.
Intrahepatic extension of pancreatic pseudocyst (Fig GI 73-35)	Low-density, round intrahepatic cystic mass or smaller, circular or tubular lucencies simulating dilated bile ducts (extension of pseudocysts along portal tracts).	The wall of the pseudocyst is initially formed by whatever tissue structures first limit its spread. Gradually, the evoked inflammatory reaction encapsulates the contents of the pseudocyst with granulation tissue and then with a fibrous wall (mature pseudocyst).
Focal fatty infiltration (Fig GI 73-36)	Single or multiple low-attenuation masses mimicking metastases.	Unlike metastases, focal fatty deposits usually do not cause local contour abnormalities, and portal and hepatic vein branches course normally through them.

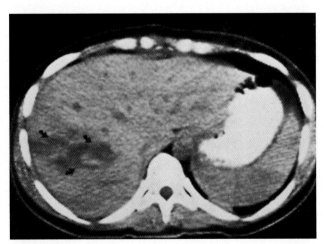

Fig GI 73-32
Hepatic laceration. CT scan after blunt trauma shows an irregular low-density plane (arrows) passing through the right lobe of the liver.[89]

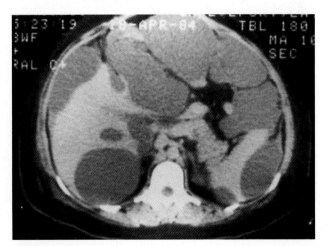

Fig GI 73-33
Biloma. Multiple intrahepatic and extrahepatic low-attenuation lesions after traumatic rupture of the biliary tree and bile peritonitis.

Condition	Imaging Findings	Comments
Hepatic infarction (Fig GI 73-37)	Well-circumscribed, peripheral, wedge-shaped area of low attenuation that is best seen on contrast-enhanced scans.	Relatively uncommon because of the liver's dual blood supply (hepatic artery, portal vein) and the tolerance of hepatocytes for low levels of oxygen.
Choledochal cyst (Fig GI 73-38)	Focal cystic mass(es).	Although they primarily involve the extrahepatic biliary tree, dilatation of the intrahepatic bile ducts may occur.

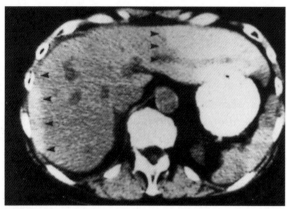

Fig GI 73-34
Radiation injury. Well-demarcated region of low attenuation corresponding to the treatment port (arrowheads).[127]

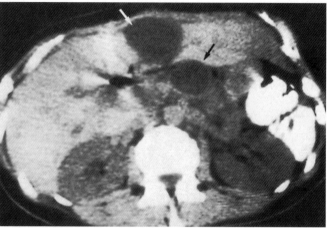

Fig GI 73-35
Intrahepatic extension of pancreatic pseudocyst. The area of decreased attenuation in the region of the falciform ligament (white arrow) is seen in association with a pseudocyst in the body of the pancreas (black arrow).[128]

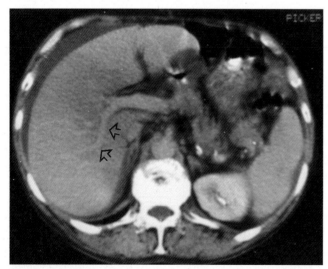

Fig GI 73-36
Focal fatty infiltration. The absence of a mass effect is seen both by the lack of contour abnormality and by the unaffected course of a portal vein branch through the area of focal fatty infiltration (arrows). Note that the margins of the lesion are poorly defined in this patient.[108]

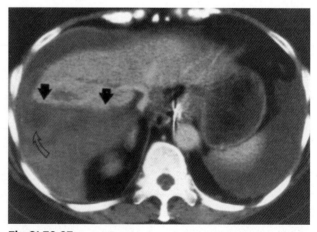

Fig GI 73-37
Hepatic infarction. Well-demarcated, wedge-shaped non-enhancing lesion in the posterior right hepatic lobe with peripheral low-attenuation components (straight arrows). Peripheral low-attenuation regions (curved arrows) could represent focal accumulations of bile and necrotic liver. Note the presence of ascites.[129]

Condition	Imaging Findings	Comments
Sarcoidosis. (Fig GI 73-39)	Coalescent granulomas may appear as multiple nodules of low attenuation.	Multiple hepatic nodules are easily mistaken for more common diseases, including metastases and lymphoma. Simultaneous involvement of the spleen is often seen.
Amyloidosis (Fig GI 73-40)	Nonspecific areas of decreased attenuation (often concomitant involvement of the spleen).	Amyloid frequently causes hepatic infiltration and enlargement, but rarely results in significant liver disease.

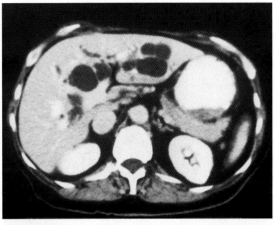

Fig GI 73-38
Choledochal cyst. Contrast-enhanced scan shows dilatation of intrahepatic bile ducts simulating multiple cystic masses.[130]

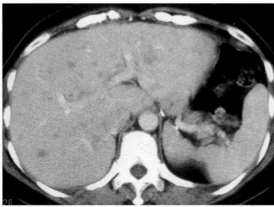

Fig GI 73-39
Sarcoidosis. Multiple irregular nodules of variable size.[131]

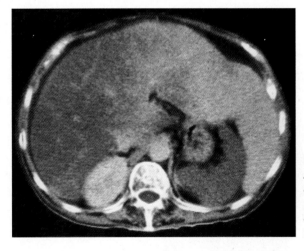

Fig GI 73-40
Amyloidosis. Contrast-enhanced scan shows low-attenuation area in the right lobe. Note that nondisplaced portal and hepatic vessels course through the low-attenuation mass, suggesting an infiltrative rather than neoplastic etiology.[132]

Hyperenhancing Focal Liver Lesions

Condition	Comments
Arterial phase	
Hepatocellular carcinoma (Fig GI 74-1)	In the early arterial phase, non-necrotic areas of a hepatocellular carcinoma appear hyperdense, as does any enhancing capsule. This is generally a transient phenomenon, and the lesion rapidly becomes isodense or hypodense. Infrequently, these tumors persist as hyperenhancing lesions during the portal vein phase.
Hemangioma (Fig GI 74-2)	Approximately 30% of hemangiomas appear as homogeneously hyperenhancing lesions in the arterial phase. Most small hemangiomas tend to be progressively hyperdense in the portal vein and equilibrium phases.

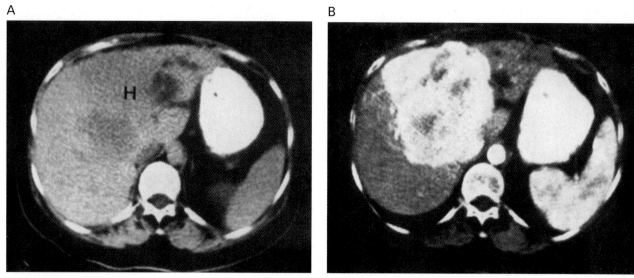

Fig GI 74-1
Hepatocellular carcinoma. (A) Noncontrast scan shows the lesion (H) as an ill-defined, low-attenuation mass. (B) Scan during peak arterial contrast shows striking enhancement throughout the mass.[133]

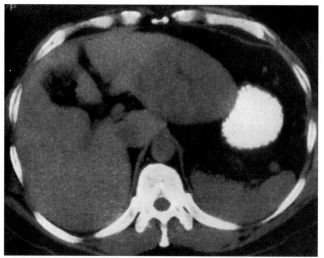

Fig GI 74-2
Hemangioma. Arterial phase scan reveals a small homogeneous, hypervascular nodule, which remained homogeneously hyperdense during the portal vein phase (not shown).[134]

Condition	Comments
Focal nodular hyperplasia (Fig GI 74-3)	On early CT scans, focal nodular hyperplasia may become hyperdense with respect to the adjacent normal liver. However, the central scar remains as a hypodense region within the mass.
Hepatocellular adenoma (Fig GI 74-4)	Hepatocellular adenomas typically demonstrate striking transient enhancement during the arterial phase. The contrast enhancement, which generally is more heterogeneous than that associated with focal nodular hyperplasia, tends to rapidly diminish on more delayed images, resulting in an isodense or even hypodense appearance during the portal phase.
Hypervascular metastases (Fig GI 74-5)	Metastases that are hyperdense during the arterial phase are uncommon lesions that usually reflect a hypervascular underlying tumor. The differential diagnosis of hyperintense metastases includes carcinoid, melanoma, pancreatic islet cell tumor, hypernephroma, pheochromocytoma, choriocarcinoma, and carcinomas of the breast and thyroid. These hypervascular metastases generally become isodense with liver before the equilibrium phase begins. Therefore, patients with these primary neoplasms should always undergo multiphasic contrast CT studies to avoid missing a metastatic liver lesion.

A   B

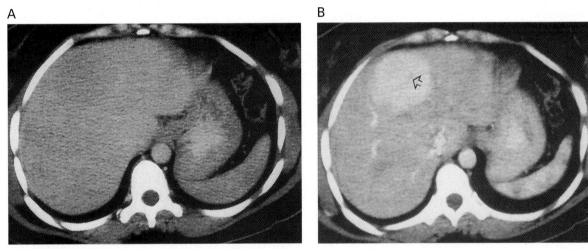

Fig GI 74-3
Focal nodular hyperplasia. (A) On the nonenhanced scan, it is very difficult to detect the lesion in the medial segment of the left hepatic lobe. (B) On the early contrast scan, the lesion is uniformly enhanced and well defined. Note the small central stellate scar (open arrow).[135]

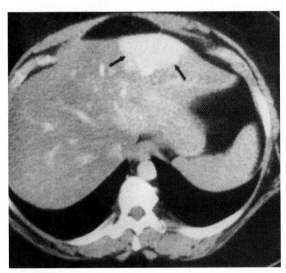

Fig GI 74-4
Hepatocellular adenoma. Early contrast scan shows marked diffuse enhancement of the lesion (arrows).[133]

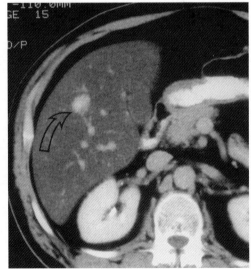

Fig GI 74-5
Metastasis. Enhancing mass (curved arrow) in the right hepatic lobe that is especially clear against the background of a diffuse fatty liver.[135]

Condition	Comments
Portal vein and/or equilibrium phases	
Hemangioma (Fig GI 74-6)	Although typically hyperenhancing during the arterial phase, hemangioma may show increased contrast enhancement relative to surrounding liver parenchyma during the portal vein or equilibrium phase.
Hepatocellular carcinoma (Fig GI 74-7)	Although typically hyperenhancing during the arterial phase, hepatocellular carcinoma may show increased contrast enhancement relative to surrounding liver parenchyma during the portal vein phase.
Focal nodular hyperplasia (Fig GI 74-8)	Although typically hyperenhancing during the arterial phase, focal nodular hyperplasia may show increased contrast enhancement relative to surrounding liver parenchyma during the portal vein phase.
Solitary fibrous tumor (Fig GI 74-9)	Solitary fibrous tumor is an unusual neoplasm of mesenchymal origin that typically affects the pleura. Several cases have been reported of liver involvement, in which this highly vascular tumor demonstrated heterogeneous and amorphous contrast enhancement during the portal vein phase and striking hyperenhancement in the equilibrium phase.
Angiomyolipoma	Angiomyolipoma is a rare benign lipomatous tumor that may show globular or linear areas with strong enhancement within a hypodense mass on scans obtained during the portal vein phase.
"Hot spot" lesion (Fig GI 74-10)	In cases of obstruction of the superior vena cava, venous collaterals to the inferior vena cava may be detected on portal vein-phase scans as geographic areas of liver parenchyma with intense opacification ("hot spot" lesion), a pattern mimicking a hypervascular lesion such as hemangioma.

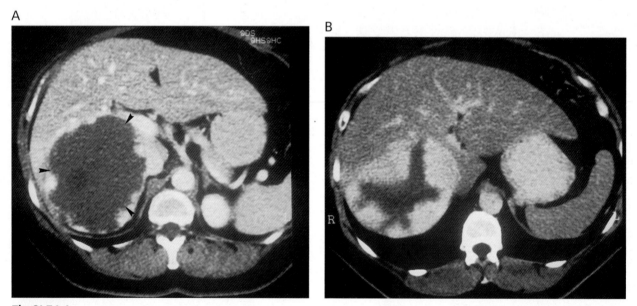

A   B

Fig GI 74-6
Hemangioma. (A) Portal vein-phase scan shows globular hyperenhancing areas in the periphery of the large lesion (arrowheads). (B) During the equilibrium phase, there is progressive peripheral pooling of contrast material.[134]

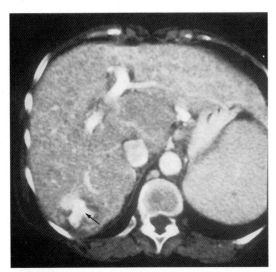

Fig GI 74-7
Hepatocellular carcinoma. Portal vein-phase study shows the hypervascular tumor with mosaic pattern (arrow).[134]

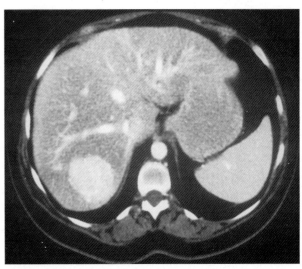

Fig GI 74-8
Focal nodular hyperplasia. Homogeneous enhancement during the portal vein phase. The lesion appears hyperdense because of the background of fatty liver parenchyma.[134]

A

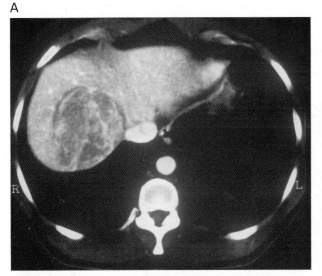

B

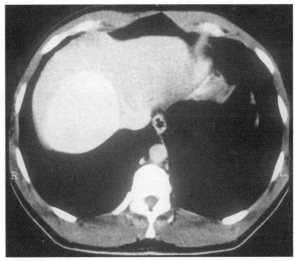

Fig GI 74-9
Solitary fibrous liver tumor. (A) Portal vein-phase scan shows heterogeneous areas of enhancement. (B) In the equilibrium phase, there is striking hyperenhancement of the lesion.[134]

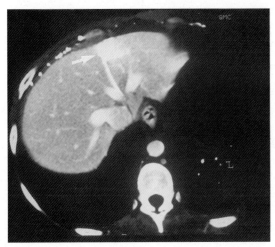

Fig GI 74-10
"Hot-spot" lesion. Geographic hyperenhancing lesion at the dome of the liver (arrow) in this patient with Hodgkin's lymphoma and superior vena cava thrombosis.[134]

Focal Cystic Lesions of the Liver

Condition	Comments
Developmental lesions Hepatic (bile duct) cyst (Figs GI 75-1 and GI 75-2)	Common benign lesion that does not communicate with the biliary tree. Solitary, or more frequently, multiple, hepatic cysts are found more often in women and are almost always asymptomatic. They appear as non-enhancing homogeneous lesions of low attenuation on CT. On MR, hepatic cysts have very low homogeneous signal intensity on T1-weighted images and very high homogeneous signal intensity on T2 images. Their extreme hyperintensity on heavily T2-weighted images allows hepatic cysts to be differentiated from metastatic disease, which appears much less intense on these sequences.
Polycystic liver disease (Fig GI 75-3)	Hepatic cysts are seen in 40% of patients with autosomal dominant polycystic disease involving the kidneys. They typical appear as multiple homogeneous cystic lesions of low attenuation on CT and with characteristic fluid-intensity on MR images. Cyst heterogeneity is consistent with intracystic hemorrhage.

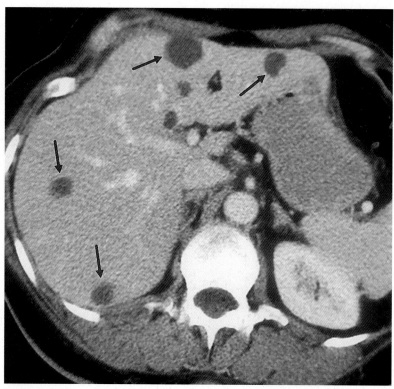

Fig GI 75-1
Hepatic cysts. Contrast CT scan shows multiple, homogeneous, rounded, well-defined, non-enhancing cystic lesions (arrows), which are consistent with simple bile duct cysts.[136]

Condition	Comments
Bile duct hamartoma (Fig GI 75-4)	Originating from embryonic bile ducts that fail to involute, these asymptomatic lesions appear as multiple small cyst-like hepatic nodules that often have a more irregular outline than simple cysts.

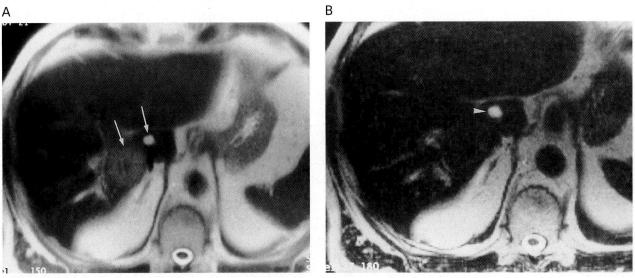

Fig GI 75-2
Differentiation between hepatic cyst and metastasis. (A) T2-weighted MR image in a patient with a history of colon carcinoma shows two high-signal-intensity lesions (arrows) in segment 1 of the liver. (B) On a heavily T2-weighted image, only the smaller lesion (arrowhead) continues to have the signal intensity of fluid. Therefore, the larger lesion represents a metastasis and the smaller lesion represents a simple bile duct cyst.[136]

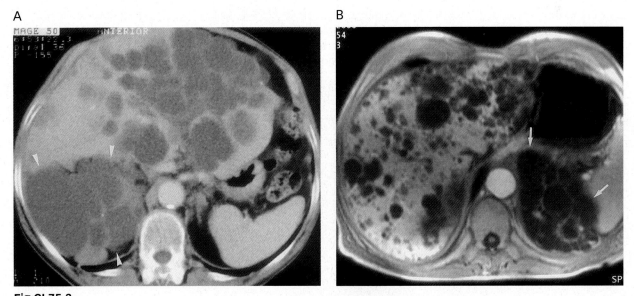

Fig GI 75-3
Polycystic disease. (A) Contrast CT scan shows multiple non-enhancing hepatic and renal cysts (arrowheads). (B) In another patient, a contrast T1-weighted MR image shows renal cysts (arrows) and the typical MR imaging appearance of hepatics cysts as homogeneous masses with well-defined borders and no enhancement of walls or contents.[136]

Condition	Comments
Caroli's disease (Fig GI 75-5)	Saccular dilatation of the intrahepatic bile ducts, which often contain calculi. CT shows hypoattenuating cystic structures of varying size that communicate with the biliary tree. A highly suggestive finding is the "central dot" sign, the presence of tiny dots with strong contrast enhancement within the dilated intrahepatic bile ducts. MR cholangiography can demonstrate the pathognomonic appearance of saccular dilated and nonobstructed intrahepatic bile ducts that communicate with the biliary tree.

A

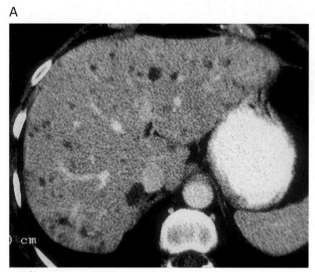

B

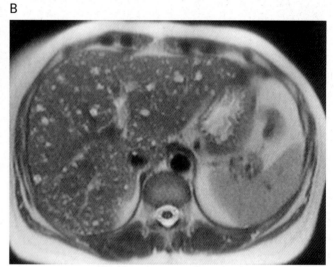

Fig GI 75-4
Bile duct hamatoma. (A) Contrast CT scan shows numerous non-enhancing cystic lesions scattered throughout the liver of this asymptomatic woman. (B) In another patient, a T2-weighted MR image shows multiple, small (<1.5 cm diameter) hyperintense nodules consistent with biliary hamartomas.[136]

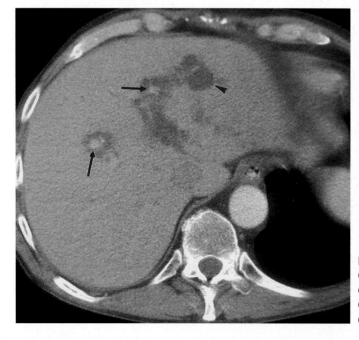

Fig GI 75-5
Caroli's disease. Contrast CT scan shows saccular dilatation of the biliary tree (arrowhead) with enhancement of central portal vein radicals (arrows), producing the central dot sign.[136]

Condition	Comments

Neoplastic lesions
  Undifferentiated
  embryonal sarcoma
  (Fig GI 75-6)
	Rare malignant tumor of older children and adolescents that appears as a solid, predominantly cystic mass with well-defined borders and occasionally a pseudocapsule separating it from normal liver tissue. There may be internal calcifications within the mass. On MR, streaky areas of high signal intensity on T1-weighted images represent intratumoral hemorrhage. The tumor generally shows heterogeneous contrast enhancement in the solid, usually peripheral, portions of the mass, especially on delayed images.

Biliary cystadenoma/ cystadenocarcinoma (Fig GI 75-7)	Cystadenomas are rare, usually slow-growing, multilocular cystic tumors that are considered premalignant lesions. They appear on CT as solitary cystic masses with a well-defined thick capsule, mural nodules, internal septa, and rarely capsular calcification. On MR, variable signal intensity on all images depends on the presence of solid components, hemorrhage, and protein content.
Cystic primary neoplasm (Fig GI 75-8)	Hepatocellular carcinoma and giant cavernous hemangioma are the two most common primary neoplasms of the liver that may rarely manifest as an entirely or partially cystic mass, usually reflecting central cystic degeneration.

A
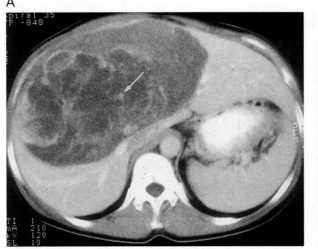

B
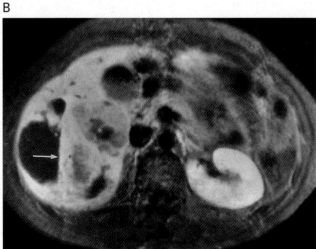

Fig GI 75-6
Undifferentiated embryonal sarcoma. (A) Contrast CT scan shows a 10-cm cystic lesion in the right lobe of the liver. Note the septa and calcifications (arrow) within the mass. (B) In a different patient, a delayed-phase contrast T1-weighted MR image shows heterogeneous enhancement of the solid portions of the lesion (arrowhead), which were hyperintense relative to normal liver on T2-weighted images.[136]

Condition	Comments
Cystic metastasis (Fig GI 75-9)	Hepatic metastases may appear cystic due to necrosis and cystic degeneration of hypervascular tumors with rapid growth (neuroendocrine tumors, sarcoma, melanoma, some types of lung and breast carcinoma) or as a manifestation of mucinous adenocarcinomas of the colon or ovary. They generally are multiple lesions with strong enhancement of the peripheral viable and irregularly defined tissue. Because ovarian metastases commonly spread via peritoneal seeding rather than hematogenously, they appear as cystic serosal implants on both the visceral peritoneal surface of the liver and the parietal peritoneum of the diaphragm, rather than as intraparenchymal masses.

A

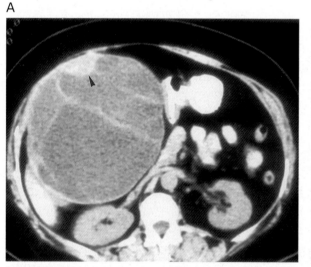

B

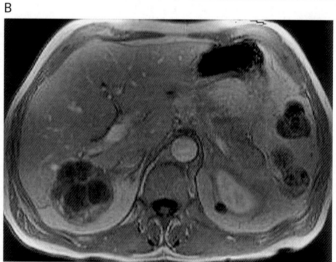

Fig GI 75-7
Biliary cystadenoma. (A) Contrast CT scan shows a 12-cm multiseptated cystic lesion in the right lobe of the liver. Note the focal papillary excrescence (arrowhead). (B) In a different patient, a contrast T1-weighted MR image shows a multiloculated mass with enhancement of the capsule and septa.[136]

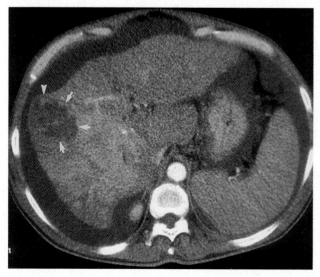

Fig GI 75-8
Cystic hepatocellular carcinoma. Contrast CT scan shows an ill-defined cystic mass in the right lobe of the liver. On this arterial-phase image, a small hypervascular nodule is seen at the periphery of the mass (arrowhead). Note the indirect signs of liver cirrhosis: atrophy of the right hepatic lobe, hypertrophy of the caudate lobe, contour irregularities, and ascites.[136]

Condition	Comments

Inflammatory lesions
  Abscess
  (Figs GI 75-10
  and GI 75-11)
	Pyogenic, amebic, or fungal abscesses may have a unilocular cystic appearance in subacute stages, when necrosis and liquefaction predominate. More acute processes may manifest as a cluster of small low-attenuation or high-signal-intensity lesions. The presence of an enhancing wall and perilesion edema can differentiate a hepatic abscess from a benign cystic liver lesion.

A

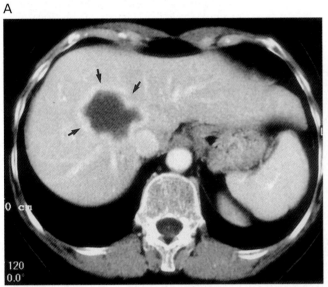

B

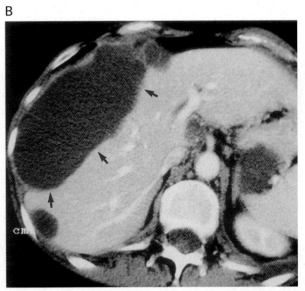

Fig GI 75-9
Cystic metastases. (A) Contrast CT scan in a patient with metastatic breast cancer shows a cystic lesion with peripheral enhancement (arrows). (B) In another patient who had ovarian cancer, there is a 7-cm elliptical cystic lesion (arrow) on the surface of the liver.[136]

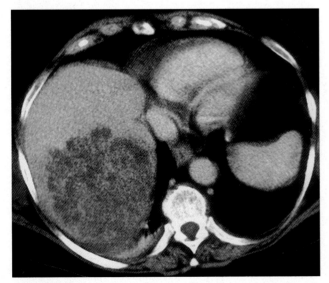

Fig GI 75-10
Pyogenic abscesses. Contrast CT scan shows a large cystic liver mass consisting of a confluent cluster of numerous tiny hepatic abscesses.[136]

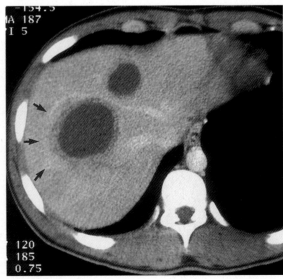

Fig GI 75-11
Amebic abscess. Contrast CT scan shows a cystic lesion with high attenuation of the surrounding normal liver parenchyma (arrows) due to hyperemia (double target sign).[136]

Condition	Comments
Hydatid cyst (Fig GI 75-12)	Cystic mass that often demonstrates coarse mural calcification and daughter cysts. On MR, the outer pericyst appears as a hypointense rim on all images because of its fibrous composition and the presence of calcifications.

Miscellaneous lesions
  Hematoma
  (Fig GI 75-13)
	Usually seconday to surgery, trauma, or hemorrhage within a solid liver neoplasm (especially hepatocellular adenoma). On CT, although acute or subacute bleeding has a higher attenuation, in the chronic stage the attenuation is identical to that of pure fluid.

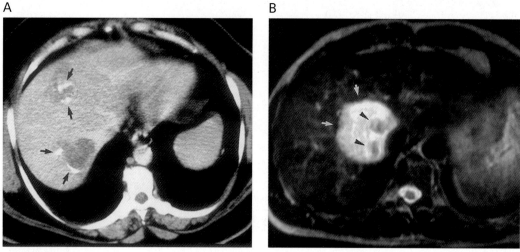

Fig GI 75-12
Hydatid cyst. (A) Contrast CT scan shows two cystic lesions with subtotally calcified walls (arrows) in the liver of a sheep raiser. (B) T2-weighted image in a different patient shows a solitary hyperintense lesion in the right lobe of the liver. Note the internal calcifications (arrowheads) and the hypointense pseudocapsule (arrows).[136]

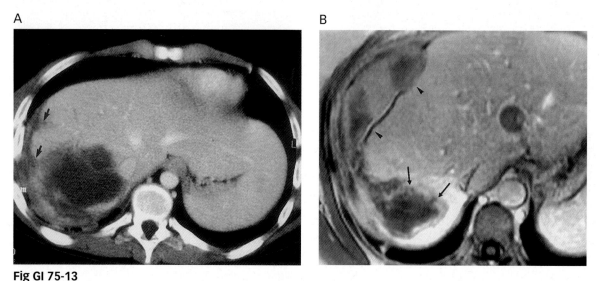

Fig GI 75-13
Hematoma. (A) Contrast CT scan in an assault victim shows a low-attenuation parenchymal hematoma in the posterior segment of the right hepatic lobe, with small coexisting irregular liver lacerations (arrows). (B) Contrast T1-weighted MR image in a young woman shows a "cystic" mass (arrows) in the right hepatic lobe with coexistent acute subcapsular hemorrhage (arrowheads), which proved to be a bleeding hepatocellular adenoma.[136]

Condition	Comments
Biloma (Fig GI 75-14)	Secondary to rupture of the biliary system, which can be spontaneous, traumatic, or iatrogenic following surgery or interventional procedures. It appears as a well-defined or slightly irregular cystic mass without septa or calcifications.
Intrahepatic pancreatic pseudocyst (Fig GI 75-15)	Well-defined homogeneous fluid-filled mass in the subcapsular region. Hemorrhage or necrotic debris within the pseudocyst causes changes in the CT attenuation or MR signal intensity.

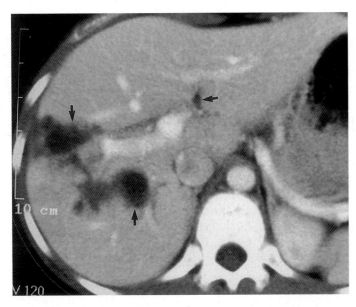

Fig GI 75-14
Biloma. Contrast CT scan shows three intrahepatic collections (arrows) without evidence of septa, capsules, or calcifications. This appearance is compatible with bilomas in this young man who experienced biliary leakage after a severe motor vehicle accident.[136]

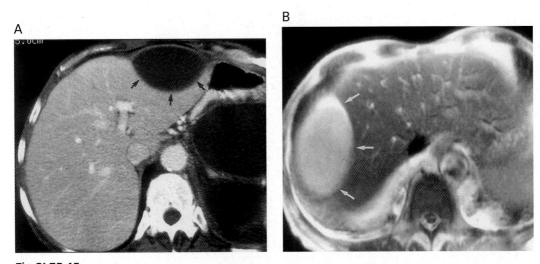

Fig GI 75-15
Intrahepatic pancreatic pseudocyst. (A) Contrast CT scan obtained 3 weeks after an episode of acute pancreatitis shows multiple intraperitoneal pseudocysts and a 5-cm cystic lesion in the left lobe of the liver (arrows). The lesion is well defined due to the presence of a capsule and has homogeneous fluid attenuation, findings that in this clinical context are pathognomonic for an intrapancreatic pseudocyst. (B) T2-weighted MR image in another patient after an episode of necrotizing pancreatitis shows a homogeneous hyperintense pseudocyst (arrows) along the right lobe of the liver.[136]

Fatty Lesions of the Liver

Condition	Comments
Benign	
Hepatic steatosis (Fig GI 76-1)	Diffuse or focal deposits of fat, typically in a periligamentous or periportal location. The diagnosis is supported by the presence of nondistorted blood vessels traversing the area. At times, however, patchy focal fat deposition or sparing may be mistaken for an infiltrative neoplasm. The use of in-phase and opposed-phase MR imaging can reliably differentiate multiple nodular steatosis from metastatic disease.
Omental packing (Fig GI 76-2)	Common postoperative appearance following hepatobiliary surgery.
Adenoma (Figs GI 76-3 and GI 76-4)	Benign, encapsulated neoplasm that most commonly occurs in young women taking oral contraceptives and often contains substantial amounts of adipose tissue. Although this may be difficult to appreciate on CT, the lipid content in hepatic adenomas is better demonstrated on chemical shift MR imaging.
Lipoma	Unusual liver tumor that appears as a well-circumscribed, uniformly hyperechoic mass on ultrasound and has the pathognomonic characteristics of a fatty lesion on CT and MR imaging.

A

B

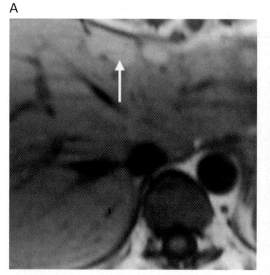
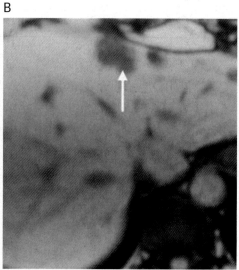

Fig GI 76-1
Focal hepatic steatosis. (A) In-phase T1-weighted MR image shows peripheral high-intensity foci (arrow). (B) On the opposed-phase image, there is a uniform decrease in the signal intensity of the foci (arrow).[137]

Condition	Comments
Angiomyolipoma (Fig GI 76-5)	Benign, unencapsulated mesenchymal tumor composed of varying proportions of smooth muscle cells, thick-walled blood vessels, and mature adipose tissue. Most commonly occurring in the kidneys, angiomyolipoma is rare in the liver. Highly echogenic on ultrasound, the appearance on CT and MR imaging depends on the amount of intratumoral fat.

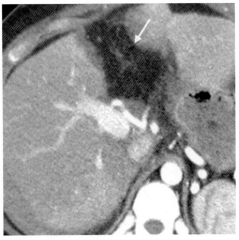

Fig GI 76-2
Omental packing. Contrast CT scan shows a hepatic pseudomass (arrow), a common postoperative finding.[137]

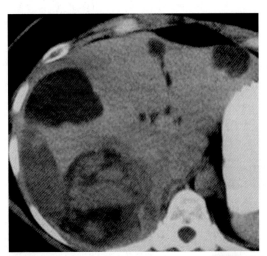

Fig GI 76-3
Hepatic adenoma. Unenhanced CT scan shows multiple fat-attenuation lesions within the liver.[137]

A   B

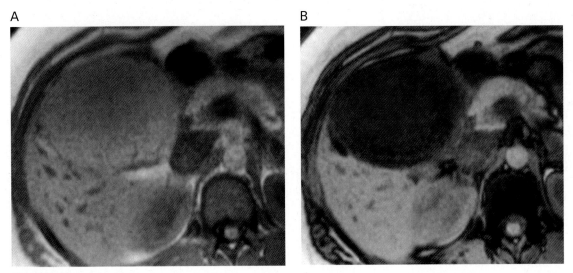

Fig GI 76-4
Hepatic adenoma. (A) In-phase T1-weighted MR image shows a large hypointense mass in the right lobe of the liver (arrow). On the out-of-phase image, there is a homogeneous decrease in the signal intensity of the fat-containing lesion.[137]

Condition	Comments
Cystic teratoma (Fig GI 76-6)	Although true liver cystic teratomas are extremely rare, intraperitoneal or retroperitoneal teratomas invading the liver are more common. The tumor frequently contains components derived from all three germ layers (ectoderm, endoderm, and mesoderm). The characteristic appearance is a heterogeneous mass containing fat, fluid and calcification; hair and proteinaceous debris may be seen within the lesion.
Adrenal rest tumor (Fig GI 76-7)	Ectopic collection of adrenocortical cells in an extra-adrenal site. Hepatic tumors are generally hypervascular subcapsular masses containing macroscopic collections of fat.
Malignant Hepatocellular carcinoma (Fig GI 76-8)	This most common primary malignant neoplasm frequently develops in a cirrhotic liver. Small (<1.5 cm), well-differentiated lesions often demonstrate diffuse fatty change, while larger tumors display more patchy areas of fat deposition.
Metastases	Although metastases to the liver usually do not contain fat, an exception is liposarcoma (primarily from the retroperitoneum or extremity), which involves the liver in about 10% of cases.

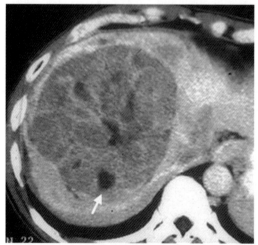

Fig GI 76-5
Angiomyolipoma. Contrast CT scan demonstrates a well-circumscribed, heterogeneous tumor of the right lobe of the liver that contains foci of fat (arrow).[137]

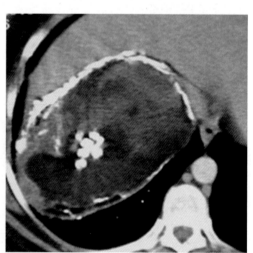

Fig GI 76-6
Hepatic invasion by a retroperitoneal teratoma. Contrast CT scan shows a predominantly fatty mass with a peripheral rim and central chunky calcification (arrow).[137]

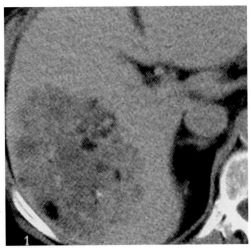

Fig GI 76-7
Adrenal rest tumor. CT scan shows a hetero-geneous lesion in the right lobe that contains macroscopic fat (arrow).[137]

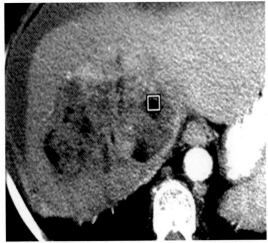

Fig GI 76-8
Hepatocellular carcinoma. Contrast CT scan shows patchy macroscopic fat deposition (□) in a large, heterogeneously enhancing hepatoma.[137]

Generalized Increased Attenuation of the Liver

Condition	Imaging Findings	Comments
Hemochromatosis (Fig GI 77-1)	Generalized increase in density of the hepatic parenchyma that contrasts sharply with the much lower density of normal intrahepatic blood vessels.	Excessive deposition of iron in body tissues with eventual fibrosis and dysfunction of the severely affected organs. May be a primary inherited disorder (excessive intestinal absorption of iron) or secondary to certain chronic anemias or repeated blood transfusions.
Glycogen storage disease (Fig GI 77-2)	Generalized increase in hepatic density or, less commonly, a generally low-density liver.	Autosomal genetic disorders of carbohydrate metabolism with various enzymatic defects. The areas of low attenuation in this condition are often nonhomogeneous and result from the fatty infiltration that occurs in long-standing glycogen storage disease.
Thorotrast deposition (Fig GI 77-3)	Generalized (often inhomogeneous) increased density of the liver (and spleen and lymph nodes).	Previously used radiographic contrast agent that is retained in endothelial cells of the liver, spleen, and adjacent lymph nodes. The alpha-emitting radionuclide has been associated with the development of hepatobiliary carcinoma, leukemia, and aplastic anemia up to 30 years after the initial injection.
Drug therapy (Fig GI 77-4)	Generalized increase in hepatic density (some also affect spleen).	Amiodarone (used to control cardiac tachyarrhythmias); gold (for treatment of rheumatoid arthritis); cisplatin (anti-cancer agent).

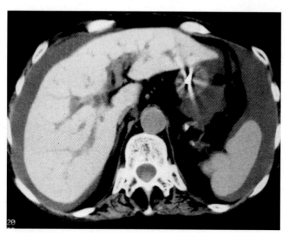

Fig GI 77-1
Hemochromatosis. Diffuse homogeneous increase in liver (and spleen) attenuation when compared with that of other soft-tissue organs. Note the hepatic and portal veins, which stand out in bold relief as low-attenuation structures against the abnormally high attenuation of the liver parenchyma.[129]

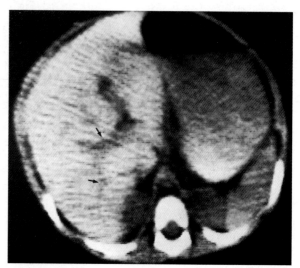

Fig GI 77-2
Glycogen storage disease. Diffuse increase in attenuation of the enlarged liver with prominent hepatic and portal venous structures (arrows).[122]

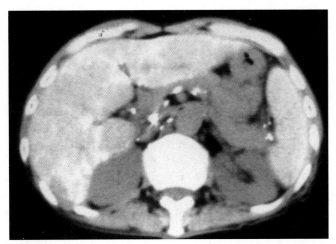

Fig GI 77-3
Thorotrast deposition. Generalized increase in the attenuation of the liver (and spleen).

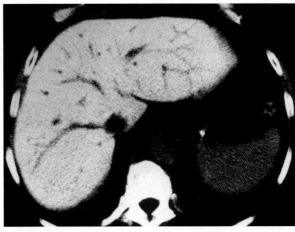

Fig GI 77-4
Amiodarone liver.[138]

Generalized Decreased Attenuation of the Liver

Condition	Imaging Findings	Comments
Fatty infiltration (Figs GI 78-1 through GI 78-3)	Generalized decrease in the attenuation value of the liver. The portal veins commonly appear as high-density structures surrounded by a background of low density caused by hepatic fat (the opposite of the normal pattern of portal veins as low-density channels on noncontrast scans).	Result of excessive deposition of triglycerides, which occurs in cirrhosis and other hepatic disorders. In normal individuals, the mean liver CT number is never lower than that of the spleen, whereas in fatty infiltration the hepatic density is much lower. In fatty infiltration of liver due to cirrhosis, there often is prominence of the caudate lobe associated with shrinkage of the right lobe.

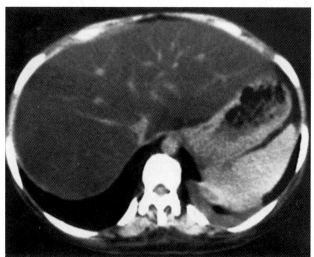

Fig GI 78-1
Fatty infiltration in cirrhosis. Generalized decrease in the attenuation value of the liver (far less than that of the spleen). The portal veins appear as high-density structures surrounded by a background of low-density hepatic fat.

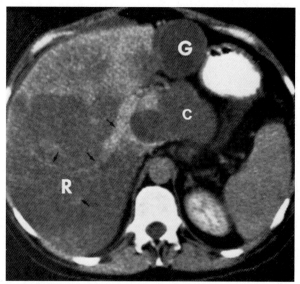

Fig GI 78-2
Patchy fatty infiltration in cirrhosis. The right (R) and caudate (c) lobes of the liver are replaced by fat to a degree that makes the density almost equal to that of the gallbladder (G). The medial segment of the left hepatic lobe has a higher CT density but contains foci of low attenuation. The spleen is large, and the caudate lobe is prominent. The portal vein (arrows) courses normally through the center of the right hepatic lobe, distinguishing fatty infiltration from a low-density tumor.[122]

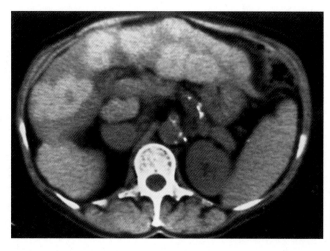

Fig GI 78-3
Regenerating nodules in cirrhosis. Multiple nodules of attenuation equal to that of normal liver are seen superimposed on a background of low-attenuation fatty infiltration. Note the calcification in the pancreas caused by chronic pancreatitis in this patient, a chronic alcoholic.

Condition	Imaging Findings	Comments
Budd-Chiari syndrome (Figs GI 78-4 and GI 78-5)	Enlarged liver with diffusely decreased attenuation (presumably due to congestion of the hepatic parenchyma).	Obstruction of hepatic venous outflow at the level of the intrahepatic venules, hepatic veins, or suprahepatic segment of the inferior vena cava. Rare condition associated with hypercoagulability states, oral contraceptives, pregnancy, invasive tumors, and congenital webs. "Flip-flop" pattern of contrast enhancement (see Fig GI 78-5).

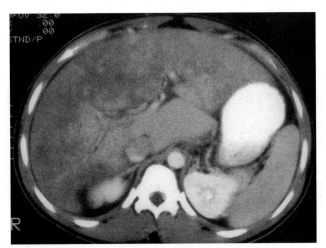

Fig GI 78-4
Budd-Chiari syndrome. Contrast scan of a woman with a coagulation disorder and hepatic vein thrombosis shows the characteristic mosaic pattern of peripheral low attenuation in both the right and left hepatic lobes. The liver is enlarged with relatively marked hypertrophy of the caudate lobe, which has a uniform attenuation.[129]

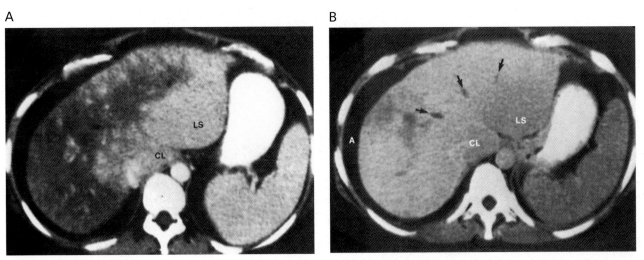

Fig GI 78-5
Budd-Chiari syndrome. Classic flip-flop pattern of hepatic contrast enhancement. (A) Initially, the normally enhancing central part of the liver, including the caudate lobe (CL) and part of the lateral segment of the left lobe (LS), appears hyperdense relative to the periphery of the liver, which enhances more slowly. (B) Later, as the contrast material washes out centrally and accretes peripherally, the central region appears relatively hypodense. Note the thrombus in the hepatic veins (arrows). (A, ascites.)[139]

Condition	Imaging Findings	Comments
Hepatic congestion (Fig GI 78-6)	Enlarged liver with diffusely decreased attenuation.	Congestive heart failure or constrictive pericarditis. Similar enhancement pattern as Budd-Chiari syndrome, though in these conditions there is marked enlargement of the inferior vena cava and hepatic veins due to backward transmission of the elevated central pressure (unlike the nonvisualized hepatic veins and small inferior vena cava seen in the Budd-Chiari syndrome).
Amyloidosis (Fig GI 78-7)	Generalized decreased density throughout the liver.	More commonly discrete areas of low attenuation within an enlarged liver.

A   B

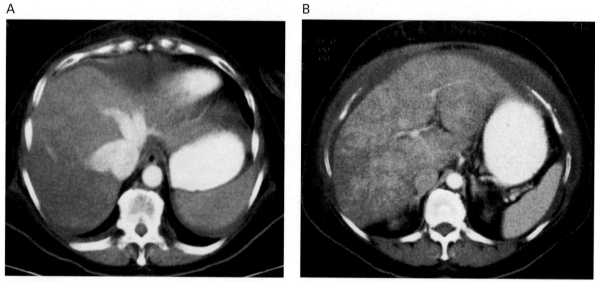

Fig GI 78-6
Congestive heart failure. (A) Early bolus-enhanced scan shows dense retrograde hepatic venous opacification. (B) Scan obtained during the vascular phase shows diffusely mottled hepatic enhancement.[140]

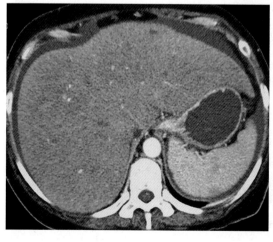

Fig GI 78-7
Amyloidosis. Diffusely enlarged liver with generalized decreased attenuation.[141]

Magnetic Resonance Imaging of the Liver

Condition	Imaging Findings	Comments
Cyst		
Simple (Fig GI 79-1)	Extremely hypointense on T1-weighted images and hyperintense on T2-weighted scans (signal intensity of water). No enhancement after contrast administration.	Intracystic hemorrhage produces high signal on T1-weighted images.
Polycystic liver disease (Fig GI 79-2)	Numerous cysts of water signal intensity.	Approximately one-third of patients with adult polycystic kidney disease have associated cysts of the liver, which do not interfere with hepatic function.
Caroli's disease (Fig GI 79-3)	Multifocal segmental dilatation of the large intrahepatic ducts, which retain their communication with the biliary tree.	In contrast, in polycystic liver disease the cysts do not communicate with the biliary tree or other cysts.

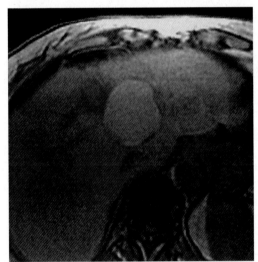

Fig GI 79-1
Hemorrhage in a simple hepatic cyst. T1-weighted image demonstrates a homogeneously hyperintense lesion, reflecting bleeding within the cyst.[142]

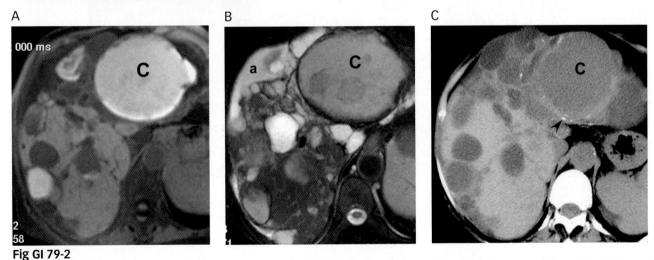

Fig GI 79-2
Polycystic liver disease. (A) T1-weighted scan shows multiple cysts (C), some of which are hyperintense due to the presence of blood. T2-weighted image shows hemorrhagic cysts and noncomplicated cysts, with the former being less hyperintense than the latter, as is typically the case. The largest hemorrhagic cyst (C) is surrounded by a hypointense rim of hemosiderin. Note also the presence of ascites. (C) Corresponding unenhanced CT scan shows the multiple hepatic cysts. Note the calcifications in the wall of the single largest cyst (C).[143]

Condition	Imaging Findings	Comments

Abscess
  Pyogenic
  (Figs GI 79-4 and GI 79-5)
	Low signal intensity on T1-weighted images and high signal intensity on T2-weighted scans.	Typically shows rim enhancement relative to the necrotic center, though small lesions (<1 cm) may enhance homogeneously, mimicking hemangioma. In many instances, this distinction can be made by demonstrating the presence of a rim of high signal around an abscess on T2-weighted images (perilesional edema). Resolution of the perilesional edema may indicate a response to therapy.

A

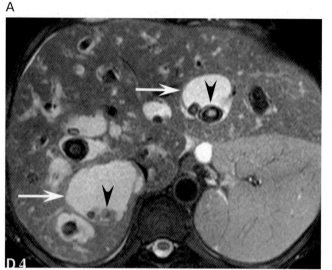

B

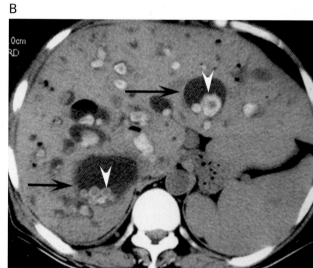

Fig GI 79-3
Caroli's disease. (A) Axial T2-weighted image shows multiple hyperintense cystic ectasias (arrows) and calculi (arrowheads). (B) Corresponding unenhanced CT scan shows multiple stones (arrowheads) within dilated bile ducts (arrows).[143]

A

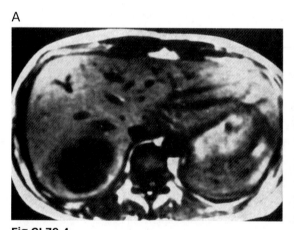

B

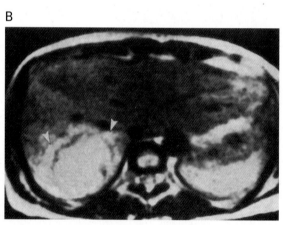

Fig GI 79-4
Pyogenic abscess with perilesional edema. (A) T1-weighted image shows a mass with fluid-like signal intensity. (B) T2-weighted image shows a thick hyperintense rim (arrowheads), representing edema, surrounding the margin of the mass.[144]

Condition	Imaging Findings	Comments
Amebic (Fig GI 79-6)	Sharply defined, well-marginated areas of low signal intensity on T1-weighted images and high signal intensity on T2-weighted scans.	Diffuse central inhomogeneity and perilesional edema are often seen on T2-weighted sequences. Successful treatment may result in the appearance of concentric rings of various signal intensities surrounding the lesion.

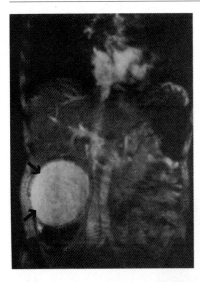

Fig GI 79-5
Pyogenic abscess. Coronal T2-weighted image shows the predominantly high-signal-intensity mass (arrows) hanging off the inferior aspect of the right hepatic lobe. Note the significant mass effect on adjacent bowel and soft tissues.[145]

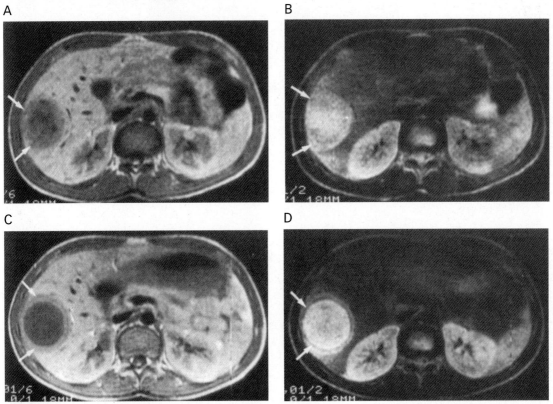

Fig GI 79-6
Amebic abscess. (A) T1-weighted image shows a heterogeneously hypointense and isointense mass in the right lobe of the liver. Note the deviation of the hepatic vasculature. An incomplete ring is seen within the wall of the abscess (arrows). (B) On the T2-weighted scan, the mass appears heterogeneously hyperintense and has an incomplete hyperintense ring (arrows). The abscess is surrounded by ill-defined zones of intermediate density. (C) After 10 days of medical treatment, a T1-weighted image shows that the abscess cavity is now homogeneously hypointense relative to liver and is bordered by a hyperintense ring surrounded by a hypointense ring (arrows). (D) T2-weighted scan taken at the same time shows the same hypointense ring about the lesion (arrows). This is bordered by a peripheral hyperintense ring that was not evident on the T1-weighted image. Note that the size of the abnormality is now the same on both images, indicating that the perifocal edema has largely resolved.[146]

Condition	Imaging Findings	Comments
Fungal (Fig GI 79-7)	Multiple, small, rounded lesions that have increased signal intensity on T2-weighted and fat-suppressed (short T1 inversion recovery) images.	Most frequently due to candidiasis in immune-compromised hosts. Fungal abscesses have variable signal intensity on conventional T1-weighted spin-echo scans.
Echinococcal (hydatid) cyst (Figs GI 79-8 through GI 79-10)	Low signal on T1-weighted images and high signal on T2-weighted scans. The rim surrounding the cyst (pericyst) has low signal on both T1- and T2-weighted images because of its fibrous component. Floating membranes within the lesion have low signal on all sequences.	The characteristic multiloculated or multicystic appearance is a distinctive feature of echinococcal disease. Although calcifications may be seen as low signal on MR, they are identified far more effectively on CT. The presence of a fat-fluid level within an echinococcal cyst indicates communicating rupture into the biliary tree.

A

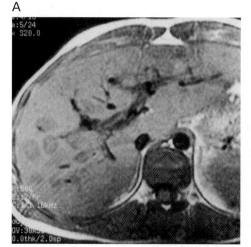

B

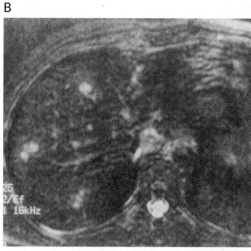

Fig GI 79-7
Fungal infection. (A) T1-weighted image shows multiple small, nodular, hypointense lesions with a "target" appearance and relatively increased central signal intensity. (B) Fat-saturated T2-weighted scan shows hyperintense nodular lesions, which correspond to the areas of hypointensity seen on the previous image. This patient with acute myelocytic leukemia showed a marked decrease in the number of liver lesions on follow-up scans.[147]

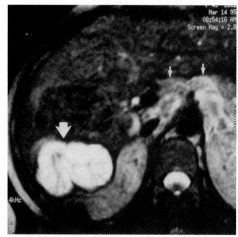

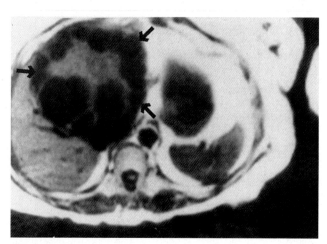

Fig GI 79-8
Echinococcal cyst. T2-weighted image shows a hyperintense mass with a capsule of lower signal intensity in the right lobe of the liver (large arrow). The hyperintense paraaortic lymphadenopathy (small arrows) was due to tuberculous infection.[147]

Fig GI 79-9
Echinococcal cyst. T1-weighted image shows a very large hydatid cyst with multiple small daughter cysts (arrows). The presence of daughter cysts may indicate early degenerative change of the mother cyst. The outer pericyst was better seen as a hypointense band on T2-weighted scans.[145]

Condition	Imaging Findings	Comments
Hemangioma (Figs GI 79-11 through GI 79-13)	Well-defined hypointense lesion on T1-weighted scans that demonstrates marked hyperintensity on T2-weighted images, on which they may contain low-intensity areas correlating with regions of fibrosis.	Hemangiomas manifest three patterns of contrast enhancement, depending on the size of the lesion. Most small (<1.5 cm) hemangiomas show uniform early enhancement, or peripheral nodular enhancement that progresses centripetally to uniform enhancement. This second pattern is commonly seen in medium-sized lesions (1.5 to 5.0 cm) and a few large (>5 cm) ones. However, most large hemangiomas demonstrate peripheral nodular enhancement, whereas the center of the lesion remains hypointense. This peripheral nodular enhancement is a useful sign for discriminating hemangiomas from metastases. However, small lesions can present a diagnostic dilemma, because a uniform pattern of enhancement is seen in both hemangiomas and vascular metastases.
Hepatocellular adenoma (Figs GI 79-14 and GI 79-15)	Heterogeneous appearance. Areas of increased signal on T1-weighted images result from the presence of fat or hemorrhage; low signal areas correspond to necrosis.	Approximately a third of hepatocellular adenomas have a peripheral rim, corresponding to a fibrous capsule, which typically is of low signal intensity on both T1- and T2-weighted scans.

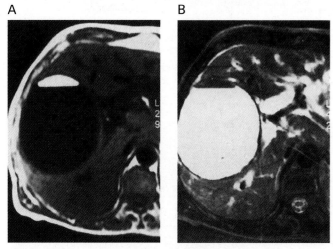

Fig GI 79-10
Echinococcal cyst. (A) T1-weighted and (B) fat-suppressed T2-weighted images show a fat-fluid level within the cyst.[148]

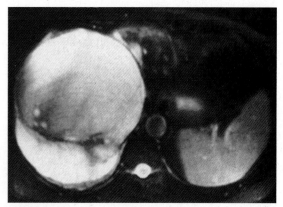

Fig GI 79-11
Giant hemangioma. T2-weighted image shows a large mass in the right lobe of the liver that has homogeneous high signal intensity, similar to that of cerebrospinal fluid. Note the band of low signal intensity, representing fibrosis, coursing horizontally through the mass.[149]

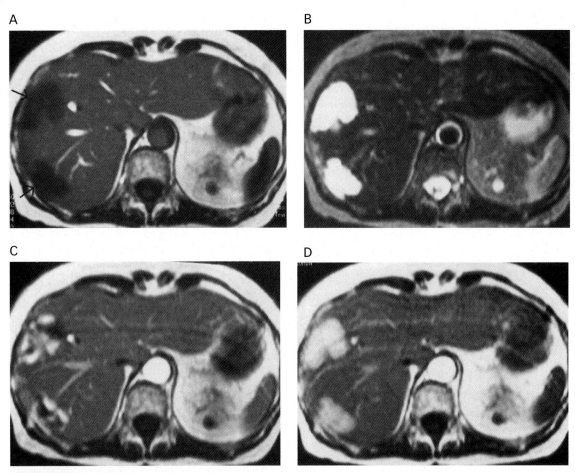

Fig GI 79-12
Hemangiomas. (A) T1-weighted image shows two hypointense, well-defined, lobulated peripheral lesions (arrows) in the right lobe of the liver. (B) On a heavily T2-weighted image, the lesions exhibit increased signal as the liver decreases in signal intensity. (C) T1-weighted image obtained within 2 minutes after contrast administration shows peripheral enhancement of the lesions. (D) Within 10 minutes after contrast, a repeat T1-weighted image demonstrates uniform, persistent enhancement of the lesions.[150]

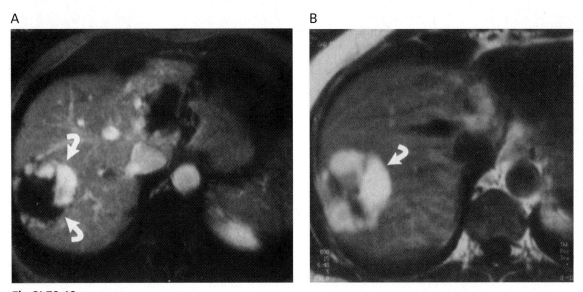

Fig GI 79-13
Hemangioma. (A) Initial T1-weighted image from a dynamic contrast study demonstrates peripheral nodular enhancement of the lesion (arrows). (B) There was progressive filling of the mass, though the central scar did not enhance.[151]

A

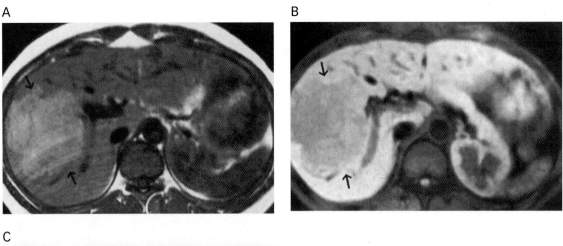

B

C

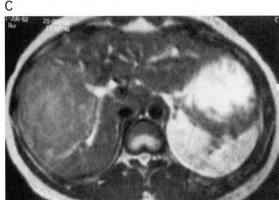

Fig GI 79-14
Hepatocellular adenoma. (A) T1-weighted image shows a mass (arrows) in the right hepatic lobe that has slightly increased signal intensity relative to the liver. (B) Fat-suppressed T1-weighted scan demonstrates the lesion (arrows) to be hypointense to the liver, indicating the fatty nature of the mass. (C) T2-weighted image shows the mass to be slightly more intense than the surrounding liver.[150]

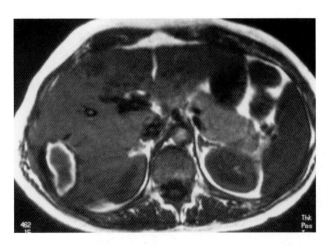

Fig GI 79-15
Hepatocellular adenoma. T1-weighted image shows a central concentric rim of high signal intensity (subacute hemorrhage) surrounding an area of low signal intensity (acute bleeding). There is also a second area of low signal intensity in the left lobe of the liver.[152]

Condition	Imaging Findings	Comments
Focal nodular hyperplasia (Fig GI 79-16)	Usually isointense or hypointense relative to the surrounding liver on T1-weighted scans and becomes slightly hyperintense or isointense on T2-weighted images.	The central scar, which is hypointense on T1-weighted scans, appears hyperintense on T2-weighted images because of its vascular channels, bile ductules, and increased edema in myxomatous tissue. After contrast administration, the enhancement profile is identical to that seen on contrast-enhanced CT scans. There is striking enhancement of the lesion during the arterial phase, followed by isointensity of the lesion relative to the hepatic parenchyma during the portal venous phase. On delayed phase imaging, the lesion demonstrates increased signal intensity relative to the liver, and the central scar exhibits high signal intensity that corresponds to the accumulation of contrast material. However, this enhancement pattern may also be seen in a well-differentiated hepatocellular carcinoma or adenoma.
Infantile hemangioendothelioma (Fig GI 79-17)	Predominantly hypointense on T1-weighted images and hyperintense on T2-weighted sequences.	Foci of hyperintense or hypointense signal on T1-weighted scans correspond to areas of hemorrhage and fibrosis, respectively.
Lipomatous tumors (Fig GI 79-18)	Lipomas demonstrate the signal intensity of fat on all sequences and do not show contrast enhancement. Angiomyolipomas usually contain a combination of fat and soft-tissue intensities.	Angiolipomas may be indistinguishable from hepatocellular carcinomas that contain fat deposits. The early phase of dynamic contrast imaging may permit differentiation between these two lesions. The fatty areas of angiomyolipomas are well vascularized and enhance early, whereas the regions of fatty change in hepatocellular carcinoma are relatively avascular and enhancement is less apparent. MR imaging with fat-suppression techniques also is useful in identifying an angiomyolipoma. Although these lesions have high signal intensity on both T1- and T2-weighted sequences, they appear hypointense to liver on images obtained with fat suppression.

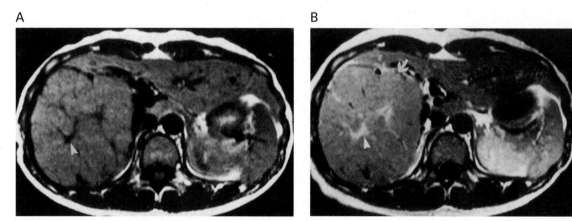

A   B

Fig GI 79-16
Focal nodular hyperplasia. (A) T1-weighted image demonstrates a large mass in the right hepatic lobe with a hypointense central scar (arrowhead). (B) On the delayed-phase contrast scan, the tumor is slightly hyperintense (arrow) relative to the surrounding liver parenchyma (prolonged enhancement), with a hyperintense central scar (arrowhead).[144]

Condition	Imaging Findings	Comments
Microhamartomas (Fig GI 79-19)	Multiple, round or irregular focal lesions of nearly uniform size scattered throughout the liver.	Often discovered incidentally, this appearance may simulate metastatic disease in a patient with a primary neoplasm (though metastases are usually more heterogeneous in size and signal intensity).
Hepatocellular carcinoma (Figs GI 79-20 and GI 79-21)	Variable appearance depending on the degree of fatty change, presence of internal fibrosis, and dominant histologic pattern of the lesion. Any surrounding capsule appears as a hypointense rim on T1-weighted images. Infrequent hemorrhage within the tumor appears hyperintense on both T1- and T2-weighted images.	After contrast administration, hepatocellular carcinomas generally demonstrate enhancement due to their hypervascularity. However, this enhancement is nonspecific and may be manifest as central, peripheral, homogeneous, or rim patterns.

A   B

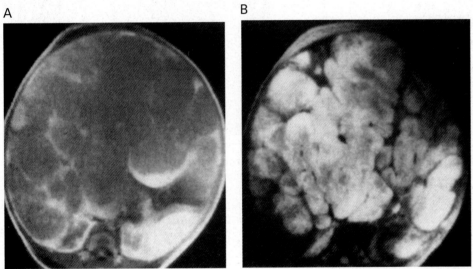

Fig GI 79-17
Infantile hemangioendothelioma. (A) T1-weighted image obtained with the patient lying in a decubitus position demonstrates a large, multinodular liver lesion with heterogeneous signal intensity that fills the abdomen. (B) T2-weighted image shows the lesion to be predominantly of high signal intensity due to its vascular nature.[150]

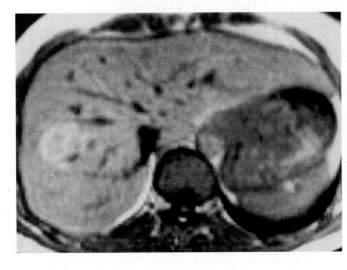

Fig GI 79-18
Lipoma. T1-weighted image demonstrates the hyperintense fatty lesion.[142]

A

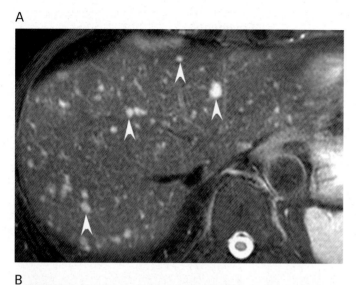

B

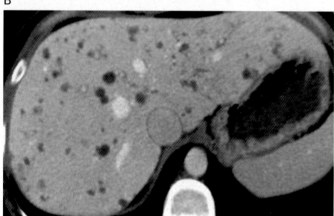

Fig GI 79-19
Biliary microhamartomas. (A) T2-weighted image shows innumerable high-signal-intensity liver lesions (arrowheads). (B) Corresponding CT scan shows multiple hypoattenuating cystic lesions in both lobes of the liver.[143]

A

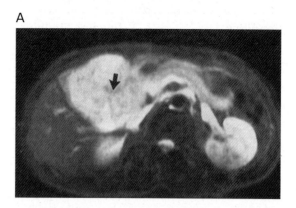

B

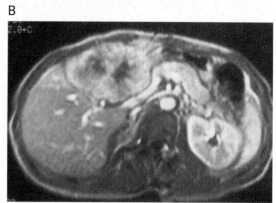

Fig GI 79-20
Hepatocellular carcinoma. (A) On a T2-weighted image, the mass has a high signal intensity, but the central scar has low signal intensity (arrow). (B) T1-weighted image after contrast shows the peripherally enhancing mass to have a central low intensity area of necrosis and scarring.[149]

A   B

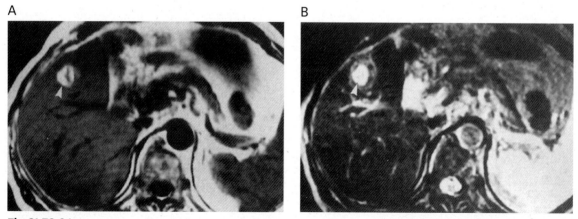

Fig GI 79-21
Hepatocellular carcinoma. Hemorrhage within the tumor (arrowheads) is hyperintense on both T1-weighted (A) and T2-weighted (B) images.[145]

Condition	Imaging Findings	Comments
Fibrolamellar carcinoma (Fig GI 79-22)	Homogeneous mass that is hypointense or isointense to normal liver on T1-weighted images and heterogeneous and isointense or slightly hyperintense on T2-weighted sequences. Any central scar is generally hypointense on all images because of its purely fibrous nature.	The enhancement pattern of the tumor parallels that on CT, with dense heterogeneous enhancement in the arterial and portal phases that becomes progressively more homogeneous on delayed images. The scar usually does not enhance and is best visualized on delayed images as the enhancement of the rest of the tumor becomes more homogeneous. Occasionally, the scar may demonstrate delayed enhancement and become either hyperintense or isointense relative to the tumor or to liver.
Hepatoblastoma (Fig GI 79-23)	Hypointense on T1-weighted images and hyperintense on T2-weighted sequences. Foci of high signal may be seen within the lesion on T1-weighted scans due to internal hemorrhage. On T2-weighted sequences, internal septa corresponding to fibrosis within the tumor appear as hypointense bands.	MR can demonstrate tumor invasion of perihepatic vessels and may be more accurate than CT in both assessing the preoperative extension of the lesion and detecting tumor recurrence after surgery.

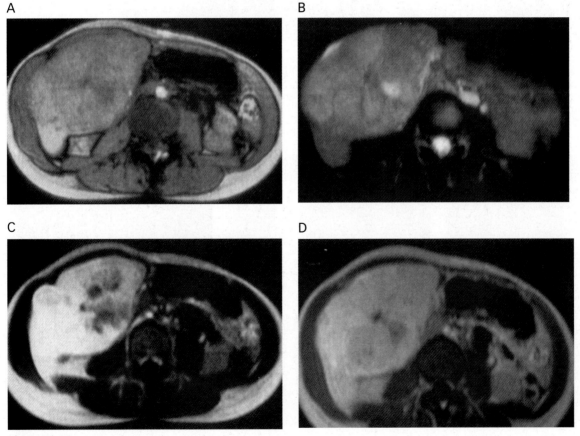

Fig GI 79-22
Fibrolamellar carcinoma. (A) T1-weighted gradient-echo image demonstrates a slightly hypointense mass with a central hypointense scar. (B) On a T2-weighted image, the mass is hyperintense and the scar remains hypointense. (C) Early and (D) delayed contrast images show that the mass initially enhances heterogeneously and then becomes increasingly homogeneous in the late phase.[153]

Condition	Imaging Findings	Comments
Intrahepatic cholangiocarcinoma (Fig GI 79-24)	Decreased signal intensity on T1-weighted images and increased signal on T2-weighted scans. The scar may appear as a central area of hypointensity on T2-weighted sequences.	The contrast enhancement pattern depends on the size of the lesion. Larger tumors (>4 cm) show peripheral enhancement that progresses centripetally and spares the central scar, a pattern that mimics hemangioma (though the degree of enhancement is usually greater in the latter). In addition, intrahepatic cholangiocarcinomas may have other features that are not associated with hemangiomas, such as satellite nodules, invasion of the portal vein, and dilatation of intrahepatic bile ducts. Smaller intrahepatic cholangiocarcinomas generally exhibit more homogeneous enhancement.

A

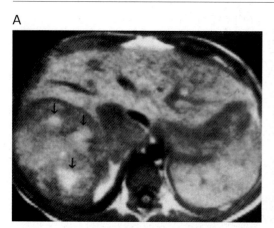

B

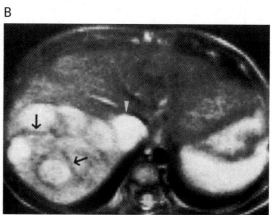

Fig GI 79-23
Hepatoblastoma. (A) T1-weighted image shows the right hepatic mass to be of predominantly low signal intensity. Areas of increased signal intensity (arrows) represent hemorrhage. (B) T2-weighted image reveals the lesion to have increased signal intensity, with hypointense bands (arrows) representing fibrotic septations. Note the hyperintense necrotic area (arrowhead) compressing the inferior vena cava.[150]

A

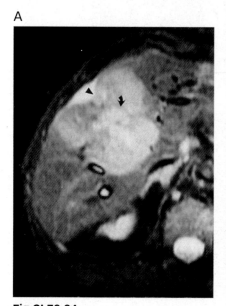

B

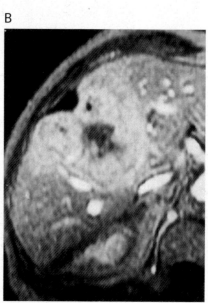

C

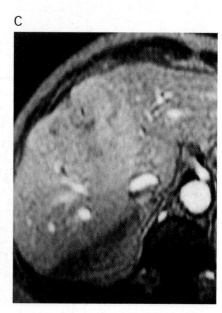

Fig GI 79-24
Intrahepatic cholangiocarcinoma. (A) STIR image shows a hyperintense well-defined tumor. The central scar is more hyperintense (arrow), and there is retraction of the liver capsule adjacent to the tumor (arrowhead). (B) After contrast administration, an acute phase scan shows enhancement at the periphery of the tumor, sparing the central scar. (C) On the delayed phase scan, there is complete, but heterogeneous, enhancement of the tumor.[154]

Condition	Imaging Findings	Comments
Biliary cystadenoma/ cystadenocarcinoma (Fig GI 79-25)	Generally mixed or low signal on T1-weighted images and predominantly high signal on T2-weighted sequences. Areas of high signal on T1-weighted scans represent hemorrhagic fluid components, whereas a low signal rim on T2-weighted scans may be due to hemorrhage in the wall of the lesion.	The variable appearance depends on the protein content of the fluid and the presence of an intra-cystic soft-tissue component. Indeed, variable signal intensity within the locules on all sequences is an important MR sign of these multiseptate hepatic lesions. As with other imaging modalities, MR cannot reliably distinguish cystadenoma from cystadenocarcinoma. Nevertheless, the presence of nodularity suggests cystadenocarcinoma (as does evidence of adenopathy or distant metastases).
Angiosarcoma (Fig GI 79-26)	Low signal intensity on T1-weighted images and predominantly high signal (with central areas of low signal) on T2-weighted sequences.	During dynamic contrast scanning, there is peripheral nodular enhancement that progresses centripetally. On delayed images, the peripheral enhancement persists, whereas the center of the lesion remains unenhanced. This appearance may reflect the presence of fibrous tissue or deoxyhemoglobin. Although this pattern may mimic that of hemangioma, the inhomogeneity of angiosarcomas on T2-weighted images is not seen in hemangiomas.

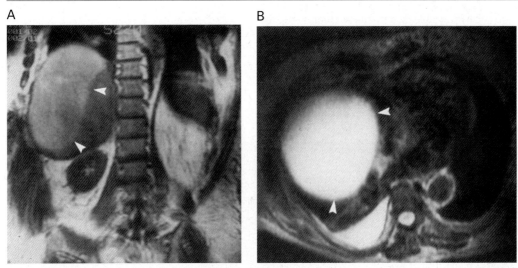

Fig GI 79-25
Biliary cystadenoma. (A) Coronal T1-weighted and (B) axial T2-weighted images demonstrate a large cystic mass (arrowheads) compressing the adjacent normal liver tissue.[120]

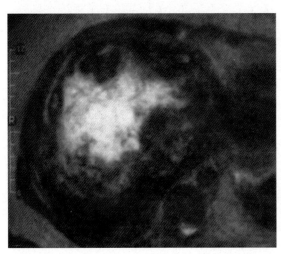

Fig GI 79-26
Angiosarcoma. T2-weighted image demonstrates heter-ogeneous high signal intensity of the central portion of a large right lobe liver mass. The peripheral areas of the lesion show only slight increased signal intensity.[155]

Condition	Imaging Findings	Comments
Undifferentiated (embryonal) sarcoma (Fig GI 79-27)	Low signal intensity on T1-weighted images and high signal intensity on T2-weighted sequences.	Signal characteristics are similar to those of cerebrospinal fluid. In some cases, foci of high signal corresponding to hemorrhage may be seen on T1-weighted scans.
Metastases (Figs GI 79-28 through GI 79-31)	Variable appearance depending on the primary tumor and the degree of necrosis, hemorrhage, and vascularity. Generally, low intensity on T1-weighted images and high signal intensity on T2-weighted sequences. Metastases with central necrosis have a distinct central region, which has even lower signal intensity on T1-weighted scans (doughnut sign), higher signal intensity on T2-weighted images (target sign), and is surrounded by a less intense rind of viable tumor. Metastases that contain considerable amounts of paramagnetic substances (mucin, fat, subacute hemorrhage, melanin, protein) may have a relatively high signal intensity on T1-weighted images. Approximately 25% of metastases, especially those from colorectal carcinoma, demonstrate a hyperintense rim or halo (viable tumor) surrounding a central hypointensity (coagulative necrosis, fibrin, and mucin).	Contrast enhancement patterns of metastases are similar to those seen on CT. Hypervascular metastases show marked early enhancement, either uniformly or as a continuous ring that fills in centrally on later images. During the portal venous phase, hypervascular metastases may become iso- or hypointense. Hypovascular metastases are seen as hypointense masses that may have an enhancing peripheral rim, which is best visualized during the arterial phase. Progressive centripetal filling in of the lesion may occur on delayed scans. At times, the peripheral rim becomes hypointense relative to the center of the lesion on delayed enhanced images (peripheral washout sign), a finding reported as highly specific for metastases.

A

B

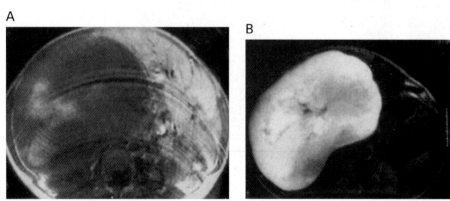

Fig GI 79-27
Undifferentiated (embryonal) sarcoma. (A) T1-weighted image shows a mass of predominantly low signal intensity containing lobulated areas of increased signal intensity that correspond to regions of hemorrhage. (B) T2-weighted image shows the mass to be heterogeneous but predominantly of high signal intensity equal to or exceeding that of cerebrospinal fluid. The central lobulated areas of markedly increased signal intensity correspond to regions of gelatinous hemorrhagic degeneration.[156]

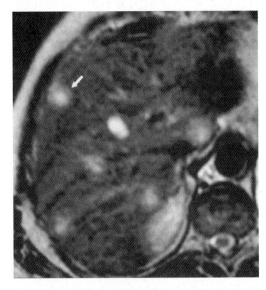

Fig GI 79-28
Metastases from colon carcinoma. T2-weighted image shows several lesions with the target sign (arrow). The periphery of the lesions (viable tumor) is relatively hypointense compared with the center (liquefactive necrosis).[157]

A

B

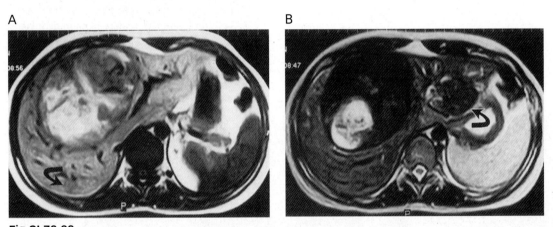

Fig GI 79-29
Hemorrhagic metastases from malignant melanoma. (A) T1-weighted image shows a well-circumscribed mass containing areas of high and low signal intensity. An ill-defined lesion is present in the posterior aspect of the right hepatic lobe (arrow). (B) T2-weighted image shows a persistent area of high signal intensity in the posterior aspect of the mass. In addition, a mass of intermediate signal intensity is identified in the left hepatic lobe (arrow). At surgery, multiple lesions were found in the liver. The dominant lesion in the right lobe contained multiple areas of hemorrhage. However, melanin could also produce high signal on T1-weighted images due to its paramagnetic characteristics.[151]

A

B

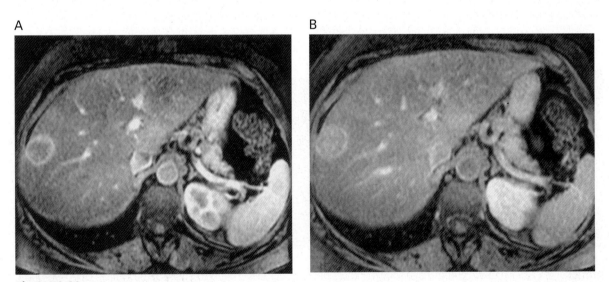

Fig GI 79-30
Metastatic uterine leiomyosarcoma. (A) During the arterial phase, the lesion has a thin enhancing rim. (B) During the portal phase, the peripheral rim is less conspicuous, and the central portion of the tumor has become progressively more enhanced.[157]

Condition	Imaging Findings	Comments
Fatty infiltration (Fig GI 79-32)	Conventional spin-echo MR imaging is relatively insensitive for detecting fatty infiltration of the liver (but other MR techniques are highly specific for documenting the presence of fat).	Proton chemical shift imaging, also known as opposed-phase gradient echo imaging, takes advantage of differences in the resonant frequency of protons in water and fat. On opposed-phase images, the fat signal is subtracted from that of water; conversely, the fat and water signals are additive on in-phase images. Therefore, lesions containing fat and water show a loss of signal on the opposed-phase images when compared with the in-phase images, clearly identifying them as containing both of these substances. Although this technique can document the presence of fat within a lesion and often avoid the need for biopsy, some primary and secondary hepatic neoplasms (including hepatocellular carcinoma) also may contain macroscopic fat and show similar changes.

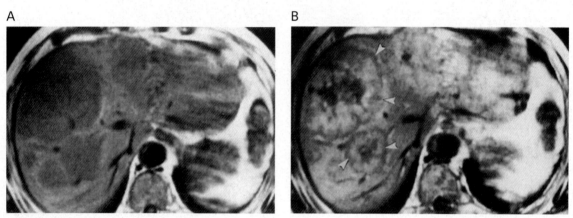

Fig GI 79-31
Metastases from colon carcinoma. (A) T1-weighted image shows multiple hypointense liver masses. (B) On a delayed-phase contrast scan, the masses demonstrate central enhancement and peripheral washout (arrowheads).[144]

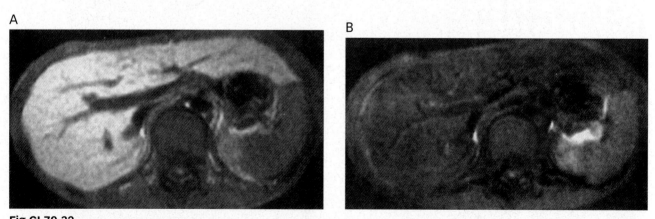

Fig GI 79-32
Fatty infiltration. (A) In-phase T1-weighted image shows homogeneously increased signal intensity of the liver. (B) Opposed-phase T1-weighted image shows reduced signal intensity of the liver, suggestive of fatty change.[158]

Condition	Imaging Findings	Comments
Hepatitis (Fig GI 79-33)	Decreased signal intensity on T1-weighted images and increased intensity on T2-weighted sequences.	Segmental atrophy may also produce abnormal signal intensity, with contrast enhancement in areas of focal confluent fibrosis.
Radiation-induced liver disease	Geographic areas of low signal intensity on T1-weighted images and high signal intensity on T2-weighted sequences.	Reflects the increased water content of hepatic tissues secondary to radiation injury.
Glycogen storage disease (Fig GI 79-34)	Increased signal intensity relative to bone marrow on T1-weighted MR images.	Reflects the accumulation of glucocerebrosides in hepatocytes.

A
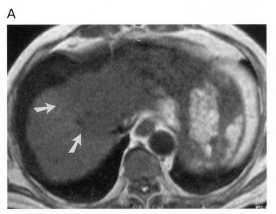

B
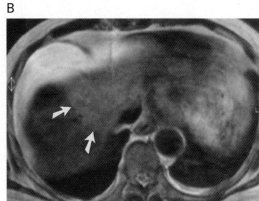

C
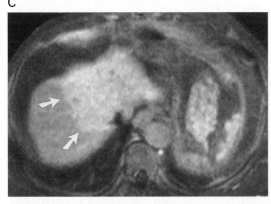

Fig GI 79-33
Hepatitis. (A) T1-weighted image reveals diffuse atrophy and irregular surface of the liver. There is decreased signal intensity of the left lobe (arrows). (B) T2-weighted image shows segmental increase in signal intensity of the left lobe (arrows). (C) Contrast T1-weighted scan demonstrates a segmental area of enhancement (arrows), probably corresponding to segmental fibrosis.[158]

A
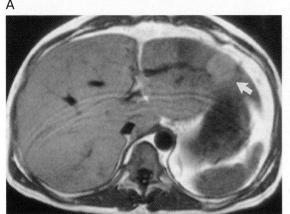

B
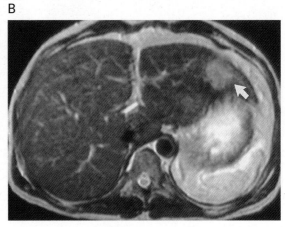

Fig GI 79-34
Glycogen storage disease. (A) T1-weighted image shows homogeneously increased signal intensity of the hepatic parenchyma compared with that of bone marrow. Note the round high-signal-intensity tumor (arrow) in the lateral segment. (B) T2-weighted image shows the high-intensity signal of the tumor (arrow).[158]

Condition	Imaging Findings	Comments
Hemochromatosis/ hemosiderosis (Fig GI 79-35 and GI 79-36)	Striking reduction in signal intensity on both T1- and T2-weighted sequences.	Appearance due to the deposition of iron within the liver in primary hemochromatosis (or within the liver, spleen, pancreas, and bone marrow in secondary hemosiderosis). In primary disease complicated by cirrhosis, the pancreas may also demonstrate decreased signal intensity.

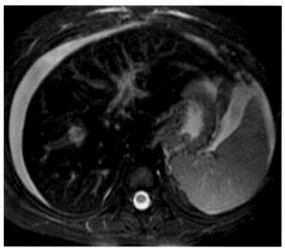

Fig GI 79-35
Hemosiderosis. T2-weighted fat-saturated image shows marked signal hypointensity in the liver in comparison with the muscles and spleen in a child who had undergone bone marrow transplantation for acute lymphoblastic leukemia. There is also evidence of ascites.[159]

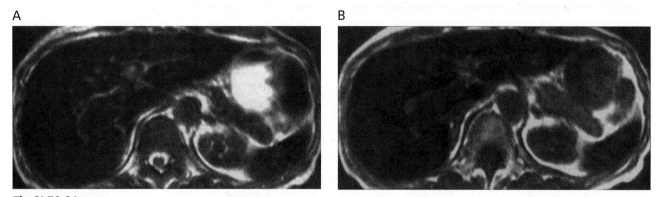

Fig GI 79-36
Hemochromatosis. (A) T2-weighted image shows decreased signal intensity of the liver, pancreas, and spleen when compared with that of paraspinal muscle. (B) T1-weighted image shows decreased signal intensity of the liver resulting from the T2 shortening effect.[158]

Condition	Imaging Findings	Comments
Sarcoidosis (Fig GI 79-37)	Coalescent granulomas may appear as multiple hypointense nodules. After a contrast agent that causes the hepatic parenchyma be very hypointense, sarcoid nodules appear as high-signal-intensity lesions.	Multiple hepatic nodules are easily mistaken for more common diseases, including metastases and lymphoma. Simultaneous involvement of the spleen is often seen.

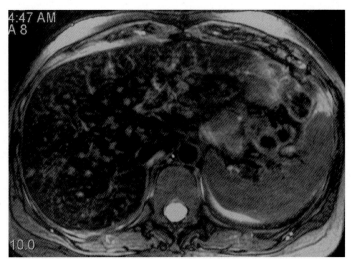

Fig GI 79-37
Sarcoidosis. T2-weighted image obtained after the administration of ferumoxidex demonstrates multiple, small, high-signal-intensity nodules throughout the liver.[160]

Perihepatic Space* on Computed Tomography

Condition	Comments

Air attenuation
  Pneumoperitoneum
  (Fig GI 80-1)
	Spontaneous pneumoperitoneum is often a result of perforation of an intraperitoneal hollow viscus that requires urgent surgical intervention. Causes include peptic ulcer disease, trauma, inflammatory disease, neoplasms, and iatrogenic procedures. Free intraperitoneal gas is often found anterior to the liver. In addition to detecting pneumoperitoneum, CT often can demonstrate mural or extraluminal changes such as bowel wall thickening and fat stranding that aids in determining the origin of the free intraperitoneal gas.

Chilaiditi syndrome	Congenital anomaly in which there is interposition of a portion of the colon (less frequently, the small bowel) between the liver and the right hemidiaphragm.

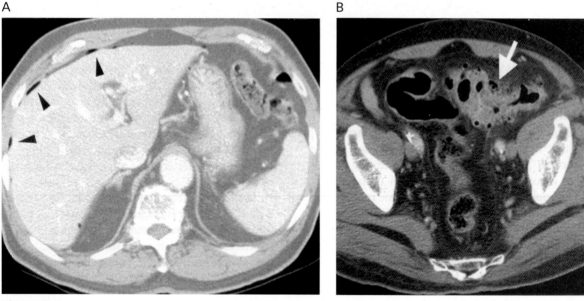

Fig GI 80-1
Pneumoperitoneum from perforated diverticulitis. (A) Contrast scan (lung window) shows free intraperitoneal gas (arrowheads) in the perihepatic space. Free intraperitoneal gas is more easily identified by using lung window settings. (B) Scan of the pelvis shows the thickened wall of the sigmoid colon (arrow) and mild pericolonic inflammatory fat stranding, findings that represent diverticulitis.

---

* The spread of inflammation and metastatic disease via peritoneal fluid to the perihepatic region is determined by the mesenteric reflections, the peritoneal recesses, and action of gravity, and hydrostatic pressure. The perihepatic ligaments may be affected by direct invasion, subperitoneal extension, or extension along lymphatics.

Condition	Comments
Fat attenuation	
Ruptured teratoma (Fig GI 80-2)	Spontaneous rupture of a cystic ovarian teratoma is rare because the lesion is usually surrounded by a thick capsule. Sudden rupture of cyst contents causes an acute peritonitis and typically appears as discontinuity of the wall of the tumor. A chronically leaking teratoma cause chronic granulomatous peritonitis, which produces a pattern of ascites, hazy omental infiltration, and an inflammatory omental mass that simulates carcinomatous or tuberculous peritonitis. The demonstration of fatty implants within the peritoneal cavity strongly suggests this diagnosis.
Lipoma/liposarcoma	Liposarcoma is one of the most common malignant tumors in the retroperitoneum, and a fatty mass in this region can be confused with a perihepatic mass. The differentiation between lipoma and liposarcoma may be extremely difficult on imaging studies.
Pseudolipoma (Fig GI 80-3)	Well-circumscribed nodule on the surface of the liver with a center of fat or soft-tissue attenuation. It is thought to arise from a detached piece of colonic fat (an epiploic appendage) that degenerates and becomes covered by a fibrous capsule before lodging between the diaphragm and the superior aspect of the liver.
Juxtacaval fat (Fig GI 80-4)	Focal collection of fat situated medially, adjacent to the lumen of the inferior vena cava near the hepatic venous confluence, which mimics a fatty mass.

A

B

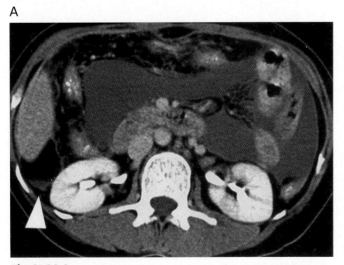
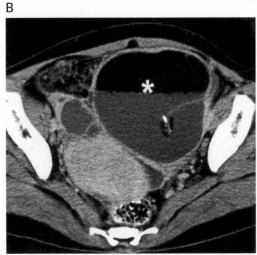

Fig GI 80-2
Ruptured ovarian teratoma. (A) Contrast scan shows a floating fat droplet (arrowhead) with a fat-fluid level in the perihepatic space and ascites in the peritoneal space. The hazy omental infiltration is suggestive of chronic granulomatous peritonitis. (B) Scan of the pelvis shows an ovarian teratoma (*) with fat attenuation and foci of calcification. (Courtesy of Y. W. Kim, M.D., Pusan Baik Hospital, Busan, Korea.)[161]

Condition	Comments
Omental infarct (Fig GI 80-5)	Relatively infrequent condition that simulates common surgical emergencies such as cholecystitis, appendicitis, or diverticulits. Usually occurring on the right, proposed etiologies include an anomalous arterial supply to the omentum, kinking of veins secondary to increased intra-abdominal pressure, and postprandial vascular congestion. On CT, it appears as a heterogeneous, fatty omental mass that contains strands of soft-tissue attenuation.
Intrahepatic omental packing (Fig GI 80-6)	This diagnosis should be suggested if there is a large fatty mass in a patient who has undergone hepatobiliary surgery, since the omentum is often used as a packing material.
Fluid attenuation Ascites (Fig GI 80-7)	An abnormal amount of intraperitoneal fluid may be caused by cirrhosis (75% of cases), peritoneal carcinomatosis, and cardiac failure. Usually of low attenuation, a perihepatic fluid collection of more than 20 H.U. suggests hemoperitoneum. The initial high attenuation of acute intraperitoneal blood decreases within several days due to clot lysis. Other causes of high-attenuation ascites include tuberculosis (high protein and cellular contents) and extravasated contrast material from the gastrointestinal or urinary tract.

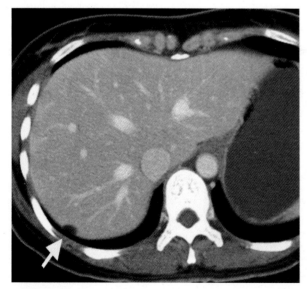

Fig GI 80-3
Pseudolipoma. Contrast scan shows a small fatty mass (arrow) in the subcapsular region of the right hepatic lobe.[161]

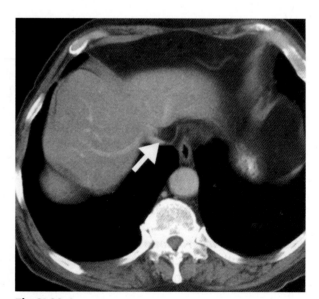

Fig GI 80-4
Juxtacaval fat. Contrast scan shows a fatty lesion (arrow) adjacent to the intrahepatic vena cava.[161]

Condition	Comments
Perihepatic infection	A perihepatic abscess is an infected fluid collection that is encapsulated by fibrinous exudates, omentum, or the adjacent visceral organs. Peritonitis is an inflammation of the serosal membrane lining the peritoneal cavity and the organs within it, while perihepatitis is the term used to refer to localized inflammation of the liver capsule.
Perihepatic abscess (Figs GI 80-8 and GI 80-9)	Subhepatic and subphrenic abscesses are 2 to 3 times greater on the right than on the left. This is a manifestation of the fact that the major route of the flow of peritoneal fluid from the pelvis is through the right paracolic gutter, since the left paracolic gutter is shallow and spread on the left is limited due to the phrenicolic ligament. Morison's pouch is the most common site of perihepatic abscess, because it is the most dependent recess. Infected material can extend around the inferior edge of the liver or laterally from Morrison's pouch to the right subphrenic space. Tuberculosis, actinomycosis, and echinococcosis are important causes of perihepatic abscesses.

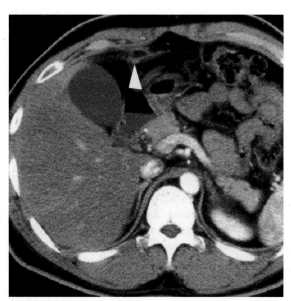

Fig GI 80-5
Omental infarct. Contrast scan shows a small, ovoid, fatty mass (arrowhead) surrounded by fat stranding around the falciform ligament.[161]

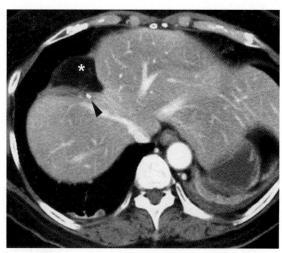

Fig GI 80-6
Omental packing. Contrast scan shows a triangular mass-like area of fat attenuation (*) with a metallic surgical clip (arrowhead), consistent with omentopexy due to surgery for hepatocellular carcinoma.[161]

Condition	Comments
Perihepatitis (Fig GI 80-10)	Enhancement of the hepatic capsule is classically described in association with pelvic inflammatory disease (Fitz-Hugh-Curtis syndrome). The typical symptoms of sudden onset of sharp right upper quadrant pain can be confused with acute cholecystitis or pleurisy. Intense enhancement along the anterior surface of the liver may be demonstrated on early-phase images (increased blood flow related to inflammation) or on delayed scans (early capsular fibrosis). Enhancement of the liver capsule may also be a manifestation of other inflammatory conditions (tuberculous peritonitis, perforated hepatic abscess, or cholecystisis), systemic lupus erythematosus, radiation, and peritoneal carcinomatosis.

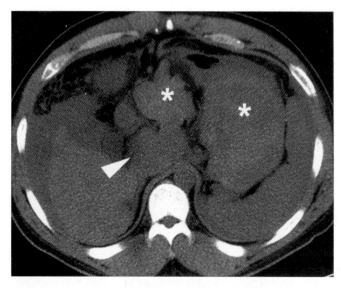

Fig GI 80-7
Hemoperitoneum. Unenhanced scan shows an exophytic mass in the caudate lobe (arrowhead). Note the high-attenuation fluid (*) around the liver and spleen.[161]

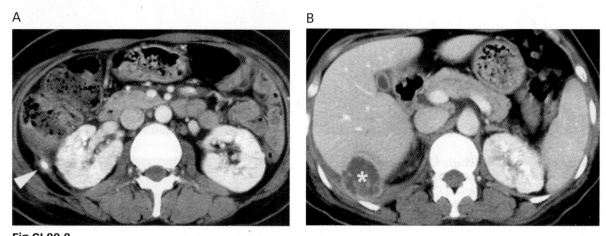

A   B

Fig GI 80-8
Appendiceal abscess. (A) Contrast scan shows calcification (arrowhead) in Morrison's pouch, a finding that represents "dropped" appendicoliths" in a patient who underwent laparoscopic appendectomy 2 months earlier. (B) More cephalad scan shows a cystic mass with wall enhancement (*). This appearance is consistent with an abscess in the posterior right subhepatic space.[161]

Condition	Comments
Peritoneal carcinomatosis (Fig GI 80-11)	Malignant seeding of the peritoneum most commonly arises from primary tumors of the ovary, colon, stomach, and pancreas. It produces large amounts of ascites, which is often loculated, and characteristic nodular peritoneal thickening and enhancement. Implants on the liver and spleen often cause scalloping of the surface by the masses. The irregular studding of the peritoneum differentiates this condition from the diffusely smooth peritoneal thickening related to tuberculous peritonitis. Calcified peritoneal carcinomatois may occur in ovarian, colon, and gastric cancer.
Pseudomyxoma peritonei (Fig GI 80-12)	Gradual accumulation of large volumes of gelatinous ascites in the peritoneal cavity related to rupture of a mucin-producing tumor of the ovary or appendix. The characteristic CT finding is hypoattenuating peritoneal implants that cause scalloping of visceral surfaces and extrinsic pressure on bowel loops.

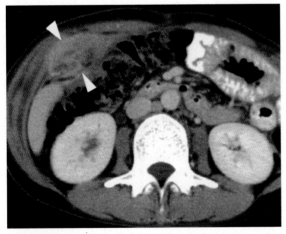

Fig GI 80-9
Actinomycosis. Contrast scan shows an inhomogeneously and avidly enhancing mass (arrowheads) with focal areas of low attenuation in the anterior right subhepatic space, findings suggestive of a small abscess.[161]

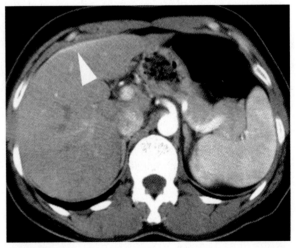

Fig GI 80-10
Fitz-Hugh-Curtis syndrome. Contrast scan (arterial phase) shows enhancement of the capsule of the left hepatic lobe (arrowhead). This capsular enhancement disappeared during the equilibrium phase. This young woman had a tubo-ovarian abscess in the left adnexal region.[161]

Condition	Comments
Subperitoneal extension (Figs GI 80-13 and GI 80-14)	The Glisson sheath, which surrounds the intrahepatic portion of the hepatic portal system, continues into the subperitoneal space of the gastrohepatic and hepatoduodenal ligaments. This permits the spread of disease not only between the intraperitoneal structures, but also between extraperitoneal and intraperitoneal sites. Gas, inflammation, tumor, or proliferative disease can extend along the subperitoneum.

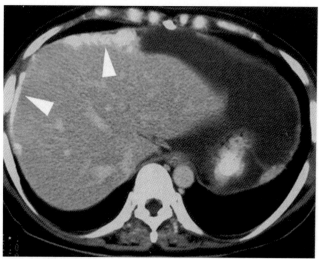

Fig GI 80-11
Peritoneal carcinomatosis. Contrast scan shows sheet-like calcified tumor plaque (arrowheads) along the right lobe of the liver secondary to serous cystadenocarcinoma of both ovaries.[161]

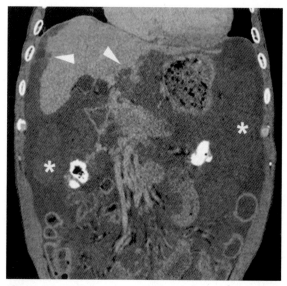

Fig GI 80-12
Pseudomyxoma peritonei. Coronal reformatted contrast image in a man with a rupture appendiceal mucocele shows multiple septated, low-attenuation masses (*) throughout the peritoneal space. Small cyst-like masses create impressions on the hepatic surface (arrowheads).[161]

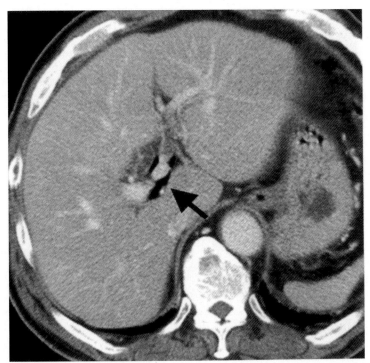

Fig GI 80-13
Emphysematous cholecystitis. Contrast scan shows that gas originating from a gallbladder perforation has diffused along the hepato-duodenal ligament to the Glisson sheath (arrow).[161]

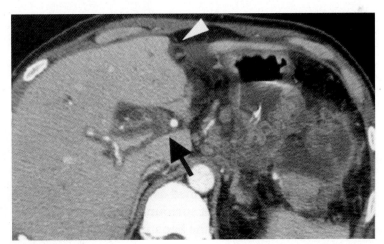

Fig GI 80-14
Pancreatitis. Contrast scan shows the inflammatory changes of pancreatitis extending upward along the portal vein (arrows) to the ligamentum teres (arrowhead). There is also a peripancreatic fluid collection.[161]

Pancreatic Masses on the Ultrasound

Condition	Imaging Findings	Comments
Pancreatic carcinoma (Figs GI 81-1 through GI 81-3)	Solid, focally enlarged lobulated mass with low-level echoes and increased sound absorption. There is often dilatation of the pancreatic duct (and common bile duct) in lesions of the head of the pancreas.	Hypoechoic pancreatic mass may be difficult to separate from a pseudomass produced by overlying bowel gas and its distal reverberation, which creates a false front and back wall. Infrequently, primary pancreatic carcinoma may appear densely hyperechoic. Other sonographic findings suggesting malignancy include liver and nodal metastases, venous compression or obstruction, and ascites.
Islet cell tumor (Fig GI 81-4)	Well-circumscribed mass that is usually indistinguishable from pancreatic carcinoma but may occasionally contain internal cystic areas.	Rare tumor, usually endocrinologically silent, and most common in the pancreatic body and tail where the greatest concentration of islets of Langerhans is located (unlike carcinoma, which most commonly affects the head of the pancreas).

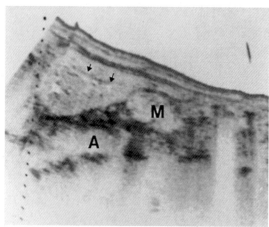

Fig GI 81-1
Carcinoma of the pancreas. Longitudinal sonogram demonstrates an irregular mass (M) with a semisolid pattern of intrinsic echoes. There is associated dilatation of the intrahepatic bile ducts (arrows). (A, aorta.)[162]

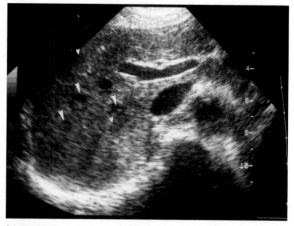

Fig GI 81-2
Pancreatic carcinoma with liver metastases. Transverse sonogram shows an enlarged liver containing multiple metastatic lesions (arrowheads).[95]

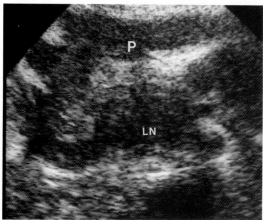

Fig GI 81-3
Pancreatic carcinoma with lymph node metastases. Diffuse enlargement of the pancreas (P) with enlarged hypoechoic paravascular lymph nodes (LN) that obscure the aorta and inferior vena cava.[95]

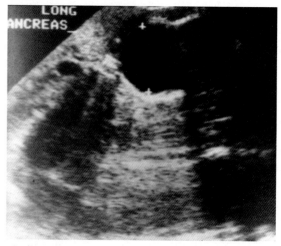

Fig GI 81-4
Islet cell tumor. This cystic mass in the head of the pancreas shows acoustic enhancement without evidence of debris.[163]

Condition	Imaging Findings	Comments
Metastases	Solid mass with variable echo pattern and increased sound absorption that may be indistinguishable from primary pancreatic carcinoma.	Metastases to the pancreatic bed primarily involve the region of the head and body (where the main lymphatic chains are located). Large masses may compress or displace the pancreas. Compared with primary carcinoma, metastases tend to be lumpier and more diffuse. They frequently are located posterior to and cause anterior displacement of the splenic and portal veins (primary carcinoma tends to be located more anteriorly and to cause posterior displacement of these vessels).
Lymphoma	Solid mass that is relatively anechoic and, when round, may initially appear to be cystic until internal echoes are demonstrated at high power or gain settings.	Primarily involves the region of the head and body (where the main lymphatic chains are located). Large masses may compress or displace the pancreas. Compared with primary carcinoma, lymphoma tends to be lumpier and more diffuse. It frequently is located posterior to and causes anterior displacement of the splenic and portal veins (primary carcinoma tends to be located more anteriorly and causes posterior displacement of these vessels).
Mucinous cystic neoplasm (Fig GI 81-5)	Multilocular or, less commonly, unilocular lesion with good through-transmission and posterior wall enhancement.	Internal septations are usually visualized and more conspicuously demonstrated on ultrasound than on CT. Nodularity and papillary projections may be demonstrated along the internal wall of the cysts.
Cystadenoma/ cystadenocarcinoma (Fig GI 81-6)	Predominantly cystic mass with septations and thick irregular walls. Relatively hypoechoic pattern with decreased sound absorption.	Uncommon tumors, usually occurring in women between ages 30 and 60. Most are located in the pancreatic body and tail, are frequently clinically silent, and can therefore attain sizes greater than 10 cm before becoming palpable. There are no specific criteria to separate benign from malignant tumors.

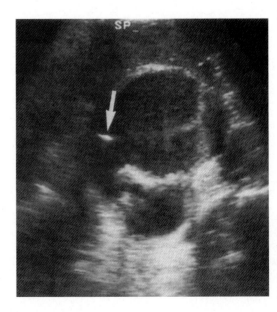

Fig GI 81-5
Mucinous cystic neoplasm. Multiloculated cystic mass with echogenic internal septa within the tail of the pancreas. Echogenic foci with shadowing that correspond to calcifications are noted along the septa (arrow). Note the low-level internal echoes.[164]

Condition	Imaging Findings	Comments
Pseudocyst (Figs GI 81-7 and GI 81-8)	Uncomplicated pseudocysts are usually anechoic with smooth walls and good sound transmission distally. They may infrequently have thick walls, be multiloculated, and contain internal debris and be difficult to differentiate from cystadenoma, cystadenocarcinoma, or abscess.	Frequent complication of acute or chronic pancreatitis. The presence of air or calcification may cause unusually bright echoes. Although most commonly located in the peripancreatic region, pseudocysts may develop apart from the pancreas (the lesser sac, or anywhere from the mediastinum to the groin).

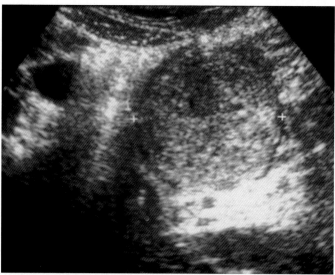

Fig GI 81-6
Serous cystadenoma. Sonogram shows a mass of low echogenicity due to the interfaces between the tiny cysts. Note the increased through transmission posterior to the mass.[165]

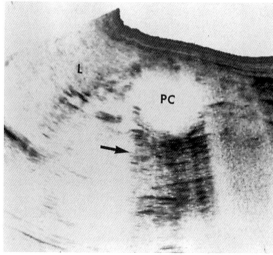

Fig GI 81-7
Pancreatic pseudocyst. Longitudinal sonogram of the right upper quadrant demonstrates an irregularly marginated pseudocyst (PC) with acoustic shadowing (arrow). (L, liver.)

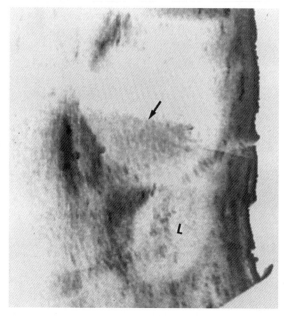

Fig GI 81-8
Pancreatic pseudocyst. An erect sonogram demonstrates a fluid-debris level (arrow) in the pseudocyst. 1(L, left kidney.)

Condition	Imaging Findings	Comments
Pancreatic abscess (Fig GI 81-9)	Complex, predominantly cystic mass, often with irregular walls and internal debris. Bright echoes in the mass (representing gas) confirm the diagnosis of an abscess.	Serious and often fatal complication in severe acute pancreatitis. Although the presence of gas in the pancreatic bed strongly suggests a pancreatic abscess, this appearance may also be demonstrated in patients with a pancreatic pseudocyst that erodes the gastrointestinal tract without forming an abscess.
Cystic fibrosis (Fig GI 81-10)	Partial or complete replacement of the pancreas by fibrofatty tissue. Atrophy of the pancreas without fibrofatty replacement may occur. Rarely, cysts of different size develop and no normal pancreatic tissue remains.	Cystic fibrosis affects the pancreas in nearly all patients, though more than 90% of the exocrine function of the pancreas must be lost before the appearance of such clinical symptoms as steatorrhea, fat intolerance, abdominal pain, and failure to thrive.

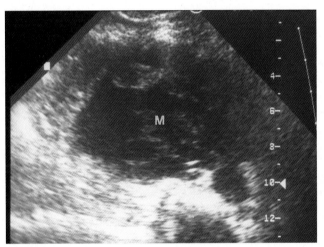

Fig GI 81-9
Pancreatic phlegmon. Transverse sonogram shows a hypoechoic mass (M) in the peripancreatic region.[95]

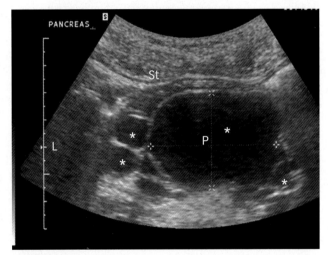

Fig GI 81-10
Cystic fibrosis. Transverse sonogram at the level of the pancreatic head (P) shows complete fibrofatty replacement of the gland with absence of normal tissue. Note the multiple cysts (*) of different sizes adjacent to the liver (L) and stomach (St).[166]

Cystic Pancreatic Masses on CT and MRI

Condition	Imaging Findings	Comments
True epithelial cyst (Fig GI 82-1)	Single, small fluid-filled structure with an imperceptible wall and no internal septa or contrast enhancement.	Multiple pancreatic cysts may be seen in von-Hippel-Lindau disease.
Pseudocyst (Figs GI 82-2 to GI 82-5)	Sharply marginated, unilocular or multilocular, fluid-density mass that is often best delineated after contrast material administration. Older cysts tend to have thicker walls that may contain calcium.	Lobulated fluid collection arising from inflammation, necrosis, or hemorrhage associated with acute pancreatitis or trauma. Because of its ability to image the entire body, CT may demonstrate pseudocysts that have dissected superiorly into the mediastinum or to other ectopic locations, such as the lumbar or inguinal region or within the liver, spleen, or kidney.

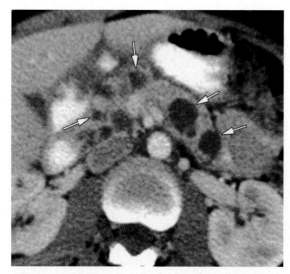

Fig GI 82-1
True epithelial cysts. Contrast CT scan shows multiple unilocular cysts (arrows) scattered throughout an otherwise healthy-looking pancreas in this patient with von Hippel-Lindau disease.[167]

A   B

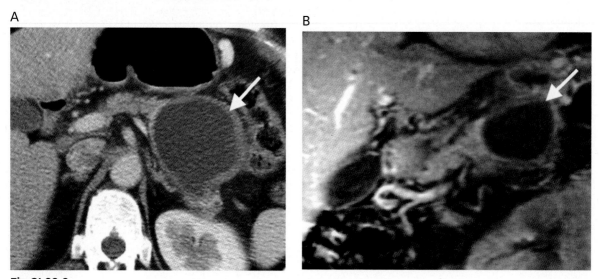

Fig GI 82-2
Pseudocyst. (A) Axial contrast CT scan demonstrate a well-defined unilocular cyst (arrow) in the tail of the pancreas. (B) T2-weighted MR image shows the cyst (arrow) with homogeneously bright signal intensity, a finding that confirms that the lesion of a fluid-filled unilocular structure.[167]

Condition	Imaging Findings	Comments
Serous cystadenoma (Fig GI 82-6)	Polycystic or microcystic pattern consisting of a collection of cysts (usually more than six) ranging from a few mm to 2 cm. Fine lobulations are common, and enhancement of septa and cyst wall may be seen. On MR, the microcysts may appear as numerous discrete foci with bright signal intensity on T2-weighted images.	The presence of a fibrous central scar, which may have a characteristic stellate pattern of calcification, is considered virtually pathognomic for serous cystadenoma.
Mucinous cystic neoplasm (Fig GI 82-7)	Mass composed of variable numbers of different-sized cysts of fluid attenuation. Multiloculated appearance with septations and sometimes calcification scattered throughout the mass	Uncommon tumors, usually occurring in women between the ages 30 and 60. Most are located in the pancreatic body and tail, are frequently clinically silent, and can therefore attain sizes greater than 10 cm before becoming palpable. Although not frequently seen, peripheral and septal calcifications are highly specific for mucinous cystic neoplasm and strongly suggestive of malignancy.

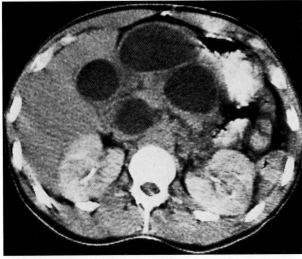

Fig GI 82-3
Multiple pancreatic pseudocysts. CT scan after the administration of contrast material demonstrates four sharply marginated, fluid-filled collections.

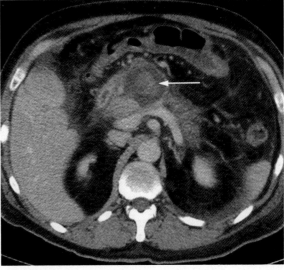

Fig GI 82-4
Hemorrhagic pseudocyst. Contrast CT scan shows a cystic mass containing an area of high attenuation (arrow), a finding consistent with recent hemorrhage.[168]

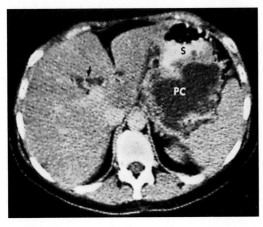

Fig GI 82-5
Ectopic pancreatic pseudocyst. The low-attenuation pseudocyst (PC) lies in the superior recess of the lesser sac posterior to the stomach (S). Note the dilated intrahepatic bile ducts (arrow).

Condition	Imaging Findings	Comments
Intraductal papillary mucinous neoplasm (IPMN) (Fig GI 82-8)	Cystic dilatation of a main or side branch pancreatic duct.	Typically occurs in elderly patients and is more common in men. Communication between the duct and the abnormal cystic structure can be shown on thin-section CT, MRI, and MRCP.

A 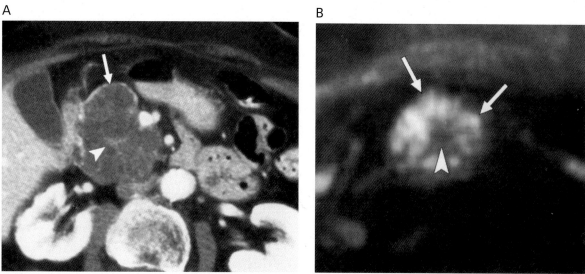 B

Fig GI 82-6
Serous cystadenoma. (A) CT scan shows a lobulated mass (arrow) of the pancreatic head with typical central scar (arrowhead) and lack of vascular encasement. (B) T2-weighted MR image shows the internal morphological features of the cyst, with high-signal-intensity microcysts (arrows) that are clearly distinguished from the dark central scar (arrowhead).[167]

A 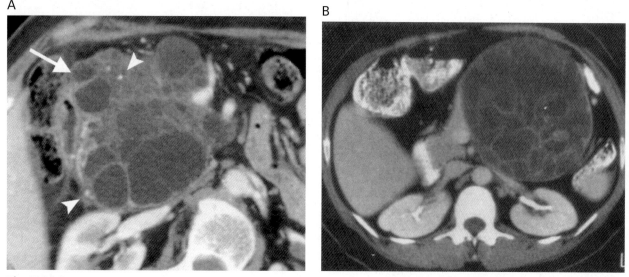 B

Fig GI 82-7
Mucinous cystic neoplasm. A contrast CT scan shows a large cystic mass (arrows) with internal septa in the head of the pancreas. The peripheral and septal calcification (arrowheads) indicate the malignant nature of the lesion. (B) In another patient, a contrast scan demonstrates a well-circumscribed, 18-cm palpable mass within the tail of the pancreas. There is enhancement on the thin external septa and peripheral wall.[164]

Condition	Imaging Findings	Comments
Other pancreatic neoplasms (Figs GI 82-9 to GI 82-12)	May manifest as a cyst containing a solid component, or as a solid tumor associated with a cystic component or cystic degeneration.	Adenocarcinoma of the pancreas, islet cell tumor, metastasis, cystic teratoma, sarcoma, solid pseudopapillary tumor, hemangioma, lympangioma, and paraganglioma.

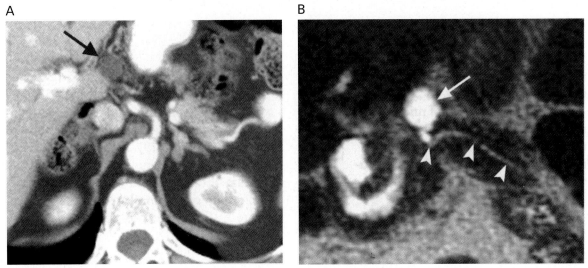

Fig GI 82-8
Intraductal IPMN. (A) Contrast CT scan shows a small cyst (arrow) in the head of the pancreas. (B) Coronal oblique MRCP shows communication between the cyst (arrow) and the main pancreatic duct (arrowheads), a finding that helped establish the diagnosis.[167]

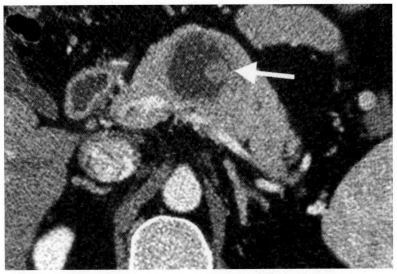

Fig GI 82-9
Islet cell tumor. CT scan in a patient with a malignant primary neuroendocrine tumor of the pancreas demonstrates a cystic lesion in the pancreatic body with peripheral mural nodules (arrows).[167]

Condition	Imaging Findings	Comments
Abscess (Fig GI 82-13)	Cystic structure containing high-attenuation debris.	Secondary infection of a pseudocyst has a high rate of morbidity and mortality and requires radiologic, endoscopic, or surgical decompression.

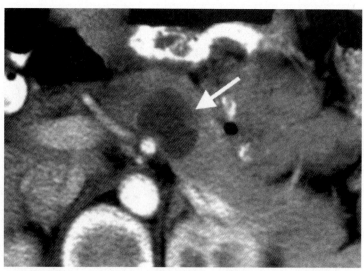

Fig GI 82-10
Pseudopapillary tumor. Contrast CT scan shows a lesion in the body of the pancreas with cystic areas and a solid component or mural nodule (arrow).[167]

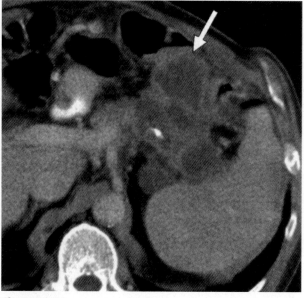

Fig GI 82-11
Pancreatic carcinoma. CT scan shows a solid tumor with cystic degeneration (arrow).[167]

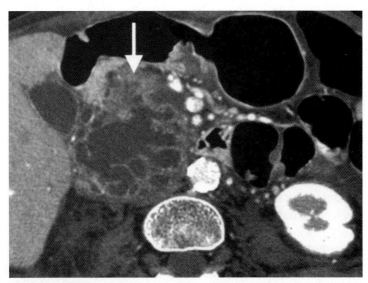

Fig GI 82-12
Malignant IPMN. CT scan demonstrates a multiseptated cyst with solid components (arrow).[167]

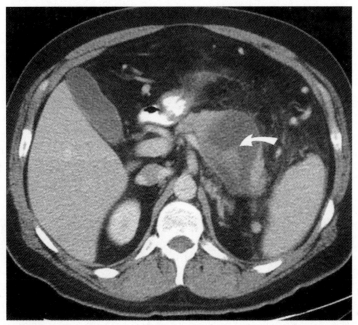

Fig GI 82-13
Pancreatic abscess. CT scan shows a heterogeneous fluid collection with low attenuation and irregular margins in the body and tail of the pancreas. Note the high-attenuation debris (arrow) within the lesion.[168]

Solid Pancreatic Masses on Computed Tomography

Condition	Imaging Findings	Comments
Pancreatic carcinoma (Figs GI 83-1 and GI 83-2)	On noncontrast studies, the tumor usually has an attenuation value similar to that of normal tissue and must alter the contour of the pancreas to be detected. On contrast studies, the relatively avascular tumor appears as an area of decreased attenuation when compared with the normal pancreas.	Some necrotic tumors have well-defined borders and a uniform low density, simulating a pseudocyst. Because a focal mass can also be seen in acute or chronic pancreatitis, a diagnosis of carcinoma requires evidence of secondary signs of malignancy such as obliteration of peripancreatic fat planes (especially posteriorly about vascular structures), lymph node enlargement, and liver metastases.

A
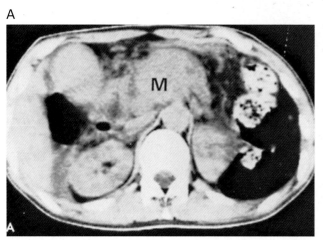

B
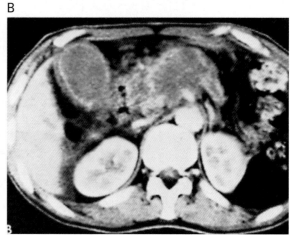

Fig GI 83-1
Pancreatic carcinoma. (A) Noncontrast scan demonstrates a homogeneous mass (M) in the body of the pancreas. (B) Contrast-enhanced scan at the time of maximum aortic contrast shows enhancement of the surrounding vascular structures and normal pancreatic parenchyma, while the pancreatic carcinoma remains unchanged and thus appears as a low-density mass.[162]

A
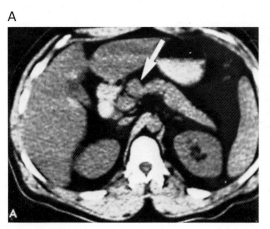

B
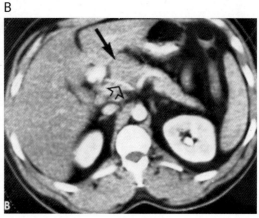

Fig GI 83-2
Pancreatic carcinoma (rapid growth and arterial encasement). (A) Initial scan demonstrates a focal change in the shape of the ventral contour of the pancreas at the junction of the body and head (arrow). There is no enlargement of the pancreatic tissue. This was initially interpreted as representing an anatomic variant. (B) Three months later, a repeat scan shows a focal tumor mass (closed arrow) in the location of the focal contour abnormality seen in (A). A dynamic CT scan after the intravenous bolus injection of contrast material demonstrates the splenic and hepatic arteries at the base of the tumor. Note that the hepatic artery (open arrow) has an irregular contour. Arteriography showed encasement by this unresectable tumor.[162]

Condition	Imaging Findings	Comments
Islet cell tumor (Figs GI 83-3 to GI 83-5)	Rapid sequential scanning after a bolus injection of contrast material can demonstrate the transient increase in contrast enhancement (tumor blush) that is characteristic of many of these tumors (it is often impossible to differentiate them from surrounding pancreatic tissue on noncontrast scans).	Most tumors are small and isodense with the uninvolved pancreas. Larger tumors may contain low-density areas due to foci of tumor necrosis. Many pancreatic islet cell tumors are malignant, and hepatic metastases may be seen on CT examination. Islet cell tumors associated with specific clinical syndromes include insulinoma (hypoglycemia, inappropriately elevated plasma levels of insulin); gastrinoma (signs and symptoms of peptic ulcer disease and elevated serum levels of gastrin); glucagonoma (diabetes mellitus, dermatitis, painful glossitis); somatostatinoma (diabetes mellitus, gallbladder disease, steatorrhea); and vipoma (massive watery diarrhea).

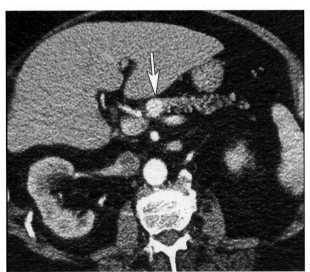

Fig GI 83-3
Insulinoma. Contrast scan demonstrates a homogeneously enhancing mass (arrow) in the neck of the pancreas in an elderly man who presented with life-threatening hyperglycemia.[170]

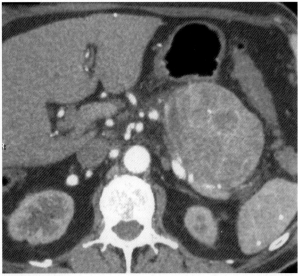

Fig GI 83-4
Vipoma. Contrast scan in an elderly man with watery diarrhea shows a huge mass with internal septa and calcification in the body and tail of the pancreas.[170]

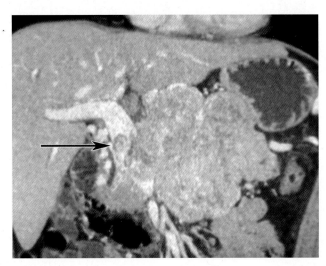

Fig GI 83-5
Islet cell tumor (nonfunctioning). Coronal CT image shows a large mass (arrow) in the left upper quadrant replacing the pancreas and invading the portal vein.[170]

Condition	Imaging Findings	Comments
Solid and papillary epithelial neoplasm (SPEN) (Fig GI 83-6)	Large, well-circumscribed, and slow-growing mass. Variety of internal appearances ranging from purely cystic to completely solid, depending on the degree of hemorrhage and necrosis of the tumor. The mass is usually surrounded by a thick, well-defined rim.	Histologically distinctive neoplasm of low malignant potential with a favorable prognosis. SPEN is typically found in young women and has a predilection for Asian and black patients.
Metastases Local invasion	Obliteration of the fat planes that normally separate the pancreas from adjacent organs.	Hepatomas and carcinoma of the stomach or gallbladder may extend directly into the pancreas. Lesions of the left adrenal and kidney may displace the tail of the pancreas, destroy surrounding fat, and occlude the splenic vein.
Hematogenous spread (Fig GI 83-7)	Predominantly round or ovoid hyperattenuating masses with smooth borders and discrete margins.	Primary tumors are most commonly renal cell or bronchogenic carcinoma. Pancreatic metastases are frequently multiple and generally show strong contrast enhancement due to hypervascularity (unlike primary pancreatic carcinomas).
Peripancreatic lymph node involvement (Fig GI 83-8)	Lobulated mass or masses impinging on the pancreas.	Enlargement of peripancreatic nodes (metastatic tumor, lymphoma, infection) can simulate pancreatic tumor. The boundary of fat between the pancreas and the nodal mass is often preserved (it may be impossible to differentiate primary pancreatic tumor from peripancreatic lymphadenopathy if the fat planes are obliterated).

A

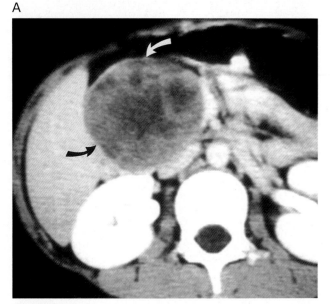

B

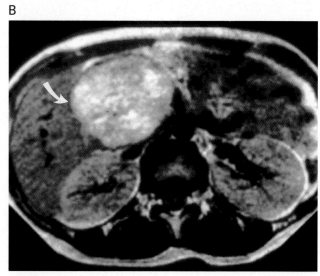

Fig GI 83-6
Solid and papillary epithelial neoplasm. (A) Contrast CT scan shows a mixed solid and cystic mass in the pancreatic head (arrows). (B) Axial T1-weighted MR image shows areas of high signal intensity due to hemorrhage within the mass (arrow).[171]

Condition	Imaging Findings	Comments
Lymphoma (Fig GI 83-9)	Lobulated mass or masses impinging on the pancreas or diffuse enlargement of the gland due to direct infiltration by lymphomatous tissue.	Lymphomatous involvement of the pancreas or peripancreatic nodes is usually part of a systemic disease in which there is also retroperitoneal and mesenteric lymphadenopathy.

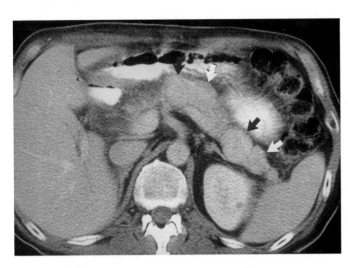

Fig GI 83-7
Metastatic renal cell carcinoma. Multiple enhancing nodular masses (arrows) in the pancreatic body and tail.[172]

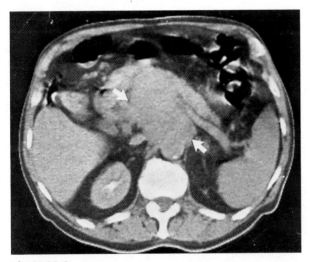

Fig GI 83-8
Peripancreatic lymph node metastases. Massive nodal enlargement (arrows) with obliteration of fat planes between the mass and the head of the pancreas.

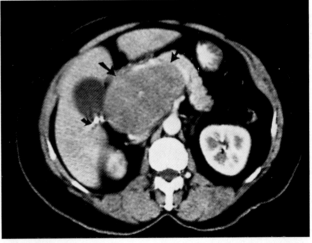

Fig GI 83-9
Lymphoma. Huge mass infiltrating the head of the pancreas (straight arrows). The curved arrow points to stones in the gallbladder.

Condition	Imaging Findings	Comments
Focal pancreatitis (acute or chronic) (Figs GI 83-10 through GI 83-12)	Focal enlargement of the head of the pancreas that may be indistinguishable from a neoplasm. The presence of evenly distributed calcifications in a focal mass strongly suggests chronic pancreatitis, though a carcinoma can arise in a pancreas that already contains calcifications from chronic inflammatory disease.	In uncomplicated acute pancreatitis, more commonly diffuse enlargement of the gland (often with a decreased attenuation value secondary to edema) or an irregular contour with indistinct margins of the gland and an increased density of the peripancreatic fat planes. In chronic pancreatitis, focal or diffuse pancreatic enlargement often represents edema in association with an acute exacerbation or fibrosis.
Pancreatic abscess (Figs GI 83-13 and GI 83-14)	Poorly defined, inhomogeneous mass that often displaces adjacent structures and generally has an attenuation value higher than that of a sterile fluid collection or pseudocyst.	The most reliable sign of an abscess is gas in the mass, though this is found in less than 50% of proven abscesses and may also occur in a patient with a pancreatic pseudocyst that erodes into the gastrointestinal tract without abscess formation. Because a pancreatic abscess often has a nonspecific CT appearance, diagnostic needle aspiration is an extremely useful adjunct for early diagnosis.

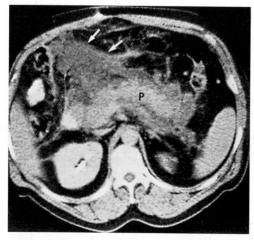

Fig GI 83-10
Acute pancreatitis. Diffuse enlargement of the pancreas (P) with obliteration of peripancreatic fat planes by the inflammatory process. Note the extension of the inflammatory reaction into the transverse mesocolon (arrows).[173]

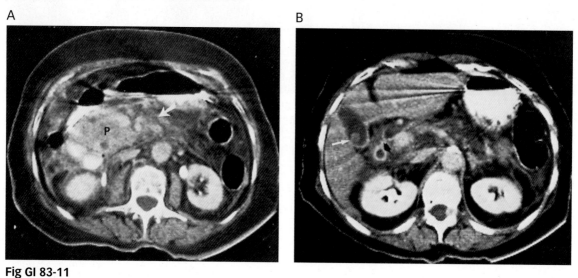

A   B

Fig GI 83-11
Acute gallstone pancreatitis. (A) There is enlargement of the head of the pancreas (P) with inflammatory reaction surrounding peripancreatic fat planes (arrow). (B) A stone (white arrow) is seen in the gallbladder and the common bile duct is enlarged (black arrow).

Condition	Imaging Findings	Comments
Cystic fibrosis (Figs GI 83-15 and GI 83-16)	Partial or complete replacement of the pancreas by fibrofatty tissue. Atrophy of the pancreas without fibrofatty replacement may occur. Rarely, cysts of different size develop and no normal pancreatic tissue remains.	Cystic fibrosis affects the pancreas in nearly all patients, though more than 90% of the exocrine function of the pancreas must be lost before the appearance of such clinical symptoms as steatorrhea, fat intolerance, abdominal pain, and failure to thrive.

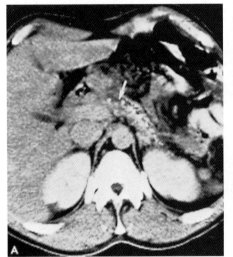

Fig GI 83-12
Chronic pancreatitis. There is pancreatic atrophy along with multiple intraductal calculi and dilatation of the pancreatic duct (arrow). The calcifications were not seen on plain abdominal radiographs.[122]

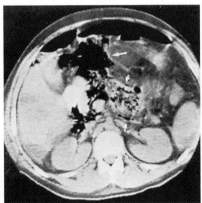

Fig GI 83-13
Pancreatic abscess. There is a gas-containing abscess (small arrows) in the pancreatic bed, with marked anterior extension (large arrow) of the inflammatory process.

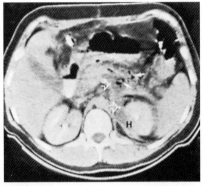

Fig GI 83-14
Pancreatic abscess after a gunshot wound. There are multiple intrapancreatic and peripancreatic gas bubbles (closed arrows), bullet fragments (open arrows), a small renal laceration, and an extrarenal hematoma (H).[89]

A

B

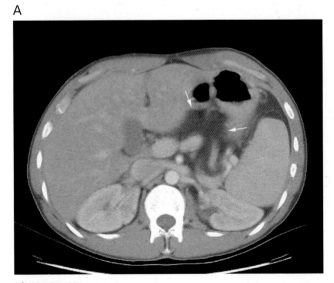

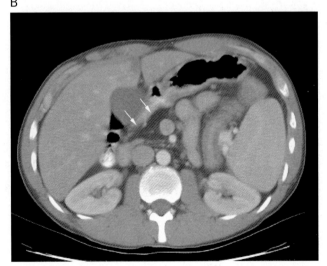

Fig GI 83-15
Cystic fibrosis. Contrast scans at the level of the pancreatic tail (A) and head (B) show complete replacement of the pancreatic parenchyma by fat (arrows). There is also enlargement of the spleen.[174]

Condition	Imaging Findings	Comments
Pancreatic and peripancreatic disease mimicking a mass (Figs GI 83-17 to 83-21)	Various appearances.	Normal unopacified bowel, anatomic variants (annular pancreas, duodenal duplication or diverticulum, intrapancreatic splenic rest, choledochal cyst), vascular lesions (superior mesenteric artery aneurysm, occlusive portal vein thrombus), neoplasm arising in an adjacent organ.

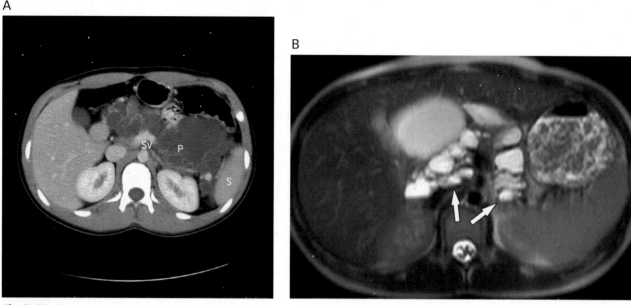

Fig GI 83-16
Pancreatic cystosis. (A) Contrast CT scan shows multiple cysts (*) in the region of the pancreas (P), which is completely replaced by fibrofatty tissue. The cyst walls have a somewhat higher attenuation than the musculature. The lesion is located along the splenic vein (Sv), and its most lateral part is situated between the left kidney (K) and the spleen (S).[175] (B) T2-weighted MR image in another patient shows innumerable cysts (arrows) replacing the pancreatic parenchyma.[174]

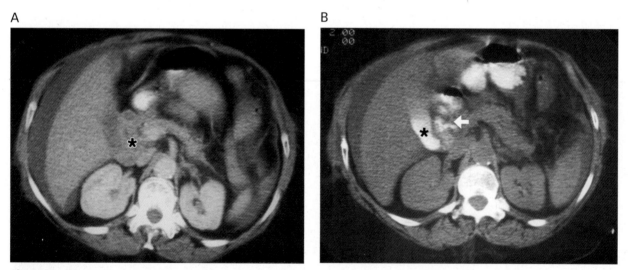

Fig GI 83-17
Normal enhanced duodenum. (A) Initial CT scan shows findings that suggest enlargement of the head of the pancreas (*). (B) Repeat scan obtained with additional contrast material shows a normal pancreatic head, with contrast material in the duodenum (arrow) and gallbladder (*).[174]

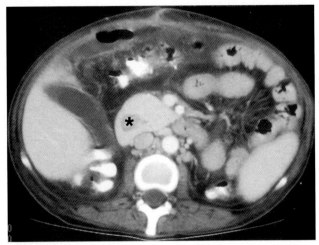

Fig GI 83-18
Annular pancreas. Pancreatic tissue surrounds the duodenum (*).[174]

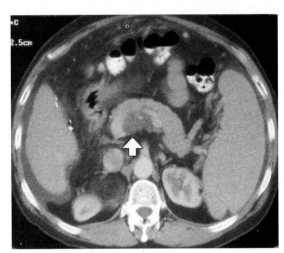

Fig GI 83-19
Venous vascular lesion. Occlusive portal vein thrombus (arrow). When this extensive, this finding may be mistaken for a mass.[174]

A

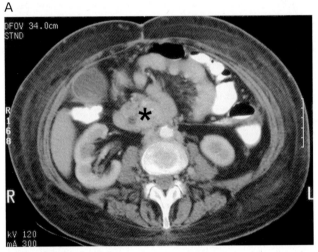

B

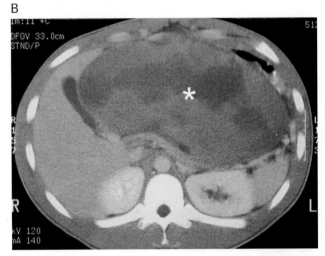

Fig GI 83-20
Mesenteric tumor-like disease. (A) Carcinoid tumor appears as a heterogeneously attenuating mass with calcifications (*) adjacent to the head of the pancreas in the root of the mesentery. (B) Desmoid tumor presents as a large, ovoid mass compressing the pancreas dorsally (*). Both of these tumors simulate lesions of pancreatic origin.[174]

A

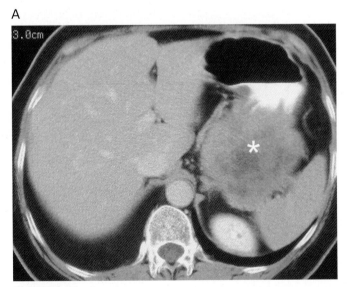

B

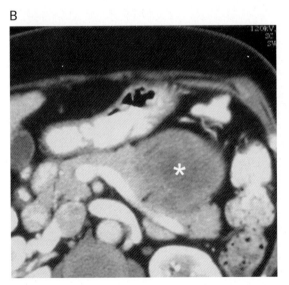

Fig GI 83-21
Gastric GIST. (A) Initial scan shows an apparent large mass (*) abutting the tail of the pancreas. (B) Focused pancreatic scan shows a sulcus between the mass (*) and the pancreatic tail (arrow), suggesting an extrapancreatic origin for the mass.[174]

Magnetic Resonance Cholangiography

Condition	Imaging Findings	Comments
Choledocholithiasis (Figs GI 84-1 and GI 84-2)	On heavily T2-weighted sequences that demonstrate the fluid-containing bile ducts as high-signal-intensity structures, biliary calculi appear as low-signal-intensity foci within the ductal system. Stones as small as 2 mm can be detected.	The primary utility of this non-invasive technique in patients with suspected choledocholithiasis may not lie in the detection of common duct stones, but rather in their exclusion as a source of abdominal pain, thus sparing the patient the risk of unnecessary endoscopic retrograde cholangiography.
Mirizzi syndrome (Fig GI 84-3)	Impacted cystic duct stone compressing the extrahepatic bile duct.	Multiplanar capability of MR cholangiography allows identification of both the obstructing calculus and the long cystic duct, which parallels the bile duct and predisposes to development of this syndrome.
Cholelithiasis (Figs GI 84-4 and GI 84-5)	Low-signal-intensity filling defects within the high-signal-intensity bile (see Figs GI 40-2 and GI 41-1) Calculi as small as 2 mm can be identified using this technique.	Although usually used to evaluate the bile ducts, MR cholangiography can image the gallbladder (either intentionally or incidentally), even in the non-fasting patient.
Malignant obstruction (Fig GI 84-6)	Narrowing of the bile duct with proximal dilatation.	Although the diagnosis is usually established with ultrasound or CT, MR cholangiography may be useful in establishing the resectability of a lesion (eg, hilar cholangiocarcinoma) by determining the proximal extent of disease (allowing immediate surgery without the need for ERCP and stent placement). This technique is also of value in delineating the biliary tract in proximal obstructions (in which ERCP may not be successful) and in distal obstructions (in which percutaneous transhepatic cholangiography may be of limited value).

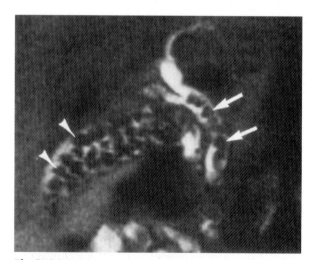

Fig GI 84-1
Biliary and gallbladder stones. Multiple calculi in both the dilated extrahepatic bile duct (arrows) and gallbladder (arrowheads).[176]

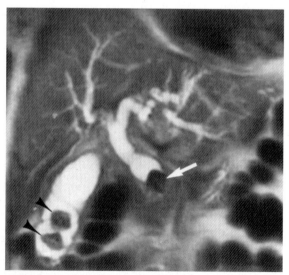

Fig GI 84-2
Impacted ampullary stone. Large obstructing calculus (white arrow) results in proximal bile duct dilatation. There are also several gallstones (black arrows).[176]

Condition	Imaging Findings	Comments
Cholangitis (Fig GI 84-7)	Variable pattern of ductal stenoses, occlusions, and irregularity.	Primary sclerosing cholangitis and AIDS cholangiopathy.

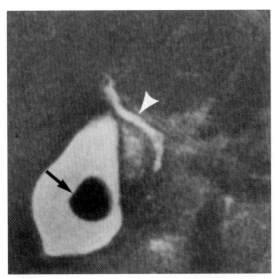

Fig GI 84-3
Gallstone. Large gallbladder calculus (black arrow) in a young man with sickle cell disease. Note the normal-caliber bile duct (white arrowhead).[176]

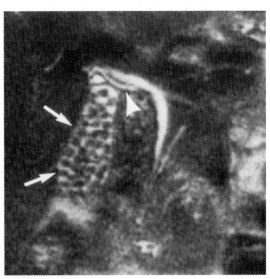

Fig GI 84-4
Multiple gallstones. Innumerable small calculi fill the gallbladder (straight arrows). The cystic duct (arrowhead) does not contain any calculi.[176]

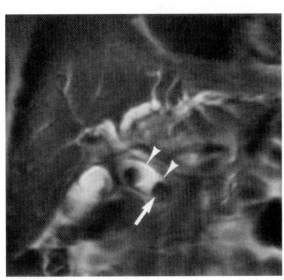

Fig GI 84-5
Mirizzi syndrome. Two calculi in the dilated cystic duct (arrowheads), which parallels the extrahepatic bile duct. The inferior calculus (arrow) eroded through the wall of the cystic duct into the extrahepatic bile duct, bridging the two structures and resulting in obstruction of the bile duct.[176]

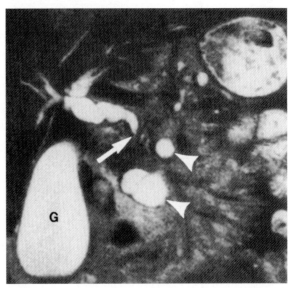

Fig GI 84-6
Pancreatic metastasis from mucinous colon carcinoma. Obstruction of the intrapancreatic segment of the bile duct (arrow). Note the dilated gallbladder (G). The enlarged lymph nodes with high signal intensity (arrowheads) represent metastases.[176]

Condition	Imaging Findings	Comments
Liver flukes (*Clonorchis sinensis*) (Fig GI 84-8)	Diffuse, uniform dilatation of the small intrahepatic ducts with no or minimal dilation of the large bile ducts and no focal obstructing lesions.	The flukes usually are not visible on images because they are very thin. However, in heavy infestation, conglomeration of organisms may result in many small, low-intensity filling defects within the intrahepatic biliary tree.
Prior biliary surgery (Figs GI 84-9 and GI 84-10)	Demonstrates post-surgical alterations of the biliary tract.	Valuable for delineating the anatomy of biliary-enteric anastomoses and complications such as anastomotic strictures, intraductal stones, and bile duct dilatation. In patients with liver transplants, MR cholangiography can visualize the biliary tract non-invasively after the biliary catheters have been removed.

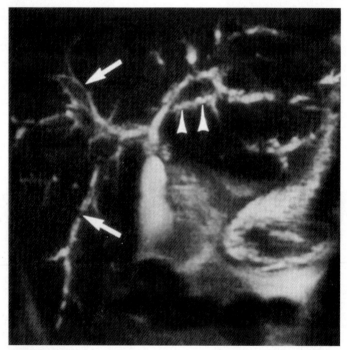

Fig GI 84-7
AIDS cholangiopathy. Multiple ductal stenoses and irregularities of the right hepatic ducts (arrows) and beading of the left hepatic ducts (arrowheads).[176]

Condition	Imaging Findings	Comments
Congenital anomalies (Figs GI 84-11 and GI 84-12)	Various appearances.	Aberrant hepatic duct, anatomic variants of cystic duct, choledochal cyst, and pancreas divisum.

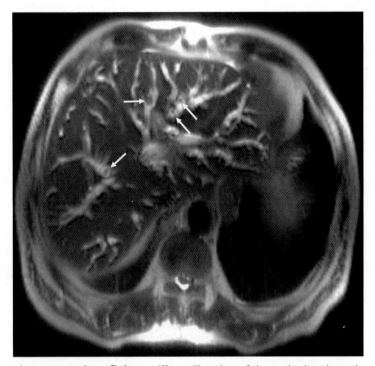

Fig GI 84-8 Liver flukes. Diffuse dilatation of the entire intrahepatic biliary ductal system. Note the filling defects (arrows) with the bile ducts due to adult flukes of *Clonorchis sinensis*.[177]

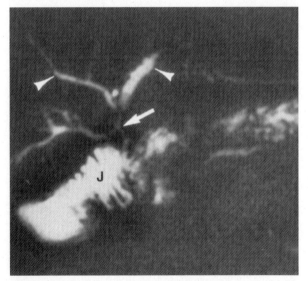

Fig GI 84-9
Stricture resulting from choledochojejunostomy after Whipple procedure for pancreatic carcinoma. Stricture of the common hepatic duct (arrow) extending to the anastomosis between the duct and the jejunum (J). The intrahepatic bile ducts are dilated (arrowheads).[176]

Condition	Imaging Findings	Comments
Gallbladder disease (Figs GI 84-13 and GI 84-14)	Various appearances.	MR cholangiography can aid in determining the presence and extent of neoplastic disease. It can detect as an incidental finding the fluid-filled Rokitansky-Aschoff sinuses within the gallbladder wall in patients with adenomyomatosis.

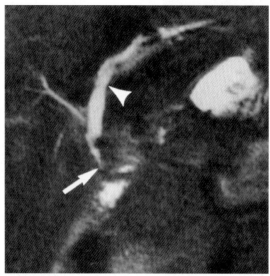

Fig GI 84-10
Bile duct obstruction secondary to transection during laparoscopic **cholecystectomy.** Stricture (arrow) of the left hepatic duct with proximal dilatation (arrowhead).[176]

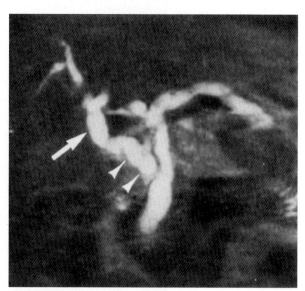

Fig GI 84-11
Aberrant right hepatic duct. The anomalous vessel (arrow) drains into the cystic duct remnant (arrowheads).[176]

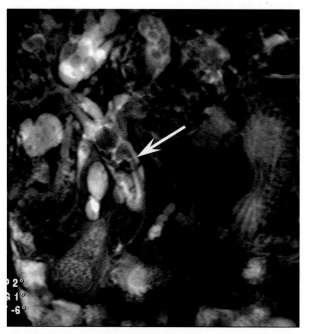

Fig GI 84-12 Choledochal cyst. Coronal image shows multiple dilated bile ducts with calculi. Multiple stones are seen within the dilated common bile duct (arrow). The cystic dilatations communicate with the major biliary tree.[178]

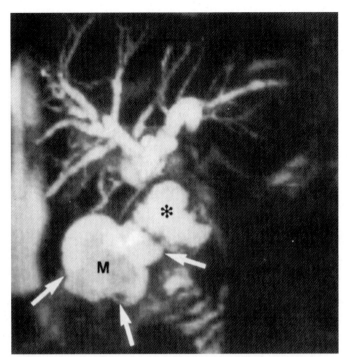

Fig GI 84-13 Gallbladder carcinoma with nodal metastases. Large mass (M) within the gallbladder (arrows) associated with a necrotic nodal metastasis (*), which resulted in proximal bile duct obstruction.[176]

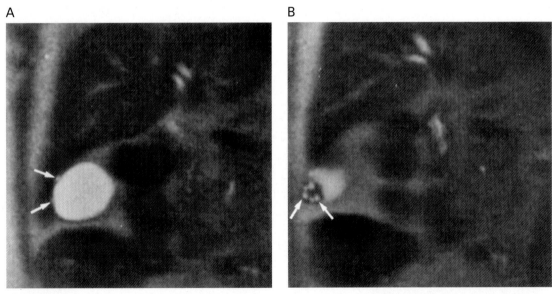

Fig GI 84-14
Adenomyomatosis. (A) Small, fluid-filled outpouchings (arrows) arise from the gallbladder, representing Rokitansky-Aschoff sinuses. (B) In the fundus of the gallbladder, there are additional fluid-filled sinuses (arrows), seen en face.[176]

Magnetic Resonance Pancreatography

Condition	Imaging Findings	Comments
Anatomic variants of the pancreatic ducts (Fig GI 85-1)	Various patterns of ductal drainage.	MR pancreatography permits non-invasive visualization of the entire normal-caliber pancreatic duct in the head and body in more than 95% of cases and the tail in almost 85%. Complete visualization of a dilated pancreatic duct is possible in virtually all cases. Demonstrates the ducts of Wirsung and Santorini as well as anomalous union of the pancreatic and bile ducts.
Congenital anomalies Pancreas divisum (Fig GI 85-2)	Separate ventral and dorsal pancreatic ducts.	Failure of fusion of the ventral anlage (that becomes the inferior pancreatic head and uncinate process) and the dorsal anlage (that becomes the superior pancreatic head and the body and tail of the gland). Although this variant may be detected incidentally in asymptomatic patients, it occurs more frequently in those who present with acute idiopathic pancreatitis.
Annular pancreas (Fig GI 85-3)	Duct within the pancreatic annulus surrounding all or part of the duodenum (usually the descending portion).	Complete annular pancreas typically presents in the neonatal period. However, patients with incomplete or partial annular pancreas may not present until adulthood (occasionally, the condition is detected incidentally). Although this anomaly can be recognized by other modalities, in the past only invasive endoscopic retrograde cholangiopancreatography has allowed definitive diagnosis.

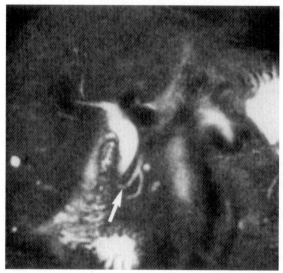

Fig GI 85-1
Anatomic variant. Persistent duct of Santorini (arrow) enters the minor ampulla and lies cephalad to the duct of Wirsung.[179]

Condition	Imaging Findings	Comments
Anomalous union of pancreatic and bile ducts (Fig GI 85-4)	Unusually long (15 mm) channel, common to the two ducts, that lies proximal to the duodenal sphincter.	Occurs in association with choledochal cysts in 33% to 83% of cases. Postulated mechanism is that the anomalous union allows reflux of pancreatic enzymes into the bile duct, thus weakening the bile duct and predisposing the patient to the development of a choledochal cyst. Also a higher incidence of gallbladder carcinoma in patients with this anomaly.

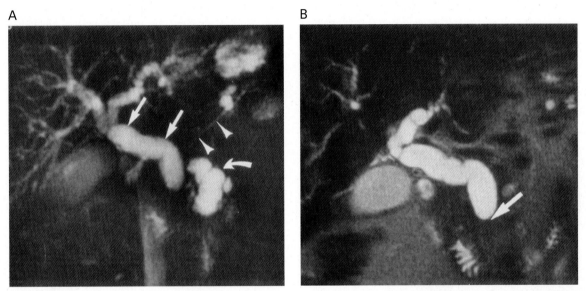

Fig GI 85-2
Pancreas divisum. (A) The distal bile duct (arrowhead) joins the ventral pancreatic duct (arrows) to enter the major ampulla. (B) The dorsal pancreatic duct (arrows) enters the minor ampulla (arrowhead) cephalad to the major ampulla. Subsequent images helped confirm the absence of communication between the central and dorsal pancreatic ducts.[180]

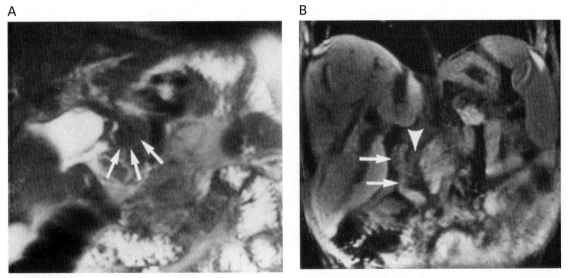

Fig GI 85-3
Annular pancreas. The lesion was detected incidentally in a 61-year-old man, in whom cannulation of the bile duct was not possible during ERCP. (A) Curvilinear duct (arrows) in the annular pancreas. (B) Coronal T1-weighted abdominal image demonstrates the annular pancreas (arrows) lying lateral to the fluid-filled duodenum (arrowhead).[179]

Condition	Imaging Findings	Comments
Sequelae of pancreatic trauma (Fig GI 85-5)	Disrupted duct and associated fluid collections.	Pancreatic duct injury may result from penetrating or blunt trauma, or be related to surgery (especially splenectomy). Acute blunt trauma usually involves the duct in the anterior portion of the body of the pancreas, which is relatively fixed and compressed against the vertebral body. If duct disruption and leakage of fluid are not recognized in the acute setting, there may be the development of a ductal stricture with proximal dilatation.
Pancreatitis (Figs GI 85-6 and GI 85-7)	In acute disease, the pancreatic duct is smooth in contour but may be slightly compressed by the edematous gland. In chronic pancreatitis, there is dilatation of the main pancreatic duct and its side branches ("chain of lakes" appearance, if severe) as well as contour irregularities, stricture formation, and intraductal calculi.	In patients who present with recurrent acute pancreatitis, MR pancreatography can suggest the cause of the disease (eg, pancreas divisum). In those with chronic inflammation, this technique is useful for depicting ductal anatomy, detecting strictures or intraductal calculi before surgery, and demonstrating complications such as pseudocysts and fistulas. Fibrosis may produce a smooth, tapered stricture in the bile duct as it traverses the pancreatic head.

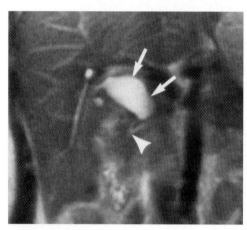

Fig GI 85-4
Anomalous union of the pancreatic and bile ducts.
The anomalous union (arrowhead) is associated with a choledochal cyst (arrows).[179]

A   B

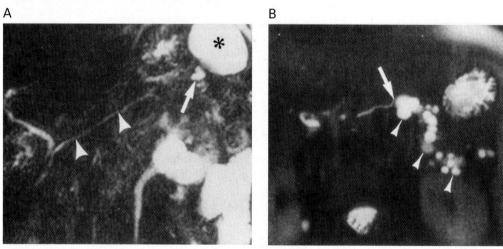

Fig GI 85-5
Pancreatic trauma. (A) Acute disruption of the pancreatic duct (arrowheads), which terminates in an 8-mm fluid collection (arrow) in the pancreatic tail. Note the large adjacent pseudocyst (*). (B) In another patient 17 years after blunt abdominal trauma, there is an abrupt point of transition between the normal pancreatic duct (arrow) and the dilated duct (arrowheads) in the body and tail of the gland.[179]

Condition	Imaging Findings	Comments
Pancreatic pseudocyst (Fig GI 85-8)	May demonstrate the ductal communication with the cystic mass.	Fewer than 50% of pseudocysts fill with contrast material when it is injected into the pancreatic duct during ERCP. Therefore, MR pancreatography and other cross-sectional techniques have a higher sensitivity for the detection of non-communicating pseudocysts. This technique also can demonstrate pseudocyst communication with adjacent organs (duodenum, stomach, spleen).
Pancreatic neoplasm (Fig GI 85-9)	Encasement and obstruction of the pancreatic (or bile) duct, which may be shown to terminate in a mass.	Approximately 90% of malignant pancreatic neoplasms are ductal in origin. Dilatation of both the pancreatic and biliary ducts ("double duct" sign) is highly suggestive for malignancy. MR pancreatography can aid in establishing resectability of the lesion and preventing unnecessary preoperative stent placement. It also can depict affected portions of the biliary tract and pancreatic duct before percutaneous intervention and radiation therapy.

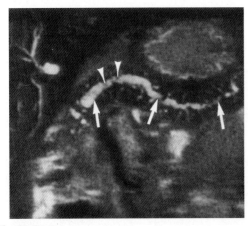

Fig GI 85-6
Chronic pancreatitis. Pancreatic duct dilatation (arrows), intraductal calculi (arrowheads), and bile duct stricture.[179]

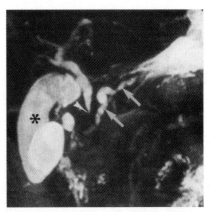

Fig GI 85-7
Chronic pancreatitis. Smooth, tapering stricture of the intrapancreatic bile duct (arrowhead), which is characteristic of this condition. The pancreatic duct (arrows) is dilated and tortuous. The gallbladder (*) is distended.[179]

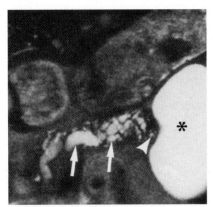

Fig GI 85-8
Pseudocyst. Dilatation of the pancreatic duct and its side branches (arrows), which terminate in a large pseudocyst (*) that is inseparable from the pancreatic tail (arrowhead). MR pancreatography was performed to delineate the ductal anatomy prior to pancreaticojejunostomy.[179]

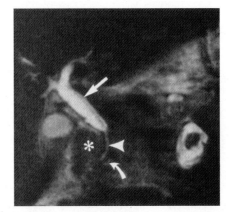

Fig GI 85-9
Carcinoma of the pancreas. The dilated extrahepatic bile duct (straight arrow) terminates in a pancreatic head mass (*). A biliary stent, which appears as a linear filling defect in the dilated bile duct, is seen to contain fluid (arrowhead) as it traverses the mass in the pancreatic head. Note the narrowing of the pancreatic duct (curved arrow) secondary to the mass.[179]

Decreased-Attenuation Masses in the Spleen

Condition	Imaging Findings	Comments
Cyst Nonparasitic (Fig GI 86-1)	Unilocular, homogenous, water-density lesion with pencil-thin margins that do not enhance after contrast material administration.	Usually congenital or traumatic in origin. Rarely secondary to pancreatitis, in which dissection of enzymes into the spleen results in an intrasplenic pseudocyst.
Echinococcal (Fig GI 86-2)	Round or oval mass with sharp margins and near-water density. The noncalcified portions of the cyst wall enhance after contrast material administration.	There may be extensive mural calcification that tends to be thick and irregular, unlike the infrequent calcification of congenital cysts that tends to be thin and smooth. Daughter cysts budding from the outer cyst wall often produce a multiloculated appearance.
Infarction (Figs GI 86-3 and GI 86-4)	Wedge-shaped area of decreased attenuation that extends to the capsule of the spleen and does not show contrast enhancement.	Chronic splenic infarction, as in sickle cell anemia, produces a shrunken spleen that often contains areas of calcification.

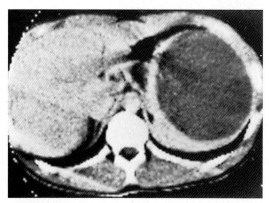

Fig GI 86-1
Congenital splenic cyst. Large, low-density mass with pencil-sharp margins filling almost all of the spleen.[181]

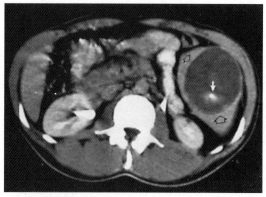

Fig GI 86-2
Echinococcal cyst. Rounded, low-density intrasplenic mass with an area of intracyst calcification (solid arrow). The cyst has pencil-sharp margins and a rim (open arrows) that is enhanced after the injection of contrast material.[181]

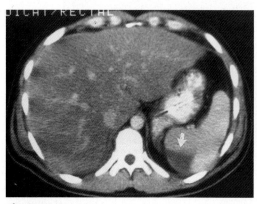

Fig GI 86-3
Infarction. Wedged-shaped, low-attenuation lesion (arrow) in the periphery of the spleen. (S, stomach; L, liver.)[95]

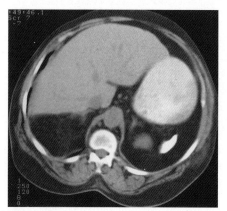

Fig GI 86-4
Autoinfarction of the spleen in a 56-year-old woman with sickle cell disease. Nonenhanced scan of the upper abdomen reveals a small, densely calcified spleen.[182]

Condition	Imaging Findings	Comments
Hematoma (Fig GI 86-5)	Initially, a hematoma may appear isodense or even slightly hyperdense on noncontrast scans when compared with normal spleen (may appear to have lower attenuation after contrast material injection as the normal spleen increases in density). As a hematoma ages (1 to 2 weeks), there is a gradual decrease in the attenuation and the nonhomogeneous appearance until the hematoma becomes homogeneous and of low attenuation.	Subcapsular hematomas appear as crescentic collections of fluid that flatten or indent the lateral margin of the spleen. Less common intrasplenic hematomas produce focal masses. The decreasing attenuation of the hematoma as it ages is the result of a decrease in hemoglobin and an increase in the water content of the hematoma.
Abscess (Figs GI 86-6 through GI 86-8)	Single or, more commonly, multiple rounded, hypodense or cystic lesions that lack a well-defined wall and do not show contrast enhancement.	Potentially life-threatening condition if appropriate therapy is postponed because of delayed diagnosis. Approximately 75% are associated with the hematogenous spread of infection, 15% with trauma, and 10% with splenic infarction. An abscess may contain gas or show layering of material or different densities in the cavity. In patients with AIDS, *Pneumocystis carinii* can occasionally disseminate from the lungs via the bloodstream to distant sites and produce multiple low-attenuation splenic lesions of varying size.
Lymphoma (Figs GI 86-9 and GI 86-10)	Single or multiple low-attenuation masses.	The spleen is involved in approximately 40% of patients at the time of initial presentation and is often the only site of involvement in patients with Hodgkin's disease. The most common CT appearance is generalized enlargement of a normal-density spleen (homogeneous lymphomatous infiltration).

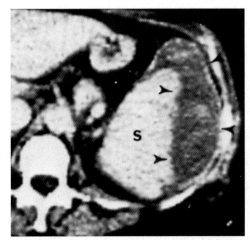

Fig GI 86-5
Traumatic subcapsular hematoma. Contrast-enhanced scan shows the hematoma as a large zone of decreased attenuation (arrowheads) that surrounds and flattens the lateral and anteromedial borders of the adjacent spleen (S).[183]

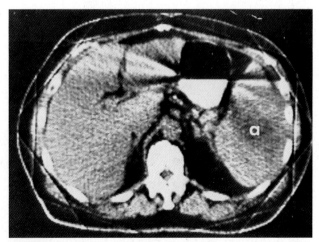

Fig GI 86-6
Traumatic subcapsular splenic abscess. The abscess (a) appears as an area of diminished attenuation in the center of spleen.[184]

Condition	Imaging Findings	Comments
Metastases (Figs GI 86-11 and GI 86-12)	Single or multiple low-attenuation lesions that may appear as ill-defined hypodense areas or as well-delineated cystic masses.	May arise from a variety of neoplasms, most commonly melanoma and carcinomas of the lung and breast. Metastatic nodules with areas of necrosis and liquefaction can contain irregularly shaped regions that approach water density.
Primary angiosarcoma (Figs GI 86-13 to GI 86-15)	Nonhomogeneous, complex mass of cystic and solid components.	The spleen is a rare site of primary malignancy. There is a variable degree of tumor enhancement after contrast material administration.

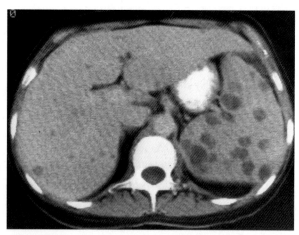

Fig GI 86-7
Fungal abscesses. Multiple low-attenuation lesions within the spleen in an immunocompromised patient.

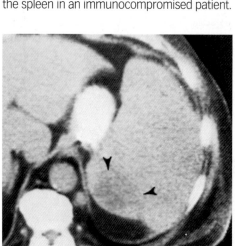

Fig GI 86-9
Lymphoma. Focal low-attenuation lesion (arrowheads) posteriorly in a markedly enlarged spleen.[183]

Fig GI 86-8
Pyogenic abscess. Enlarged spleen containing a massive amount of air. The presence of perisplenic air and fluid indicates rupture of the spleen (straight solid arrow). The inflammation extends into the adjacent perisplenic fat (open arrow). Note the retroperitoneal air adjacent to the right adrenal gland (curved solid arrow).[182]

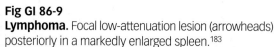

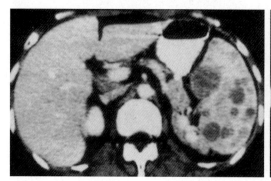
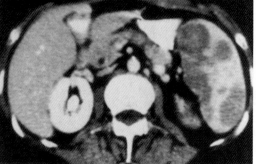

Fig GI 86-10
Lymphoma. Multiple discrete low-attenuation lesions in an enlarged spleen.[126]

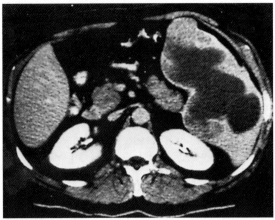

Fig GI 86-11
Metastases from melanoma. Multiple confluent lesions, with necrotic central areas showing a cystic appearance. The liver is not involved.[89]

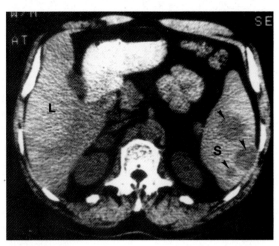

Fig GI 86-12
Metastases. Three discrete low-attenuation lesions (arrowheads) in the spleen (S). (L, liver.)[95]

A

B

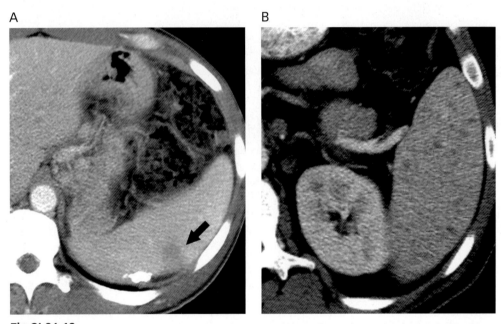

Fig GI 86-13
Kaposi's sarcoma. (A) Contrast CT scan shows an ill-defined, wedge-shaped hypoattenuating lesion (arrow) in the spleen. Note also the enhancing enlarged nodes in the region of the lesser curvature of the stomach. (B) In another patient, there are multiple tiny nodules in the spleen. (Courtesy of Diego Aguirre, M.D., Department of Radiology, Fundacion Santa Fe de Bogota, Bogota, Columbia.)[185]

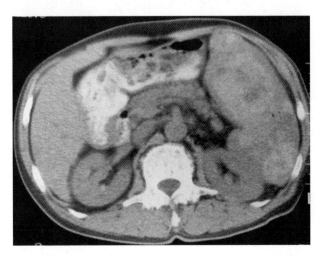

Fig GI 86-14
Angiosarcoma. Noncontrast scan shows multiple splenic masses that have increased attenuation reflecting previous hemorrhage.[182]

Condition	Imaging Findings	Comments
Benign tumors (Figs GI 86-16 to GI 86-20)	Single or multiple low-attenuation masses.	Hemangioma, hamartoma, lymphangioma, inflammatory pseudotumor.
Intrasplenic pseudocyst (Fig GI 86-21)	Single or multiple low-attenuation lesions typically associated with other CT findings of pancreatitis (enlargement of the pancreas with ill-defined margins, obliteration of peripancreatic fat planes, calcification).	Develops in 1% to 5% of patients with pancreatitis due to direct extension of a pancreatic pseudocyst or from the digestive effects of pancreatic enzymes on splenic vessels or parenchyma along the splenorenal ligament. In the absence of other CT criteria indicating pancreatitis, it may be impossible to differentiate an intrasplenic pseudocyst from other nonparasitic cysts of the spleen.

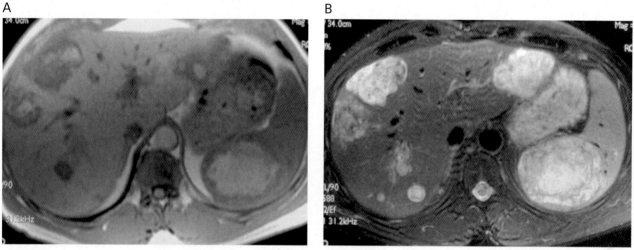

Fig GI 86-15
Angiosarcoma with liver metastases. (A) Axial T1-weighted MR image shows a dominant splenic mass with a central area of high signal intensity, a finding consistent with hemorrhage. The liver metastases also demonstrate high-signal-intensity hemorrhage. (B) T2-weighted MR image shows mixed high signal intensity in the splenic mass and liver metastases.[186]

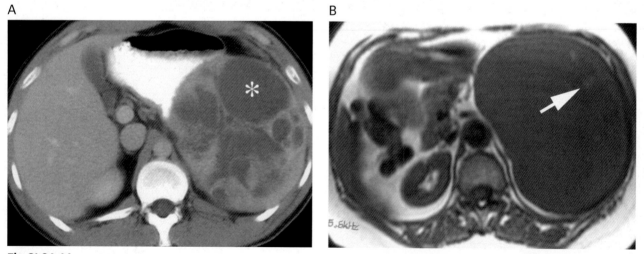

Fig GI 86-16
Cavernous hemangioma. (A) Contrast scan shows a well-defined intrasplenic mass with peripheral enhancement surrounding areas of nonenhancement (*). (B) In another patient, an axial T1-weighted MR image shows a large hypointense mass completely replacing the spleen. Several foci of high signal intensity (arrow) within the mass probably represent hemorrhage.[187]

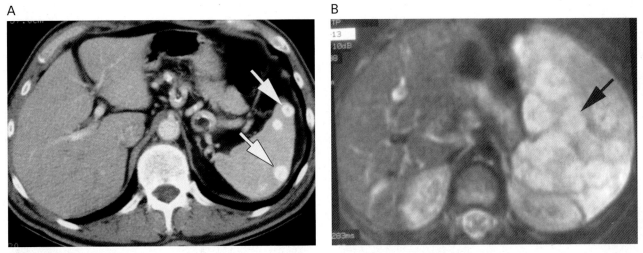

Fig GI 86-17
Multiple hemangiomas. (A) Contrast scan shows multiple densely enhancing masses (arrows). (B) In a young boy with Klippel-Trebaunay syndrome and worsening left upper quadrant pain, an axial T2-weighted MR image shows several high-intensity masses (arrow).[187]

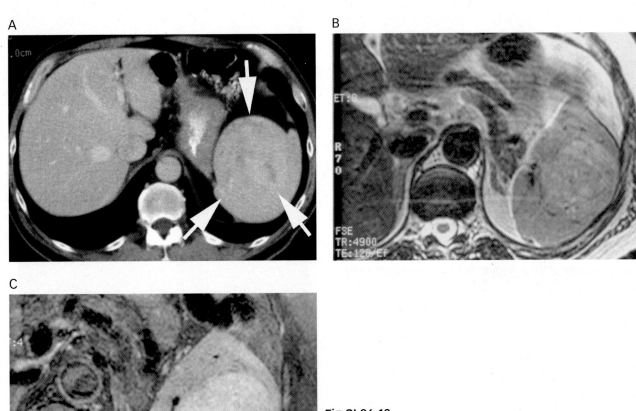

Fig GI 86-18
Hamartoma. (A) Contrast CT scan shows heterogeneous enhancement of the mass (arrows), which was discovered incidentally. (B) In another patient, a T2-weighted MR image shows a mass that is slightly hyperintense relative to the normal splenic parenchyma. (C) A T1-weighted image after contrast administration shows homogeneous enhancement of the mass.[187]

Condition	Imaging Findings	Comments
Sarcoidosis (Fig GI 86-22)	Multiple low-attenuation nodules.	This pattern develops in up to 15% of cases. Abdominal and thoracic adenopathy frequently accompanies hepatosplenic nodules in patients with sarcoidosis, though about 25% of patients have normal chest radiographs and no evidence of enlarged abdominal lymph nodes.

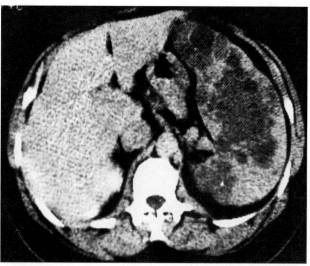

Fig GI 86-19
Lymphangiomatosis. Low-density, nonenhancing cystic areas within an enlarged spleen. Note the calcification in the posterior aspect of the spleen.[188]

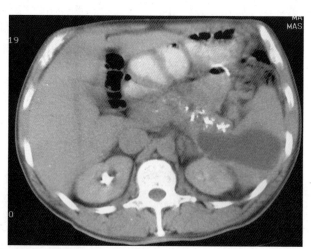

Fig GI 86-21
Intrasplenic pseudocyst. Enhanced scan demonstrates extension of a pancreatic tail pseudocyst into the spleen. Note the mild peripancreatic inflammation and extensive pancreatic calcification.[182]

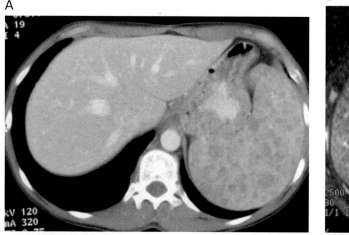

A

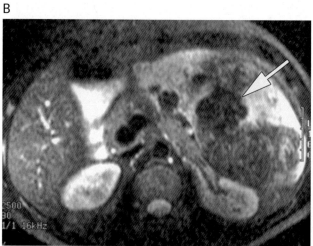

B

Fig GI 86-20
Littoral cell angioma. (A) Contrast CT scan shows an enlarged spleen containing innumerable hypoattenuating masses. (B) In a different patient, a T2-weighted MR image shows multiple hypointense masses (arrow) adjacent to the normally bright splenic parenchyma.

Condition	Imaging Findings	Comments
Gaucher's disease (Fig GI 86-23)	Multiple low-attenuation nodules.	Enzymatic deficiency that results in an abnormal accumulation of glucocerebrosides in the reticuloendothelial tissue of the bone marrow, liver, and spleen.
Peliosis (Fig GI 86-24)		Rare entity characterized by the presence of widespread blood-filled cystic spaces within the splenic parenchyma. Although the etiology of this generally asymptomatic condition is unknown, it may be associated with malignant hematologic diseases (Hodgkin's disease, myeloma), disseminated malignancy, tuberculosis, the use of anabolic and contraceptive steroids, prior Thorotrast injection, and certain viral infections.

A
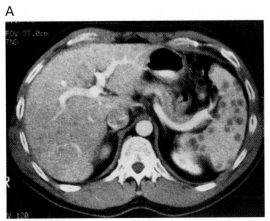

B
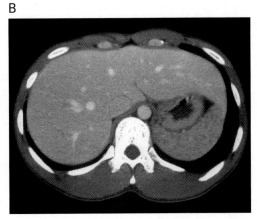

Fig GI 86-22
(A) Sarcoidosis. Contrast-enhanced scan in an asymptomatic man obtained during the hepatic parenchymal phase shows multiple discrete nodules throughout the spleen. The liver nodules are faintly visualized.[113] (B) In this patient, there are innumerable small hypoattenuating nodules.[189]

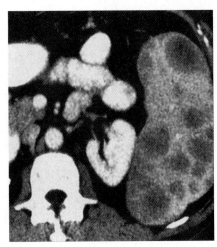

Fig GI 86-23
Gaucher's disease. Multiple discrete nodules of decreased enhancement corresponding to local deposits of glucocerebroside in reticuloendothelial cells.[190]

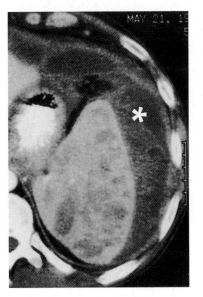

Fig GI 86-24
Peliosis. Multiple rounded, low-attenuation lesions of different sizes throughout the splenic parenchyma. Preoperatively, these lesions were thought to be intrasplenic hematomas. The hemoperitoneum (*) occurred secondary to trauma and was unrelated to the splenic peliosis.[191]

Splenic Lesions on Magnetic Resonance Imaging

Condition	Imaging Findings	Comments
Cyst		
Nonparasitic (Fig GI 87-1)	Unilocular, homogeneous lesion that has the signal intensity of water on all pulse sequences, pencil-thin margins, and no contrast enhancement.	Most common benign focal splenic mass. Usually congenital or traumatic in origin.
Echinococcal (Fig GI 87-2)	Single or multiple masses with near-water signal intensity. Noncalcified portions of the cyst wall may show contrast enhancement.	Daughter cysts may be seen budding from the outer cyst wall. CT is superior to MRI for demonstrating the characteristic mural calcification.
Infarction	Perfusion defect on delayed contrast-enhanced images	A typical feature is the rim sign of capsular enhancement that is caused by blood supply from capsular vessels.
Hematoma (Fig GI 87-3)	High signal intensity on T1-weighted images during the acute phase.	Old, healed hematomas are commonly hypointense on both T1- and T2-weighted images.
Abscess		
Bacterial (Fig GI 87-4)	Single or multiple cyst-like masses that typically show peripheral and perilesional contrast enhancement.	Usually larger than fungal abscesses, they are frequently associated with endocarditis.
Fungal (Fig GI 87-5)	Multiple small lesions that appear hyperintense on T2-weighted, fat-saturation images.	Most frequently seen in immunocompromised patients. They usually do not show peripheral enhancement in the acute stage because of the immunocompromised state of these patients, or in the chronic stage because of fibrotic changes.

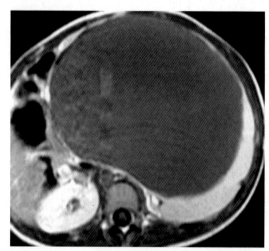

Fig GI 87-1
Epithelial cyst. Contrast T1-weighted image shows a huge homogeneous, nonenhancing mass that causes lateral displacement of the normal splenic parenchyma.[192]

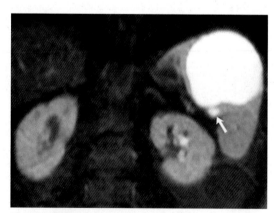

Fig GI 87-2
Echinococcal cyst. T2-weighted coronal image shows a septated hyperintense lesion. The small peripheral cyst represents a daughter cyst (arrow).[192]

Condition	Imaging Findings	Comments
Hemangioma (Fig GI 87-6)	Small, well-defined, homogeneous lesion that is hypo- or isointense to splenic parenchyma on T1-weighted images and usually hyperintense on T2-weighted images. Characteristic peripheral enhancement with centripetal, delayed progression.	Second most common focal lesion and the most common benign tumor of the spleen. Smaller hemangiomas may show homogeneous enhancement on immediate postcontrast images, remaining enhanced on delayed studies. Large hemangiomas are heterogeneous with areas of hemorrhage and thrombosis.

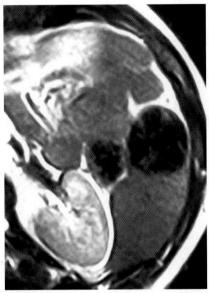

Fig GI 87-3
Hematoma. Axial T2-weighted image shows a round, hypointense mass in the anterior portion of the spleen, representing an old, healed hematoma.[192]

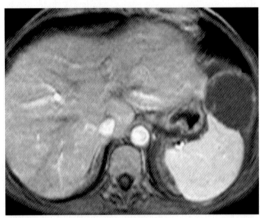

Fig GI 87-4
Bacterial abscess. Contrast T1-weighted, fat-saturated image shows peripheral enhancement of a huge cyst-appearing lesion in a man with endocarditis.[192]

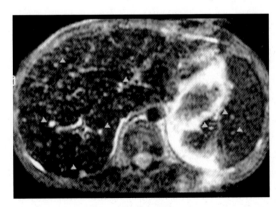

Fig GI 87-5
Fungal abscess. T2-weighted, fat-saturated image shows multiple, round, hyperintense lesions in the liver and spleen (arrowheads) representing *Candida* microabscesses.[192]

Condition	Imaging Findings	Comments
Lymphangioma (Fig GI 87-7)	Multicystic lesion, though some of the cysts may be hyperintense on T1-weighted images because of the proteinaceous or hemorrhagic contents.	Although malignant degeneration of lymphangioma is rare, MRI can show intracystic solid components.

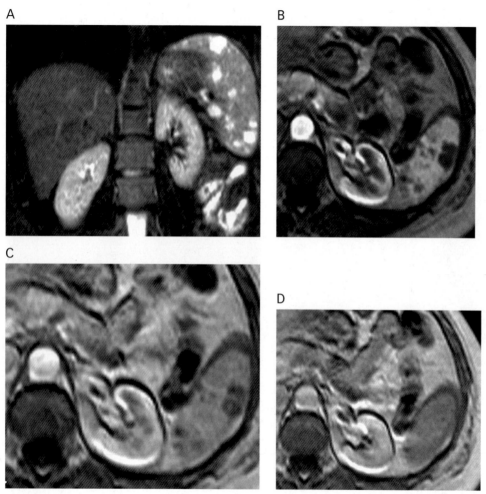

Fig GI 87-6
Hemangioma. (A) Coronal fat-saturated T2-weighted image shows multiple hyperintense splenic nodules. (B) Immediate, (C) one minute, and (D) delayed T1-weighted images after contrast administration shows the progressive centripetal enhancement pattern that is typical of hemangioma. By the final image, the nodules have become almost completely isointense to the splenic parenchyma.

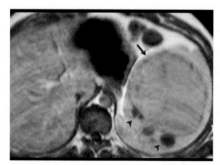

Fig GI 87-7
Lymphangioma. Contrast T1-weighted image shows a sub-capsular multilocular mass with hypoitense (arrowheads) and hyperintense (arrow) nonenhancing areas, revealing their cystic nature. The hyperintense areas were secondary to proteinaceous content.

Condition	Imaging Findings	Comments
Hamartoma (Fig GI 87-8)	Sharply defined, rounded solid lesion with heterogeneous hyperintensity on T2-weighted images.	On delayed postcontrast images, a hamartoma typically shows relatively uniform and intense enhancement with central hypovascular areas.
Lymphoma (Fig GI 87-9)	Multiple focal lesions, diffuse splenic involvement or, infrequently, a single mass. Generally isointense to splenic parenchyma on both T1- and T2-weighted images. Immediate postcontrast images show hypovascular nodules, which usually become rapidly isointense to the spleen.	Most common splenic malignancy. Lymphoma can be hypointense on T2-weighted images, unlike metastases, which rarely exhibit this appearance.

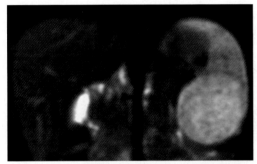

Fig GI 87-8
Hamartoma. Coronal fat-saturated T2-weighted image shows a heterogeneous hyperintense mass in the inferior pole of the spleen.

A   B

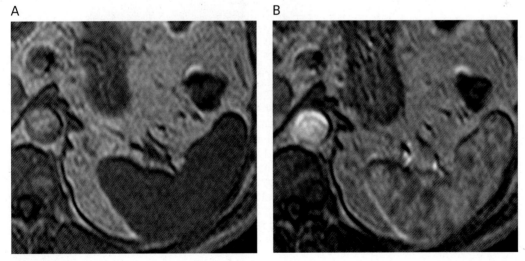

Fig GI 87-9
Lymphoma. Immediate postcontrast T1-weighted image (A) shows multiple small hypovascular nodules that are not detectable on a delayed scan (B). The precontrast image (not shown) appeared normal.

Condition	Imaging Findings	Comments
Metastases (Fig GI 87-10)	Usually isointense on unenhanced sequences. They may be hyperintense on T2-weighted images when necrosis or cystic changes are present. Hemorrhagic or melanoma metastases can have high signal on T1-weighted images.	The T2-hyperintensity and high signal on T1-weighted images can help distinguish metastases from lymphoma, which rarely shows necrosis or hemorrhage.
Angiosarcoma	Multiple nodular heterogeneous masses with intense and heterogeneous enhancement.	Rare primary malignancy of the spleen.
Intrahepatic pseudocyst (Fig GI 87-11)	Single or multiple lesions that usually have a more heterogeneous appearance than true cysts.	Develops from direct extension of a pancreatic pseudocyst or from the digestive effects of pancreatic enzymes on splenic vessels or parenchyma along the splenorenal ligament.

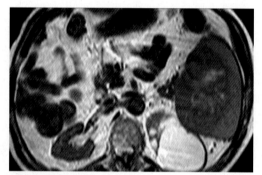

Fig GI 87-10
Metastasis (colon cancer). T2-weighted image shows a heterogeneous mass with central hyperintense areas representing regions of necrosis.

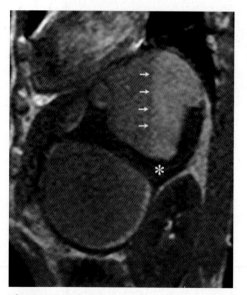

Fig GI 87-11
Intrasplenic pseudocyst. Sagittal unenhanced T1-weighted image shows a bilobulated mass surrounding and extending to the spleen (*). Note the presence of a fluid-fluid level within the superior component of the mass with hyperintense signal of the dependent compartment, indicating its hemorrhagic content.

Condition	Imaging Findings	Comments
Miscellaneous conditions (Fig GI 87-12)	Multiple nodules.	Storage diseases (Gaucher, Niemann-Pick), peliosis, sarcoidosis.

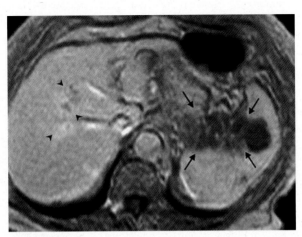

Fig GI 87-12
Peliosis. Immediate postcontrast T1-weighted image in a patient with disseminated tuberculosis shows a multicystic mass (arrows) with septal and peripheral enhancement. Note the several liver lesions with peripheral enhancement (arrowheads), which were not detectable on the unenhanced image (not shown).

Peritoneal and Omental Abnormalities

Condition	Imaging Findings	Comments
Diffuse infiltrative lesions		
Peritoneal carcinomatosis (Fig GI 88-1)	Peritoneal thickening, seeding nodules, and omental infiltration. Ascites is present in more than 70% of cases. These findings are not specific for peritoneal carcinomatosis and can be seen in other diffuse infiltrative lesions.	Metastatic peritoneal tumors most commonly originate from the ovary, stomach, pancreas, colon, uterus, and bladder. Hematogenous metastases frequently develop from malignant melanoma, as well as from primary breast and lung carcinoma.
Tuberculous peritonitis (Fig GI 88-2)	Relatively smooth peritoneum with minimal thickening and pronounced enhancement, mesenteric involvement with macronodules (5 mm), a thin omental line (fibrous wall covering the infiltrated omentum), mesenteric lymphadenopathy with low-attenuation centers, and calcifications.	Caused by hematogenous spread of pulmonary tuberculosis or rupture of an involved mesenteric node, usually in an immunocompromised patient. The uncommon fibrotic type of tuberculous peritonitis is characterized by loculated ascites, large omental masses, and separation or fixation of bowel loops.
Malignant peritoneal mesothelioma (Fig GI 88-3)	Variable appearance that may include ascites, irregular or nodular peritoneal thickening, a stellate pattern of the mesentery, bowel wall thickening, and scalloping of or mass effect on adjacent abdominal organs.	Unusual condition that accounts for 12% to 30% of mesotheliomas. The condition is associated with heavy exposure to asbestos, and has a long latent period. Pleural calcifications or plaques are present in more then 50% of cases, but calcified peritoneal plaques are unusual.

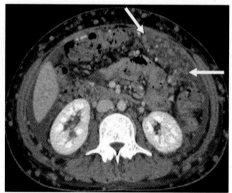

Fig GI 88-1
Peritoneal carcinomatosis. Hematogenous dissemination of malignant melanoma causes multiple nodules in the peritoneal space, including the omentum (arrows), retroperitoneal spaces, and the subcutaneous fat layer of the abdomen.[193]

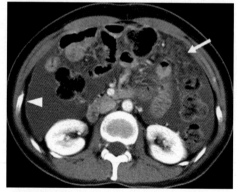

Fig GI 88-2
Tuberculous peritonitis. Large amount of ascites with even peritoneal thickening (arrowhead) and diffuse omental infiltration (arrow) without associated lymphadenopathy. The initial clinical impression was carcinomatosis.[193]

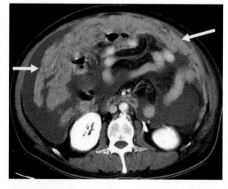

Fig GI 88-3
Malignant peritoneal mesothelioma. Diffuse platelike mass in the greater omentum (arrows), massive ascites, and peritoneal thickening.[193]

Condition	Imaging Findings	Comments
Pseudomyxoma peritonei (Fig GI 88-4)	Extensive low-attenuation material throughout the peritoneal cavity, omentum, and mesentery, which frequently appears loculated and has irregular septations. Scalloping of visceral surfaces, especially the liver, is diagnostic. Calcification of the mucinous material may occur with chronic disease.	Intraperitoneal accumulation of gelatinous mucinous material that arises from a ruptured benign or malignant mucus-producing tumor of the appendix, ovary, pancreas, stomach, colon, or urachus.
Lymphomatosis (Fig GI 88-5)	Soft-tissue attenuation mass that often surrounds mesenteric vessels. A characteristic finding is associated retroperitoneal and mesenteric lymphadenopathy. Omental involvement causes smudging and caking rather than a discrete nodular pattern.	Unlike other peritoneal malignant diseases, lymphomatous involvement is curable without surgery. However, the diagnosis is difficult on CT because the appearance closely mimics peritoneal carcinomatosis and tuberculous peritonitis.

A

B

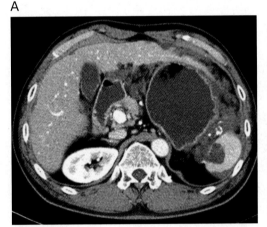
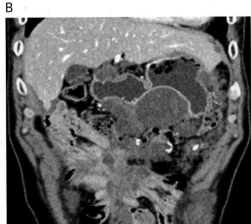

Fig GI 88-4
Pseudomyxoma peritonei. (A) Axial and (B) coronal scans show multiple low-attenuation masses in the omentum and peritoneal cavity. There is curvilinear or punctuate calcifications of the seeding nodules; scalloping of the liver, spleen, and stomach; and small bowel adhesions from mesenteric infiltration.[193]

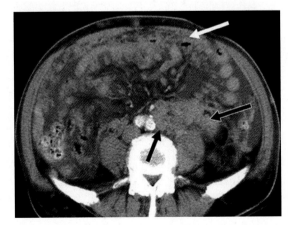

Fig GI 88-5
Lymphomatosis. Innumerable seeding nodules in the peritoneal cavity and omentum (white arrow) with evidence of ascites. Multiple enlarged lymph nodes with conglomeration (black arrows) are seen in the retroperitoneal spaces.[193]

Condition	Imaging Findings	Comments
Cirrhosis/portal hypertension	Edema of the mesentery, omentum, or retro-peritoneum.	One of the most common causes of diffuse omental infiltrative lesions. The appearance varies from a mild infiltrative haze to the presence of mass-like lesions with discrete margins.
Systemic disorders (Figs GI 88-6 and GI 88-7)	Nonspecific appearance of soft-tissue infiltration or masses that may be associated with ascites.	Amyloidosis, eosinoiphilic gastroenteritis, extra-medullary hematopoiesis, and sarcoidosis.
Solid/cystic mass lesions Primary neoplasm (Figs GI 88-8 to GI 88-10)	Benign tumors are usually well circumscribed, while malignant lesions typically have indistinct margins and invade into surrounding structures. Both types can appear complex, with cystic and solid elements.	Must less common than secondary processes. They include lipoma, leiomyoma, fibroma, neuro-fibroma, GIST, cystic mesothelioma, malignant fibrous histiocytoma, hemangiopericytomas, leio-myosarcoma, liposarcoma fibrosarcoma, desmo-plastic small round cell tumor, and primary papillary serous carcinoma.

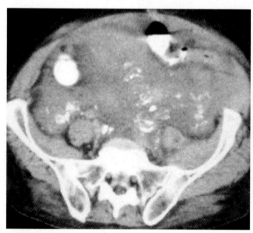

Fig GI 88-6
Amyloidosis. Extensive peritoneal soft-tissue infiltration and multifocal coarse calcifications.[194]

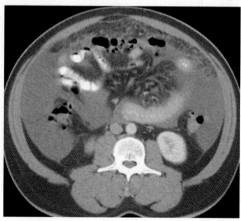

Fig GI 88-7
Sarcoidosis. Diffuse soft-tissue thickening involving the mesentery, omentum, and parietal peritoneum.[194]

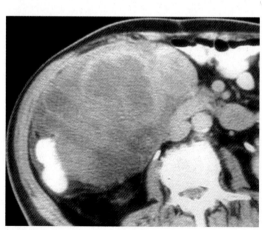

Fig GI 88-8
GIST. Large, heterogenous, omentum-based mass.[195]

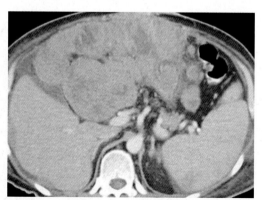

Fig GI 88-9
Malignant fibrous histiocytoma. Large, heterogeneous soft-tissue peritoneal mass.[195]

Condition	Imaging Findings	Comments
Secondary neoplasm (Figs GI 88-11 and GI 88-12)	Large, heterogenous mass associated with thickened peritoneum.	Far more common than primary tumors, they may have metastasized by direct spread, peritoneal seeding, or hematogenous spread.
Predominantly cystic/ developmental lesions (Fig GI 88-13)	Single or multiloculated fluid-filled mass with a thin wall and occasional septa.	Cystic lymphangioma, enteric duplication cyst, enteric cyst, mesothelial cyst, and extrapancreatic pseudocyst. Vessels are often seen coursing between multiloculated cysts of a lymphangioma.

A

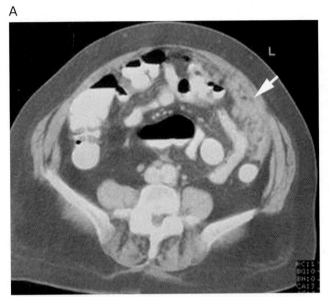

B

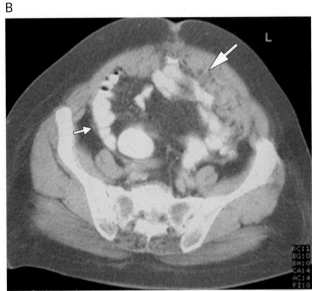

Fig GI 88-10
Primary serous papillary carcinoma. (A) Omental cake in the left lower quadrant displaces adjacent loops of large and small bowel. (B) In this lower image, there is lace-like omental infiltration (large arrow) with irregular nodular thickening of the peritoneum (small arrow). The mesenteric fat is normal and there is no lymphadenopathy or ascites.[196]

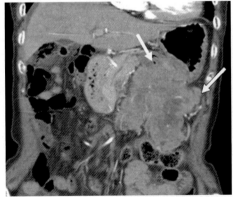

Fig GI 88-11
Metastasis. Large lobulated mass (arrows) in the left upper quadrant of the abdomen representing an exophytic carcinoma extending directly from the greater curvature of the stomach.[193]

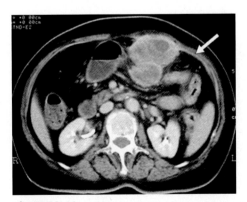

Fig GI 88-12
Metastasis. Large, lobulated, heterogeneous mass in the mid-abdomen, inferior to the stomach. The thickened peritoneum (arrow) adjacent to the mass is suggestive of a malignant lesion, which in this case was an ovarian carcinoma.[193]

Condition	Imaging Findings	Comments
Infectious processes (Fig GI 88-14)	Initially may appear as a low-attenuation, loculated fluid collection. As an abscess matures, the surrounding peritoneal membrane thickens and shows marked contrast enhancement. Gas bubbles are pathognomonic, but seen in less than one-third of cases. A gas-fluid level indicates fistulization to the intestinal lumen. Paragonimiasis can produce multiple, small, often densely calcified nodules scattered in the peritoneal cavity.	May develop from perforation (ulcer, diverticulis) or secondary to an adjacent inflammation (pancreatitis, pericholecystitis) or surgery. Common locations include the right subphrenic space, the subhepatic space, and the pouch of Douglas. Oral contrast is often necessary to differentiate a fluid-containing intestinal loop from an abscess.
Miscellaneous lesions Omental infarction (Fig GI 88-15)	Variable appearance ranging from subtle, focal, hazy soft-tissue infiltration of the omentum to a more extensive, masslike fullness that can resemble infiltration from more ominous causes. A pattern of whirling fatty tissue around a vascular structure may be a specific finding.	Most commonly related to torsion secondary to a hernia, a focus of inflammation, previous laparotomy, or a tumor. Frequently occurring on the right, the nonspecific clinical appearance may be difficult to distinguish from acute appenditicits or cholecystitis.

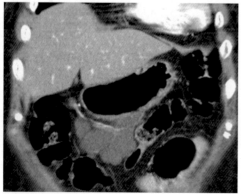

Fig GI 88-13
Lymphangioma. Coronal contrast scan shows a lobulated cystic mass in the greater omentum inferior to the gastric antrum.[193]

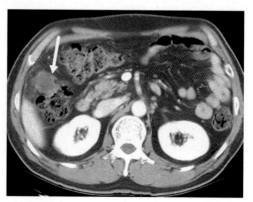

Fig GI 88-14
Paragonimiasis. Multifocal ill-defined cystic lesions and several nodules (arrow) in the omentum on the right side of the abdomen.[193]

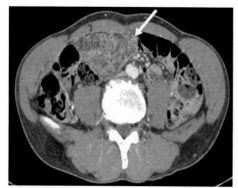

Fig GI 88-15
Omental infarction. Localized fatty infiltration and congestion with a secondary mass (arrow) in the right lower aspect of the anterior abdomen.[193]

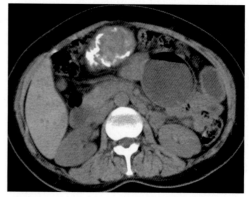

Fig GI 88-16
Foreign-body granuloma. Large, well-circumscribed mass with dense calcification in the anterior mid-abdomen, an appearance suggestive of a foreign-body granuloma or organizing hematoma. After contrast injection, the mass showed no enhancement. The patient had a palpable mass for 10 years that developed soon after a Caesarian section.[193]

Condition	Imaging Findings	Comments
Foreign body granuloma (Fig GI 88-16)	Well-circumscribed mass that may have dense calcification and a characteristic spongiform pattern with gas bubbles.	Adhesions and a thick capsule that develops around a retained laparotomy sponge and may manifest as acute or delayed nonspecific symptoms. An exudative response may lead to complications of fistula or abscess formation.
Hematoma	Acute intraperitoneal hemorrhage has high attenuation (>30–80 HU). In the chronic stage (1–2 weeks), the collection has decreased attenuation (0–20 HU).	Most common causes are blunt trauma (especially to the spleen or liver), intestinal perforation with vascular erosion, spontaneous rupture of a vascular tumor (hepatic adenoma, cavernous hemangioma, hepatoma, angiosarcoma), extrauterine pregnancy, and excessive coagulation or bleeding disorder.
Hernia (Fig GI 88-17)	May contain varying amounts of fat, soft-tissue, and gas-filled loops of bowel.	Sagittal and coronal reformations are of value for demonstrating hernia orifices, retained organs, and complications.
Sclerosing encapsulating peritonitis (Fig GI 88-18)	Dilated small bowel at the center of the abdomen, encased within a thick fibrocollagenous membrane (as in a cocoon).	Rare benign cause of acute or subacute intestinal obstruction.
Tumor-like conditions (Fig GI 88-19)	Focal soft-tissue masses that mimic peritoneal malignancy.	Aggressive fibromatosis (intra-abdominal desmoid), inflammatory pseudotumor, retractile mesenteritis, Castleman's disease.

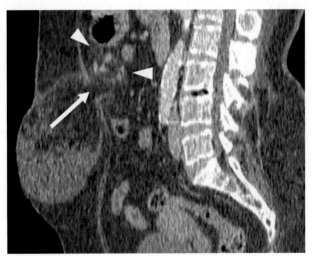

Fig GI 88-17
Ventral hernia. Sagittal scan shows herniation of omental fat through a defect (arrow) in the anterior abdominal wall. Focal ill-defined lesions with increased attenuation (arrowheads) in the omental fat adjacent to the abdominal wall defect are suggestive of omental fat infarction secondary to vascular compromise.[193]

A

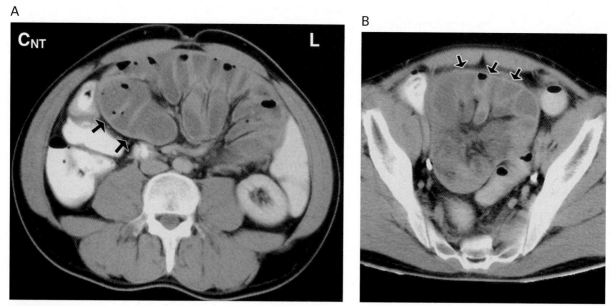

Fig GI 88-18
Sclerosing encapsulating peritonitis. (A, B) Sequential images show dilated small bowel loops in the center of the abdomen encapsulated within thick fibrous membranes (arrows).[197]

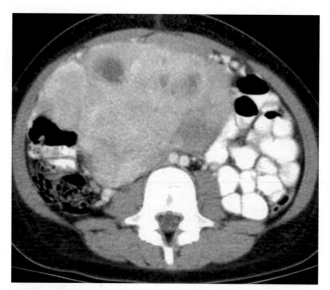

Fig GI 88-19
Inflammatory pseudotumor. The huge mass suggests a peritoneal malignancy.[194]

Hemoperitoneum

Blood usually has a higher attenuation than other body fluids, though its CT appearance may vary depending on the age, extent, and location of the hemorrhage. Because of its high protein content, unclotted extravasated blood generally measures 30 to 45 HU. However, this may be reduced in a patient with anemia (decreased serum hematocrit level) or in a hemorrhage that is more than 48 hours old. Clotted blood has an attenuation of 45 to 70 HU. Therefore, on CT images, the highest-attenuation hematoma (sentinel clot) is that closest to the site of bleeding, while the lower attenuation unclotted blood is located farther from the source. The sentinel clot sign is valuable for identifying the dominant source of hemoperitoneum in patients with multiple injuries from trauma. Active arterial extravasation of contrast material has an attenuation value higher than that of free or clotted blood.

Condition	Comments
Trauma	
Solid organ injury (Figs GI 89-1 and GI 89-2)	The spleen is the most frequently injured organ (40%) in blunt abdominal trauma. Injuries to the liver account for 20%, though the liver is the single most commonly injured organ when blunt and penetrating trauma are combined. Visceral injuries are conveniently divided into intraparenchymal contusion or hematoma, subcapsular hematoma, laceration, fracture, and vascular pedicle injury.
Bowel and mesenteric injury (Fig GI 89-3)	Found in about 5% of those who undergo surgery for blunt abdominal trauma, these injuries may be difficult to detect clinically since abdominal rigidity, pain, and decreased bowel sounds are apparent in only one-third of patients at initial presentation. Active extravasation of contrast can be seen if there is mesenteric vessel injury.
Iatrogenic (Fig GI 89-4)	Any surgical procedure performed within the peritoneal cavity may be complicated by hemoperitoneum.
Bleeding diathesis (Fig GI 89-5)	Anticoagulation therapy, blood dyscrasia.
Tumor-associated hemorrhage (Figs GI 89-6 and GI 89-7)	Although uncommon, any primary or metastatic tumor can rupture and bleed into the peritoneal cavity. The most common cause of nontraumatic hepatic hemorrhage is a hypervasvular neoplasm such as hepatocellular carcinoma or adenoma. Although common, hemangiomas are not associated with nontraumatic hemoperitoneum. Lung carcinoma, renal cell carcinoma, and melanoma are the metastatic lesions that most often cause hemoperitoneum.

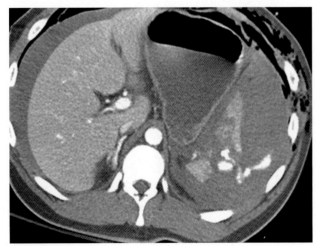

Fig GI 89-1
Acute arterial extravasation. Contrast CT scan shows active bleeding from a splenic rupture due to blunt trauma.[198] Note the sentinel clot sign produced by serpiginous areas of high attenuation surrounded by lower attenuation areas of hematoma.

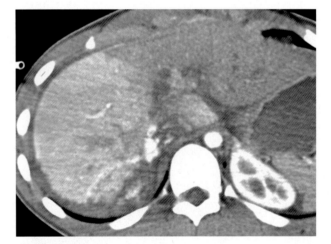

Fig GI 89-2
Liver avulsion. Large liver laceration with active extravasastion and hemoperitoneum following motor vehicle accident. At surgery, the liver was totally avulsed from the inferior vena cava, leaving the latter open at the level of the diaphragm.[198]

Condition	Comments
Gynecologic conditions (Figs GI 89-8 and GI 89-9)	The reproductive tract is the most common source of spontaneous hemoperitoneum in women of childbearing age. The most frequent causes are ectopic pregnancy and ruptured ovarian cyst. Endometriosis and uterine rupture causing peritoneal bleeding are much less common occurrences.
Vascular source (Fig GI 89-10)	A ruptured aortic aneurysm tends to cause retroperitoneal hemorrhage, though extremely large leaks occasionally result in bleeding into the peritoneal cavity. Splenic artery aneurysms, which account for 60% of visceral artery aneurysms are four times as common in women and the rate of rupture is especially increased during pregnancy. Other vascular sources for hemoperitoneum include hepatic artery aneurysms and pseudoaneuryms of the hepatic, splenic, and gastroduodenal arteries complicating pancreatitis.

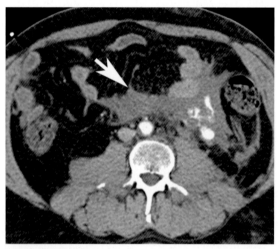

Fig GI 89-3
Mesenteric tear. Active extravasation from jejunal mesenteric vessels with associated jejunal injury and mesenteric hemorrhage indicated by a triangular region of hemoperitoneum (arrow).[198]

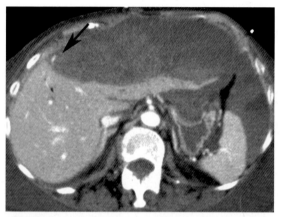

Fig GI 89-4
Hematoma after a pancreatoduodenectomy (Whipple's operation). Large abdominal hematoma that involves the left perihepatic and perisplenic space, with evidence of active extravasation (arrow).[198]

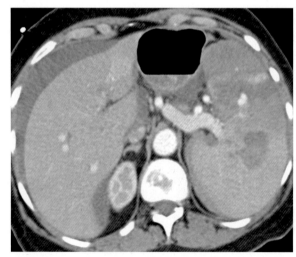

Fig GI 89-5
Splenic rupture in polycythemia vera. Pooling of contrast material in a huge spleen. Multiple splenic pseudo-aneurysms were subsequently treated with embolization.[198]

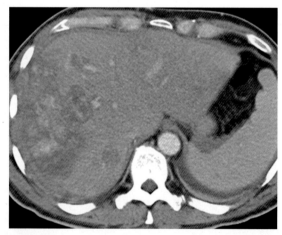

Fig GI 89-6
Ruptured hepatic angiosarcoma. Heterogeneous low-attenuation lesion in the right hepatic lobe, with evidence of increased vascularity, active extravasation, and hemoperitoneum. The high-attenuation material adjacent to the lesion represents perihepatic blood secondary to capsular rupture.[198]

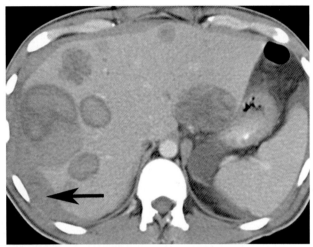

Fig GI 89-7
Hemorrhagic liver metastases (testicular choriocarci-noma). There are multiple hemorrhagic hepatic masses with central high attenuation. Hemoperitoneum (arrow) is seen adjacent to the largest lesion.[198]

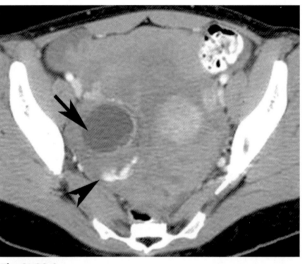

Fig GI 89-8
Ruptured hemorrhagic ovarian cyst. Adnexal cyst with an internal hematocrit level (arrow), surrounded by a pelvic hemorrhage. A curvilinear focus of extravasation (arrowhead) that is visible posterior to the cyst was found at surgery to represent acute bleeding from an internal iliac artery branch.[198]

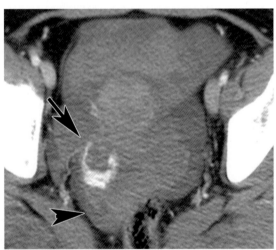

Fig GI 89-9
Ectopic pregnancy. Hemorrhagic right adnexal mass corresponds to an ectopic gestational sac with associated active extravasation (arrow) and blood in the cul-de-sac (arrowhead). (Courtesy of Alvaro Huete, M.D., Santiago, Chile.).[198]

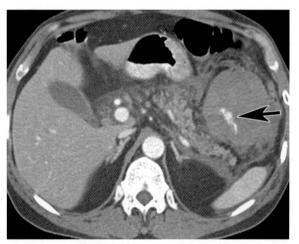

Fig GI 89-10
Hemorrhagic pancreatitis. Hematoma in the gastrocolic ligament with a focus of active extravasation (arrow). The bleeding vessel, a pancreatic branch of the splenic artery, was successfully embolized.[198]

Fatty Lesions in the Abdomen and Pelvis on Computed Tomography

Condition	Comments
Liver (Fig GI 90-1)	Angiomyolipomas consist of fat and blood vessels and appear as well-defined low-attenuation hepatic masses. Intratumoral areas of denser angiomuscular tissue may show strong enhancement. Lipomas are encapsulated tumors composed of adipose tissue that are sharply marginated and do not enhance. Fatty infiltration produces focal or generalized areas of low attenuation within the liver.
Pancreas (Figs GI 90-2 to GI 90-5)	Pancreatic lipomatosis is the term for fatty deposits in the parenchyma, which may occur in obese and diabetic patients with varying levels of pancreatic insufficiency. On contrast studies, a focal deposition of fat interposed between normal pancreatic parenchyma may mimic a hypoattenuating cystic or solid neoplasm. In advanced disease, especially in patients with cystic fibrosis, the entire pancreatic parenchyma is replaced by fat, and the fluid-filled pancreatic duct may even appear as a linear density.
Gastrointestinal tract (Figs GI 90-6 to GI 90-8)	Lipomas are submucosal fatty masses than can occur anywhere in the bowel. The presence of higher attenuation areas raises the possibility of liposarcoma, though this is rarely seen in the gastrointestinal tract. In epiploic appendagitis, there is a paracolonic oval fatty mass (the infarcted or inflamed appendix epiploica) surrounded by a well-circumscribed hyperattenuating rim (inflamed visceral peritoneal lining). Intussusceptions typically contains some mesentery attached to the involved segments of the bowel and may be led by a fatty mass (lipoma).

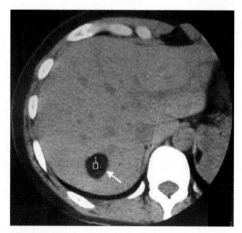

Fig GI 90-1
Hepatic angiomyolipoma. Well-defined oval mass (arrow) with an attenuation value of fatty tissue (−57 H) in a woman with an echogenic nodule suggestive of hemangioma detected on ultrasound.[199]

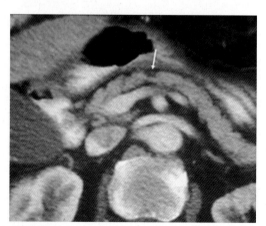

Fig GI 90-2
Focal fatty infiltration of the pancreas. Hypoattenuating pancreatic mass (arrow) that does not deform the border and has typical fatty density.[199]

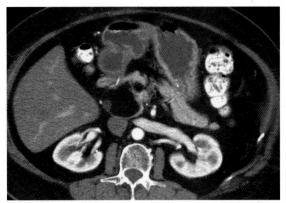

Fig GI 90-3
Lipoma of the pancreas. Large, homogeneous, fat-attenuation mass within the pancreatic head (arrows) with lateral displacement of the common bile duct (arrowhead).[200]

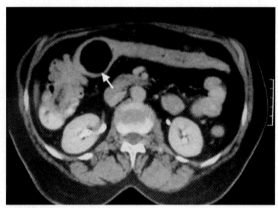

Fig GI 90-4
Pancreatic lipomatosis. Complete replacement of the parenchyma by fatty tissue with marked glandular atrophy. Note the dense acini (arrows) separated by increased fatty tissue.[199]

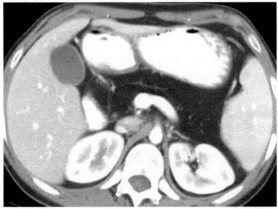

Fig GI 90-5
Fatty replacement of the pancreas. In a patient with cystic fibrosis, pancreatic tissue is virtually completely replaced by tissue with fat attenuation (arrowheads). Note the thin linear density of the main pancreatic duct.[200]

Fig GI 90-6
Colonic lipoma. Characteristic fat-attenuation mass (arrow) in the proximal part of the transverse colon.[199]

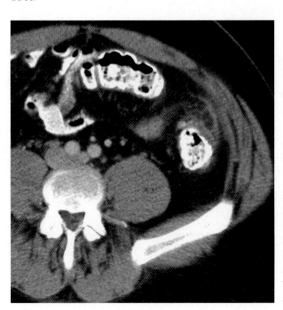

Fig GI 90-7
Epiploic appendagitis. Ovoid mass of fat attenuation (open arrow) anterior to the descending colon. The mass is surrounded by a hyperattenuating rim. A central high-attenuation dot was seen on images obtained superiorly (not shown). Note the moderate fat stranding (arrowhead) and the mild focal thickening of the adjacent colonic wall (solid arrow).[200]

Condition	Comments
Mesentery (Figs GI 90-9 and GI 90-10)	Mesenteric panniculitis is a rare inflammatory and fibrotic process in which the mesenteric vessels are surrounded and separated by a fatty mass and small well-differentiated nodules are seen in the mesentery. This "misty mesentery" appearance can also be produced by any process that infiltrates the mesentery, such as hemorrhage, edema, or tumor (lymphoma). Cavitating mesenteric lymph node syndrome is a complication of celiac disease in which very low attenuation in the cavitary masses may mimic fat.
Omentum (Fig GI 90-11)	Infarction may develop due to torsion or spontaneous venous thrombosis. CT demonstrates a large, cake-like mass centered in the omentum.
Herniation of abdominal and pelvic fat (Fig GI 90-12)	Inguinal hernias are the most common. Indirect hernias originate lateral to the inferior epigastric vessels, while direct hernias arise medially. Femoral hernias are more common in women. Less common hernias include spigelian (through the linea semilunaris), lumbar, and perineal.

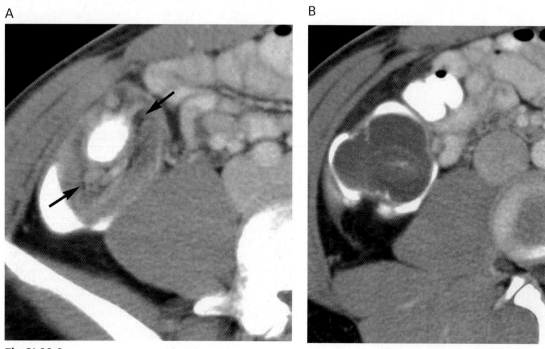

A   B

Fig GI 90-8
Intussusception led by a lipoma. (A) Small amount of mesenteric fat between the walls of the intussusceptum and the intussuscipiens (arrows). (B) More superior image shows a leading lipoma (arrowhead).[200]

Condition	Comments
Adrenal (Figs GI 90-13 to GI 90-15)	Myelolipomas are composed of mature fat cells associated with proliferating hematopoietic cells, which produce heterogeneous attenuation within the predominantly fatty mass. High-attenuation regions may reflect hemorrhage or calcifications. Adenomas are common tumors that usually are small and nonfunctional and detected as incidental findings. Hyperfunctional adenomas can produce Cushing's and Conn's syndromes.

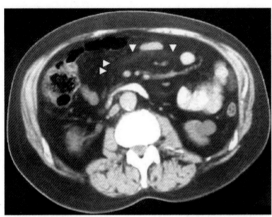

Fig GI 90-9
Mesenteric panniculitis. Discrete increase (arrowheads) in density of fatty tissue surrounding mesenteric vessels without evidence of vascular displacement. Note the thin halo of normal fatty tissue surrounding the mesenteric vessels.[199]

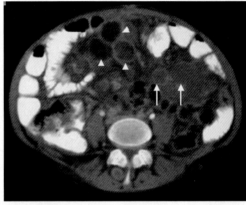

Fig GI 90-10
Cavitating mesenteric lymph node syndrome.
Multiple, round, fluid-attenuation masses with thin walls (arrows) in the mesentery. Some of the masses have lower attenuation values (arrowheads), indicating the presence of fatty material.[199]

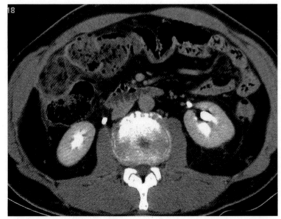

Fig GI 90-11
Omental infarction. Inhomogeneous, round, high-attenuation fatty mass in the greater omentum (arrows). The mass is anterior to the ascending colon and exerts mass effect on it. There is mild adjacent wall thickening (arrowhead).[200]

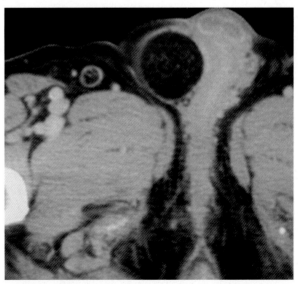

Fig GI 90-12
Inguinal hernia. Well-defined fatty mass within the inferior aspect of the right inguinal canal (arrow), representing herniation of intra-abdominal fat.[200]

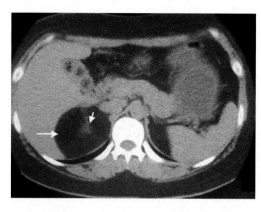

Fig GI 90-13
Adrenal myelolipoma. Large, heterogeneous right adrenal mass (long arrow) with a more dense area in the center (short arrow) and fatty attenuation (-102 H) in the periphery.[199]

A

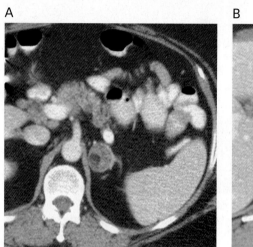

B

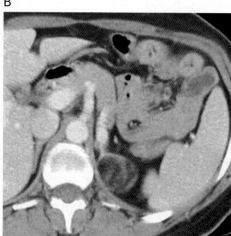

Fig GI 90-14
Adrenal myelolipoma. (A) Well-defined mass with predominantly soft-tissue attenuation in the left adrenal gland. Note the nodule of fat attenuation (arrow). (B) In another patient, a contrast scan shows a heterogeneous mass (arrows) with fatty and enhancing soft-tissue components. The presence of fat permits a reliable diagnosis of a benign myelolipoma despite the soft-tissue elements.[200]

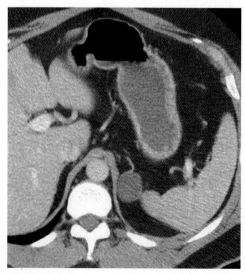

Fig GI 90-15
Adrenal adenoma. Low-attenuation mass in the left adrenal gland (arrow).[200]

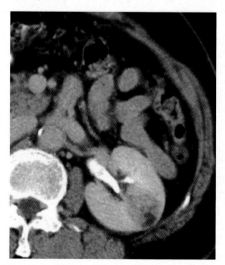

Fig GI 90-16
Renal angiomyolipoma. Heterogeneous mass in the lateral portion of the left kidney. The mass is predominantly of soft-tissue attenuation and resembles a renal cell carcinoma. However, the presence of focal areas of fat attenuation (arrows) permits confident diagnosis of an angiomyolipoma.[200]

Condition

Kidney
(Figs GI 90-16 to GI 90-20)

Comments

Angiomyolipomas are composed of abnormal blood vessels, mature fat, and smooth muscle that present as a heterogeneous fatty mass. A characteristic finding is linear or serpentine vascular structures traversing the lesion. Hemorrhage within the tumor may obscure its fatty nature. Uncommon renal lipomas are composed exclusively of adipose tissue and thus appear as sharply defined low-attenuation masses with no internal components or enhancement. Renal sinus lipomatosis is an excessive accumulation of fat that produces characteristic low-attenuation about the renal pelvis. Replacement lipomatosis, related to parenchymal atrophy secondary to chronic ureteral obstruction or a staghorn calculus, is essentially an advanced type of renal sinus lipomatosis.

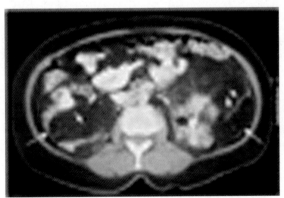

Fig GI 90-17
Bilateral renal angiomyolipomas. Bilateral low-attenuation masses (long arrows) projecting to the perinephric space in this patient with tuberous sclerosis. Note the serpentine vascular structures (short arrows) located within the lesions.[199]

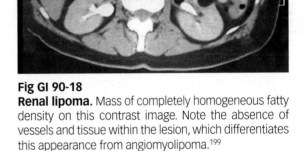

Fig GI 90-18
Renal lipoma. Mass of completely homogeneous fatty density on this contrast image. Note the absence of vessels and tissue within the lesion, which differentiates this appearance from angiomyolipoma.[199]

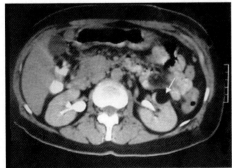

Fig GI 90-19
Renal sinus lipomatosis. Extensive fatty deposition in the left renal sinus (arrow) that surrounds and compresses the collecting system. The thickness of the renal parenchyma is slightly reduced (arrowheads). Of incidental note are thin calcifications in the gallbladder.[199]

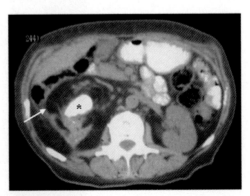

Fig GI 90-20
Replacement lipomatosis. Generous fatty infiltration (arrow) of both the right renal parenchyma and perinephric space. Note the calcified staghorn calculus (*) in the renal pelvis.[199]

Condition	Comments
Ovary (Figs GI 90-21 and GI 90-22)	Fat attenuation within an ovarian mass, with or without calcification, is consistent with a mature cystic teratoma. There may be a fat-water interface and the tumor may contain teeth or a hairy mass. Lipomas and leiomyosarcomas are extremely rare.
Retroperitoneum (Figs GI 90-23 and GI 90-24)	Liposarcoma is the most common retroperitoneal neoplasm in an adult. Differentiated tumors contain a substantial amount of fat and appear as heterogenous low-attenuation masses.

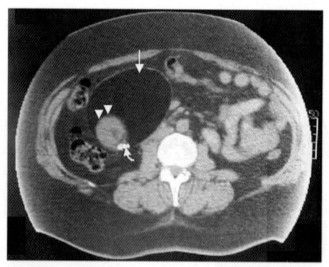

Fig GI 90-21
Ovarian teratoma. Large mass containing components of the three germ layers. It consists of low-attenuation fatty tissue (straight arrow), teeth (curved arrow), and structures with attenuation similar to that of the abdominal musculature (arrowheads).[199]

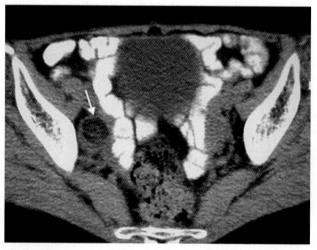

Fig GI 90-22
Ovarian lipoma. Well-defined tumor in the right adnexal region that has smooth margins (arrow) and the attenuation of fat.[199]

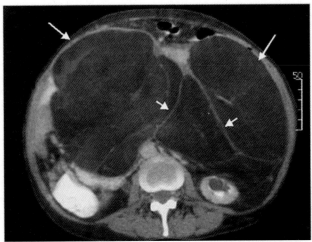

Fig GI 90-23
Retroperitoneal liposarcoma. There is a huge tumor mass (long arrows) with heterogeneous fatty attenuation that has septa (short arrows) and well-defined lobular contours. There is mass effect on adjacent structures, such as the left kidney, but no evidence of infiltration.[199]

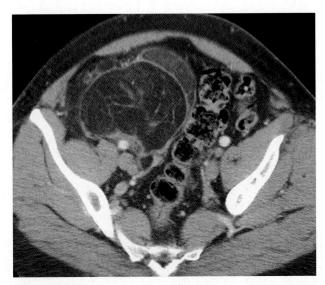

Fig GI 90-24
Retroperitoneal liposarcoma. The coarse, thickened septa (arrow) in this heterogeneous, fat-attenuation mass are suggestive of a well-differentiated tumor.[200]

Inferior Vena Cava (IVC) Filling Defects

Condition	Comments
Artifact	Delayed images showing resolution of the filling defect are usually sufficient to confirm the artifactual nature of these pseudolesions. At times, it may be necessary to perform flow-sensitive or delayed contrast-enhanced MRI sequences.
Pseudothrombosis (Fig GI 91-1)	This most common IVC filling defect seen on CT is caused by laminar flow of enhanced blood from the renal veins streaming parallel to the column of unopacified blood returning from the lower body.
Others (Fig GI 91-2)	Artifactual filling defects may also result from poorly enhanced blood, such as from an accessory hepatic vein, flowing into an opacified IVC, or from laminar reflux of opacified blood from the heart into the IVC (usually related to right heart disease or a high contrast injection rate). The rare "pseudolipoma," which refers to a partial volume artifact of juxtacaval fat above the caudate lobe rather than a true intraluminal lesion, is common in patients with chronic liver disease.
Benign filling defect (Figs GI 91-3 and GI 91-4)	By far the most common true filling defect of the IVC. It may be idiopathic or reflect a hypercoagulable state (oral contraceptive use, antiphospholipid syndrome, vascular injury, paraneoplastic syndrome, coagulopathy), venous stasis (immobility, heart failure, external compression), or a foreign body (IVC filter or venous catheter).

A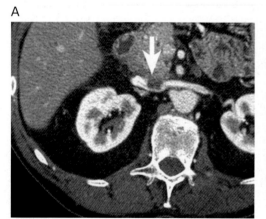

B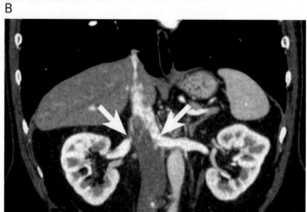

Fig GI 91-1
Laminar flow artifact. (A) Axial enhanced CT image shows a filling defect (arrow) caused by inflow of opacified blood from the renal veins mixing with poorly opacified blood in the IVC. (B) Curved multiplanar image reveals opacified blood from the renal veins streaming into the IVC (arrows), illustrating how the axial image can show an apparent IVC filling defect.[201]

Condition	Comments
Malignant filling defect (Figs GI 91-5 and GI 91-6)	Cancers can extend directly into the IVC from adjacent organs or occasionally arise as primary malignancies of the IVC. Neoplasms that commonly extend directly into the IVC include renal cell, hepatocellular, and adrenocortical carcinoma. At times, invasion may be secondary to metastases to the lung and kidney and retroperitoneal lumph nodes or from pancreatic carcinoma or Wilms' tumor. Primary intraluminal sarcomas are rare. Factors that distinguish malignant from bland thrombus include the presence of a contiguous adjacent mass and enhancement of the filling defect. However, malignancy predisposes to thrombosis due to hypercoagulability, and a bland downstream thrombus may coexist with a malignant thrombus more superiorly in the ICV.

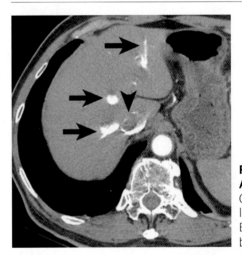

Fig GI 91-2
Artifact due to high injection rate. Early arterial phase CT image shows an IVC filling defect (arrowhead) due to laminar flow of refluxed contrast from the hepatic veins. Bright enhancement in the hepatic veins (arrows) is seen because of reflux of contrast from the heart.[201]

A   B

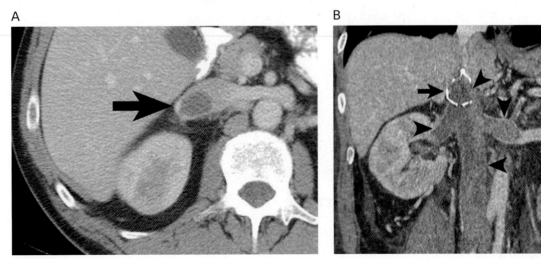

Fig GI 91-3
Bland thrombus. (A) Axial enhanced CT image before IVC filter placement shows bland thrombus (arrow) in the IVC. (B) Coronal multiplanar image reconstructed from CT data after IVC filter placement shows extension of bland thrombus into both renal veins (arrowheads) and the infrahepatic portion of the IVC. Note the IVC filter (arrow) and decreased enhancement of the right kidney due to hypoperfusion.[201]

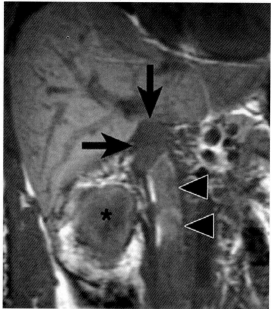

Fig GI 91-4
Bland and tumor thrombus. Coronal T1-weighted MR image reveals bland thrombus (arrowheads) that formed inferior relative to tumor thrombus (arrows) in the infrahepatic portion of the IVC. The low-signal-intensity lesion in the right kidney (*) represented renal cell carcinoma.[201]

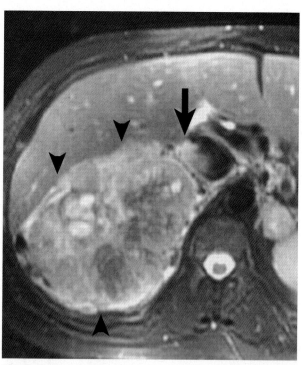

Fig GI 91-5
Renal cell carcinoma. Axial T2-weighted MR image with fat saturation shows a large, right renal mass (arrowheads) with heterogeneous high signal intensity. Note the tumor thrombus in the adjacent portion of the IVC (arrow).[201]

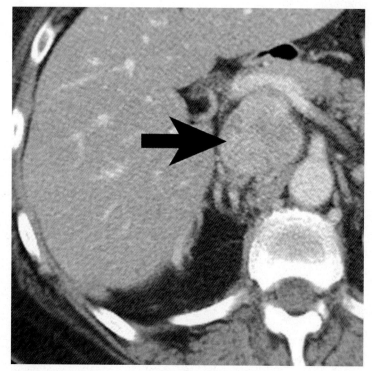

Fig GI 91-6
Leiomyosarcoma. Contrast CT scan demonstrates a heterogeneously enhancing mass (arrow) that arose in the IVC.[201]

Sources

1. Reprinted with permission from "Functional Disorders of the Pharyngoesophageal Junction" by WB Seaman, *Radiologic Clinics of North America* (1967;7:113–119), Copyright ©1967, WB Saunders Company.
2. Reprinted with permission from "A Roentgen-Anatomic Correlation" by JL Clements et al, *American Journal of Roentgenology* (1974;121: 221–231), Copyright ©1974, American Roentgen Ray Society.
3. Reprinted with permission from "Symptomatic Congenital Ectopic Gastric Mucosa in the Upper Esophagus" by SM Williams et al, *American Journal of Roentgenology* (1987;148:147–148), Copyright ©1987, American Roentgen Ray Society.
4. Nyugen KT, Kosiuk J, Place C, et al. Two unusual causes of dysphagia: a pictorial essay. *J Can Assoc Radiol* 1987;38:42.
5. Willing S, El Gammal T. Thoracic osteophyte producing dysphagia in a case of diffuse idiopathic skeletal hypertrophy. *Am J Gastroenterol* 1983;78:381.
6. Reprinted with permission from "Transverse Folds in the Human Esophagus" by VK Gohel et al, *Radiology* (1978;128:303–308), Copyright ©1978, Radiological Society of North America Inc.
7. Reprinted with permission from "Candida Esophagitis: Accuracy of Radiographic Diagnosis" by MS Levine, AJ Macones, and I Laufer, *Radiology* (1985;154:581–587), Copyright ©1985, Radiological Society of North America Inc.
8. Shortsleeve MJ, Levine MS. Herpes esophagitis in otherwise healthy patients: clinical and radiographic findings. *Radiology* 1992;182:859.
9. Balthazar EJ, Megibow AJ, Hulnick DH. Cytomegalovirus esophagitis and gastritis in AIDS. *AJR Am J Roentgenol* 1985;144:1201.
10. Goodman P, Pinero SS, Rance RM, et al. Mycobacterial esophagitis in AIDS. *Gastrointest Radiol* 1989;14:103.
11. Ghahremani GG, Gore RM, Breuer RI, et al. Esophageal manifestations of Crohn's disease. *Gastrointest Radiol* 1982;7:199.
12. Bova JG, Dutton NE, Goldstein HM, et al. Medication-induced esophagitis: diagnosis by double-contrast esophagography. *AJR Am J Roentgenol* 1987;148:731.
13. Agha FP. The esophagus after endoscopic injection sclerotherapy. Acute and chronic changes. *Radiology* 1984;153:37.
14. Luedtke P, Levine MS, Rubesin S, et al. Radiologic Diagnosis of Benign Esophageal Strictures: A Pattern Approach. *RadioGraphics* 2003;23:897–909.
15. Levine MS, Rubesin SE. Diseases of the Esophagus: Diagnosis with Esophagography. *Radiology* 2005;237:414–427.
16. Zimmerman SL, Levine MS, Rubesin SE, et al. Idiopathic Eosinophilic Esophagitis in Adults. The Ringed Esophagus. *Radiology* 2005; 236:159–165.
17. Reprinted with permission from "Calcified Primary Tumors of the Gastrointestinal Tract" by GG Ghahremani, MA Meyers, and RB Port, *Gastrointestinal Radiology* (1978;2:331–339), Copyright ©1978, Springer-Verlag.
18. Plavsic BM, Robinson AE. Intraluminal esophageal diverticulum caused by ingestion of acid. *AJR Am J Roentgenol* 1992;159: 765–766.
19. Reprinted with permission from "Crohn's Disease of the Stomach: The 'Ram's Horn' Sign" by J Farman et al, *American Journal of Roentgenology* (1975;123:242–251), Copyright ©1975, American Roentgen Ray Society.
20. Reprinted with permission from "Phlegmonous Gastritis" by MA Turner, MC Beachley, and B Stanley, *American Journal of Roentgenology* (1979;133:527–528), Copyright ©1979, American Roentgen Ray Society.
21. Levy AD, Sobin LH. Gastrointestinal Carcinoids: Imaging Features with Clinicopathologic Comparison. *RadioGraphics* 2007;27: 237–257.
22. Reprinted with permission from "An Evaluation of Nissen Fundoplication" by J Skucas et al, *Radiology* (1976;118:539–543), Copyright ©1976, Radiological Society of North America Inc.
23. Reprinted with permission from "Nonfundic Gastric Varices" by T Sos, MA Meyers, and HA Baltaxe, *Radiology* (1972;105:579–580), Copyright ©1972, Radiological Society of North America Inc.
24. Macpherson RI. Gastrointestinal tract duplications: clinical, pathologic, etiologic, and radiologic considerations. *RadioGraphics* 1993;13: 1063–1080.
25. Reprinted with permission from "Elevated Lesions in the Duodenal Bulb Caused by Heterotopic Gastric Mucosa" by R Langkamper et al, *Radiology* (1980;137:621–624), Copyright ©1980, Radiological Society of North America Inc.
26. Buck JL, Elsayed AM. Ampullary tumors: radiologic–pathologic correlation. *RadioGraphics* 1993;13:193–212.
27. Reprinted with permission from "Chronic Idiopathic Intestinal Pseudo-Obstruction" by JE Maldonado et al, *American Journal of Medicine* (1970;49:203–212), Copyright ©1970, Technical Publishing Company.
28. Reprinted from *Radiology of the Newborn and Young Infant* by LE Swischuk with permission of Williams & Wilkins Company, ©1980.
29. Ekberg O, Sjostrom B, Brahme F. Radiological findings in *Yersinia ileitis. Radiology* 1977;15:123.
30. Matsui T, Iida M, Murakami M, et al. Intestinal anisakiasis: clinical and radiologic features. *Radiology* 1985;157:299.
31. Reprinted with permission from "Tumors of the Small Intestine" by CA Good, *American Journal of Roentgenology* (1963;89:685–705), Copyright ©1963, American Roentgen Ray Society.
32. Gedgaudas-McClees RK. *Handbook of Gastrointestinal Imaging.* New York: Churchill-Livingstone, 1987.
33. Ko YT, Lim JH, Lee DH, et al. Small intestinal bezoar: sonographic detection. *Abdom Imaging* 1993;18:271–272.
34. Zalev AH, Gardiner GW. Crohn's disease of the small intestine with polypoid configuration. *Gastrointest Radiol* 1991;16:18–20.
35. Tada S, Iida M, Matsui T, et al. Amyloidosis of the small intestine: findings on double-contrast radiographs. *AJR Am J Roentgenol* 1991;156:741–744.
36. Reprinted with permission from "The Roentgen Diagnosis of Retractile Mesenteritis" by AR Clemett and DG Tracht, *American Journal of Roentgenology* (1969;107:787), Copyright ©1969, American Roentgen Ray Society.
37. Reprinted with permission from "Giant Duodenal Ulcers" by RL Eisenberg, AR Margulis, and AA Moss, *Gastrointestinal Radiology* (1978;2:347–353), Copyright ©1978, Springer-Verlag.
38. Reprinted with permission from "Intraluminal Duodenal Diverticulum" by JCH Laudan and GI Norton, *American Journal of Roentgenology* (1963;90:756–760), Copyright ©1963, American Roentgen Ray Society.
39. Nakano H, Jaramillo E, Watanabe M, et al. Intestinal tuberculosis: findings on double-contrast barium enema. *Gastrointest Radiol* 1992;17:108–114.
40. Reprinted with permission from "Cecal Diverticulitis in Young Patients" by JF Norfray et al, *Gastrointestinal Radiology* (1980;5:379–382), Copyright ©1980, Springer-Verlag.
41. Reprinted with permission from "Typhoid Fever" by RS Francis and RN Berk, *Radiology* (1974;112:583–585), Copyright ©1974, Radiological Society of North America Inc.
42. Marn CS, Yu BFB, Nostrant TT, et al. Idiopathic cecal ulcer: CT findings. *AJR Am J Roentgenol* 1989;153:761–763.
43. Nakamura S, Iida M, Tominaga M, et al. *Salmonella* colitis: assessment with double-contrast barium enema examination in seven patients. *Radiology* 1992;184:537–540.

44. Reprinted with permission from "Nonspecific Ulcers of the Colon Resembling Annular Carcinoma" by GA Gardiner and CR Bird, *Radiology* (1980;137:331–334), Copyright ©1980, Radiological Society of North America Inc.

45. Reprinted with permission from "Colitis in the Elderly: Ischemic Colitis Mimicking Ulcerative and Granulomatous Colitis" by RL Eisenberg, CK Montgomery, and AR Margulis, *American Journal of Roentgenology* (1979;133:1113–1118), Copyright ©1979, American Roentgen Ray Society.

46. Reprinted with permission from "Caustic Colitis Due to Detergent Enema" by SK Kim, C Cho, and EM Levinsohn, *American Journal of Roentgenology* (1980;134:397–398), Copyright ©1980, American Roentgen Ray Society.

47. Puy-Montbrun T, Delechenault P, Ganansia R, et al. Rectal stenosis due to Veganine suppositories. *Gastrointest Radiol* 1990;15:169–170.

48. Levy AD, Sobin LH. Gastrointestinal carcinoids: imaging features with clinicopathologic comparison. *RadioGraphics* 2007;27:237–257.

49. Reprinted with permission from "Value of the Pre-Operative Barium Enema Examination in the Assessment of Pelvic Masses" by RK Gedgaudas et al, *Radiology* (1983;146:609–616), Copyright ©1983, Radiological Society of North America Inc.

50. Reprinted with permission from "Lymphoid Follicular Pattern of the Colon in Adults" by FM Kelvin et al, *American Journal of Roentgenology* (1979;133:821–825), Copyright ©1979, American Roentgen Ray Society.

51. Reprinted with permission from "Plain Film Findings in Severe Pseudomembranous Colitis" by RJ Stanley et al, *Radiology* (1976;118:7–11), Copyright ©1976, Radiological Society of North America Inc.

52. Reprinted with permission from "Double Tracking in the Sigmoid Colon" by JT Ferrucci et al, *Radiology* (1976;120:307–312), Copyright ©1976, Radiological Society of North America Inc.

53. Levy A, Murakata L, Abbott RM, Rohrmann CA. Benign Tumors and Tumorlike Lesions of the Gallbladder and Extrahepatic Bile Ducts: Radiologic-Pathologic Correlation. *RadioGraphics* 2002;22:387–413.

54. Reprinted with permission from "Cholangiographic Findings in Cholangiolitic Hepatitis" by DA Legge et al, *American Journal of Roentgenology* (1971;113:16–20), Copyright ©1971, American Roentgen Ray Society.

55. Reprinted with permission from "Congenital Hepatic Fibrosis Associated with Renal Tubular Ectasia" by I Unite et al, *Radiology* (1973;109:565–570), Copyright ©1973, Radiological Society of North America Inc.

56. Reprinted with permission from "Recurrent Pyogenic Cholangitis in Chinese Immigrants" by CS Ho and DE Wesson, *American Journal of Roentgenology* (1974;122:368–374), Copyright ©1974, American Roentgen Ray Society.

57. Takeyama N, Gokan T, Ohgiya Y, et al. CT of Internal Hernias. *RadioGraphics* 2005;25:997–1015.

58. Wojtasek DA, Codner MA, Nowak EJ. CT diagnosis of cecal herniation through the foramen of Winslow. *Gastrointest Radiol* 1991;16:77–79.

59. Wechsler RJ, Kurtz AB, Needleman L, et al. Cross-sectional imaging of abdominal wall hernias. *AJR Am J Roentgenol* 1989;153:517–521.

60. Aguirre DA, Santosa AC, Casola G, Sirlin CB. Abdominal Wall Hernias: Imaging Features, Complications, and Diagnostic Pitfalls at Multi-Detector Row CT. *RadioGraphics* 2005;25:1501–1520.

61. Lee GHL, Cohen AJ. CT imaging of abdominal hernias. *AJR Am J Roentgenol* 1993;161:1209–1213.

62. Maglinte DDT, Alvarez SZ, Ng AC, et al. Patterns of calcifications and cholangiographic findings in hepatobiliary tuberculosis. *Gastrointest Radiol* 1988;13:331–335.

63. Reprinted with permission from "Plain Film Roentgenographic Findings in Alveolar Hydatid Disease: *Echinococcus multilocularis*" by WM Thompson, DP Chisholm, and R Tank, *American Journal of Roentgenology* (1972;116:345–358), Copyright ©1972, American Roentgen Ray Society.

64. Reprinted with permission from "Calcifications in the Liver" by JJ Dariak, M Moskowitz, and KR Kattan, *Radiologic Clinics of North America* (1980;18:209–219), Copyright ©1980, WB Saunders Company.

65. Baker SR, Broker MH, Charnsangavej C, et al. Calcification in the portal vein wall. *Radiology* 1984;152:18.

66. Reprinted with permission from "Radiodense Liver in Transfusion Hemochromatosis" by WL Smith and F Quattromani, *American Journal of Roentgenology* (1977;128:316–317), Copyright ©1977, American Roentgen Ray Society.

67. Paige ML, Ghahremani GG, Brosnan JJ. Laminated radiopaque enteroliths: diagnostic clues to intestinal pathology. *Am J Gastroenterol* 1987;82:432.

68. Reprinted with permission from "Calcification in an Insulinoma of the Pancreas" by EL Wolf et al, *American Journal of Gastroenterology* (1984;79:559–561), Copyright ©1976, Williams & Wilkins.

69. Reprinted with permission from "Differential Diagnosis of Pancreatic Calcification" by EJ Ring et al, *American Journal of Roentgenology* (1973;117:446–452), Copyright ©1973, American Roentgen Ray Society.

70. Reprinted with permission from "An Early Rim Sign in Neonatal Adrenal Hemorrhage" by PW Brill, IH Krasna, and H Aaron, *American Journal of Roentgenology* (1976;127:289–291), Copyright ©1976, American Roentgen Ray Society.

71. Reprinted from *Radiology of the Kidney* by AJ Davidson with permission of WB Saunders Company, ©1985.

72. Reprinted with permission from "Calcified Renal Masses: A Review of Ten Years' Experience at the Mayo Clinic" by WW Daniel et al, *Radiology* (1972;103:503–508), Copyright ©1972, Radiological Society of North America Inc.

73. Reprinted with permission from "Gonadoblastoma: An Ovarian Tumor with Characteristic Pelvic Calcifications" by EQ Seymour et al, *American Journal of Roentgenology* (1976;127:1001–1002), Copyright ©1976, American Roentgen Ray Society.

74. Ney C, Friedenberg RM. *Radiographic Atlas of the Genitourinary System*. Philadelphia: Lippincott, 1981.

75. Baker SR, Elkin M. *Plain Film Approach to Abdominal Calcifications*. Philadelphia: WB Saunders, 1983.

76. Reprinted with permission from "Calcification in Undifferentiated Abdominal Malignancies" by MK Dalinka et al, *Clinical Radiology* (1975;26:115–119), Copyright ©1975, Royal College of Radiologists.

77. Ba-Ssalamah A, Prokop M, Uffmann M, et al. Dedicated Multi-detector CT of the Stomach: Spectrum of diseases. *RadioGraphics* 2005;23:625–644.

78. Fishman EK, Urban BA, Hruban RH. CT of the stomach: spectrum f disease. *RadioGraphics* 1996;16:1035–1054.

79. Insko EK, Levine MS, Birnbaum BA, Jacobs JE. Benign and malignant lesions of the stomach: evaluation of CT criteria for differentiation. *Radiology* 2003;228:166–171.

80. Jayaraman MV, Mayo-Smith WW, Movson JE, et al. CT of the duodenum: an overlooked segment gets its due. *RadioGraphics* 2001;21:S147–S160.

81. Wittenberg J, Harisinghani MG, Jhaveri K, et al. Algorithmic approach to CT diagnosis of the abnormal bowel wall. *RadioGraphics* 2002;22:1093–1109.

82. Hoeffel C, Crema MD, Belkacem A. Multi-detector row CT: spectrum of disease involving the ileocecal area. *RadioGraphics* 2006;26:1373–1390.

83. Levine DS, Navarro OM, Chaudry, et al. Imaging the complications of bone marrow transplantation in children. *RadioGraphics* 2007;27:307–324.

84. Lucey BC, Stuhlfaut JW, Soto JA. Mesenteric lymph nodes seen at imaging: causes and significance. *RadioGraphics* 2005;25:351–365.

85. Yenarkarn P, Thoeni RF, Hanks D. Case 107: Lymphoma of the Mesentery. *Radiology* 2007;242:628–631.

86. Pickhardt PJ, Bhalla S. Unusual nonneoplastic peritoneal and subperitoneal conditions: CT findings. *RadioGraphics* 2005;25:719–730.

87. Levy A, Murakata L, Abbott RM, Rohrmann CA. Benign tumors and tumorlike lesions of the gallbladder and extrahepatic bile ducts: radiologic-pathologic correlation. *RadioGraphics* 2002;22:387–413.

88. Hanbidge AE, Buckler PM, O'Malley ME, Wilson SR. Imaging evaluation for acute pain in the right upper quadrant. *RadioGraphics* 2004;24:1117–1133.

89. Reprinted from *Alimentary Tract Radiology*, ed 3, by AR Margulis and HJ Burhenne (Eds) with permission of The CV Mosby Company, St Louis, ©1983.

90. Reprinted with permission of "Caroli's Disease: Sonographic Findings" by CA Mittelstaedt et al, *American Journal of Roentgenology* (1980;134:585–587), Copyright ©1980, American Roentgen Ray Society.

91. Esensten M, Ralls PW, Colletti P, et al. Posttraumatic intrahepatic biloma: sonographic diagnosis. *AJR Am J Roentgenol* 1983;140:303–305.

92. Mortele KJ, Segatto E, Ros P. The infected liver: Radiologic-pathologic correlation. *RadioGraphics* 2004;24:937–955.

93. Levy A, Murakata L, Abbott RM, Rohrmann CA. Benign tumors and tumorlike lesions of the gallbladder and extrahepatic bile ducts: radiologic-pathologic correlation. *RadioGraphics* 2002;22:387–413.

94. Athey PA, Sax SL, Lamki N, et al. Sonography in the diagnosis of hepatic artery aneurysms. *AJR Am J Roentgenol* 1986;147:725–727.

95. Krebs CA, Giyanani VL, Eisenberg RL. *Ultrasound Atlas of Disease Processes*. Norwalk: Appleton & Lange, 1993.

96. Reprinted from *Ultrasonography of Digestive Diseases* by FS Weill, The CV Mosby Company, St Louis, with permission of the author, ©1982.

97. Hanbidge AE, Buckler PM, O'Malley ME, Wilson SR. Imaging evaluation for acute pain in the right upper quadrant. *RadioGraphics* 2004;24:1117–1133.

98. Reprinted with permission from "Ultrasonography and Computed Tomography in the Evaluation of Hepatic Microabscesses in the Immunosuppressed Patient" by PW Callen, RA Filly, and FS Marcus, *Radiology* (1980;136:433–434), Copyright ©1980, Radiological Society of North America Inc.

99. Pedrosa I, Saiz A, Arrazola J, et al. Hydatid disease: radiologic and pathologic features and complications. *RadioGraphics* 2000;20:793–817.

100. Mortele KJ, Segatto E, Ros P. The infected liver: radiologic-pathologic correlation. *RadioGraphics* 2004;24:937–955.

101. Bude RO, Bowerman RA. Case 20: Biliary ascariasis. *Radiology* 2000;214:844–947.

102. Marn CS, Bree RL, Silver TM. Ultrasonography of the liver: technique and focal and diffuse disease. *Radiol Clin North Am* 1991;29:1151–1168.

103. Reprinted with permission from "Infantile Hemangioendothelioma of the Liver" by AH Dachman et al, *American Journal of Roentgenology* (1983;140:1091–1096), Copyright ©1983, American Roentgen Ray Society.

104. Brandt DJ, Johnson CD, Stephens DH, et al. Imaging of fibrolamellar hepatocellular carcinoma. *AJR Am J Roentgenol* 1988;151:295–299.

105. Ros PR, Buck JL, Goodman ZD, et al. Intrahepatic cholangiocarcinoma: radiologic-pathologic correlation. *Radiology* 1988;167:689–693.

106. Choi BI, Lim JH, Han MC. Biliary cystadenoma and cystadenocarcinoma: CT and sonographic findings. *Radiology* 1989;171:57–61.

107. Prasad SR, Hanlin W, Rosas H, et al. Fat-containing lesions of the liver: radiologic-pathologic correlation. *RadioGraphics* 2005;25:321–331.

108. Baker MK, Wenker JC, Cockerill EM, et al. Focal fatty infiltration of the liver: diagnostic imaging. *RadioGraphics* 1985;5:923–939.

109. Courtesy of Diego Aguirre, M.D., Fundacion Santa Fe de Bogota, Bogota, Columbia in Restrepo CS, Martinez S, Lemos JA, et al.

110. Kurtz AB, Rubin CS, Cooper HS, et al. Ultrasound findings in hepatitis. *Radiology* 1980;136:717–723

111. Eisenberg RL. *Clinical Imaging: An Atlas of Differential Diagnosis*. Gaithersburg: Aspen, 1992.

112. Weill FS. *Ultrasonography of Digestive Diseases*. St Louis: CV Mosby, 1982.

113. Hanbidge AE, Buckler PM, O'Malley ME, Wilson SR. Imaging evaluation for acute pain in the right upper quadrant. *RadioGraphics* 2004;24:1117–1133.

114. Reprinted with permission from "Hepatic Cysts: Treatment with Alcohol" by WJ Bean and BA Rodan, *American Journal of Roentgenology* (1985;144:237–241), Copyright ©1985, American Roentgen Ray Society.

115. Brancatelli G, Federle MP, Vilgrain V, et al. Fibropolycystic liver disease: CT and MR imaging findings. *RadioGraphics* 2005;25:659–670.

116. Reprinted with permission from "Variable CT Appearance of Hepatic Abscesses" by RA Halvorsen et al, *American Journal of Roentgenology* (1984;142:941–947), Copyright ©1984, American Roentgen Ray Society.

117. Hanbidge AE, Buckler PM, O'Malley ME, Wilson SR. Imaging evaluation for acute pain in the right upper quadrant. *RadioGraphics* 2004;24:1117–1133.

118. Pedrosa I, Saiz A, Arrazola J, et al. Hydatid disease: radiologic and pathologic features and complications. *RadioGraphics* 2000;20:793–817.

119. Mortele KJ, Segatto E, Ros P. The Infected liver: radiologic-pathologic correlation. *RadioGraphics* 2004;24:937–955.

120. Lim JH, Kim SY, Park CM. Parasitic diseases of the biliary tract. *AJR Am J Roentgenol* 2007;188:1596–1603.

121. Restrepo CS, Martinez S, Lemos JA, et al. Imaging Manifestations of Kaposi Sarcoma. *RadioGraphics* 2006;26:1169–1183.

122. Reprinted from *Computed Tomography of the Body* by AA Moss, G Gamsu, and HK Genant (Eds) with permission of WB Saunders Company, ©1983.

123. Mendez-Uriburu L, Ahualli J, Mendez-Uriburu J, et al, CT Appearances of intraabdominal and intrapelvic fatty lesions. *AJR Am J Roentgenol* 2004;183:933–943.

124. Lucaya J, Enriquez G, Amat L, et al. Computed tomography of infantile hepatic hemangioendothelioma. *AJR Am J Roentgenol* 1985;144:821–826.

125. Buetow PC, Buck JL, Ros PR, et al. Malignant vascular tumors of the liver: radiologic-pathologic correlation. *RadioGraphics* 1994;14:153–166.

126. Fishman EK, Kuhlman JE, Jones RJ. CT of lymphoma: spectrum of disease. *RadioGraphics* 1991;11:647–669.

127. Unger EC, Lee JKT, Weyman PJ. CT and MR imaging of radiation hepatitis. *J Comput Assist Tomogr* 1987;11:264–268.

128. Murphy BJ, Casillas J, Ros PR, et al. The CT appearance of cystic masses in the liver. *RadioGraphics* 1989;9:307–322.

129. Foley WD, Jochem RJ. Computed tomography: focal and diffuse liver disease. *Radiol Clin North Am* 1991;29:1213–1234.

130. Savader SJ, Benenati JF, Venbrux AC, et al. Choledochal cysts: classification and cholangiographic appearance. *AJR Am J Roentgenol* 1991;156:327–331.

131. Koyama T, Ueda H, Togashi K, et al. Radiologic manifestations of sarcoidosis in various organs. *RadioGraphics* 2004;24:87–104.

132. Suzuki S, Takizawa K, Nakajima Y, et al. CT findings in hepatic and splenic amyloidosis. *J Comput Assist Tomogr* 1986;10:332–334.

133. Moss AA, Gamsu G, Genant HK, eds. *Computed Tomography of the Body with Magnetic Resonance Imaging*. Philadelphia: WB Saunders, 1992.

134. Valls C, Andia E, Sanchez A, et al. Hyperenhancing focal liver lesions: Differential diagnosis with helical CT. *AJR Am J Roentgenol* 1999;173:605.

135. Foley WD, Jochem RJ. Computed tomography: focal and diffuse liver disease. *Radiol Clin North Am* 1991;29:1213.

136. Mortele KJ, Ros P. Cystic focal liver lesions in the adult: differential CT and MR imaging features. *RadioGraphics* 2001;21:895–910.

137. Prasad SR, Hanlin W, Rosas H, et al. Fat-containing lesions of the liver: radiologic-pathologic correlation. *RadioGraphics* 2005;25: 321–331.

138. Keenan WB. The diagnosis: amiodarone toxicity. *Radiology Today* 1994 (January);17.

139. Gore RM, Levine MS, Lauger I, eds. *Textbook of Gastrointestinal Radiology*. Philadelphia: WB Saunders, 1994.

140. Moulton JS, Miller BL, Dodd GD, et al. Passive hepatic congestion in heart failure: CT abnormalities. *AJR Am J Roentgenol* 1988;151: 932–939.

141. Georgiades CS, Neyman EG, Barish MA, Fishman EK. Amyloidosis: Review and CT Manifestations. *RadioGraphics* 2004;24:405–416.

142. Mathieu D, Vilgrain V, Mahfouz AE, et al. Benign liver tumors. *Magn Reson Imaging Clin N Am* 1997;5:255.

143. Brancatelli G, Federle MP, Vilgrain V, et al. Fibropolycystic liver disease: CT and MR imaging findings. *RadioGraphics* 2005;25: 659–670.

144. Ito K, Honjo K, Fujita, et al. Liver neoplasms: diagnostic pitfalls in cross-sectional imaging. *RadioGraphics* 1996;16:273.

145. Mergo PJ, Ros PR. MR imaging of inflammatory disease of the liver. *Magn Reson Imaging Clin N Am* 1997;5:367.

146. Elizondo G, Weissleder R, Stark DD, et al. Amebic liver abscess: diagnosis and treatment evaluation with MR imaging. *Radiology* 1987;165:795.

147. Kawamoto S, Soyer PA, Fishman EK, Bluemke DA. Nonneoplastic liver disease: Evaluation with CT and MR imaging. *RadioGraphics* 1998;18:827.

148. Montero JBM, Garcia A, Lafuente JL, et al. Fat-fluid level in hepatic hydatid cyst: A new sign of rupture into the biliary tree? *AJR Am J Roentgenol* 1996;167:91.

149. Buetow PC, Pantongrag-Brown L, Buck JL. Focal nodular hyperplasia of the liver: radiologic-pathologic correlation. *RadioGraphics* 1996;16:369.

150. Powers C, Ros PR, Stoupis C, et al. Primary liver neoplasms: MR imaging with pathologic correlation. *RadioGraphics* 1994;14:459.

151. Horton KM, Bluemke DA, Hruben RH, et al. CT and MR imaging of benign hepatic and biliary tumors. *RadioGraphics* 1999;19:431.

152. Casillas VJ, Amendola MA, Gascue A, et al. Imaging of nontraumatic hemorrhagic hepatic lesions. *RadioGraphics* 2000;20:363.

153. McLarney JK, Rucker PT, Bender GN, et al. Fibrolamellar carcinoma of the liver: Radiologic-pathologic correlation. *RadioGraphics* 1999;19:453.

154. Soyer P, Bluemke DA, Reichle R, et al. Imaging of intrahepatic cholangiocarcinoma. 1. Peripheral cholangiocarcinoma. *AJR Am J Roentgenol* 1995;165:1427.

155. Buetow PC, Midkiff RB. Primary malignant neoplasms in the adult. *Mag Reson Imaging Clin N Am* 1997;5:289.

156. Buetow PC, Buck JL, Pantongrag-Brown, et al. Undifferentiated (embryonal) sarcoma of the liver. Pathologic basis of imaging findings in 28 cases. *Radiology* 1997;203:779.

157. Sica GT, Ji H, Ros PR. CT and MR imaging of hepatic metastases. *AJR Am J Roentgenol* 2000;174:691.

158. Tani I, Kurihara Y, Kawaguchi A, et al. MR imaging of diffuse liver disease. *AJR Am J Roentgenol* 2000;174:965.

159. Levine DS, Navarro OM, Chaudry, et al. Imaging the complications of bone marrow transplantation in children. *RadioGraphics* 2007;27: 307–324.

160. Koyama T, Ueda H, Togashi K, et al. Radiologic manifestations of sarcoidosis in various organs. *RadioGraphics* 2004;24:87–104.

161. Kim S, Kim TU, Lee JW, et al. The perihepatic space: comprehensive anatomy and CT features of pathologic conditions. *RadioGraphics* 2007;27:129–143.

162. Reprinted from *Diagnostic Imaging in Internal Medicine* by RL Eisenberg with permission of McGraw-Hill Book Company, ©1985. Courtesy of Gretchen AW Gooding, MD.

163. Ros PR, Hamrick-Turner JE, Chiecho MV, et al. Cystic masses of the pancreas. *RadioGraphics* 1992;12:673–686.

164. Buetow PC, Rao P, Thompson LDR. Mucinous cystic neoplasms of the pancreas: Radiologic-pathologic correlation. *RadioGraphics* 1998;18:433–439.

165. Kim YH, Saini S, Sahani D, et al. Imaging diagnosis of cystic pancreatic lesions: Pseudocyst versus Nonpseudocyst. *RadioGraphics* 2005;25:671–685.

166. Van Rijn RR, Schilte PPM, Wiarda BM, et al. Case 113: Pancreatic cystosis. *RadioGraphics* 2007;243:598–602.

167. Sahani DV, Kadavigere R, Saokar A, et al. Cystic pancreatic lesions: a simple imaging-based classification system for guiding management. *RadioGraphics* 2005;25:1471–1484.

168. Kim YH, Saini S, Sahani D, et al. Imaging diagnosis of cystic pancreatic lesions: Pseudocyst versus Nonpseudocyst. *RadioGraphics* 2005;25:671–685.

169. Buetow PC, Rao P, Thompson LDR. Mucinous cystic neoplasms of the pancreas: Radiologic-pathologic correlation. *RadioGraphics* 1998;18:433–439.

170. Horton KM, Hriban RH, Yeo C, Fishman EH. Multi-detector row CT of pancreatic islet cell tumors. *RadioGraphics* 2006;26:453–464.

171. Kim YH, Saini S, Sahani D, et al. Imaging diagnosis of cystic pancreatic lesions: Pseudocyst versus Nonpseudocyst. *RadioGraphics* 2005;25:671–685.

172. Klein KA, Stephens DH, Welch TJ. CT characteristics of metastatic disease of the pancreas. *RadioGraphics* 1998;18:369–378.

173. Reprinted with permission from "Computed Tomography of Mesenteric Involvement in Fulminant Pancreatitis" by RB Jeffrey, MD Federle, and FC Laing, *Radiology* (1983;147:185–192), Copyright ©1983, Radiological Society of North America Inc.

174. Robertson MB, Choe KA, Joseph PM. Review of the abdominal manifestations of cystic fibrosis in the adult patient. *RadioGraphics* 2006;26:679–690.

175. Van Rijn RR, Schilte PPM, Wiarda BM, et al. Case 113: Pancreatic cystosis. *Radiology* 2007;243:598–602.

176. Fulcher AS, Turner MA, Capps GW. MR cholangiography: Technical advances and clinical applications. *RadioGraphics* 1999;19:25.

177. Lim JH, Kim SY, Park CM. Parasitic diseases of the biliary tract. *AJR Am J Roentgenol* 2007;188:1596–1603.

178. Brancatelli G, Federle MP, Vilgrain V, et al. Fibropolycystic liver disease: CT and MR imaging findings. *RadioGraphics* 2005;25: 659–670.

179. Fulcher AS, Turner MA. MR pancreatography: A useful tool for evaluating pancreatic disorders. *RadioGraphics* 1999;19:5.

180. Fulcher AS, Turner MA. MR cholangiography: Technical advances and clinical applications. *RadioGraphics* 1999;19:25.

181. Reprinted with permission from "Computed Tomography of the Spleen" by J Piekarski et al, *Radiology* (1980;135:683–689), Copyright ©1980, Radiological Society of North America Inc.

182. Rabushka LS, Kawashima A, Fishman EK. Imaging of the spleen: CT with supplemental MR examination. *RadioGraphics* 1994;14: 307–332.

183. Reprinted from *Computed Body Tomography* by JKT Lee, SS Sagel, and RJ Stanley (Eds) with permission of Raven Press, New York, ©1988.

184. Reprinted with permission from "Sonography of Splenic Abscess" by S Pawar et al, *American Journal of Roentgenology* (1982;138: 259–262), Copyright ©1982, American Roentgen Ray Society.

185. Restropo CS, Martinez S, Lemos JA, et al. Imaging Manifestations of Kaposi's sarcoma. *RadioGraphics* 2006;26:1169–1185.

186. Abbott RM, Levy A, Aguilera NS, et al. Primary vascular neoplasms of the spleen: radiologic-patholigc correlation. *RadioGraphics* 2004;24:1137–1163.

187. Abbott RM, Levy A, Aguilera NS, et al. Primary vascular neoplasms of the spleen: radiologic-patholigc correlation. *RadioGraphics* 2004;24:1137–1163.

188. Pistoia F, Markowitz SK. Splenic lymphangiomatosis: CT diagnosis. *AJR Am J Roentgenol* 1988;150:121–122.

189. Koyama T, Ueda H, Togashi K, et al. Radiologic manifestations of sarcoidosis in various organs. *RadioGraphics* 2004;24:87–104.

190. Urban BA, Fishman EK. Helical CT of the spleen. *AJR Am J Roentgenol* 1998;170:997.

191. Urrutia M, Mergo PJ, Ros LH, et al. Cystic masses of the spleen: Radiologic-pathologic correlation. *RadioGraphics* 1196;16:107.

192. Luna A, Ribes R, Caro P, et al. MRI of focal splenic lesions without and with dynamic gadolinium enhancement. *AJR Am J Roentgenol* 2006;186:1533–1547.

193. Yoo EY, Kim JH, Kim M-J, et al. Greater and lesser omentum: normal anatomy and pathologic processes. *RadioGraphics* 2007;27:707–720.

194. Pickhardt PJ, Bhalla S. Unusual nonneoplastic peritoneal and subperitoneal conditions: CT findings. *RadioGraphics* 2005;25:719–730.

195. Pickhardt PJ, Bhalla S. Primary neoplasms of peritoneal and subperitoneal origin: CT findings. *RadioGraphics* 2005;25:983–995.

196. Demir MK, Aker FV, Koskal N. Case 98: Primary Serous Papillary Carcinoma of the Peritoneum. *Radiology* 2006;240:905–909.

197. Demir MK, Akinci O, Onur E, Koskal N. Case 108: Sclerosing Encapsulating Peritonitis. *Radiology* 2007;242:939–939.

198. Lubner M, Menias C, Rucker C, et al. Blood in the Belly: CT Findings of Hemoperitoneum. *RadioGraphics* 2007;27:109–125.

199. Mendez-Uriburu L, Ahualli J, Mendez-Uriburu J, et al. CT Appearances of Intraabdominal and Intrapelvic Fatty Lesions. *AJR Am J Roentgenol* 2004;183:933–943.

200. Pereira JM, Sirlin CB, Pinto PS, Casola G. CT and MR imaging of extrahepatic fatty masses of the abdomen and pelvis: techniques, diagnosis, differential diagnosis, and pitfalls. *RadioGraphics* 2005;25:69–85.

201. Kaufman LB, Yeh BM, Breiman, et al. Inferior vena cava filling defects on CT and MRI. *AJR Am J Roentgenol* 2005;185:717–726.

4

Genitourinary Patterns

Misplaced, Displaced, or Absent Kidney

Condition	Imaging Findings	Comments
Unilateral renal agenesis (solitary kidney) (Fig GU 1-1)	Filling of the renal fossa with bowel loops (sharply outlined gas or fecal material in the plane of the renal fossa on nephrotomography). The contralateral kidney usually shows compensatory hypertrophy.	Rare anomaly that is associated with a variety of other congenital malformations. It is essential to exclude a nonfunctioning, diseased kidney by ultrasound or CT. After nephrectomy, the renal outline is generally preserved on plain films if the perinephric fat is left in situ.
Renal ectopia (Figs GU 1-2 and GU 1-3)	Abnormally positioned kidney that can be found in various locations. The ectopic kidney usually functions, though the nephrogram and pelvocalyceal system may be obscured by overlying bone and fecal contents.	Includes pelvic kidney, intrathoracic kidney, and crossed ectopia (the ectopic kidney lies on the same side as the normal kidney and is usually fused with it). Whenever only one kidney is seen on excretory urography, a full view of the abdomen is essential to search for an ectopic kidney.
Nephroptosis	Excessive caudal movement of a mobile kidney (especially the right) when the patient goes from supine to erect position. There may be associated changes in the ureter (angulation at the ureteropelvic junction, loops, kinks, and tortuosity).	Most commonly occurs in thin females. If a ptotic kidney becomes fixed in its dropped state, permanent ureteral kinking causes impaired drainage, increased hydronephrosis, and a greater chance of infection.
Malrotation (Fig GU 1-4)	Often bizarre appearance of the renal parenchyma, calyces, and pelvis that may suggest a pathologic condition in an otherwise normal kidney.	Unilateral or bilateral anomaly. When the renal pelvis is situated in an anterior or lateral position, the upper part of the ureter often appears to be displaced laterally, suggesting an extrinsic mass. The elongated pelvis of a malrotated kidney may mimic obstructive dilatation.

B

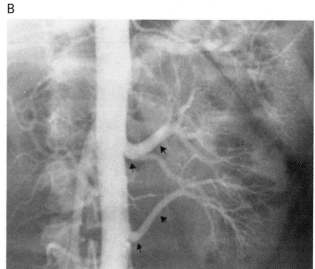

A

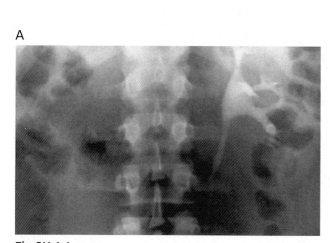

Fig GU 1-1
Solitary kidney. (A) Excretory urogram demonstrates a normal left kidney with no evidence of right renal tissue. (B) Aortogram shows two renal arteries to the left kidney (arrows) and no evidence of a right renal artery, thus confirming the diagnosis of unilateral renal agenesis.

Condition	Imaging Findings	Comments
Horseshoe kidney (Fig GU 1-5)	Characteristic urographic features include vertical or reversed longitudinal axes of the kidneys (upper poles tilted away from the spine), demonstration on the nephrogram phase of a parenchymal isthmus (if present) connecting the lower poles, and projection of the lower calyces medial to the upper calyces on frontal views. The large and flabby pelves may simulate an obstruction.	Most common type of fusion anomaly. Both kidneys are malrotated, and their lower poles are joined by a band of normal renal parenchyma (an isthmus) or connective tissue. True ureteropelvic junction obstruction may develop because of the unusual course of the ureter, which arises high in the renal pelvis, passes over the isthmus, and may kink at the ureteropelvic junction.

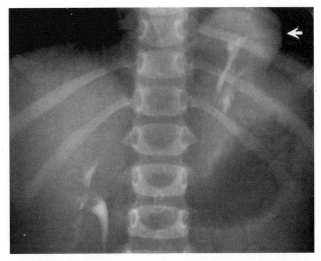

Fig GU 1-3
Intrathoracic kidney (arrow).

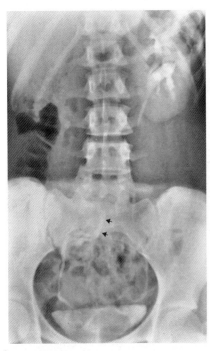

Fig GU 1-2
Pelvic kidney. The arrows point to the collecting system.

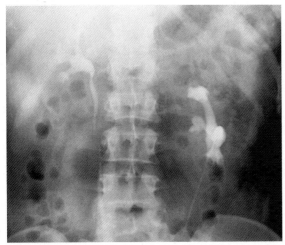

Fig GU 1-4
Malrotation of the left kidney. Note the apparent lateral displacement of the upper ureter and the elongation of the pelvis.

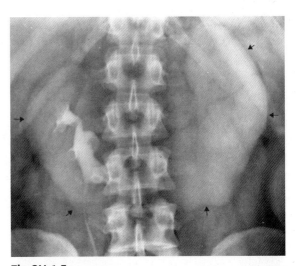

Fig GU 1-5
Horseshoe kidney (arrows). The prolonged nephrogram and delayed calyceal filling on the left are caused by an obstructing stone at the ureteropelvic junction on that side.

Condition	Imaging Findings	Comments
Hepatomegaly/splenomegaly (Fig GU 1-6)	Downward displacement of a kidney.	Liver enlargement almost always causes downward displacement of the right kidney.
Intra- or extrarenal masses Downward displacement (Fig GU 1-7)	Direction of displacement of the kidney depends on the type of underlying mass.	Adrenal tumor or hemorrhage; large upper pole intrarenal mass. Splenomegaly infrequently causes downward and medial displacement of the left kidney.
Upward displacement (Fig GU 1-8)		Small liver (high right kidney in advanced cirrhosis with a shrunken liver); Bochdalek's hernia (intrathoracic kidney); lower pole intrarenal mass.
Medial displacement (Fig GU 1-9)		Splenomegaly; large extracapsular or subcapsular renal mass (hematoma, lipoma).
Lateral displacement		Lymphoma; lymph node metastases; retroperitoneal sarcoma; expansion of a peripelvic mass (cyst, tumor, abscess, hydronephrosis); aortic aneurysm; adrenal tumor; pancreatic tumor or pseudocyst.

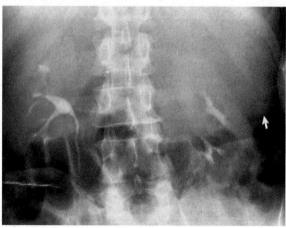

Fig GU 1-6
Splenomegaly. Downward displacement of the left kidney. The arrow points to the inferior margin of the spleen.

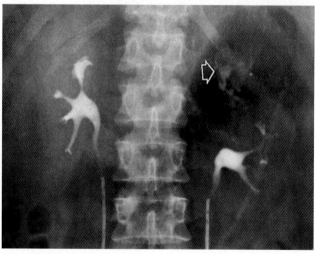

Fig GU 1-7
Calcified adrenal teratoma (arrow). Downward displacement of the left kidney.

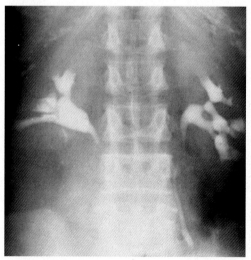

Fig GU 1-8
Renal cell carcinoma. Upward displacement of the right kidney and distortion of the collecting system by the large lower pole mass.

Condition	Imaging Findings	Comments
Transplanted kidney (Fig GU 1-10)	Kidney overlies the ilium.	Evidence of surgical clips or markers.

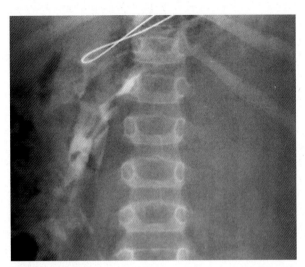

Fig GU 1-9
Wilms' tumor. Massive displacement of the left kidney across the midline by a huge mass filling much of the left side of the abdomen.

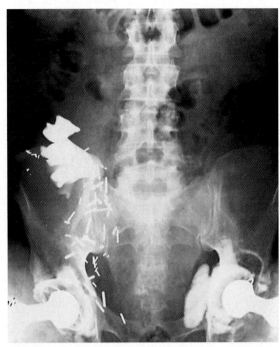

Fig GU 1-10
Kidney transplant.

Unilateral Small, Smooth Kidney

Condition	Imaging Findings	Comments
Renal ischemia (Fig GU 2-1)	Small, smooth kidney. Unilateral delayed appearance and excretion of contrast material with subsequent hyperconcentration. There may be ureteral notching (due to collateral arteries) and vascular calcification.	Chronic ischemia (usually arteriosclerosis or fibromuscular hyperplasia) causes tubular atrophy and shrinkage of glomeruli. Often associated with hypertension, which is likely if the right kidney is at least 2 cm shorter than the left or if the left kidney is at least 1.5 cm shorter than the right. May be bilateral if there is generalized renal arteriosclerosis.
Chronic (total) renal infarction (Fig GU 2-2)	Global shrinkage of the kidney with absent opacification. There may be a peripheral rim of opacified cortex during the nephrogram phase (probably reflects viable renal cortex perfused by perforating collateral vessels from the renal capsule).	Renal occlusion is most commonly secondary to an embolism from the heart. A decrease in renal size is detectable within 2 weeks and reaches its maximum extent by 5 weeks. Compensatory enlargement of the contralateral kidney (in individuals young enough to provide this reserve).
Radiation nephritis (Fig GU 2-3)	Progressive ischemic atrophy and decreased function produce a unilateral small, smooth kidney with some decrease in renal function.	Diffuse renal ischemia and vasculitis are due to inclusion of the kidney in the radiation field. Tends to become apparent after a latent period of 6 to 12 months. The threshold dose is approximately 2300 rads over a 5-week period.

A
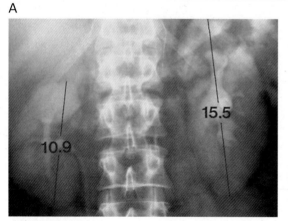

B
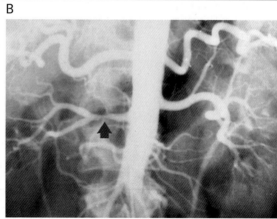

Fig GU 2-1
Renal ischemia associated with hypertension. Diminished size of the right kidney (A) due to renal artery stenosis (B) (arrow).

A
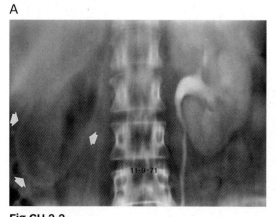

B
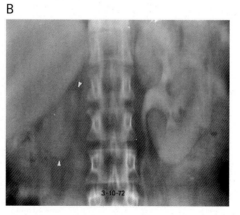

Fig GU 2-2
Renal infarction due to acute renal artery occlusion. (A) An initial nephrotomogram demonstrates a thin cortical rim surrounding the right kidney (arrows), reflecting viable renal cortex perfused by perforating collateral vessels from the renal capsule. (B) Four months later, a repeat nephrotomogram shows a marked decrease in the size of the atrophic right kidney (arrowheads).[1]

Condition	Imaging Findings	Comments
Congenital hypoplasia (Fig GU 2-4)	Small, smooth kidney with five or fewer calyces and an enlarged contralateral kidney (compensatory hypertrophy). Generally good function with a normal relation between the amount of parenchyma and the size of the collecting system.	Miniature replica of a normal kidney. Must be differentiated from an acquired atrophic kidney due to vascular or inflammatory disease (may require angiographic demonstration of the aortic orifice of the renal artery, which is small in a hypoplastic kidney but of normal size in an atrophic kidney).
Postobstructive atrophy	Small, smooth kidney with dilated calyces, a thin cortex, and usually effaced papillae. Compensatory hypertrophy of the contralateral kidney depending on the age of the patient, duration of the process, and severity of functional impairment.	Generally appears after surgical correction of urinary tract obstruction. Atrophy probably results from a combination of increased hydrostatic pressure on renal tissue and ischemia from the compression of intrarenal arteries and veins.
Postinflammatory atrophy (acute bacterial nephritis)	Uniform decrease in renal size with smooth or minimally irregular contour.	Unusual form of severe gram-negative bacterial infection in adult patients with altered host resistance (especially diabetes mellitus). The kidney becomes smoothly enlarged with decreased function in the acute phase, then shows a rapid return of function and global loss of tissue over a few weeks after the initiation of appropriate antibiotic therapy.
Reflux atrophy	Small, smooth kidney with dilated calyces, a thin cortex, and effaced papillae.	Structural kidney damage caused by vesicoureteral reflux with resulting increased hydrostatic pressure and tissue ischemia. Unlike reflux nephropathy, there is no infection or focal scarring. The appearance persists after spontaneous or surgical resolution of the vesicoureteral reflux.

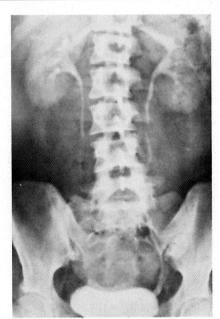

Fig GU 2-3
Radiation nephritis. Excretory urogram 5 years after radiation therapy for abdominal lymphoma shows that the left kidney has shrunk markedly. Delayed film showed no contrast material in the collecting system. Although a large left paraspinous mass deviates the axis of the left kidney, ultrasound revealed no obstruction; the intensity of the nephrogram excludes long-standing obstructive atrophy.[2]

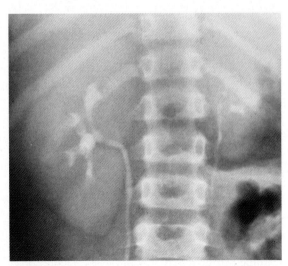

Fig GU 2-4
Congenital hypoplasia. The small left kidney, a miniature replica of a normal kidney, has good function and a normal relation between the amount of parenchyma and the size of the collecting system. Note the compensatory hypertrophy of the right kidney.

Unilateral Small, Scarred Kidney

Condition	Imaging Findings	Comments
Reflux nephropathy (chronic atrophic pyelonephritis) (Fig GU 3-1)	Unifocal or multifocal reduction in parenchymal thickness (most frequently in the upper pole). Cortical depression overlying retracted papilla whose calyx is secondarily smoothly dilated. May be bilateral (but usually asymmetric).	Related to chronic pyelonephritis and vesicoureteral reflux. By the teenage years, the lesions are fully developed and are no longer progressive unless there are complicating factors (stone formation, obstruction, neurogenic bladder). Cortical depressions must be differentiated from fetal lobulation (which occurs between calyces rather than directly over them). In children, reflux nephropathy may inhibit growth of all or a portion of the affected kidney.
Lobar infarction (Fig GU 3-2)	Initially, local failure of calyceal filling with a triangular nephrographic defect whose base is in the subcapsular region. After approximately 4 weeks, a wide-based cortical depression develops with a normal underlying papilla and calyx. May be multifocal or bilateral.	Usually caused by cardiac embolism (mitral stenosis and atrial fibrillation, infective endocarditis, or mural thrombus overlying a myocardial infarct). In the less common total infarction (occlusion of a main renal artery), the kidney does not function, often has a peripheral rim of opacified cortex, and progressively shrinks after 2 to 3 weeks.

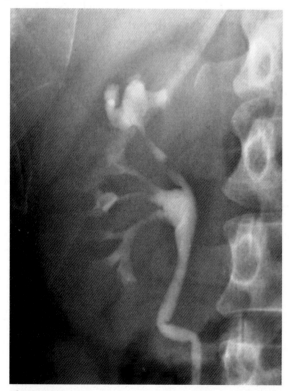

Fig GU 3-1
Chronic atrophic pyelonephritis. Focal reduction in parenchymal thickness involving the upper pole of the right kidney.

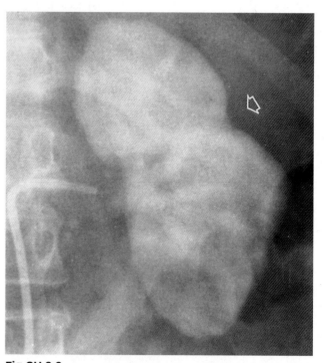

Fig GU 3-2
Segmental renal infarction. Film from the nephrogram phase of a selective arteriogram demonstrates a typical peripheral triangular defect with its base in the subcapsular region (arrow).

Condition	Imaging Findings	Comments
Renal tuberculosis (Fig GU 3-3)	Scarring with retraction of the underlying papilla (indistinguishable from reflux nephropathy) or a small, calcified nonfunctioning kidney (autonephrectomy).	Bizarre array of calyceal deformities with papillary destruction, stricture formation (pelvocalyceal system and ureter), and often calcified masses. Bilateral in approximately 25% of cases.

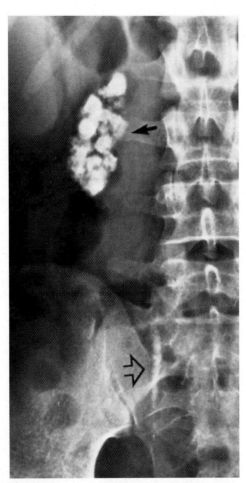

Fig GU 3-3
Tuberculous autonephrectomy. Plain film shows coarse irregular calcification that retains a reniform shape (black arrow). Note also the tuberculous calcification of the distal right ureter (open arrow).[3]

Unilateral Large, Smooth Kidney

Condition	Imaging Findings	Comments
Obstructive uropathy (Fig GU 4-1)	Unilateral (or bilateral) large, smooth kidney with a dilated pelvocalyceal system and delayed contrast material excretion. Prolonged hydronephrosis causes diffuse narrowing of the renal parenchyma.	Acute urinary obstruction is most commonly associated with the passage of a calculus or blood clot. Causes of chronic obstruction include benign and malignant tumors of the ureter and adjacent organs, inflammatory strictures and masses, and retroperitoneal tumor or fibrosis.
Renal vein thrombosis (see Fig GU 13-4)	Unilateral large, smooth kidney. Little or no opacification in acute thrombosis. Some contrast material excretion if venous occlusion is partial or is accompanied by adequate collateral formation. The collecting system is attenuated by surrounding interstitial edema.	May be a primary event in severely dehydrated infants and children. In adults, most often a complication of another renal disease (amyloidosis, membranous glomerulonephritis, pyelonephritis), trauma, or extension of thrombus or tumor from the inferior vena cava. If unresolved, may produce renal infarction and a small, smooth, nonfunctioning kidney. Enlargement of collateral pathways for renal venous flow causes extrinsic indentations on the pelvis and ureter.
Acute arterial infarction	Unilateral large, smooth, nonopacified kidney. A retrograde pyelogram shows a normal pelvocalyceal system that is effaced by surrounding interstitial edema. Characteristic cortical rim of contrast (peripheral cortex that continues to be perfused by capsular collateral arteries).	Follows embolic, thrombotic, or traumatic occlusion of a renal artery. After 2 to 3 weeks, the kidney begins to shrink and eventually becomes small in the late stage.

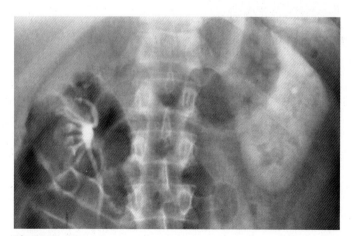

Fig GU 4-1
Obstructive uropathy. Acute urinary obstruction causes a large, smooth left kidney with delayed contrast excretion and prolonged nephrogram.

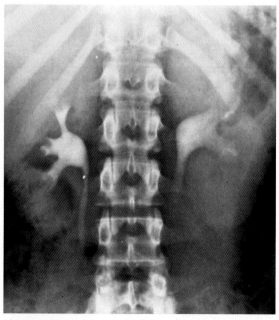

Fig GU 4-2
Acute pyelonephritis. Generalized enlargement of the left kidney with decreased density of contrast material in the collecting system.

Condition	Imaging Findings	Comments
Acute pyelonephritis (Fig GU 4-2)	Unilateral global enlargement of the kidney with decreased and delayed contrast material excretion and mild dilatation of the collecting system. There is often focal polar swelling and calyceal compression. Characteristic wedge-shaped zones of diminished enhancement radiating from the collecting system to the renal surface on CT.	Primarily affects women 15 to 40 years of age and is most commonly due to *Escherichia coli*. The most severe form (acute bacterial nephritis) occurs in patients with altered host resistance (diabetes mellitus, immunosuppressant therapy). In uncomplicated acute pyelonephritis, the radiographic abnormalities revert to normal after appropriate therapy. In severe disease, there may be marked parenchymal wasting and a small, smooth kidney.
Compensatory hypertrophy (Fig GU 4-3)	Unilateral smooth, large kidney that is normal in all respects except for its size and the thickness of the renal parenchyma. The pelvocalyceal system and ureter may appear distended (high urinary flow rate).	Response to congenital absence, surgical removal, or disease of the contralateral kidney. The ability of the kidney to undergo compensatory hypertrophy diminishes with age (some state that it does not occur after age 30). After surgical removal of the opposite kidney, the contralateral kidney reaches its maximum size in approximately 6 months.
Duplicated pelvocalyceal system (Fig GU 4-4)	Unilateral (or bilateral) large, smooth kidney. Normal function and appearance of the duplex pelvocalyceal system.	Represents earlier than normal dichotomous branching of the ureteral bud. The two branches encounter a greater mass of metanephric blastema than otherwise would have occurred (causing a larger than normal amount of renal parenchyma associated with the duplex collecting system).

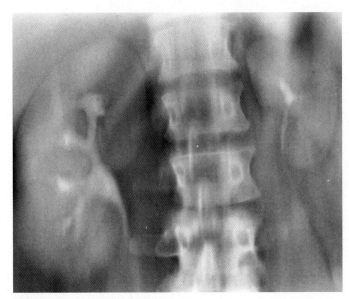

Fig GU 4-3
Compensatory hypertrophy. Markedly enlarged right kidney in a patient with a hypoplastic left kidney.

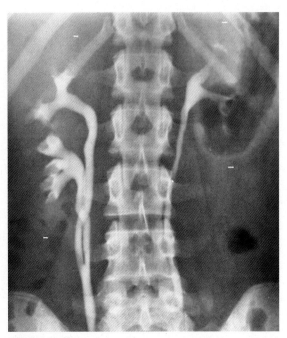

Fig GU 4-4
Duplicated right pelvocalyceal system.

Unilateral Large, Multilobulated Kidney

Condition	Imaging Findings	Comments
Xanthogranulomatous pyelonephritis (Fig GU 5-1)	Unilateral nonfunctioning kidney with multi-focal enlargement and an obstructing radiopaque calculus at the ureteropelvic junction. There is obstructive dilatation of the collecting system on retrograde pyelography. In the tumefactive form, single or multiple irregular inflammatory masses distort the opacified collecting system or renal margins (simulates renal abscess or neoplasm).	Nodular replacement of renal parenchyma by large lipid-filled macrophages (foam cells) that develop in chronically infected kidneys. May cause multiple small nodules coalescing to form several large masses, a single granulomatous mass, or diffuse replacement of the renal parenchyma. CT shows the characteristic fatty consistency of the xanthogranulomatous mass.
Multicystic dysplastic kidney (Fig GU 5-2)	Unilateral, multilobulated, nonfunctioning mass in the area normally occupied by the kidney. Thin curvilinear calcification may outline cyst walls. The vascularized walls of individual cysts may become slightly opaque during urography (cluster-of-grapes sign). Usually there is compensatory hypertrophy of the contralateral kidney.	Nonhereditary congenital dysplasia, usually asymptomatic, in which the kidney is composed almost entirely of large thin-walled cysts with only little solid renal tissue. Most common cause of an abdominal mass in the newborn. Other manifestations include an atretic ureter with a blind proximal end (on retrograde pyelography) and an absent or severely atretic renal artery. Ultrasound can differentiate the disorganized pattern of cysts and the lack of renal parenchyma and reniform contour in multicystic kidney disease from the precise organization of symmetrically positioned fluid-filled spaces in hydronephrosis.

A

B

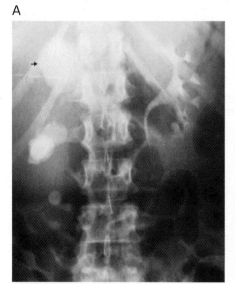
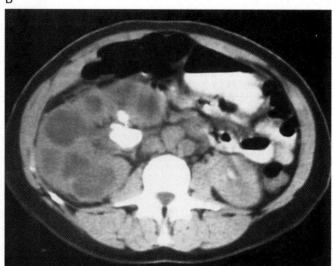

Fig GU 5-1

Xanthogranulomatous pyelonephritis. (A) Excretory urogram shows a unilateral nonfunctioning right kidney with several large radiopaque calculi at the ureteropelvic junction and in the proximal ureter. The arrow points to an opacified gallbladder. (B) CT scan shows the characteristic fatty consistency of the multiple xanthogranulomatous masses. Note the dense zone at the ureteropelvic junction.

Condition	Imaging Findings	Comments
Malacoplakia	Unilateral multifocal kidney enlargement with diminished or absent contrast material excretion. Multiple granulomas produce a mass effect on the pelvocalyceal system. No calcification.	Rare inflammation of renal parenchyma characterized by cortical and medullary granulomatous masses containing large mononuclear cells with abundant cytoplasm. Usually associated with *Escherichia coli* infection. Approximately 75% of cases are multifocal, and 50% are bilateral. Malacoplakia of the urinary tract most commonly affects the bladder.

A   B

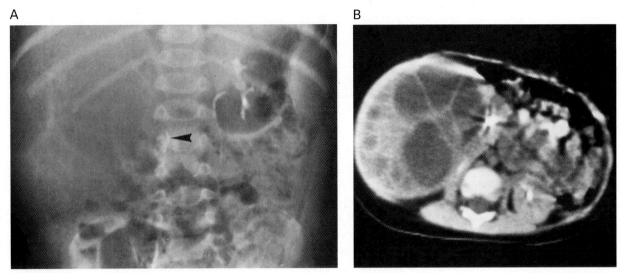

Fig GU 5-2
Segmental multicystic dysplastic kidney involving only the medial portion of the right kidney. (A) Excretory urogram shows a large multiloculated renal mass displacing the opacified collecting system (arrowhead) over the spine. (B) Enhanced CT scan confirms the intrarenal multiloculated mass.[4]

Bilateral Small, Smooth Kidneys

Condition	Imaging Findings	Comments
Generalized arteriosclerosis (Fig GU 6-1)	Bilaterally small kidneys that may be smooth or show focal depressions (scars) representing infarctions. Uniform loss of cortical thickness but normal nephrogram, papillae, and pelvocalyceal system. Increased radiolucency in the renal pelvis is due to proliferation of renal sinus fat.	Generalized arteriosclerosis involving most of the interlobar and arcuate arteries causes uniform shrinkage of both kidneys. A similar appearance may develop in scleroderma, chronic tophaceous gout, and polyarteritis (due to the accelerated atherosclerotic or necrotic arterial lesions associated with these diseases). Usually not detected before age 50.
Nephrosclerosis (benign and malignant) (Fig GU 6-2) (see Fig GU 14-2)	Radiographic appearance of benign nephrosclerosis is similar to that of arteriosclerotic kidney disease. In malignant nephrosclerosis, there is invariably diminished opacification of the kidneys. Occasionally there may be subcapsular bleeding (concave, inward displacement of the parenchyma).	Benign nephrosclerosis consists of thickening and subendothelial hyalinization of afferent arterioles associated with hypertension. In malignant nephrosclerosis, there is accelerated or malignant hypertension with proliferative endarteritis. It is controversial whether the elevated blood pressure is the cause or the result of the afferent arteriolar lesion.
Atheroembolic renal disease	Radiographic appearance similar to that of malignant nephrosclerosis.	Caused by the dislodgment from the aorta of multiple atheromatous emboli that occlude intrarenal arteries. May be spontaneous or result from external trauma or from a direct insult to the aorta during surgery or catheter manipulation.
Chronic glomerulonephritis (Figs GU 6-3 and GU 6-4)	Globally small kidneys with smooth contours, normal calyces and papillae, and occasional peripelvic fat proliferation. The density of the nephrogram and pelvocalyceal system varies with the severity of the disease. There may be cortical calcification (best seen on CT)	Develops weeks or months after an episode of acute glomerulonephritis (not always poststreptococcal). Associated with progressive hypertension and renal failure. Approximately 50% of patients eventually develop the nephrotic syndrome.
Papillary necrosis (see Figs GU 16-1 and GU 16-2)	Bilateral globally shrunken kidneys with impaired function sometimes occur in severe disease (most patients have normal-sized kidneys). Earlier signs include papillary enlargement followed by disruption (tract formation, cavitation, papillary slough). Sloughed, eventually calcified, papillae may cause urinary tract obstruction and predispose to infection.	Bilateral small, smooth kidneys primarily occur in papillary necrosis associated with analgesic abuse. Small kidneys are not reported in papillary necrosis due to diabetes mellitus or sickle cell disease. Usually unilateral if papillary necrosis is secondary to noninfected urinary tract obstruction, renal vein thrombosis, or trauma.

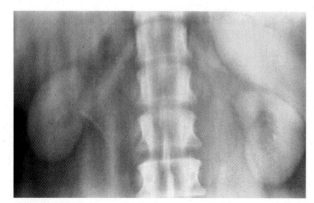

Fig GU 6-1
Generalized arteriosclerosis.

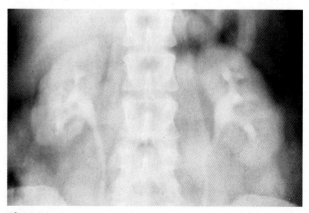

Fig GU 6-2
Benign nephrosclerosis. Bilaterally small kidneys with several shallow infarct scars. The pelvocalyceal systems and renal opacification are normal.[5]

Condition	Imaging Findings	Comments
Hereditary nephropathy Hereditary chronic nephritis (Alport's syndrome)	Small, smooth kidneys with impaired excretion of contrast material.	Distinctive histologic feature of fat-filled macrophages (foam cells), especially in the corticomedullary junction. Males are affected by a more severe form of renal disease and usually die before age 50. No hypertension. Most patients also have nerve deafness and ocular abnormalities.
Medullary cystic disease (see Fig GU 10-5)	Normal or small kidneys with smooth contour and impaired excretion of contrast material. Large medullary cysts may produce sharply defined radiolucent defects on nephrotomography (best seen on CT). The cysts are usually too small to cause pelvocalyceal displacement or lobulation of the renal contour.	Variable number of often very small cysts in the corticomedullary junction and medulla. More often involves females. Clinical findings include anemia, polyuria, hyposthenuria, and salt wasting. No hypertension.
Amyloidosis (late)	Typically causes smooth enlargement of both kidneys. In long-standing disease, amyloid kidneys become small with preservation of their normal contours and pelvocalyceal relations.	Shrinkage of the kidneys presumably occurs as a result of ischemic atrophy of nephrons induced by the involvement of renal blood vessels by amyloid deposits.
Arterial hypotension	Bilateral small, smooth kidneys with their nephrograms becoming progressively denser over time or remaining unchanged.	May be secondary to shock or a reaction to contrast material. Once the hypotension is reversed, the urogram usually reverts to normal.

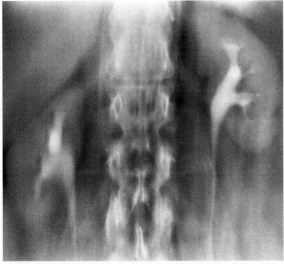

Fig GU 6-3
Chronic glomerulonephritis. Nephrotomogram shows bilateral small, smooth kidneys. The uniform reduction in parenchymal thickness is particularly apparent in the right kidney. Note that the pelvocalyceal system is well opacified and without the irregular contours and blunted calyces seen in chronic pyelonephritis.

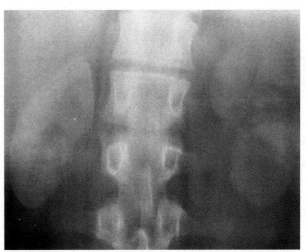

Fig GU 6-4
Chronic glomerulonephritis. Plain film tomogram shows bilateral small, smooth kidneys with diffuse fine calcification in the renal parenchyma.

Bilateral Large, Smooth Kidneys

Condition	Imaging Findings	Comments
Proliferative or necrotizing disorders		
Acute glomerulo-nephritides (Fig GU 7-1)	Bilateral large kidneys (may be of normal size) with global parenchymal thickening and smooth contours. The nephrogram is homogeneously faint or normal. The pelvocalyceal system is normal, though opacification is often faint (ultrasound is the most efficacious test to show that the calyces are not dilated and thus not obstructed).	Kidneys may remain enlarged or normal throughout the course of illness. If the disease progresses to a chronic stage (especially in the poststreptococcal type), the kidneys become bilaterally small with smooth contours. (Note: A patient with renal failure must be well hydrated before a contrast examination is performed.)
Glomerular abnormality in multisystem diseases	Nonspecific findings of acute glomerular disease (large, smooth, nonobstructed kidneys with or without impaired excretion of contrast material).	Specific extrarenal findings vary depending on the underlying disease (see below).
Polyarteritis nodosa (Fig GU 7-2)	Multiple small aneurysms that most often arise at arterial bifurcations and predominantly involve small arteries of the kidneys, mesentery, liver, pancreas, heart, muscles, and nerves.	Necrotizing inflammation involving all layers of the walls of arterioles and small arteries. Hypertension and hematuria are common. Rupture of an intrarenal aneurysm may cause renal infarction or perinephric or parenchymal hematoma.
Systemic lupus erythematosus (see Figs C 33-4 and C 34-9)	Subluxation and malalignment of joints without erosions (eg, boutonnière and swan neck deformities). Pleural and pericardial effusions. Patchy infiltrates at lung bases.	Connective tissue disorder primarily involving young or middle-aged women. Probably an immune complex disease. Characteristic butterfly rash.
Wegener's granulomatosis (see Fig C 9-14)	Granulomatous lesions in the kidneys, upper respiratory tract (especially the paranasal sinuses), and lungs (multiple pulmonary nodules that often cavitate).	Necrotizing vasculitis and granulomatous inflammation. Renal involvement in more than 90% of patients (primarily focal or acute glomerulonephritis).

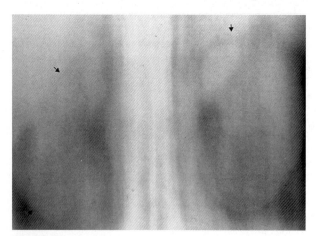

Fig GU 7-1
Acute glomerulonephritis. Nephrotomogram demonstrates bilateral large kidneys with smooth contours (arrows). The nephrographic density, although faint, was maximal at this time. The calyces were never visualized.[5]

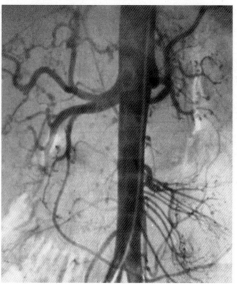

Fig GU 7-2
Polyarteritis nodosa. An aortogram demonstrates innumerable small aneurysms arising from vessels throughout the abdomen. The aorta and its major branches are spared.

Condition	Imaging Findings	Comments
Allergic angiitis	Fleeting, patchy pulmonary consolidations with nonsegmental distribution. Confluent densities may cavitate.	Necrotizing vasculitis separated from polyarteritis nodosa because of prominent eosinophilia, the presence of perivascular granulomas, lung involvement, and clinical association with bronchial asthma (except for pulmonary manifestations, organ involvement is similar to that of polyarteritis nodosa).
Goodpasture's syndrome (see Fig C 2-11)	Pulmonary hemorrhage causing patchy airspace consolidation (especially in the perihilar region, simulating pulmonary edema) followed by a reticular pattern that initially clears. Repeated attacks cause interstitial deposition of hemosiderin and progressive interstitial fibrosis.	Most likely an autoimmune disease with circulating antibodies to the glomerular and alveolar basement membranes. Usually occurs in young men.
Henoch-Schönlein purpura (Fig GU 7-3)	Bleeding into joints and the gastrointestinal tract (regular thickening of small bowel folds with separation of loops).	Acute vasculitis characterized by purpura, nephritis, abdominal pain, and joint pain. Most commonly occurs in the first two decades and frequently develops several weeks after a streptococcal infection. Usually self-limited.
Thrombotic thrombocytopenic purpura	Bilateral large, smooth kidneys.	Hemolytic anemia, hemorrhage, and oliguric or anuric renal failure occur as a result of arterial thrombosis and proliferative lesions of the glomerular epithelium.
Diabetic glomerulosclerosis (Fig GU 7-4)	Wide spectrum of radiographic changes in diabetes mellitus.	Nodular sclerosis of renal glomeruli and arterioles (Kimmelstiel-Wilson syndrome) may occur in chronic diabetics and lead to the development of the nephrotic syndrome or chronic renal failure.

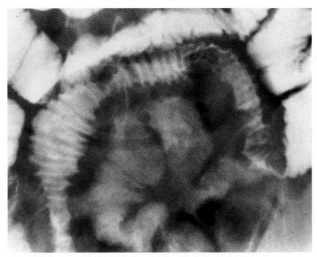

Fig GU 7-3
Henoch-Schönlein purpura. Hemorrhage and edema in the intestinal wall cause regular thickening of small bowel folds.

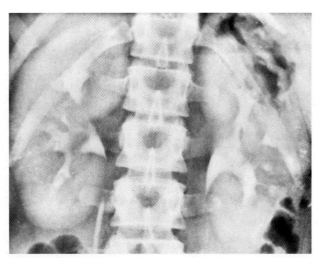

Fig GU 7-4
Diabetic glomerulosclerosis with nephrotic syndrome and chronic renal failure. An excretory urogram demonstrates bilateral large, smooth kidneys with normal calyces.[2]

Condition	Imaging Findings	Comments
Subacute infective endocarditis	Focal or diffuse glomerulonephritis	Diffuse glomerulonephritis that is indistinguishable from other types of immune complex diseases. Small emboli may produce a focal glomerulitis, whereas large emboli to the kidneys may cause infarction. The spleen is frequently involved, and petechial skin lesions are common.
Abnormal protein deposition Amyloidosis (Fig GU 7-5)	Bilateral large, smooth kidneys with normal or impaired opacification and normal pelvocalyceal systems. With time, the kidneys decrease in size and eventually become small.	Kidneys affected in more than 80% of patients with amyloidosis secondary to chronic suppurative or inflammatory disease. Renal involvement in approximately 35% of patients with primary amyloidosis. May be complicated by renal vein thrombosis (produces decreased kidney opacification).
Multiple myeloma	Bilateral large, smooth kidneys with reduced opacification. The pelvocalyceal system is normal but often diffusely attenuated in patients with severe renal involvement. In late stages, the kidneys may eventually shrink.	Abnormal proteins precipitated in the tubules cause renal insufficiency in up to 50% of cases. Diffuse renal infiltration of plasma cells is rare. Renal function may also be compromised by impaired renal blood flow (increased blood viscosity) and nephrocalcinosis due to hypercalcemia. (Note: A patient with renal failure must be well hydrated before a contrast examination is performed.)
Abnormal fluid accumulation Acute tubular necrosis	Bilateral large, smooth kidneys with characteristic immediate and prolonged increased nephrogram (increasingly dense nephrogram in 25% of cases) that may persist for more than 1 day. The pelvocalyceal system is faintly or not opacified and is usually globally attenuated because of increased parenchymal thickness.	Reversible renal failure with or without oliguria that follows exposure of the kidney to certain toxic agents (mercury, ethylene glycol, carbon tetrachloride, bismuth, arsenic, urographic contrast material) or to a period of prolonged severe ischemia (shock, crush injury, burns, transfusion reaction, severe dehydration, renal transplantation, aortic resection). Usually reversible, but may require temporary dialysis. The proximal convoluted tubules may rarely calcify after recovery.

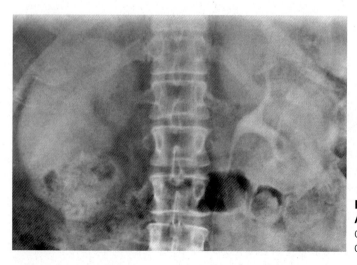

Fig GU 7-5
Amyloidosis. Bilateral large, smooth kidneys. Decreased opacification and prolonged nephrogram on the right are secondary to superimposed ureteral obstruction.

Condition	Imaging Findings	Comments
Acute cortical necrosis (Fig GU 7-6)	Bilateral large, smooth kidneys with poor opacification. Normal pelvocalyceal systems on retrograde studies. Classic appearance of punctate or linear (tramline) calcification confined to the renal cortex develops within approximately 1 month.	Very uncommon form of acute renal failure in which there is patchy or universal necrosis of the renal cortex with sparing of the medulla. May be associated with severe burns, multiple fractures, internal hemorrhage, transfusions of incompatible blood, and especially complications of pregnancy (abruptio placentae, septic abortion, or placenta previa).
Other conditions Leukemia (Fig GU 7-7)	Bilateral large, smooth kidneys with nephrographic and pelvocalyceal density varying from normal to markedly depressed. The collecting systems may be attenuated by neoplastic cell infiltration.	Most common malignant cause of bilateral global renal enlargement. More frequent in children with acute leukemia, especially of the lymphocytic type. Superimposed hemorrhage may produce a focal parenchymal mass, a subcapsular collection of blood, or obstructive or nonobstructive clots in the renal pelvis or ureters.
Acute interstitial nephritis	Bilateral large, smooth kidneys with normal to diminished opacification. There is a return to normal appearance after withdrawal of the offending drug.	Inflammatory cell infiltration representing a complication of exposure to certain drugs (most commonly methicillin; also phenindione, diphenylhydantoin, sulfonamides, ampicillin, and cephalothin). Probably represents an allergic or idiosyncratic reaction rather than direct drug nephrotoxicity.

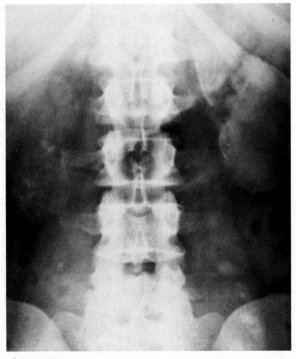

Fig GU 7-6
Bilateral acute renal cortical necrosis. There is punctate calcification in the right kidney and a peripheral rim of calcification surrounding the left kidney.

Condition	Imaging Findings	Comments
Acute urate nephropathy	Bilateral large, smooth kidneys with unopacified pelvocalyceal systems and increasing nephrographic density.	Flooding of nephrons with large amounts of uric acid crystals (which deposit in the collecting tubules and interstitium). Most commonly a complication of therapy of leukemia, lymphoma, myeloproliferative disorders, or polycythemia vera (cytotoxic agents release large amounts of nucleoprotein that is metabolized to uric acid). (Note: Contrast material may be dangerous in these patients because of its uricosuric effect.)
Acromegaly (Fig GU 7-8)	Bilateral large, smooth kidneys with normal structure and function.	Manifestation of the generalized organomegaly.
Nephromegaly associated with other diseases	Bilateral large, smooth kidneys with normal structure and function.	Hepatic cirrhosis (especially in patients with marked fatty changes in the liver); hyperalimentation (increase in the fluid compartments of the kidney related to the hyperosmolality of administered solutions); diabetes mellitus (even in the absence of diabetic glomerulosclerosis); hemophilia; Fabry disease (lipid deposition in the renal parenchyma).
Sickle cell disease (homozygous)	Bilateral large, smooth kidneys. Eventually there is impaired concentration of contrast material and dilated pelvocalyceal systems and ureters.	Reflects vascular dilatation, engorgement of vessels, glomerular enlargement, interstitial edema, and increased renal blood flow. Lobar infarction may develop. Papillary necrosis is more common in patients with heterozygous disease.

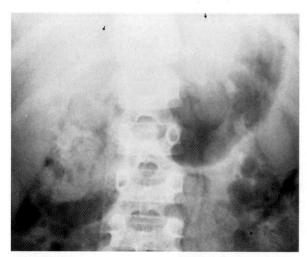

Fig GU 7-7
Chronic leukemia. Diffuse infiltration of leukemic cells has caused bilateral enlargement of the kidneys (arrows).

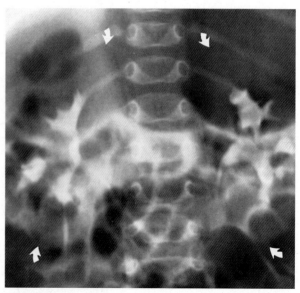

Fig GU 7-8
Acromegaly. Bilateral enlargement of well-functioning kidneys. The arrows point to the superior and inferior margins of the kidneys, both of which are approximately five vertebral bodies in length.

Condition	Imaging Findings	Comments
Bilateral duplication	Bilateral long, smooth kidneys (normal width). Two pelvocalyceal systems on both sides.	May mimic a neoplasm if one of the collecting systems is obstructed and nonfunctioning.
Physiologic response to contrast material and diuretics	Bilateral large, smooth kidneys with normal structure and function.	Vasodilatation or diuresis may increase renal size, presumably because of volume expansion of the vascular tree, tubular lumens, or interstitial fluid space. Renal area may increase up to 35% (mean increase, only 5%).
Bilateral hydronephrosis	Bilateral large, smooth kidneys with dilated pelvocalyceal systems and delayed excretion. Prolonged hydronephrosis causes diffuse parenchymal narrowing and small, smooth kidneys.	May be congenital or acquired (bladder outlet obstruction or an inflammatory mass obstructing both ureters).

Bilateral Large, Multifocal Kidneys

Condition	Imaging Findings	Comments
Adult polycystic kidney disease (Figs GU 8-1 and GU 8-2)	Bilateral large kidneys with multilobulated contours. The pelvic and infundibular structures are elongated, effaced, and often displaced around larger cysts to produce a crescentic outline. Characteristic mottled nephrogram (Swiss cheese pattern) due to the presence of innumerable lucent cysts of various sizes throughout the kidneys. Plaques of calcification occasionally occur in the cyst walls.	Inherited disorder in which many progressively growing cysts cause lobulated enlargement of the kidneys and progressive renal impairment (presumably due to cystic compression of nephrons that causes localized intrarenal obstruction). Approximately 35% of patients have associated cysts of the liver (they do not interfere with hepatic function). About 10% have one or more saccular (berry) aneurysms of cerebral arteries (may rupture and produce fatal subarachnoid hemorrhage). Hypertension is common. Patients tend to be asymptomatic during the first three decades of life (early diagnosis is made by chance or as the result of a specific search prompted by a positive family history).
Acquired cystic kidney disease	Bilateral large kidneys with multilobulated contours and no renal function. Requires ultrasound or CT for detection.	Multiple cyst formation occurs in chronically failed kidneys of patients undergoing long-term hemodialysis. The degree of enlargement may approach that of adult polycystic kidney disease. The process may reverse after successful renal transplantation.
Lymphoma	Bilaterally enlarged kidneys with multifocal bulges of renal contours and displacement of the pelvocalyceal systems. There may be a single mass in one kidney or a normal urogram (lymphomatous nodules too small to displace the collecting structures or distort the renal contour). Opacification of the kidneys progressively diminishes as the lymphomatous masses grow, coalesce, and replace nephrons.	Renal involvement occurs much more frequently in non-Hodgkin's lymphoma than in Hodgkin's disease. Usually asymptomatic unless there is a palpable mass, hypertension (mass impressing renal artery or causing renal vein occlusion), or obstructive uropathy (ureteral encasement by lymphomatous tissue in the retroperitoneum). Radiation or chemotherapy may produce uric acid nephropathy or radiation nephritis.

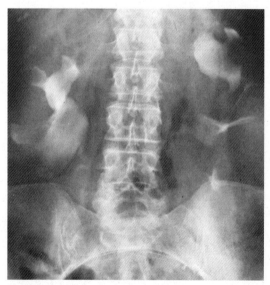

Fig GU 8-1
Adult polycystic kidney disease. Excretory urogram shows marked multifocal enlargement of both kidneys, focal displacement of the collecting structures, and normal opacification.[5]

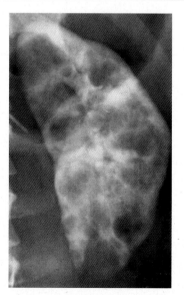

Fig GU 8-2
Adult polycystic kidney disease. Nephrogram phase from selective arteriography of the left kidney demonstrates innumerable cysts ranging from pinhead size to 2 cm. The opposite kidney had an identical appearance.[6]

Focal Renal Mass

Condition	Imaging Findings	Comments
Normal variant	Focal "mass" on the surface of a kidney that may be confused with a neoplasm.	Fetal lobulation (prominence of the centrilobar cortex where two adjacent lobes abut); dromedary hump; hilar bulge (prominence of the suprahilar region of the left kidney that may cause focal displacement of the upper pole collecting system).
Column of Bertin (Fig GU 9-1)	Focal "mass" apparently arising from the surface of the kidney with compression and splaying of the pelvocalyceal system. May simulate a true neoplasm.	Mass of normal cortical tissue in the renal parenchyma. Most commonly develops at the junction of the middle and upper thirds of a duplex kidney. The correct diagnosis can be made by radionuclide scanning, which reveals normal or even increased uptake of isotope in the pseudo-tumor in contrast to decreased uptake in other renal masses.

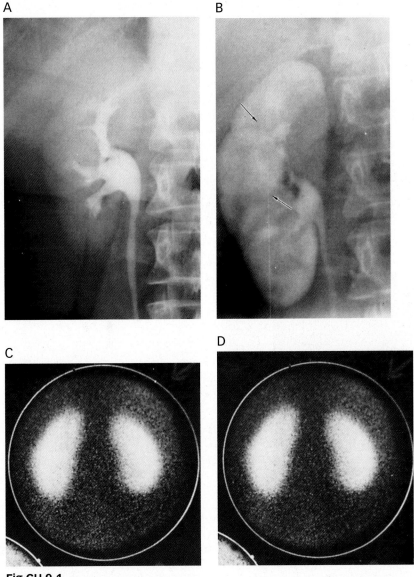

Fig GU 9-1
Column of Bertin. (A) Excretory urogram shows displacement of the upper calyceal system of the right kidney. (B) Film from the nephrotomogram phase of a selective right renal arteriogram shows the large column (arrows), which appears denser than the medullary substance. Renal scans (C, D) show normal-functioning parenchyma.[7]

Condition	Imaging Findings	Comments
Simple renal cyst (Figs GU 9-2 and GU 9-3)	Focal contour expansion of the kidney outline on the nephrogram. The cortical margin appears as a very thin, smooth radiopaque rim about the bulging lucent cyst (beak sign). A thickened wall suggests bleeding into a cyst, cyst infection, or a malignant lesion. When a simple cyst is completely embedded in the kidney parenchyma, the thin rim and beak are absent, and the renal size and contour are normal. A renal cyst causes focal displacement of adjacent portions of the pelvocalyceal system, with the collecting structures remaining smooth and attenuated rather than shaggy and obliterated as with a malignant neoplasm.	Unifocal fluid-filled mass that is usually unilocular, though septa sometimes divide the cyst into chambers that may or may not communicate with each other. Cysts vary in size and may occur at single or multiple sites in one or both kidneys. Thin curvilinear calcification occurs in approximately 3% of simple cysts (not pathognomonic of a benign process as 20% of masses with this appearance are malignant). Ultrasound or CT can unequivocally demonstrate a simple renal cyst. Cyst puncture is necessary if there is an atypical appearance or a strong clinical suspicion of abscess, or if the patient has hematuria or hypertension.
Malignant neoplasm (Figs GU 9-4 through GU 9-6)	Focal mass with indistinct outlines and a density similar to that of normal parenchyma (unlike the classic radiolucent mass with sharp margins and a thin wall representing a benign cyst). Necrotic neoplasms may appear cystic, though they are usually surrounded by thick, irregular walls. Initially, there is elongation of adjacent calyces, followed by distortion, narrowing, or obliteration of part or all of the collecting system due to progressive tumor enlargement and infiltration. Large tumors may partially obstruct the pelvis or upper ureter and cause proximal dilatation or even a nonfunctioning kidney.	Renal cell carcinoma (hypernephroma) is the most common malignant renal neoplasm, predominantly occurring in patients over age 40. Approximately 10% of hypernephromas contain calcification (usually located in reactive fibrous zones about areas of tumor necrosis). Of all masses containing calcium in a nonperipheral location, almost 90% are malignant (peripheral curvilinear calcification is more suggestive of a benign cyst, but a hypernephroma can have a calcified fibrous pseudocapsule and present an identical radiographic appearance). Bilateral carcinomas occur in approximately 2% of cases (especially in von Hippel-Lindau disease). Nephroblastoma (Wilms' tumor) is common in children. Sarcomas, metastases, and invasive transitional cell carcinoma are rare.

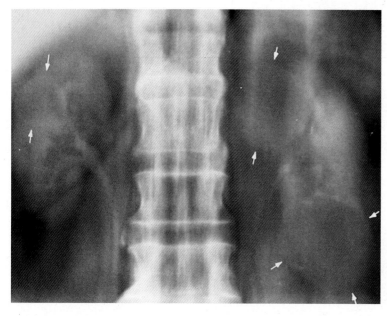

Fig GU 9-2
Renal cysts. Nephrotomogram demonstrates bilateral renal cysts (arrows).

Condition	Imaging Findings	Comments
Benign neoplasm (Figs GU 9-7 through GU 9-9)	Unifocal renal mass enlarging the kidney and causing distortion and displacement of the adjacent portion of the pelvocalyceal system. No tumor calcification or irregular obliteration of the pelvocalyceal system as in malignant disease. Fat in an angiomyolipoma may produce a well-defined area of mottled radiolucency on plain films.	Most common benign tumor of the kidney is hamartoma (angiomyolipoma), which develops in a large percentage of patients with tuberous sclerosis in whom involvement is usually multifocal and bilateral. Angiomyolipomas typically appear as intensely echogenic masses on ultrasound and have a high fat content on CT. Other benign tumors include adenoma (usually small, asymptomatic, and discovered incidentally), reninoma (uncommon benign tumor of juxtaglomerular cells associated with increased renin secretion and hypertension), and mesenchymal tumors (fibroma, lipoma, leiomyoma, and angioma).

A

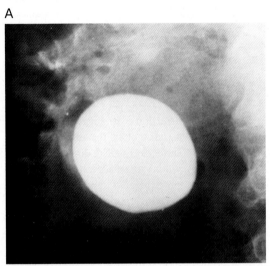

B

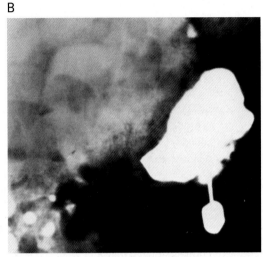

Fig GU 9-3
Renal cyst puncture. (A) The instillation of contrast material shows the smooth inner wall characteristic of a benign cyst. (B) In another patient, the introduction of contrast material reveals the markedly irregular inner border of a necrotic renal cell carcinoma.

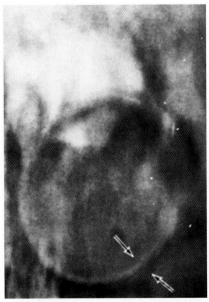

Fig GU 9-4
Renal cell carcinoma. Nephrotomogram demonstrates a lucent, well-demarcated renal mass with a thick wall (arrows).[8]

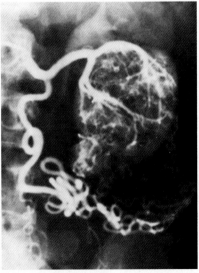

Fig GU 9-5
Renal cell carcinoma. Left renal arteriogram demonstrates a large hypervascular mass with striking enlargement of capsular vessels.

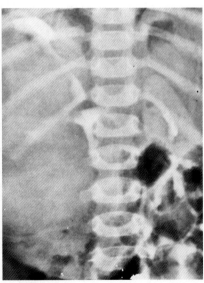

Fig GU 9-6
Wilms' tumor. Huge mass in the right kidney distorts and displaces the pelvocalyceal system.[2]

Condition	Imaging Findings	Comments
Renal/perirenal abscess (Fig GU 9-10)	Focal, usually polar, renal mass that may displace or efface adjacent portions of the pelvocalyceal system. In a chronic abscess, a nephrographic radiolucent defect in the well-defined mass corresponds to a central collection of necrotic tissue (thick-walled cavity with an irregular inner margin). Perirenal infection causes partial or complete obscuration of the renal outline, loss of the psoas margin, immobility of the kidney with respiration, and lumbar scoliosis concave to the side of involvement. The demonstration of extraluminal gas around or inside the kidney is virtually pathognomonic of renal or perirenal abscess.	Most renal and perirenal abscesses occur by direct extension from renal pelvic infection, especially if there is a calculus obstructing the ureter or pelvis. Since the introduction of antibiotics, renal abscess is infrequently due to direct or hematogenous spread of an extraurinary infection. A renal abscess usually does not spread to the contralateral side because the medial fascia surrounding the kidney is closed and the spine and great vessels act as natural deterrents. An inflammatory process can extend around the entire kidney, though it usually is most pronounced on the dorsal and superior aspects where the renal fascia is open and the surrounding tissues offer little resistance. The radiographic appearance may be indistinguishable from that of a renal neoplasm.
Focal hydronephrosis	Increased renal length and a localized bulge in contour. Sharply marginated lucency corresponds to the dilated calyces filled with nonopacified urine seen during the nephrogram phase. The obstructed area slowly opacifies as contrast material passes into the dilated, urine-filled system (may require films as late as 24 to 36 hours after injection). Nonobstructed calyces draining the remainder of the kidney opacify normally, though they may be displaced by the mass effect of the hydronephrotic segment.	Caused by obstruction to drainage of one portion of the kidney (most often the upper pole of a kidney with partial or complete duplication of the collecting system). May reflect congenital ureteropelvic duplication with an ectopic ureterocele or be the result of infection (especially tuberculosis). Retrograde or antegrade pyelography may be of value to visualize precisely the point of obstruction (if not determined on delayed films).

A
B

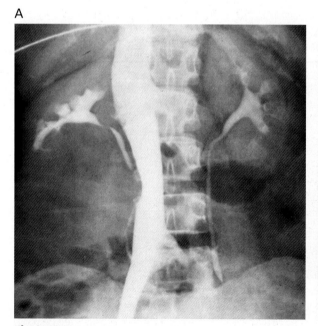
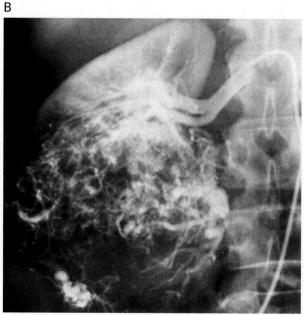

Fig GU 9-7
Renal hamartoma. (A) A combined excretory urogram and inferior vena cavagram shows a large mass in the lower pole of the right kidney with displacement but no invasion of the pelvocalyceal system and inferior vena cava. (B) Arteriography shows the mass to be hypervascular. The overall radiographic appearance is indistinguishable from that of renal cell carcinoma.

Condition	Imaging Findings	Comments
Multilocular cyst	Unifocal mass, usually in a polar location, that produces a sharply defined lucent nephrographic defect and often displaces the pelvocalyceal system. Calcification and faint septa may be detected.	Uncommon unilateral mass composed of multiple cysts of various sizes and adjoining primitive cellular elements. May be detected as a palpable mass in infants. May represent a form of congenital cystic dysplasia or a benign renal neoplasm. Differs from multicystic (dysgenetic) kidney in that it is unilateral, involves only a segment of an otherwise normal kidney, and has no associated abnormalities of the ureter or renal artery.
Congenital arteriovenous malformation	Unifocal mass, most commonly in a parapelvic or medullary location, which impresses the pelvocalyceal system. Cirsoid vascular channels occasionally produce multinodular impressions on the pelvocalyceal system. Curvilinear calcification may form in the walls of the mass.	Most commonly cirsoid (multiple coiled vascular channels grouped in a cluster). The much rarer cavernous form is composed of a single well-defined artery feeding into a single vein. Usually presents with hematuria and may produce an abdominal bruit.
Xanthogranulomatous pyelonephritis (see Fig GU 5-1)	Unifocal or multifocal masses with displacement of nondilated calyces and normal or diminished opacification. Calcification is common.	Nodular replacement of renal parenchyma by large lipid-filled macrophages (foam cells) that develops in chronically infected kidneys. Most commonly appears as a unilateral nonfunctioning kidney with multifocal enlargement and an obstructing radiopaque calculus at the ureteropelvic junction. May simulate a renal neoplasm (CT shows the characteristic fatty consistency of the xanthogranulomatous mass).
Subcapsular hematoma	Nonopacifying mass between opacified renal parenchyma and the renal capsule that flattens and compresses the underlying renal parenchyma. May extrinsically compress the pelvocalyceal system and even result in a nonfunctioning kidney.	Post-traumatic or spontaneous (often associated with neoplasm, arteriosclerosis, or polyarteritis nodosa). A large subcapsular hematoma may produce hypertension (Page kidney).

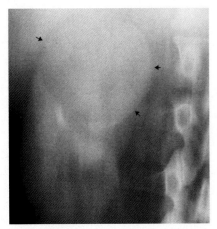

Fig GU 9-8
Renal adenoma. A nephrotomogram shows the tumor to be a smooth, relatively lucent mass (arrows) that is indistinguishable from a cyst.

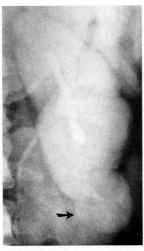

Fig GU 9-9
Reninoma. Small mass (arrow) arising from the lower pole of the left kidney.[9]

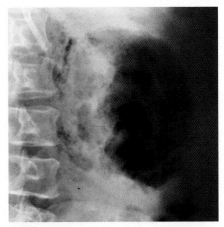

Fig GU 9-10
Renal abscess. Large amounts of extraluminal gas in and around the left kidney.

Cystic Diseases of the Kidneys

Condition	Imaging Findings	Comments
Simple renal cyst (Fig GU 10-1)	Focal contour expansion of the renal outline on the nephrogram phase. The cortical margin appears as a very thin, smooth radiopaque rim about the bulging lucent cyst (beak sign). A thickened wall suggests bleeding into the cyst, cyst infection, or a malignant lesion. Thin curvilinear calcification is seen in approximately 3% of cases (not pathognomonic of a benign process, as 20% of masses with this appearance are malignant).	Unifocal, fluid-filled mass. Usually unilocular, though septa sometimes divide the cyst into chambers that may or may not communicate with each other. Cysts vary in size and may occur at single or multiple sites in one or both kidneys. Ultrasound or CT scans unequivocally demonstrate simple renal cysts. Cyst puncture is necessary if there is an atypical appearance or a strong clinical suspicion of an abscess or if the patient has hematuria or hypertension.
Parapelvic cyst	Hilar mass displacing the kidney laterally and rotating it on its anteroposterior axis. Occasionally compresses hilar fat to produce a thin, lucent fat line separating the cyst from the adjacent renal parenchyma.	Extraparenchymal cyst occurring in the region of the renal hilum. Most parapelvic cysts lie lateral to the renal pelvis and can spread, elongate, and compress adjacent calyces (may even cause obstruction).
Adult polycystic kidney disease	Bilateral large kidneys with a multilobulated contour. The pelvic and infundibular structures are elongated, effaced, and often displaced around larger cysts to produce a crescentic outline. The characteristic mottled, "Swiss cheese" nephrogram is due to the presence of innumerable lucent cysts of various sizes throughout the kidneys. Plaques of calcification occasionally occur in cyst walls.	Inherited disorder in which many progressively growing cysts cause lobulated enlargement of the kidneys and progressive renal impairment. Approximately 35% of patients have associated cysts of the liver (they do not interfere with hepatic functions). About 10% have one or more saccular (berry) aneurysms of the cerebral arteries (may rupture and produce fatal subarachnoid hemorrhage). Hypertension is common.
Infantile polycystic kidney disease (Fig GU 10-2)	Kidneys appear as large soft-tissue masses occupying much of the abdomen and displacing the stomach and bowel. Smooth cortical margins (unlike the adult form). If there is sufficient renal function, urography results in a nephrogram with a streaky pattern of alternating dense and lucent bands reflecting contrast material puddling in elongated cystic spaces that radiate perpendicular to the cortical surface.	Rare, usually fatal, autosomal recessive disorder that manifests itself at birth by diffusely enlarged kidneys, renal failure, and maldevelopment of intrahepatic bile ducts. In the childhood form, renal abnormality is usually milder but is associated with severe congenital hepatic fibrosis and portal hypertension.

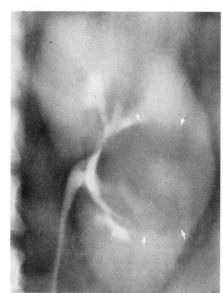

Fig GU 10-1
Simple renal cyst. Nephrotomogram shows the smooth-walled, fluid-filled mass (arrows).

Condition	Imaging Findings	Comments
Medullary sponge kidney (renal tubular ectasia) (Fig GU 10-3)	Ectatic tubules appear either as fine linear striations of contrast producing a brush border pattern or as more cystic dilatation simulating a cluster of grapes. Plain radiographs often demonstrate small, smoothly rounded calculi occurring in clusters or in a fan-like arrangement in the papillary tip of one or more renal pyramids.	Cystic dilatation of distal collecting tubules in the renal pyramids. The ectatic changes may be limited to a single pyramid, but are usually more extensive and bilateral (often asymmetric). Renal function is preserved, though tubular stasis predisposes to calculus formation and pyelonephritis. Generally asymptomatic, except when medullary calculi become dislodged and produce renal colic or hematuria.
Multicystic dysplastic kidney (Fig GU 10-4)	Unilateral, multilobulated, nonfunctioning mass in the area normally occupied by the kidney. There may be thin curvilinear calcification outlining cyst walls. The vascularized walls of individual cysts may become slightly opaque during urography to produce the cluster-of-grapes sign (round lucent cysts separated from each other by slightly opacified septa). Usually there is compensatory hypertrophy of the contralateral kidney.	Nonhereditary congenital dysplasia (usually asymptomatic) in which the kidney is composed almost entirely of large thin-walled cysts with little solid renal tissue. Most common cause of an abdominal mass in the newborn. Other manifestations include an atretic ureter with a blind proximal end (on retrograde pyelography) and an absent or severely atretic renal artery. Ultrasound can differentiate the disorganized pattern of cysts and lack of renal parenchyma and reniform contour in multicystic kidney disease from the precise organization of symmetrically positioned fluid-filled spaces in hydronephrosis.

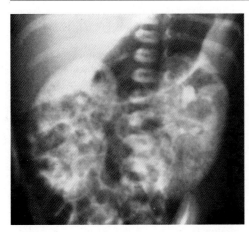

Fig GU 10-2
Infantile polycystic kidney disease. Excretory urogram in a young boy with large, palpable abdominal masses demonstrates renal enlargement with characteristic streaky densities leading to the calyceal tips. There is only minimal distortion of the calyces.

A

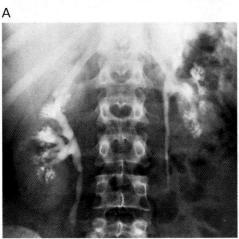

B

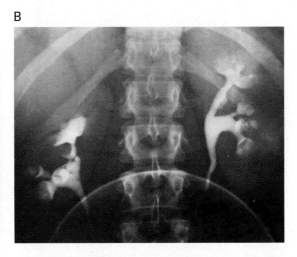

Fig GU 10-3
Medullary sponge kidney. (A) Excretory urogram demonstrates multiple small, smoothly rounded calculi occurring in clusters in the papillary tips of multiple renal pyramids. (B) In another patient, the ectatic tubules appear as fine linear striations of contrast producing the characteristic brush border pattern.

Condition	Imaging Findings	Comments
Calyceal cyst or diverticulum (pyelogenic cyst)	Sharply defined, often spherical cystic space. Delayed urographic opacification occurs by retrograde filling through a narrow channel that typically arises from a calyceal fornix.	Possible causes include a parenchymal cyst draining into a calyx, a ruptured cortical abscess, and dilatation of a renal tubule or the blind end of a branching wolffian duct.
Medullary cystic disease (Fig GU 10-5)	Normal or small kidneys with smooth contours and impaired excretion of contrast material. A large medullary cyst may produce a sharply defined radiolucent defect on a nephrotomogram (best seen on CT). The cysts are usually too small to cause pelvocalyceal displacement or lobulation of the renal contours.	Hereditary nephropathy consisting of a variable number of cysts (often very small) in the corticomedullary junction and medulla. More often involves females. Clinical findings include anemia, polyuria, hyposthenuria, and salt wasting. No hypertension.
Multilocular cyst	Unifocal mass that is usually in a polar location. Sharply defined lucent nephrographic defect. Calcification and faint septa may be detected. Often, displacement of the pelvocalyceal system.	Uncommon unilateral mass composed of multiple cysts of various sizes and adjoining primitive cellular elements. May be detected as a palpable mass in infants. Represents either a form of congenital cystic dysplasia or a benign renal neoplasm. Differs from multicystic (dysgenetic) kidney in that a multilocular cyst is unilateral, involves only a segment of an otherwise normal kidney, and has no associated abnormality of the ureter or renal artery.
Perinephric cyst (pararenal pseudocyst, urinoma)	Elliptical soft-tissue mass in the flank with upward and lateral displacement of the lower pole of the kidney, medial displacement of the ureter, and often obstructive hydronephrosis. Usually reduced or absent excretion of contrast material. Infrequently, evidence of extravasation into the mass.	Most cases result from accidents, operative trauma, or renal transplantation. In infants and children, congenital obstruction of the urinary tract may be a factor. Most common clinical finding is a palpable flank mass (usually a normal urinalysis and no fever).

A
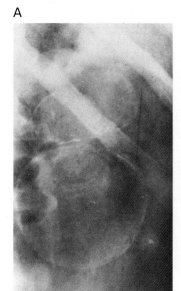

B
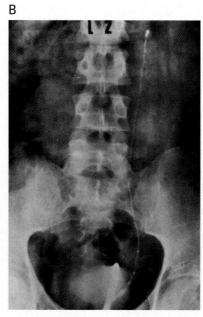

Fig GU 10-4
Multicystic dysplastic kidney. (A) Plain film of the abdomen demonstrates multiple thin, curvilinear calcifications outlining the cysts. (B) Retrograde pyelogram shows atresia of the proximal ureter.[10]

Condition	Imaging Findings	Comments
Acquired cystic kidney disease	Bilateral large kidneys with multilobulated contours and no renal function. Requires ultrasound or CT for detection.	The development of multiple cysts occurs in the chronically failed kidneys of patients undergoing long-term hemodialysis. The degree of enlargement may approach that of adult polycystic kidney disease. The process may reverse after successful renal transplantation.
Echinococcal cyst	Thick-walled cyst with nonhomogeneous lucency. Often produces narrowing or even obstruction of an adjacent calyx. There may be a permanent or intermittent communication between the cyst and the calyceal system.	Usually a solitary cyst, predominantly in the polar region, that may have a calcified wall. Communication with the collecting system almost always occurs through the calyx rather than directly to the pelvis.
Congenital cortical cystic disease	Kidneys usually appear normal. A large cortical cyst may cause a focal contour bulge or calyceal distortion.	In young infants with congenital heart disease and the trisomy syndromes, numerous small cysts may occur along the capsular surface and outline fetal fissures (no functional or clinical abnormality). In tuberous sclerosis, the cysts are of tubular origin, and severe involvement may lead to hypertension and renal failure.
Cystic dysplasia (associated with lower urinary tract obstruction)	Rarely detected on excretory urography (accompanying hydronephrosis obscures evidence of the multiple cortical cysts).	Rarely recognized as a clinical entity but relatively common on pathologic examination of the kidneys in children with lower urinary tract obstruction in fetal life (especially boys with congenital urethral valves). The increased pressure presumably results in malformation of the renal parenchyma and the development of numerous cortical cysts, especially beneath the capsule. Mild involvement is apparently compatible with a normal life span.

A   B   C

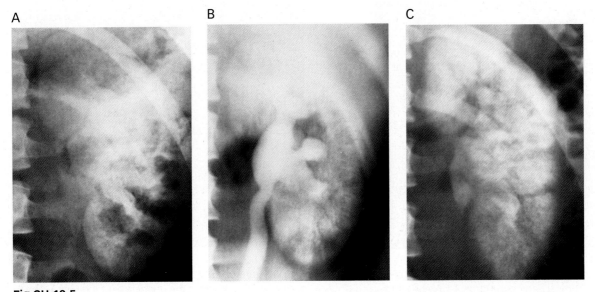

Fig GU 10-5
Medullary cystic disease. (A) A 4-minute radiograph from an excretory urogram shows a normal-sized kidney with a smooth margin, delayed contrast excretion, and a poor but homogeneous nephrogram over the entire kidney. (B) Tomogram taken at 10 minutes shows opacification of the collecting system with mild blunting of the calyces. The nephrogram is composed of many streaky collections of contrast material radiating from the calyces to the periphery. (C) Radiograph taken at 120 minutes shows a high-density nephrogram confined to the medulla. This is probably caused by accumulation of contrast material in dilated tubules. The cortex and the columns of Bertin are recognizable as radiolucent areas.[11]

Depression or Scar in the Renal Margin

Condition	Imaging Findings	Comments
Fetal lobulation	Slight notching of the renal contour that is located between normal calyces. May be multifocal or bilateral.	Common normal variant. The notches represent points at which the centrilobar cortex of one lobe abuts that of an adjacent lobe.
Splenic impression	Flattening of the upper lateral margin of the left kidney.	The impression on the renal contour is probably made by the spleen during development of the left kidney. There is often an associated bulge lower on the lateral margin of the kidney (dromedary hump).
Renal infarction (Fig GU 11-1; see Fig GU 3-2)	Wide-based cortical depression with normal underlying papilla and calyx. May be multifocal or bilateral.	Usually caused by cardiac embolism (mitral stenosis and atrial fibrillation, infective endocarditis, or mural thrombus overlying a myocardial infarct).
Chronic atrophic pyelonephritis (Fig GU 11-2; see Fig GU 3-1)	Cortical depression overlying a retracted papilla, whose calyx is secondarily smoothly dilated. May be bilateral (but usually is asymmetric).	Related to chronic pyelonephritis and vesicoureteral reflux. Cortical depressions must be differentiated from fetal lobulation (which occurs between calyces rather than directly overlying them).
Tuberculosis (see Fig GU 3-3)	Single or multiple cortical depressions that may give the renal surface an irregular appearance.	May produce a pattern indistinguishable from that of chronic atrophic pyelonephritis.

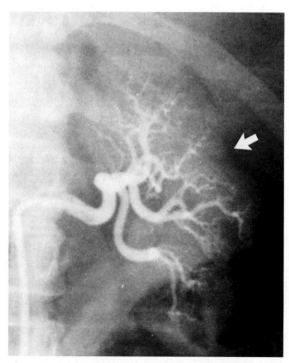

Fig GU 11-1
Renal infarction. Selective left renal arteriogram shows a wide-based cortical depression (arrow) reflecting an infarct scar. Note the tortuosity and rapid tapering of interlobar arteries and their branches that is characteristic of arteriolar nephrosclerosis.

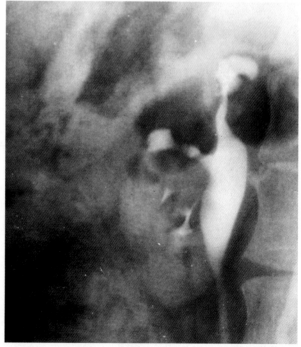

Fig GU 11-2
Chronic pyelonephritis. Focal areas of parenchymal loss and calyceal clubbing in the upper pole of the right kidney.[12]

Renal Pseudotumors (Normal Structures)

Condition	Imaging Findings	Comments
Dromedary hump (Fig GU 12-1)	Bulge on the lateral border of the left kidney just below its interface with the spleen.	Postulated to result from flattening of the developing left kidney by the fetal spleen, as the entity rarely occurs in the right kidney. Usually a normal thickness of renal parenchyma between the underlying calyx and the overlying renal capsule.
Fetal lobulation (see Fig GU 12-1)	Nodular cortical outline with multiple sharp cortical indentations that typically occur between underlying calyces.	Prominence of the centrilobar cortex where two adjacent lobes abut. Lobulation is normal at birth but usually disappears after 5 years.
Column of Bertin (see Fig GU 9-1)	Focal "mass" apparently arising from the surface of the kidney with compression and splaying of the pelvocalyceal system.	Mass of normal cortical tissue located within the renal parenchyma that may simulate a true neoplasm. Most commonly develops at the junction of the middle and upper thirds of a duplex kidney.
Hilar lip (Figs GU 12-2 and GU 12-3)	Localized bulge in the medial aspect of the renal contour immediately above or below the hilum.	Extra infolding of normally thicker parenchyma at either pole results in a redundancy of renal cortex that produces a pseudotumor. This phenomenon is most common in the suprahilar region of the left kidney.

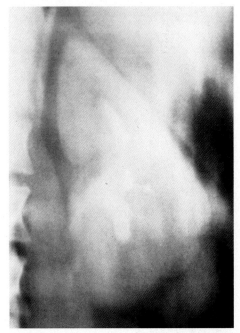

Fig GU 12-1
Dromedary hump. There is flattening of the upper two-thirds of the lateral border of the left kidney, most likely from splenic pressure. Note also the multiple fetal lobulations in the lower third of the lateral renal contour.[4]

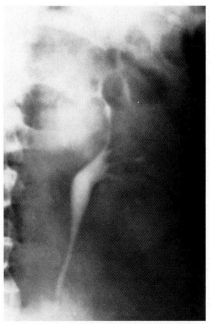

Fig GU 12-2
Suprahilar pseudotumor. Overgrowth of the renal parenchyma in the suprahilar area impresses the upper infundibulum laterally. The density of this area is similar to that of the remainder of the cortical nephrogram.[4]

Condition	Imaging Findings	Comments
Renal sinus lipomatosis (Fig GU 12-4)	Large deposits of fat-density material that may be associated with stretching and elongation of the pelvocalyceal system.	The increased fat deposition may be related to the normal aging process, in which gradual loss of renal parenchyma is accompanied by shrinkage of the kidney away from the hilar structures and the stimulation of fat deposition. Abnormal amounts of sinus fat may develop in response to renal tissue loss resulting from infection, trauma, and infarction. Prominent sinus fat also may be seen in patients with severe obesity.
Malrotation (see Fig GU 1-4)	Often bizarre appearance of the renal parenchyma, calyces, and pelvis that may suggest a pathologic condition in an otherwise normal kidney.	Unilateral or bilateral anomaly. When the renal pelvis is situated in an anterior or lateral position, the upper part of the ureter appears to be displaced laterally, suggesting an extrinsic mass. The elongated pelvis of a malrotated kidney may mimic obstructive dilatation.
Vascular impression	Occasionally presents as a discrete hilar mass without producing a characteristic extrinsic defect on the renal pelvis.	Normal or anomalous arteries and veins and their major or peripheral branches. A discrete hilar (parapelvic) mass may be produced when a vessel makes an abrupt turn so that its long axis comes to lie in an anteroposterior plane for part of its course. Tomography with the patient in an oblique position usually shows that the mass has disappeared; in equivocal cases, renal arteriography may be required.

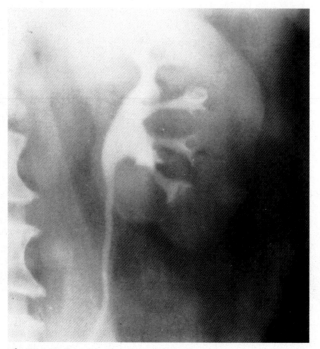

Fig GU 12-3
Infrahilar pseudotumor. Lobular mass projecting from the kidney in the region of the infrahilar area represents a cortical pseudotumor.[4]

Condition	Imaging Findings	Comments
Superimposed abdominal shadows	Renal pseudotumor.	Unusual-shaped spleen, accessory spleen, gallbladder, fluid-filled duodenal bulb, or gastric fundus.
Focal hypertrophy (regenerated nodule)	Renal pseudotumor.	Acquired condition in which attempts at compensatory hypertrophy in diseased kidneys are limited to islands of still healthy renal tissue interposed between large segments of scarred kidney. Underlying disorders include chronic pyelonephritis, glomerulonephritis, trauma, and ischemia.

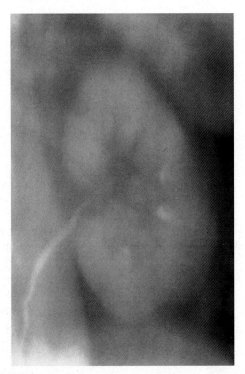

Fig GU 12-4
Renal sinus lipomatosis. Nephrotomography demonstrates the extensive sinus fat around the renal pelvis. The fat infiltrates around the infundibula and peripheral calyces.[4]

Persistent or Increasingly Dense Nephrogram

Condition	Imaging Findings	Comments
Acute extrarenal obstruction (Fig GU 13-1)	Unilateral (rarely bilateral) increasingly dense nephrogram that may have striations. Delayed and decreased excretion of contrast material into a dilated (hydronephrotic) collecting system.	Most common cause of an increasingly dense nephrogram. Usually due to a ureteral calculus or blood clot and associated with symptoms of ureteral colic.
Renal ischemia (see Fig GU 14-3)	Unilateral increasingly dense nephrogram. Delayed and decreased excretion of contrast material, decreased kidney size, and often notching of the ipsilateral proximal ureter.	Severe stenosis of the main renal artery causes diminished renal perfusion pressure and the development of arterial collaterals.
Hypotension/shock	Bilateral increasingly dense nephrograms. Decreased or absent excretion of contrast material.	Diminished perfusion pressure of both kidneys. Once normal blood pressure is restored, there is rapid pelvocalyceal opacification and a return to normal nephrographic density. Most commonly an adverse reaction to contrast material during urography (kidney size decreased compared to scout film).
Acute tubular necrosis	Bilateral immediate and persistent dense nephrograms (may be increasingly dense). Decreased or absent excretion of contrast material.	Causes include severe ischemia (shock, crush injuries, burns, transfusion reactions) and exposure to toxic agents (carbon tetrachloride, ethylene glycol, mercury, bismuth, arsenic). An uncommon cause is contrast material nephrotoxicity (dose-related and potentiated by pre-existing dehydration, low-flow states, and chronic renal disease, especially diabetic nephropathy).
Acute tubular blockage	Bilateral increasingly dense or persistent dense nephrograms. Decreased excretion of contrast material into nondilated collecting systems.	Causes include multiple myeloma, urate nephropathy, amyloidosis, hemo- or myoglobulinuria, sulfonamide therapy, and massive precipitation of Tamm-Horsfall protein (may be a complication of contrast material given to severely dehydrated infants and children).

A

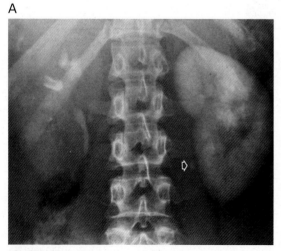

B

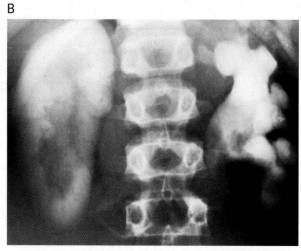

Fig GU 13-1
Acute urinary tract obstruction. (A) Excretory urogram demonstrates a prolonged nephrogram on the left with fine cortical striations (alternating radiolucent and radiopaque lines) and no calyceal filling. An arrow points to the obstructing stone in the proximal left ureter. (B) In another patient, there is a prolonged and intensified obstructive nephrogram of the right kidney. On the left, there is marked dilatation of the pelvocalyceal system but no persistent nephrogram, reflecting an intermittent chronic obstruction on this side.

Condition	Imaging Findings	Comments
Acute bacterial nephritis (severe pyelonephritis) (Fig GU 13-2)	Unilateral immediate and persistent dense nephrogram. Minimal or absent excretion of contrast material.	Most often seen with acute suppurative pyelonephritis, especially in patients with diabetes mellitus.
Acute glomerulonephritis (Fig GU 13-3)	Bilateral increasingly dense nephrograms.	Probably reflects reduced glomerular perfusion due to obliterative changes in the renal microvasculature.
Acute renal vein thrombosis (Fig GU 13-4)	Unilateral increasingly dense nephrogram. Decreased or absent excretion of contrast material.	Most frequently occurs in children who are severely dehydrated. In adults, generally a complication of another renal disease (chronic glomerulonephritis, amyloidosis, pyelonephritis), trauma, extension of thrombus from the inferior vena cava, and direct invasion or extrinsic pressure secondary to a renal tumor.
Acute papillary necrosis (see Fig GU 16-1)	Increasingly dense nephrogram. Characteristic central or eccentric cavitation of papillae or complete sloughing of papillary tips (may calcify).	Unusual presentation due to tubular obstruction by necrotic papillary tips. Underlying causes include analgesic abuse (especially phenacetin), sickle cell anemia, diabetes, and pyelonephritis.

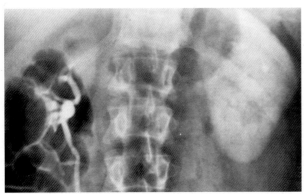

Fig GU 13-2
Acute bacterial nephritis. Persistent dense nephrogram on the left with minimal opacification of the collecting system.

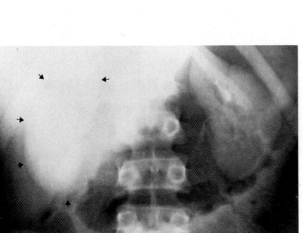

Fig GU 13-3
Acute renal failure. Film from an excretory urogram 20 minutes after the injection of contrast material shows bilateral persistent nephrograms with no calyceal filling.

Fig GU 13-4
Acute renal vein thrombosis. Film of the right kidney taken 5 minutes after the injection of contrast material shows a dense nephrogram (arrows) and the absence of calyceal filling.

Diminished Concentration of Contrast Material in the Pelvocalyceal System

Condition	Comments
Bilateral	
Overhydration/inadequate dehydration	Causes dilution of the contrast material (the kidneys may be entirely normal).
Polyuria	Excretion of large volumes of hypotonic urine due to diuretic therapy, diabetes insipidus (lack of antidiuretic hormone secreted by the posterior lobe of the pituitary gland), diabetes mellitus, and intrinsic renal diseases.
Renal failure (uremia) (Fig GU 14-1)	Severely decreased renal function due to a variety of underlying causes.
Nephrosclerosis (Fig GU 14-2)	Long-standing hypertension causes narrowing of extra- and intrarenal arteries with prolonged intrarenal circulation time and decreased excretion of contrast material.
Technical	Injection of an inadequate dose of contrast material.
Unilateral	
Urinary tract obstruction	Elevated pressure in the dilated collecting system causes diminished filtration of contrast material. Delayed parenchymal opacification compared with the nonobstructed kidney, with the nephrogram eventually becoming more dense than normal because of a decreased rate of flow through the tubules (enhanced water resorption by the nephrons and greater concentration of the contrast material).

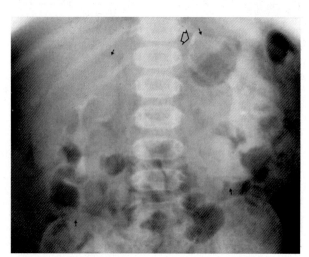

Fig GU 14-1
Nephrotic syndrome causing renal failure. Excretory urogram demonstrates striking enlargement of both kidneys. (Solid arrows point to the tips of the upper and lower poles of the kidneys.) There is decreased opacification of both collecting systems. Of incidental note is calcification in the left adrenal gland (open arrow).

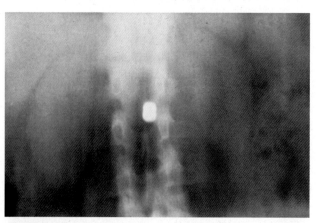

Fig GU 14-2
Malignant nephrosclerosis. Nephrotomogram obtained 5 minutes after the injection of contrast material shows minimum opacification of small, smooth kidneys.[5]

Condition	Comments
Renal parenchymal infection	Most commonly due to tuberculosis (obstruction of the pelvocalyceal system or ureter, autonephrectomy, or severe narrowing of the renal artery).
Trauma	Spasm of the pelvocalyceal system. Decreased renal function may result in failure to detect extravasation of poorly opacified urine.
Renal artery stenosis involving opposite kidney (Fig GU 14-3)	On rapid-sequence studies, the affected kidney demonstrates delayed appearance and excretion of contrast material. Eventually, increased water reabsorption produces an increased concentration of contrast material on the affected side, making the normal side appear to have diminished concentration.

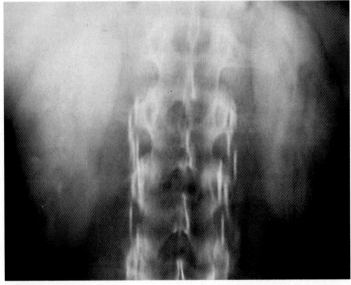

Fig GU 14-3
Renovascular hypertension. A film from a rapid-sequence urogram obtained 3 minutes after the injection of contrast material shows no calyceal opacification on the left in a patient with left renal artery stenosis.

Solitary or Multiple Filling Defects in the Pelvocalyceal System

Condition	Imaging Findings	Comments
Calculus (Figs GU 15-1 and GU 15-2)	Round or oval, frequently mobile filling defect. Often multiple and bilateral. A large calculus may form a cast of the pelvocalyceal system (staghorn calculus). If the obstruction is acute, the increased intrapelvic pressure may permit little or no glomerular filtration and produce the radiographic appearance of a delayed but prolonged nephrogram and the lack of calyceal filling on the affected side.	More than 80% of renal calculi are radiopaque and detectable on plain abdominal radiographs. These typically develop secondary to hyperparathyroidism, renal tubular acidosis, hyperoxaluria, or any cause of increased calcium excretion in the urine (20% are idiopathic). Radiodense calcium stones are often invisible in the midst of opaque urine. Completely lucent calculi are composed of uric acid or urates, xanthine, or matrix concentrations. Struvite (magnesium ammonium phosphate) stones are moderately radiopaque with variable internal density (found mainly in women with chronic urinary tract infection). Cystine calculi are mildly opaque.
Blood clot (Fig GU 15-3)	Single or multiple nonopaque filling defects. Asymptomatic unless it causes pelvocalyceal obstruction. Usually becomes significantly smaller or disappears within 2 weeks (though rarely a residual fibrin mass that may eventually calcify).	Causes of urinary tract bleeding include trauma, tumor, instrumentation, nephritis and vasculitis, rupture of arterial aneurysm, vascular malformation, bleeding disorder, and anticoagulant therapy.
Air	Single or multiple, round, freely movable filling defects that are not associated with any signs of obstruction. Must be differentiated from superimposed intestinal gas that projects at least partially outside the urinary tract in different positions or on subsequent films.	Causes include instrumentation (retrograde pyelogram), trauma, surgery, ureterointestinal anastomosis, and vesicovaginal fistula. Rarely a manifestation of emphysematous pyelonephritis in diabetics (also gas in the renal parenchyma and perirenal soft tissues).

A   B

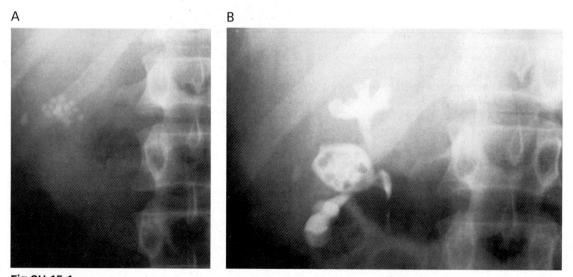

Fig GU 15-1
Cystine stones. (A) Plain film shows multiple radiopaque calculi. (B) Excretory urogram demonstrates the stones as lucent filling defects in the opacified renal pelvis.

Condition	Imaging Findings	Comments
Transitional cell carcinoma (Figs GU 15-4 and GU 15-5)	Single or multiple, smooth or irregular filling defect. Characteristic stippled pattern reflects trapping of small amounts of contrast material in the interstices of papillary tumor fronds. May develop stippled calcific deposits visible on CT. A wide area of superficial spreading occasionally causes an irregular mucosal pattern and thickening of the pelvocalyceal wall.	Usually occurs in patients 50 to 70 years of age and presents with hematuria and pain. The tumor is infrequently palpable (unless it causes chronic obstruction and pronounced hydronephrosis). Primary squamous cell carcinoma and sarcomas rarely cause pelvocalyceal filling defects.
Benign tumor	Single or multiple filling defects.	Mesenchymal tumor; papilloma; hemangioma; fibrous ureteral polyp.

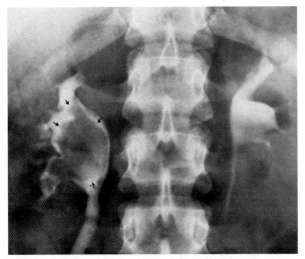

Fig GU 15-2
Xanthinuria. A large lucent stone (arrows) almost fills the right pelvocalyceal system.

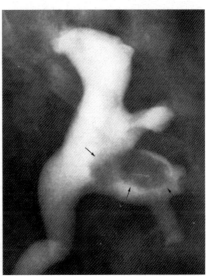

Fig GU 15-3
Blood clot. Large filling defect with a smooth contour (arrows). A CT scan showed the attenuation value of the blood clot to be 62 H, a density higher than that of transitional cell carcinoma but lower than that of a nonopaque stone.[13]

A

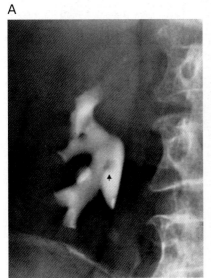

B

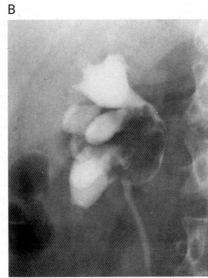

Fig GU 15-4
Transitional cell carcinoma of the renal pelvis in two patients. (A) A small filling defect (arrow) in the renal pelvis simulates a blood clot, stone, fungus ball, or sloughed papilla. (B) A huge mass fills virtually all the renal pelvis.

Condition	Imaging Findings	Comments
Sloughed papilla (Fig GU 15-6)	Triangular lucent filling defect with the remaining calyx having a round, saccular, or club-shaped configuration. A sloughed papilla may stay in place and become calcified (typically ring-shaped with a lucent center) or pass down the ureter (simulating a stone and even causing obstruction).	Usually develops in a patient with renal papillary necrosis due to analgesic abuse (less frequently secondary to severe urinary tract infection, obstruction, or acute bacterial nephritis).
Fungus ball (mycetoma) (Fig GU 15-7)	Single or multiple, large nonopaque mass that often fills the renal pelvis and may cause obstruction. Contrast material may fill the interstices to produce a lacelike radiodense pattern.	Most mycetomas are caused by *Candida albicans*. *Aspergillus* is the second most common organism. Usually there is involvement of the renal parenchyma (hematogenous dissemination), with the fungus ball forming from mycelia shed into the pelvis.
Cholesteatoma	Single round mass or multiple stringy filling defects with indistinct margins. Contrast material extends into concentric laminations to produce an onion skin pattern of alternating density and lucency.	Unusual form of tissue slough resulting from keratinizing squamous metaplasia of the uroepithelium. Generally associated with chronic infection and impaired urinary drainage. Approximately half the patients have calculi.
Aberrant papilla	Oval or round filling defect in a major infundibulum without any signs of obstruction.	Papilla without a calyx. Must be differentiated from a normal calyx seen end-on (which appears normal when viewed in profile on other projections).

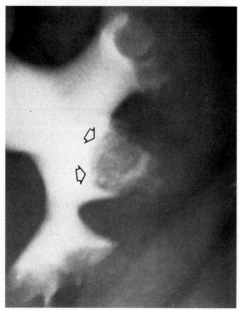

Fig GU 15-5
Transitional cell carcinoma of the renal pelvis. A small filling defect occupies an interpolar calyx (arrows). Although the defect might at first be mistaken for a large but otherwise normal papilla, the many small contrast stipples and the suggestively irregular border make its neoplastic nature evident.[14]

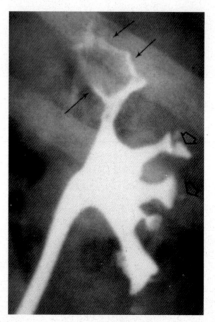

Fig GU 15-6
Sloughed papillae in papillary necrosis. A ring of contrast material (long arrows) surrounds a triangular lucent filling defect, which represents an almost complete papilla that has been separated from the rest of the renal parenchyma. The short arrows point to less severe extension of contrast material from the calyces into the papillae.[7]

Condition	Imaging Findings	Comments
Inspissated pus/ necrotic debris	Irregular filling defect.	Pyelonephritis of suppurative, xanthogranulo-matous, or tuberculous origin. There may also be mucosal ulceration, irregularity, and scarring from the infectious process.
Pyelitis cystica (see Fig GU 18-6)	Multiple, small, sharply defined, unchanging filling defects in the pelvocalyceal system.	Multiple, small cysts in the pelvic wall that typically develop in older women with chronic urinary tract infection.
Acute pyelonephritis (Fig GU 15-8)	Linear striations in the renal pelvis (and proximal ureter).	Probably reflects acute mucosal edema.
Leukoplakia	Localized or generalized irregularity of the pelvocalyceal wall.	Squamous metaplasia of transitional cells that develops in patients with a history of chronic infection. Unlike cholesteatoma, leukoplakia is smaller and is frequently associated with carcinoma. Coexisting calculi occur in approximately 50% of patients.
Blood vessels/vascular malformation	Varying pattern of single or multiple, intra-luminal or extrinsic filling defects.	Normal renal artery or major branch (solitary, extrinsic defect); arterial collaterals (multiple, small marginal defects, especially in the proximal ureter); aneurysm or arteriovenous fistula; renal vein thrombosis; venous collaterals.
Extrinsic compression (see Section GU 17)	Generalized narrowing of part or all of the pelvo-calyceal system.	Peripelvic or parenchymal cyst impinging on the renal pelvis; renal sinus lipomatosis.

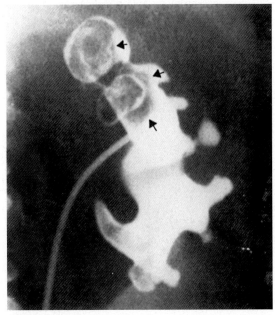

Fig GU 15-7
Fungus ball in renal candidiasis. Retrograde pyelo-gram demonstrates a large filling defect (arrows) in the left renal pelvis.[15]

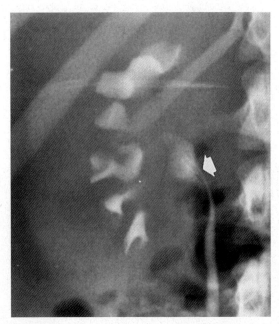

Fig GU 15-8
Acute pyelonephritis. Linear striations (arrow) in the right renal pelvis.

Clubbing or Destruction of Renal Calyces

Condition	Imaging Findings	Comments
Papillary necrosis (Fig GU 16-1)	Cavitation of the central portion of the papilla or complete sloughing of the papillary tip. The cavitation may be central or eccentric with its long axis paralleling that of the papilla. The cavity varies from long and thin to short and bulbous, and the margins may be sharp or irregular. With sloughing, the remaining calyx has a round, saccular, or club-shaped configuration, and there is a ring of contrast material surrounding the triangular lucent filling defect that represents the sloughed necrotic tissue (which may calcify or pass down the ureter).	Ischemic coagulative necrosis involving various amounts of the medullary papillae and pyramids. Most often occurs in patients with diabetes, pyelonephritis, urinary tract infection or obstruction, sickle cell disease, or phenacetin abuse. The earliest radiographic sign (often overlooked on excretory urography) is a cleavage plane that develops in a zone of ischemia and communicates with the calyx, producing a faint streak of contrast material oriented parallel to the long axis of the papilla and usually extending from the fornix (also can arise in the papillary tip).
Tuberculosis (Fig GU 16-2)	Initially, irregularity of one or several papillae or calyces (indistinguishable from papillary necrosis from other causes). Progressive destruction produces large irregular cavities. Fibrosis and stricture formation in the pelvocalyceal system cause narrowing or obstruction of the infundibulum to the affected calyx.	Other characteristic radiographic manifestations in the advanced stage of hematogenously spread tuberculosis include cortical scarring and parenchymal atrophy (simulating chronic bacterial pyelonephritis); focal intrarenal masses mimicking neoplasms (tuberculous granulomas that do not communicate with the collecting system); a densely calcified, nonfunctioning shrunken kidney (autonephrectomy); and ureteral changes (corkscrew and pipe stem ureter).
Chronic pyelonephritis (Fig GU 16-3)	Clubbed, dilated calyces are caused by retraction of papillae and most frequently involve the poles. Depressed cortical scars typically develop over involved calyces.	May be unifocal or multifocal, unilateral or bilateral (but usually asymmetric). End stage of vesicoureteral reflux and recurrent urinary tract infection in childhood.
Hydronephrosis (Fig GU 16-4)	Dilatation of the entire pelvocalyceal system. The kidneys may be small and smooth (postobstructive renal atrophy).	Most commonly the result of one prolonged or several intermittent episodes of obstruction. Nonobstructive hydronephrosis may be due to reflux, bacterial endotoxins, pregnancy, or nephrogenic diabetes insipidus.
Localized caliectasis	Calyceal dilatation due to the obstruction of an infundibulum.	Causes include neoplasm (renal cell or transitional cell carcinoma), tuberculosis, inflammatory stricture, calculus, and anomalous vessel.

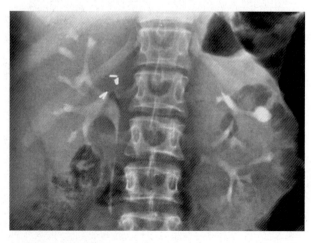

Fig GU 16-1
Papillary necrosis. Generalized saccular or club-shaped configuration of both calyces bilaterally in a patient with sickle cell disease.

Condition	Imaging Findings	Comments
Congenital megacalyces	Dilated calyces that often have a polygonal or faceted appearance. The renal cortex and kidney size are normal. Bilateral in approximately 20% of cases.	Congenital nonobstructive enlargement of calyces due to malformations of the renal papillae that are probably secondary to temporary intrauterine obstruction.
Medullary sponge kidney (tubular ectasia) (Fig GU 16-5)	Broadening, increased cupping, and distortion of calyces. The ectatic tubules appear as fine linear striations of contrast producing a brush border pattern. With increasing dilatation, the tubules become more cystic and simulate a cluster of grapes. Plain films often demonstrate multiple, small, smoothly rounded calculi occurring in clusters or in a fan-like arrangement in the papillary tip of one or more renal pyramids.	Cystic dilatation of distal collecting tubules in the renal pyramids. The ectatic changes may be limited to a single pyramid, but are usually more extensive and bilateral (though often asymmetric). Although renal function is preserved, tubular stasis predisposes to calculus formation and pyelonephritis. Generally asymptomatic, except when medullary calculi become dislodged and produce renal colic or hematuria.

A

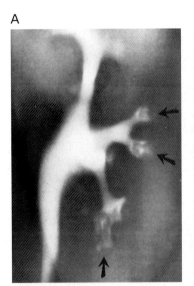

B

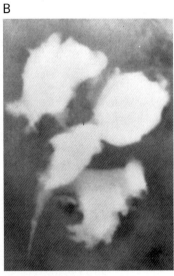

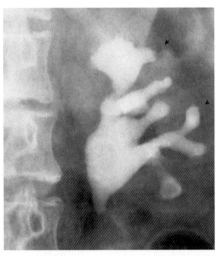

Fig GU 16-2
Active tuberculosis causing papillary destruction (arrows). (A) Early. (B) Advanced.[3]

Fig GU 16-3
Chronic pyelonephritis. Diffuse rounded clubbing of multiple calyces with atrophy and thinning of the overlying renal parenchyma. The arrows indicate the outer margin of the kidney.

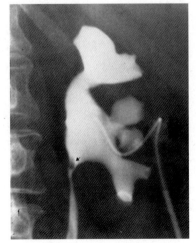

Fig GU 16-4
Hydronephrosis. Dilatation of the entire pelvocalyceal system proximal to an obstructing cryptococcus fungus ball (arrow) at the ureteropelvic junction.

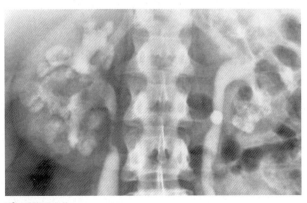

Fig GU 16-5
Medullary sponge kidney. Caliectasis with medullary calculi throughout both kidneys.

Effaced Pelvocalyceal System

Condition	Imaging Findings	Comments
Extrinsic compression		
Global enlargement of renal parenchyma	Bilateral large, smooth kidneys with effaced pelvocalyceal systems (see Section GU 7).	Excessive renal bulk occurs with cellular infiltration or proliferation, deposition of abnormal proteins, or accumulation of interstitial edema or blood.
Renal sinus mass or masslike abnormality	Unilateral large, smooth kidney with effaced pelvocalyceal system (see Section GU 4).	Renal vein occlusion; acute arterial infarction; acute bacterial nephritis.
Renal sinus lipomatosis (Fig GU 17-1)	Elongation and attenuation of the pelvocalyceal system caused by the accumulation of an excessive amount of fat-density material in the renal sinus (diagnosis easily confirmed on CT).	Often a normal variant in an obese person or a reflection of the loss of kidney parenchyma due to ischemia, infarction, or infection. May mimic single or multiple peripelvic masses.
Parapelvic cysts (Fig GU 17-2)	Elongation and attenuation of the pelvocalyceal system by multiple or multiloculated water-density cysts.	Can be differentiated from renal sinus lipomatosis by ultrasound or CT. A single parapelvic cyst causes focal displacement and smooth effacement of the adjacent portion of the pelvocalyceal system.
Hemorrhage into renal sinus	Attenuation of the pelvocalyceal system with impaired excretion of contrast material.	Spontaneous hemorrhage into the renal sinus may be a self-limited complication of anticoagulant therapy.

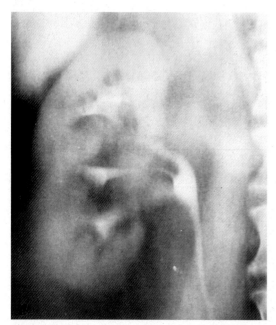

Fig GU 17-1
Renal sinus lipomatosis. Nephrotomogram shows increased radiolucency (fat) around the renal sinuses and calyces causing stretching and elongation of the pelvocalyceal system.[7]

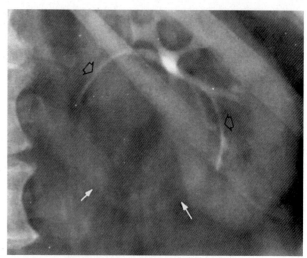

Fig GU 17-2
Renal cyst. Smooth displacement of the attenuated lower pole calyces (open arrows). The solid arrows indicate the inferior extent of the cyst.

Condition	Imaging Findings	Comments
Spasm/inflammation Infection	Generalized effacement of the pelvocalyceal system.	Acute pyelonephritis and acute bacterial nephritis (may result from spasm of smooth muscles of the collecting system wall, swelling of the kidney, or paralysis of smooth muscle due to bacterial endotoxins). Uroepithelial tuberculosis produces submucosal granulomas and mucosal ulcerations that render the collecting system nondistensible.
Hematuria	Generalized effacement of the pelvocalyceal system. The appearance reverts to normal as the bleeding ceases.	Upper urinary tract bleeding (from the kidney or directly from uroepithelial structures) irritates pelvocalyceal smooth muscles.
Infiltrating malignant uroepithelial tumor (Figs GU 17-3 and GU 17-4)	Generalized effacement of the pelvocalyceal system associated with a nodular mucosal pattern.	Most commonly a transitional cell carcinoma that grows superficially or infiltrates deeply over a large portion of the pelvocalyceal system.
Oliguria	Unilateral or bilateral collapse of the pelvocalyceal system.	Low-flow states such as water deprivation, renal ischemia, and oliguric renal failure.

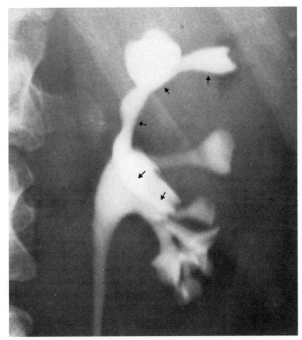

Fig GU 17-3
Renal hamartoma. Large mass distorting and displacing the pelvocalyceal system (arrows).

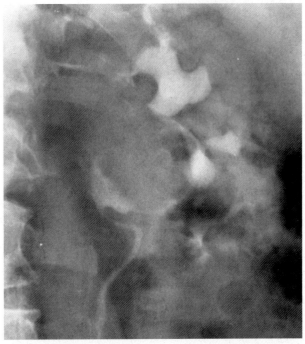

Fig GU 17-4
Transitional cell carcinoma of the renal pelvis. A large mass distorts the pelvocalyceal system and causes deviation of the ureter.

Filling Defects in the Ureter

Condition	Imaging Findings	Comments
Calculus (Fig GU 18-1)	Round or oval filling defect that tends to become impacted in areas of normal anatomic narrowing (ureteropelvic and ureterovesical junctions and the site where the ureter crosses the sacrum and the iliac vessels).	Extremely common and clinically associated with hematuria and ureteral colic. Approximately 80% of ureteral calculi are radiopaque.
Blood clot (Fig GU 18-2)	Single or multiple nonopaque filling defects of various sizes and shapes that may cause temporary ureteral obstruction. They typically become much smaller or disappear within several weeks.	Causes of urinary tract bleeding include trauma, tumor, instrumentation, nephritis and vasculitis, rupture of an arterial aneurysm, vascular malformation, bleeding disorder, and anticoagulant therapy.
Air bubble	Single or multiple, round, freely movable filling defects that are not associated with any signs of obstruction.	Air bubbles are most commonly introduced into the ureter (and pelvocalyceal system) during a retrograde study. Other causes include trauma, surgery, infection, and fistula. Must be distinguished from superimposed intestinal gas, which projects at least partially outside the ureter in different positions or on subsequent films.
Blood vessels and vascular malformations (Fig GU 18-3)	Various patterns of single or multiple extrinsic defects.	Normal renal artery or major branch (solitary); arterial or venous collaterals (multiple, small marginal defects, especially in the proximal ureter, related to renal artery stenosis or renal vein thrombosis); ovarian vein syndrome (solitary compression of the right ureter at the S1 level after several pregnancies).

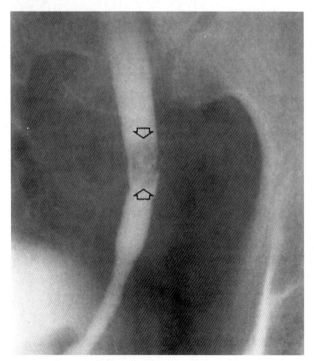

Fig GU 18-1
Nonopaque ureteral calculus (arrows).

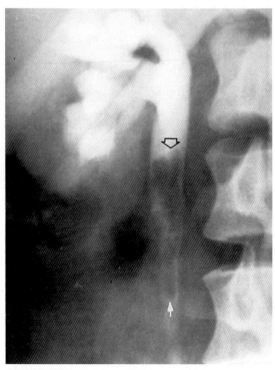

Fig GU 18-2
Blood clot in a proximal ureter (arrows).

Condition	Imaging Findings	Comments
Transitional cell carcinoma (Figs GU 18-4 and GU 18-5)	Smooth or irregular shaggy filling defect. Characteristic stippled pattern represents the trapping of small amounts of contrast material in the interstices of papillary tumor fronds. Lesions that are predominantly infiltrating may produce short or long strictures.	Usually occurs in patients 50–70 years of age and presents with hematuria and pain. May reflect metastatic seeding from a more proximal lesion of the urogenital tract. There is often localized dilatation of the ureter below the level of the expanding intraluminal tumor, in contrast to ureteral collapse distal to an obstructing stone.
Ureteral polyp	Elongated, smoothly marginated filling defect that is generally located in the proximal ureter.	Usually occurs in patients 20 to 40 years of age. Intermittent pain is common, whereas hematuria and ureteral obstruction are rare.
Papilloma	Round, irregular, often multiple filling defects most commonly located in the lower ureter. Frequently causes ureteral obstruction.	Although histologically benign, papillomas often recur and therefore may be considered as low-grade malignancies. Associated tumors may occur in the bladder.
Mesenchymal tumor	Single, small, smooth filling defect.	Fibroma; lipoma; hamartoma; hemangioma (bleeding tendency); fibroepithelial polyp (often multiple).
Metastases	Irregular narrowing of the ureteral lumen. Extension of the lesion may produce an intra-luminal mass.	Metastases to the ureter from distant sources are rare and generally a late event (other evidence of distant metastases is usually present). They may arise from almost any organ in the body but have been reported with slightly greater frequency from tumors of the prostate, stomach, breast, lung, and colon. Metastases may occur at any site along the ureter and frequently are seen in both ureters. Many malignant lesions, particularly the lymphomas, cause displacement of the ureters (due to retroperitoneal nodal metastases) without actual invasion.

A

B

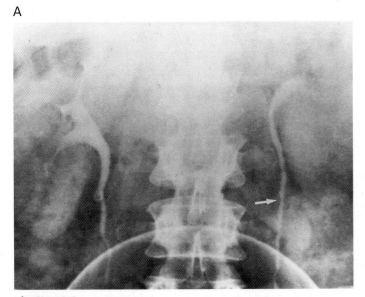
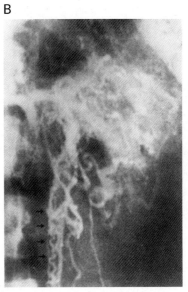

Fig GU 18-3
Renal vein thrombosis. (A) Excretory urogram shows characteristic notching (arrow) of the upper ureter. There is enlargement of the left kidney with poor calyceal function due to compression from parenchymal engorgement. (B) In another patient with renal vein thrombosis and ureteral notching, a venogram demonstrates exuberant periureteral collaterals (arrows).[16]

Condition	Imaging Findings	Comments
Ureteritis cystica (Fig GU 18-6)	Multiple, small, smooth, rounded lucent filling defects that primarily involve one or both proximal ureters. There may also be involvement of the pelvocalyceal system and bladder.	Multiple inflammatory cysts that typically develop in older women, usually in association with chronic urinary tract infection. A single cyst may simulate a transitional cell tumor (but persists unchanged over many years).
Tuberculosis (Fig GU 18-7)	Diffuse irregularity of the ureteral wall simulating multiple filling defects. As the disease heals, there are usually multiple areas in which ureteral strictures alternate with dilated segments (beaded, or corkscrew, appearance).	Almost always tuberculous involvement of the kidney. In advanced disease, the ureter becomes thickened, fixed, and aperistaltic (pipe stem ureter). Often, there is irregular calcification of the vas deferens and seminal vesicles.
Schistosomiasis (see Fig GI 58-1)	Multiple filling defects in the distal ureter, almost always associated with a similar process in the bladder.	Usually caused by *Schistosoma haematobium*. Characteristic calcification of the bladder wall.
Malacoplakia (Fig GU 18-8)	Smooth, single or multiple, round or oval filling defects that predominantly occur in the distal ureter. May produce a scalloped appearance and occasionally a stricture.	Uncommon chronic inflammatory disease that primarily affects women, most of whom have a history of recurrent or chronic urinary tract infection. Malacoplakia more frequently involves the bladder.
Sloughed papilla/ inspissated pus/ tissue debris	Irregular filling defect that may cause ureteral obstruction.	Papillary necrosis; necrotizing tumor; necrotizing pyelonephritis (especially in diabetics); pyonephrosis.
Endometriosis	Single or multiple filling defects in the distal ureter below the pelvic brim. May cause ureteral stricture or extrinsic ureteral compression.	Uncommon condition presenting with pain or cyclic urinary symptoms, including hematuria in a woman in the childbearing years. Often a history of previous gynecologic or abdominal surgery.

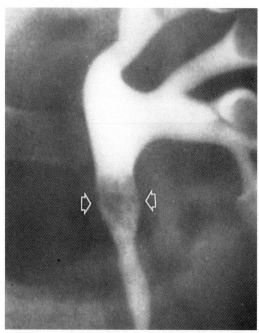

Fig GU 18-4
Transitional cell carcinoma of the ureter. The presence of stippling throughout this proximal ureteral filling defect (arrows) and the suggestive papillary contour of its proximal and distal margins allow the correct diagnosis to be made preoperatively.[14]

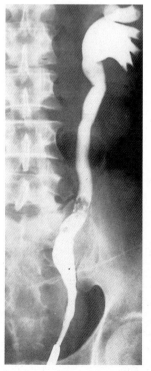

Fig GU 18-5
Transitional cell carcinoma of the midureter. Irregular stricture with proximal ureteral and pelvocalyceal dilatation.

Condition	Imaging Findings	Comments
Benign ureteral stricture	Usually a smooth, conical narrowing. If short and eccentric, may occasionally simulate an extrinsic defect.	May be congenital or secondary to trauma, surgery, instrumentation, stone passage, inflammation, or radiation therapy.
Compression or invasion from adjacent malignancy or nodes	Extrinsic defect that may be smooth or irregular.	Direct extension of retroperitoneal or pelvic malignancy or extrinsic compression by enlarged lymph nodes.
Ureteral diverticulum	Localized extrinsic compression by a cystic lesion that causes slightly delayed opacification.	Very rare solitary (occasionally multiple) out-pouching along the course of the ureter. An enlarged diverticulum due to infection, stone formation, or obstruction may make an extrinsic impression on the adjacent ureter.
Ureteral spasm and peristalsis	May simulate a localized filling defect or vascular notching.	Transitory appearance, unlike a true ureteral filling defect.

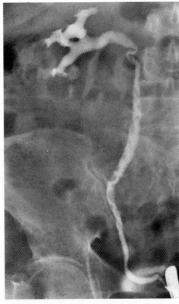

Fig GU 18-6
Ureteritis cystica. Multiple, small, smooth lucent filling defects in the contrast-filled ureter and pelvis in a patient with chronic urinary tract infection.

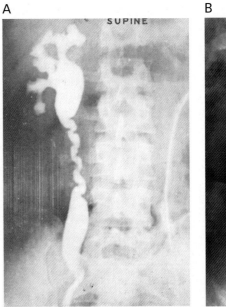
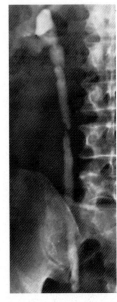

Fig GU 18-7
Ureteral tuberculosis. (A) Segmental areas of dilatation and constriction produce a corkscrew, or beaded, pattern.[7] (B) Thickening and fixation of the ureter (pipe stem ureter).[17]

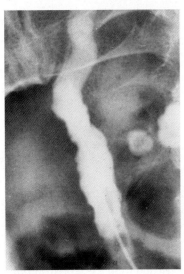

Fig GU 18-8
Malacoplakia of the ureter. Magnified view of the distal right ureter shows multiple filling defects simulating ureteritis cystica.[18]

Obstruction of the Ureter

Condition	Imaging Findings	Comments
Calculus (Fig GU 19-1)	Approximately 80% are radiopaque enough to be seen on plain films. Often oval with its long axis paralleling the course of the ureter. A calculus most commonly lodges in the lower portion of the ureter, especially at the ureterovesical junction and the pelvic brim. A nonopaque ureteral calculus appears as a lucent filling defect on excretory urography (retrograde pyelography may be necessary to demonstrate a ureteral calculus if renal function is insufficient).	Ureteral calculi are extremely common, and their detection is clinically important. An obstructing distal calculus must be differentiated from far more common phleboliths, which are spherical and located in the lateral portion of the pelvis below a line joining the ischial spines (ureteral calculi are situated medially above the interspinous line). Calculi produce characteristic posterior shadowing on ultrasound and high attenuation values on CT.
Stricture Congenital ureteropelvic junction (UPJ) obstruction (Fig GU 19-2)	Sharply defined UPJ narrowing with dilatation of the pelvocalyceal system that persists even when the patient is placed in a position favoring gravity drainage of the pelvis. Late manifestations of long-standing UPJ obstruction include wasting of kidney substance, diminished parenchymal and pelvocalyceal opacification, and the "rim" sign (nephrogram of remaining renal parenchyma rimming the dilated calyces).	May be caused by an intrinsic stenosis of the ureter or by extrinsic compression of the UPJ by a crossing blood vessel or fibrous band. Most patients have no demonstrable anatomic abnormality, and the decreased urine flow through the UPJ is secondary to abnormal muscle development, inadequate distensibility, or a deficiency of transmitter substance at nerve endings. UPJ obstruction is especially common in patients with horseshoe and incompletely rotated kidneys. Characteristic kinks, angulations, and "high insertions" of the ureter are most likely the result rather than the cause of pelvic distention.

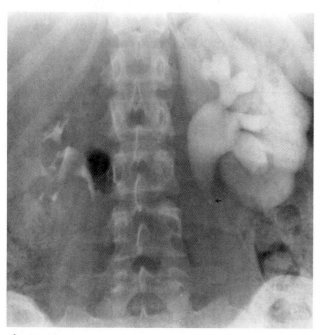

Fig GU 19-1
Obstructing ureteral calculus. Excretory urogram demonstrates a prolonged nephrogram and marked dilatation of the collecting system and pelvis proximal to the obstructing stone (arrow).

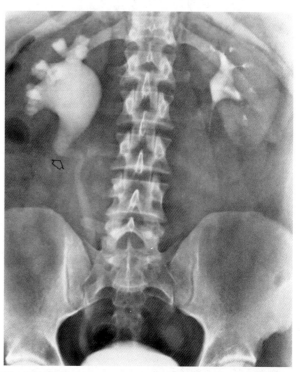

Fig GU 19-2
Congenital ureteropelvic junction (UPJ) obstruction.
Note the characteristic kink or angulation at the UPJ (arrow).

Condition	Imaging Findings	Comments
Tuberculosis	Healing produces multiple areas of ureteral stricture alternating with dilated segments to produce a beaded, or corkscrew, appearance. In advanced disease, the wall of the ureter becomes thickened and fixed with no peristalsis (pipe stem ureter) and a straight course to the bladder.	Ureteral obstruction is a late manifestation, which is almost always associated with renal tuberculosis. There is often a contracted bladder with a thickened wall. Calcification of the ureter and bladder is infrequent.
Schistosomiasis (see Fig GI 58-1)	Stricture, aperistalsis, and calcification (usually linear) of the distal ureter.	Almost always associated with dense calcification of the bladder wall.
Postsurgery/ instrumentation (Fig GU 19-3)	Localized narrowing of the ureter.	Causes include accidental ligation of the ureter, edema of the ureteral wall, and instrumental perforation (most heal rapidly and without sequelae if less than 50% of the ureteral circumference is involved and there is no distal obstruction). Postsurgical abscess, hematoma, or urinoma may cause diffuse narrowing and displacement of the ureter by extrinsic compression.
Radiation therapy (Fig GU 19-4)	Ureteral narrowing that gradually develops several months to years after treatment. Most commonly occurs just above the ureterovesical junction after pelvic irradiation (eg, for uterine carcinoma).	Most commonly occurs if the ureter was originally involved with malignancy. A radiation-induced stricture may be impossible to differentiate from tumor recurrence.

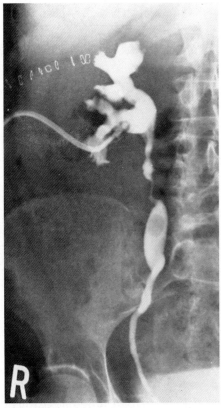

Fig GU 19-3
Postsurgery stricture. Fibrotic narrowing of the proximal ureter secondary to stone removal.

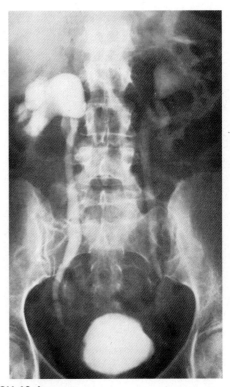

Fig GU 19-4
Radiation cystitis causing ureteral obstruction. After external and intracavitary radiotherapy for cervical cancer, an excretory urogram shows the bladder wall to be thickened and bladder opacity to be reduced. Narrowing of the distal ureters causes bilateral hydronephrosis.[4]

Condition	Imaging Findings	Comments
Post-traumatic	During surgery, one or both ureters may be sectioned, causing nonfunction of the involved kidney or formation of a local abscess.	Cutting or ligating the ureters usually produces prompt symptoms, and the presence of anuria for 8 to 10 hours after major pelvic surgery should suggest the possibility of bilateral ureteral injury. Kinking, crushing, or clamping of the vascular supply to the ureters may not produce evidence of injury until several weeks after surgery, when necrosis of the ureteral wall may occur leading to fistulization. Unilateral injury that does not produce anuria may not be recognized. External trauma rarely injures the ureters, as they lie deep in the retroperitoneal area adjacent to the lumbar spine and are well protected throughout their course.
Adjacent inflammatory disease	Extrinsic narrowing and displacement of one or both ureters (most often the pelvic portion).	Causes include diverticulitis, Crohn disease, appendiceal abscess, and postoperative abscess.
Invasion or compression by extrinsic malignancy		
Retroperitoneal tumor	Extrinsic compression, encasement, or invasion causing often irregular narrowing of the proximal ureter. The affected ureter is usually displaced laterally (rarely medially).	Most frequently lymphoma or metastases (pancreas, melanoma, colon). Primary retroperitoneal tumors (eg, liposarcoma) are much less common.
Pelvic tumor (Fig GU 19-5)	Extrinsic narrowing and often irregularity of the distal ureter. The ureter is typically straightened or displaced medially.	Causes include carcinoma of the cervix or other pelvic organ (direct extension or lymph node metastases) and pelvic lymphoma.

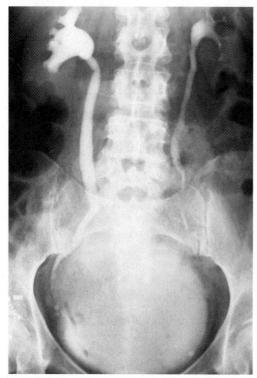

Fig GU 19-5
Pelvic tumor. Dilatation of the right ureter and pelvis due to partial obstruction by a large ovarian mass.

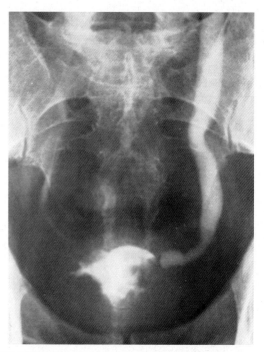

Fig GU 19-6
Bladder cancer causing left ureteral obstruction. Contrast material opacifies the distal left ureter to the point of obstruction. The tumor involves the ureteral orifice and produces a "pseudoureterocele" appearance.[4]

Condition	Imaging Findings	Comments
Bladder carcinoma (Fig GU 19-6)	Unilateral or bilateral obstruction of the distal ureters.	Most common with infiltrating tumors, especially those arising in the trigone. The distal ureters may also be obstructed by lymph node metastases.
Cystitis (Fig GU 19-7)	Unilateral or bilateral obstruction of the distal ureters.	In acute cystitis, there is compression of the intramural portion of the ureters by edema and inflammation. In chronic cystitis, the ureterovesical junction is obstructed by fibrosis or an inflammatory mass.
Ureterocele Simple (Fig GU 19-8)	Unilateral or bilateral, round or oval density of opacified urine (in the dilated distal segment of the ureter) separated from opacified urine in the bladder by a thin (2- to 3-mm) radiolucent halo representing the wall of the prolapsed ureter and the bladder mucosa (cobra head sign).	Cystic dilatation of the distal intravesical segment of the ureter with protrusion into the bladder lumen. Probably caused by congenital or acquired stenosis of the ureteral orifice that predisposes to infection and stone formation, both of which may aggravate the degree of obstruction.
Ectopic (Fig GU 19-9)	Ureteral obstruction with hydronephrosis or nonvisualization of the upper segment of a duplicated collecting system.	If the ectopic ureteral orifice is stenotic, proximal distention of the ureter under the submucosa of the bladder produces a characteristic eccentric filling defect at the base of the bladder.

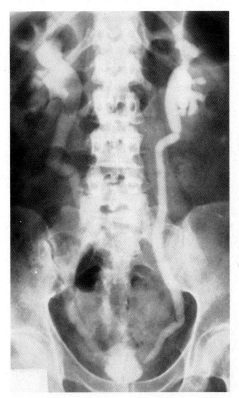

Fig GU 19-7
Severe interstitial cystitis. Bilateral ureteral obstruction and marked contraction of the bladder secondary to severe interstitial cystitis due to systemic lupus erythematosus in a young woman on steroids. The bladder capacity was reduced to approximately 1 ounce.[4]

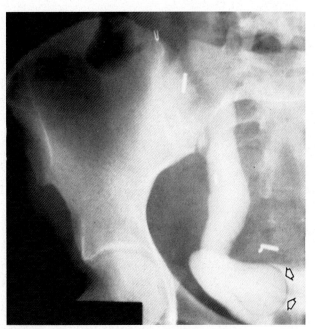

Fig GU 19-8
Simple ureterocele (arrows).

Condition	Imaging Findings	Comments
Blood clots	Irregular radiolucent filling defects that may produce temporary (usually incomplete) obstruction.	Causes of bleeding include trauma, tumor, instrumentation, vascular malformation, hemorrhagic inflammation, bleeding disorder, and anticoagulant therapy.
Vascular compression		
Renal artery	Extrinsic tubular impression, usually with mild dilatation of the more proximal ureter but rarely significant obstruction.	Normal and aberrant renal arteries in the proximal ureter; iliac vessels in the lower ureter (L5-S1 level).
Ovarian vein syndrome	Extrinsic compression of the right ureter at the S1 level producing mild to moderate obstruction.	Caused by a markedly dilated ovarian vein or possibly by locally induced periureteral fibrosis that develops after several pregnancies.
Aneurysm of abdominal aorta or iliac artery	Extrinsic compression with localized or diffuse lateral displacement of the ureter above the pelvic brim.	The aneurysm is most commonly of arteriosclerotic origin and is often calcified. Ureteral obstruction may also be due to dissecting or mycotic aneurysms.
Retrocaval ureter (Fig GU 19-10)	Abrupt medial swing of the right ureter, which usually lies over or medial to the vertebral pedicles at the L4-L5 level.	Developmental defect of the inferior vena cava. Compression of the ureter between the inferior vena cava and the posterior abdominal wall often causes narrowing or obstruction of the ureter with progressive hydronephrosis.

A

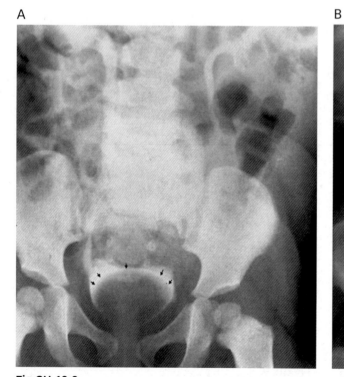

B

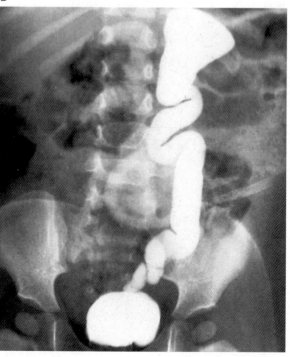

Fig GU 19-9
Ectopic ureterocele. (A) Excretory urogram demonstrates a large lucency (arrows) filling much of the bladder. There is slight downward and lateral displacement of the visualized collecting system on the left. (B) Cystogram shows contrast material refluxing to fill the markedly dilated collecting system draining the upper pole of the left kidney. Note the severe dilatation and tortuosity of the ureter.

Condition	Imaging Findings	Comments
Transitional cell carcinoma of the ureter (Fig GU 19-11)	Smooth or irregular filling defect. Infiltrating carcinoma usually appears as an irregular stricture with overhanging margins (occasionally concentric smooth narrowing with tapering edges that may be difficult to differentiate from ureteral narrowing due to an inflammatory process, calculus, or extrinsic compression).	Rare manifestation. There may be characteristic localized dilatation of the distal ureter, in contrast to the ureteral collapse distal to an obstructing stone. Retrograde pyelography may demonstrate the typical meniscus appearance of the superior border of the contrast column (wine glass sign outlining the lower margin of the tumor).
Benign ureteral tumor	Smooth or irregular filling defect in the ureter. Obstruction is rare, except with papilloma.	Papillomas occur in older patients (50 to 70 years of age), often involve the lower third of the ureter, and tend to produce short filling defects with shaggy and irregular margins and no pedicle. Polyps generally affect young adults, primarily involve the upper third of the ureter, and appear as long, narrow filling defects that have smooth margins and are frequently pedunculated. Submucosal mesenchymal tumors also occur.
Benign pelvic mass (Fig GU 19-12)	Extrinsic narrowing and lateral deviation of one or both pelvic ureters.	Causes include uterine fibroid, ovarian cyst, enlarged uterus (pregnancy or postpartum), and occasionally a markedly distended rectosigmoid colon.

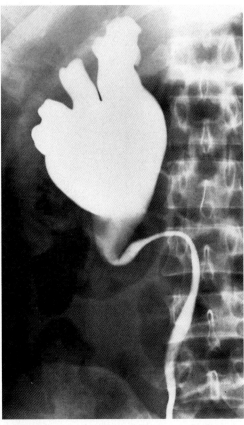

Fig GU 19-10
Retrocaval ureter. Note the medial swing of the right ureter distal to the ureteropelvic junction.

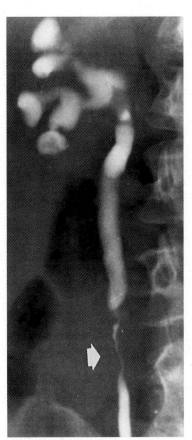

Fig GU 19-11
Transitional cell carcinoma of the ureter. Irregular stricture (arrow) causing proximal ureteral and pelvocalyceal dilatation.

Condition	Imaging Findings	Comments
Pelvic lipomatosis (see Fig GU 22-4)	Bilateral, symmetric medial displacement and compression of the ureters. Increased radiolucency in the pelvis is caused by the excessive deposition of fat (easily confirmed on CT).	Benign condition with increased deposition of normal, mature adipose tissue in the extraperitoneal pelvic soft tissues around the urinary bladder, rectum, and prostate. Almost all reported cases have been in men. Elevation, elongation, and compression of the rectosigmoid colon and the pear-shaped bladder along with widening of the retrorectal space.
Retroperitoneal fibrosis (Fig GU 19-13)	Smooth and conical narrowing and frequently medial deviation of both ureters between L4 and S2 with proximal ureteral dilatation.	Fibrosing inflammatory process enveloping but not invading retroperitoneal structures. Although the etiology is unknown, many cases are associated with drug ingestion (eg, methysergide, ergot derivatives, phenacetin, and methyldopa). May coexist with similar fibrotic processes in other sites (fibrosing mediastinitis, sclerosing cholangitis, retro-orbital pseudotumor, retractile mesenteritis, Riedel's thyroiditis).
Retroperitoneal abscess/hematoma	Extrinsic compression and lateral displacement of the ureter (and kidney). A retroperitoneal gas collection is diagnostic of an abscess. Calcification suggests a tuberculous psoas abscess.	An abscess may originate from spondylitis (especially tuberculous), perinephric abscess, urinary tract infection, pancreatitis, or a perforated duodenum or be a complication of retroperitoneal surgery. A hematoma may be caused by trauma, ruptured aortic aneurysm, bleeding disorder, or anticoagulant therapy or be a complication of surgery.

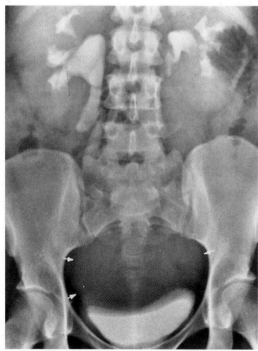

Fig GU 19-12
Hydronephrosis of pregnancy. Excretory urogram performed 3 days postpartum demonstrates bilateral large kidneys with dilatation of the ureters and pelvocalyceal systems, especially on the right. The large pelvic mass (arrows) indenting the superior surface of the bladder represents the uterus, which is still causing extrinsic pressure on the ureters.

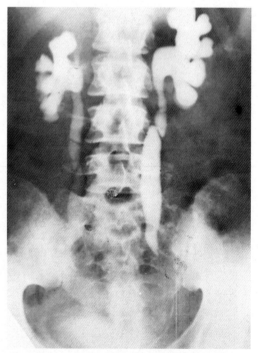

Fig GU 19-13
Retroperitoneal fibrosis. Marked bilateral hydronephrosis with bilateral ureterectasis above the level of the sacral promontory. Below this point, both ureters, where visualized, appear to be normal in caliber. No definite ureteral deviation is seen. An excretory urogram performed 1 year previously was entirely normal.[7]

Condition	Imaging Findings	Comments
Papillary necrosis with sloughed papilla	Irregular filling defect simulating an obstructing ureteral stone.	Evidence of papillary necrosis involving other papillae and calyces.
Inspissated pus	Irregular filling defect simulating an obstructing ureteral stone.	Ureteral obstruction is due to a mass of pus from a proximal infectious process. A similar appearance may be caused by tissue debris from a necrotic tumor.
Bladder diverticulum	Single (if congenital) or multiple outpouchings from the bladder that occasionally are large enough to obstruct the distal ureter by extrinsic compression.	Congenital diverticula are usually located near the ureteral orifice and more commonly cause urinary infection and vesicoureteral reflux. Acquired diverticula are usually multiple and result from obstruction of the bladder outlet or urethra. A "Hutch" diverticulum in a paraplegic occurs above and lateral to the ureteral orifice and often produces an obstructed ureter just above the bladder ("notch" sign).
Herniation of ureter	Abnormal course of a redundant ureter that may lead to obstruction.	May be congenital (in femoral, inguinal, sciatic, or internal hernia) or secondary to pelvic surgery.
Endometriosis	Extrinsic obstruction of the distal ureter, usually below the pelvic brim. May produce an intraluminal mass or a stricture and mimic a ureteral tumor.	Uncommon condition in which heterotopic foci of endometrium occur in extrauterine locations. Cyclical urinary symptoms (including hematuria) in women of childbearing age.
Amyloidosis	Narrowing, rigidity, and partial obstruction of the ureter.	Caused by a localized accumulation of amyloid in primary or secondary disease.
Ureteral valve (Fig GU 19-14)	Sharp horizontal obstruction that usually involves the distal ureter.	Transverse folds or redundant ureteral mucosa that may be either congenital or secondary to chronic inflammation.

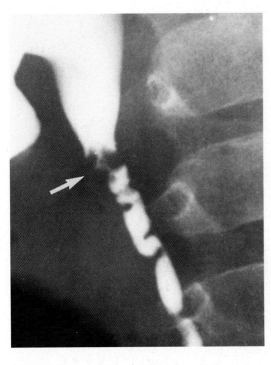

Fig GU 19-14
Obstructing valve (arrow) at the ureteropelvic junction. Retrograde study shows smooth infoldings below the valve representing fetal folds, which usually regress as the child grows.[19]

Ureterectasis

Condition	Imaging Findings	Comments
Ureteral obstruction (Figs GU 20-1 and GU 20-2; see Section GU 19)	Ureteral dilatation proximal to the point of obstruction. Most often unilateral, but may be bilateral due to an extrinsic lesion.	Causes include calculus, tumor, stricture (congenital, traumatic, surgical, radiation, inflammatory), ureterocele, and extrinsic compression (malignancy, inflammation, pelvic lipomatosis, retroperitoneal fibrosis, pregnancy).
Vesicoureteral reflux (Fig GU 20-3)	Generalized dilatation of one or both ureters (and pelvocalyceal systems) occurring with severe reflux.	Most common in children. The relation between reflux and urinary tract infection is controversial, though the combination of the two can produce severe renal scarring as well as dilated and.tortuous ureters that may require reimplantation.
Obstruction of urethra or bladder outlet (see Figs GU 19-9 and GU 26-1)	Bilateral dilatation of the ureters and pelvocalyceal systems. If the obstruction is chronic, the bladder is usually dilated and has trabeculation and diverticula.	Causes include posterior urethral valves, ectopic ureterocele, prostatic hypertrophy or carcinoma, stricture, and diverticulum.
Postobstructive hydronephrosis and hydroureter	Unilateral or bilateral dilatation of the pelvocalyceal system and ureter without evidence of obstruction.	Results from one prolonged or several intermittent episodes of obstruction.
Congenital ureterectasis	Diffuse or segmental dilatation of the ureter (most commonly the lower third) with a normal pelvocalyceal system and no demonstrable ureteral abnormality.	Congenital, nonprogressive malformation of the ureteral wall.

A

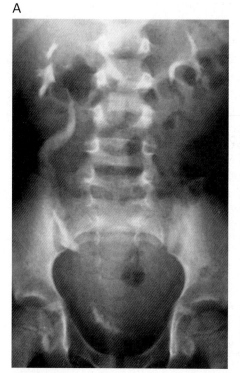

B

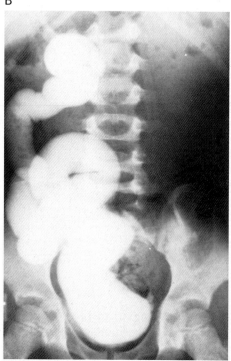

Fig GU 20-1

Complete duplication with ureteral obstruction. (A) Excretory urogram demonstrates dilatation and lateral displacement of the right ureter. Ureteral duplication was not suspected. (B) A delayed film after a voiding cystogram demonstrates contrast material filling a dilated and tortuous ureter to the upper segment. This ureter, which was not seen on the excretory urogram, has laterally displaced the ureter to the lower segment.[20]

Condition	Imaging Findings	Comments
Congenital megaloureter	Functional, smoothly tapered narrowing of the juxtavesical segment with minimal to extensive dilatation (up to 5 cm in diameter) of the pelvic ureter. Vigorous, nonpropulsive peristaltic waves in the dilated segment are similar to those in esophageal achalasia. Bilateral in 20% to 40% of cases.	Represents failure of the juxtavesical segment of the ureter to transmit peristaltic waves (no demonstrable ureteral obstruction and a relaxed, opened, nonrefluxing ureteral orifice). Usually diagnosed in adults, either as an incidental finding or in a patient with vague lower quadrant pain. May remain unchanged for years, but if infection or decompensation occurs, the condition may progress to produce massive dilatation of the entire ureter and collecting system.
Infection	Dilatation of the lower third of the ureter is a relatively common result of urinary tract infection (especially recurring cystitis).	Probably related to smooth muscle paralysis in the urinary tract due to bacterial endotoxins. Mild to moderate dilatation of the ureter and pelvocalyceal system may occur in acute pyelonephritis.
Neurogenic bladder (see Figs GU 22-2 and GU 23-1)	Unilateral or bilateral dilatation of the ureter and pelvocalyceal system. The bladder may be large and flaccid or contracted with mural trabeculation and diverticula formation.	Disease or injury involving the spinal cord or peripheral nerves supplying the bladder. Causes include congenital anomalies (spina bifida, myelomeningocele, sacral agenesis), spinal cord trauma or tumor, syphilis, and diabetes mellitus.

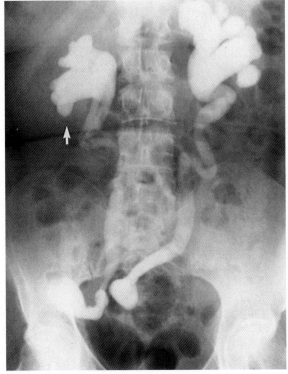

Fig GU 20-2
Ileal conduit stenosis. Drainage film from an ileal loopogram shows bilateral hydronephrosis, right lower pole parenchymal scarring (arrow), and failure of the conduit to empty.[21]

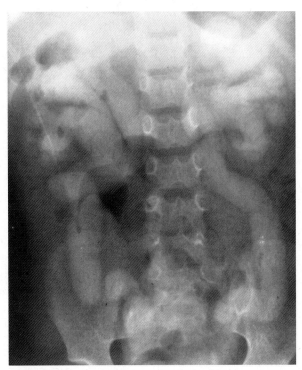

Fig GU 20-3
Vesicoureteral reflux. Voiding cystogram in a young girl shows bilateral reflux with gross dilatation of the upper tracts.

Condition	Imaging Findings	Comments
Chagas disease	Bilateral ureteral dilatation, usually with dilatation of the bladder.	Destruction of myenteric plexuses due to infection by the protozoan *Trypanosoma cruzi* (endemic to South America and Central America).
Diabetes insipidus	Bilateral dilatation of the ureters and pelvocalyceal systems. There often is an overdistended bladder.	Continual overloading of the urinary tract in nephrogenic diabetes insipidus (no tubular response to endogenous or exogenous antidiuretic hormone). Rare in pituitary diabetes insipidus.
Absent abdominal musculature (Eagle-Barrett, or prune belly, syndrome) (Fig GU 20-4)	Diffuse dilatation of the ureters, pelvocalyceal systems, and bladder.	Rare congenital condition, occurring almost exclusively in males. Bulging of the flanks (due to a lack of support by abdominal muscles) is a characteristic finding on plain films.

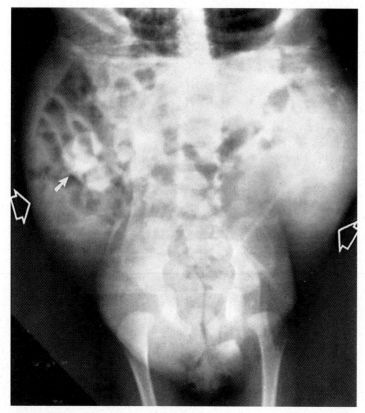

Fig GU 20-4
Prune belly syndrome. Pronounced bulging of the flanks (open arrows). The patient had multiple genitourinary anomalies, including hydronephrosis of the right collecting system (small arrow).

Deviation of the Ureter

Condition	Comments
Lateral ureteral deviation	Position of the ureter 1 cm or more lateral to the tip of an adjacent transverse process.
Retroperitoneal lymphadenopathy (Figs GU 21-1 and GU 21-2)	Lymphoma, metastases, or, less commonly, infection. Lateral deviation of both kidneys or the abdominal segments of both ureters suggests lymphoma or, in a male, metastases from a testicular neoplasm.
Other retroperitoneal masses	Primary neoplasm (neurofibroma, lipoma, fibrosarcoma, liposarcoma); extension from primary tumor of the spine; hematoma; inflammatory mass (eg, abscess).
Aortic aneurysm/tortuosity (Fig GU 21-3)	Often contains intramural calcium. Usually displaces the left ureter, though an aneurysm that primarily projects to the right occasionally can cause lateral displacement of the right ureter. Because of adhesions between the aorta and the ureters, lateral displacement of one ureter is often accompanied by medial displacement of the other. Tortuosity or aneurysm of the common iliac artery also can displace the ureter laterally.

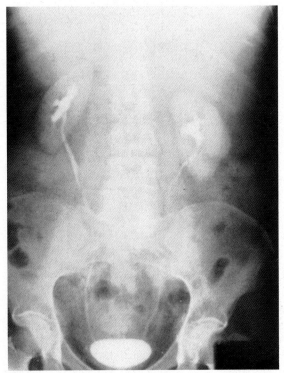

Fig GU 21-1
Hodgkin's lymphoma. Lateral displacement of both upper ureters, secondary to enlarged paracaval and para-aortic lymph nodes. Note also the splenomegaly and inferior displacement of the left kidney.[4]

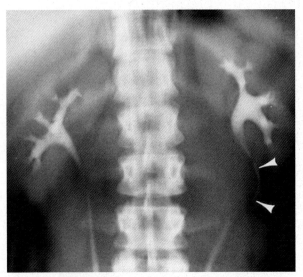

Fig GU 21-2
Retroperitoneal metastases from left testicular seminoma. Nephrotomogram shows lateral displacement of the proximal left ureter (arrowheads).[4]

Condition	Comments
Malrotated or horseshoe kidney (see Fig GU 1-4)	When the renal pelvis is situated in an anterior or a lateral position, the upper part of the ureter often appears displaced laterally, suggesting an extrinsic mass. The elongated pelvis of the malrotated kidney may mimic obstructive dilatation; in horseshoe kidney, true ureteropelvic junction obstruction may develop because of the unusual course of the ureter.
Prominent psoas muscle	Typically occurs bilaterally in muscular young men. The ureter proceeds caudally along the lateral edge of the widening muscle for several inches before swerving medially to pass along the anterior surface of the muscle.
Benign pelvic mass (see Fig GU 19-1)	Causes include uterine fibroid, ovarian cyst, enlarged uterus (pregnancy or postpartum), hematocolpos, and occasionally a markedly distended rectosigmoid colon.
Ureteric hernia (Fig GU 21-4)	Uncommon entity; 90% occur in inguinal or femoral hernias.
Medial ureteral deviation	Ureter situated medial to the adjacent lumbar pedicles. Medial deviation is possible if the ureter overlies the pedicle, and likely if there is 5 cm or less distance between the ureters.

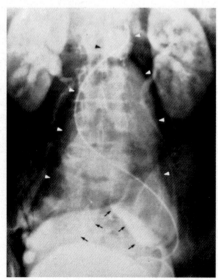

Fig GU 21-3
Aortic and common iliac aneurysms. Aortography faintly opacifies massively dilated vessels (arrowheads) because of contrast dilution. The deviated ureters typically follow the lateral borders of the aortic and common iliac artery aneurysms. The medial borders of the common iliac aneurysms are indicated (arrows).[4]

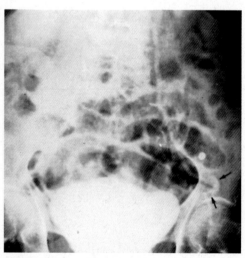

Fig GU 21-4
Ureterosciatic hernia. Excretory urogram demonstrates a "horizontal curlicue" or horizontal looping of the left ureter in the region of the greater sciatic foramen (arrows).[22]

Condition	Comments
Proximal or midureter	
Renal or retroperitoneal mass	Although ureteral displacement is more commonly lateral, medial deviation can result from a benign or malignant neoplasm, hematoma, or abscess.
Retrocaval ureter (see Fig GU 18-7)	Abrupt medial swing of the ureter, which usually lies over or medial to the vertebral pedicles at the L4-L5 level. This developmental defect of the vena cava, rather than the ureter itself, occurs almost exclusively on the right. Compression of the ureter between the inferior vena cava and posterior abdominal wall often causes narrowing or obstruction of the ureter with progressive hydronephrosis.
Severe pyelectasis	Marked dilatation of the renal pelvis (eg, ureteropelvic junction obstruction) causes the kidney to rotate about its long axis, with the upper ureter becoming anterior and medial. This appearance may mimic a retrocaval ureter, though this can be excluded by demonstration of the anterior location of the ureter on a radiograph obtained in the lateral projection.
Retroperitoneal fibrosis (Fig GU 21-5)	Dilatation of the proximal urinary tract with narrowing, straightening, and frequently medial deviation of both ureters between L4 and S2. In this disorder of unknown etiology (many cases have been associated with drug ingestion, principally methysergide for migraine), the fibrosing inflammatory process envelops the retroperitoneal structures but usually does not invade them.

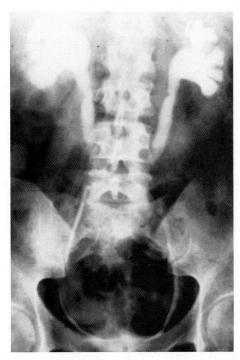

Fig GU 21-5
Retroperitoneal fibrosis. Bilateral retrograde pyelogram shows dilatation of the collecting systems and ureters to the level of the L4–L5 disk space with medial deviation of the ureters.[4]

Condition	Comments
Distal (pelvic) ureter	
Pelvic lymphadenopathy	Primarily lymphoma or metastases.
Pelvic hematoma	Usually associated with pelvic fractures.
Pelvic lipomatosis (Fig GU 21-6)	Bilateral, symmetric medial displacement and compression of the ureters. Characteristic increased radiolucency in the pelvis is caused by the excessive deposition of normal, mature adipose tissue around the urinary bladder, rectum, and prostate. Almost all reported cases have been in men.
Bladder diverticulum (Fig GU 21-7)	Characteristic smoothly rounded medial deviation of the lower ureter down to its entrance into the bladder. The reason for the deviation is obvious if the diverticulum is opacified during urography. Unlike other causes of medial deviation of the pelvic segment of the ureter, with bladder diverticulum the terminal segment of the ureter is displaced all the way down to the trigone, rather than having a normal position as it approaches and enters the bladder.
Vascular causes	Aneurysm or tortuosity of the hypogastric artery; markedly enlarged collateral veins in patients with obstruction of the inferior vena cava.

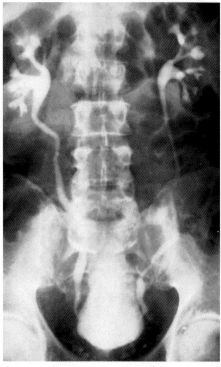

Fig GU 21-6
Pelvic lipomatosis. Medial deviation of the ureters associated with mild distal ureteral obstruction. The characteristic pear-shaped bladder is elevated by perivesical fat.[4]

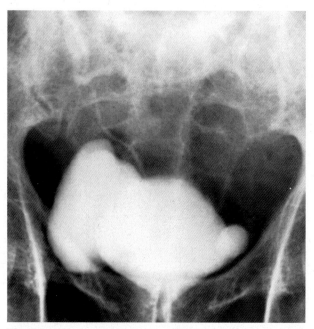

Fig GU 21-7
Bladder diverticulum. Medial displacement of the distal right ureter by the large diverticulum. Note the small left-sided diverticulum.[4]

Condition	Comments
Abdominoperineal resection	After this procedure and other types of operations on the descending colon and sigmoid, the lower segments of the ureter swing medially in the region of the pelvic inlet. Despite the prominent medial deviation, there is no obstruction; deviation of a similar degree by extrinsic masses, such as enlarged lymph nodes, tends to be associated with some degree of ureteral obstruction.
Cystocele or uterine prolapse (Fig GU 21-8)	Low position of the bladder causes symmetric medial displacement of the pelvic ureters.
Adnexal mass	Inflammatory or neoplastic process.
Neoplasm of bony pelvis	Lesion arising from the lateral bony wall (eg, chondrosarcoma) with an associated mass extending into the pelvis can cause medial displacement of the ureter.

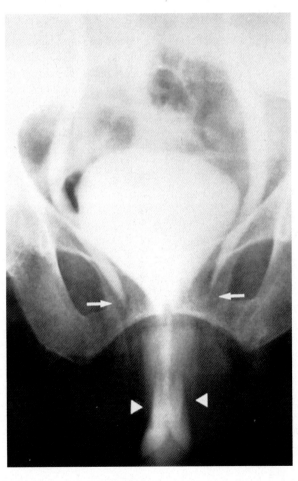

Fig GU 21-8
Cystocele. Coned view shows the medially displaced distal ureters compressed at the level of the levator sling (arrows). The ureterovesical junctions are several centimeters lower (arrowheads).[4]

Small Urinary Bladder

Condition	Imaging Findings	Comments
Transitional cell carcinoma (infiltrating)	Asymmetric bladder contraction with an irregular, thickened wall and mural filling defects. Localized tumor infiltration causes marked bladder deformity. There is often unilateral or bilateral ureteral obstruction.	The wall of the urinary bladder is the most common site of transitional cell cancer. Plain radiographs may demonstrate punctate, coarse, or linear calcifications that are usually encrusted on the surface of the tumor but occasionally lie within it (see Fig GI 58-4).
Cystitis (Fig GU 22-1)	Small bladder with trabeculation and mural irregularities in chronic disease or severe acute cystitis. There may be associated filling defects (fungus balls, blood clots). Characteristic mural and luminal gas in emphysematous cystitis.	Acute inflammation of the urinary bladder generally does not produce any radiographically detectable abnormality (the wall may be thickened and irregular because of severe mucosal and intramural edema with spasm).
Neurogenic bladder (Fig GU 22-2)	Small, spastic, heavily trabeculated bladder with an irregular thickened wall and diverticula formation. May have a pointed dome (pine tree bladder).	Disease or injury involving the spinal cord or peripheral nerves supplying the bladder. Causes include spinal neoplasm or trauma, syphilis, diabetes mellitus, and congenital anomalies (spina bifida, myelomeningocele, sacral agenesis). A neurogenic bladder can also be large and atonic with little trabeculation.
Extrinsic bladder compression (Figs GU 22-3 and GU 22-4)	Bilaterally symmetric narrowing, elevation, and elongation of the bladder, often resulting in a teardrop- or pear-shaped configuration.	Causes include pelvic hematoma (associated with pelvic fractures), pelvic lipomatosis (fat density compressing the bladder), pelvic edema (inferior vena caval occlusion), and pelvic neoplastic or inflammatory disease.
After surgery or radiation therapy	Small bladder with a smooth or irregular surface.	Radiation cystitis develops several months to several years after irradiation (especially intracavitary).

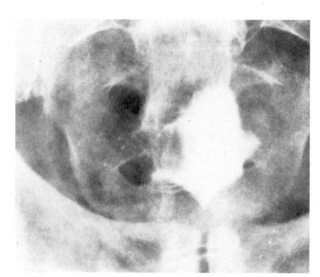

Fig GU 22-1
Cyclophosphamide (Cytoxan) cystitis. Six months after repeated cycles of cyclophosphamide therapy, the bladder volume is greatly reduced and the bladder wall appears ulcerated and edematous.[2]

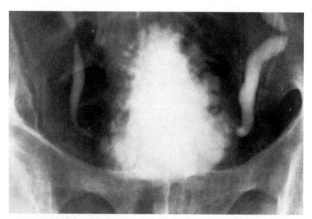

Fig GU 22-2
Neurogenic bladder. Small, spastic, trabeculated bladder with a pointed dome.[23]

Condition	Imaging Findings	Comments
Schistosomiasis (see Fig GI 58-1)	Small, fibrotic bladder with characteristic mural calcification. The calcification is initially most apparent and extensive at the base of the bladder, but may surround the bladder completely. There may be ureteral calcification (parallel dense lines, especially in the pelvic portion of the ureter).	Blood fluke with a snail host. The irritative effect of ova passing through or lodging in the wall of the bladder stimulates an inflammatory response (granuloma formation, obliterative vasculitis, progressive fibrosis). The development of squamous cell carcinoma of the bladder is a frequent complication (especially in Egypt).
Tuberculosis	Initially, thickening and trabeculation of the bladder wall. Later there is a progressive decrease in bladder capacity and a smoother wall. Eventually, the bladder virtually disappears and the ureters seem to enter directly into the urethra. Calcification is infrequent in the bladder but common in the vas deferens.	Almost invariably associated with renal and ureteral involvement. There may be reflux and, occasionally, dilatation of one or both ureters and pelvocalyceal systems secondary to bladder muscular hypertrophy that produces ureteral constriction.

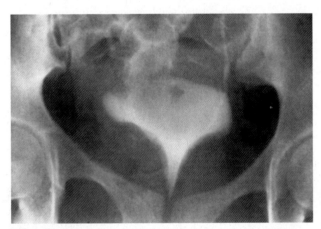

Fig GU 22-3
Pelvic hematoma. Symmetric narrowing of the base of the bladder.

A
B

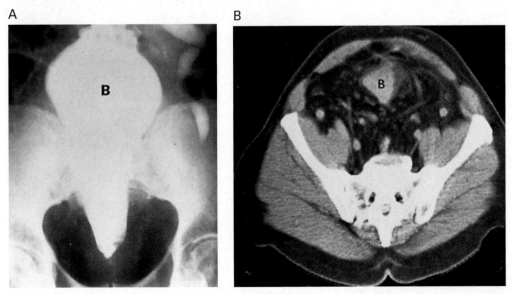

Fig GU 22-4
Pelvic lipomatosis. (A) Excretory urogram demonstrates bilateral hydronephrosis, displacement of the left ureter, and an abnormal pear-shaped urinary bladder (B). (B) A CT scan reveals that the compressed bladder (B) is surrounded by low-density fat, confirming the diagnosis of pelvic lipomatosis.

Large Urinary Bladder

Condition	Imaging Findings	Comments
Obstruction of bladder outlet or urethra (see Figs GU 19-9 and GU 26-1)	Dilated bladder with trabeculation and diverticula formation. With prolonged obstruction, the bladder may become thin walled and atonic.	Causes include prostatic hypertrophy or carcinoma, stricture, diverticulum, posterior urethral valve, and ectopic ureterocele. Congenital bladder neck obstruction is a controversial entity.
Neurogenic bladder (Figs GU 23-1 and GU 23-2)	Dilatation of a smooth, thin-walled, atonic bladder with little or no trabeculation.	Suggests underlying diabetes, tabes dorsalis, or syringomyelia. Differs from a spastic neurogenic bladder, which is small and heavily trabeculated.
Bladder prolapse (Fig GU 23-3)	Bladder dilatation caused by outlet obstruction. The base of the bladder projects below the inferior margin of the symphysis pubis (may be evident only in the upright position).	After childbirth, the bladder and anterior vaginal wall may prolapse into the vaginal cavity (cystocele). May be associated with incontinence.
Chagas disease	Dilatation of the bladder and both ureters.	Destruction of myenteric plexuses due to infection by the protozoan *Trypanosoma cruzi* (endemic to South America and Central America).
Megacystis syndrome	Large, smooth-walled bladder with bilateral or unilateral ureteral reflux occurring either at low pressure or only during voiding. The bladder neck and proximal urethra commonly fail to funnel and distend normally during voiding.	Most commonly occurs in childhood, especially in girls. The bladder trigone is twice or triple the normal size, and the ureteral orifices are gaping. Postvoiding films show no significant bladder residual.

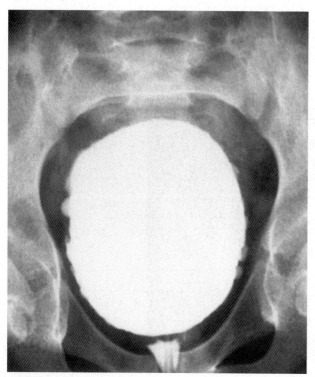

Fig GU 23-1
Neurogenic bladder. Large, atonic bladder in a child with traumatic paralysis of the lower extremities.

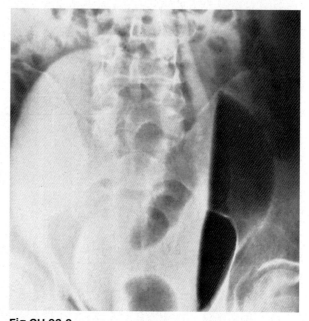

Fig GU 23-2
Neurogenic bladder in diabetes. Lateral decubitus view shows the massively enlarged, atonic bladder containing an air-urine level secondary to severe vesical infection by a gas-forming organism.

Condition	Imaging Findings	Comments
Diabetes insipidus	Dilatation of the bladder and both ureters.	Continual overloading of the urinary tract in nephrogenic diabetes insipidus (no tubular response to endogenous or exogenous antidiuretic hormone). Rare in pituitary diabetes insipidus.
Absent abdominal musculature (Eagle-Barrett, or prune belly, syndrome) (see Fig GU 20-4)	Diffuse dilatation of the bladder, ureters, and pelvocalyceal systems.	Rare congenital condition that occurs almost exclusively in males. Bulging of the flanks (due to a lack of support by the abdominal muscles) is a characteristic finding on plain films.
Psychogenic/drug-induced	Smooth-walled, markedly distended bladder with normal function.	No underlying neurologic disease. May be associated with the use of tranquilizers and muscle relaxants.

A   B

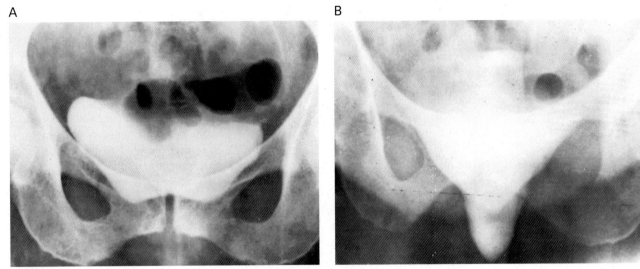

Fig GU 23-3
Cystocele. (A) Supine view. The lowermost portion of the bladder is visualized slightly below the upper edge of the symphysis pubis, a finding that is consistent with that in a cystocele. (B) Upright position. Contrast material is well below the symphysis pubis, indicating a marked cystocele. Note the superimposed urethrocele.

Single or Multiple Filling Defects in the Urinary Bladder

Condition	Imaging Findings	Comments
Calculus (Fig GU 24-1)	Single or multiple filling defects that vary in size from tiny concretions, each the size of a grain of sand, to an enormous single calculus occupying the entire bladder lumen. Most are circular or oval, but they can be amorphous, laminated, or even spiculated. Calculi frequently occur in bladder diverticula, lying in an unusual position close to the lateral pelvic wall or having a dumbbell shape with one end lodged in the diverticulum and the other projecting into the bladder.	Stone formation in the bladder is primarily a disorder of elderly men who have obstruction or infection of the lower urinary tract. Frequently associated lesions include bladder outlet obstruction, urethral stricture, neurogenic bladder, bladder diverticulum, and cystocele. Upper urinary tract stones that migrate down the ureter are occasionally retained in the bladder.
Blood clot	Irregular intraluminal filling defects of various sizes. Large clots may occupy almost the entire bladder lumen but are still completely surrounded by contrast material (unlike tumors). Blood clots often change in size and shape or disappear over several days.	Common causes of bleeding (originating from the kidneys or the bladder itself) include tumor, trauma, instrumentation, vascular malformation, hemorrhagic inflammation, bleeding disorder, and anticoagulant therapy.
Air bubble	Smooth, round, freely movable intraluminal defect. A large amount can produce an air-fluid level on a film obtained with a horizontal beam. There may be associated intramural gas (linear streaks or small round lucencies) in emphysematous cystitis.	Causes of air in the bladder include instrumentation, surgery, penetrating trauma, fistulas to gas-containing hollow organs, and emphysematous cystitis (usually in diabetic patients). Both intraluminal and intramural gas must be differentiated from superimposed bowel gas.
Instrument	Opaque or nonopaque intraluminal filling defect.	Most commonly, the inflated balloon of a Foley catheter.

A

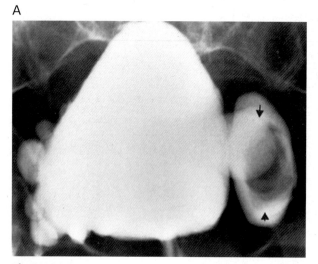

B

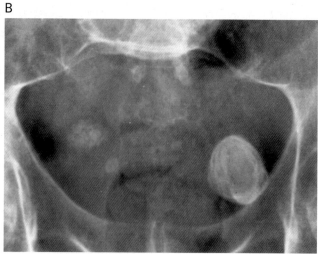

Fig GU 24-1
Bladder calculi. (A) Excretory urogram demonstrates a large stone (arrows) in a left-sided bladder diverticulum. (B) Plain radiograph of the pelvis shows the laminated stone and multiple smaller calculi that were obscured by contrast material in the right-sided bladder diverticula on the contrast-filled view.

Condition	Imaging Findings	Comments
Neoplasm		
Transitional cell carcinoma (Fig GU 24-2)	Single or multiple polypoid defects that arise from the bladder wall and are fixed in position (unlike a calculus, blood clot, or air). May produce only focal bladder wall thickening and rigidity. Punctate, coarse, or linear calcification is occasionally encrusted on the surface of the tumor (rarely lying within it).	Predominantly involves men over age 50. Hematuria, frequency, and dysuria are the most common presenting symptoms. Tumors originating near the ureteral orifices may cause early ureteral obstruction. May be associated with other transitional tumors of the pelvocalyceal system or ureter. Because urography can detect only approximately 60% of symptomatic bladder carcinomas, all patients with lower urinary tract hematuria should undergo cystoscopy.
Polyp	Single or multiple filling defects that may be pedunculated and movable.	Common tumor consisting of a fibrous stalk with a covering of normal transitional epithelium.
Papilloma	Solitary or multiple polypoid defects with smooth or irregular margins. May be pedunculated. No evidence of bladder wall invasion.	Benign, frond-like tumor that usually arises on the trigone. Often recurs and therefore may be considered as a low-grade malignancy.
Metastases	Direct extension of tumor causes an extrinsic defect with irregular margins. Hematogenous metastases produce solitary or multiple filling defects with smooth or irregular margins. Noninvading pelvic lymph node metastases cause a smooth extrinsic impression on the bladder wall.	Direct extension from primary carcinomas of the prostate, uterus, rectosigmoid, cervix, or ovary. Hematogenous metastases (rare) from lung, breast, and stomach tumors and melanoma. Bladder tumors may also be secondary to papillary tumors of the kidney or ureter and clear cell adenoma of the kidney.
Lymphoma	Direct invasion from perivesical lymphoma causes an irregular defect. Lymph node enlargement without invasion (more common) causes an extrinsic impression. There may be single or multiple well-circumscribed foci limited to the bladder wall.	Primary lymphoma of the bladder is extremely rare. Secondary involvement is not uncommon with advanced lymphoma. Diffuse infiltration or localized bladder masses occasionally occur in leukemia.

B

A

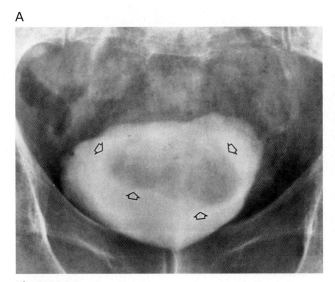
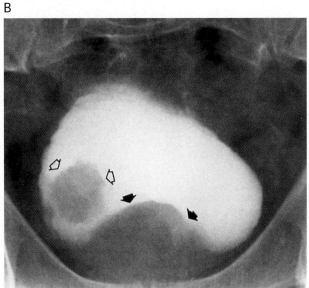

Fig GU 24-2

Transitional cell carcinoma. (A) Large, irregular filling defect (arrows) in the bladder. (B) In another patient, the irregular tumor (open arrows) is associated with a large filling defect (closed arrows), representing benign prostatic hypertrophy, at the base of the bladder.

Condition	Imaging Findings	Comments
Mesenchymal tumor	Various patterns (small polypoid filling defect to large, often fungating, mass). May be pedunculated.	Impossible to differentiate benign from malignant varieties unless there is evidence of wall invasion. Histologic types include leiomyoma, neurofibroma, hemangioma, fibroma, pheochromocytoma, and rhabdomyosarcoma (most common bladder tumor in children and often termed *sarcoma botryoides*).
Prostatic enlargement (Figs GU 24-3 and GU 24-4)	Smooth or irregular extrinsic filling defect of varying size at the base of the bladder. If a chronic process, there is trabeculation of the bladder wall and diverticula formation. Bladder outlet obstruction causes dilatation of the pelvocalyceal system and the ureter. The distal ureters often have a fishhook deformity (due to elevation of the trigone).	Most common causes are benign prostatic hypertrophy and carcinoma of the prostate. Although the contour of the filling defect is usually more irregular in carcinoma, benign hypertrophy and carcinoma usually cannot be differentiated unless there is evidence of tumor invasion into neighboring structures or distal metastases.
Simple ureterocele (Fig GU 24-5)	Round or oval density of opacified urine (in the dilated distal segment of the ureter) separated from opacified urine in the bladder by a thin (2–3 mm) radiolucent halo representing the wall of the prolapsed ureter and the bladder mucosa (cobra head sign).	Cystic dilatation of the distal intravesical segment of the ureter with protrusion into the bladder lumen. Often an incidental finding, but may predispose to obstruction, infection, and stone formation. May be unilateral or bilateral.
Ectopic ureterocele (see Fig GU 19-9)	Smooth or lobulated, usually eccentric filling defect at the base of the bladder. Associated with a duplicated collecting system (ureterocele arises from the ureter draining the upper segment, which is nonfunctioning or hydronephrotic).	Congenital lesion generally found in children (especially females). The ectopic ureter enters the bladder wall near its normal site of insertion. Instead of communicating with the lumen, the ectopic ureter continues for a variable distance before opening into the bladder neck or posterior urethra. If the orifice is stenotic, proximal distention of the ureter under the submucosa of the bladder produces the eccentric filling defect.

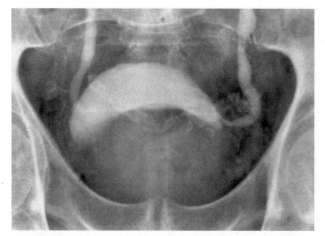

Fig GU 24-3
Benign prostatic hypertrophy. Large, smooth filling defect at the base of the bladder. Note the fishhook appearance of the distal ureters and the calcification in the vas deferens.

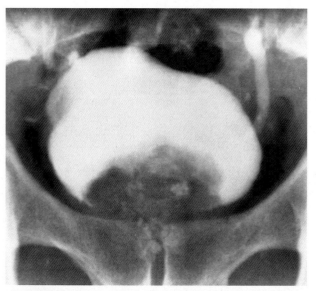

Fig GU 24-4
Carcinoma of the prostate. Elevation of and markedly irregular impression on the floor of the contrast-filled bladder.

Condition	Imaging Findings	Comments
Endometriosis (Fig GU 24-6)	Smooth, round or lobulated, extrinsic or intrinsic filling defect (usually located on the posterior wall).	Uncommon condition that presents with pain or cyclic urinary symptoms, including hematuria. Often a history of previous gynecologic or abdominal surgery.
Amyloidosis	Irregular, lobulated filling defect.	Very rare manifestation of primary or secondary disease.
Schistosomiasis (see Fig GI 58-1)	Single or multiple discrete filling defects (may produce a honeycomb appearance).	Usually caused by *Schistosoma haematobium*. Characteristic calcification of the bladder wall.
Fungus ball	Single large or multiple small filling defects that often contain gas that produces a mottled appearance. Contrast material occasionally enters the fungus ball and accentuates its laminated appearance.	Most often caused by *Candida albicans* in patients with debilitating diseases, diabetes mellitus, or prolonged antibiotic or steroid therapy.
Cystitis (Figs GU 24-7 and GU 24-8)	Various patterns of irregular wall thickening and mural or mucosal filling defects. Intraluminal or intramural gas in emphysematous cystitis. Multiple cysts project into the lumen in cystitis cystica. There may be amorphous calcification.	Multiple conditions, including hemorrhagic cystitis ("honeymoon cystitis"), interstitial cystitis (chronic inflammation in women), granulomatous cystitis (complication of chronic granulomatous disease of childhood or secondary to extension of Crohn's disease or granulomatous prostatitis), radiation cystitis, tuberculous cystitis, and cyclophosphamide (Cytoxan) cystitis.
Cystitis cystica/cystitis glandularis (Fig GU 24-9)	Lobulated contour of the bladder that contains nodular masses of varying size and number.	Common chronic reactive inflammatory disorders in which metaplasia of theurothelium is incited by irritants such as infection, calculi, outlet obstruction, or even tumor.

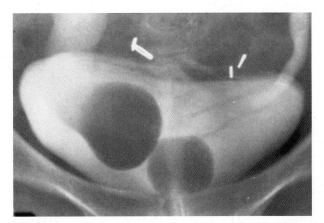

Fig GU 24-5
Bilateral simple ureteroceles.

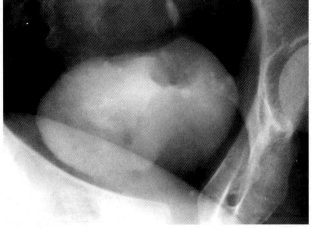

Fig GU 24-6
Endometriosis. Right posterior oblique view of the bladder shows an irregular, rounded filling defect along the posterior dome.[24]

Condition	Imaging Findings	Comments
Malacoplakia (Fig GU 24-10)	Smooth, single or multiple, round or oval filling defects that are most commonly located on the bladder floor. The radiographic pattern may suggest a neoplastic process or severe cystitis.	Uncommon chronic inflammatory disease that predominantly affects women, most of whom have a history of recurrent or chronic urinary tract infection. There may also be ureteral involvement (general dilatation with multiple filling defects or a scalloped appearance and occasionally a stricture).
Intramural hematoma	Smooth or irregular mural defect. There may be associated intraluminal filling defects (blood clots).	Follows surgery, trauma, or instrumentation.
Foreign body	Opaque or nonopaque filling defect.	Foreign material may become the nidus for calculus formation.

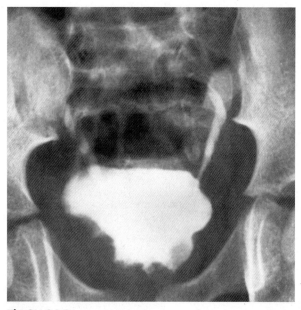

Fig GU 24-7
Cystitis. Irregular, lobulated filling defects (representing intense mucosal edema) at the base of the bladder.

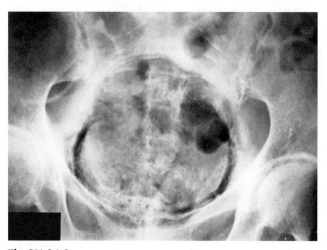

Fig GU 24-8
Emphysematous cystitis. Plain film of the pelvis shows radiolucent gas in the wall of the bladder.[7]

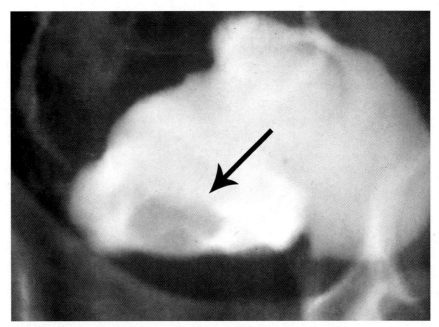

Fig GU 24-9
Cystitis cystica and cystititis glandularis. Oblique view shows a nodular filling defect (arrow) in a lobulated bladder.[24]

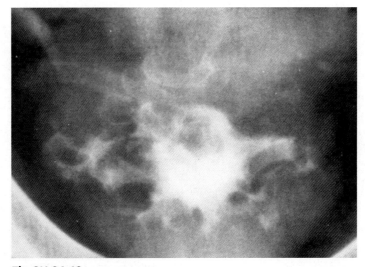

Fig GU 24-10
Malacoplakia. Postvoiding excretory urogram shows multiple smooth, nodular filling defects.[18]

Gas in the Bladder Lumen or Wall

Condition	Imaging Findings	Comments
Emphysematous cystitis (Fig GU 25-1)	Intraluminal gas associated with a ring of lucent gas outlining all or part of the bladder wall.	Inflammatory cystitis that most often occurs in diabetic patients and is caused by gas-forming bacteria.
Iatrogenic	Intraluminal gas.	Follows cystoscopy, surgery, or trauma.
Bladder fistula (Figs GU 25-2 through GU 25-4)	Intraluminal gas.	Fistula formation between the intestinal or genital tract (or both) and the urinary tract. Major underlying causes include diverticulitis (approximately 50%); carcinomas of the colon, rectum, bladder, cervix, and uterus; and Crohn's disease. Less frequent causes include trauma, radiation therapy, foreign bodies, and abscesses.
Fungus ball in bladder	Soft-tissue mass containing gas (contrast material may enter the fungus ball and further accentuate its laminated appearance).	Composed of layers of mycelia separated by air and proteinaceous material. Usually due to infection by *Candida albicans*, especially in severely debilitated patients undergoing prolonged antibiotic or steroid therapy. Gas results from the chemical action of fungi on glucose in the urine (producing CO_2 and butyric and lactic acid).

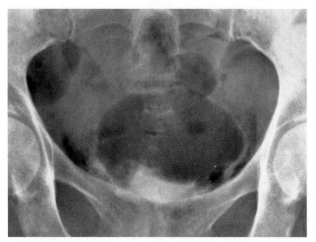

Fig GU 25-1
Emphysematous cystitis. Large amount of air in the bladder. Note the small clusters of air in the wall of the bladder in this patient with severe infection complicating diabetes.

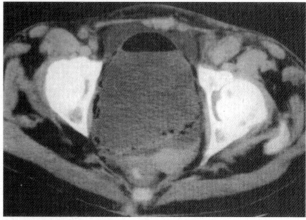

Fig GU 25-2
Emphysematous cystitis. CT scan shows gas in the bladder wall and lumen of a diabetic patient with Escherichia coli infection.[25]

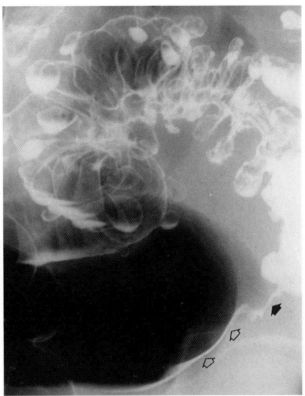

Fig GU 25-3
Colovesical fistula in diverticulitis. Barium enema examination demonstrates contrast material in the fistulous tract
(solid arrow) between the sigmoid colon and the bladder.
Barium can also be seen lining the base of the gas-filled
bladder (open arrows).

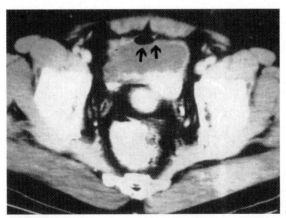

Fig GU 25-4
Colovesical fistula secondary to diverticulitis. CT scan
shows gas in the bladder (arrows).[25]

Urinary Tract Obstruction Below the Bladder in Children

Condition	Imaging Findings	Comments
Meatal stenosis	Distal urethral narrowing, often with severe proximal dilatation.	Much more common in males. May be congenital or secondary to infection or trauma. Often associated with hypospadiac openings.
Urethral stricture	Smooth narrowing of the urethral lumen of varying length (multiple in approximately 10% of cases).	Almost all congenital strictures occur in boys and are located in the bulbomembranous portion. Most commonly iatrogenic (instrumentation or repair of hypospadias) or due to trauma (straddle injury or kick).
Posterior urethral valve (Fig GU 26-1)	Elongation and dilatation of the posterior urethra with a characteristic thin, sail-like lucent defect representing the bulging valve.	Thin transverse membrane, found almost exclusively in males, that causes outlet obstruction and may lead to severe hydronephrosis and renal damage. The bladder neck often appears narrow (although it is usually normal in width) because of the disparity in size between it and the urethra bulging posteriorly beneath it. Anterior urethral valves are extremely rare.

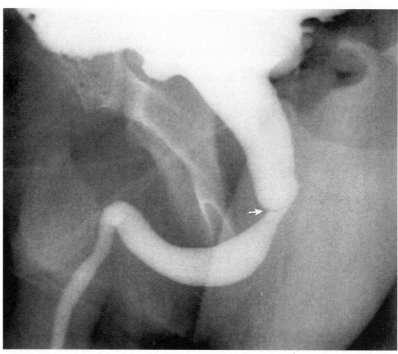

Fig GU 26-1
Posterior urethral valve. Voiding cystourethrogram shows the spinnaker-sail shape of the valve (arrow). Distally, the caliber of the bulbous urethra is normal.[26]

Condition	Imaging Findings	Comments
Ectopic ureterocele (see Fig GU 19-9)	Smooth or lobulated, usually eccentric filling defect at the base of the bladder associated with a duplicated collecting system (the ureterocele arises from the ureter draining the upper segment, which is nonfunctioning or hydronephrotic).	Congenital lesion in which the ectopic ureter enters the bladder wall near its normal site of insertion. Instead of communicating with the lumen, the ureter continues for a variable distance before opening into the bladder neck or posterior urethra. If the orifice is stenotic, proximal distention of the ureter under the submucosa of the bladder produces the eccentric filling defect.
Foreign body	Single or, less frequently, multiple filling defects that are usually radiopaque.	In addition to causing urinary tract obstruction, a foreign body may be the nidus for calculus formation.
Congenital bladder neck obstruction	Small, narrowed bladder neck. There may occasionally be an anterior or posterior indentation, diaphragm, or collar at the bladder neck opening and failure of funneling during voiding.	Controversial entity with such postulated causes as muscular hypertrophy, fibrous ring, and bladder neck dyskinesia.
Urethral diverticulum	Tubular, round or oval, smooth outpouching that is separate from the urethra but communicates with it.	Diverticulum of the urethra distal to the external sphincter is an uncommon but important cause of urinary obstruction in male children.
Congenital urethral duplication	Accessory urethra may be completely duplicated, join the main urethra distally, or end blindly.	Extremely rare anomaly that almost always occurs in males.
Hypertrophy of verumontanum	Round or oval filling defect in the prostatic urethra.	Rare cause of obstruction that is probably transient and may be the result of maternal estrogen stimulation near term. May be secondary to inflammatory lesions of the urethra and bladder in older boys and men.
Hydrometrocolpos	Extrinsic pressure narrowing of the urethra with proximal dilatation of the bladder and ureters.	Rare congenital anomaly associated with obstruction of the vaginal outlet and secondary dilatation of the vagina and uterus by retained nonsanguinous secretions.

Calcification of the Vas Deferens

Condition	Comments
Diabetes mellitus (Fig GU 27-1)	Most common cause. There is generally bilaterally symmetric calcification in the muscular elements of the vasa with the lumens remaining widely patent.
Degenerative change (aging) (Fig GU 27-2)	Appearance identical to that of vas deferens calcification in a diabetic patient, but develops in individuals with no evidence of diabetes or other predisposing factor. Calcification presumably occurs with greater frequency and at a younger age in diabetic men because this disease accelerates the degenerative process.
Tuberculosis	Inflammation causes partial or complete thrombosis of the lumen of the vas deferens, resulting in intraluminal calcification. The calcification is more frequently unilateral and irregular than in the noninflammatory form (diabetes, degenerative change).
Other infections	Inflammatory intraluminal calcification, often unilateral and irregular like tuberculosis, can develop in gonorrhea, syphilis, schistosomiasis, and chronic nonspecific urinary tract infection.

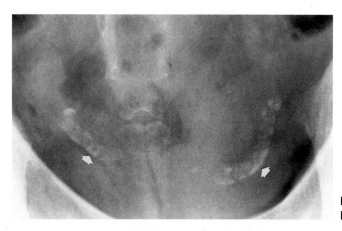

Fig GU 27-1
Diabetes mellitus.

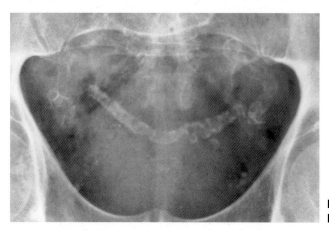

Fig GU 27-2
Degenerative change of aging.

Anechoic (Cystic) Renal Masses

Condition	Comments
Simple renal cyst (Fig GU 28-1)	Thin-walled, fluid-filled anechoic mass with strongly enhancing posterior wall.
Adult polycystic kidney disease (Fig GU 28-2)	Enlarged kidneys containing many anechoic areas of variable size representing multiple cysts. Often associated hepatic and pancreatic cysts.
Parapelvic cyst (Fig GU 28-3)	Medially placed fluid-filled anechoic mass with an echogenic wall. The cyst displaces the pelvocalyceal echo complex, but does not separate it as would be expected in hydronephrosis. Unlike hydronephrosis, the calyces are not dilated nor do they communicate with the mass.
Hydronephrosis (Fig GU 28-4)	Early mild hydronephrosis appears as a small central sonolucent area (representing the dilated fluid-filled collecting system). As the obstruction of the urinary system progresses, there is separation of the normal echo complex of the collecting system. Eventually, the calyces become completely effaced and the normal kidney is completely replaced by an anechoic hydronephrotic sac.

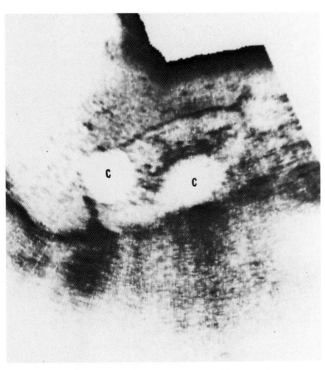

Fig GU 28-1
Simple renal cysts. Anechoic fluid-filled masses (C) with strongly enhanced posterior walls.

Condition	Comments
Multicystic dysplastic kidney (Fig GU 28-5)	Nonhereditary developmental anomaly, thought to result from an obstruction early in embryonic life, that typically presents in the neonatal period as a palpable abdominal mass. It is usually unilateral, but can be bilateral or segmental and may be associated with a hypoplastic or atretic renal artery, renal vein, ureter, and renal pelvis. Pathologically, the renal tissue is replaced by large cysts connected by fibrous tissue. The characteristic sonographic appearance is normal or enlarged kidneys with lobulated contours containing numerous cysts of varying sizes and shapes.
Medullary cystic disease	Multiple anechoic cystic structures (often very small) in the corticomedullary junction and the medulla. Clinical findings include anemia, polyuria, hyposthenuria, salt wasting, and renal failure.
Lesions that may mimic renal cyst (Fig GU 28-6)	An anechoic cystic pattern can be produced not only by liquids but also by any tissues or substances that acoustically behave like a liquid. For example, uniform gelatin-like clots, abscesses consisting only of leukocytes without debris, and unclotted blood (as in hematomas and intrarenal vascular malformations and aneurysms) all show cystic patterns. A few solid lesions also occasionally produce a pattern that so closely simulates a cyst that only the most scrupulous and meticulous technique can differentiate them. In addition to vascular anomalies, hematomas, and abscesses, other lesions that may mimic renal cysts on ultrasound include urine collections (localized hydronephrosis, urinoma), cysts containing small mural tumors, and necrotic and hemorrhagic tumors.

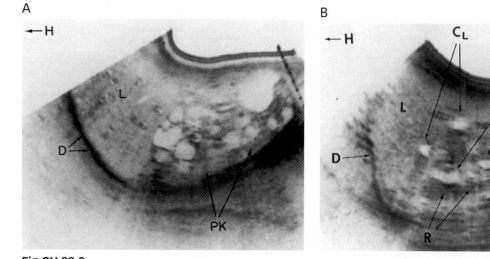

Fig GU 28-2
Adult polycystic kidney disease. (A) Parasagittal sonogram of the right kidney (PK) shows a random distribution of multiple cysts that vary dramatically in size. The normal reniform contour is maintained. (B) Parasagittal sonogram in a young, asymptomatic member of the family shows multiple cysts (C_R, C_L) in the right kidney (R) and liver (L). (D, diaphragm; H, head.)[2]

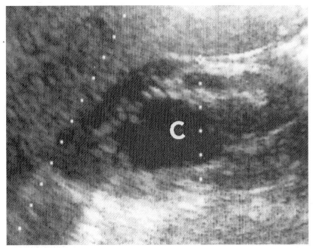

Fig GU 28-3
Parapelvic cyst (C). Fluid-filled collection that displaces but does not separate the pelvocalyceal echo complex.

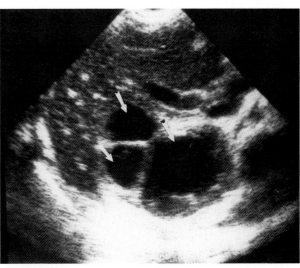

Fig GU 28-4
Hydronephrosis. Obstructed renal pelvis and calyces produce the sonographic pattern of multiple communicating cystic structures (arrows).[25]

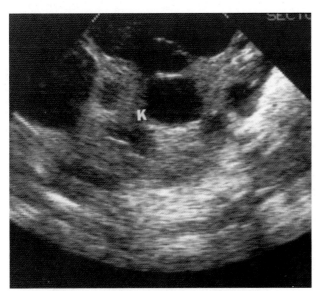

Fig GU 28-5
Multicystic dysplastic kidney. Sagittal sonogram demonstrates the cystic kidney (K). Note the absence of communication between the cystic structures.[27]

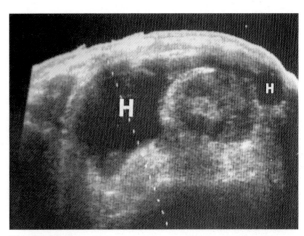

Fig GU 28-6
Hematoma. Extensive anechoic collection (H) about a renal transplant.

Complex Renal Masses

Condition	Comments
Renal neoplasm (Fig GU 29-1)	Although they usually produce a solid pattern, renal cell carcinomas that are partly cystic or those associated with a large amount of hemorrhage assume fluidlike characteristics that acoustically may overshadow their basically solid nature. A similar appearance is seen with a neoplasm that has become necrotic and contains debris that is jellylike and acts as a homogeneous sound-transmitting medium. With meticulous technique, low-level internal echoes are almost always detectable. In questionable cases, needle aspiration of the mass may be necessary to confirm the correct diagnosis.
Cyst (Figs GU 29-2 and GU 29-3)	Multilocular or multiple cysts placed very close together (eg, polycystic disease) may produce an overall complex mass, although each clear space actually represents an individual cyst. Cysts containing debris (infected cysts) or clot (hemorrhagic cysts) are also complex. Dysplastic kidney (the most common cause of an abdominal mass in the newborn) produces a disorganized cystic pattern with lack of renal parenchyma and reniform contour (unlike the precise organization of symmetrically positioned fluid-filled spaces in hydronephrosis due to congenital ureteropelvic junction obstruction).

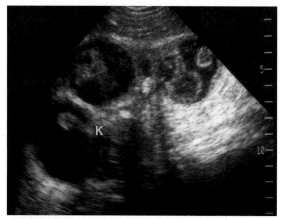

Fig GU 29-1
Leukemic infiltration. Sagittal sonogram of the kidney (K) shows multiple complex masses with cystic and solid components.[27]

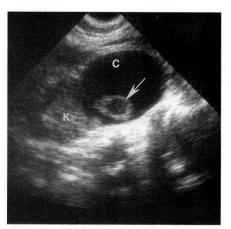

Fig GU 29-2
Renal cyst with a blood clot. Sagittal sonogram of the kidney (K) shows that the cyst (C) contains a blood clot (arrow).[27]

Condition	Comments
Abscess (Figs GU 29-4 through GU 29-6)	Variable pattern that may be primarily solid or cystic with a well-defined or poorly defined wall that is generally not as smooth as that of an uncomplicated cyst. Characteristically contains low-level echoes representing inflammatory debris. A fluid-debris level may sometimes be noted. The mass may contain highly echogenic areas (usually peripherally located) due to gas formation within the abscess.

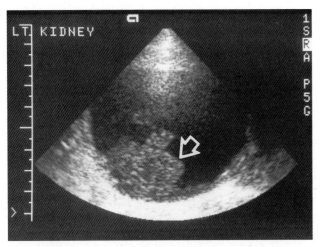

Fig GU 29-3
Renal cyst with malignancy. Enlarged sonogram demonstrates the solid renal tumor (arrow) within the cyst.[27]

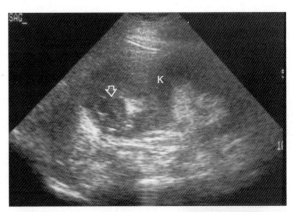

Fig GU 29-4
Renal abscess. Sagittal sonogram of the kidney (K) reveals a complex mass (arrow) in the upper pole.[27]

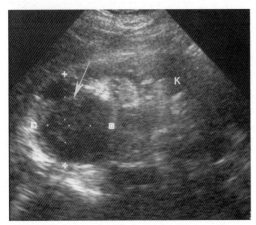

Fig GU 29-5
Renal abscess. Enlarged sonogram of the kidney (K) shows an irregular mass containing low-level echoes (arrow).[27]

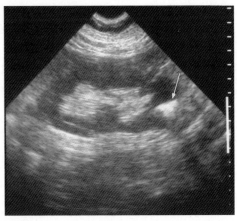

Fig GU 29-6
Renal abscess. Sagittal sonogram of the kidney demonstrates a peripheral, high-echogenic cluster of echoes (arrow) representing gas formation in the abscess.[27]

Condition	Comments
Hematoma/ hemorrhagic infarct (see Fig GU 35-4)	Hematomas may demonstrate fragments of clot, and, although predominantly cystic, their walls tend to be less smooth than those of uncomplicated renal cysts. Hemorrhagic infarcts (as in renal vein thrombosis) produce a complex pattern (especially during the acute phase) that is due to areas of hemorrhage and necrosis. A thrombus may occasionally be seen in the renal vein. In contrast, ischemic infarcts secondary to renal artery stenosis tend to appear normal on ultrasound.
Hydronephrosis/ pyonephrosis (Figs GU 29-7 and GU 29-8)	Internal echoes may occur from the edges of dilated calyceal rims and fornices, converting the fluid pattern of hydronephrosis to an apparently complex one. If the urine in an obstructed kidney is heavily infected (pyonephrosis), the degree of echogenicity is increased.

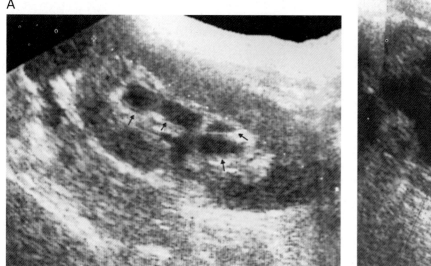
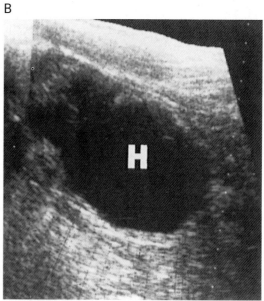

Fig GU 29-7
Hydronephrosis. (A) In a patient with moderate disease, the dilated calyces and pelvis appear as echo-free sacs (arrows) separated by septa of compressed tissue and vessels. (B) In a patient with severe hydronephrosis, the intervening septa have disappeared, leaving a large fluid-filled sac (H) with no evidence of internal structure and no normal parenchyma apparent at its margins.

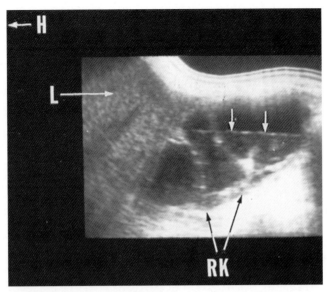

Fig GU 29-8
Pyonephrosis. Parasagittal sonogram of the right kidney (RK)
demonstrates marked hydronephrosis and a characteristic fluid
level (arrows). The fluid level indicates sediments in the renal
collecting system and is a typical finding of pyonephrosis. (H,
head; L, liver).[2]

Solid Renal Masses

Condition	Comments
Renal cell carcinoma (Figs GU 30-1 through GU 30-3)	Solid mass with numerous internal echoes and no evidence of acoustic enhancement. There is often an irregular or poorly defined interface with the remaining normal parenchyma. May contain sonolucent areas representing hemorrhage, necrosis, or cystic degeneration. Bright echoes around or within the mass may represent circumferential or intratumoral calcification. Extension of tumor into the renal vein or inferior vena cava can be easily detected.

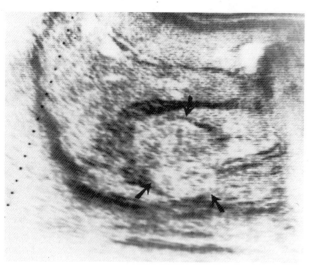

Fig GU 30-1
Renal cell carcinoma. Echo-filled solid mass (arrows) with no posterior enhancement.

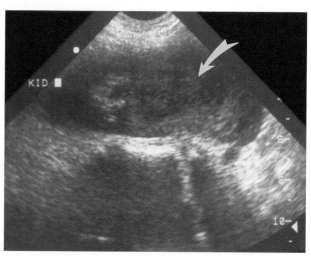

Fig GU 30-2
Renal cell carcinoma. Solid hypoechoic mass (arrow) in the inferior half of the kidney (KID) that disrupts the collecting system and distorts the renal outline.[27]

A

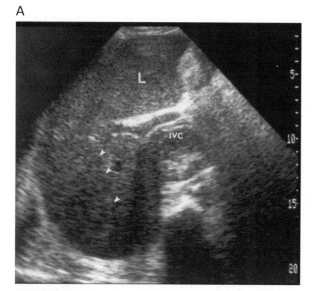

B

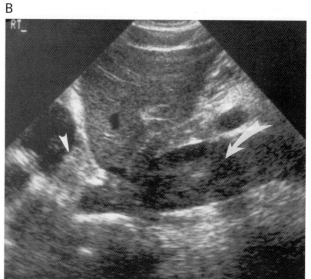

Fig GU 30-3
Renal cell carcinoma with venous extension. (A) Transverse sonogram reveals a thrombus in the inferior vena cava (IVC) and metastatic deposits (arrowheads) in the liver (L). (B) Sagittal scan identifies the distended IVC containing thrombus (large arrow) that extends into the right atrium (arrowhead).[27]

Condition	Comments
Angiomyolipoma (Figs GU 30-4 and GU 30-5)	Single or multiple renal masses that are extremely echogenic (probably because of the numerous fatty-fibrous interfaces with the lesion). Although most occur as isolated, unilateral kidney lesions in otherwise normal persons, these benign tumors also develop in a large percentage of patients with tuberous sclerosis, in whom the involvement is usually multifocal and bilateral. The characteristic high fat content of an angiomyolipoma can be well demonstrated by CT. However, sonography is unreliable in diagnosing an angiomyolipoma, because up to a third of small renal cell carcinomas have an identical appearance.
Other benign tumors (Fig GU 30-6)	Benign tumors tend to be small and well encapsulated and rarely produce clinical symptoms. They include adenoma, lipoma, fibroma, oncocytoma, and hemangioma. The tissue characteristics depend on the cellular constituents of the tumor.
Wilms' tumor (Figs GU 30-7 and GU 30-8)	Mass of generally homogeneous increased echogenicity that may contain relatively sonolucent areas due to cystic necrosis.

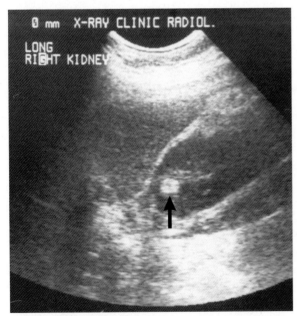

Fig GU 30-4
Angiomyolipoma. Sonography of the right kidney in an asymptomatic woman demonstrates a highly echogenic mass (arrow).[28]

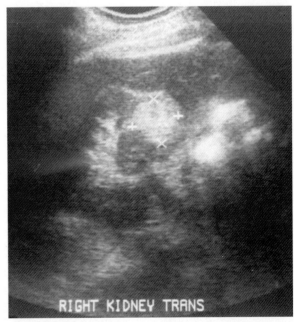

Fig GU 30-5
Renal cell carcinoma mimicking angiomyolipoma.
Ultrasound shows a small echogenic mass.[28]

Condition	Comments
Metastases (Fig GU 30-8)	Single or multiple focal renal lesions or diffuse infiltration of the kidney can be caused by metastases from carcinoma of the lung, breast, stomach, contralateral kidney, and choriocarcinoma. Metastases to the kidneys usually occur only in patients with widely disseminated malignancy. The patient is typically asymptomatic, though there may be renal enlargement, pain, hematuria, and decreased renal function. The echogenicity of the metastases varies widely depending on the primary lesion.
Leukemia (Fig GU 30-9)	Diffusely enlarged kidneys with increased echogenicity. Loss of the corticomedullary demarcation but preservation of the renal sinus echo pattern.

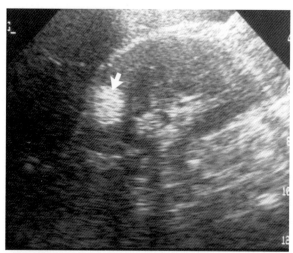

Fig GU 30-6
Adenoma. Highly echogenic mass (arrow) in the upper pole of the kidney.[27]

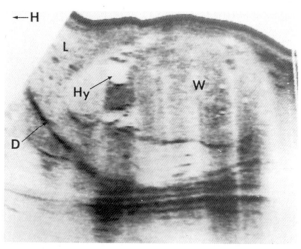

Fig GU 30-7
Wilms' tumor. Parasagittal supine sonogram demonstrates a huge mass (W) involving the lower pole of the right kidney and resulting in hydronephrosis of the upper collecting system (Hy). Wilms' tumors tend to have a moderately low internal echogenicity and, as in this patient, often contain multiple tiny cystic spaces. The large mass dramatically displaces the liver (L). (D, diaphragm; H, head.)[2]

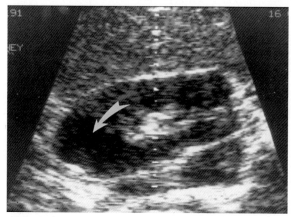

Fig GU 30-8
Metastases. Infiltration of the upper pole of the kidney (arrow) by metastatic spindle cell carcinoma.[27]

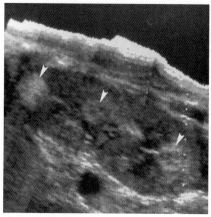

Fig GU 30-9
Leukemia. Multiple echogenic deposits representing infiltration (arrowheads).[29]

Condition	Comments
Lymphoma (Fig GU 30-10)	Characteristically produces a mass effect with one or several areas of decreased echogenicity because it is composed of tissue of fairly uniform type so that there is little difference in specific acoustic impedance between adjacent internal structures.
Infantile polycystic kidney disease	Innumerable ectatic renal tubules ("cysts") in the large kidneys are so small that their lumens are not resolved by ultrasound. Instead, the interfaces produced by the walls of these tubules cause increased echogenicity throughout the parenchyma of the kidney. Increased echoes from ectatic tubules in the cortex as well as in the medulla cause a loss of the normal sharp distinction between the medullary and cortical areas and its replacement by a homogeneous parenchyma of increased echoes.
Calcified renal mass	Mural calcification, usually in the wall of a cyst but occasionally in the wall of a hematoma or abscess, can cause marked reflection of sound that prevents the through-transmission of enough sound to define the far wall. Correlation with plain radiographs is essential to document the presence of calcification causing this appearance.

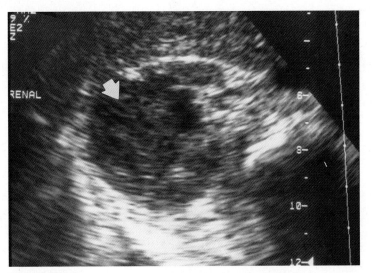

Fig GU 30-10
Lymphoma. Transverse sonogram demonstrates a hypoechoic mass (arrow) in the kidney.[27]

Cystic Renal Masses on Computed Tomography

Condition	Imaging Findings	Comments
Benign renal cyst (Figs GU 31-1 and GU 31-2)	Sharply delineated, near–water attenuation lesion with a very thin wall, no internal septations, and no contrast enhancement.	Most common unifocal mass of the kidney. A renal cyst may have a high attenuation due to hemorrhage into the cyst, calcification of the cyst wall, infection, leakage of contrast material into the cyst by a communication with the collecting system or by diffusion, or image degradation by high-density streak artifacts.
Parapelvic cyst (Fig GU 31-3)	Appearance identical to that of a simple, benign, renal parenchymal cyst though it is located adjacent to the renal sinus.	May be difficult to distinguish from a dilated or an extrarenal pelvis on nonenhanced scans. After administration of contrast material, the unenhanced parapelvic cyst is easily detected adjacent to contrast-filled hilar collecting structures.
Polycystic kidney disease (Fig GU 31-4)	Multiple cysts in lobulated and enlarged kidneys.	Splaying and distortion of the renal collecting system. Hepatic or pancreatic cystic disease can be demonstrated in approximately one-third of patients.

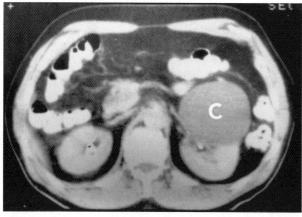

Fig GU 31-1
Benign renal cyst. Nonenhancing left renal mass (C) with a sharply marginated border and a thin wall.

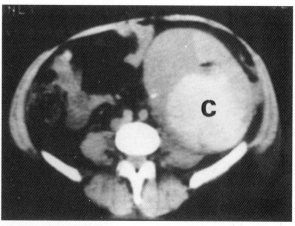

Fig GU 31-2
Benign renal cyst. High attenuation in the cyst (C) represents hemorrhage.

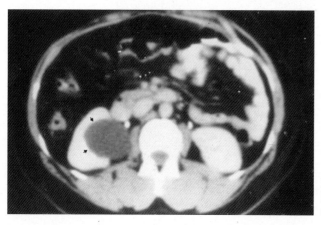

Fig GU 31-3
Parapelvic cyst. Well-marginated water-density mass (arrows).

Condition	Imaging Findings	Comments
Multicystic dysplastic kidney	Entire kidney consists of numerous cystic masses that vary in size.	No functioning renal parenchyma is detectable after administration of contrast material (unlike multilocular cystic nephromas or unilateral polycystic disease).
Multilocular renal cyst	Multiple fluid-filled cysts separated by thick septa and sharply demarcated from normal renal parenchyma.	Rare condition. May contain peripheral or central calcification with a circular, stellate, flocculent, or granular pattern.
Multilocular cystic nephroma (Fig GU 31-5)	Multiloculated cystic mass (indistinguishable from cystic renal cell carcinoma).	Uncommon benign neoplasm characterized by multiple noncommunicating cysts that do not contain hemorrhagic material and are contained within a well-defined capsule. Usually found in males under age 4 and in middle-aged females.

B

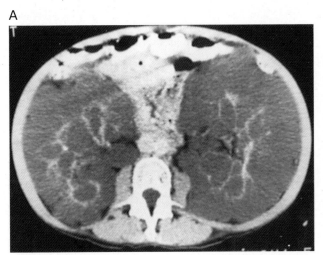
A

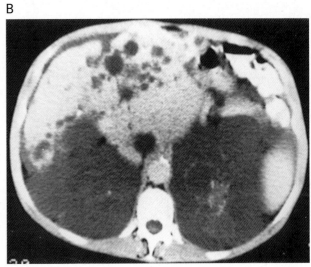

Fig GU 31-4
Polycystic disease. (A) Rim of contrast enhancement in the severely thinned renal parenchyma about the innumerable large renal cysts. (B) Scan at a higher level also shows diffuse cystic involvement of the liver.

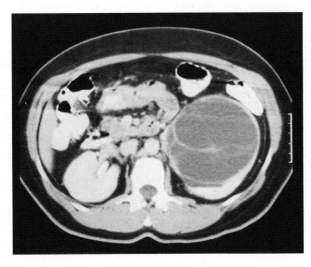

Fig GU 31-5
Multilocular cystic nephroma. The thick-walled, non-enhancing left renal mass contains irregular internal septations.[28]

Condition	Imaging Findings	Comments
Cystic renal cell carcinoma (Fig GU 31-6)	Multiloculated cystic mass.	Septations within the mass usually show some contrast enhancement, unlike the generally nonenhancing margins of a multilocular cystic nephroma.
Lesions that may mimic renal cyst (Figs GU 31-7 and GU 31-8)	Low-attenuation masses that often have somewhat more irregular margins than a simple cyst.	Necrotic tumor; hematoma; abscess; vascular anomaly; urine collections (localized hydronephrosis, urinoma).

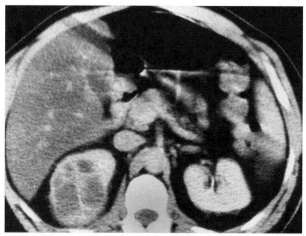

Fig GU 31-6
Cystic clear-cell renal carcinoma. Contrast scan shows enhancement of portions of this multilocular cystic mass, which contains thick septations.[28]

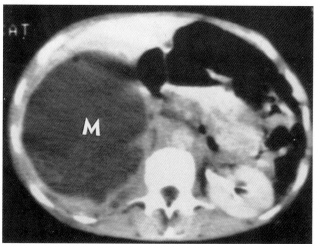

Fig GU 31-7
Necrotic renal cell carcinoma. The huge nonenhancing, cyst-like mass (M) has irregular margins (especially on its medial and posterior aspects).

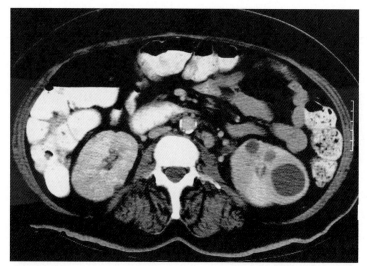

Fig GU 31-8
Renal abscesses. Multiple nonenhancing lesions in the left kidney of an insulin-dependent diabetic woman with fever of unknown origin, leukocytosis, pyuria, and urine cultures positive for *Escherichia coli.*[28]

Focal Solid Renal Masses on Computed Tomography

Condition	Imaging Findings	Comments
Renal cell carcinoma (hypernephroma) (Fig GU 32-1)	Renal contour abnormality that is frequently irregularly shaped, poorly demarcated from normal parenchyma, and has an attenuation value near that of normal renal tissue (unlike a simple cyst that is smooth, sharply demarcated, and has a uniform attenuation value near that of water).	After the injection of contrast material, a solid renal neoplasm demonstrates a small but definite increase in density that is probably due primarily to vascular perfusion (unlike a simple cyst, which shows no change in attenuation value). However, this increased density is much less than that of the surrounding normal parenchyma, which also tends to concentrate the contrast material, and thus the renal neoplasm becomes more apparent on contrast-enhanced scans.
Angiomyolipoma (hamartoma) (Figs GU 32-2 and GU 32-3)	Single or multiple renal masses having zones of different density ranging from −150 H (fat) to +150 H (calcification). After contrast injection, portions of the tumor may be enhanced, though fatty tissue in areas of necrosis does not increase in density.	Although the CT diagnosis of angiomyolipoma is highly specific, renal lipoma, liposarcoma, or retroperitoneal liposarcoma invading the kidney cannot be absolutely excluded. If the diagnosis is in doubt, ultrasound can demonstrate the highly echogenic foci characteristic of fat rather than fluid or nonfatty solid tissue.
Renal oncocytoma (Fig GU 32-4)	Homogeneous mass that is only slightly less dense than renal parenchyma after injection of contrast material. The tumor is sharply separated from the normal cortex and does not invade the calyceal system or adjacent structures.	Rare benign renal tumor thought to originate from proximal tubular epithelial cells. May be impossible to differentiate from a renal adenoma or renal cell carcinoma without additional diagnostic studies (angiography, radionuclide scanning).

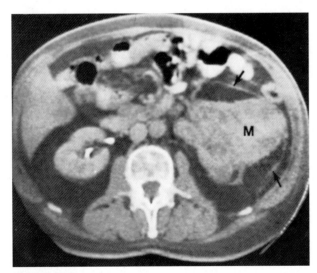

Fig GU 32-1
Renal cell carcinoma. Large mass (M) of the left kidney with thickening of Gerota's fascia (arrows).[30]

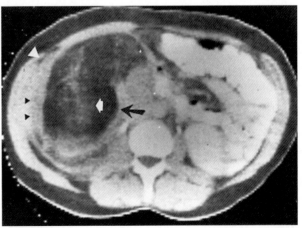

Fig GU 32-2
Angiomyolipoma. Fatty mass (long arrow) intermixed with (short arrow) and surrounded by (arrowheads) areas of tissue density, representing intratumoral and perinephric hemorrhage, respectively.[31]

Condition	Imaging Findings	Comments
Lymphoma (Figs GU 32-5 and GU 32-6)	Various patterns, including bilaterally enlarged kidneys without demonstrable masses; multiple focal, nodular, solid masses that have decreased density on postcontrast scans; focal, irregular, solitary, solid intrarenal masses; dilatation of intrarenal collecting structures produced by diffuse interstitial infiltration of the kidneys; and perirenal disease extending into the renal pelvis.	Renal involvement by lymphoma is commonly found at postmortem examination (30% to 50%), but is seldom detected by conventional urographic studies. Multiple parenchymal nodules are by far the most common manifestation of renal lymphoma. Bilateral involvement occurs in approximately 75% of cases.
Metastases	Solid mass indistinguishable from a primary renal malignancy.	Most commonly from primary tumors of the lung, breast, stomach, colon, cervix, or pancreas. Leukemic infiltrations may produce bilateral renal enlargement and intrarenal masses.
Transitional cell carcinoma (Figs GU 32-7 and GU 32-8)	After intravenous injection of contrast material, the tumor appears as a pelvic filling defect with a smooth, lobulated, or irregular margin.	Small pelvic tumors that do not produce hydronephrosis or invade the peripelvic fat are usually not detected on precontrast CT scans.

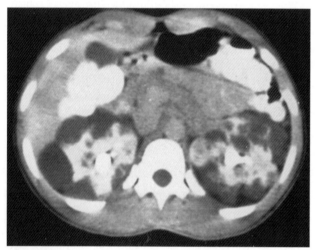

Fig GU 32-3
Multiple renal hamartomas in tuberous sclerosis. Innumerable low-attenuation masses in both kidneys.

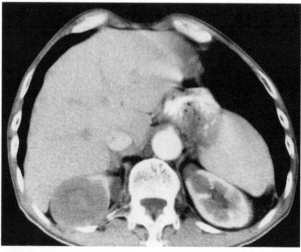

Fig GU 32-4
Renal oncocytoma. Well-defined, homogeneous mass in the upper pole of the right kidney. (Small cysts are present bilaterally.)[28]

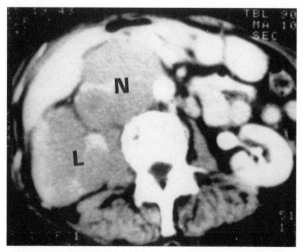

Fig GU 32-5
Lymphoma. The right kidney is completely replaced by a lymphomatous mass (L). Note the extensive nodal involvement (N).

Condition	Imaging Findings	Comments
Wilms' tumor (Figs GU 32-9 and GU 32-10)	Large, at least partially intrarenal mass that usually has a central density lower than that of normal renal parenchyma, whereas the periphery of the tumor is virtually isodense.	Most common primary malignant renal tumor of childhood. Renal vein thrombosis or tumor extension, which occurs in up to 10% of cases, may be demonstrated as a low-density intraluminal defect after injection of contrast material.
Infection Acute pyelonephritis (focal bacterial nephritis) (Fig GU 32-11)	Single or multiple, poorly marginated masses of decreased density.	After injection of contrast material, there may be a characteristic striated appearance of regularly oriented zones of increased density in the affected kidney.

A   B

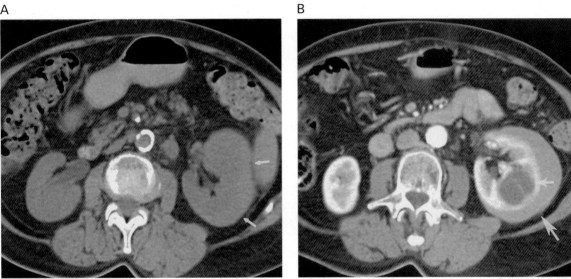

Fig GU 32-6
Lymphoma. (A) Initial unenhanced scan shows an enlarged kidney with subcapsular soft-tissue attenuation (arrows) and an ill-defined lesion posteriorly. (B) Contrast scan confirms the presence of both subcapsular and parenchymal masses (arrows).[32]

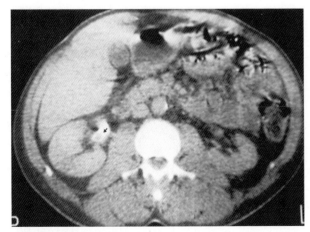

Fig GU 32-7
Transitional cell carcinoma. Filling defect (arrow) in the opacified renal pelvis.

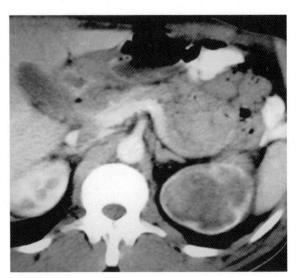

Fig GU 32-8
Transitional cell carcinoma. Diffuse tumor infiltration of the left kidney with preservation of its reniform contour.[33]

Condition	Imaging Findings	Comments
Renal abscess (Figs GU 32-12 and GU 32-13)	Often well-defined mass of decreased density that typically has a thick, irregular wall.	After injection of contrast material, there is a variable pattern of wall enhancement. May be difficult to distinguish from a centrally necrotic renal cell carcinoma.
Xanthogranulomatous pyelonephritis (Fig GU 32-14)	Multiple nonenhancing, round areas of decreased attenuation that may be of a characteristic fatty consistency.	Unusual nodular replacement of renal parenchyma by large lipid-filled macrophages (foam cells) that may develop in chronically infected kidneys. Typically a large calculus in the renal pelvis or collecting system and absence of contrast material excretion in the kidney or an area of focal involvement.

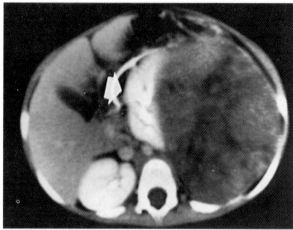

Fig GU 32-9
Wilms' tumor. Large low-density mass pushing the functioning portion of the left kidney (arrow) across the midline.

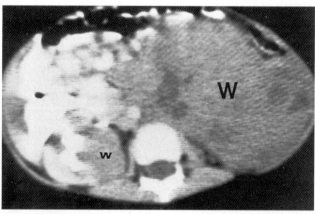

Fig GU 32-10
Bilateral Wilms' tumor. Huge left renal mass (W) that crosses the midline. There is also a small separate mass (w) in the right kidney.[33]

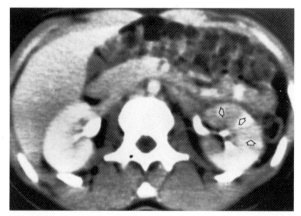

Fig GU 32-11
Acute pyelonephritis. Postcontrast scan shows characteristic low-density striations (arrows) in the left kidney.

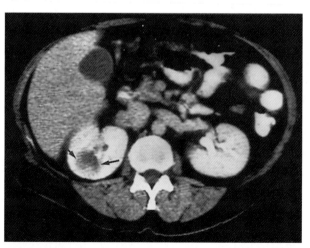

Fig GU 32-12
Renal abscess. Contrast-enhanced CT scan through both kidneys demonstrates a discrete low-density area (arrows), which proved to be an abscess on diagnostic needle aspiration.

Condition	Imaging Findings	Comments
Infarction (Fig GU 32-15)	Low-attenuation, often wedge-shaped mass.	Frequently, a higher attenuation subcapsular rim on contrast-enhanced scans.
Hematoma Intrarenal (Fig GU 32-16)	Focal area of decreased attenuation in the kidney.	After contrast injection, there is decreased enhancement of the hematoma compared with the normal renal parenchyma.

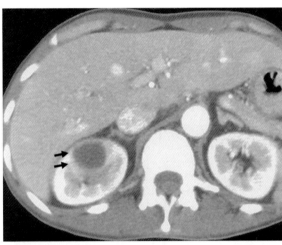

Fig GU 32-13
Renal abscess. Cystic lesion with adjacent renal parenchymal edema (arrows), representing a *Staphylococcus aureus* abscess in a patient with acquired immunodeficiency syndrome.[32]

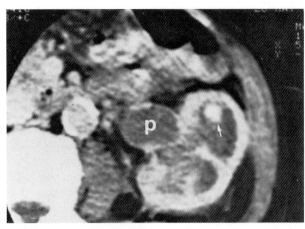

Fig GU 32-14
Xanthogranulomatous pyelonephritis. The renal pelvis (p) and intrarenal collecting structures are filled with low-density pus. Note the prolonged opacification of the left renal cortex and the high-density focus (arrow) representing a renal calculus.[34]

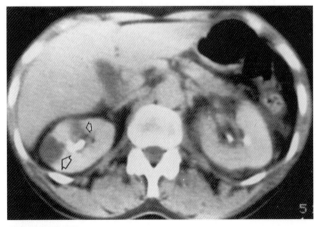

Fig GU 32-15
Infarction. Two wedge-shaped areas of decreased attenuation (arrows) in the right kidney.

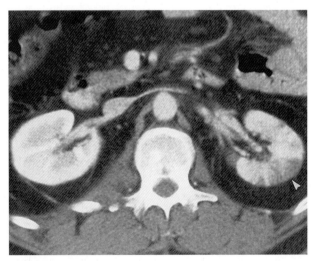

Fig GU 32-16
Renal contusion. Contrast scan demonstrates a focal area of decreased enhancement in the interpolar region of the left kidney (arrowhead).[35]

Condition	Imaging Findings	Comments
Subcapsular (Fig GU 32-17)	Lenticular low-density fluid collection with flattening of the renal parenchyma.	Shortly after injury, a subcapsular hematoma has a higher density than the surrounding kidney because of the fresh extravasation of blood. Follow-up scans show that the hematoma diminishes in intensity as it liquefies.
Multiple severe renal lacerations ("shattered kidney") (Figs GU 32-18 and GU 32-19)	Devitalized renal fragments, severe compromise in contrast excretion, extensive hemorrhage, and active arterial bleeding.	Catastrophic injury generally requiring surgical exploration and often nephrectomy. At times, intra-arterial embolization may salvage the kidney.

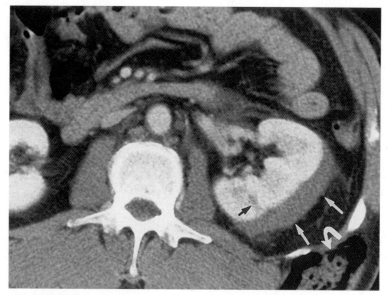

Fig GU 32-17
Subcapsular hematoma. Contrast scan demonstrates a subcapsular fluid collection (straight white arrows) flattening the posterolateral contour of the left kidney. There is minimal cortical laceration (black arrow). Note also the subcutaneous emphysema in the left side of the back (curved arrow). A chest tube had been inserted for a left pneumothorax (not shown).[35]

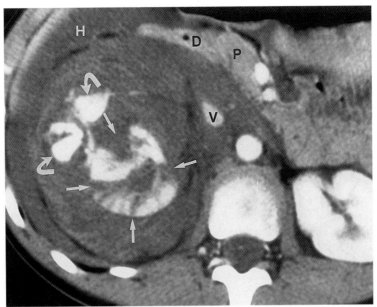

Fig GU 32-18
Multiple renal lacerations. Contrast scan shows several deep lacerations of the interpolar region of the right kidney (straight arrows) associated with areas of active arterial extravasation (curved arrows) Note the anterior displacement of the duodenum (D), pancreas (P), and inferior vena cava (V). A hemoperitoneum (H) is seen in Morrison's pouch.[35]

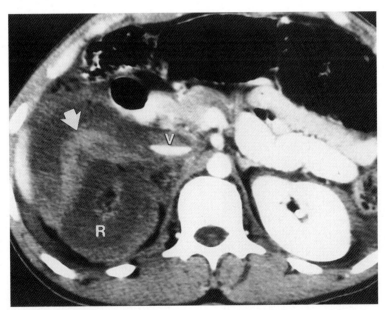

Fig GU 32-19
Shattered kidney. Contrast scan demonstrates a devitalized upper pole of the right kidney due to segmental infarction (RP). Note the perinephric hyperattenuating blood clot (arrow). Flattening of the inferior vena cava (V) indicates hypovolemic shock.[35]

Renal Sinus Abnormalities

Condition	Imaging Findings	Comments
Non-neoplastic Lipomatosis (Fig GU 33-1)	Increase in the fatty tissue enveloping the vascular structures in the renal sinus.	The quantity of renal fat in the renal pelvis normally and gradually increases with age and obesity. Proliferation of sinus fat also occurs abnormally in association with processes causing destruction or atrophy of renal tissue, as well as with increased exogenous or endogenous steroids.
Replacement lipomatosis (Fig GU 33-2)	Mass-like proliferation of renal sinus fat associated with markedly atrophied renal parenchyma. A staghorn calculus is often present.	Sequella of severe renal atrophy or destruction, usually due to chronic calculus disease with resultant hydronephrosis and inflammation. This process may mimic a fat-containing neoplasm originating in the renal sinus, but there is no evidence of focal mass effect on the intrarenal collecting system.
Cysts (Fig GU 33-3)	Peripelvic cysts may mimic hydronephrosis on unenhanced studies. However, after contrast administration, the enhanced collecting systems are displaced and compressed by the water-attenuation sinus cysts. A parapelvic cyst appears as a larger, single lesion with water attenuation.	Single or multiple benign extraparenchymal peripelvic cysts confined to the renal pelvis are common, frequently bilateral, asymptomatic, and thought to be of lymphatic origin. Single parapelvic cysts originate in the medial renal parenchymal tissue and protrude into the renal pelvis.
Vascular lesions (Fig GU 33-4)	On contrast scans, tortuous, dilated vascular structures within a mass-like lesion. MR shows signal voids, and Doppler ultrasound demonstrates a characteristic high-flow pattern.	Renal artery aneurysm, arteriovenous malformation, or renal vein varix can involve the renal sinus and appear as a parapelvic or peripelvic lesion.

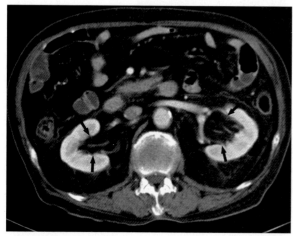

Fig GU 33-1
Renal sinus lipomatosis. Contrast CT scan shows proliferation of fat (arrows) in both renal sinuses in an asymptomatic 76-year-old man.[36]

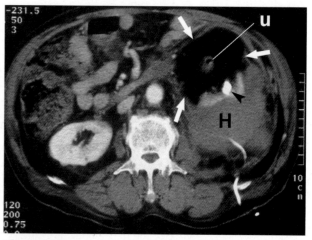

Fig GU 33-2
Replacement lipomatosis. Contrast CT scan shows a tumor-like mass of fat (arrows) occupying the left renal sinus and surrounding the left ureter (u). The left renal parenchyma is markedly atrophied in associated with a large stone (arrowhead). The large amount of subcapsular hematoma (H) reflects hemorrhage complicating insertion of a nephrostomy tube for stone extraction.[36]

Condition	Imaging Findings	Comments
Inflammatory lesions (Fig GU 33-5)	Lobulated masslike lesion with focal areas of high attenuation representing hemorrhage or debris.	Primary inflammatory lesions involving the renal sinus are rare. Much more common is extension of a renal inflammatory process into the renal sinus and perinephric space.
Hemorrhage	Acute hemorrhage has a higher attenuation than normal fluid.	Generally a complication of anticoagulant therapy, though it can be secondary to trauma.
Urinoma (see Fig 37.2)	Extravasation of contrast material confirms the diagnosis.	Usually associated with ureteral obstruction secondary to stone disease, which results in rupture of the collecting system.

A   B

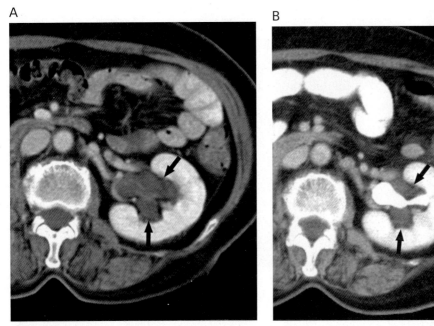

Fig GU 33-3
Renal sinus cyst. (A) Contrast-enhanced CT scan obtained during the nephrographic phase shows low-attenuation cystic lesions (arrows) in the left renal sinus. This finding could be misinterpreted as hydronephrosis. (B) Delayed scan during the excretory phase shows the cysts (arrows) in the renal sinus, an appearance different from that of hydronephrosis. The enhanced calyces are stretched and attenuated but not obstructed by the cysts.[36]

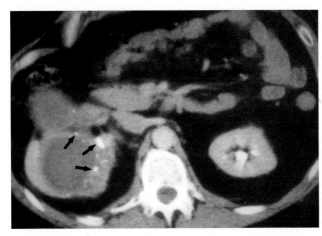

Fig GU 33-4
Renal artery aneurysm. CT scan demonstrates a large, lobulated, mass-like lesion with soft-tissue attenuation and rim calcifications (arrows) in the right renal sinus.[36]

Condition	Imaging Findings	Comments
Neoplastic Tumor of the renal pelvis (Figs GU 33-6 through GU 33-8)	A small lesion appears as a central solid mass in the renal pelvis that expands to compress the renal sinus fat. Larger masses obliterate the renal sinus fat and infiltrate into the surrounding parenchyma.	Malignant tumors arising from the renal pelvis constitute 5% of urinary tract neoplasms. About 90% are transitional cell carcinomas, with the rest being of squamous cell origin. These tumors are centered in the renal pelvis and secondarily invade the renal sinus fat and renal parenchyma. The presence of a renal stone with a large infiltrating tumor is suggestive of squamous cell carcinoma.

A

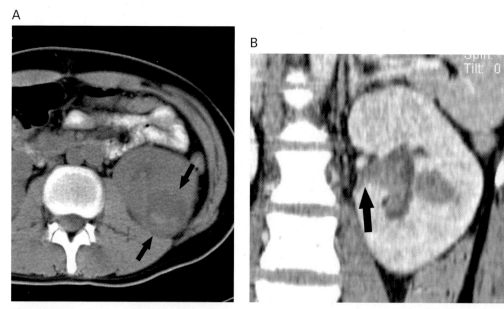

B

Fig GU 33-5
Aspergillosis. (A) Unenhanced CT scan shows a lobulated mass (arrows) with focal internal high attenuation that simulates hemorrhage within the lesion. (B) Contrast coronal reformatted image demonstrates the poorly enhancing, low-attenuation mass-like renal parenchymal lesion, which extends to the renal sinus (arrow). The nephrectomy specimen showed a hemorrhagic mass due to focal invasive aspergillosis, which may be difficult to differentiate from a tumor.[36]

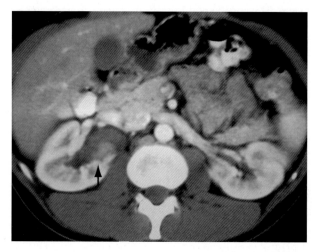

Fig GU 33-6
Transitional cell carcinoma. Contrast CT scan demonstrates a sessile filling detect (arrow) expanding into the renal sinus fat.[37]

Condition	Imaging Findings	Comments
Primary tumor of mesenchymal origin (Fig GU 33-9)	In general, a relatively well-circumscribed mass with its epicenter in the renal sinus and surrounded by attenuated renal parenchyma. The renal pelvis is stretched over the tumor and there may be hydronephrosis.	Primary mesenchymal renal tumors are rare, but may develop in the renal sinus space as well as in the renal capsule and renal parenchyma. Benign tumors include hemangioma, fibroma, leiomyoma, angiomyolipoma, neurogenic tumor, and teratoma. Malignant renal neoplasms include leiomyosarcoma, fibrosarcoma, liposarcoma, hemangiopericytoma, and malignant fibrous histiocytoma.
Tumor of the renal parenchyma projecting into the renal sinus (Fig GU 33-10)	A mass extending from the renal parenchyma to invade the renal sinus produces a filling defect and often results in hydronephrosis or calyceal displacement.	Renal cell carcinomas commonly extend into the renal sinus. Three-dimensional CT or MRI helps delineate the precise location of the renal mass and its relationship to the collecting system and renal vessels. Benign multilocular cystic nephroma also often herniates into the renal sinus.
Retroperitoneal tumor extending into the renal sinus (Fig GU 33-11)	Bulky retroperitoneal mass that envelops and surrounds the normal constituents of the renal sinus, often with contiguous spread to the perinephric space. Lymphomatous masses are typically homogeneous with minimal enhancement, but considerably less than normal renal parenchyma.	Because the renal sinus is a medial extension of the perinephric space, any retroperitoneal tumor can extend to the renal sinus. The most common is lymphoma. A characteristic feature of lymphoma is continued patency of the renal vessels despite tumor encasement.

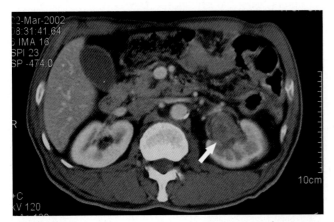

Fig GU 33-7
Transitional cell carcinoma. Contrast CT scan shows an ill-defined, low-attenuation mass (arrow) obliterating the renal sinus fat.[36]

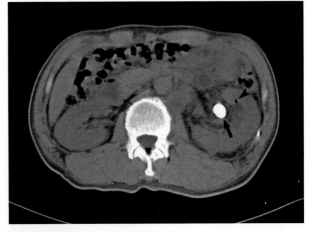

Fig GU 33-8
Squamous cell carcinoma. CT scan demonstrates a high-attenuation stone in the left renal pelvis. A tiny amount of gas (arrowhead), due to a previously performed percutaneous nephrostomy, in seen in the renal sinus.[36]

Condition	Imaging Findings	Comments
Metastasis (Fig GU 33-12)	Soft-tissue attenuation mass in the renal sinus, often with obstructive hydronephrosis.	Metastases to sinus lymph nodes may reflect a generalized retroperitoneal process or be a manifestation of isolated involvement, such as with primary gonadal tumors.

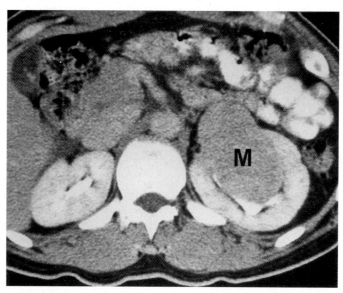

Fig GU 33-9
Hemangiopericytoma. Contrast CT scan shows a large, well-defined mass (M) with soft-tissue attenuation occupying the central portion of the left renal sinus and compressing the enhanced pelvocalyceal system.[38]

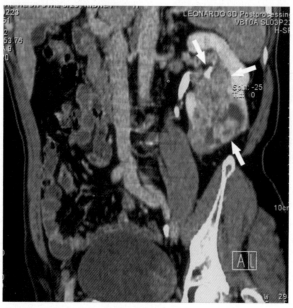

Fig GU 33-10
Extension of renal cell carcinoma. Contrast coronal reformatted CT scan shows tumor involvement of the renal sinus and the extent of the renal cell carcinoma (arrow).[36]

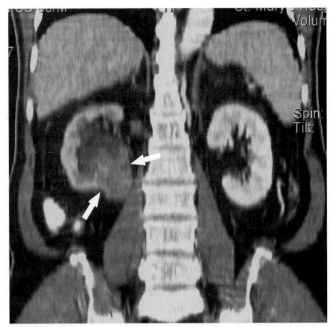

Fig GU 33-11
Extension of retroperitoneal lymphoma. Contrast coronal reformatted CT scan demonstrates a large, relatively homogeneous retroperitoneal mass (arrows) extending to the renal sinus and causing mild hydronephrosis of the right kidney.[36]

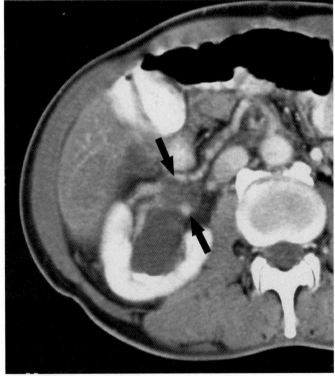

Fig GU 33-12
Metastases. Contrast CT scan shows a soft-tissue attenuation mass (arrows), representing metastastic lymphadenopathy from colon cancer, which extends into the right renal sinus and causes obstructive hydronephrosis.[36]

Perinephric Mass on Computed Tomography and Magnetic Resonance Imaging

Condition	Comments
Tumors	
Renal cell carcinoma (Fig GU 34-1)	Although a common neoplasm, perinephric spread is unusual and typically seen in bulky tumors.
Lymphoma (Fig GU 34-2)	Generally a manifestation of widespread disease (primary renal lymphoma is rare). It usually appears as a homogeneous, hypervascular, mildly enhancing lesion associated with obstructive encasement of retroperitoneal vessels.
Post-transplantation lymphoproliferative disorder	Associated with Epstein-Barr virus infection, it is a complication in 2% of solid organ recipients. In kidney transplants, it typically occurs in the renal hilum as a hypointense lesion on both T1- and T2-weighted images and has minimal contrast enhancement.
Metastases	Although metastases to the kidney are often found at autopsy, generally in patients with widely disseminated disease, they are infrequently detected on imaging.
Retroperitoneal tumors (Fig GU 34-3)	Perinephric involvement may result from direct spread by contiguous extension, especially from sarcomas and bulky primary renal tumors.
Fluid	
Hematoma (Fig GU 34-4)	Nontraumatic perinephric hematomas may develop secondary to bleeding diathesis, ruptured aortic aneurysm, polycystic disease, angiomyolipoma, or renal cell carcinoma.
Urinoma (Fig GU 34-5)	Extravasation of contrast material may be detected in patients with perinephric urinoma related to trauma or rupture a fornix of an obstructed renal pelvis.
Abscess	An abscess in the perinephric region may result from a urinary tract infection or infection of a preexisting perinephric hematoma or urinoma. Prediposing factors include diabetes and immunosuppressive therapy.
Lymphangiomatosis	Unilocular or multilocular thin-walled perinephric cysts representing a rare benign malformation of the perinephric lymphatic system.

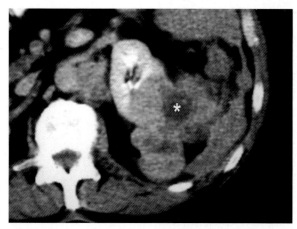

Fig GU 34-1
Renal cell carcinoma. Contrast CT scan demonstrates a large heterogeneous and necrotic mass (asterisk) invading the perinephric space. Significant thickening of the renal fascia is also seen.[39]

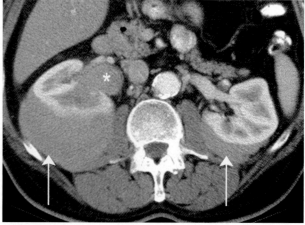

Fig GU 34-2
Non-Hodgkin's lymphoma. Contrast CT scan shows bilateral perinephric (arrows) and right peripelvic (asterisk) masses.[39]

Condition	Comments
Inflammation Xanthogranulomatous pyelonephritis (Fig GU 34-6)	Perinephric extension of a locally aggressive tumorlike renal mass, usually associated with renal stones, obstructive hydronephrosis, and chronic infection.
Pancreatitis	Fluid may dissect between fascial planes to the right perinephric space in inflammations of the head or neck of the pancreas and to the left perinephric space if there is inflammatory involvement of the pancreatic tail.

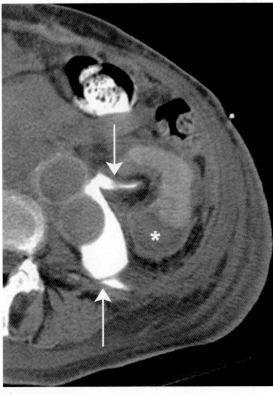

Fig GU 34-3
Retroperiotoneal liposarcoma. Contrast CT scan shows a large heterogeneous, predominantly fat-containing mass (arrows) in the right upper quadrant, which invades the perinephric space and renal hilum.[39]

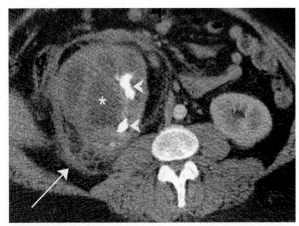

Fig GU 34-4
Hematoma. CT in a patient with acute flank pain demonstrates a perirenal hematoma (arrow) originating from a ruptured angiomyolipoma (asterisk).[39]

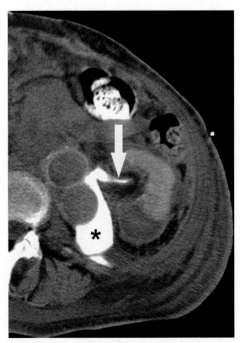

Fig GU 34-5
Urinoma. Delayed contrast CT scan shows excreted contrast material passing from the left renal pelvis (arrow) into a perinephric fluid collection (asterisk), confirming the diagnosis. The patient developed flank pain after aortic aneurysm repair.[39]

Condition	Comments
Proliferative disease	
Extramedulary hemtopoiesis (Fig GU 34-7)	Develops in patients with chronic anemia, leukemia and other blood dyscrasias, or marrow replacement by tumor or overgrowth of bone.
Retroperitoneal fibrosis	Low signal-intensity mass on both T1- and T2-weighted MR images (low-attenuation on CT), which infiltrates the retroperitoneum and encases the major vessels. Isolated perinephric involvement rarely occurs.
Others (Fig GU 34-8)	Rossi-Dorfman disease (benign systemic histiocytic proliferation) and Erdheim-Chester disease (lipoid granulomatosis).

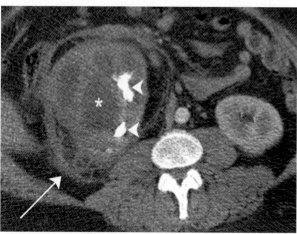

Fig GU 34-6
Xanthogranulomatous pyelonephritis. Contrast CT scan shows an enlarged right kidney with an abscess-like low-attenuation cavity (asterisk) in the right hilum. The staghorn calculus (arrowhead) was also seen on unenhanced images. The inflammatory process extends to the perinephric space (arrow).[39]

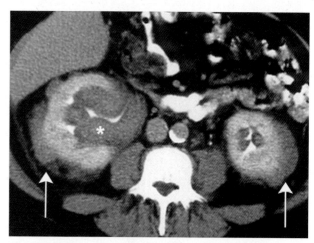

Fig GU 34-7
Extramedullary hematopoiesis. Contrast-enhanced CT scan shows a large hypodense, hypervascular mass encasing the right renal hilum and distorting the collecting system (asterisk). There is involvement of the perirenal space bilaterally (arrows). Note the preservation of the contours of the kidneys.[39]

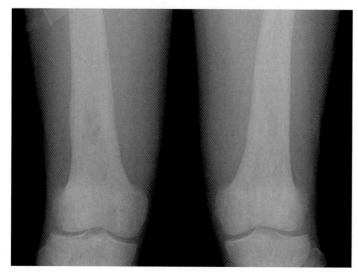

Fig GU 34-8
Erdheim-Chester disease. Contrast CT scan shows a left perinephric hypovascular mass (arrow) associated with fat stranding and moderate hydronephrosis (asterisk).[39]

Condition	Comments
Subcapsular disease	
Renal cortical necrosis (Fig GU 34-9)	Usually a complication of obstetric catastrophe, there is destruction of the cortex of the kidney with sparing of the renal medulla. On CT, there is normal medullary enhancement but no enhancement of the renal cortex, except for a thin subcapsular rim.
Nephroblastomatosis (Fig GU 34-10)	Multiple or diffuse embryonal nephroblastic rests, precursors of Wilms' tumors, that produce well-defined round or ovoid foci in the periphery of the renal cortex.

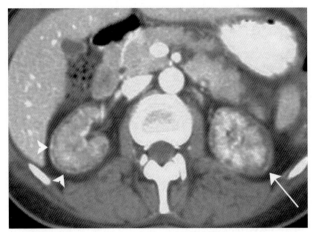

Fig GU 34-9
Cortical necrosis. In this patient with acute renal failure following severe antepartum hemorrhage, a contrast CT scan demonstrates a lack of enhancement of the renal cortex (arrow) but normal renal medulla enhancement. Note the slight enhancement of the renal capsule (arrowheads).[39]

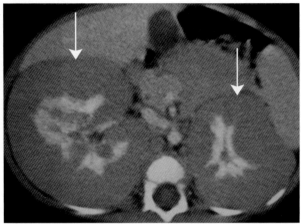

Fig GU 34-10
Nephroblastomatosis. Contrast CT scan shows bilateral enlargement of the kidneys caused by hypodense, non-enhancing, cortical soft-tissue masses (arrows). Note the distortion of the renal parenchyma centrally.[39]

Increased Renal Cortical Echogenicity with Preservation of Medullary Sonolucency*

Condition	Comments
Renal parenchymal disease (Figs GU 35-1 and GU 35-2)	Acute and chronic glomerulonephritis; systemic lupus erythematosus; nephrosclerosis; diabetic nephropathy; acute tubular necrosis; renal cortical necrosis; Alport's syndrome; renal transplant rejection.
Deposition disorders	Amyloidosis; leukemic infiltration.
Diffuse nephrocalcinosis	Deposition of calcium salts, primarily in the renal cortex, causes diffuse high echogenicity of this region. If the calcification is predominantly medullary, there is a reversed pattern with the medulla appearing extremely echogenic.
Normal variant	Corticomedullary differentiation is exaggerated in normal kidneys when there is enhanced amplification of echoes due to passage of the sound beam through a medium of low attenuation between the kidney and the transducer (eg, fluid-filled gallbladder, ascites, or cystic mass anterior to the liver).

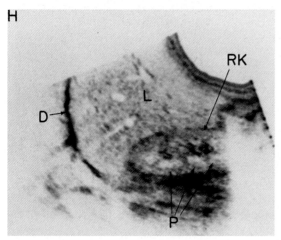

Fig GU 35-1
Chronic renal failure. Parasagittal sonogram of the right kidney (RK) shows that the echogenicity of renal cortical tissue has increased to such an extent that it is now greater than that of the hepatic parenchyma (L). The renal medullary pyramids (P) are clearly visible in the right kidney. (D, diaphragm; H, head.)[2]

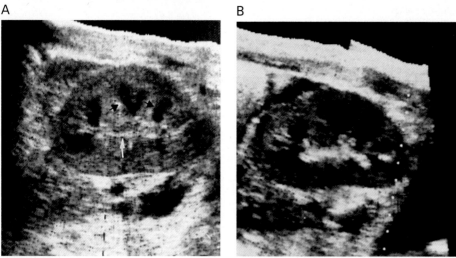

Fig GU 35-2
Renal transplant rejection. (A) Sagittal supine sonogram shows enlargement of the renal transplant with increased sonolucency of the medullary pyramids (black arrows) and thinning of the central echogenic hilar structures (white arrow). (B) Another patient with markedly dilated medullary pyramids of an enlarged renal allograft.[40]

---

*Pattern: Exaggeration of the normal separation between cortex and medulla. Increased renal parenchymal echogenicity correlates with the degree of interstitial (not glomerular) change and the deposition of collagen or calcium.

Focal or Diffuse Distortion of Normal Renal Anatomy and Elimination of Corticomedullary Definition

Condition	Comments
Focal acute bacterial nephritis (lobar nephronia) (Fig GU 36-1)	Inflammatory infiltrate appears as a renal mass displacing adjacent calyces. It is more lucent than renal cortical tissue and may be difficult to differentiate from an abscess. Unlike an abscess, focal acute bacterial nephritis does not have accentuation of the far wall, does not contain shifting debris, and lacks a sharp or rounded contour. After appropriate antibiotic therapy, there is rapid resolution of the process (an abscess cavity tends to persist).
Chronic atrophic pyelonephritis (Fig GU 36-2)	Focal increase in echoes (representing parenchymal scarring) in the involved area of the cortex and medulla.
Healing renal infarct	Focal increase in echoes (representing parenchymal scarring) in the involved area of the cortex and medulla.
Infantile polycystic kidney disease	Generalized increase in parenchymal echoes with loss of corticomedullary definition (can even be diagnosed in utero by means of these criteria).

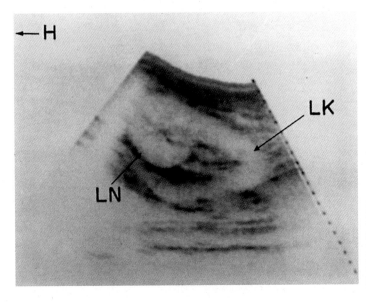

Fig GU 36-1
Focal acute bacterial nephritis. Prone parasagittal sonogram of the left kidney (LK) demonstrates acute focal bacterial nephritis (LN) as focal prominence of the renal parenchyma with poor definition of medullary pyramids in the upper pole. (H, head.)[2]

Condition	Comments
Congenital hepatic fibrosis with tubular ectasia	Nephromegaly with generalized increase in parenchymal echoes and loss of corticomedullary definition. Usually associated with high-level echoes in the liver representing hepatic fibrosis.
End-stage renal disease (Figs GU 36-3 and GU 36-4)	Some renal parenchymal disorders originally classified as type I can occur as type II abnormalities late in the course of the disease when the kidney is small and demonstrates high-intensity echoes throughout its substance (making differentiation between cortex and medulla no longer possible).

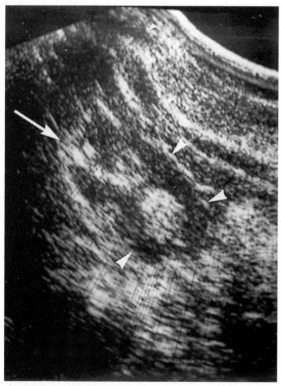

Fig GU 36-2
Chronic atrophic pyelonephritis. Prone sonogram of the kidney (arrowheads) shows a focal loss of renal parenchyma and extension of the calyces peripherally from the renal sinus to the renal margin. Note the associated focal area of increased echogenicity due to fibrosis (arrow) in the upper pole.[12]

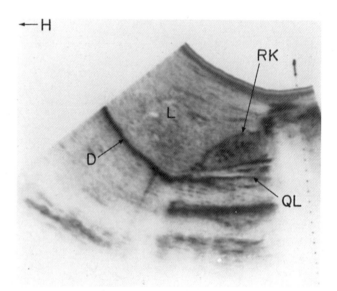

Fig GU 36-3
Renal failure due to chronic glomerulonephritis. Parasagittal sonogram demonstrates a tiny right kidney (RK) with marked thinning of the renal parenchyma. The echogenicity of the renal tissue greatly exceeds that of the adjacent liver (L). The medullary pyramids are no longer distinguishable. Scans of the left kidney showed similar findings. (D, diaphragm; H, head; QL, quadratus lumborum muscle.)[2]

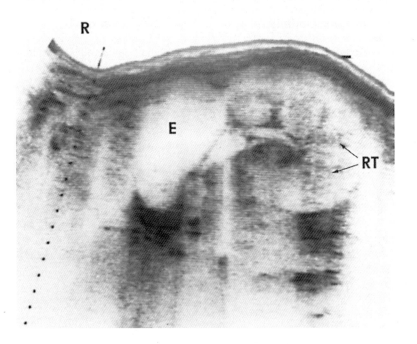

Fig GU 36-4
Renal transplant rejection. Transverse sonogram shows that the renal transplant (RT) has become huge and has lost its corticomedullary definition. The renal vascular pedicle is compressed as it enters the renal hilum. An effusion (E), sometimes seen with acute transplant rejection, is noted medial to the kidney (R, right.).[2]

Fluid Collections Around the Transplanted Kidney

Condition	Imaging Findings	Comments
Lymphocele (Fig GU 37-1)	Well-defined cystic area that often contains numerous internal septations.	Localized accumulation of lymph in the extraperitoneal space that occurs either as a result of interruption of the recipient's lymphatics or secondary to leakage of lymph from the surface of the transplanted kidney. Lymphocele is the most common type of extraurinary fluid collection, seen in 1% to 15% of renal transplant patients. Generally a late complication in patients who have had a prior episode of graft rejection.
Urinoma (Fig GU 37-2)	Purely cystic extraurinary fluid collection. Often accompanied by hydronephrosis secondary to compression of the ureter. Rarely contains internal septations.	Early post-transplant complication that develops because of extravasation from the collecting system. The urinary leak may result from poor surgical technique at the ureteroneocystostomy site or ureteral necrosis due to a compromised blood supply, or it may be a manifestation of ureteral graft rejection. Radionuclide demonstration of a urinary leak confirms the diagnosis.
Abscess (Fig GU 37-3)	Complex mass that typically contains numerous internal echoes (caused by septa and debris) and has relatively poorly defined borders (inflammation and edema around the lesion). Debris in an abscess may shift with changes in patient position.	Early complication that produces unexplained postoperative fever. Increased isotope uptake on ^{67}Ga scintigraphy confirms the presence of an abscess, though a false-positive scan may be produced by wound healing or rejection.

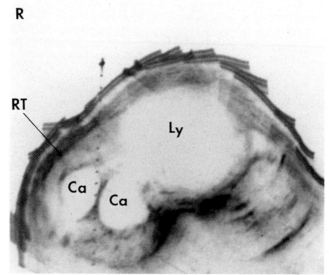

Fig GU 37-1
Lymphocele. Transverse sonogram of the right iliac fossa shows a large lymphocele (Ly) obstructing the transplanted kidney (RT) and causing gross dilatation of the calyces (Ca) and slight thinning of the overlying renal parenchyma. A small amount of ascites is seen adjacent to the lymphocele. (R, right.)[2]

Condition	Imaging Findings	Comments
Hematoma (Fig GU 37-4)	Acute hematoma produces a well-defined, hypoechoic or anechoic extraurinary fluid collection. An old hematoma appears as a complex mass containing echogenic and cystic components (may be difficult to distinguish from an abscess).	Small, clinically insignificant hematomas are frequently seen in the immediate postoperative period. A large hematoma may develop because of graft rupture or injury to the vascular pedicle of the transplanted kidney.

A
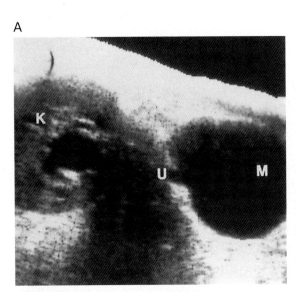

B
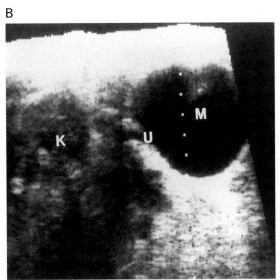

Fig GU 37-2
Urinoma. (A) Sagittal and (B) transverse sonograms show the large sonolucent mass (M) connected by the ureter (U) to the renal transplant (K).[27]

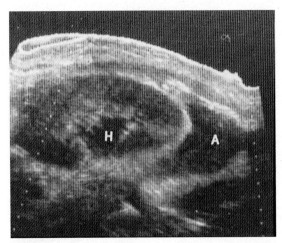

Fig GU 37-3
Abscess. Complex mass with internal echoes (A) adjacent to the transplanted kidney. Note the hydronephrosis (H).

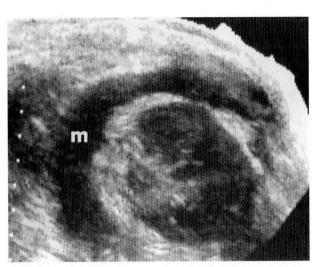

Fig GU 37-4
Hematoma. Hypoechoic fluid collection (m) about the transplanted kidney.

Adrenal Masses on Computed Tomography

Condition	Imaging Findings	Comments
Cushing's syndrome Functioning cortical adenoma (Fig GU 38-1)	Solid mass that may have a low attenuation value due to a high lipid content.	Found in 10% to 15% of patients with Cushing's syndrome. May be impossible to differentiate from adrenal carcinoma (found in approximately 5% of patients with Cushing's syndrome).
Adrenal hyperplasia (Figs GU 38-2 and GU 38-3)	Diffuse, bilateral adrenal enlargement with preservation of shape (may have a nodular component).	Associated CT findings in patients with Cushing's syndrome are an abnormally low attenuation value of the liver resulting from hepatic fat depositionand an increase in retroperitoneal and subcutaneous fat.
Aldosteronoma (Fig GU 38-4)	Contour abnormality (often small). Often contains a large amount of fat that produces a low attenuation value.	Aldosteronomas tend to be much smaller than the large cortical adenomas in patients with Cushing's syndrome. Low-attenuation tumors may be difficult to distinguish from retroperitoneal fat.
Carcinoma (Figs GU 38-5 and GU 38-6)	Often bilateral solid masses that frequently contain low-density areas resulting from necrosis or prior hemorrhage.	Usually grows slowly and can become extremely large before producing symptoms. Because lymphatic and hepatic metastases are common at the time of initial presentation, CT scans at multiple abdominal levels should be performed before a resection is attempted.
Metastases (Figs GU 38-7 through GU 38-9)	Masses of soft-tissue density that vary considerably in size and are frequently bilateral.	Common site of metastatic disease (especially from primary tumors of the lung, breast, thyroid, colon, and melanoma). May appear nonhomogeneous or even cystic if tumor necrosis has occurred.

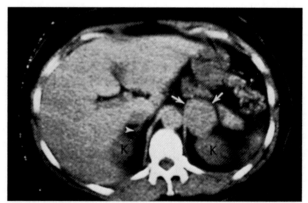

Fig GU 38-1
Cushing syndrome due to functioning cortical adenoma. A 4-cm mass in the left adrenal gland (arrows) is seen posterior to the tail of the pancreas and anterior to the kidney (K). The arrowhead points to the normal right adrenal gland.[30]

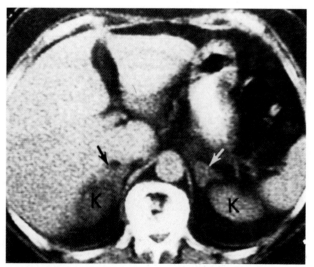

Fig GU 38-2
Cushing syndrome due to adrenal hyperplasia. Although the adrenal glands are enlarged (arrows), their normal configuration is maintained. (K, kidneys.)[30]

Condition	Imaging Findings	Comments
Nonfunctioning adenoma (Figs GU 38-10 and GU 38-11)	Smooth, well-defined mass with low attenuation reflecting its lipid content.	About 30% of adenomas do not contain sufficient lipid to have low attenuation on CT. To make the critical distinction between adenoma and metastasis, delayed scans can be obtained to evaluate the washout of contrast material. Loss of 50% of the attenuation value of the adrenal mass at delayed CT is specific for an adenoma; less than 50% washout could reflect either a metastasis or an atypical adenoma.

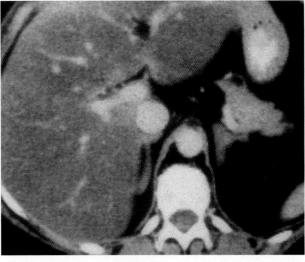

Fig GU 38-3
Cushing's syndrome due to adrenal hyperplasia. There is thickening of the limbs of the left adrenal gland but a normal right adrenal gland. The prominent intra-abndominal fat and hepatic steatosis are typical findings in this disease.[41]

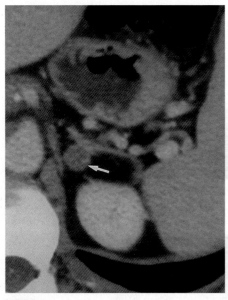

Fig GU 38-4
Aldosteronoma. There is a well-circumscribed left adrenal mass (arrow).[41]

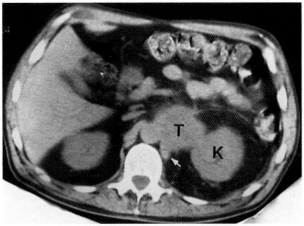

Fig GU 38-5
Adrenal carcinoma. Large soft-tissue tumor (T) invading the anteromedial aspect of the left kidney (K) and left crus of the diaphragm (arrow).[42]

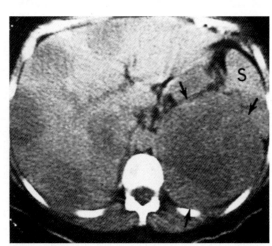

Fig GU 38-6
Adrenal carcinoma causing adrenogenital syndrome. Large mass in the left upper quadrant (arrows) displacing the spleen (S) anteriorly. Multiple round metastases are present in the liver.[43]

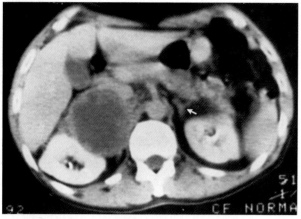

Fig GU 38-7
Metastasis. Huge irregular low-attenuation mass representing an adrenal metastasis from oat cell carcinoma of the lung. The left adrenal gland (arrow) is normal.

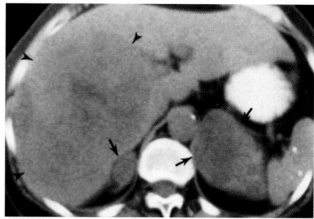

Fig GU 38-8
Metastases. Bilateral adrenal metastases (arrows) in a patient with colonic carcinoma. A large liver metastasis (arrowheads) is also present.[30]

A   B

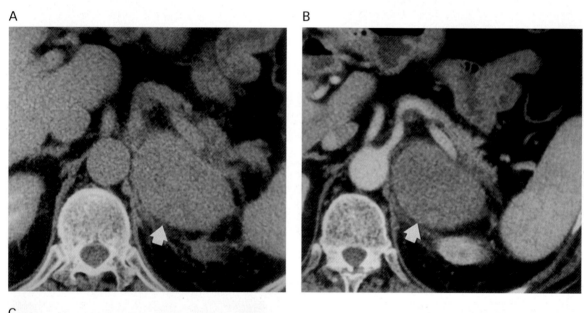

C

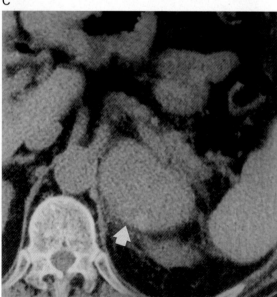

Fig GU 38-9
Metastasis. Typical attenuation and washout pattern of metastasis. (A) Unenhanced scan in a man with lung cancer shows an enlarged left adrenal gland (arrow) with irregular margins and attenuation of 40 HU. (B) On the dynamic enhanced phase image, there is only a minimal increase in attenuation to 53 HU. (C) On the 10-minute delayed image of the left adrenal gland (arrow), there is persistent enhancement (56 HU). The lack of significant washout is consistent with an adrenal metastasis.[41]

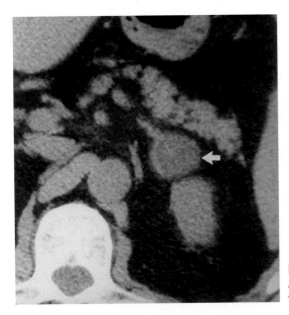

Fig GU 38-10
Adenoma. Smooth, well-defined left adrenal mass (arrow) with typical low attenuation.[41]

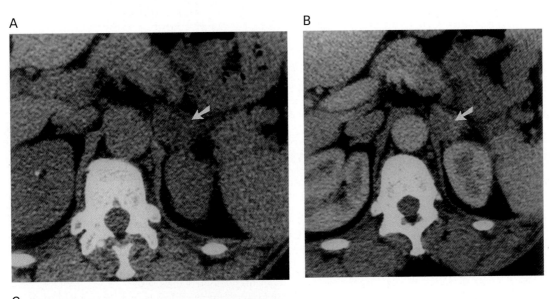

A

B

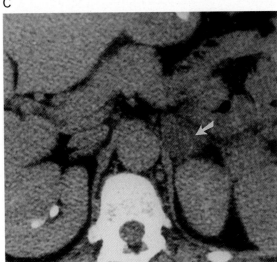

C

Fig GU 38-11
Adenoma. Typical attenuation and washout pattern of adenoma. (A) Unenhanced scan in a woman with a history of breast cancer shows a left adrenal mass (arrow) with an attenuation of 4 HU, consistent with an adenoma. (B) On the dynamic enhanced phase image, the adrenal gland (arrow) enhances vigorously to 54 HU. (C) On the 10-minute delayed image, the attenuation of the left adrenal gland (arrow) is 23 HU (lower than that of the normal right adrenal gland, kidneys, and liver). The greater than 50% washout is diagnostic of an adenoma and confirms the finding on the initial unenhanced scan.[41]

Condition	Imaging Findings	Comments
Myelolipoma/adenolipoma (Fig GU 38-12)	Well-circumscribed mass that has an attenuation value in the range of fat and frequently contains areas of calcification.	Rare tumors that may be indistinguishable from cortical adenomas and aldosteronomas, which also can have low attenuation values as a result of their high fat content.
Pheochromocytoma (Figs GU 38-13 and GU 38-14)	Usually a unilateral (10% are bilateral) adrenal mass of soft-tissue density. May have an attenuation value less than that of liver or renal parenchyma and simulate a thick-walled cystic lesion.	If the adrenal glands are normal despite strong clinical suspicion of a pheochromocytoma, the rest of the abdomen and pelvis should be examined to detect the approximately 10% of tumors that are ectopic. The examination may be expanded to the neck and chest if the abdomen and pelvis are normal.
Neuroblastoma	Soft-tissue or fatty mass that often contains calcification and may have cystic components.	Computed tomography can detect calcification that is not readily apparent on conventional radiography. It also can easily demonstrate hepatic, skeletal, and pulmonary metastases for accurate staging as well as assess the response to treatment and detect recurrent disease.
Lymphoma (Fig GU 38-15)	Often bilateral renal masses.	Non-Hodgkin's lymphoma is the most common subtype. Bilateral in 50% of cases, adrenal lymphoma is usually associated with retroperitoneal adenopathy or other sites of metastases.
Adrenal hemorrhage (Fig GU 38-16)	Increased attenuation if the hemorrhage is acute.	Secondary to trauma (80%), systemic anticoagulant therapy, sepsis, or stress such as surgery.
Adrenal cyst	Rounded, low-density mass. Rim of calcification occurs in approximately 15% of cases.	Most commonly a pseudocyst, which results from degenerative necrosis and hemorrhage into an adrenal mass. Other types of cysts include parasitic, epithelial, and endothelial (lymphangiectatic, angiomatous, and hamartomatous).
Hydatic cyst (Fig GU 38-17)	Variable appearance ranging from purely cystic or solid lesion to a complex cystic mass with septa and intraluminal daughter cyst.	Rare manifestation of disseminated echinococcal disease. The imaging features depend on the stage of evolution of the disease.

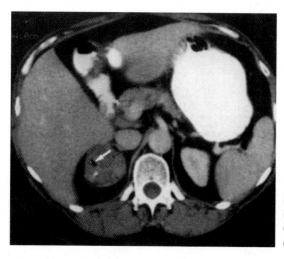

Fig GU 38-12
Myelolipoma. Incidentally discovered right adrenal mass containing a small amount of fat (arrow). Note the calcification within the lesion.[44]

Condition	Imaging Findings	Comments
Lymphangioma (Fig GU 38-18)	Cystic mass with internal septa.	Usually an incidental finding, though symptoms (flank pain, nausea, vomiting) may result from local compression.
Hemangioma (Fig GU 38-19)	Hypoattenuating mass that may contain necrotic areas and phleboliths.	Rare and generally asymptomatic, though a large mass may cause symptoms.

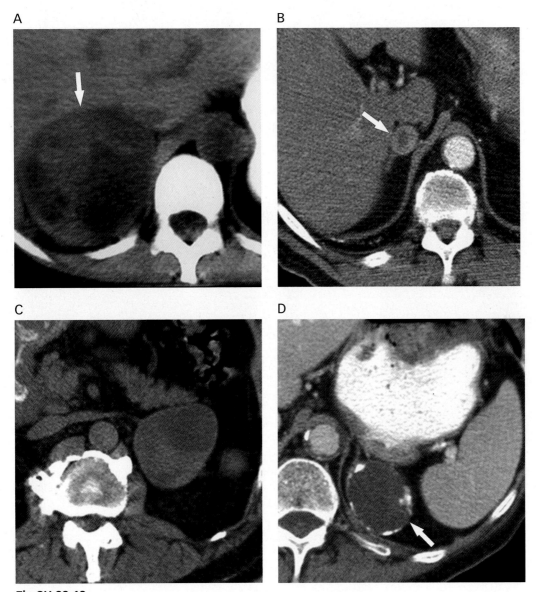

Fig GU 38-13
Pheochromocytoma (spectrum of appearances). (A) Unenhanced scan shows a heterogeneously attenuating mass in the right adrenal gland (arrow). (B) Contrast scan shows a mass in the right adrenal gland (arrow) with peripheral enhancement and a central area of low attenuation due to necrosis. (C) Unenhanced scan shows a mass with cystic and solid components in the left adrenal gland. (D) Contrast scan shows a cystic adrenal lesion with a calcified rim (arrow).[45]

A

B

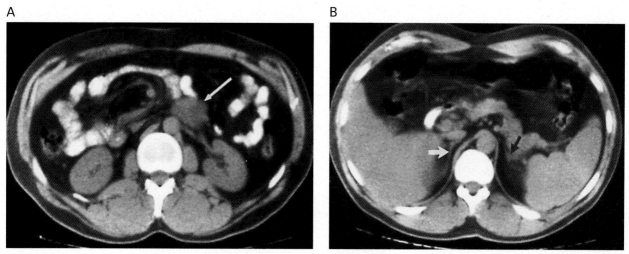

Fig GU 38-14
Ectopic pheochromocytoma. (A) Soft-tissue mass (arrow) adjacent to the aorta and in front of the left renal vein. (B) Scan taken at a higher level demonstrates that both the right and the left adrenal glands are normal (arrows).[46]

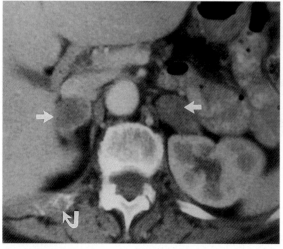

Fig GU 38-15
Lymphoma. Bilateral adrenal masses (straight arrows). Note the destructive lymphomatous lesion involving the right rib (curved arrow).[41]

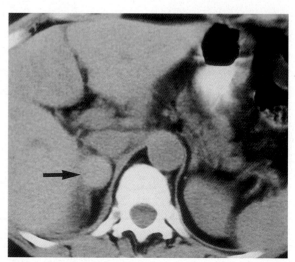

Fig GU 38-16
Hemorrhage. Unenhanced scan obtained two days after motor vehicle accident shows an enlarged right adrenal mass (arrow) with an attenuation value of 53 HU. The mass was not present on CT scans acquired at admission (not shown).[41]

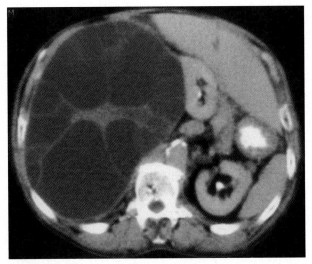

Fig GU 38-17
Hydatid cyst. Large mass filled with daughter cysts that produce a honeycomb appearance.[47]

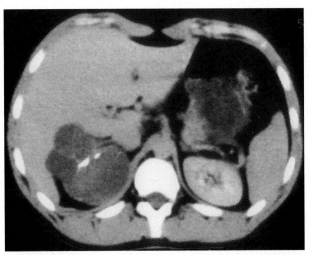

Fig GU 38-18
Lymphangioma. Lobulated cystic mass with calcified septa.[47]

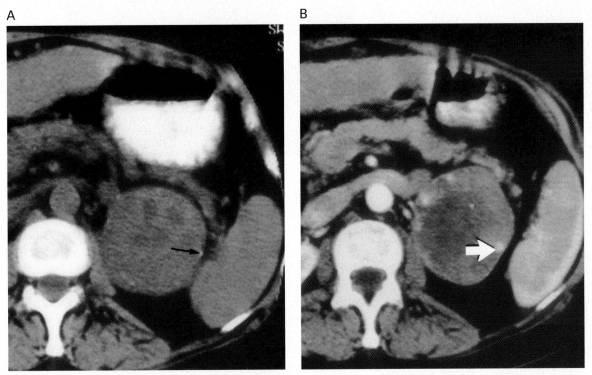

Fig GU 38-19
Hemangioma. Scans (A) before and (B) after contrast injection show a well-circumscribed soft-tissue mass with punctate calcification (arrow in A) and peripheral nodular enhancement (arrow in B).[47]

Adrenal Masses on Magnetic Resonance Imaging

Condition	Imaging Findings	Comments
Adenoma (Figs GU 39-1 and GU 39-2)	Typically either slightly hypointense or isointense relative to the liver on T1-weighted images and slightly hyperintense or isointense to hepatic parenchyma on T2-weighted images.	Hyperfunctioning adrenal adenomas may cause Cushing's syndrome or aldosteronism (Conn syndrome). Nonfunctioning adrenal adenomas are usually detected incidentally and may simulate metastases when they occur in patients with cancer. Chemical shift imaging, which is used to detect lipid within an organ, is the most sensitive method for making the critical differentiation between adenomas and metastases. On out-of-phase images, there is signal drop-off in lipid-containing adenomas, which appear darker than on in-phase images. Conversely, adrenal metastases do not contain lipid and there is no significant signal loss on out-of-phase images.

A
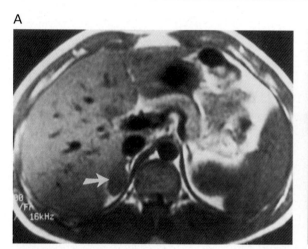
B
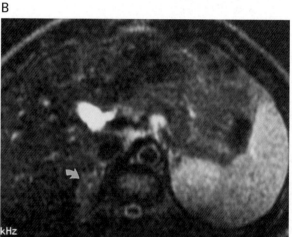

Fig GU 39-1
Adenoma. (A) T1-weighted image (no fat saturation) shows a right adrenal mass (arrow) with a signal intensity similar to that of the liver. (B) T2-weighted image shows that the signal intensity of the mass (arrow) remains similar to that of the liver. This pattern is typical for adrenal adenomas, which tend to be equal to the liver in signal intensity on all pulse sequences.[48]

A
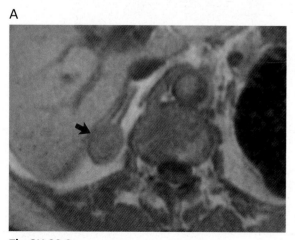
B
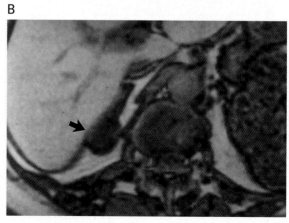

Fig GU 39-2
Chemical shift imaging in adenoma. (A) T1-weighted in-phase image demonstrates a right adrenal mass (arrow) that was previously detected in a woman with breast cancer. (B) On the out-of-phase image, there is a signal drop off in the adrenal gland (arrow), which is diagnostic of an adenoma.[49]

Condition	Imaging Findings	Comments
Adrenal hyperplasia	Signal intensity closely follows that of the normal adrenal gland.	CT is preferable for demonstrating the diffuse bilateral adrenal enlargement with preservation of shape that is characteristic of this disorder.
Carcinoma (Fig GU 39-3)	Large mass that is heterogeneous on both T1- and T2-weighted images due to the presence of internal hemorrhage and necrosis.	Rare tumor that is usually large at the time of diagnosis and can manifest as a hyperfunctioning mass. Multiplanar MR imaging (especially sagittal and coronal projections) is valuable in demonstrating tumor invasion of adjacent organs and direct extension into the inferior vena cava.
Metastases (Figs GU 39-4 and GU 39-5)	Usually bilateral, metastases typically have low signal intensity on T1-weighted images, high signal intensity on T2-weighted images, and show progressive contrast enhancement.	Most common malignant lesions involving the adrenal gland. The most important feature differentiating metastases from adenomas is the lack of signal loss on out-of-phase images.

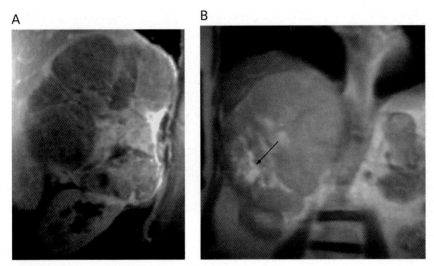

A   B

Fig GU 39-3
Carcinoma. (A) Sagittal T1-weighted and (B) coronal T2-weighted contrast images show a large mass involving the right adrenal gland. The mass exhibits heterogeneous low signal intensity on the T1-weighted image and high signal intensity with a heterogeneous enhancement pattern and areas of necrosis (arrow in B) on the T2-weighted image.[50]

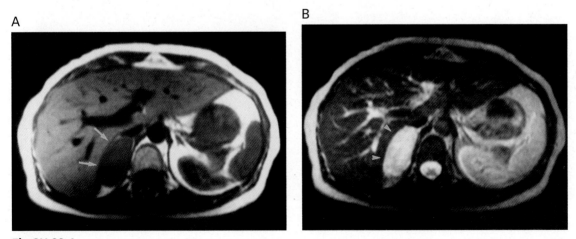

A   B

Fig GU 39-4
Metastasis (breast carcinoma). (A) T1-weighted image (no fat saturation) shows a large right adrenal mass (arrows) that is nondescriptly hypointense relative to the liver. (B) T2-weighted image shows that the lesion (arrowheads) has become hyperintense relative to the liver, conforming with the typical appearance of an adrenal metastasis.[48]

Condition	Imaging Findings	Comments
Pheochromocytoma (Fig GU 39-6)	Characteristically a pronounced increase in signal intensity relative to liver on T2-weighted images.	Multiplanar imaging capability of MR is of value in searching for extra-adrenal pheochromocytomas, which may lie anywhere along the sympathetic chain.
Myelolipoma (Fig GU 39-7)	Fat-containing regions within the tumor have a signal intensity identical to that of subcutaneous and retroperitoneal fat on all pulse sequences.	The appearance of a myelolipoma depends on the relative amount of fat contained within the tumor. If necessary, fat saturation techniques may be performed to prove the fatty nature of the lesion.
Hemorrhage (Figs GU 39-8 and GU 39-9)	Varying appearance that reflects the evolutionary stages of hemorrhage on MR imaging.	May be spontaneous, traumatic, or related to anticoagulation. Neonatal adrenal hemorrhage may be related to the trauma of delivery, septicemia, asphyxia, or abnormal clotting factors.

A   B

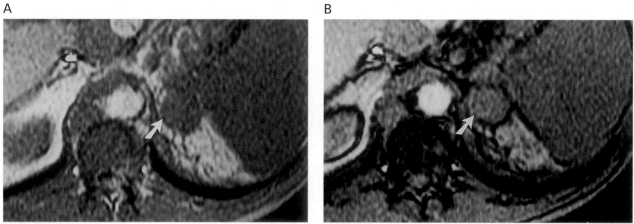

Fig GU 39-5
Chemical shift imaging in metastasis. (A) T1-weighted in-phase image demonstrates a left adrenal mass (arrow) in a man with lung cancer. (B) On the out-of-phase image there is no significant signal loss in the adrenal gland compared with that of the spleen, consistent with a metastasis.[49]

A   B

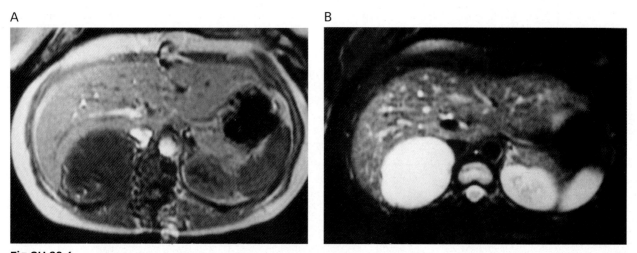

Fig GU 39-6
Pheochromocytoma. (A) T1-weighted GRE image shows a large right adrenal mass that is hypointense relative to the liver. (B) Fat saturation T2-weighted scan shows marked hyperintensity of the adrenal lesion due to the long T2 relaxation time classically reported for pheochromocytomas.[48]

Condition	Imaging Findings	Comments
Cyst (Fig GU 39-10)	Contents have the typical appearance of fluid (hypointense on T1-weighted images and hyperintense on T2-weighted images).	Epithelialized cysts are the most common type of adrenal cystic lesions.
Pseudocyst (Fig GU 39-11)	Complex appearance with septations, blood products, or a soft-tissue component secondary to hemorrhage or hyalinized thrombus.	Representing about 40% of cystic lesions of the adrenal, pseudocysts typically arise after an episode of adrenal hemorrhage and do not have an epithelial lining. They may also result from degenerative necrosis and hemorrhage into an adrenal mass.

A
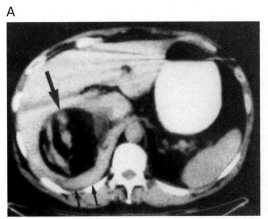
B
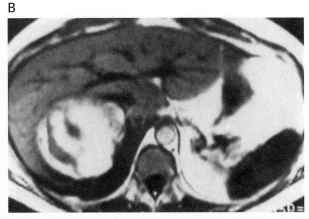

Fig GU 39-7
Myelolipoma. (A) CT scan shows a mass in the right adrenal gland (large arrow) with surrounding hemorrhage (small arrows) that was more predominant on sections obtained at lower levels. (B) T1-weighted image (no fat saturation) at an identical unit shows hyperintense signal corresponding to fat within the lesion. Areas of hemorrhage can be differentiated from fat by comparing the appearances on non–fat saturation and fat saturation images.[48]

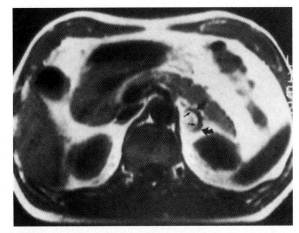

Fig GU 39-8
Subacute hematoma. T1-weighted image (no fat saturation) obtained 6 weeks after a motor vehicle accident shows the concentric rim sign, suggestive of a subacute hematoma. The outer dark rim (large arrows) is thought to be due to hemosiderin deposition; the inner bright ring (small arrows) is thought to represent methemoglobin accumulation. The center of the hemorrhagic adrenal lesion is of intermediate signal intensity. This sign dates the hemorrhage to at least 3 weeks after the inciting incident.[48]

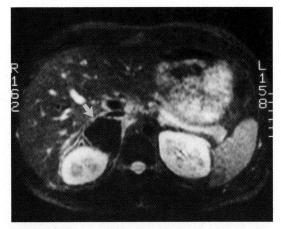

Fig GU 39-9
Chronic hematoma. T2-weighted image with fat saturation shows a uniformly hypointense right adrenal mass (arrow), consistent with hemosiderin deposition.[48]

Condition	Imaging Findings	Comments
Lymphangioma (Fig GU 39-12)	Thin-walled cystic lesion with low signal intensity on T1-weighted images and high signal intensity on T2-weighted images. No substantial internal enhancement.	Rare, asymptomatic lesion similar to lymphangiomas arising elsewhere.
Lymphoma (Fig GU 39-13)	Low signal intensity on T1-weighted images and heterogeneous high signal on T2-weighed images. Minimal progressive contrast enhancement.	Lymphoma (especially non-Hodgkin's) occasionally involves the adrenal gland and in bilateral in 50% of patients.

A
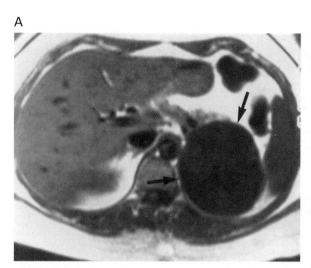

B
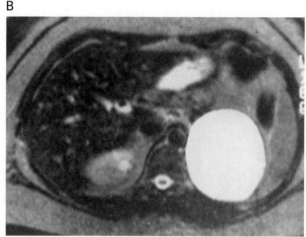

Fig GU 39-10
Cyst. (A) T1-weighted image shows a large left–right adrenal mass (arrows) that is hypointense relative to the liver. (B) T2-weighted image shows that the lesion has a markedly long T2 characteristic of a cyst. The diagnosis was subsequently confirmed by ultrasound.[44]

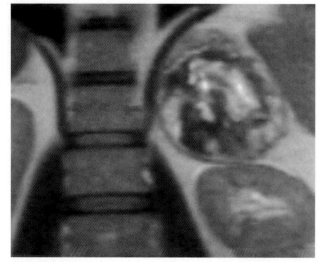

Fig GU 39-11
Pseudocyst. (A) Coronal T2-weighted image shows a left adrenal mass with areas of signal intensity similar to that of blood.[50]

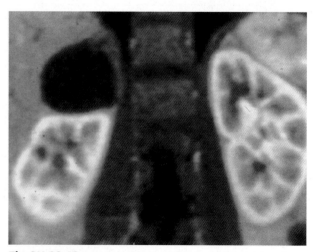

Fig GU 39-12
Lymphangioma. Coronal T1-weighted image shows a typical well-circumscribed area of low signal intensity.[50]

Condition	Imaging Findings	Comments
Neuroblastoma (Fig GU 39-14)	Heterogeneous low signal intensity on T1-weighted images and high signal intensity on T2-weighted images, with evidence of contrast enhancement. Areas of intratumoral hemorrhage typically have high signal intensity on T1-weighted images.	Second most common pediatric abdominal mass (after Wilms' tumor). Neuroblastomas arise from the neural crest in the adrenal medulla or along the sympathetic chain.

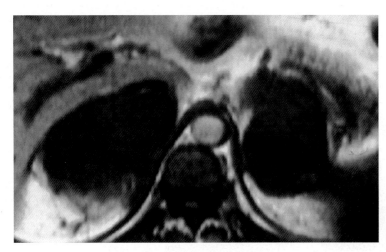

Fig GU 39-13
Lymphoma. Axial T1-weighted image shows bilateral lymphomatous deposits as areas of low signal intensity.[50]

A

B

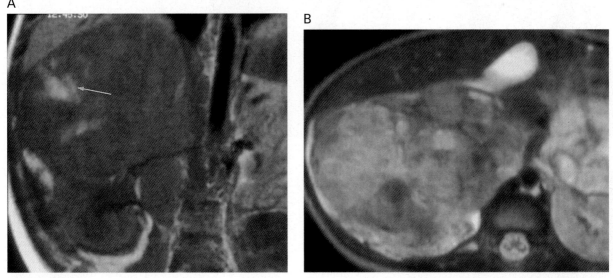

Fig GU 39-14
Neuroblastoma. (A) Coronal T1-weighted image shows a right adrenal tumor that is predominantly hypointense and contains areas of high-signal-intensity hemorrhage (arrow). (B) On the T2-weighted image, the tumor is hyperintense. (Courtesy of Marilyn Siegel, M.D., Mallinckrodt Institute of Radiology, Washington University, St. Louis, MO.)[50]

Bladder Masses on Computed Tomography and Magnetic Resonance Imaging

Condition	Imaging Findings	Comments
Neoplasms		
Transitional cell carcinoma (Figs GU 40-1 and GU 40-2)	Single or multiple polypoid masses that show contrast enhancement. May produce only focal bladder wall thickening or invade the surrounding tissues. Punctate, coarse, or linear calcification (5%) typically encrusts the surface of the mass rather than lying within it. On T1-weighted MR images, urine is dark and the bladder wall and tumor are of intermediate signal intensity. T1-weighted sequences are ideal for detection of extravesical infiltration into high-signal fat. On T2-weighted images, the intermediate-signal tumor contrasts with the high signal intensity of urine and low signal intensity of muscle. These sequences are best for evaluating tumor depth, differentiating tumor from fibrosis, and detecting invasion of surrounding organs and marrow metastases.	Most common urinary tract cancer in the United State and Europe, it occurs most frequently in older men. The underlying cause is direct prolonged contact of the bladder urothelium with urine containing carcinogens, predominantly from cigarette smoking (implicated in up to half the cases). There is also a well-documented link with a variety of occupational and environmental chemicals. Most urothelial tumors are located at the bladder base (80%); 60% are single and more than half measure less than 2.5 cm. They often are multicentric, with synchronous and metachronous tumors of the bladder and the upper urinary tract.

A

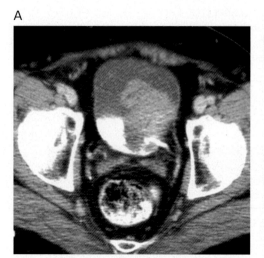

B

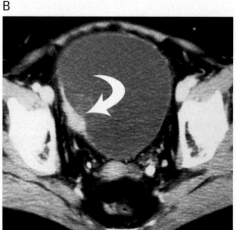

C

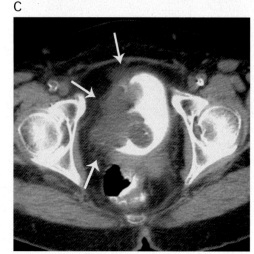

Fig GU 40-1
Transitional cell carcinoma. (A) CT scan shows a large, lobular mass within the bladder. (B) In another patient, the tumor appears as an enhancing area of focal wall thickening (arrow). (C) In a third patient, a large bladder mass is associated with irregular soft-tissue stranding (arrows) from tumor invasion into the perivesical fat.[51]

Condition	Imaging Findings	Comments
Squamous cell carcinoma (Figs GU 40-3 and GU 40-4)	Nonspecific findings of a single enhancing bladder mass or focal or diffuse wall thickening. Muscle invasion is common and extravesical spread may be extensive, involving surrounding organs and the abdominal wall.	Although accounting for less than 5% of bladder neoplasms in the United States, it represents more than half of bladder cancers in parts of the world where schistosomiasis is endemic. Other risk factors include chronic irritation from in-dwelling catheters, bladder calculi, and chronic infection. Paraplegic patients, who may have all these risk factors, are at increased risk.

A

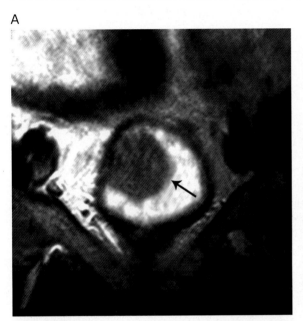

B

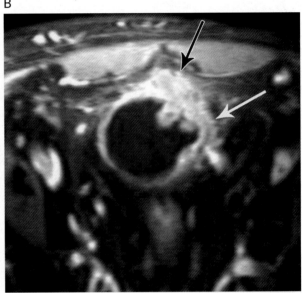

Fig GU 40-2
Transitional cell carcinoma. (A) Coronal T2-weighted MR image shows an intermediate-signal-intensity mass (arrow) within the bright urine-filled bladder. The hyperintense bladder wall is intact. (B) Axial contrast-enhanced T1-weighted image in another patient shows tumor invasion into the perivesical fat (arrows).[51]

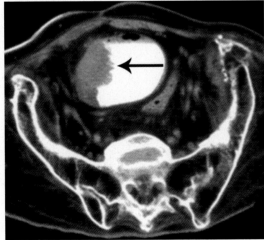

Fig GU 40-3
Squamous cell carcinoma. CT cystogram shows an irregular mass involving the lateral wall of the bladder. Note the loss of trabecular structure in the bones and fatty infiltration of the muscles in this paraplegic patient.[51]

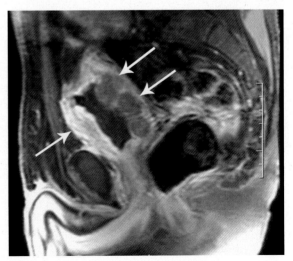

Fig GU 40-4
Squamous cell carcinoma. Sagittal enhanced and fat-suppressed T1-weighted MR image shows thickening of the anterior and posterior walls of the bladder (arrows), which represented chronic inflammatory changes with diffuse invasive malignancy.[51]

Condition	Imaging Findings	Comments
Adenocarcinoma (Fig GU 40-5)	Usually contains solid and cystic (mucin) elements. CT is most sensitive for detecting calcification, which is common and tends to be peripheral.	Uncommon bladder neoplasm (<2%) that is classically associated with bladder exstrophy and a persistent urachus. Other risk factors include chronic mucosal irritation and urinary diversion procedures. Urachal carcinomas are usually located at the dome of the bladder, in or slightly off the midline. Most adenocarcinomas are aggressive lesions that demonstrate early extravesical spread.
Metastases	Various patterns depending on the source of spread.	Most commonly the result of direct invasion from adjacent pelvic neoplasms (colon, prostate, or rectum). Less frequently, bladder metastases may develop from hematogenous or lymphangitic spread of cancers from the stomach, breast, or lung. A late manifestation of cancer, when bladder metastases are detected there is usually evidence of a locally invasive adjacent primary neoplasm or other signs of a distant primary tumor.
Small cell/neuroendocrine tumor (Fig GU 40-6)	Large, polypoid or nodular lesion with patchy contrast enhancement that may have an ulcerated surface and most often involves the lateral walls of the bladder. Central necrosis and cystic change may be seen.	Rare, highly aggressive tumors that are frequently associated with a history of cigarette smoking. CT may demonstrate local invasion, lymphadenopathy, and diffuse peritoneal metastases.

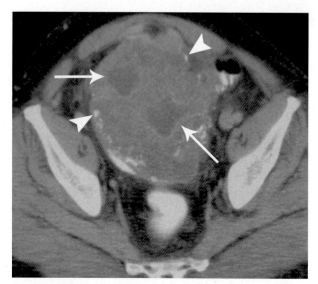

Fig GU 40-5
Urachal adenocarcinoma. CT scan shows a large, predominantly solid, midline mass with peripheral calcifications (arrowheads). Within the mass are scattered low-attenuation areas (arrows), which represent mucin.[51]

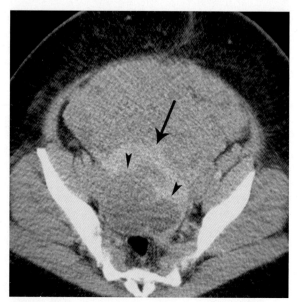

Fig GU 40-6
Small cell carcinoma. CT scan shows a large soft-tissue mass that fills the pelvis and surrounds the uterus (arrows). Note the scalloping of the posterior uterine wall (arrowheads).[51]

Condition	Imaging Findings	Comments
Other tumors (Fig GU 40-7)	Various appearances.	Leiomyoma, leiomyosacroma, carcinoid, rhabdomyosarcoma, neurofibroma, paragangioma, and lymphoma.
Non-neoplastic masses Inflammatory pseudotumor (pseudosarcomatous fibromyxoid tumor) (Fig GU 40-8)	Single mass that may be exophytic or polypoid and ulcerated. Intramural solid and cystic variants also occur. On T2-weighted MR images, the lesion may be heterogeneous, with a central hyperintense component (necrotic tissue) surrounded by a low-signal-intensity periphery. Ring-like enhancement is often seen on both CT and MRI.	Non-neoplastic proliferation of spindle and inflammatory cells with myxoid components that may be locally aggressive and mimic malignancy clinically and on imaging studies.
Endometriosis (Fig GU 40-9)	Nonspecific bladder filling defect typically located posteriorly. MRI generally shows hemorrhagic foci with high signal intensity (representing blood) on T1-weighted images. Homogeneous or peripheral enhancement.	Although the urinary tract is not usually involved with endometriosis, the bladder is the most commonly affected site. Cyclic hematuria is highly suggestive of the diagnosis, but occurs in only 20% of cases.
Malacoplakia (Fig GU 40-10)	Various patterns of single or multiple lesions (polypoid, vascular, or solid) or circumferential wall thickening, associated with vesicoureteric reflux and dilatation of the upper urinary tract.	The bladder is the part of the urinary tract most frequently affected by this rare chronic granulomatous condition. Occurring primarily in women, it is more common in diabetic or immune-compromised individuals. At times, malacoplakia may be extremely aggressive, invading the perivesical space and even causing bone destruction.

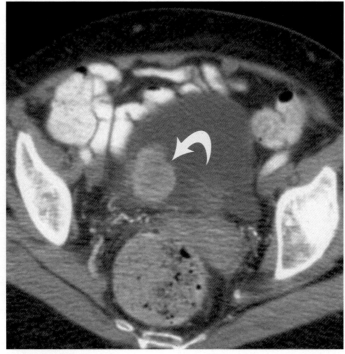

Fig GU 40-7
Carcinoid. Contrast CT demonstrates a nonspecific solid, polypoid, enhancing mass (arrow) in the bladder.[51]

Condition	Imaging Findings	Comments
Cystitis cystica/ cystitis glandularis	Hypervascular polypoid mass. On T2-weighted MR images, the lesion has predominantly low signal intensity with a central branching high signal pattern that shows the most contrast enhancement.	Common chronic reactive inflammatory disorders that occur in the setting of chronic irritation. Cystitis glandularis also develops in association with pelvic lipomatosis and bladder exstrophy. Unlike in transitional cell carcinoma, the muscle layer remains intact.

A
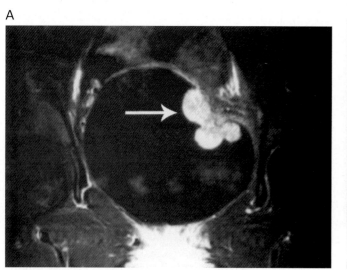

B
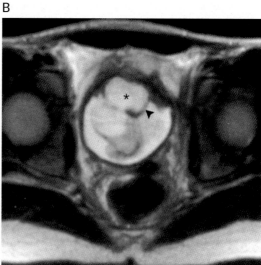

Fig GU 40-8
Inflammatory pseudotumor. (A) Coronal fat-suppressed T1-weighted MR image shows a polypoid mass projecting into the bladder lumen (arrows). Axial T2-weighted image in another patient shows a lobulated polypoid mass arising from the anterior wall of the bladder. Note the central hyperintensity (*) and low peripheral signal intensity (arrowhead).[52]

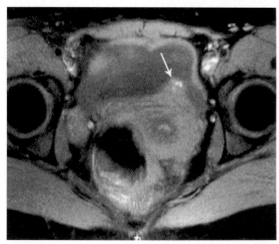

Fig GU 40-9
Endometriosis. Fat-suppressed T1-weighted MR image shows high-signal-intensity foci (arrow) within a soft-tissue mass in the vesicouterine space, projecting into the bladder lumen posteriorly.[52]

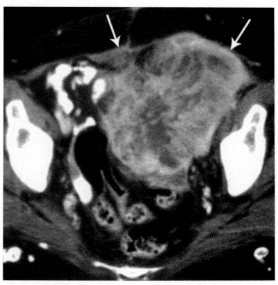

Fig GU 40-10
Malacoplakia. Contrast CT scan through the upper pelvis shows a large, irregularly enhancing mass (arrows) that is contiguous with the bladder.[52]

Condition	Imaging Findings	Comments
Schistosomiasis (Fig GU 40-11)	Fibrotic, thick-walled bladder with typical curvilinear calcifications.	Uncommon in the United States, infestation with this parasite is a major health problem in developing parts of the world and may be seen in immigrants, especially from Africa. The characteristic calcification in chronic disease represents large numbers of calcified eggs within the bladder wall.
Crohn's disease (Fig GU 40-12)	CT shows gas within the bladder, focal irregularity of the wall (most commonly on the right), and tethering of thickened adjacent bowel.	The most frequent cause of fistulization between inflamed small and large bowel and the bladder. The presence of oral contrast in the bladder is diagnostic of a fistula between the bowel and bladder. Other signs of pelvic Crohn's disease may include fibrofatty proliferation, infiltration of fat, phlegmon, and lymphadenopathy.
Diverticulitis (Fig GU 40-13)	CT shows thickening of the bladder wall with gas in the bladder lumen, as well as an adjacent inflamed colon with diverticula and pericolonic fat stranding.	Cystitis and colovesical fistulas (typically involving the left wall of the bladder) are relatively common complications of diverticulitis.
Radiation and chemotherapy cystitis (Figs GU 40-14 and GU 40-15)	Focal or diffuse irregular thickening of the bladder wall in acute cystitis. In chronic disease, the small fibrosed bladder has a thick wall and there is usually resultant hydronephrosis.	Severe hemorrhagic cystitis may develop after chemotherapy or irradiation of the bladder. This may be complicated by fistula formation, which may appear clinically as pneumaturia or fecaluria and on imaging studies as gas within the bladder.

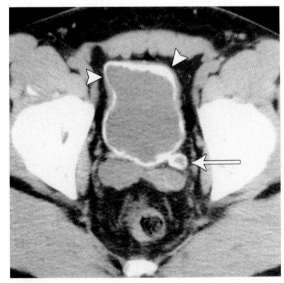

Fig GU 40-11
Schistosomiasis. CT scan demonstrates curvilinear calcification in the bladder wall (arrowheads), which also extends to the distal left ureter (arrow).[52]

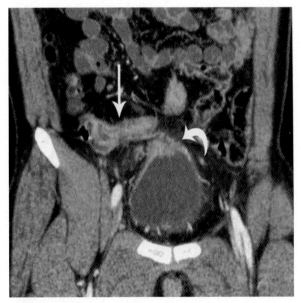

Fig GU 40-12
Crohn's disease. Contrast coronal CT reformation shows thickening of the wall of the distal small bowel (straight arrow) and the adjacent bladder (curved arrow). A small bowel series (not shown) showed a fistula connecting the abnormal segment of ileum to the bladder.[52]

Condition	Imaging Findings	Comments
Extrinsic masses (Figs GU 40-16 and GU 40-17)	Various patterns depending on the specific underlying cause.	Extrinsic masses protruding into the bladder may mimic an intravesical mass. These include masses of prostatic, uterine, or ovarian origin, extramedullary hematopoiesis; urachal cyst or tumor, paraganglionic tissue, hamartoma, amyloidosis, and vascular malformations.

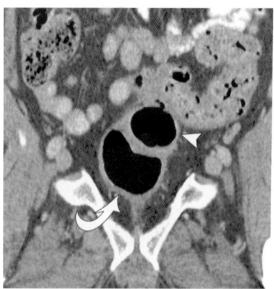

Fig GU 40-13
Diverticulitis. Coronal CT reformation shows a thick-walled, gas-filled abscess (arrowhead) immediately adjacent to the bladder. There is diffuse thickening of the bladder wall (arrow).[52]

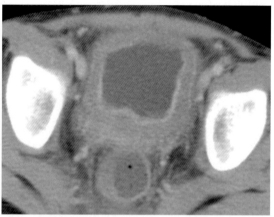

Fig GU 40-14
Chemotherapy cystitis. CT scan shows marked thickening and increased mucosal enhancement of the bladder after cyclophosphamide therapy following bone marrow transplantation in a child with acute lymphoblastic leukemia.[53]

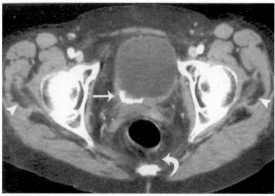

Fig GU 40-15
Radiation cystitis (chronic). CT scan shows focal thickening and calcification of the right wall of the bladder (straight arrow). There is subtle widening of the presacral space (curved arrow) and fatty infiltration of the pelvic musculature (arrowheads).[52]

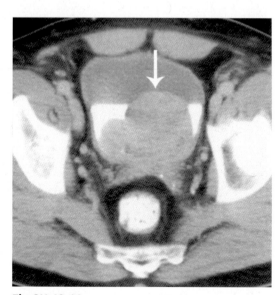

Fig GU 40-16
Benign prostatic hypertrophy. CT scan shows a large, smooth, lobular mass bulging into the base of the bladder (arrow). Despite its large size, this "mass" proved to be benign hypertrophy of the prostate.[52]

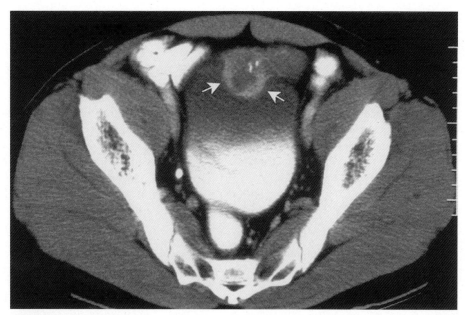

Fig GU 40-17
Urahcal adenocarcinoma. CY shows a cystic mass (arrows) at the anterior dome of the bladder.[54]

Urethral Disease

Condition	Imaging Findings	Comments
Trauma Blunt (Figs GU 41-1 and GU 41-2)	Various patterns of extravasation of contrast material. In type I injury, the posterior urethra is stretched, but the continuity of the urethra is maintained.	Posterior urethral injury is usually caused by a crushing force to the pelvis (eg, high-speed automobile accident) and is associated with pelvic fractures. Anterior urethral injury generally results from a straddle pelvic injury and is most often isolated. When there is blood in the meatus, which is present in about half of significant urethral injuries, retrograde urethrography should be performed immediately to assess for urethral injury.
Penetrating (Fig GU 41-3)	Extravasation of contrast material at the site of injury.	Usually secondary to gunshot or knife wounds, or from the insertion of a foreign body into the external meatus.
"Penile fracture" (Fig GU 41-4)	Extravasation of contrast material in the penile urethra adjacent to the site of a corpus cavernosal injury.	Rupture of the corpus cavernosa from trauma to the erect penis. An uncommon injury, it generally occurs during strenuous sexual activity. Fluoroscopic observation after contrast injection into the corpora cavernosum may show the exact site of a tunica albuginea tear, which may not be evident at surgery.
Postirradiation	Narrowing or fistulization	Urethritis, urethral stricture, and urethral fistula may develop following radiation therapy.

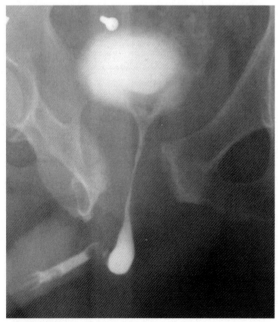

Fig GU 41-1
Blunt trauma. Stretching of the posterior urethra with diatasis of the pubic symphysis.[55]

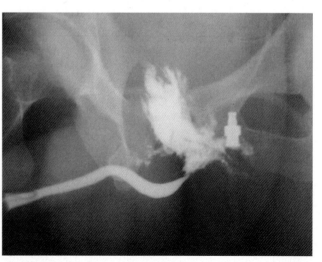

Fig GU 41-2
Blunt trauma. Extensive extravasation of contrast material without flow into the prostatic urethra or bladder due to complete rupture of the posterior urethra. A fracture of the right pubic ramus was diagnosed.[55]

Condition	Imaging Findings	Comments
Postsurgery	Extravasation of contrast material at the bulbous urethra and bulbomembranous junction.	Urethral injury and disruption is a complication of simultaneous kidney–pancreas transplantation with bladder drainage in male patients. The underlying cause is thought to be activated proteolytic exocrine enzymes from the transplanted pancreas.
Acquired inflammatory disease		
Gonococcal and other urethritis (Figs GU 41-5 and GU 41-6)	Irregular narrowing (stricture) or extensive extravasation (fistula). For suspected periurethral abscess, ultrasound can demonstrate its presence and CT or MRI are of value in assessing its extent and complications such as fasciitis and Fournier gangrene.	Gonorrheal infection remains the leading reportable sexually transmitted disease in adults in the United States, though nongonococcal urethritis (especially *Chlamydia*) is increasing in frequency. The diagnosis of acute infection is usually made on the basis of clinical and laboratory findings, and imaging studies are not necessary for uncomplicated urethritis. Serious complications requiring imaging include urethral stricture, periurethral abscess, and periurethral fistula.
Condyloma accuminata (Fig GU 41-7)	Multiple papillary filling defects in the anterior urethra.	Soft, sessile, squamous papillomas on the penile glands and shaft caused by viral infection. Also known as "venereal warts," in up to 5% of male patients they may extend to the prostatic urethra and bladder. The diagnostic procedure of choice is voiding cystourethrography, because retrograde urethrography may result in retrograde seeding.
Tuberculosis	Anterior urethral stricture associated with multiple fistulas.	Rare urinary tract manifestation of tuberculosis. Genital disease is a descending infection, and renal tuberculosis is usually evident. Rupture of a prostatic abscess into surrounding structures may lead to the development of fistulas to the urethra.

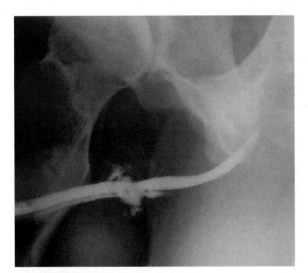

Fig GU 41-3
Penetrating injury. Extravasation of contrast material from the penile urethra following a gunshot wound.[55]

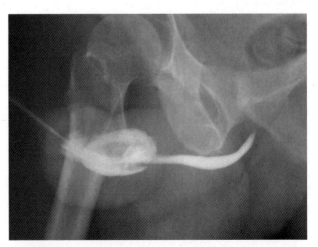

Fig GU 41-4
Penile fracture. Extravasation of contrast material in the penile urethra adjacent to the site of a corpus cavernosal injury.[55]

Condition	Imaging Findings	Comments
Diverticula (Fig GU 41-8)	Variety of shapes and configurations, a neck that can be wide or narrow, and either communicating or not communicating with the urethra.	Occurring in about 1.5% of women, they are thought to be acquired secondary to rupture of dilated and infected periurethral glands. Another common cause is disruption of the periurethral fascia during bladder neck suspension surgery for stress incontinence, which results in focal posterior urethral prolapse. MRI is more sensitive than voiding cystourethrography for detecting urethral diverticula.
Calculi (Fig GU 41-9)	Rounded filling defects in the urethra. Calcified stones may be detectable on a preprocedure scout film of the lower abdomen.	Most urethral calculi are small stones expelled from the bladder during voiding. A stone occasionally may be large enough to lodge at a point of urethral narrowing, such as the membranous urethra. Primary stone formation may rarely occur in the presence of a urethral stricture or diverticulum.
Tumors (Figs GU 41-10 and GU 41-11)	Intraluminal mass or irregular narrowing. Fistula formation may complicate malignant disease.	Both benign and malignant urethral tumors are infrequent in women and rare in men.

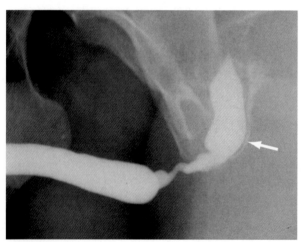

Fig GU 41-5
Gonococcal urethral stricture. Irregular, beaded narrowing of a segment of the distal bulbous urethra with opacification of the left Cowper duct (arrow).

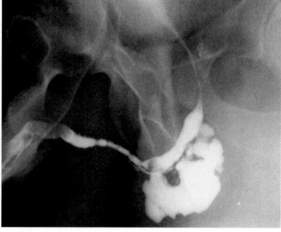

Fig GU 41-6
Gonococcal urethral stricture with periurethral abscess. Long segment of irregular, beaded narrowing in the bulbous urethra with opacification of the Littré glands (arrow). Note the irregular periurethral cavity originating from the ventral aspect of the bulbous urethra.[55]

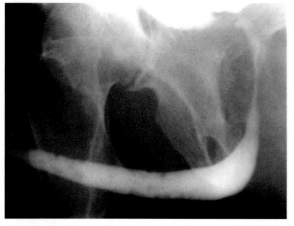

Fig GU 41-7
Condyloma acuminata. Multiple small filling defects in the anterior urethra.[55]

A

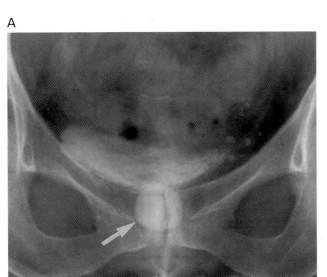

B

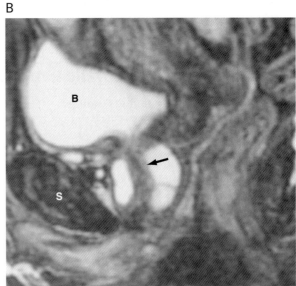

Fig GU 41-8
Urethral diverticulum. (A) Postvoiding image obtained during excretory urography demonstrates a contrast-filled urethral diverticulum (arrow). (B) T2-weighted MR image shows a large diverticulum surrounding the urethra (arrow), with a septum that results in an impression at the bladder base (female prostate sign). B, bladder; S, pubic symphysis.[55]

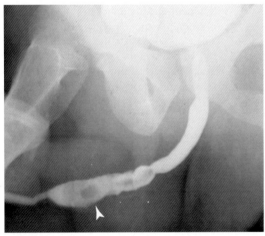

Fig GU 41-9
Calculi associated with urethral stricture. The stones (arrowhead) lie in a segment of an anterior urethral stricture.[55]

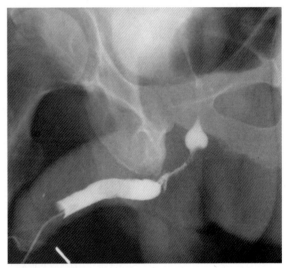

Fig GU 41-10
Squamous cell carcinoma. Irregular stricture of the bulbous urethra.[55]

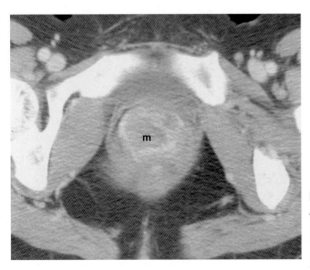

Fig GU 41-11
Adenocarcinoma of the urethra. Contrast CT scan in a woman with previous hysterectomy shows an inhomogeneous soft-tissue mass of the urethra (m) representing a high-grade tumor.[55]

Cystic Retroperitoneal Mass

Condition	Imaging Findings	Comments
Non-neoplastic cysts		
Pancreatic pseudocyst (Fig GU 42-1)	Round or oval fluid collection with a thin or thick wall.	Although most often peripancreatic, encapsulated collections of pancreatic fluid can be seen in ectopic locations in the abdomen, mediastinum, or pelvis. The diagnosis is suggested when other signs of acute pancreatitis are present.
Nonpancreatic pseudocyst	Unilocular or multilocular fluid-filled mass with a thick wall.	Rare lesion that has a thick fibrous wall and contains hemorrhage, pus, or serous fluid. Unlike a pancreatic pseudocyst, it is not associated with high levels of amylase or lipase in the cystic fluid.
Lymphocele (Fig GU 42-2)	Low-attenuation mass. A negative attenuation value due to fat within the fluid is rare but strongly suggestive of this diagnosis.	Fluid-filled cyst without an epithelial lining that occurs in up to 25% of patients following radical retroperitoneal lymphadenectomy. It also may develop after renal transplant surgery. Retroperitoneal lymphoceles may cause venous obstruction with subsequent edema and thromboembolic complications.
Urinoma (Fig GU 42-3)	Fluid collection with water attenuation. After contrast administration, the attenuation can increase progressively as contrast-enhanced urine enters the urinoma.	Encapsulated collection of chronically extravasated urine. Although typically in the perirenal space, they may be seen in other locations, possibly due to disruption of a more inferior part of the ureter. Urinary extravasation may be secondary to obstruction or to such nonobstructive causes as abdominal trauma and injury to the collecting system during surgery or diagnostic instrumentation.
Hematoma (Fig GU 42-4)	The appearance depends on the time that has elapsed since the traumatic event. Acute or subacute blood has a higher attenuation than does pure fluid due to clot formation. A chronic hematoma has decreased attenuation because of the breakdown of blood products.	Retroperitoneal hematomas may be associated with trauma, ruptured abdominal aortic aneurysm, anticoagulant therapy, or blood dyscrasia.

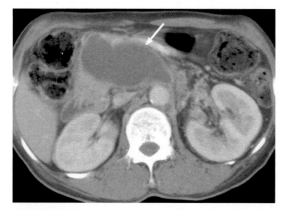

Fig GU 42-1
Pancreatic pseudocyst. Thin-walled fluid collection in the anterior pararenal space (arrow).[56]

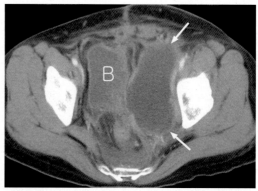

Fig GU 42-2
Lymphocele. Hypoattenuating cystic mass located in the obturator space (arrows) and compressing the urinary bladder (B) in this woman who three months previously had undergone a radical hysterectomy for cervical cancer.[56]

Condition	Imaging Findings	Comments
Neoplastic		
Cystic lymphangioma (Fig GU 42-5)	Large, thin-walled multiseptate cystic mass. The attenuation varies from fluid to fat.	Congenital benign tumor due to failure of the developing lymphatic tissue to establish normal communication with the remainder of the lymphatic system. They are unusual in the retroperitoneum, with most occurring in the head or neck.
Lymphangioleiomyoma (Fig GU 42-6)	Large, thin- or thick-walled multiseptate cystic mass containing low-attenuation material.	Found almost exclusively in premenopausal women, it results from the proliferation of smooth muscle cells in lymphatic vessels that causes obstructive changes and cystic collections of chylous material. The lesion is similar to cystic lymphangioma, though this process consists of endothelium-lined spaces without muscle cells.

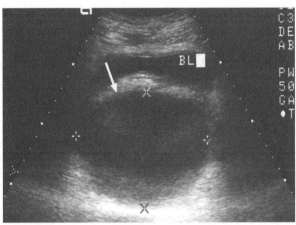

Fig GU 42-3
Urinoma. Large fluid collection with ring enhancement in the presarcal space (arrow) in a woman who had undergone radical hysterectomy for cervical cancer.[56]

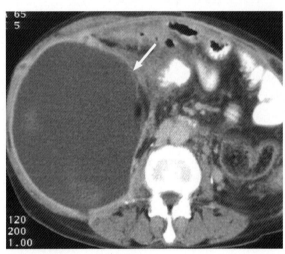

Fig GU 42-4
Hematoma. Huge cystic mass with thin walls in the right retroperitoneal space (arrow).[56]

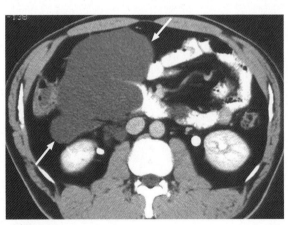

Fig GU 42-5
Cystic lymphangioma. Lobulated cystic mass in the anterior pararenal space. The third portion of the duodenum is compressed by the mass.[56]

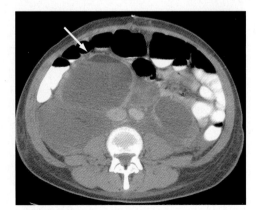

Fig GU 42-6
Lymphangioleiomyoma. Large cystic retroperitoneal masses fill the lower abdomen. Note the fat-fluid level (arrow).[57]

Condition	Imaging Findings	Comments
Mucinous cystadenoma (Fig GU 42-7)	Homogeneous unilocular cystic mass.	Early diagnosis of this rare lesion is important because of its malignant potential.
Cystic teratoma (Fig GU 42-8)	Complex mass containing a well-circumscribed fluid component, adipose tissue, and calcification.	Most commonly diagnosed in asymptomatic newborn females or young girls, these cystic tumors are composed of well-differentiated derivations from at least two of the three germ layers (ectoderm, mesoderm, endoderm). Cystic teratomas are likely benign; solid teratomas are more often malignant.
Cystic mesothelioma	Nonspecific, thin-walled, multilocular cystic lesion.	Rare benign neoplasm of mesothelial origin that usually occurs in the serous surface lining of the pelvic viscera but may develop in the retroperitoneum. Unlike malignant mesothelioma, cystic mesothelioma is not related to prior asbestos exposure.
Mullerian cyst (Fig GU 42-9)	Unilocular or multilocular thin-walled cyst containing clear fluid.	Extremely rare urogenital cyst that typically occurs in women during the child-bearing age.
Epidermoid cyst (Fig GU 42-10)	Unilocular, thin-walled cystic mass with fluid attenuation.	Rare, congenital, usually asymptomatic lesion arising in the presacral region, usually in middle-aged women.
Tailgut cyst (Fig GU 42-11)	Multicystic lesion with an attenuation value varying from water to soft tissue.	Rare, congenital lesion that arises from vestiges of the embryonic hindgut and occurs between the rectum and sacrum. It is more common in women and usually appears in middle age. Malignant degeneration can cause loss of discrete margins and involvement of contiguous structures.

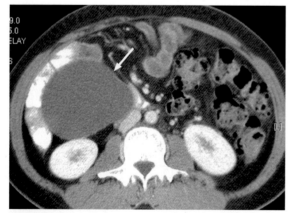

Fig GU 42-7
Mucinous cystadenoma. Large mass of homogeneously low attenuation in the right anterior pararenal space (arrow).[56]

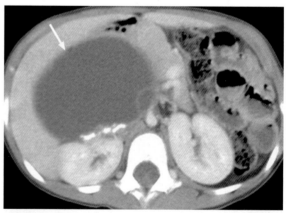

Fig GU 42-8
Cystic teratoma. Well-defined hypoattenuating mass with internal septa and calcifications in the right anterior pararenal space (arrow).[56]

Condition	Imaging Findings	Comments
Bronchogenic cyst	Rounded, well-circumscribed, low-attenuation cyst. It can be misdiagnosed as a solid mass if it appears hyperattenuating due to the protein contents of the lesion.	Although most occur in the mediastinum, they may rarely be found in a retroperitoneal location.
Cystic change in solid neoplasm (Fig GU 42-12)	Cystic mass with an irregular wall or a soft-tissue mass with a central area of low attenuation. Rarely, there may be internal hemorrhage with subsequent liquefaction and formation of a fibrous capsule, presenting an appearance that mimics a cystic mass.	Paragangioma, neurogenic tumor.

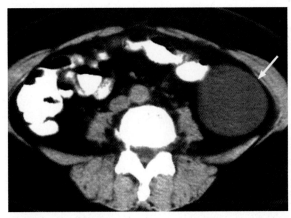

Fig GU 42-9
Mullerian cyst. Well-defined cystic mass in the left retroperitoneal space (arrow).[56]

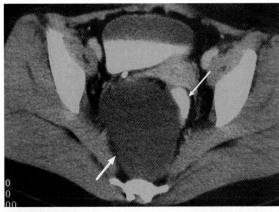

Fig GU 42-10
Epidermoid cyst. Well-defined hypoatttenuating mass in the pelvic retroperitoneum (thick arrow). There is anterior displacement of the rectum (thin arrow).[56]

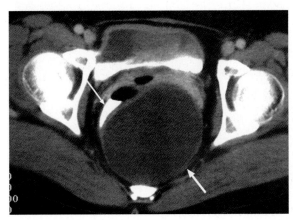

Fig GU 42-11
Tailgut cyst. Well-defined, thin-walled multicystic mass in the presacral space (thin arrows). The rectum is compressed and anteriorly displaced (thick arrow).[56]

Condition	Imaging Findings	Comments
Pseudomyxoma retroperitonei (Fig GU 42-13)	Multicystic masses with thick walls or septa that displace and distort adjacent structures. Curvilinear or punctuate mural calcifications may occur.	Rare accumulation of gelatinous material secondary to rupture of a mucinous lesion in a retrocecal appendix and fixation of the lesion to the posterior abdominal wall. The process is more commonly seen in the peritoneal cavity, where it is related to rupture of a mucinous lesion of the appendix or ovary.
Perianal mucinous carcinoma (Fig GU 42-14)	Multiple conglomerate cystic masses, which represent mucus pools, surround the anus and rectum.	Rare malignancy that may arise from an anal fistula, anal duct, or duplicated duct. It spreads around the anal canal and extends into the perianal soft tissue, while the overlying anorectal mucosa remains intact.

A

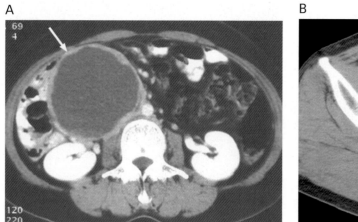

B

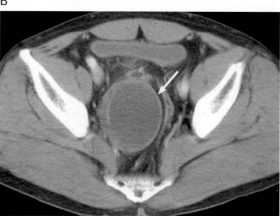

Fig GU 42-12
Cystic change in solid neoplasm. (A) Paraganglioma appears as a cystic mass with irregular walls in the right anterior pararenal space (arrow). (B) Neurilemoma appears as a cystic mass in the pelvic retroperitoneum (arrow).[56]

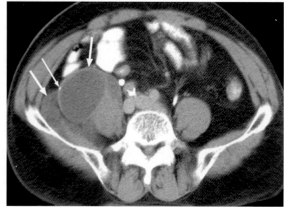

Fig GU 42-13
Pseudomyxoma retroperitonei (from rupture of a mucinous cystadenocarcinoma of the appendix). Lobulated low-attenuation masses in the right lower quadrant (thick arrows), mass effect on the right psoas muscles and right ureter, and a tiny wall calcification (thin arrow).[56]

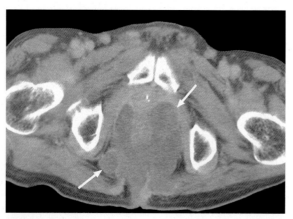

Fig GU 42-14
Perianal mucinous adenocarcinoma. Thin-walled collection in the anterior pararenal space (arrow).[56]

Cystic-Appearing Pelvic Masses

Condition	Comments
Follicular cyst (Fig GU 43-1)	Unruptured, enlarged graafian follicle that is often found incidentally in asymptomatic patients of reproductive age. Larger cysts occasionally may become palpable and cause pelvic pain. Although most follicular cysts regress spontaneously, hemorrhage into a cyst may cause symptoms of an acute abdomen and lead to emergency surgery.
Paraovarian cyst (Fig GU 43-2)	Arises from remnants of the wolffian duct system, which courses within the mesovarium. Like ovarian epithelial tumors and endometriomas, paraovarian cysts do not demonstrate the cyclical regression and growth associated with physiologic ovarian cysts.
Corpus luteum cyst (Fig GU 43-3)	Typically larger and more symptomatic than follicular cysts, corpus luteum cysts develop after continued hemorrhage or lack of resolution of the corpus luteum. Low-level echoes may develop within the cysts because of acute hemorrhage.
Theca lutein cyst (Fig GU 43-4)	Largest of the physiologic ovarian cysts that classically occur when human chorionic gonadotropin (HCG) levels are abnormally increased (as in gestational trophoblastic disease and the ovarian hyperstimulation syndrome caused by treatment with infertility drugs). Usually bilateral and multilocular.
Polycystic ovary disease (Fig GU 43-5)	Complex endocrinologic disorder associated with chronic anovulation in which there is the development of numerous small subcapsular follicular cysts with a thickened and fibrotic ovarian capsule. The individual cysts can be easily seen on transvaginal sonography, but are often too small to be demonstrated on transabdominal studies. The combination of enlarged polycystic ovaries and obesity, oligomenorrhea, and hirsutism is termed the Stein-Leventhal syndrome, in which there is an increased risk for the development of endometrial and possibly breast carcinoma.
Hydrosalpinx (Fig GU 43-6)	Unilateral or bilateral dilatation of the fallopian tubes that develops as a consequence of tubal adhesions secondary to pelvic inflammatory disease. Massive tubal distention may produce an appearance indistinguishable from that of other large cystic adnexal masses.
Serous cystadenoma (Fig GU 43-7)	Benign ovarian tumor. May contain an occasional septum.

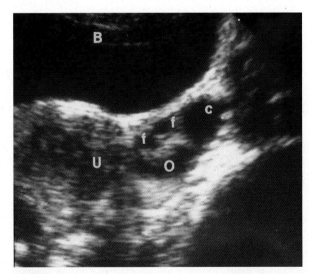

Fig GU 43-1
Follicular cysts. Endovaginal scan demonstrates multiple anechoic masses (f) within the ovary (O). (B, bladder; C, corpus luteum cyst; U, uterus.)[27]

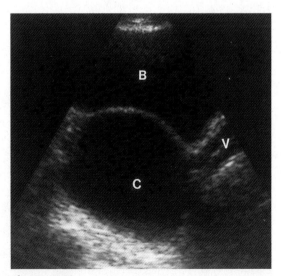

Fig GU 43-2
Paraovarian cyst. Sagittal sonogram demonstrates the cyst (C) superior to the vagina (V). The uterus had been removed. (B, bladder.)[27]

A

B

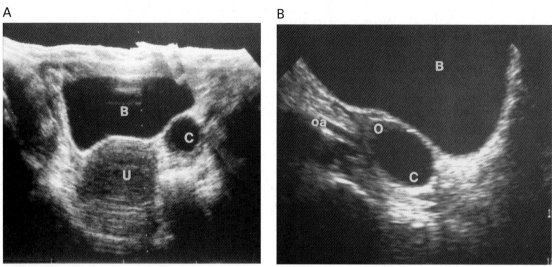

Fig GU 43-3
Corpus luteum cyst. (A) Transverse and (B) sagittal sonograms show the smooth-walled anechoic cyst (C) in the left ovary (O). (B, bladder; oa, ovarian artery.)[27]

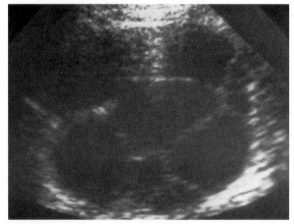

Fig GU 43-4
Theca lutein cyst. Multiseptated cystic structure in the adnexal region.[58]

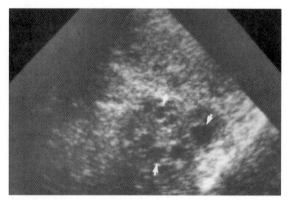

Fig GU 43-5
Polycystic ovary disease. Typical appearance of multiple subcapsular follicular cysts (arrows).[58]

A

B

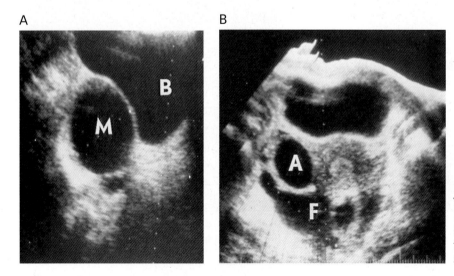

Fig GU 43-6
Tubo-ovarian abscess. (A) Large sonolucent mass (M) posterior to the bladder (B). (B) In another patient, there is fluid in the cul-de-sac (F) posterior to the cystic abscess (A).

Condition	Comments
Endometrioma (Fig GU 43-8)	Endometriosis can produce a broad spectrum of ultrasound appearances, one of which is an almost completely sonolucent mass.
Hydrocolpos (Figs GU 43-9 and GU 43-10)	Large, tubular, midline retrovesical mass in a newborn girl with an imperforate hymen. Retained secretions and cellular debris may produce internal echoes. If not discovered in the newborn period, the genital tract obstruction tends to go unnoticed until menarche, when it becomes a hematometrocolpos.

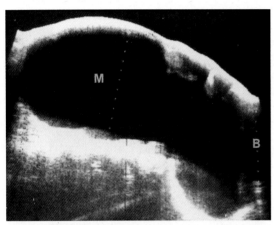

Fig GU 43-7
Serous cystadenoma. Sagittal sonogram shows a large cystic pelvoabdominal mass (M). (B, bladder.)[27]

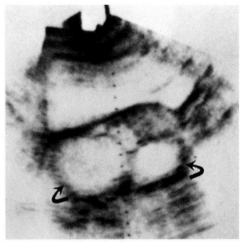

Fig GU 43-8
Endometrioma. Several sonolucent masses (arrows), simulating multiple follicular cysts, arising from the ovary.[59]

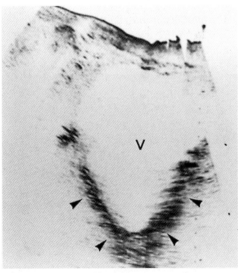

Fig GU 43-9
Hydrocolpos. Postvoiding midsagittal sonogram of a newborn girl shows a large cystic area (V) with good through-transmission of sound (arrowheads).[60]

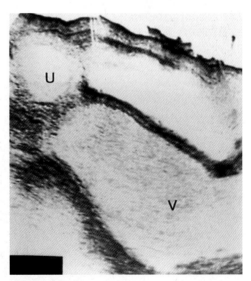

Fig GU 43-10
Hematometrocolpos. Longitudinal pelvic sonogram in a 15-year-old girl with primary amenorrhea and pain demonstrates marked distention of the vagina (V) and uterus (U).[60]

Complex Pelvic Masses

Condition	Comments
Cystadenocarcinoma/ mucinous cystadenoma (Figs GU 44-1 and GU 44-2)	Typically appears as a large cystic mass with well-defined internal septa. The number and arrangement of the internal septa do not appear to correlate with whether the mass is benign or malignant. In general, however, the more solid and irregular the areas in the mass, the more likely that it represents a malignant tumor. Other findings suggesting underlying malignancy include ascites, hepatic metastases (usually relatively hypoechoic masses in the liver), and peritoneal implants.
Dermoid cyst (Fig GU 44-3)	Complex, predominantly solid mass containing high-level echoes arising from hair or calcification in the mass. This highly echogenic nature may make it difficult to delineate the mass completely or to distinguish it from surrounding gas-containing loops of bowel. As with other ovarian tumors, the more irregular and solid the internal components of the mass, the more likely that it is malignant.
Endometrioma (Figs GU 44-4 and GU 44-5)	May appear as a predominantly cystic mass with some thickness or irregularity of the wall and a variable amount of solid internal components related to clot formation and retraction, fibrosis, and liquefaction.

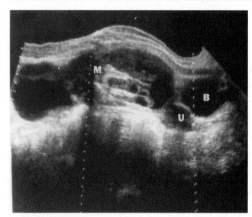

Fig GU 44-1
Cystadenocarcinoma. Sagittal sonogram shows a complex multilocular mass (M) separate from the uterus (U). (B, bladder.)[61]

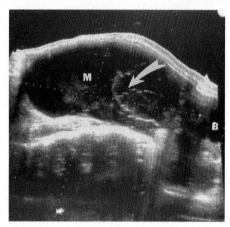

Fig GU 44-2
Mucinous cystadenocarcinoma. Sagittal sonogram of the pelvis shows a predominantly cystic mass (M) that contains some septations (arrow). (B, bladder.)[27]

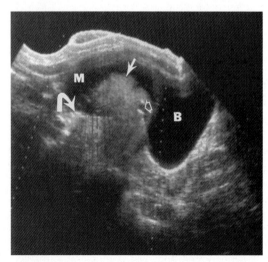

Fig GU 44-3
Dermoid cyst. Sagittal sonogram of the pelvis shows a mass (M) that exhibits the "tip of the iceberg" sign (straight arrow), a fat-fluid level (curved arrow), and calcifications (open arrow). (B, bladder.)[61]

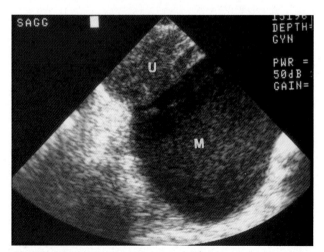

Fig GU 44-4
Endometrioma. Sagittal endovaginal scan shows the predominantly cystic mass (M) containing low-level echoes representing hemorrhage in the dependent portion. (U, uterus.)[27]

Condition	Comments
Tubo-ovarian abscess (Fig GU 44-6)	Complex adnexal mass that often has a thick and irregular wall or contains echoes or fluid levels representing the layering of purulent debris. Free pelvic fluid suggests superimposed peritonitis. The free fluid may become loculated into a peritoneal abscess, especially in the cul-de-sac (the most dependent portion of the peritoneal space in the supine patient). Some abscesses have a very echogenic appearance due to small gas bubbles produced by gas-forming organisms.

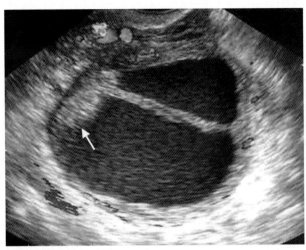

Fig GU 44-5
Edometrioma. In addition to low-level echoes within it, the lesion has thick septations and a soft-tissue component caused by clot formation (arrow).[62]

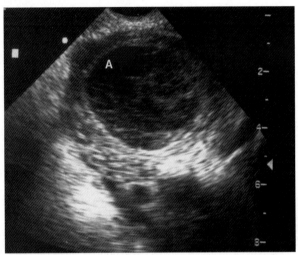

Fig GU 44-6
Pelvic inflammatory disease. Endovaginal scan shows an abscess (A) that contains low-level echoes and is surrounded by a well-defined wall.[27]

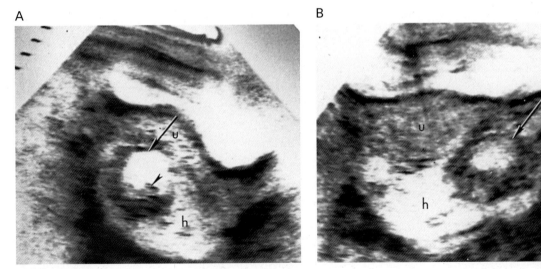

Fig GU 44-7
Ectopic pregnancy. (A) Sagittal and (B) transverse sonograms show an extrauterine gestational sac (arrows) on the left with a fetus in it (arrowhead). Note the complex cystic mass (h), which represents a hematoma, in the cul-de-sac. No fetal heart activity was noted. (U, uterus.)[63]

Condition	Comments
Ectopic pregnancy (Figs GU 44-7 through GU 44-9)	Extrauterine, extraovarian adnexal mass. More than 95% of ectopic pregnancies occur in the fallopian tubes, especially the isthmic and ampullary portions. More than half the patients with this complication of pregnancy have a history or pathologic evidence of pelvic inflammatory disease, which appears to provide an environment receptive to tubal implantation. Often associated with urine or plasma levels of HCG that are substantially lower for the expected date of gestation than those in patients with normal intrauterine pregnancies. The classic ultrasound appearance consists of an enlarged uterus that does not contain a gestational sac and is associated with an irregular adnexal mass, an "ectopic fetal head," or fluid in the cul-de-sac. The incidence of coexisting ectopic and intrauterine pregnancies is only 1 in 30,000.
Molar pregnancy (Fig GU 44-10)	Proliferative disease of the trophoblast that may manifest as a complete or partial hydatidiform mole, invasive mole, or choriocarcinoma. A hydatidiform mole, the most common form of gestational trophoblastic disease, is noninvasive and usually manifests in the second and third trimesters. This type of mole distends and fills the endometrial cavity without invading the myometrium. Ultrasound shows a uterus that is enlarged for gestational age and is filled with multiple small, hyperechoic areas with good posterior acoustic enhancement. The cysts represent grossly swollen villi from trophoblastic hyperplasia. During the first trimester, the molar tissue may appear as a homogeneously echogenic endometrial mass.
Hemorrhagic corpus luteum cyst (Fig GU 44-11)	Complex adnexal mass that may be associated with intraperitoneal blood if rupture has occurred. May be extremely difficult to distinguish from ectopic pregnancy, though in most cases the complex mass can be shown to be located within the ovary rather than separate from both the uterus and the ovary, as in an ectopic pregnancy. Corpus luteum cysts may be associated with early intrauterine pregnancies and elevated levels of human chorionic gonadotropin.
Ovarian torsion (Fig GU 44-12)	Usually occurs secondary to an underlying ovarian abnormality, such as ovarian cyst or tumor, that causes the ovarian pedicle to completely or partially rotate on its axis. The resulting interruption of arterial and venous circulation produces vascular engorgement in the ovarian parenchyma that may eventually lead to hemorrhagic infarction.

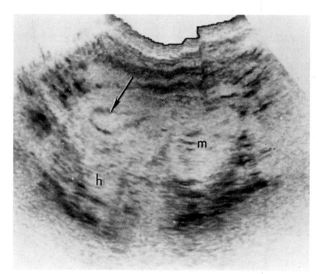

Fig GU 44-8
Pseudogestational sac in ectopic pregnancy. Transverse sonogram shows a sac-like structure with no fetal pole (arrow) in the uterus. There is also a solid collection in the cul-de-sac (h) and a left adnexal mass (m).[63]

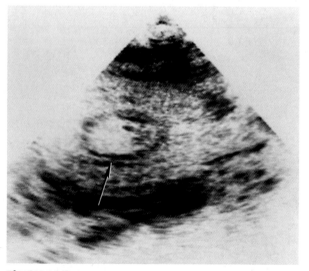

Fig GU 44-9
Double decidual sac in ectopic pregnancy. Transverse sonogram shows a second line (arrow) parallel to a portion of the decidual sac.[63]

Condition	Comments
Trophoblastic disease (Figs GU 45-10 and GU 45-11)	Spectrum of pregnancy-related disorders ranging from a benign hydatidiform mole to the more malignant and frequently metastatic choriocarcinoma. Typically appears as a large, soft-tissue solid mass of placental (trophoblastic) tissue filling the uterine cavity and containing echoes of low to moderate amplitude. Numerous small cystic fluid-containing spaces are scattered throughout the lesion. Multiple larger sonolucent areas represent degeneration or internal hemorrhage in the molar tissue.

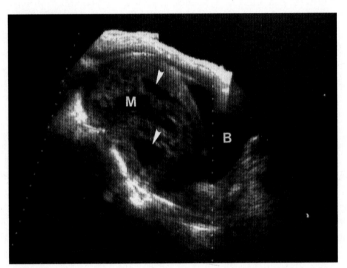

Fig GU 45-11
Trophoblastic disease. Sagittal sonogram shows a uterine mass (M) containing irregular cystic areas (arrowheads) representing degeneration or internal hemorrhage in the molar tissue. (B, bladder.)[27]

Magnetic Resonance Imaging of the Female Pelvis

Condition	Imaging Findings	Comments
Leiomyoma (fibroid) of the uterus (Figs GU 46-1 through GU 46-3)	Well-circumscribed mass that has medium to low signal intensity on T1-weighted images and is usually hypointense to adjacent myometrium or endometrium on T2-weighted images. Central or diffuse areas of increased signal intensity on T2-weighted images are seen with degeneration (hyaline, mucinous, hemorrhagic, or myxomatous).	Most accurate modality for assessing the number, location, and size of leiomyomas, especially in women who plan to have uterine-preserving myomectomies. MRI can help differentiate between a uterine leiomyoma (which is potentially removable) and adenomyosis (which requires hysterectomy). This modality also is valuable in distinguishing subserosal leiomyomas from other solid pelvic masses when sonography is indeterminate.
Adenomyosis (Figs GU 46-4 and GU 46-5)	On T2-weighted images, typically a poorly marginated mass of low signal intensity that has an irregular and indistinct border with the adjacent myometrium. There usually is diffuse thickening of the junctional zone. On T1-weighted images, no abnormality may be apparent. Small foci of high signal intensity on both T1- and T2-weighted images may result from hemorrhage within endometrial islands in the lesion.	A common disease in women over age 30, adenomyosis refers to the presence of endometrial tissue deep within the myometrial wall. Adenomyosis often coexists with uterine fibroids. Because it involves the myometrium diffusely, adenomyosis is a nonresectable condition that usually is treated by hysterectomy.
Congenital uterine anomalies (Figs GU 46-6 and GU 46-7)	On T2-weighted images, the septum of a septate uterus appears as a thin, hypointense fibrous band separating the adjacent endometrial cavities (which have high signal intensity). In a bicornuate uterus, there is a deep external notch in the fundus of the uterus and a thick or double medium-intensity band of myometrium between the two endometrial cavities.	MRI frequently can differentiate between septate and bicornuate uterus without the need for laparoscopy. This distinction is critical, because a septate uterus can be corrected easily in an outpatient setting with transvaginal resection of the septum. A bicornuate uterus is not always repaired (but if it is, a laparotomy is required).

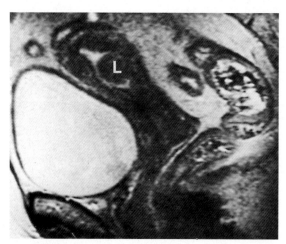

Fig GU 46-1
Submucosal leiomyoma of the uterus. Sagittal T2-weighted image shows a well-circumscribed hypointense leiomyoma (L) almost completely surrounded by endometrium.[65]

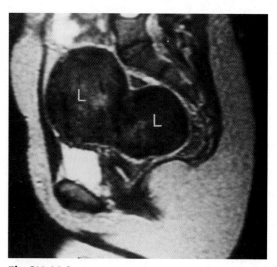

Fig GU 46-2
Subserosal leiomyomas of the uterus. Sagittal T2-weighted image shows two large subserosal leiomyomas (L), which appear as well-defined hypointense lesions along the superior surface of the uterus.[65]

Condition	Imaging Findings	Comments
Endometrial carcinoma (Figs GU 46-8 through GU 46-11)	On T2-weighted images, an intact hypointense junctional zone around the high-intensity lesion indicates that the tumor is limited to the endometrium. Measuring the depth of high-intensity tumor within the surrounding hypointense myometrium can determine whether the invasion is superficial or deep.	Gadolinium can substantially increase the sensitivity of MR imaging for assessing the depth of tumor invasion. The tumor does not enhance as much as the surrounding myometrium and thus has low- or intermediate-signal intensity when compared with the well-enhanced myometrium and the hypointense endometrial cavity. Myometrial invasion can be detected as intermediate-signal tumor within the high-signal myometrium.

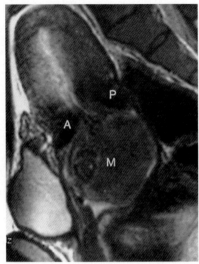

Fig GU 46-3
Prolapsing leiomyoma. Sagittal T2-weighted image shows a large submucosal leiomyoma (M) splaying apart the anterior (A) and posterior (P) lips of the cervix and protruding through the external cervical os. Before imaging, the clinical suspicion based on physical examination was carcinoma of the cervix.[66]

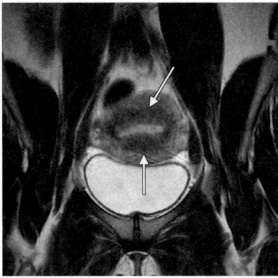

Fig GU 46-4
Diffuse adenomyosis. Coronal T2-weighted image shows markedly diffuse enlargement of the junctional zone (arrows) replacing normal myometrium.[67]

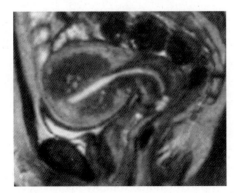

Fig GU 46-5
Adenomyosis. Sagittal T2-weighted image demonstrates oval areas of thickened junctional zone containing a few hyperintense foci that are characteristic of this condition.[66]

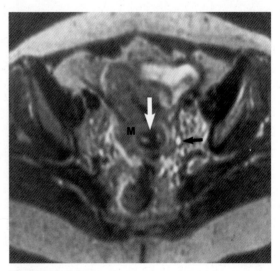

Fig GU 46-6
Septate uterus. Axial T2-weighted image at the miduterine (small arrow) level shows a single uterine horn with two endometrial canals divided by a septum (large arrow). (M, myometrium.)[68]

Condition	Imaging Findings	Comments
Cervical carcinoma (Figs GU 46-12 and GU 46-13)	High-intensity mass within the hypointense cervical stroma on T2-weighted images. An intact ring of hypointense stroma surrounding the lesion indicates that the tumor is confined to the cervix. Pericervical or parametrial extension is indicated if the tumor completely involves the hypointense cervical stroma or spreads outside it.	Multiplanar imaging capability of MRI may permit an accuracy rate for tumor staging higher than that of clinical palpation. In addition to demonstrating extension into the pericervical and parametrial tissue, MR can define tumor size and location as well as involvement of the uterus, pelvic side wall, bladder, and rectum.

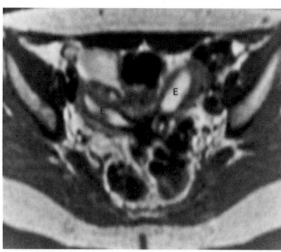

Fig GU 46-7
Bicornuate uterus. Axial T2-weighted image shows two uterine horns of similar size with functioning endometrium (E).[68]

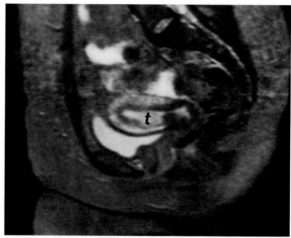

Fig GU 46-8
Endometrial carcinoma (superficially invasive). Sagittal T2-weighted image shows tumor (t) causing segmental disruption of the junctional zone, with tumor confined to the inner half of the myometrium.[65]

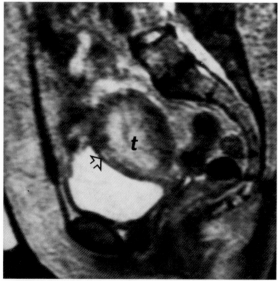

Fig GU 46-9
Endometrial carcinoma (superficially invasive). Sagittal T2-weighted scan shows tumor (t) extending to the outer half of the myometrium (arrow).[65]

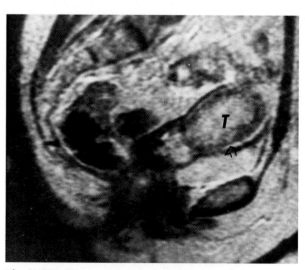

Fig GU 46-10
Endometrial carcinoma (deeply invasive). Sagittal T2-weighted image shows tumor (T) extending to the outer half of the myometrium (arrow).[66]

A

B

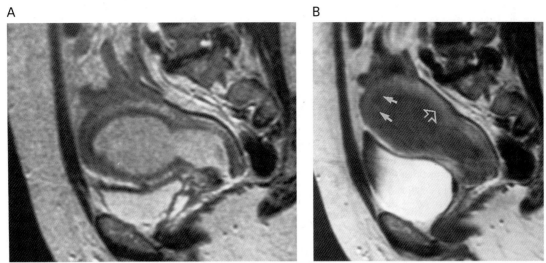

Fig GU 46-11
Endometrial carcinoma (value of gadolinium). (A) Sagittal T2-weighted image shows a markedly enlarged endometrial cavity with intact junctional zone (suggesting a stage 1A tumor confined to the myometrium). (B) Sagittal gadolinium-enhanced T1-weighted scan at the same level (bladder contains more urine) shows intermediate-intensity tumor invading the junctional zone and myometrium of the fundus (solid arrows), which was proved at surgery to represent stage 1C tumor (invasion to more than 50% of the endometrium). Note the normal high-intensity enhancement of the posterior myometrium (open arrow).[69]

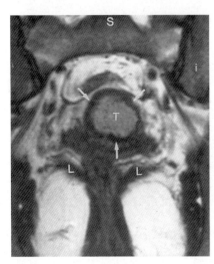

Fig GU 46-12
Cervical carcinoma without full-depth stromal invasion. Coronal T2-weighted image through the cervix demonstrates a thin, intact, low-signal-intensity rim (arrows), representing residual cervical stroma surrounding the medium-signal-intensity tumor (T), which expands the cervix. Identification of this intact rim has high predictive value for excluding invasion into the parametrial and paracervical areas. The sacrum (S), iliac bones (i), and levator ani muscles (L) are labeled for orientation.[66]

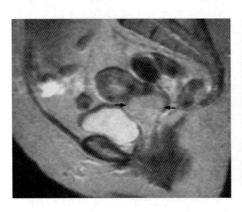
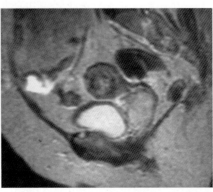

Fig GU 46-13
Cervical carcinoma. Sagittal T2-weighted images show the high-intensity tumor (arrows) extending into the proximal vagina but not invading the bladder wall.[69]

Condition	Imaging Findings	Comments
Ovarian cyst (Figs GU 46-14 and GU 46-15)	Well-circumscribed adnexal mass with homogeneously low signal on T1-weighted images and high signal on T2-weighted images (similar to characteristics of urine on all pulse sequences).	Hemorrhagic cysts tend to have high signal intensity on both T1- and T2-weighted images.
Dermoid cyst (cystic teratoma) (Fig GU 46-16)	Fatty component is isointense relative to subcutaneous fat on all pulse sequences. Components other than fat have a wide variety of signal intensities.	Chemical shift imaging, fat suppression, and the demonstration of intratumoral fat-fluid levels are useful in differentiating a dermoid cyst from hemorrhagic adnexal lesions.
Endometriosis (Fig GU 46-17)	Variable signal intensity patterns reflecting the age of the hemorrhagic fluid. Some are hyperintense on T1-weighted images and hypointense on T2-weighted studies. Others are hyperintense on both sequences (methemoglobin). In some cases, a hypointense hemosiderin rim may be detected on T2-weighted images.	Although MRI is accurate in helping to characterize an adnexal mass as an endometrioma, this modality is not able to routinely identify small implants and adhesions. Therefore, laparoscopy remains the primary procedure for the diagnosis and staging of endometriosis.

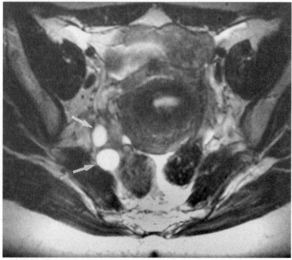

Fig GU 46-14
Simple ovarian cysts. Axial T2-weighted image shows two well-defined, homogeneous high-signal-intensity corpus luteum cysts (arrows) in the right ovary.[70]

Fig GU 46-15
Hemorrhagic ovarian cyst. Axial T1-weighted image demonstrates a well-defined homogeneous high-signal-intensity mass (arrows). Similar high signal intensity was also seen on T2-weighted images. Spontaneous resolution occurred, differentiating it from an endometrioma.[68]

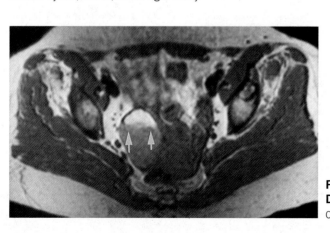

Fig GU 46-16
Dermoid cyst. Axial T2-weighted image shows an oval right ovarian mass containing a fat-fluid level (arrows).[69]

Condition	Imaging Findings	Comments
Polycystic ovary (Fig GU 46-18)	On T2-weighted images, characteristic appearance of a hyperintense ring of peripheral high-intensity cysts (similar to a string of pearls) surrounding low-signal-intensity central stroma.	Complex endocrinologic disorder associated with chronic anovulation in which there is the development of numerous small subcapsular follicular cysts with a thickened and fibrotic ovarian capsule.
Carcinoma of the ovary (Figs GU 46-19 and GU 46-20)	Solid components often have low to intermediate signal on T1-weighted images and variable signal on T2-weighted images (ranging from intermediate to high).	MRI has had relatively little impact on staging, as this type of cancer spreads primarily through peritoneal dissemination, and MRI often cannot identify small peritoneal implants. A diagnosis of malignancy can be made if the study identifies involvement of adjacent pelvic organs, intraperitoneal metastases, retroperitoneal lymphadenopathy, or distant metastases.

A

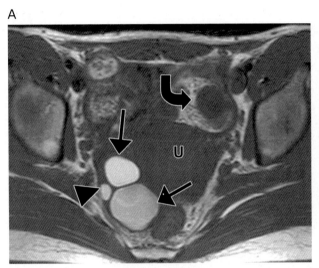

B

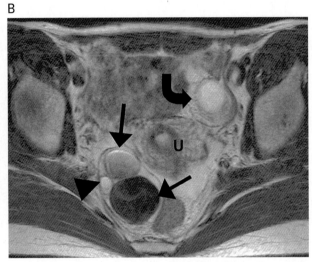

Fig GU 46-17
Endometrial (chocolate) cysts. (A) Axial T1-weighted image shows multiple cysts in the right ovary. All three cysts are hyperintense (straight arrows, arrowhead), indicating that the adnexal mass is not due to fat as in a dermoid. (B) On the T2-weighted image, one of the cysts is hyperintense (arrowhead) and the other two are hypointense (straight arrows). U = uterus; curved arrow = left ovary.[71]

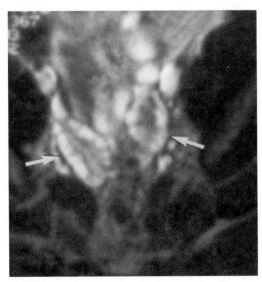

Fig GU 46-18
Polycystic ovaries. Coronal T2-weighted image demonstrates bilateral ovarian enlargement (arrows) with rims of multiple, small high-intensity subcapsular follicles and abundant central stroma.[68]

Condition	Imaging Findings	Comments
Serous carcinoma (Figs GU 46-21 and GU 46-22)	Intermediate to high signal intensity on T2-weighted images.	Characteristic pattern of intracystic or exophytic projections in the papillary form of the tumor.
Metastases to the ovaries (Fig GU 46-23)	Various patterns.	The most common extragenital neoplasms that metastasize by hematogenous or lymphatic spread to the ovaries are primary tumors of the intestines, stomach, and breast.
Fibrothecoma (Fig GU 46-24)	Variable appearance depending on the relative amounts of spindle cells, collagen, edema, and cyst formation.	Most common solid benign tumor of the ovary.
Brenner tumor (Fig GU 46-25)	Extensive low signal on T2-weighted images, reflecting the abundant fibrous content.	Sharply circumscribed, almost always benign tumors characterized by a nest of transitional cells scattered through the stromal component. Brenner tumors are frequently associated with mucinous cystic tumors in the same ovary.

A

B

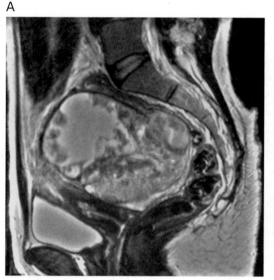
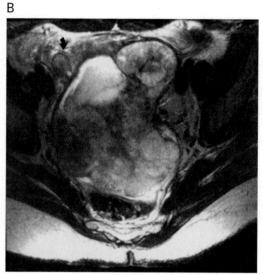

Fig GU 46-19
Carcinoma of the ovary. (A) Sagittal T2-weighted image shows a large cystic and solid mass located above the uterus and anterior to the rectum. Note that the mass does not seem to be arising from either of these structures. (B) T2-weighted axial image demonstrates the extensive solid components of the mass. Again, the mass does not appear to arise from the rectum and it obliterates the left ovary. Note that the right ovary shows no evidence of tumor (arrow).[70]

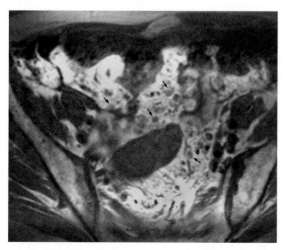

Fig GU 46-20
Peritoneal and mesenteric implants from ovarian carcinomatosis. T1-weighted image shows numerous very small nodules studding the sigmoid and small bowel mesenteries and omentum (arrows).[70]

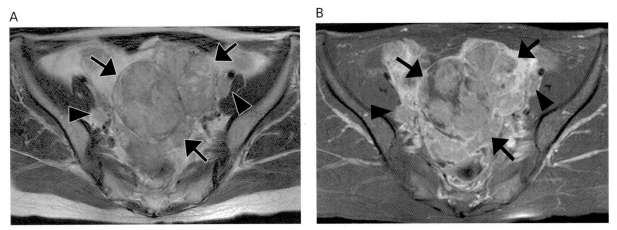

Fig GU 46-21
Serous carcinoma. T1-weighted contrast image with fat suppression shows a solid nodular, enhancing mass (arrows). Note the enlargement of external iliac lymph nodes bilaterally (arrowheads), which is a strong indicator of malignancy.[71]

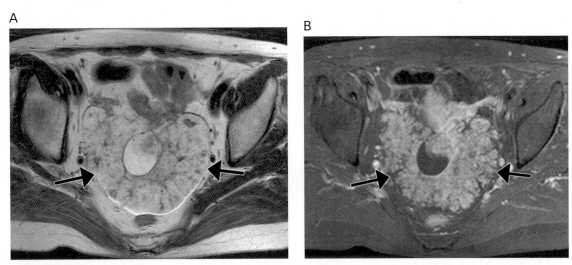

Fig GU 46-22
Serous papillary carcinoma. (A) Axial T2-weighted images shows a cystic and solid mass (arrows). (B) Contrast-enhanced, fat-suppressed T1-weighted image shows the characteristic exophytic projections of the tumor (arrows).[71]

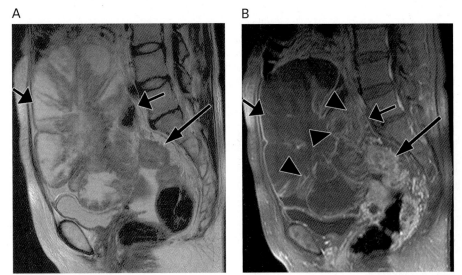

Fig GU 46-23
Metastases to the ovaries. (A) T2-weighted and (B) contrast-enhanced, fat-suppressed T1-weighted images show a multicystic right ovarian mass (short arrows) with a solid component. The irregular thick septa and solid component enhance on the post-contrast image (arrowheads). A rectal tumor (long arrow) in seen.[71]

Condition	Imaging Findings	Comments
Pelvic congestion syndrome (Fig GU 46-26)	Dilated, tortuous tubular structures that contain variable signal intensity depending on the rate of flow within them.	Common cause of pelvic pain that results from dilated, tortuous, and congested veins produced by retrograde flow through incompetent valves in ovarian veins.
Gartner cyst (Fig GU 46-27)	Often high signal intensity on T1-weighted images because of the proteinaceous nature of the cystic fluid. Low signal intensity on fat-suppressed images.	Remant of the mesonephric (wolffian) duct. Most cysts are small and typically paravaginal in the anterolateral position. A large cyst can cause urethral or even ureteric obstruction.
Periurethral cyst (Fig GU 46-28)	Cystic mass that has low signal intensity on T1-weighted images and high signal intensity on T2-weighed scans.	Congenital dilatation of a periurethral gland, which is often asymptomatic. Symptomatic infection can result in urethral diverticula. MR is superior to transvaginal ultrasound for demonstrating lesions in the urethra and periurethral region.

A

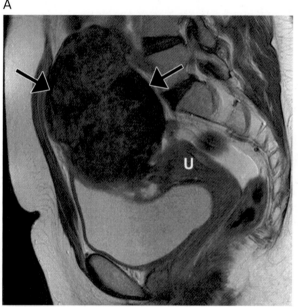

B

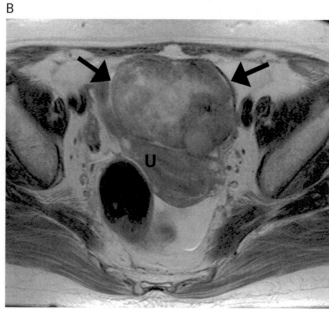

Fig GU 46-24
Fibrothecoma. (A) Sagittal T2-weighted image shows a hypointense solid mass (arrows), reflecting the fibrotic mature of the lesion. U = uterus. (B) Axial T2-weighted image in another patient shows a heterogeneous solid mass (arrows) with intermediate to high signal intensity. There is ascites in the cul-de-sac. The uterus is enlarged, an abnormal finding in this post-menopausal woman.[71]

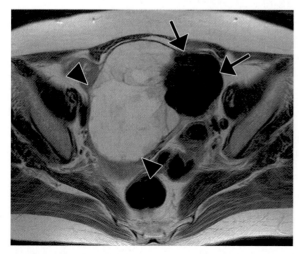

Fig GU 46-25
Brenner tumor. T2-weighted axial image shows a solid mass (arrows) that is sharply demarcated and has low signal intensity. In addition, there is a multicystic mass (arrowheads) that represents a mucinous cystadenoma.[71]

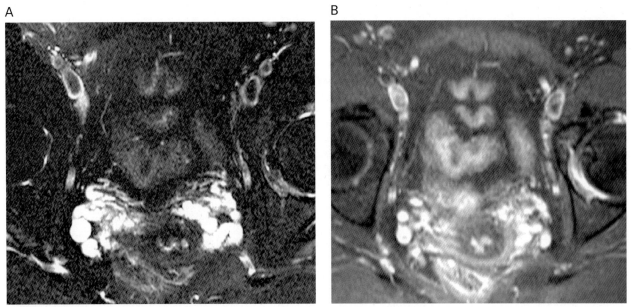

Fig GU 46-26
Pelvic congestion syndrome. (A) Coronal T2-weighted image and (B) T1-weighted contrast image with fat-suppression demonstrate severely congested pelvic veins.[67]

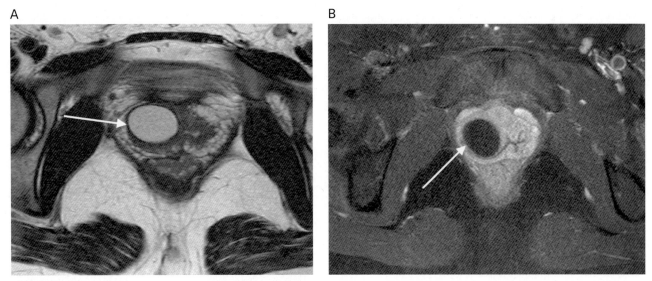

Fig GU 46-27
Gartner cyst. (A) Axial T2-weighted image and (B) T1-weighted contrast image with fat-suppression show the cystic mass.[67]

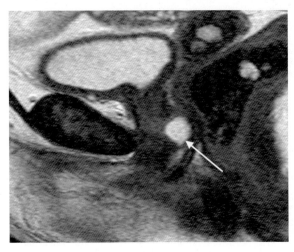

Fig GU 46-28
Periurethral cyst. Sagittal T2-weighted image shows the cystic mass (arrow).[67]

Diffusely Enlarged Uterus on Magnetic Resonance Imaging

Condition	Imaging Findings	Comments
Pregnancy-related changes Postpartum uterus	Normal uterine enlargement tends to persist longer after caesarean section than after vaginal delivery due to the delay in involution. Uterine volume decreases more rapidly in women who breast feed.	The normal zonal anatomy is usually not identifiable for about 6 weeks after vaginal delivery and as much as 6 months after caesarean section.
Delay of involution (Figs GU 47-1 and GU 47-2)	Hematomas demonstrate variable signal intensity and lack of enhancement. The presence of air bubbles in the uterine cavity and homogeneous cervical enhancement suggests intrauterine infection.	One of the most common causes of a uterus that is larger than expected after delivery. Among the underlying factors are fetal problems (excess amniotic fluid, multiple gestations), prolonged labor, intrauterine remnants (clots, placenta, debris), leiomyomas, uterine anomalies, and intrauterine infection.
Retained placenta fragments and retained products of conception (Figs GU 47-3 and GU 47-4)	Retained placental tissue has high signal intensity on T2-weighted images and shows prominent contrast enhancement. Associated hematoma exhibits variable signal intensity on all sequences and does not enhance.	The typical presentation of retained placenta is a large and soft uterus, prolonged bleeding delivery after dilatation and curettage, and an elevated level of human chorionic gonadotropin.

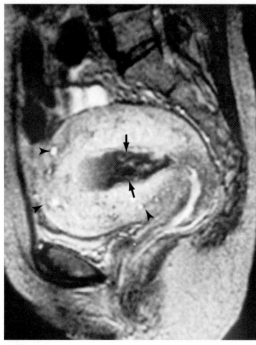

Fig GU 47-1
Delayed uterine involution. Sagittal T2-weighted MR image 10 days after vaginal delivery shows that the uterus is still enlarged. The myometrium has high signal intensity with prominent vessels (arrowheads). Low-signal-intensity fluid is seen in the endometrial cavity (arrows), a finding indicative of blood products.[73]

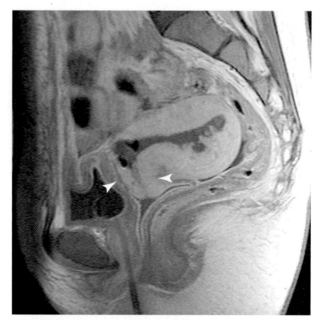

Fig GU 47-2
Postpregnancy endometritis. Sagittal contrast T1-weighted MR image in a woman who experienced septic shock 3 weeks after caesarean section shows intense enhancement of the uterus with particularly prominent cervical enhancement (arrowheads). The cervix does not usually enhance so intensely unless it is significantly inflamed. The fluid seen in the endometrial cavity was found to be pus related to infection by methicillin-resistant *Staphylococcus aureus*.[73]

Condition	Imaging Findings	Comments
Hormonal causes		The most important hormonal factors resulting in uterine enlargement are increased serum levels of estrogen, progesterone, and gonadotropin. Uterine exposure to these hormones can be endogenous (hormone-producing tumor) or exogenous.
Exogenous estroprogesterone (Fig GU 47-5)	The myometrium appears swollen and globular with high signal intensity, whereas the endometrium can become atrophic due to muscle hypertrophy, sinusoidal dilatation, and edema.	Estroprogesterone (oral contraceptive pill) is also used for the treatment of dysmenorrhea. The imaging findings are more pronounced in women taking higher concentrations of the hormone.
Exogenous tamoxifen (Fig GU 47-6)	Heterogeneous endometrial hyperplasia. There may be multiple cysts or latticelike enhancement of the endometrium on post-contrast images.	This widely used treatment for breast cancer may also be associated with such endometrial abnormalities as hyperplasia, polyps, and carcinoma.
Endogenous hormones (Fig GU 47-7)	Findings similar to those with tamoxifen use.	The presence of a hormone-producing tumor should be considered when there is both an enlarged uterus and an adnexal mass.

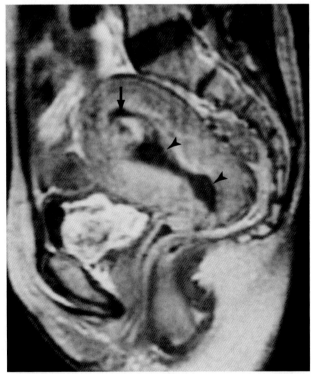

Fig GU 47-3
Retained placenta. Sagittal contrast T1-weighted MR image shows marked enhancement of the lesion protruding into the uterine cavity (arrow). The nonenhancing area in the lesion corresponds to a clot. Arrowhead = blood in the uterine cavity.[73]

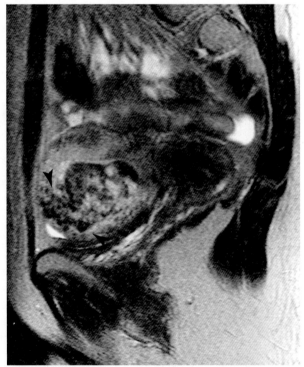

Fig GU 47-4
Retained products of conception. Sagittal T2-weighted MR image shows numerous signal voids with ill-defined borders (arrows) in the anterior uterine wall.[73]

Condition	Imaging Findings	Comments
Vascular lesions		Uterine enlargement can result from prominently engorged vessels or myometrial edema.
Ateriovenous malformations	Characteristic cluster of serpentine flow-related signal voids within a thick myometrium.	Tangle of vessels possessing the histologic characteristics of both arteries and veins without an intervening capillary network. Probably acquired following trauma, they can be associated with such conditions as normal uterine pregnancy, miscarriage, abortion, ectopic pregnancy, endometrial cancer, and choriocarcinoma.
Pelvic congestion syndrome (Fig GU 47-8)	In addition to uterine enlargement and engorged arcuate vessels in the myometrium, there typically are varicose veins around the uterus and ovaries with retrograde filling of ovarian veins.	Vague symptoms, including chronic pelvic pain, associated with dilated ovarian and pelvic veins resulting from left renal vein reflux.
Adenomyosis (Figs GU 47-9 and GU 47-10)	Diffuse or focal widening of the junctional zone in an enlarged uterus with diffuse or focal low signal on T2-weighted images. Bright spots on T1- or T2-weighted images correspond to heterotopic endometrial tissue, cystic dilatation of endometrial glands, or hemorrhagic foci.	Benign invasion of the endometrium into the myometrium with reactive overgrowth of the musculature. Striations of high signal intensity radiating from the endometrium indicate benign endometrial invasion. However, blending of these fine striations with the myometrium (pseudo-widening of the endometrium) can resemble invasion by uterine malignancy.

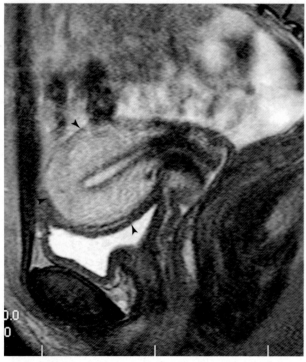

Fig GU 47-5
Estroprogesterone. Sagittal T2-weighted MR image shows a globular uterine corpus (arrowheads), a myometrium with increased signal intensity (higher than that of a normal uterus in a reproductive-age woman), and an atrophic endometrium.[73]

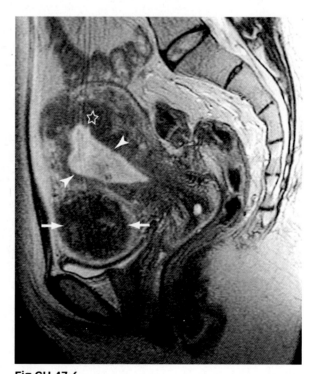

Fig GU 47-6
Tamoxifen. Sagittal T2-weighted MR image shows thickened endometrium (arrowheads) and myometrium. The heterogeneous endometrial thickening is consistent with hyperplasia. The thickened junctional zone in the posterior urethra (star) is indicative of adenomyosis. A leiomyoma (arrow) is present in the anterior uterine wall.[73]

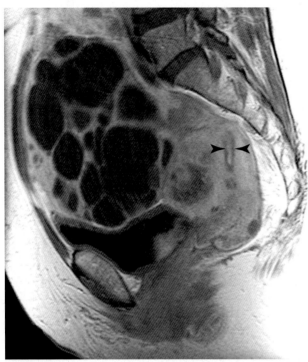

Fig GU 47-7
Granulosa cell tumor. Sagittal contrast T1-weighted MR image shows marked enhancement of the endometrium (arrowheads), which is indicative of cystic hyperplasia. The ovarian wall and septa also demonstrate significant enhancement. After surgery, the estradiol level returned to normal.[73]

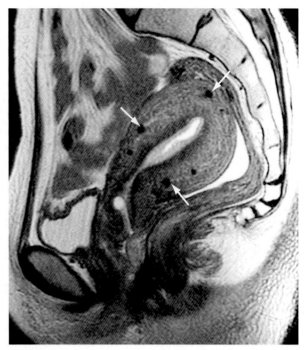

Fig GU 47-8
Pelvic congestion syndrome. Sagittal T2-weighted MR image shows a thickened myometrium with numerous dilated signal voids (arrows).[73]

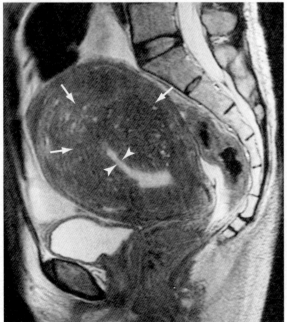

Fig GU 47-9
Adenomyosis. Sagittal T2-weighted MR image shows indistinct zonal anatomy. Widening of the junctional zone is clearly seen in the region around the distorted endometrium (arrowheads). The myometrium has decreased signal with tiny spots of high signal intensity (arrows).[73]

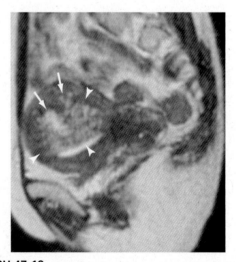

Fig GU 47-10
Adenomyosis (pseudo-widening of the endometrium). Sagittal T2-weighted MR image shows a heterogeneous area of high signal intensity (arrowheads) within the myometrium that protrudes into the uterine cavity. The interface between the lesion and the myometrium is indistinct. Fine hyperintense striations (arrows) extend into the myometrium, producing an appearance that is an extreme example of pseudo-widening of the endometrium.[73]

Condition	Imaging Findings	Comments
Neoplasms		
Multiple nodule pattern (Figs GU 47-11 through GU 47-13)	Leiomyomas typically have low signal intensity with a speckled appearance on T2-weighted images. In diffuse leiomyomatosis, innumerable low-to-intermediate signal intensity nodules blend into one another and virtually replace the uterine parenchyma. The rare leiomyosarcoma appears either as a prominently enlarged uterus with multiple sarcomatous nodules or as extensive invasion.	Leiomyomas are by far the most common uterine tumor. Leiomyosarcomas are rare and can enlarge extremely rapidly after their initial presentation. Necrotic areas within this malignant lesion appear as slightly high signal intensity on T1-weighted images and as heterogeneous areas on T2-weighted images.
Diffuse myometrial involvement (Fig GU 47-14)	Various patterns. A band of low signal intensity within the area of myometrial invasion, which is either sharply demarcated or diffusely infiltrated on T2-weighted images, is highly suggestive of low-grade stromal sarcoma.	Endometrial stromal sarcoma, hematological malignancies, metastatic disease.
Intrauterine device (Fig GU 47-15)	Band of low signal intensity.	A chronic excess of prostaglandin, the release of which is stimulated by an intrauterine device, is thought to lead to progressive myometrial hypertrophy and the observation that women with these devices generally have a larger uterus.

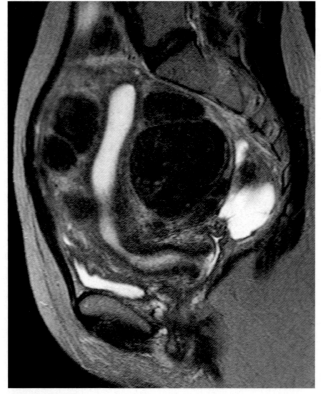

Fig GU 47-11
Multiple leiomyomas. Sagittal T2-weighted MR image shows a diffusely enlarged uterus containing several fatty lesions with clear margins and distinctive low signal intensity.[73]

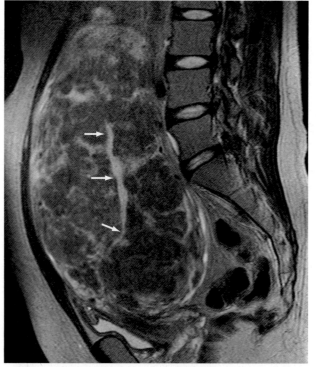

Fig GU 47-12
Diffuse leiomyomatosis. Sagittal T2-weighted MR image demonstrates a prominently enlarged uterus with innumerable leiomyomas that appear to blend with one another. The endometrium (arrows) is markedly elongated and distorted by the multiple submucosal nodules.[73]

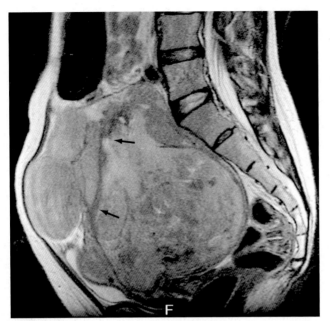

Fig GU 47-13
Leiomyosarcoma. Sagittal T2-weighted MR image shows an enlarged, irregularly shaped uterus. The tumor occupies the endometrial cavity (arrows). Note the proiminent nodules (m) in the anterior wall.[73]

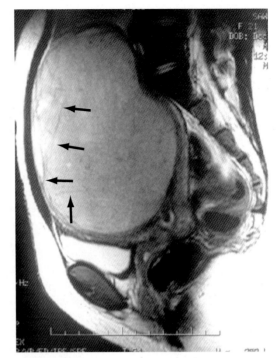

Fig GU 47-14
Endometrial stromal sarcoma. Sagittal T2-weighted image shows a huge tumor that replaces the endometrial cavity (arrowheads) and infiltrates the myometrium. Bands of low signal intensity (arrows) are seen in the infiltrated myometrium. These bands corresponded to preserved bundles of myometrium at histologic examination of this low-grade tumor.[73]

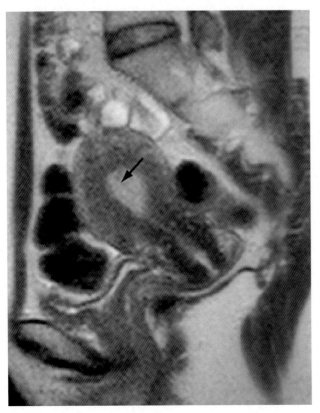

Fig GU 47-15
Intrauterine device. The IUD (arrow) appears as a band of low signal intensity in the endometrium of a globular uterus.[73]

The Endometrium

Condition	Comments
Normal menstrual changes (Figs GU 48-1 through GU-48-3)	During menstruation, the endometrium appears as a thin, echogenic line (1–4 mm in thickness). Intraluminal blood or sheets of sloughed endometrium may be identified. Once the proliferative phase of the menstrual cycle (days 6–14) begins, the endometrium becomes thicker (5–7 mm) and more echogenic relative to the myometrium, reflecting the development of glands, blood vessels, and stroma. In the late proliferative (periovulatory) phase, the endometrium thickens (up to 11 mm) and develops a multilayered appearance with an echogenic basal layer and hypoechoic inner functional layer, separated by a thin echogenic median layer arising from the central interface or luminal content. The layered appearance usually disappears 48 hours after ovulation. During the secretory phase, the endometrium becomes even thicker (7–16 mm) and more echogenic (probably due to stromal edema and glands distended with mucus and glycogen).
Pregnancy (Figs GU 48-4 through GU 48-7)	The normal gestational sac can be seen at 4.5 weeks gestation and should be visualized when greater than 5 mm in length. The yolk sac should be visualized at 5–6 weeks gestation, and an embryo may be seen before 6 weeks. One sign indicating a normal intrauterine pregnancy at an early stage is the intradecidual sign, which occurs when the sac is too small to indent or deform the central endometrial echo. Another is the double decidual sac sign, which appears as a hypoechoic line interposed between two hyperechoic rings about the sac (due to apposition of the endometrial walls). An intrauterine finding of ectopic pregnancy (seen in 10–20% of cases) is the pseudogestational sac. This may range in appearance from anechoic fluid to echogenic material (termed a decidual cast) in the uterine cavity. An empty gestational sac may represent a blighted ovum. Absent fetal cardiac activity when the crown-to-rump length is greater than 5 mm is indicative of embryonic demise.
Postpartum Normal appearance	The endometrial cavity measures less than 2 cm in anteroposterior diameter. The wall of the cavity may have a variable appearance, ranging from smooth, well-defined borders to irregular, heterogeneous linings. Small echogenic foci within the endometrial cavity may merely reflex retained membranes and clots not completely expelled with the placenta. Tiny central echoes representing intrauterine gas may be seen in up to 20% of healthy women in the postpartum period; clot and debris are seen in about 25%. However, persistent thickening of the endometrial cavity suggests retained products of conception (see below).

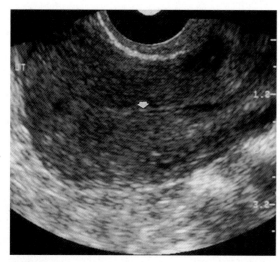

Fig GU 48-1
Normal premenopausal endometrium. A sagittal image of the uterus obtained during menstruation shows a thin endometrial lining (arrow) with a trace of fluid.[72]

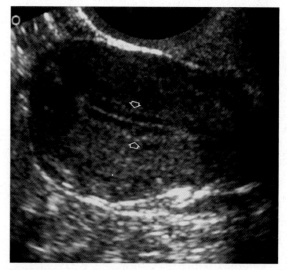

Fig GU 48-2
Normal premenopausal endometrium. Sagittal image of the uterus obtained during the late proliferative phase of the menstrual cycle demonstrates the endometrium with a multilayered appearance (arrows).[72]

Condition	Comments
Endometritis (Fig GU 48-8)	The most common cause of fever in the postpartum period, it complicates 2 to 3% of vaginal deliveries and up to 85% of caesarean sections. It also is associated with prolonged labor, premature rupture of membranes, retained clots, and retained products of conception. Ultrasound shows a thickened, heterogeneous endometrium with intracavitary fluid and characteristic multiple echogenic foci representing intrauterine gas.

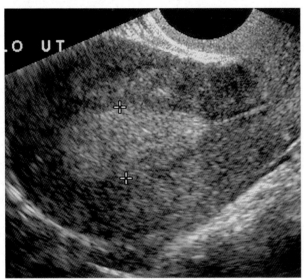

Fig GU 48-3
Normal premenopausal endometrium. Sagittal image of the uterus obtained during the secretory phase of the menstrual cycle shows a thickened, echogenic endometrium (cursors).[72]

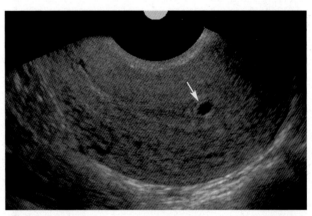

Fig GU 48-4
Intradecidual sign. Transvaginal image of a retroflexed uterus. Note the echogenic ring (arrow) eccentrically located in the endometrium that abuts the interface between the anterior and posterior endometrium. (Courtesy Deborah Levine, MD, Boston, MA.)

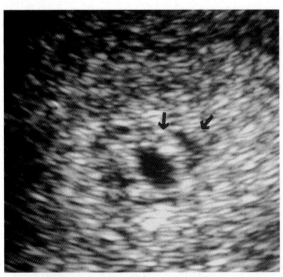

Fig GU 48-5
Double decidual sac sign. Sonogram of an early intrauterine pregnancy demonstrates two hyperechoic rings (arrows). The inner ring represents the combined chorion-decidua capsularis, and the outer ring represents the decidua parietalis.[72]

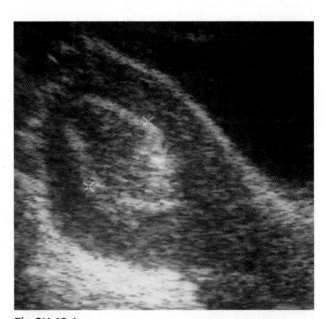

Fig GU 48-6
Decidual cast. Transabdominal image reveals echogenic material within the endometrium (cursors).[72]

Condition	Comments
Retained products of conception (Fig GU 48-9)	Ultrasound shows echogenic material within the endometrial canal. Calcifications may develop at a later stage. Urinary atony and retained products of conception are the most common causes of postpartum hemorrhage. Uterine atony is seen in the immediate postpartum period, while retained products of conception usually causes hemorrhage or infection at a later date. A normal-appearing uterus and endometrial cavity in the presence of postpartum hemorrhage indicates urinary atony, whereas an echogenic intracavitary mass is suggestive of retained products of conception.

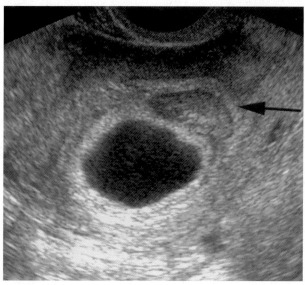

Fig GU 48-7
Blighted ovum. Sonogram shows the gestational sac with no visible embryo or yolk sac. A small subchorionic hematoma is noted (arrow).[72]

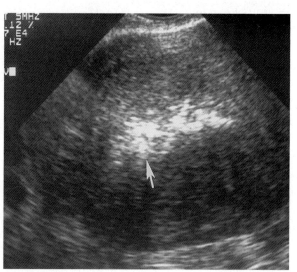

Fig GU 48-8
Endometritis. Multiple echogenic foci within the endometrium (arrow) represent gas.[72]

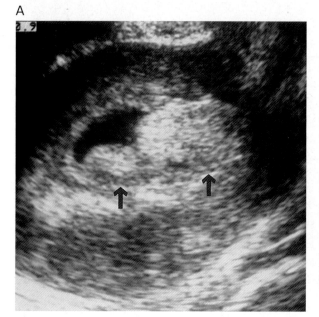

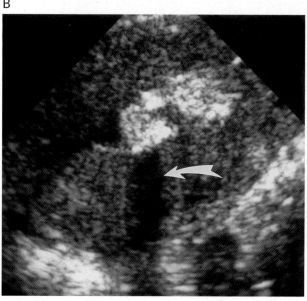

Fig GU 48-9
Retained products of conception. (A) Echogenic material within the endometrial canal (arrows). (B) Echogenic material with posterior acoustic shadowing (arrow) is consistent with calcified retained products of conception.[72]

Condition	Comments
Postmenopausal	
Normal appearance (Fig GU 48-10)	The endometrium is thin, homogeneous, and echogenic. A double-layer thickness (< 5 mm) without focal thickening generally excludes significant disease and is consistent with atrophy.
Endometrial polyps (Fig GU 48-11)	This common cause of postmenopausal bleeding is most frequently seen in women receiving tamoxifen. They are best seen at sonohysterography, where they appear as echogenic, smooth, intracavitary masses outlined by fluid. Although often appearing as nonspecific endometrial thickening, polyps are often identified as focal masses with the endometrial canal.
Submucosal fibroids (Fig GU 48-12)	A cause of postmenopausal bleeding, uterine leiomyomas are benign soft-tissue tumors that occur in women of all ages. Although their size and frequency decrease with age, they may grow until menopause and then involute. Fibroids typically are hypoechoic solid masses, which may be heterogeneous or hyperechoic, depending on the degree of degeneration and calcification. Submucosal fibroids may distort the uterine cavity with varying degrees of intracavitary extension, which is best visualized at sonohysterography. Determining the intracavitary extent of a leiomyoma is important for surgical management because hysteroscopic myomectomy can be performed if more than half the volume of the mass is within the endometrial canal.
Endometrial hyperplasia (Fig GU 48-13)	Abnormal proliferation of endometrial stroma and glands, which represents a spectrum of endometrial changes ranging from glandular atypia to frank neoplasia. Biopsy is required for a definitive diagnosis of this process, which is thought to precede up to one-third of endometrial carcinoma. Ultrasound shows diffusely smooth or, less commonly, focal hyperechoic endometrial thickening. Asymmetric thickening with surface irregularity may produce an appearance that is suspicious for cancer.

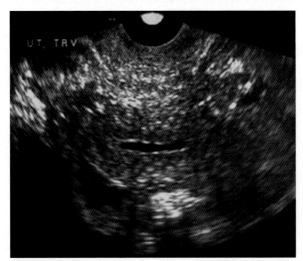

Fig GU 48-10
Postmenopausal endometrial atrophy. The endometrium has thin walls and is outlined with fluid.[72]

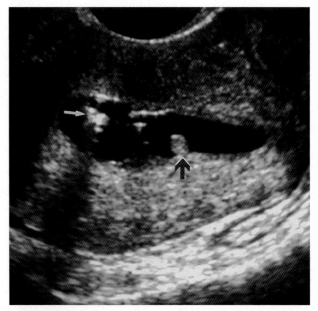

Fig GU 48-11
Endometrial polyp. Sonohysterogram reveals a small polyp attached by a stalk to the endometrium (black arrow). An echogenic focus in the endometrial cavity (white arrow) represents injected air.[72]

Condition	Comments
Endometrial adenocarcinoma (Fig GU 48-14)	Although the most common invasive gynecologic malignancy, due to early detection and treatment it is not a leading cause of cancer deaths. It produces nonspecific heterogeneity and irregular endometrial thickening. Demonstration of irregularity of the endometrium–myometrium border indicates invasive disease. The detection of an intrauterine fluid collection in a postmenopausal woman, although possibly related to cervical stenosis, should raise concern for endometrial (or cervical) carcinoma.

A

B

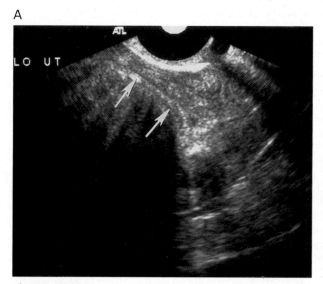
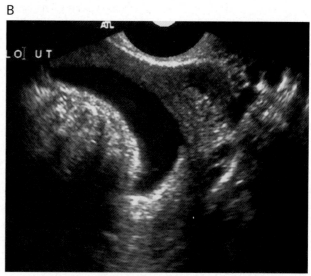

Fig GU 48-12
Submucosal fibroid. (A) Transvaginal sonogram shows a uterine mass (arrows) with posterior acoustic shadowing. (B) Sono-hysterogram demonstrates the submucosal location of the mass, a finding that is consistent with an echogenic fibroid.[72]

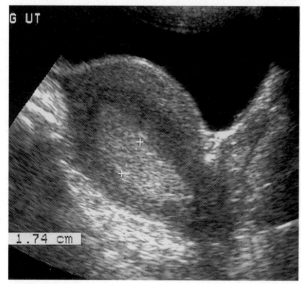

Fig GU 48-13
Endometrial hyperplasia. There is diffuse thickening of the endometrium.[72]

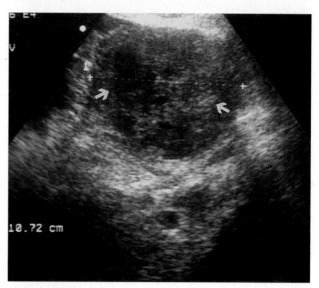

Fig GU 48-14
Endometrial adenocarcinoma. Heterogeneous endometrial mass (arrows) that is difficult to distinguish from the myometrium. Cursors indicate the entire transverse width of the uterus.[72]

Complications of Pregnancy

Condition	Imaging Findings	Comments
Blighted ovum (Fig GU 49-1)	Large, often irregularly shaped gestational sac with no evidence of fetal echoes.	Blighted ovum (anembryonic pregnancy) is the term for an abnormal pregnancy in which the embryo either develops abnormally or has failed to develop. The gestational sac may develop normally even without any embryo in the uterus, and a yolk sac is usually present. Although of unknown cause, blighted ovum generally is associated with an abnormal karyotype (primarily autosomal trisomy, triploidy, or monosomy X).
Abortion		Premature termination of pregnancy.
Incomplete (Fig GU 49-2)	Large, distorted sac containing retained products of conception and either fetal parts or no evidence of an embryo.	Retention of some of the products of conception within the uterus (portions of nonviable fetus and/or placenta, membranes, and blood clot).
Missed (Fig GU 49-3)	Retention of nonviable pregnancy within the uterus for at least 2 months.	This type of abortion generally occurs in the late first trimester when the uterus is smaller than expected for the stage of pregnancy.
Incompetent cervix (Fig GU 49-4)	Abnormal dilatation of a shortened endocervical canal with protrusion of fluid-containing membranous tissue.	Premature dilatation of the endocervical canal before the onset of labor. Generally occurs in the second trimester without any vaginal bleeding or labor pain, and it may recur with subsequent pregnancies. Predisposing factors include cervical trauma (dilatation and curettage, cone biopsy), abortion (with laceration and cauterization), and congenital normal variations.

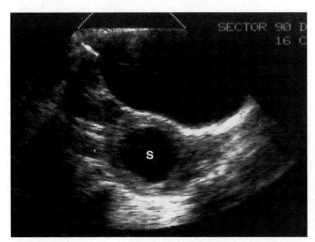

Fig GU 49-1
Blighted ovum. Sagittal scan identifies an enlarged gestational sac (S) without fetal echoes.[27]

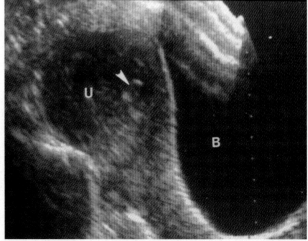

Fig GU 49-2
Incomplete abortion. Enlarged sagittal sonogram of the uterus (U) shows the retained products of conception and a nonviable fetus (arrowhead). (B, bladder.)[27]

Condition	Imaging Findings	Comments
Ectopic pregnancy (Figs GU 49-5 through GU 49-7)	Extrauterine gestational sac containing a live embryo is most definitive sonographic sign (but is present in less than 5% of cases). An irregular adnexal mass and blood in the cul-de-sac are other important findings, as is the adnexal ring sign (sac-like extrauterine structure that develops when the lining of the fallopian tube surrounding the ectopic sac expands and becomes more echogenic due to trophoblastic reaction). Pseudogestational sac (surrounded by a single echogenic layer of decidua) representing blood in the endometrial cavity may be seen in the uterus in ectopic pregnancy (rather than the "double decidual sac sign" of an intrauterine pregnancy).	Potentially life-threatening disorder that is a leading cause of maternal death. More than 95% of ectopic pregnancies occur within the fallopian tubes, especially in patients with evidence of prior pelvic inflammatory disease. The demonstration of a normal-appearing intrauterine pregnancy (embryo with fetal cardiac activity; yolk sac; or gestational sac) virtually excludes an ectopic pregnancy, as co-existing intrauterine and extrauterine pregnancies occur in only 1 of 30,000 cases.

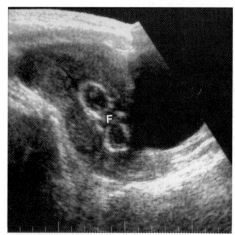

Fig GU 49-3
Missed abortion. Sagittal scan of the uterus shows a nonviable fetus (F) and no definable placenta.[27]

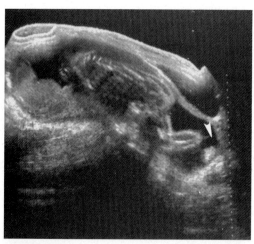

Fig GU 49-4
Incompetent cervix. Sagittal sonogram shows a shortened endocervical canal (arrowhead).[27]

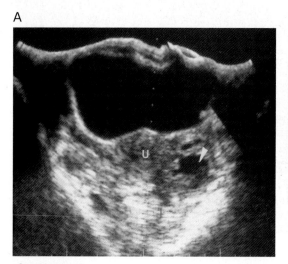
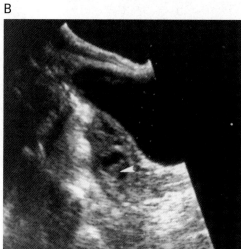

Fig GU 49-5
Ectopic pregnancy. (A) Transverse sonogram demonstrates the ectopic gestational sac in the left adnexa (arrowhead), outside the uterus (U). (B) Sagittal sonogram of the left adnexa identifies the gestational sac and the fetal pole (arrowhead).[27]

Condition	Imaging Findings	Comments
Trophoblastic disease (Fig GU 49-8)	Large solid mass of placental (trophoblastic) tissue filling the uterine cavity and containing echoes of low to moderate amplitude. Typically contains multiple tiny cystic areas scattered throughout the lesion.	Spectrum of pregnancy-related disorders ranging from a benign hydatidiform mole to the more malignant and frequently metastatic chorio-carcinoma. The level of β-HCG can be used to diagnose, monitor treatment response, and follow up trophoblastic disease (though it may take up to 4 months for the level to return to normal after the tumor has been evacuated).
Placenta previa (Figs GU 49-9 and GU 49-10)	Abnormal positioning of the echogenic placenta so that a portion either partially or completely covers the cervical os.	A low-lying placenta is common during the second trimester, but the majority converts to a normal position by the time of delivery. The most common clinical presentation is painless vaginal bleeding, primarily in the third trimester.

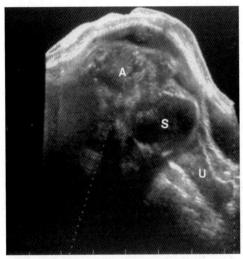

Fig GU 49-6
Ectopic pregnancy. Sonogram demonstrates a late abdominal pregnancy with the skull (S) and abdomen (A) of the fetus outside the uterus (U).[27]

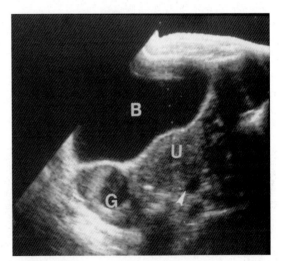

Fig GU 49-7
Ectopic pregnancy. Transverse sonogram of the pelvis shows fluid in the cul-de-sac (arrowhead) in addition to the uterus (U) and the ectopic gestational sac (G). (B, bladder.)[27]

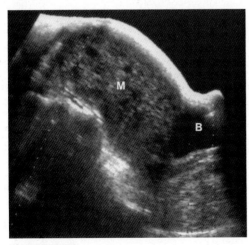

Fig GU 49-8
Trophoblastic disease. Sagittal sonogram of the pelvis shows a large mass (M) with cystic spaces filling the uterus. (B, bladder.)[27]

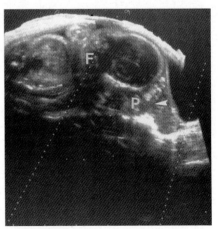

Fig GU 49-9
Placenta previa (total). Sagittal midline sonogram in the last trimester shows the placenta (P) completely covering the internal cervical os (arrowhead). (F, fetus.)[27]

Condition	Imaging Findings	Comments
Abruptio placentae (Fig GU 49-11)	Hematoma with varying echotexture (depending on its age) that most commonly occurs in a subchorionic location because of an abruption at the edge of the placenta. Retroplacental hemorrhage occurs with more central abruption.	Premature separation of a normally positioned placenta from the myometrium that may cause vaginal bleeding, pelvic or abdominal pain, fetal distress, and coagulopathy disorders. May range from clinically silent to severe and life-threatening hemorrhage. Occurs in 1% of pregnancies and is associated with premature labor and delivery and a perinatal mortality rate of 15% to 25%. Risk factors include maternal hypertension, smoking, and cocaine abuse.
Co-existent pelvic mass (Figs GU 49-12 and GU 49-13)	Combination of a fetus and a mass in the uterus or ovary.	Primarily leiomyoma or cystadenoma. Leiomyomas situated in the lower uterine segment predispose to obstructed labor; abortions are more prevalent in patients with multiple fibroids and those located in the body of the uterus. Cystadenomas often show significant growth during pregnancy; pedunculated tumors may undergo torsion, and rupture may occur.

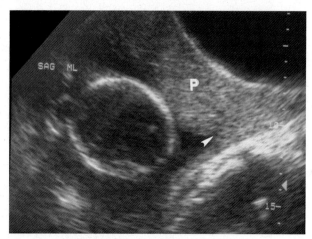

Fig GU 49-10
Placenta previa (partial). Sagittal sonogram shows the placenta (P) partially covering the cervical os (arrowhead).[27]

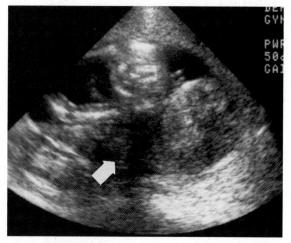

Fig GU 49-11
Abruptio placentae. Transverse sonogram shows abruptio with hematoma formation (arrow).[27]

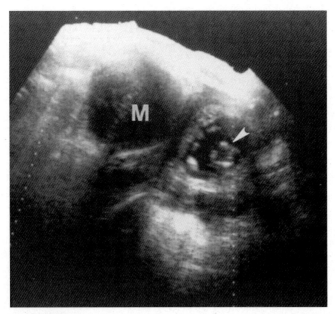

Fig GU 49-12
Coexisting leiomyoma. Sagittal sonogram demonstrates the pregnant uterus (arrowhead) and the hypoechoic mass (M).[27]

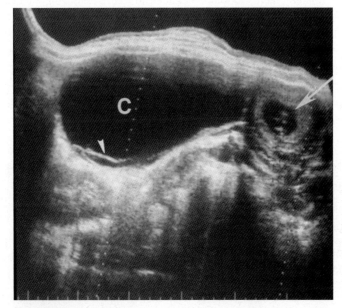

Fig GU 49-13
Coexisting cystadenoma. Sagittal sonogram shows a large cystic mass (C) with septation (arrowhead) and a viable pregnancy.[27]

Fluid Collection in the Scrotum

Condition	Imaging Findings	Comments
Hydrocele (Figs GU 50-1 and GU 50-2)	Echo-free zone with strong posterior sound transmission. The wall shows various degrees of thickness and may contain calcific deposits. The underlying testis is well visualized and is smoothly surrounded by fluid, except on its posterior surface where the testis is attached to the epididymis.	Abnormal accumulation of serous fluid between the tunica vaginalis and its contents. May be congenital (because of a direct communication with the abdominal cavity as a result of failure of the processus vaginalis to close) or secondary to an adjacent disease process (epididymitis, tuberculosis, trauma, mumps). Septations in a hydrocele suggest hemorrhage or infection. Internal echoes represent fibrous bodies that originate from a detached villous projection or from the tunica vaginalis.
Varicocele (Fig GU 50-3)	Tubular, serpiginous, anechoic fluid collection in the region of the epididymis just proximal to the upper pole of the testicle. The multicystic pattern reflects the bag-of-worms appearance of a varicocele on physical examination.	Dilatation and tortuosity of the veins of the pampiniform plexus that are most commonly observed on the left side of the scrotum. Primary varicoceles are predominantly seen in young boys. Secondary varicoceles usually result from obstruction of the renal vein, spermatic vein, or inferior vena cava.
Spermatocele (Fig GU 50-4)	Echo-free fluid collection that can be differentiated from a hydrocele because of its anatomic location (a spermatocele is located in the epididymis and displaces the testicle anteriorly, whereas a hydrocele usually surrounds the testicle anteriorly).	Retention cyst of small tubules that originates at the head of the epididymis and is often bilateral. Echogenic material in a spermatocele may represent sediment composed of cellular debris, fat, or spermatozoa.

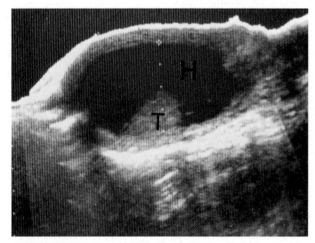

Fig GU 50-1
Hydrocele. The normal testis (T) is surrounded by a large, anechoic hydrocele (H).

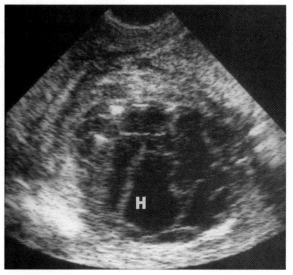

Fig GU 50-2
Multilocular hydrocele. Transverse scan shows a complicated hydrocele (H) with thin septations.[27]

Condition	Imaging Findings	Comments
Cyst (Fig GU 50-5)	Anechoic, well-defined structure with a sharp wall and good through-transmission of sound.	Testicular cysts are more common than previously believed and are often detected as an incidental finding. May be congenital or post-traumatic, though the precise etiology is unclear. Epididymal cysts are secondary to intrinsic cystic dilatation of the epididymal tubules and are filled with serous fluid.

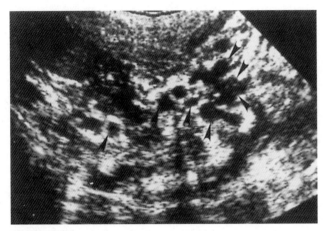

Fig GU 50-3
Varicocele. Real-time scan demonstrates multiple lucent tubular structures (arrowheads).[27]

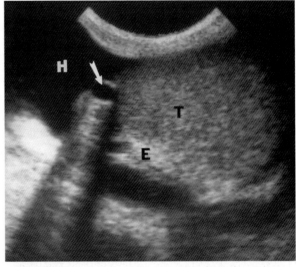

Fig GU 50-4
Spermatocele. Sagittal scan of the scrotum shows an anechoic mass (arrow) in the head of the epididymis. (E, body of epididymis; H, hydrocele; T, testis.)[27]

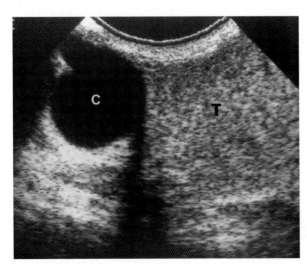

Fig GU 50-5
Epididymal cyst. Sagittal scan shows an anechoic mass (C) in the head of the epididymis. (T, testis.)[27]

Sources

1. Reprinted with permission from "The Cortical Rim Sign in Renal Infarction" by GJ Paul and TF Stephenson, *Radiology* (1977;122:338), Copyright ©1977, Radiological Society of North America Inc.

2. Reprinted from *Uroradiology: An Integrated Approach* by GW Friedland et al (Eds) with permission of Churchill Livingstone Inc, ©1983.

3. Reprinted with permission from "Genitourinary Tuberculosis" by AK Tonkin and DM Witten, *Seminars in Roentgenology* (1979;14:305–318), Copyright ©1979, Grune & Stratton Inc.

4. Reprinted from *Clinical Urography: An Atlas and Textbook of Urological Imaging* by HM Pollack (Ed) with permission of WB Saunders Company, ©1990.

5. Reprinted from *Radiologic Diagnosis of Renal Parenchymal Disease* by AJ Davidson with permission of WB Saunders Company, ©1977.

6. Reprinted with permission from "Polycystic Kidney Disease" by MA Bosniak and MA Ambos, *Seminars in Roentgenology* (1975;10: 133–143), Copyright ©1975, Grune & Stratton Inc.

7. Reprinted from *Radiographic Atlas of the Genitourinary System* by C Ney and RM Friedenberg with permission of JB Lippincott Company, ©1981.

8. Reprinted with permission from "The Thick-Wall Sign: An Important Finding in Nephrotomography" by MA Bosniak and D Faegenburg, *Radiology* (1965;84:692–698), Copyright ©1965, Radiological Society of North America Inc.

9. Reprinted with permission from "The Radiology of Juxtaglomerular Tumors" by NR Dunnick et al, *Radiology* (1983;147:321–326), Copyright ©1983, Radiological Society of North America Inc.

10. Reprinted with permission from "The Radiological Diagnosis of Congenital Multicystic Kidney: 'Radiological Triad'" by M Kyaw, *Clinical Radiology* (1974;25:45–62), Copyright ©1974, Royal College of Radiologists.

11. Reprinted with permission from "Early Medullary Cystic Disease" by FA Burgener and RF Spataro, *Radiology* (1979;130:321–322), Copyright ©1979, Radiological Society of North America Inc.

12. Reprinted with permission from "Ultrasonic Characteristic of Chronic Atrophic Pyelonephritis" by CJ Kay et al, *American Journal of Roentgenology* (1979;132:47–53), Copyright ©1979, American Roentgen Ray Society.

13. Reprinted with permission from "Diagnostic Value of CT Numbers in Pelvocalyceal Filling Defects" by RA Parienty et al, *Radiology* (1982;145:743–747), Copyright ©1982, Radiological Society of North America Inc.

14. Reprinted with permission from "The 'Stipple Sign': Urographic Harbinger of Transitional Cell Neoplasms" by GK McLean, HM Pollack, and MP Banner, *Urologic Radiology* (1979;1:77–83), Copyright ©1979, Springer-Verlag.

15. Reprinted with permission from "Fungus Balls in the Renal Pelvis" by RA Boldus, RC Brown, and DA Culp, *Radiology* (1972;102:555–557), Copyright ©1972, Radiological Society of North America Inc.

16. Reprinted with permission from "Renal Vein Thrombosis: Occurrence in Membranous Glomerulonephropathy and Lupus Nephritis" by WG Bradley et al, *Radiology* (1981;139:571–576), Copyright ©1981, Radiological Society of North America Inc.

17. Reprinted from *Clinical Urography* by DM Witten, GH Myers, and BC Utz with permission of WB Saunders Company, ©1977.

18. Reprinted with permission from "Malakoplakia of the Urinary Tract" by GB Elliott, PJ Maloney, and JG Clement, *American Journal of Roentgenology* (1972;116:830–837), Copyright ©1972, American Roentgen Ray Society.

19. Reprinted with permission from "Valves of the Ureter" by KW Albertson and LB Talner, *Radiology* (1972;103:91), Copyright ©1972, Radiological Society of North America Inc.

20. Reprinted with permission from "Lateral Ureteral Displacement: Sign of Nonvisualized Duplication" by AD Amar, *Journal of Urology* (1971;105:638–641), Copyright ©1971, Williams & Wilkins Company.

21. Reprinted with permission from "The Radiology of Urinary Diversions" by MP Banner et al, *Radiographics* (1984;4:885–913), Copyright ©1984, Radiological Society of North America Inc.

22. Reprinted with permission from "Hernias of the Ureters—An Anatomic-Roentgenographic Study" by HM Pollack, GL Popky, and ML Blumberg, *Radiology* (1975;117:275–281), Copyright ©1975, Radiological Society of North America Inc.

23. Reprinted from *Radiology of the Urinary System* by M Elkin with permission of Little, Brown & Company, ©1980.

24. Wong-You-Cheong JJ, Woodward PJ, Manning MA, Sesterhenn IA. Inflammatory and Nonneoplastic bladder masses: Radiologic-Pathologic Correlation. *RadioGraphics* 2006;26:1847–1868.

25. "Genitourinary Tract Gas: Imaging Evaluation" by RC Joseph et al, *RadioGraphics* (1996;16:295).

26. Reprinted with permission from "Posterior Urethral Valves" by GW Friedland et al, *Clinical Radiology* (1976;27:367–373), Copyright ©1976, Royal College of Radiologists.

27. Reprinted from *Ultrasound Atlas of Disease Processes* by CA Krebs, VL Giyanani, and RL Eisenberg, with permission of Appleton & Lange, ©1993.

28. "Imaging of Renal Masses" by NS Curry, *Radiologist* (1995;2:73–81).

29. Reprinted from *Ultrasound Home Study Course* by CA Krebs, with permission of the American Society of Radiologic Technologists, ©1990.

30. Reprinted from *Computed Body Tomography* by JKT Lee, SS Sagel, and RJ Stanley (Eds) with permission of Raven Press, New York, ©1983.

31. Reprinted with permission from "Angiomyolipoma: Ultrasonic-Pathologic Correlation" by DS Hartman et al, *Radiology* (1981;139: 451–458), Copyright ©1981, Radiological Society of North America Inc.

32. Rucker CM, Menias CO, Bhalla S. Mimics of renal colic: alternative diagnoses at unenhanced helical CT. *RadioGraphics* 2004;24: S11–S33.

33. Browne RFJ, Meehan CP, Colville J, et al. Transitional Cell carcinoma of the upper urinary tract: spectrum of imaging findings. *Radio-Graphics*. 2005;25:1609–1627.

34. Reprinted from *Computed Tomography of the Body* by AA Moss, G Gamsu, and HK Genant (Eds) with permission of WB Saunders Company, ©1983.

35. Kawashima A, Sandler CM, Corl FM, et al. Imaging of renal trauma: a comprehensive review. *RadioGraphics* 2001;21:557–574.

36. Rha SE, Byun JY, Jung SE, et al. The renal sinus: pathologic spectrum and multimodality imaging approach. *RadioGraphics* 2004;24: S117–S131.

37. Browne RFJ, Meehan CP, Colville J, et al. Transitional cell carcinoma of the upper urinary tract: spectrum of imaging findings. *Radio-Graphics* 2005;25:1609–1626.

38. Choi YJ, Hwang TK, Kang SJ, et al. Hemangiopericytoma of renal sinus expanding to the renal hilum: an unusual presentation causes misinterpretation as transitional cell carcinoma. *J Korean Med Sci* 1996;11:351–355.

39. Westphalen A, Yeh B, Gayyum A, et al. Differential diagnosis of perinephric masses on CT and MRI. *AJR*. 2004;183:1697–1792.

40. Reprinted with permission from "Renal Ultrasound: Test Your Interpretation" by RL Eisenberg et al, *Radiographics* (1982;2:153–178), Copyright ©1982, Radiological Society of North America Inc.

41. Mayo-Smith WW, Boland GW, Noto RB, Lee MJ. State-of-the-art adrenal imaging. *RadioGraphics* 2001;21:995–1012.

42. Reprinted from *Diagnostic Imaging in Internal Medicine* by RL Eisenberg with permission of McGraw-Hill Book Company, ©1985. Courtesy of Nolan Karstaedt, MD, and Neil Wolfman, MD.

43. Reprinted with permission from "Computed Tomography of the Adrenal Gland" by N Karstaedt et al, *Radiology* (1978;129:723–730), Copyright ©1978, Radiological Society of North America Inc.

44. "Magnetic Resonance Imaging of the Adrenal Gland" by GW Boland and MJ Lee, *Critical Reviews in Diagnostic Imaging* (1995;36:115–174).

45. Blake MA, Kalra M, Maher MM, et al. Pheochromocytoma: an imaging chameleon. *RadioGraphics* 2004;24:S87–S99.

46. Reprinted with permission from "Pheochromocytoma: Value of Computed Tomography" by TJ Welch et al, *Radiology* (1983;148: 501–503), Copyright ©1983, Radiological Society of North America Inc.

47. Otal P, Escourrou G, Mazerolles C, et al. Imaging features of uncommon adrenal masses with histopathologic correlation. *Radio-Graphics* 1999;19:569–581.

48. "State-of-the-Art MR Imaging of the Adrenal Gland" by MJ Lee, WW Mayo-Smith, PF Hahn, et al, *Radiographics* (1994;14:1015–1029).

49. Mayo-Smith WW, Boland GW, Noto RB, Lee MJ. State-of-the-art adrenal imaging. *Radiographics* 2001;21:995–1012.

50. Elsayes KM, Mukundan G, Narra VR, et al. Adrenal masses: MR imaging features with pathologic correlation. *RadioGraphics* 2004;24: S73–S86.

51. Wong-You-Cheong JJ, Woodward PJ, Manning MA, Sesterhenn IA. Neoplasms of the urinary bladder: radiologic-pathologic correlation. *RadioGraphics*. 2006;26:553–580.

52. Wong-You-Cheong JJ, Woodward PJ, Manning MA, Sesterhenn IA. Inflammatory and nonneoplastic bladder masses: radiologic-pathologic correlation. *RadioGraphics* 2006;26:1847–1868.

53. Levine DS, Navarro OM, Chaudry, et al. Imaging the complications of bone marrow transplantation in children. *RadioGraphics* 2007;27: 307–324.

54. Mengiardi B, Wiesner W, Stoffel F, et al. Case 44: adenocarcinoma of the urachus. *Radiology* 2002;222:744–747.

55. Kawashima A, Sandler CM, Wasserman NF, et al. Imaging of urethral disease: a pictorial review. *RadioGraphics* 2004;24:S195–S216.

56. Yang DM, Jung DH, Kim H, et al. Retroperitoneal cystic masses: CT, Clinical and pathologic findings and literature review. *RadioGraphics* 2004;24:1353–1365.

57. Attili AK, Kazerooni. Case 116: Lymphangioleiomyomatosis. *Radiology* 2007;244:303–308.

58. "Ovarian Masses Revisited: Radiologic and Pathologic Correlation" by CL Sutton, CD McKinney, JE Jones, et al, *Radiographics* (1992;12: 853–877).

59. Reprinted from *Ultrasonography in Obstetrics and Gynecology* by PW Callen (Ed) with permission of WB Saunders Company, ©1983.

60. Reprinted with permission from "Pediatric Gynecologic Radiology" by CK Grimes, DM Rosenbaum, and JA Kirkpatrick, *Seminars in Roentgenology* (1982;17:284–301), Copyright ©1982, Grune & Stratton Inc.

61. Reprinted from *Gynecology Sonography Home Study Course* by CA Krebs, with permission of the American Society of Radiologic Technologists, ©1990.

62. Kuligowska E, Deeds L, Lu K. Pelvic pain: overlooked and under-diagnosed gynecologic conditions. *RadioGraphics* 2005;25:3–20.

63. Reprinted with permission from "Ectopic Pregnancy: Sonographic-Pathologic Correlations" by BA Spirt et al, *Radiographics* (1984;4: 821–848), Copyright ©1984, Radiological Society of North America Inc.

64. Nalaboff KM, Pellerito JS, Ben-Levi, E. Imaging the endometrium: disease and normal variants. *RadioGraphics* 2001;21:1409–1424.

65. "Magnetic Resonance Imaging of the Uterus" by R Kier, *MRI Clinics of North America* (1994;2:189–210).

66. "MRI of the Female Pelvis: An Overview" by MD Patel, *Applied Radiology* (1994;31–38).

67. Kuligowska E, Deeds L, Lu K. Pelvic pain: overlooked and under-diagnosed gynecologic conditions. *RadioGraphics* 2005;25:3–20.

68. "MR Imaging of the Female Pelvic Region" by MC Olson, HV Posniak, CM Tempany, and CM Dudiak, *RadioGraphics* (1992;12:445–465).

69. "MRI of the Female Pelvis: When and How?" by MJ Lee and IC Yoder, *The Radiologist* (1994;1:201–207).

70. "Magnetic Resonance Imaging of the Ovary" by EK Outwater and ML Schiebler, *MRI Clinics of North America* (1994;2:245–274).

71. Imaoka I, Wada A, Kaji Y, et al. Developing an MR imaging strategy for diagnosis of ovarian masses. *RadioGraphics* 2006;26:1431–1448.

72. Nalaboff KM, Pellerito JS, Ben-Levi E. Imaging the endometrium: disease and normal variants. *RadioGraphics* 2001;21:1409–1424.

73. Kido A, Togashi K, Koyama T, et al. Diffusely enlarged uterus: evaluation with MR imaging. *RadioGraphics* 2003;23:1423–1439.

5

Skeletal Patterns

Localized Osteoporosis

Condition	Comments
Disuse atrophy (immobilization) (Fig B 1-1)	To maintain osteoblastic activity at normal levels, bones must be subjected to a normal amount of stress and muscular activity. Within a few weeks after the fracture of a bone, localized osteoporosis becomes detectable, especially distal to the site of injury. The cortical margin of an involved bone never completely disappears (unlike bone destruction due to disease). Similar disuse atrophy due to immobilization follows neural or muscular paralysis.
Sudeck's atrophy (reflex sympathetic dystrophy) (Fig B 1-2) ·	Rapid development of painful osteoporosis after relatively trivial injury. Probably of neurovascular origin, Sudeck's atrophy most often involves the hands and feet with a mottled, irregular osteoporosis that primarily affects the periarticular region. The juxta-articular cortex may become extremely thin but remains intact, unlike in an arthritic process.
Inflammatory disease (Fig B 1-3)	Localized osteoporosis often is the first (though nonspecific) radiographic manifestation of inflam-matory diseases such as osteomyelitis, tuberculosis, and rheumatoid arthritis. In pyogenic infections, bone destruction typically precedes osteoporosis, whereas in tuberculosis the reverse is true. Periarticular demineralization is a classic early sign of rheumatoid arthritis.
Burn, frostbite, electric shock (Fig B 1-4)	Bone demineralization, most marked where soft-tissue damage was greatest, is an early radio-graphic finding that may persist for a prolonged period.
Tumor (Figs B 1-5 and B 1-6)	Most commonly metastases and multiple myeloma. Also primary benign and malignant bone tumors.
Shoulder-hand syndrome	Radiographic appearance simulates that of Sudeck's atrophy. Shoulder pain and stiffness combined with pain, swelling, and vasomotor phenomena in the hand after an acute illness (especially myocardial infarction, in which the left side is usually involved).

A

B

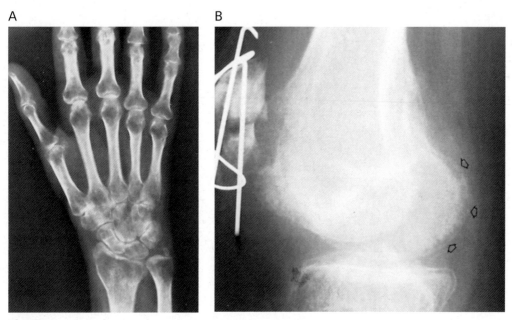

Fig B 1-1
Disuse osteoporosis. (A) Severe periarticular demineralization follows prolonged immobilization of the extremity. (B) In a patient with a fractured patella, there is pronounced subcortical demineralization in the distal femur. The cortical margin (arrows) remains intact.

Condition	Comments
Regional migratory osteoporosis (transitory osteoporosis)	Osteoporosis after the development of severe pain about a major joint (especially the hip, knee, or ankle) in a middle-aged or elderly adult. Often termed *transitory demineralization of the femoral head,* as the hip is most frequently involved. Self-limited but disabling disorder that heals completely in 2 to 4 months.

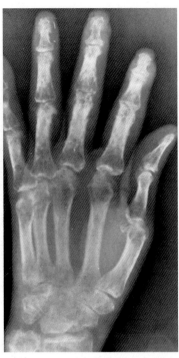

Fig B 1-2
Sudeck's atrophy. Patchy osteoporosis predominantly affecting the periarticular regions. Endosteal scalloping and intracortical striations are evident even without magnification films.

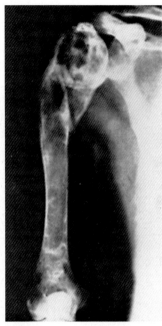

Fig B 1-4
Electrical injury. Comminuted fracture of the head and shaft of the humerus associated with mottled decalcification of the humeral head. The cortex of the humerus is thin, and the medullary cavity is widened. Discrete areas of rarefaction can be seen in the shaft and distal metaphyseal region.[1]

A   B

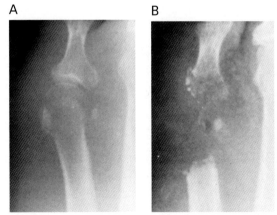

Fig B 1-3
Staphylococcal osteomyelitis. (A) Initial film of the first metatarsophalangeal joint shows soft-tissue swelling and periarticular demineralization due to hyperemia. (B) Several weeks later, there is severe bony destruction about the metatarsophalangeal joint.

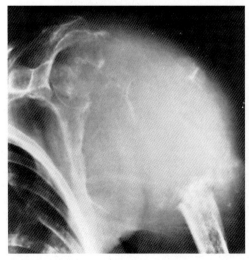

Fig B 1-5
Metastases to bone. Osteolytic (blowout) metastasis to the humerus from carcinoma of the kidney.

Condition	Comments
Osteoporosis circumscripta (Paget's disease) (Figs B 1-7 and B 1-8)	Early lytic phase of Paget's disease of the skull, in which an area of sharply demarcated radiolucency represents the destructive phase that primarily involves the outer table and spares the inner table. Deossification begins in the frontal or occipital area and slowly spreads to encompass the major portion of the calvarium. Irregular islands of sclerosis and diploic thickening during the reparative process result in the characteristic mottled, cotton-wool appearance. In long bones, the destructive phase typically begins at one edge of the bone and extends along the shaft for a variable distance to produce a sharply demarcated, V-shaped area of deossification (blade-of-grass appearance).
Diabetes mellitus (Fig B 1-9)	May produce severe localized osteoporosis mimicking bone destruction. There is often a substantial amount of bone restitution after conservative therapy.

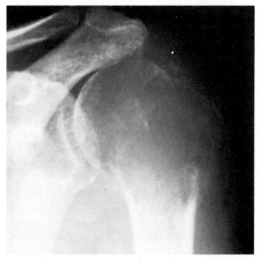

Fig B 1-6
Solitary plasmacytoma of the humeral head. The highly destructive lesion has expanded the bone and broken through the cortex.

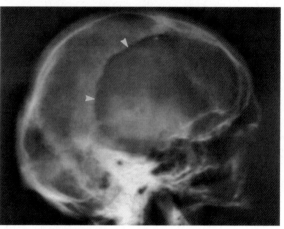

Fig B 1-7
Osteoporosis circumscripta. Well-defined area of osteolysis in the frontal and occipital regions of the skull (arrowheads) in Paget's disease.[2]

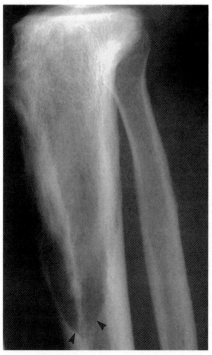

Fig B 1-8
Blade-of-grass appearance. Frontal view of the knee in a patient with Paget's disease shows a large osteolytic area that begins in the subchondral portion of the proximal tibia and has a sharp inferior margin (arrowheads).[2]

Condition	Comments
Avascular necrosis (Fig B 1-10)	Initially, avascular necrosis of cancellous bone causes localized demineralization. With healing, necrotic bone is replaced by new bone that is irregular in architecture and of greater density. When avascular necrosis involves the articular surface, the initial radiographic change is a crescent of lucency.
Hemophilia	Articular hemorrhage initially results in marked periarticular osteoporosis due to local hyperemia and disuse. As cartilage is destroyed, sclerosis of adjacent bone occurs with superimposed osteophytic and other degenerative changes.

A
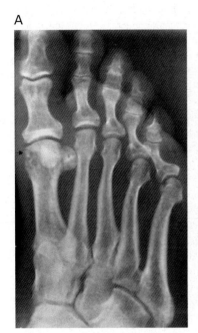
B
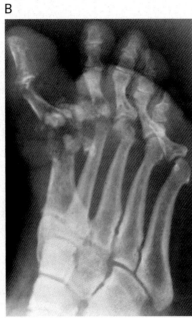

Fig B 1-9
Acute osteomyelitis in diabetes. (A) Initial film of the foot in a diabetic patient with a soft-tissue infection shows minimal hyperemic osteoporosis about the head of the first metatarsal with some loss of the sharp cortical outline (arrow). (B) One month later, there is severe bone destruction involving not only the head of the first metatarsal but also the rest of the big toe and the second and third metatarsophalangeal joints.

A
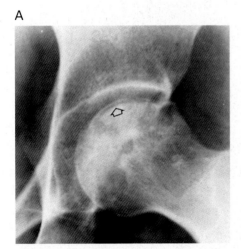
B
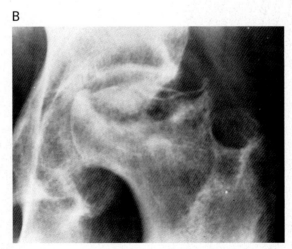

Fig B 1-10
Avascular necrosis of the femoral head. (A) An arc-like radiolucent cortical band (crescent sign) (arrow) in the femoral head represents a fracture line. (B) Eventually, there is a combination of lytic and sclerotic areas with severe flattening of the femoral head.

Generalized Osteoporosis

Condition	Comments
Osteoporosis of aging (senile or postmenopausal osteoporosis) (Fig B 2-1)	Most common form of generalized osteoporosis. As a person ages, the bones lose density and become more brittle, fracturing more easily and healing more slowly. Many elderly persons are also less active and have poor diets that are deficient in protein. Females are affected more often and more severely than males, as postmenopausal women have deficient gonadal hormone levels and decreased osteoblastic activity.
Drug-induced osteoporosis (Fig B 2-2)	Patients receiving large doses of steroids over several months often develop generalized osteoporosis. Patients treated with 15,000 to 30,000 U of heparin for 6 months or longer also may develop generalized osteoporosis (possibly due to a direct local stimulating effect of heparin on bone resorption).
Deficiency states Protein deficiency (or abnormal protein metabolism)	Inability to produce adequate bone matrix in such conditions as malnutrition, nephrosis, diabetes mellitus, Cushing's syndrome, and hyperparathyroidism. Also patients with severe liver disease (hepatocellular degeneration, large or multiple liver cysts or tumors, biliary atresia). Pure dietary protein deficiency is rare in developed countries.

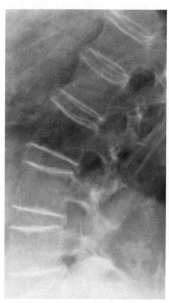

Fig B 2-1
Osteoporosis of aging. Generalized demineralization of the spine in a postmenopausal woman. The cortex appears as a thin line that is relatively dense and prominent (picture-frame pattern).

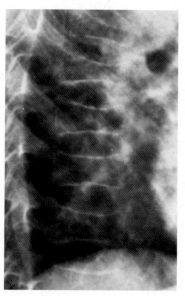

Fig B 2-2
Steroid therapy. Lateral view of the thoracic spine in a patient on high-dose steroid therapy for dermatomyositis demonstrates severe osteoporosis with thinning of cortical margins and biconcave deformities of vertebral bodies.

Condition	Comments
Vitamin C deficiency (scurvy) (Fig B 2-3)	Deficiency of ascorbic acid causes abnormal function of osteoblasts and defective osteogenesis. Characteristic radiographic findings include widening and increased density of the zone of provisional calcification (the "white line" of scurvy); marginal spur formation (Pelken's spur); demineralization of epiphyseal ossification centers that are surrounded by a dense, sharply demarcated ring of calcification (Wimberger's sign); and subperiosteal hemorrhage along the shafts of long bones (calcification of elevated periosteum and hematoma is a radiographic sign of healing).
Intestinal malabsorption	Underlying mechanism in such conditions as sprue, scleroderma, pancreatic disease (insufficiency, chronic pancreatitis, mucoviscidosis), Crohn's disease, decreased absorptive surface of the small bowel (resection, bypass procedure), infiltrative disorders of the small bowel (eosinophilic enteritis, lactase deficiency, lymphoma, Whipple's disease), and idiopathic steatorrhea.
Endocrine disorders (Fig B 2-4)	Hypogonadism (especially Turner's syndrome and menopause); adrenocortical abnormality (Cushing's syndrome, Addison's disease); non-endocrine steroid-producing tumor (eg, oat cell carcinoma); diabetes mellitus; pituitary abnormality (acromegaly, hypopituitarism); thyroid abnormality (hyperthyroidism and hypothyroidism).

A

B

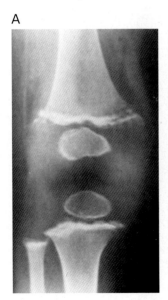
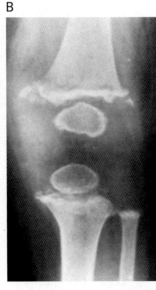

Fig B 2-3
Scurvy. (A and B) Frontal views of both knees demonstrate widening and increased density of the zone of provisional calcification, producing the characteristic white line of scurvy. Note also the submetaphyseal zone of lucency and the characteristic marginal spur formation (Pelken's spur). The epiphyseal ossification centers are surrounded by a dense, sharply demarcated ring of calcification (Wimberger's sign).

Condition	Comments
Neoplastic disorders (Figs B 2-5 and B 2-6)	Diffuse cellular proliferation in the bone marrow with no tendency to form discrete tumor masses may produce generalized skeletal deossification simulating postmenopausal osteoporosis in adults with multiple myeloma or diffuse skeletal metastases and in children with acute leukemia. Pressure atrophy produces cortical thinning and trabecular resorption.

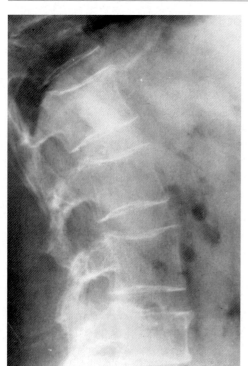

Fig B 2-4
Cushing's syndrome due to adrenal hyperplasia. Marked demineralization and an almost complete loss of trabeculae in the lumbar spine. The vertebral end plates are mildly concave, and the intervertebral disk spaces are slightly widened. Note the compression of the superior end plate of L4.[3]

B

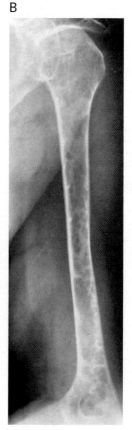

A

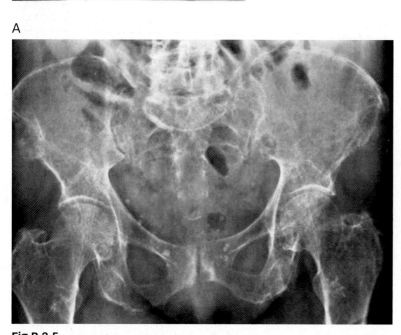

Fig B 2-5
Multiple myeloma. (A) Diffuse skeletal deossification involving the pelvis and proximal femurs. (B) Generalized demineralization of the humerus with thinning of the cortices.

Condition	Comments
Anemia (Fig B 2-7)	Extensive marrow hyperplasia widens medullary spaces and thins cortices in such conditions as thalassemia and sickle cell anemia. Severe iron deficiency can produce a similar appearance.
Collagen disease (Fig B 2-8)	Rheumatoid arthritis; ankylosing spondylitis; systemic lupus erythematosus; scleroderma; dermatomyositis. Usually associated with characteristic joint changes.
Osteogenesis imperfecta (Fig B 2-9)	Inherited generalized disorder of connective tissue with multiple fractures, hypermobility of joints, blue sclerae, poor teeth, deafness, and cardiovascular disorders such as mitral valve prolapse or aortic regurgitation. Osteogenesis imperfecta congenita develops in utero and appears at birth as bowing and deformity of the extremities due to multiple fractures (death in utero or soon after birth is usually caused by intracranial hemorrhage in these infants with paper-thin skulls). In the less severe tarda form, the disorder is first noted during childhood or young adulthood because of an unusual tendency for fractures, loose-jointedness, and the presence of blue sclerae. Fractures often heal with exuberant callus formation that may simulate a malignant tumor and cause bizarre deformities.

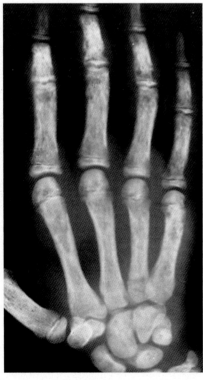

Fig B 2-6
Leukemia. Patchy areas of deossification throughout the metacarpals and phalanges.

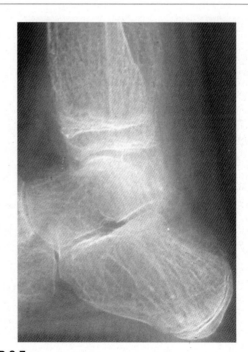

Fig B 2-7
Thalassemia. Lateral view of the ankle demonstrates pronounced widening of the medullary spaces with thinning of the cortices. Note the absence of normal modeling due to the pressure of the expanding marrow space. Localized radiolucencies simulating multiple osteolytic lesions represent tumorous collections of hyperplastic marrow.

Condition	Comments
Neuromuscular diseases and dystrophies (Fig B 2-10)	Decreased muscular tone leading to osteoporosis, bone atrophy with cortical thinning, scoliosis, and joint contractures occurs in congenital disorders and such acquired conditions as spinal cord disease and immobilization for chronic disease or major fracture. Lack of the stress stimulus of weight bearing is the underlying cause of the generalized disuse atrophy termed *space flight osteoporosis*.
Homocystinuria	Inborn error of methionine metabolism that causes a defect in the structure of collagen or elastin and a radiographic appearance similar to that of Marfan's syndrome. Striking osteoporosis of the spine and long bones (extremely rare in Marfan's syndrome).
Lipid storage diseases (Fig B 2-11)	Gaucher's disease and Niemann-Pick disease. Accumulation of abnormal quantities of complex lipids in the bone marrow produces a generalized loss of bone density and cortical thinning.
Hemochromatosis	Iron-storage disorder often associated with diffuse osteoporosis of the spine and vertebral collapse. Approximately half the patients have a characteristic arthropathy that most frequently involves the small joints of the hand. Hepatosplenomegaly and portal hypertension are common.

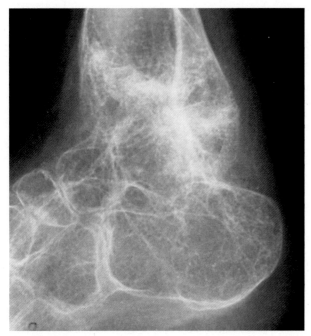

Fig B 2-8
Juvenile rheumatoid arthritis. Lateral view of the ankle demonstrates severe demineralization of bone. Note the pronounced narrowing of the joints involving the talus and other tarsal bones.

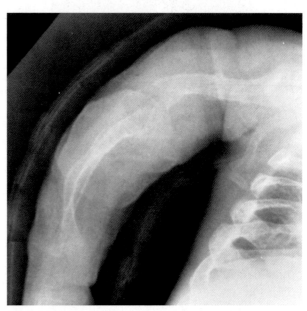

Fig B 2-9
Osteogenesis imperfecta. Pronounced osteoporosis and cortical thinning of all bones with evidence of previous fractures and resultant deformities.

Condition	Comments
Hemophilia (see Fig B 10-19)	Multiple episodes of hemarthrosis may cause hyperemia combined with atrophy of bone and muscle, resulting in severe osteoporosis. Radiographic signs suggestive of hemophilia include abnormally large or prematurely fused epiphyses, widening and deepening of the intercondylar notch of the femur, and squaring of the inferior border of the patella.
Idiopathic juvenile osteoporosis	Rare condition characterized by the abrupt onset of generalized or focal bone pain in children 8 to12 years of age. The disease is usually self-limited with spontaneous radiologic and clinical improvement.

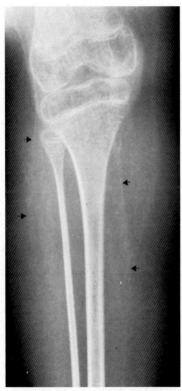

Fig B 2-10
Muscular dystrophy. Thin, demineralized bones of the lower leg. The increased lucency, representing fatty infiltration in muscle bundles, makes the fascial sheaths appear as thin shadows of increased density (arrows) surrounded by fat.

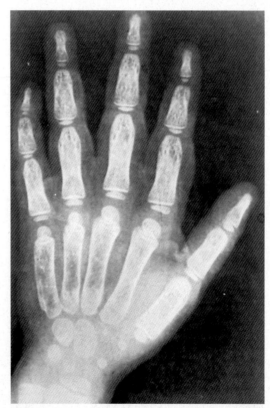

Fig B 2-11
Niemann-Pick disease. Diffuse widening of the metacarpals and phalanges with thin cortices and coarsened trabeculae.[4]

Osteomalacia

Condition	Comments
Deficient absorption of calcium or phosphorus Rickets (Fig B 3-1)	Systemic disease of infancy and childhood in which calcification of growing skeletal elements is defective because of a deficiency of vitamin D in the diet or a lack of exposure to ultraviolet radiation (sunshine). Most common in premature infants and usually develops between 6 and 12 months of age. Classic radiographic signs include cupping and fraying of metaphyseal ends of bone with disappearance of normally sharp metaphyseal lines; delayed appearance of epiphyseal ossification centers, which have blurred margins (unlike the sharp outlines in scurvy); and excessive osteoid tissue in the sternal ends of ribs producing characteristic beading (rachitic rosary).
Malabsorption states	Primary small bowel disease (sprue, Crohn's disease, lymphoma, small bowel fistula, amyloidosis); pancreatic insufficiency (exocrine) or inflammation; hepatobiliary disease (biliary atresia or acquired chronic biliary obstruction); postoperative gastric or small bowel resection; mesenteric disease; cathartic abuse.
Dietary calcium deficiency	Extremely rare.

A
B

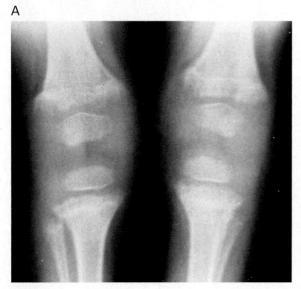
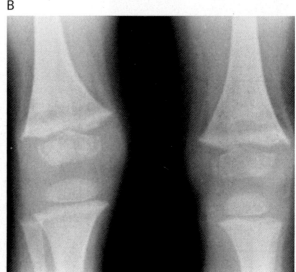

Fig B 3-1
Rickets. (A) Initial film shows severe metaphyseal changes involving the distal femurs and proximal tibias and fibulas. Note the pronounced demineralization of the epiphyseal ossification centers. **(B)** After vitamin D therapy, there is remineralization of the metaphyses and an almost normal appearance of the epiphyseal ossification centers.

Condition	Comments
Excessive renal excretion of calcium or phosphorus	
Renal tubular acidosis (Fig B 3-2)	Kidney is unable to excrete an acidic urine (below pH 5.4) because the distal nephron cannot secrete hydrogen against a concentration gradient. This can lead to cation wasting (calcium and potassium) and so-called "renal rickets." Usually there is very dense and extensive renal parenchymal calcification, often associated with staghorn calculi.
Vitamin D–resistant rickets	Hereditary disorder (X-linked dominant) with diminished proximal tubular resorption of phosphorus. May also reflect an end-organ resistance to vitamin D.
Fanconi's syndrome	Multiple defects of renal tubular resorption that may be inherited (autosomal recessive) or acquired secondary to such conditions as Wilson's disease, multiple myeloma, and lead or cadmium intoxication. Characterized by hypophosphatemia and large amounts of glucose, amino acids, and protein in the urine.
Hyperparathyroidism (Fig B 3-3)	Excessive secretion of parathyroid hormone leads to a generalized disorder of calcium, phosphorus, and bone metabolism resulting in elevated serum calcium and phosphate. May be primary (adenoma, carcinoma, or generalized hyperplasia of all glands; parathormone-like secretion by nonparathyroid tumor) or secondary (more common and most often due to chronic renal failure). Classic radiographic signs include subperiosteal bone resorption, generalized osteosclerosis (including rugger-jersey spine), brown tumors, salt-and-pepper skull, and soft-tissue calcification. Increased incidence of nephrocalcinosis, urinary tract calculi, pancreatitis, peptic ulcer, and gallstones.

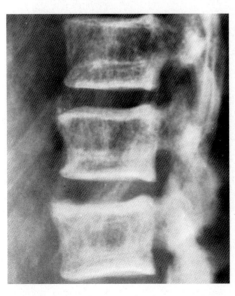

Fig B 3-2
Rickets due to renal tubular disorder. Striking thickening of the cortices of the vertebral bodies with increased trabeculation of spongy bone.

Condition	Comments
Hypophosphatasia (Fig B 3-4)	Inherited (autosomal recessive) metabolic disorder in which a low level of alkaline phosphatase leads to defective mineralization of bone. Hypophosphatasia discovered in utero or during the first few days of life is generally fatal, with the calvarium and many bones of the skeleton uncalcified. If the condition develops later, the radiographic appearance closely resembles that of rickets with large unossified areas in the skull simulating severe widening of sutures. High incidence of fractures and bone deformities.
Wilson's disease (Fig B 3-5)	Rare familial disorder in which impaired hepatic excretion of copper results in toxic accumulation of the metal in the liver, brain, and other organs. Characteristic pigmentation of the cornea (Kayser-Fleischer ring). Approximately half the patients demonstrate skeletal changes.
Anticonvulsant drug therapy	Prolonged use of anticonvulsants (eg, dilantin) and many tranquilizers stimulates hepatic enzymatic activity, resulting in accelerated degradation of biologically active vitamin D_3 to inactive metabolites.
Fibrogenesis imperfecta and axial osteomalacia	Extremely rare conditions of older individuals in which acquired vitamin D resistance leads to osteomalacia in both the axial and appendicular bones (fibrogenesis imperfecta) or only the axial skeleton (axial osteomalacia).

A

B

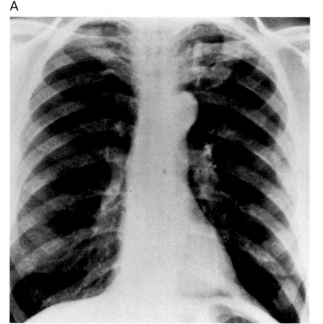
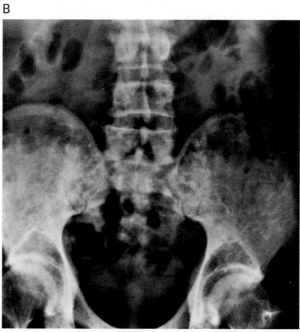

Fig B 3-3
Hyperparathyroidism. Views of **(A)** the chest and **(B)** the abdomen show generalized bony demineralization with striking prominence of residual trabeculae (especially in the ribs).

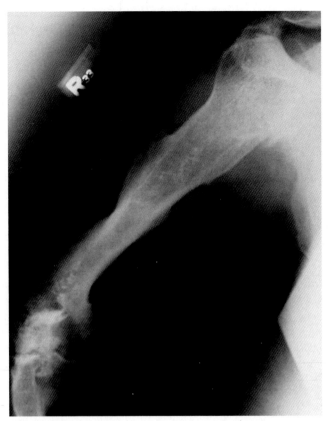

Fig B 3-4
Hypophosphatasia. Osteomalacia of the arm with ossification of the deltoid and other muscle insertions. Severe manifestations of the condition in a 43-year-old man, 4 feet 9 inches tall.[5]

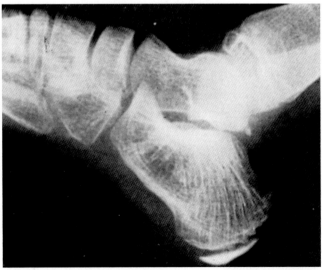

Fig B 3-5
Wilson's disease. Lateral view of the ankle and foot demonstrates marked demineralization, thinning of the cortex, and coarsening of the trabecular pattern, all best seen in the os calcis.[6]

Solitary or Multiple Osteosclerotic Bone Lesions

Condition	Imaging Findings	Comments
Bone island	Single or multiple areas of dense compact bone that most commonly occur in the pelvis and upper femurs. Sharply demarcated lesion, though the margins often display thorny radiation giving a brush border appearance.	Asymptomatic and completely benign. Almost half enlarge over a period of years and many show activity on radionuclide bone scans (must be distinguished from osteoblastic metastases).
Osteoma (see Fig SK 1-9)	Well-circumscribed, extremely dense round lesion (rarely larger than 2 cm). Most often arises in the outer table of the skull, paranasal sinuses (especially frontal and ethmoid), and mandible.	Benign hamartomatous lesion consisting exclusively of osseous tissue. Osteomas (often multiple) are associated with soft-tissue tumors and multiple premalignant colonic polyps in Gardner's syndrome.
Osteoid osteoma (Fig B 4-1)	Small, round or oval lucent nidus (less than 1 cm in diameter) surrounded by a large, dense sclerotic zone of cortical thickening. Although usually located in the cortex, the nidus may be in an intramedullary or subperiosteal position and be difficult to detect.	Benign bone tumor that usually develops in young men. Classic clinical symptom is local pain that is worse at night and dramatically relieved by aspirin. At times, the dense sclerotic reaction may obscure the nidus on conventional radiographs and require tomography (conventional or computed) for demonstration. Surgical excision of the nidus is essential for cure (it is not necessary to remove the reactive calcification).
Osteoblastic metastases (Figs B 4-2 and B 4-3)	Single or multiple ill-defined areas of increased density that may progress to complete loss of normal bony architecture. Varies from a small, isolated round focus of sclerotic density to a diffuse sclerosis involving most or all of a bone (eg, ivory vertebral body).	Osteoblastic metastases are most commonly secondary to lymphoma and carcinomas of the breast and prostate. Other primary tumors include carcinomas of the gastrointestinal tract, lung, and urinary bladder. Osteoblastic metastases are generally considered to be evidence of slow growth in a neoplasm that has allowed time for reactive bone proliferation.

A

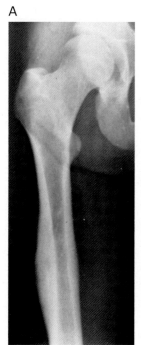

B

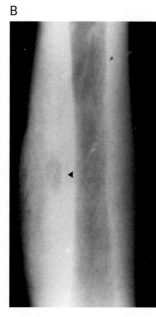

Fig B 4-1
Osteoid osteoma. (A) Full and (B) coned views of the midshaft of the femur demonstrate a dense sclerotic zone of cortical thickening laterally, which contains a small oval lucent nidus (arrowhead).

Condition	Imaging Findings	Comments
Osteochondroma (exostosis) (Figs B 4-4 through B 4-6)	Projection of bone that initially grows outward at a right angle to the host bone. As the lesion grows, the pull of neighboring muscles and tendons orients the tumor parallel to the long axis of the bone and pointed away from the nearest joint. Typically there is blending of the cortex of an osteochondroma with that of normal bone. In flat bones, an osteochondroma appears as a relatively localized area of amorphous, spotty calcification.	Benign projection of bone with a cartilaginous cap that probably represents a local dysplasia of cartilage at the epiphyseal growth plate. The lesion arises in childhood or adolescence and continues to grow until fusion of the closest epiphyseal line. Most commonly develops in the metaphyseal region of a long bone (eg, femur, tibia, or humerus). Rapid growth or the development of localized pain suggests malignant degeneration to chondrosarcoma. There are multiple and bilateral osteochondromas in hereditary multiple exotoses (diaphyseal aclasis).

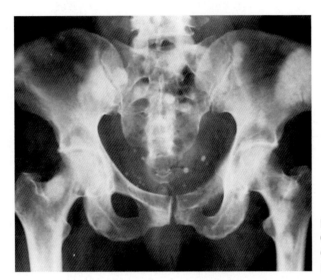

Fig B 4-2
Osteoblastic metastases. Multiple areas of increased density involving the pelvis and proximal femurs representing metastases from carcinoma of the urinary bladder.

A

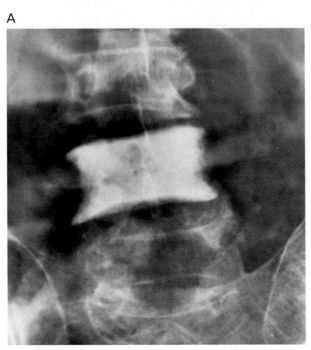

B

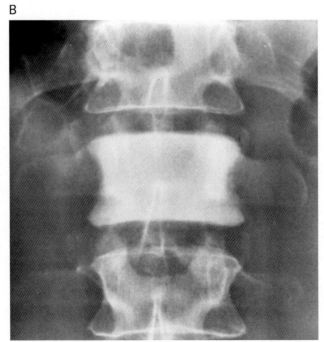

Fig B 4-3
Ivory vertebrae. (A) Carcinoma of the prostate. (B) Lymphoma.

Condition	Imaging Findings	Comments
Callus formation	Localized increase in bone density about a healed or healing fracture.	Callus formation about a rib fracture may simulate a pulmonary nodule and necessitate oblique views or chest fluoroscopy for differentiation.
Bone infarct in shaft (Fig B 4-7)	Densely calcified area in the medullary cavity. May be sharply limited by a dense sclerotic zone or be associated with serpiginous dense streaks extending from the central region of calcification.	Underlying causes include occlusive vascular disease, sickle cell anemia, collagen disease, chronic pancreatitis, Gaucher's disease, and radiation therapy.

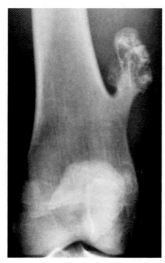

Fig B 4-4
Osteochondroma of the distal femur. The long axis of the tumor is parallel to that of the femur and pointed away from the knee joint.

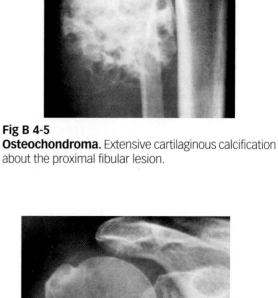

Fig B 4-5
Osteochondroma. Extensive cartilaginous calcification about the proximal fibular lesion.

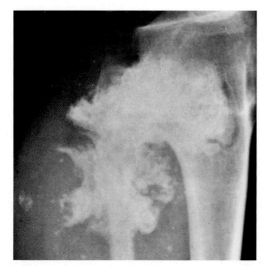

Fig B 4-6
Multiple exostoses with sarcomatous degeneration. A chondrosarcoma from one of the many exostoses in this patient appears as a large soft-tissue mass with amorphous calcification.

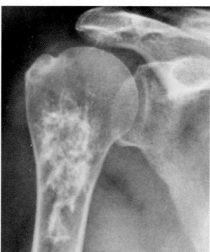

Fig B 4-7
Bone infarct. Densely calcified area in the medullary cavity of the humerus with dense streaks extending from the central region.

Condition	Imaging Findings	Comments
Avascular necrosis involving articular end of bone (Fig B 4-8)	Advanced stage consisting of lytic and sclerotic areas with flattening and irregularity of joint surfaces leading to early secondary degenerative changes (especially in weight-bearing joints).	Most commonly involves the femoral head. May affect the proximal half of the navicular after a fracture. Also can occur in any disorder associated with medullary bone infarcts or be secondary to steroid therapy or Cushing's disease.
Healed or healing benign bone lesion	Initially lytic bone lesion may become sclerotic spontaneously or with appropriate therapy.	Fibrous cortical defects, nonossifying fibromas, and bone cysts may spontaneously regress. Brown tumors in primary hyperparathyroidism become sclerotic after removal of the parathyroid adenoma. Even some lytic metastases may become osteoblastic after irradiation, chemotherapy, or hormone therapy.
Osteomyelitis Chronic or healed osteomyelitis (Fig B 4-9)	Thickening and sclerosis of bone with irregular outer margin surrounding a central ill-defined area of lucency. The cortex may become so dense that the medullary cavity is difficult to demonstrate.	Reactivation of infection may appear as recurrence of deep soft-tissue swelling, periosteal calcification, or the development of lytic abscess cavities in the bone.
Brodie's abscess (Fig B 4-10)	Well-circumscribed lytic area surrounded by an irregular zone of dense sclerosis.	Chronic bone abscess of low virulence that never had an acute stage. Painful lesion often simulating an osteoid osteoma.
Garré's sclerosing osteomyelitis (Fig B 4-11)	Exuberant sclerotic reaction without any bone destruction, sequestration, or periosteal response.	Rare, chronic nonsuppurative infection of bone due to an organism of low virulence.
Paget's disease (Fig B 4-12)	In the reparative stage, there is a mixed lytic and sclerotic pattern with cortical thickening and enlargement of affected bone. In the sclerotic stage, there may be uniform areas of increased bone density (eg, ivory vertebra in the spine and cotton-wool appearance in the skull).	Purely sclerotic phase is less common than the combined destructive and reparative stages. Ivory vertebra may simulate osteoblastic metastases or Hodgkin's disease, though in Paget's disease the vertebra is also expanded in size.

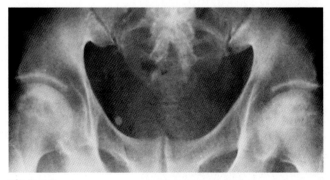

Fig B 4-8
Avascular necrosis. Sclerotic changes in the femoral heads bilaterally.

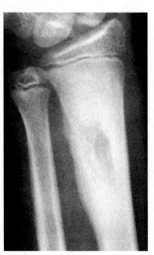

Fig B 4-9
Chronic osteomyelitis. Ill-defined area of lucency in the distal radial shaft is almost obscured by the sclerotic periosteal new bone formation.

Condition	Imaging Findings	Comments
Mastocytosis (Fig B 4-13)	Scattered, well-defined sclerotic foci simulating blastic metastases. There may also be diffuse osteosclerosis mimicking myelofibrosis.	Caused by diffuse deposits of mast cells in the bone marrow. Episodic release of histamine from mast cells causes pruritus, flushing, tachycardia, asthma, and headaches and an increased incidence of peptic ulcers. There is often hepatosplenomegaly, lymphadenopathy, and pancytopenia.

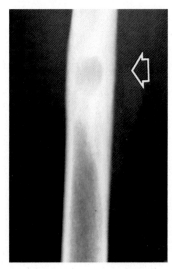

Fig B 4-10
Brodie's abscess. Well-circumscribed lucent lesion completely fills the femoral medullary canal and is surrounded by dense endosteal sclerosis and cortical thickening (arrow).[7]

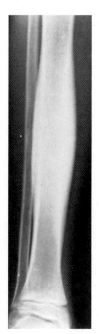

Fig B 4-11
Garré's sclerosing osteomyelitis. Exuberant sclerotic reaction in the midshaft of the tibia without evidence of bone destruction.

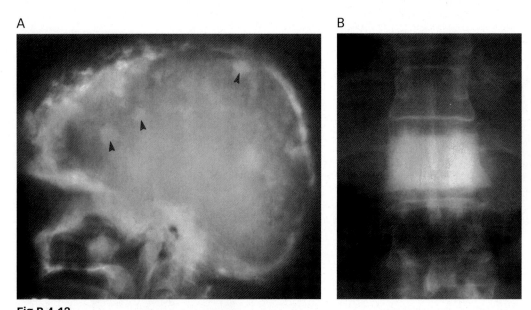

Fig B 4-12
Paget's disease. (A) Cotton-wool skull. Lateral radiograph shows diffuse calvarial thickening with several areas of focal sclerosis (arrowheads). (B) Ivory vertebra. Frontal radiograph shows diffuse sclerosis in the T10 vertebral body.[2]

Condition	Imaging Findings	Comments
Fibrous dysplasia	Dense, spotty, or linear calcification simulating medullary bone infarct.	Infrequent manifestation of long-standing disease.
Primary bone sarcoma (Figs B 4-14 and B 4-15)	Sclerosing forms may contain extremely dense new bone.	Osteogenic sarcoma; chondrosarcoma; Ewing's sarcoma.
Osteopoikilosis (Fig B 4-16)	Multiple sclerotic foci (2 mm to 2 cm) producing a typical speckled appearance.	Rare asymptomatic hereditary condition that primarily involves the small bones of the hands and feet, the pelvis, and the epiphyses and metaphyses of long bones.

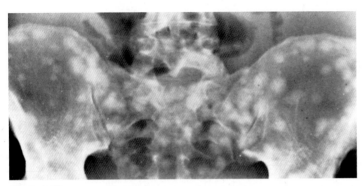

Fig B 4-13
Mastocytosis. Multiple scattered, well-defined sclerotic foci in the pelvis simulate blastic metastases.

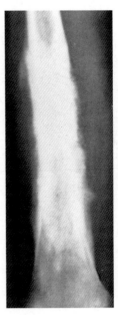

Fig B 4-14
Ewing's sarcoma. Sunburst pattern of horizontal spicules of dense bone.

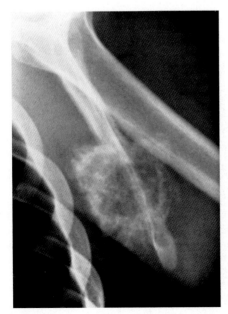

Fig B 4-15
Chondrosarcoma. Ill-defined, calcium-containing mass near the angle of the scapula.

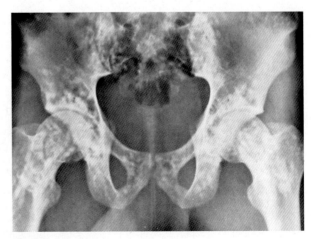

Fig B 4-16
Osteopoikilosis. Innumerable small, well-circumscribed areas of increased density throughout the pelvis and proximal femurs.

Condition	Imaging Findings	Comments
Osteopathia striata (Fig B 4-17)	Dense longitudinal lines in tubular bones. Ilial involvement produces linear densities radiating from the acetabulum and fanning out to the iliac crest (sunburst pattern).	Rare, asymptomatic bone disorder reflecting an error in internal bone modeling.
Congenital stippled epiphyses (chondrodysplasia punctata) (Fig B 4-18)	Multiple punctate calcifications occurring in epiphyses before the normal time for appearance of ossification centers. Most commonly involves the hips, knees, shoulders, and wrists.	Rare condition. Affected bones may be shortened or the process may regress and leave no deformity. The densities may disappear by age 3 or may gradually increase in size and coalesce to form a normal-appearing single ossification center.

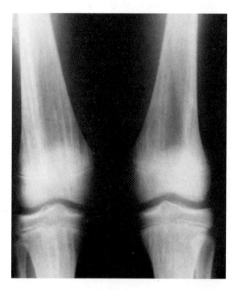

Fig B 4-17
Osteopathia striata. Dense longitudinal striations in the distal femur and proximal tibia.

A   B

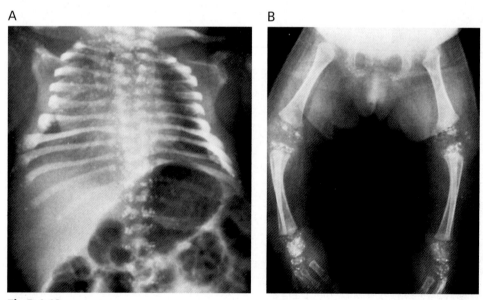

Fig B 4-18
Congenital stippled epiphyses. Multiple small punctate calcifications of various sizes involve virtually all the epiphyses in views of (A) the chest and upper abdomen and (B) the lower extremities.

Condition	Imaging Findings	Comments
Multiple myeloma (see Fig B 5-13)	Generalized patchy or uniform bone sclerosis.	Very rare manifestation. Scattered, slow-growing osteoblastic lesions with dense plasmacytic infiltrates and normal laboratory findings may be termed *plasma-cell granuloma*.
Tuberous sclerosis	Dense sclerotic foci most often affecting the bones of the cranial vault and the pedicles and posterior portions of the vertebral bodies.	Rare inherited disorder presenting with clinical triad of convulsive seizures, mental deficiency, and adenoma sebaceum. Associated with renal and intracranial hamartomas and characteristic scattered intracerebral calcifications.
Syphilis/yaws (Fig B 4-19)	Gumma formation causes an ill-defined lytic area surrounded by extensive dense bony proliferation and exuberant periosteal new bone formation.	Chronic osteomyelitis caused by spirochete (*Treponema*) infection.
Osteitis condensans ilii	Zone of dense sclerosis along the iliac side of the sacroiliac joint. Usually bilateral and symmetric, though there may be some variation in density between the two sides. Unlike ankylosing spondylitis, in osteitis condensans ilii the sacrum is normal and the sacroiliac joint space is preserved.	Occurs almost exclusively in women during the childbearing period, usually after pregnancy. May represent a reaction to the increased stress to which the sacroiliac region is subjected during pregnancy and delivery, as a similar type of sclerotic reaction (osteitis pubis) may be seen in the pubic bone adjacent to the symphysis in women who have borne children. The condition is usually asymptomatic and self-limited and is rarely detectable in women past 50.

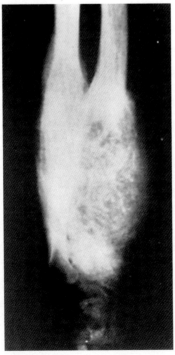

Fig B 4-19
Yaws. Expanding inflammatory process with surrounding sclerosis involving the right forearm.[8]

Generalized Osteosclerosis

Condition	Imaging Findings	Comments
Myelosclerosis (myelofibrosis, myeloid metaplasia) (Fig B 5-1)	Approximately half the patients have a widespread, diffuse increase in bone density (ground-glass appearance) that primarily affects the spine, ribs, and pelvis but can also involve the long bones and skull. Uniform obliteration of fine trabecular margins of ribs results in sclerosis simulating jail bars crossing the thorax.	Hematologic disorder in which gradual replacement of marrow by fibrosis produces a varying degree of anemia and a leukamoid blood picture. Most commonly idiopathic, though a large percentage of patients have antecedent polycythemia vera. Extramedullary hematopoiesis causes massive splenomegaly, often hepatomegaly, and sometimes tumor-like masses in the posterior mediastinum. Patchy osteosclerosis in long bones may produce a mottled appearance suggesting a destructive malignancy.
Osteoblastic metastases (Fig B 5-2)	Generalized diffuse osteosclerosis.	Primarily lymphoma and carcinomas of the prostate and breast.
Paget's disease (Fig B 5-3)	Diffuse osteosclerosis may develop in advanced stage of polyostotic disease.	Although the radiographic appearance may simulate that of osteoblastic metastases, characteristic cortical thickening and coarse trabeculation should suggest Paget's disease.
Sickle cell anemia (Fig B 5-4)	Diffuse sclerosis with coarsening of the trabecular pattern may be a late manifestation.	More commonly generalized osteoporosis due to marrow hyperplasia. Also characteristic "fish vertebrae" and a high incidence of acute osteomyelitis (often caused by *Salmonella* infection). Splenomegaly and extramedullary hematopoiesis are common.

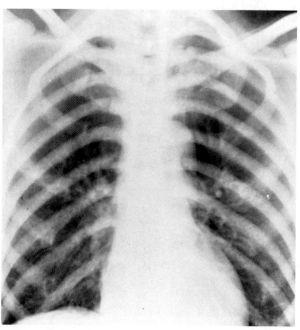

Fig B 5-1
Myelosclerosis. Diffuse uniform sclerosis of the bones of the thorax produces an appearance of jail bars.

Condition	Imaging Findings	Comments
Osteopetrosis (Albers-Schönberg disease, marble bones) (Fig B 5-5)	Symmetric, generalized increase in bone density involving all bones. Lack of modeling causes widening of metaphyseal ends of tubular bones. In the spine, characteristic "bone-within-a-bone" appearance (a miniature bone inset in each vertebral body) and "sandwich vertebrae" (increased density at end plates).	Rare hereditary bone dysplasia in which failure of the resorptive mechanism of calcified cartilage interferes with its normal replacement by mature bone. Varies in severity and age of clinical presentation from a fulminant, often fatal condition at birth to an essentially asymptomatic form that is an incidental radiographic finding. Although radiographically dense, the involved bones are brittle, and fractures are common even with trivial trauma. Extensive extramedullary hematopoiesis (hepatosplenomegaly and lymphadenopathy).
Pyknodysostosis (Fig B 5-6)	Diffuse, dense, sclerotic bones. Unlike osteopetrosis, the medullary cavity is preserved, and there is no metaphyseal widening. Characteristically, there is mandibular hypoplasia with loss of the normal mandibular angle and craniofacial disproportion.	Rare hereditary bone dysplasia. Patients have short stature but hepatosplenomegaly is infrequent. Numerous wormian bones may simulate cleidocranial dysostosis.

A   B

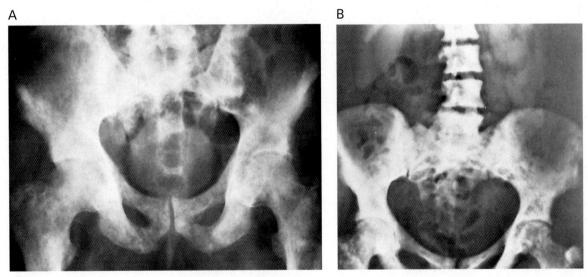

Fig B 5-2
Osteoblastic metastases. (A) Carcinoma of the prostate. (B) Carcinoma of the breast.

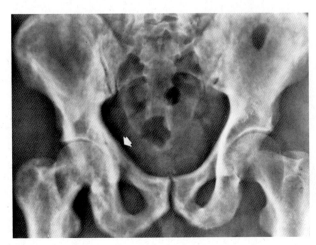

Fig B 5-3
Paget's disease. Diffuse sclerosis with cortical thickening involving the right femur and both iliac bones. Note the characteristic thickening and coarsening of the iliopectineal line (arrow) on the involved right side.

Condition	Imaging Findings	Comments
Melorheostosis (Fig B 5-7)	Irregular sclerotic thickening of the cortex, usually confined to one side of a single bone or to multiple bones of one extremity. Sclerosis begins at the proximal end of the bone and extends distally, resembling wax flowing down a burning candle.	Rare disorder, usually occurring in childhood, that typically presents with severe pain sometimes associated with limitation of motion, contractures, or fusion of an adjacent joint. Involvement of the hands and wrists may produce multiple small sclerotic islands of dense bone simulating osteopoikilosis.

A

B

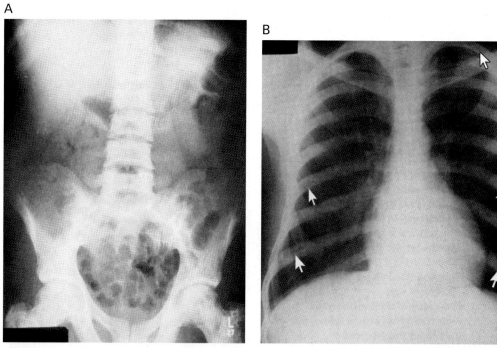

Fig B 5-4
Sickle cell anemia. (A) Patchy sclerosis of the pelvic bone and vertebrae, caused by medullary infarction and dystrophic calcification. (B) In another young patient, there is dense sclerosis of the rib cage with some areas of lucency (arrows).[9]

A

B

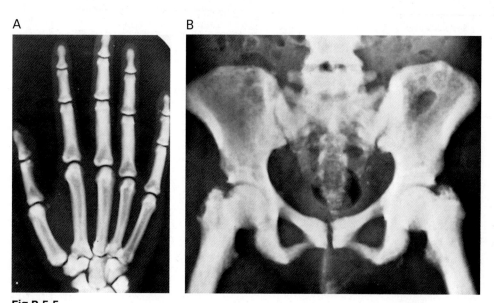

Fig B 5-5
Osteopetrosis. (A) Striking sclerosis of the bones of the hand and wrist. (B) Generalized increased density of the lower spine, pelvis, and hips in a 74-year-old woman with the tarda form of the condition.

Condition	Imaging Findings	Comments
Generalized cortical hyperostosis (van Buchem's syndrome)	Diffuse symmetric sclerosis of the skull, mandible, clavicles, ribs, and diaphyses of long bones.	Rare dysplasia in which diaphyseal sclerosis is accompanied by thickening of the endosteal surface of the cortex, which causes widening of the cortex but does not increase the diameter of the bone.
Fluorosis (Fig B 5-8)	Dense skeletal sclerosis most prominent in the vertebrae and pelvis. Obliteration of individual trabeculae may cause affected bones to appear chalky white. There is often calcification of interosseous membranes and ligaments (iliolumbar, sacrotuberous, and sacrospinous).	Fluorine poisoning may result from drinking water with a high concentration of fluorides, industrial exposure (mining, smelting), or excessive therapeutic intake of fluoride (treatment of myeloma or Paget's disease). There is usually also periosteal roughening and articular bone deposits in long bones at sites of muscular and ligamentous attachments.
Engelmann-Camurati disease (progressive diaphyseal dysplasia) (Fig B 5-9)	Endosteal and periosteal cortical thickening cause fusiform enlargement and sclerosis of long bones. Primarily involves the diaphyses, sparing the epiphyses and metaphyses.	Rare bone disorder associated with a neuromuscular dystrophy that causes a peculiar wide-based, waddling gait. Encroachment on the medullary canal may cause anemia and secondary hepatosplenomegaly.
Mastocytosis (see Fig B 4-12)	May present with diffuse osteosclerosis that often is not sharply demarcated from normal bone and intermingles with osteolytic areas. Another appearance is scattered, well-defined sclerotic foci simulating osteoblastic metastases.	Caused by diffuse deposits of mast cells in the bone marrow. Episodic release of histamine from mast cells causes pruritus, flushing, tachycardia, asthma, headaches, and an increased incidence of peptic ulcers. Often hepatosplenomegaly, lymphadenopathy, and pancytopenia.

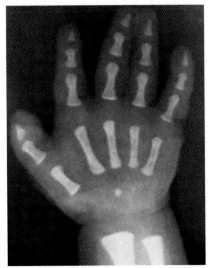

Fig B 5-6
Pyknodysostosis. Generalized increase in density with cortical thickening of the bones of the hand. The distal phalanges are hypoplastic, and the terminal tufts are absent.

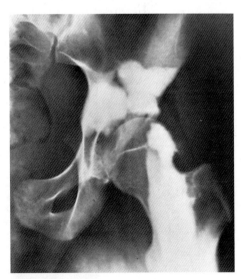

Fig B 5-7
Melorheostosis. Dense cortical sclerosis involves the proximal femur and the lower portion of the ilium.

Condition	Imaging Findings	Comments
Hypervitaminosis D/ idiopathic hypercalcemia	Generalized sclerosis and cortical thickening. Typically there are dense transverse metaphyseal bands (increase in depth of provisional zones of calcification).	Hypervitaminosis D results from excessive intake over a few days to several years. Idiopathic hypercalcemia is the result of excessive vitamin D intake, hypersensitivity to vitamin D, or an inborn error of cholesterol metabolism producing sterol intermediates with vitamin D–like properties. Causes renal calcification and renal failure.

A
B

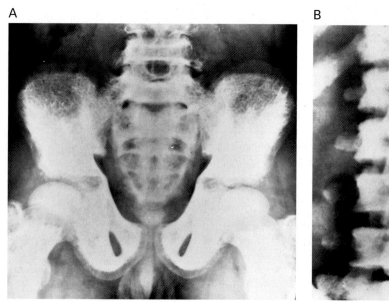

Fig B 5-8
Fluorosis. (A) Dense skeletal sclerosis with obliteration of individual trabeculae causes the pelvis and proximal femurs to appear chalky white. **(B)** Diffuse vertebral sclerosis in another patient.[10]

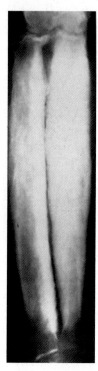

Fig B 5-9
Progressive diaphyseal dysplasia. Dense endosteal and periosteal cortical thickening causes fusiform enlargement and increased density of the midshafts of the radius and ulna.

Condition	Imaging Findings	Comments
Polyostotic fibrous dysplasia (Fig B 5-10)	Diffuse homogeneous ground-glass density involving multiple bones. May cause marked sclerosis and thickening of facial bones, often with obliteration of sinuses and orbits, producing a leonine appearance (leontiasis ossea).	Proliferation of fibrous tissue in the medullary cavity. Often there are localized pigmentations (café au lait spots) that tend to have an irregular outline ("coast-of-Maine"), unlike the smoothly marginated lesions in neurofibromatosis. Approximately one-third of females also demonstrate precocious puberty (Albright's syndrome).
Renal osteodystrophy (Fig B 5-11)	Generalized osteosclerosis, often combined with soft-tissue calcification, is one manifestation.	Represents a skeletal response to chronic renal disease of any origin. In primary hyperparathyroidism, sclerosis is generally associated with healing.
Craniometaphyseal dysplasia	Generalized diaphyseal sclerosis (but metaphyseal lucency) that eventually progresses to more normal mineralization. Lack of modeling of tubular bones and often sclerosis of the base of the skull and the mandible.	Rare hereditary disorder in which failure of normal tubulation of bone is combined with hypertelorism, a broad flat nose, and defective dentition.
Congenital syphilis (Fig B 5-12)	Diffuse cortical thickening and increased density of the shafts of long bones.	Most common radiographic appearance of late-stage disease that reflects periosteal reaction to underlying gummas.

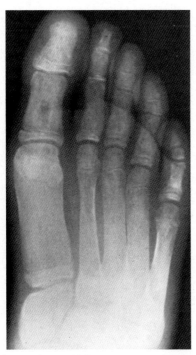

Fig B 5-10
Polyostotic fibrous dysplasia. The bones of the feet show a smudgy, ground-glass appearance of the medullary cavities with failure of normal modeling.

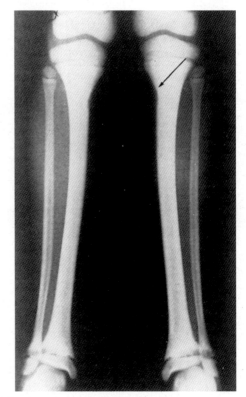

Fig B 5-11
Renal osteodystrophy. Sclerosis of the long bones in a boy with chronic glomerulonephritis, renal rickets, and secondary hyperparathyroidism. In addition to the increased skeletal density, note the widened zone of provisional calcification at the ankles and the subperiosteal resorption along the medial margins of the upper tibial shafts (arrow).

Condition	Imaging Findings	Comments
Metaphyseal abnormalities (see Section B 21)	Dense, transverse metaphyseal bands.	Most commonly a manifestation of lead intoxication. Also caused by phosphorus or bismuth poisoning, cretinism, treated leukemia, and healed rickets or scurvy.
Hypoparathyroidism/ pseudohypoparathyroidism	Band-like increase in density in long bones, usually localized to the metaphyseal area (probably reflects an abnormality in enchondral bone formation).	More frequent radiographic manifestations are cerebral calcification (especially involving the basal ganglia, the dentate nuclei of the cerebellum, and the choroid plexus) in hypoparathyroidism and shortening of the fourth and fifth metacarpals plus calcific or bony deposits in the skin or subcutaneous tissues in pseudohypoparathyroidism.
Gaucher's disease	Diffuse osteosclerosis may develop in the reparative stage. More common manifestations include Erlenmeyer flask deformity with ground-glass pattern and aseptic necrosis of the femoral head.	Inborn error of metabolism characterized by accumulation of abnormal quantities of complex lipids in the reticuloendothelial cells of the spleen, liver, and bone marrow.
Multiple myeloma (Fig B 5-13)	Uniform sclerosis of bone.	Very rare manifestation.
Hereditary hyperphosphatasia (Fig B 5-14)	Generalized widening and increased density of bone is one manifestation (especially in adults). In children, there is more commonly bowing and thickening of long bones with a varying pattern of density and thickness of the cortices.	Rare hereditary disease associated with elevated serum alkaline phosphatase. Thickening of the calvarium with patchy sclerosis may simulate the cotton-wool appearance of Paget's disease.

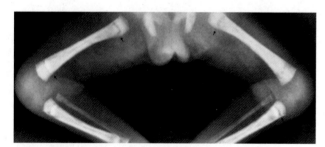

Fig B 5-12
Congenital syphilis. Diffuse sclerosis with transverse bands of lucency (arrows) in the diaphyses of the femurs and tibias.

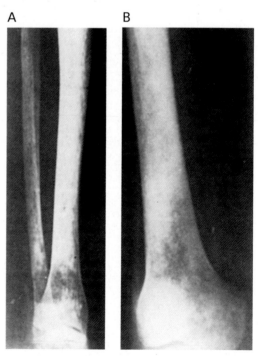

Fig B 5-13
Sclerotic myeloma. Views of (A) the leg and (B) the femur demonstrate diffuse and nodular sclerosis. Cortical thickening of the tibia encroaches on the medullary canal. Similar changes were evident in the pelvis.[11]

Condition	Imaging Findings	Comments
Infantile cortical hyperostosis (Caffey's disease) (see Fig B 8-8)	Massive cortical thickening, widening, and sclerosis of bone with laminated periosteal reaction in the healing phase. Primarily involves the mandible, scapula, clavicle, ulna, and ribs.	Now uncommon disease characterized by hyperirritability, soft-tissue swelling, periosteal new bone formation, and cortical thickening of underlying bones. The onset is always before the age of 5 months. Scapular lesion (usually unilateral) may be mistaken for a malignant tumor.
Physiologic osteosclerosis of newborns	Extremely dense and sclerotic skeleton (may mimic osteopetrosis).	Normal variant (especially in prematures). Usually disappears within a few weeks.

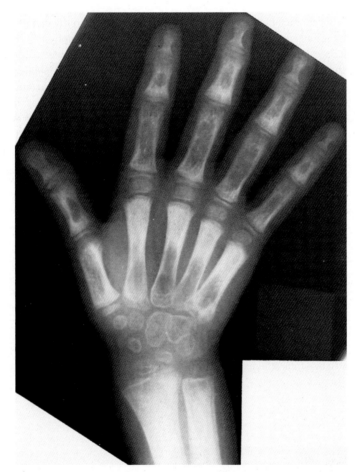

Fig B 5-14
Hereditary hyperphosphatasia. Areas of sclerosis about the metacarpals and middle phalanges associated with thinning of the cortices. The proximal phalanges show diffuse deossification.

Bubbly Lesions of Bone

Condition	Imaging Findings	Comments
Fibrous dysplasia (monostotic) (Fig B 6-1)	Well-defined lucent area (varies from completely radiolucent to homogeneous ground-glass density depending on the amount of fibrous or osseous tissue deposited in the medullary cavity). Primarily involves long bones (especially the femur and tibia), ribs, and facial bones. Often there is local expansion of bone with endosteal erosion of the cortex (predisposes to pathologic fractures).	Proliferation of fibrous tissues in the medullary cavity, usually beginning during childhood. The most common cause of an expansile focal rib lesion. In severe and long-standing disease, affected bones may be bowed or deformed ("shepherd's crook" deformity of the femur). Malignant degeneration is extremely rare in fibrous dysplasia.
Giant cell tumor (Figs B 6-2 and B 6-3)	Eccentric, lucent metaphyseal lesion that may extend to the immediate subarticular cortex of a bone but does not involve the joint. Expansion toward the shaft produces a well-demarcated lucency, often with cortical expansion but without a sclerotic shell or border. Typically involves the distal femur, proximal tibia, distal radius, or ulna.	Lytic lesion in the end of a long bone of a young adult after epiphyseal closure. Usually asymptomatic, but may be associated with intermittent dull pain and a palpable tender mass and predispose to pathologic fracture. Approximately 20% are malignant (best seen as tumor extension through the cortex and an associated soft-tissue mass on CT). There is much overlap in the radiographic appearance of benign and malignant lesions.
Fibrous cortical defect (Fig B 6-4)	Small, often multilocular, eccentric lucency that causes cortical thinning and expansion and is sharply demarcated by a thin, scalloped rim of sclerosis. Initially round, the defect soon becomes oval with its long axis parallel to that of the host bone.	Not a true neoplasm, but rather a benign and asymptomatic small focus of cellular fibrous tissue causing an osteolytic lesion in the metaphyseal cortex of a long bone (most frequently the distal femur). One or more fibrous cortical defects develop in up to 40% of all healthy children. Most regress spontaneously and disappear by the time of epiphyseal closure. A persistent and growing lesion is termed *nonossifying fibroma* (see below).
Nonossifying fibroma (Fig B 6-5)	Multilocular, eccentric lucency that causes cortical thinning and expansion and is sharply demarcated by a thin, scalloped rim of sclerosis.	Results from continued proliferative activity of a fibrous cortical defect and is seen in older children and young adults.

A

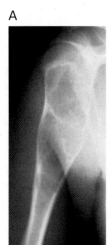

B

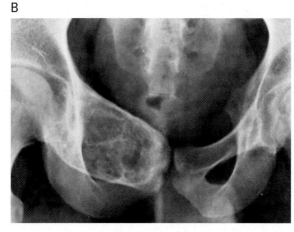

Fig B 6-1
Fibrous dysplasia. Views of (A) the humerus and (B) the ischium in two different patients show expansile lesions containing irregular bands of sclerosis, giving them a multilocular appearance.

Condition	Imaging Findings	Comments
Simple bone cyst (Figs B 6-6 and B 6-7)	Expansile lucent lesion that is sharply demarcated from adjacent normal bone. May contain thin septa (scalloping of underlying cortex) that produce a multiloculated appearance. Tends to have an oval configuration with its long axis parallel to that of the host bone.	True fluid-filled cyst with a wall of fibrous tissue. Begins adjacent to the epiphyseal plate and appears to migrate down the shaft (in reality, the epiphysis has migrated away from the cyst). Bone cysts arise in children and adolescents and most commonly involve the proximal humerus and femur. Often presents as a pathologic fracture that may show the fallen fragment sign (fragments of cortical bone are free to fall to the dependent portion of the fluid-filled cyst, unlike a bone tumor that has a firm tissue consistency).

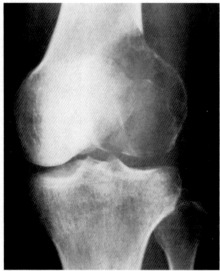

Fig B 6-2
Giant cell tumor of the distal femur. Typical eccentric lucent lesion in the metaphysis extends to the immediate subarticular cortex. The surrounding cortex, though thinned, remains intact.

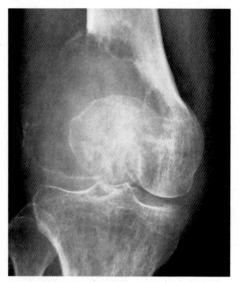

Fig B 6-3
Malignant giant cell tumor. The tumor has caused cortical disruption, extends outside the host bone, and has an ill-defined margin.

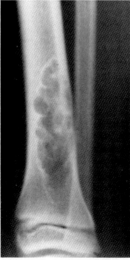

Fig B 6-4
Fibrous cortical defect. Multilocular, eccentric lucency in the distal tibia. Note the thin, scalloped rim of sclerosis.

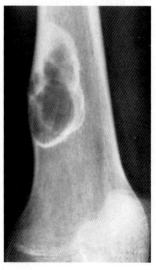

Fig B 6-5
Nonossifying fibroma. Multilocular, eccentric lucency with a sclerotic rim in the distal femur.

Condition	Imaging Findings	Comments
Aneurysmal bone cyst (Fig B 6-8)	Expansile, eccentric, cyst-like lesion causing marked ballooning of thinned cortex. Light trabeculation and septation in the lesion may produce a multiloculated appearance. Periosteal reaction may develop. Primarily involves the metaphyses of long bones (especially the femur and tibia) and the posterior elements of vertebrae.	Not a true neoplasm or cyst, but rather numerous blood-filled arteriovenous communications. Most frequently occurs in children and young adults and presents with mild pain of several months' duration, swelling, and restriction of movement. May extend beyond the axis of the host bone and form a visible soft-tissue mass that, when combined with a cortex so thin that it is invisible on plain radiographs, may be mistaken for a malignant bone tumor.
Enchondroma (Figs B 6-9 and B 6-10)	Well-marginated lucency arising in the medullary canal (usually near the epiphyses) that expands bone locally and often causes thinning and endosteal scalloping of the cortex (may lead to pathologic fracture with minimal trauma). Primarily involves the small bones of the hands and feet. Characteristic calcifications (varying from minimal stippling to large, amorphous areas of increased density) develop in the lucent matrix.	Common benign cartilaginous tumor that is most frequently found in children and young adults. Usually asymptomatic and discovered either incidentally or when a pathologic fracture occurs. The development of severe pain or radiographic growth of the lesion with loss of marginal definition, cortical disruption, and local periosteal reaction suggests malignant degeneration (increased incidence the closer the tumor is to the axial skeleton). Multiple enchondromatosis is termed *Ollier's disease*.

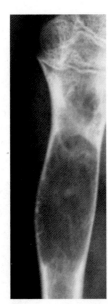

Fig B 6-6
Simple bone cyst in the proximal humerus. The cyst has an oval configuration, with its long axis parallel to that of the host bone. Note the thin septa that produce a multiloculated appearance.

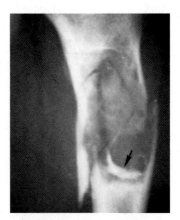

Fig B 6-7
Fallen fragment sign. After pathologic fracture, a cortical bone fragment (arrow) lies free in a subtrochanteric bone cyst.[12]

Condition	Imaging Findings	Comments
Central chondrosarcoma (Fig B 6-11)	Localized lucent area of osteolytic destruction in the metaphyseal end of a bone. When the rate of tumor growth exceeds that of bone repair, the margins of the lesion become irregular and ill defined and the tumor extends to cause cortical destruction and invasion of soft tissues. The cartilaginous tissue in a chondrosarcoma can be easily recognized by the amorphous punctate, flocculent, or "snowflake" calcifications that are seen in approximately two-thirds of central tumors.	Malignant tumor of cartilaginous origin that may originate de novo or in a pre-existing cartilaginous lesion (osteochondroma, enchondroma). The tumor is about half as common as osteogenic sarcoma, develops at a later age (half the patients are more than 40 years old), grows more slowly, and metastasizes later. Central chondrosarcoma may also appear as an aggressive, poorly defined osteolytic lesion that blends imperceptibly with normal bone and can expand to replace the entire medullary cavity (may simply be a later phase of the first, benign-appearing type).

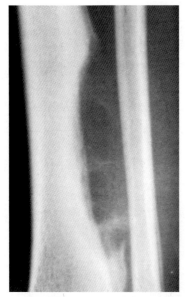

Fig B 6-8
Aneurysmal bone cyst of the tibia. Expansile, eccentric, cystic lesion with multiple fine internal septa. Because the severely thinned cortex is difficult to detect, the tumor resembles a malignant process.

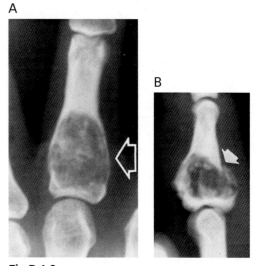

Fig B 6-9
Enchondroma. (A) Well-demarcated tumor (arrow) expands the bone and thins the cortex. (B) Pathologic fracture (arrow).

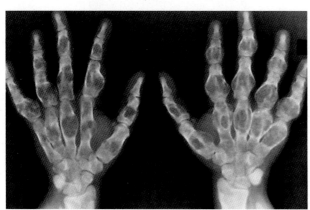

Fig B 6-10
Multiple enchondromatosis. View of both hands demonstrates multiple globular and expansile lucent filling defects involving all the metacarpals and the proximal and middle phalanges.

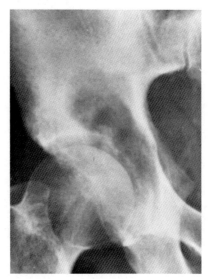

Fig B 6-11
Central chondrosarcoma. Irregular and ill-defined lytic lesion of the lower ilium.

Condition	Imaging Findings	Comments
Brown tumor (Fig B 6-12)	Single or multiple focal lytic areas that are generally well demarcated and often cause expansion of bone. Primarily involves the mandible, pelvis, ribs, and femur.	True cyst representing intraosseous hemorrhage in patients with hyperparathyroidism (especially the primary type). Usually there is other radiographic evidence of hyperparathyroidism. A large cyst may simulate malignancy or lead to pathologic fractures and bizarre deformities.
Localized myeloma (solitary plasmacytoma) (Figs B 6-13 and B 6-14)	Expansile, often trabeculated lucency that predominantly involves the ribs, long bones, and pelvis. A highly destructive tumor may expand or balloon bone before it breaks through the cortex. In the spine, an affected vertebral body may collapse or be destroyed.	Infrequent condition in which a single plasma cell tumor presents as an apparently solitary destructive bone lesion with no evidence of the major disease complications usually associated with multiple myeloma. Generally develops into typical multiple myeloma (diffuse lytic lesions) within 1 to 2 years.
Metastasis (Figs B 6-15 and B 6-16)	Single large metastatic focus appearing as an expansile, trabeculated lesion (blowout metastasis).	Typically secondary to carcinomas of the kidneys and thyroid. Most lytic metastases are irregular, poorly defined, and multiple.
Lymphoma (Fig B 6-17)	Single or multiple lytic defects. There may be endosteal scalloping of the cortex.	Mottled pattern of destruction and sclerosis may simulate hematogenous metastases.

B

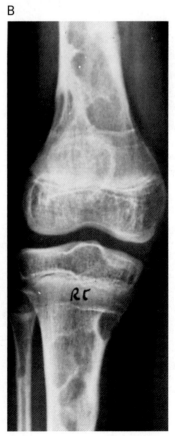

A

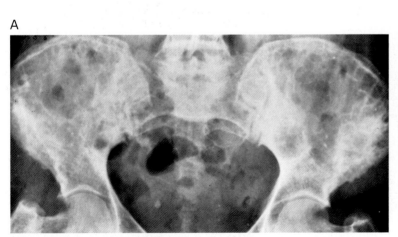

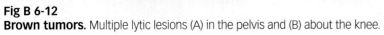

Fig B 6-12
Brown tumors. Multiple lytic lesions (A) in the pelvis and (B) about the knee.

Condition	Imaging Findings	Comments
Langerhans cell histiocytosis (Fig B 6-18)	Usually a well-defined medullary lucency (rapidly growing lesions may have indistinct, hazy borders) that predominantly affects the skull, pelvis, femur, and spine. There is often endosteal scalloping and local or extensive periosteal reaction. Characteristic finding is a peculiar beveled contour of the lesion that produces a "hole-within-a-hole" effect.	In the skull, typically produces one or more small punched-out areas that originate in the diploic space, expand and perforate both the inner and outer tables, and often contain a central bone density (button sequestrum). In the spine, generally spotty destruction in a vertebral body that proceeds to collapse the vertebra into a thin flat disk (vertebra plana).

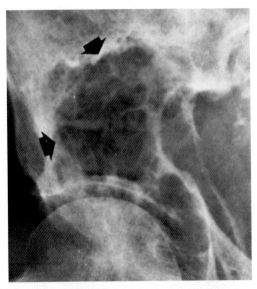

Fig B 6-13
Solitary plasmacytoma of the ilium (arrows). Some residual streaks of bone remain in this osteolytic lesion, producing a soap-bubble appearance.

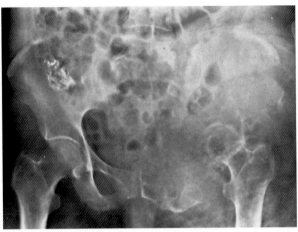

Fig B 6-14
Solitary plasmacytoma. Highly destructive tumor that has obliterated virtually all of the left half of the pelvis.

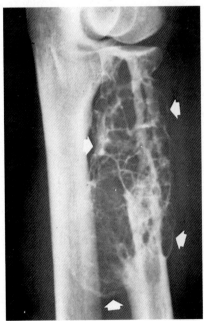

Fig B 6-15
Renal cell carcinoma metastatic to bone. Typical expansile bubbly lesion (arrows) in the proximal shaft of the radius.

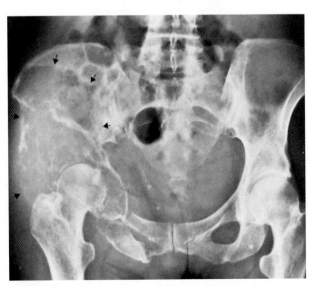

Fig B 6-16
Metastatic thyroid carcinoma. Large area of entirely lytic, expansile destruction (arrows) involves the left ilium.

Condition	Imaging Findings	Comments
Osteoblastoma (Fig B 6-19)	Well-circumscribed, eccentric, and expansile lucency that may break through the cortex to produce a soft-tissue component surrounded by a thin calcific shell.	Rare bone neoplasm that most often arises in adolescence. Approximately half involve the vertebral column (most frequently the neural arches and processes). The remainder affects the long bones or the small bones of the hands and feet. Although predominantly lytic, osteoblastomas may have some internal calcification, and their aggressive appearance often simulates that of a malignant lesion.
Chondroblastoma (Fig B 6-20)	Eccentric, round or oval lucency in an epiphysis that often has a thin sclerotic rim and may contain flocculent calcification. May also involve the greater trochanter of the femur and the greater tuberosity of the humerus.	Rare, benign cartilaginous tumor of the epiphysis that occurs in children and young adults (most frequently males) before enchondral bone growth ceases.
Chondromyxoid fibroma (Fig B 6-21)	Eccentric, round or oval lucency arising in the metaphysis of a long bone. The overlying cortex is usually bulging and thinned, and the inner border is generally thick and sclerotic, often with scalloped margins. Approximately 50% involve the tibia (the remainder affect the pelvis and other bones of the extremities).	Uncommon benign bone tumor originating from cartilage-forming connective tissue and predominantly occurring in young adults. Calcification is infrequent (unlike chondroblastoma and other cartilaginous bone lesions).

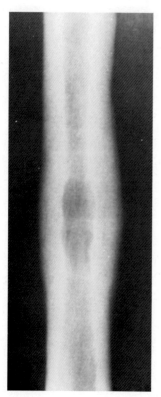

Fig B 6-17
Lymphoma. There is a focal lytic defect with endosteal scalloping of the cortex.

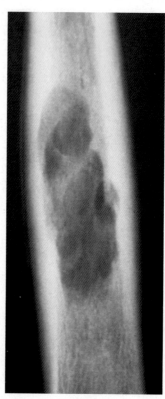

Fig B 6-18
Langerhans cell histiocytosis. Bubbly osteolytic lesion in the femur, with scalloping of the endosteal margins and a thin layer of periosteal response.

Condition	Imaging Findings	Comments
Epidermoid inclusion cyst	Well-circumscribed lucency in a terminal phalanx that may cause thinning, expansion, or even loss of the cortical margin.	Unlike an enchondroma, usually a history of penetrating trauma and no stippled calcification.
Intraosseous ganglion (Fig B 6-22)	Well-defined lucency with a sclerotic margin adjacent to the articular surface.	Most commonly involves the proximal tibia (near the attachment of the cruciate ligaments, and the head and neck of the femur, and the medial malleolus.
Lipoma	Expansile lucency with a thinned cortex. May break through the cortex and have an adjacent soft-tissue component.	Rare tumor that arises in the calcaneus, skull, ribs, or extremities.
Glomus tumor	Central well-circumscribed lucency that primarily involves the distal aspect of the terminal phalanx of a finger.	May mimic an enchondroma, but a glomus tumor is painful. A subungual glomus tumor may cause pressure erosion at that site.
Ossifying fibroma	Smooth, round, or expansile mass involving the skull, face, or mandible.	Rare tumor that may be associated with reactive bone sclerosis or calcification of the tumor matrix.
Adamantinoma	Large loculated, expansile lucent mass that usually involves the midportion of the tibia.	Rare tumor that primarily affects adolescents and young adults. The histologic pattern resembles ameloblastoma of the mandible. Often recurs and may metastasize.
Fungal infection (Fig B 6-23)	Focal area of lytic destruction (often multiple).	Coccidioidomycosis; blastomycosis. Sclerosis and periosteal reaction may develop.
Echinococcal cyst	Large, central radiolucent area associated with endosteal scalloping and expansion. May show cortical breakthrough and a soft-tissue mass.	Usually monostotic and predominantly involves the pelvis, spine, and long bones.

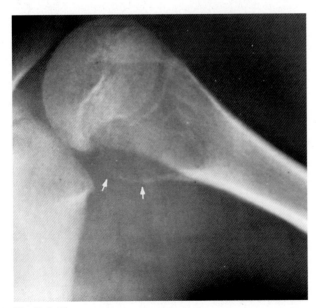

Fig B 6-19
Osteoblastoma. Expansile, eccentric mass in the proximal humerus causes thinning of the cortex (arrows).

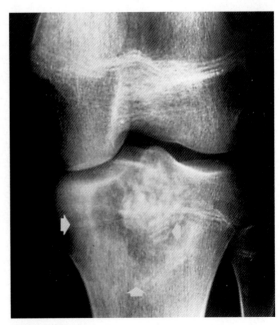

Fig B 6-20
Chondroblastoma. Osteolytic lesion containing calcification (arrows) in the epiphysis. Note the open epiphyseal line.[13]

Condition	Imaging Findings	Comments
Hemophilic pseudotumor (Fig B 6-24)	Central or eccentric lucent lesion, often with a large adjacent soft-tissue hemorrhage. There may be cortical erosion suggesting a sarcoma.	Extensive local area of intraosseous hemorrhage that most commonly involves the femur, pelvis, tibia, and small bones of the hands.
Cystic osteomyelitis (tuberculosis)	Single or multiple small oval lucencies lying in the long axis of a bone and having well-defined margins with sclerosis. Primarily involves the skull, shoulder, pelvic girdles, and axial skeleton.	Rare manifestation of disseminated tuberculosis. In children (who are more commonly affected), the lesions usually affect the peripheral skeleton, are symmetric in distribution, and are unaccompanied by sclerosis.
Desmoplastic fibroma	Osteolytic lesion that destroys medullary bone with cortical erosion and expansion. Generally has an aggressive appearance simulating that of a malignant tumor.	Extremely rare benign neoplasm characterized by abundant collagen formation. Most commonly involves the pelvis, mandible, humerus, tibia, and scapula.
Hemangioma (Fig B 6-25; see Fig SP 2-3)	Lucent area with delicate bony trabeculation. Most commonly occurs near the end of a tubular or flat bone.	Rare manifestation. Much more commonly produces multiple coarse linear striations running vertically in a demineralized vertebral body or a sunburst pattern of osseous spicules radiating from a central lucency in the skull.

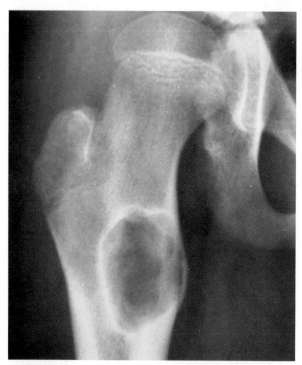

Fig B 6-21
Chondromyxoid fibroma. Ovoid, eccentric metaphyseal lucency with thinning of the overlying cortex and a sclerotic inner margin.

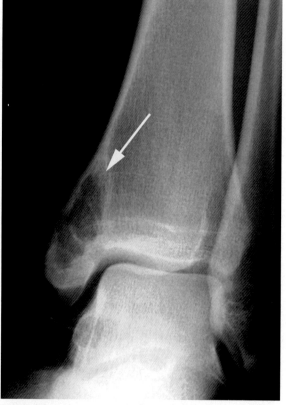

Fig B 6-22
Intraosseous ganglion cyst. Lucent lesion with sclerotic margin (arrow) in the medial malleolus.[14]

Condition	Imaging Findings	Comments
Angiomatous lesion (Fig B 6-26)	Single or (more frequently) multiple lucent metaphyseal lesions, which often have a sclerotic margin and are sometimes associated with a soft-tissue mass.	Rare congenital malformation consisting of endothelium-lined structures that may be lymphatic channels (lymphangiomatosis) or blood vascular channels (hemangiomatosis). Usually there is widespread involvement of multiple long bones, flat bones, and the skull.

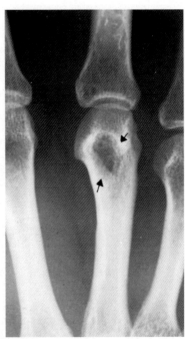

Fig B 6-23
Coccidioidomycosis. Typical well-marginated, punched-out lytic defect in the head of the third metacarpal (arrows).[15]

A

B

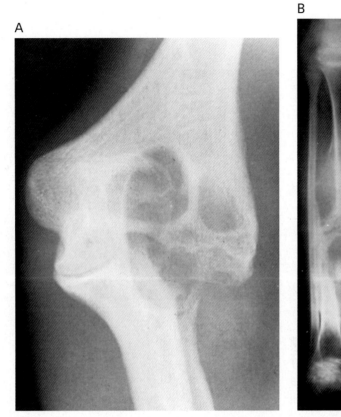

Fig B 6-24
Hemophilia. (A) Large subchondral cysts about the elbow. (B) Destructive, expansile lesion of the lower tibial shaft.[16]

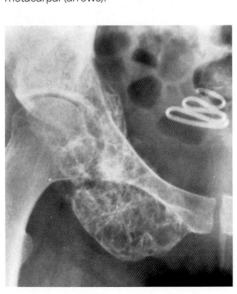

Fig B 6-25
Hemangioendothelioma. Expansile lucency containing delicate bony trabeculation.

Condition	Imaging Findings	Comments
Sarcoidosis (Fig B 6-27)	Single or multiple, sharply circumscribed, punched-out areas of lucency, primarily involving the small bones of the hands and feet. There may be cortical thinning, expansion, or destruction.	Perivascular granulomatous infiltration in the haversian canals destroys the fine trabeculae, producing a mottled or lace-like coarsely trabeculated pattern.
Pigmented villonodular synovitis (PVNS) (Fig 6-28).	Lucent lesion extending to the articular surface.	Protrusion of proliferative synovium infrequently produces a synovial cystic mass that can mimic a giant cell tumor.

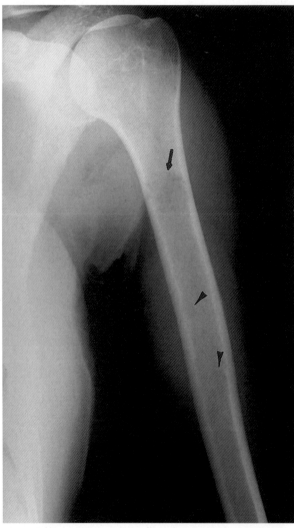

Fig B 6-26
Cystic angiomatosis. Lytic lesion in the proximal left humerus (arrow) with relatively well-defined lobular margins and minimal marginal sclerosis. Additional lytic lesions (arrowheads) are in the midhumeral diaphysis. Multiple lesions were seen elsewhere in the axial and proximal appendicular skeleton.[17]

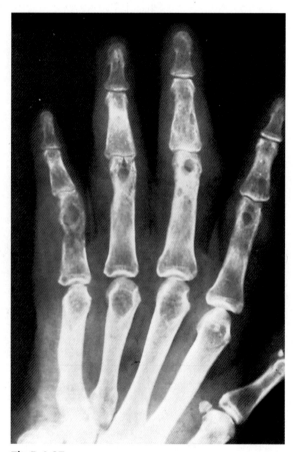

Fig B 6-27
Sarcoidosis. Multiple osteolytic lesions throughout the phalanges, having a typical punched-out appearance. The apparent air density in the soft tissues is a photographic artifact.

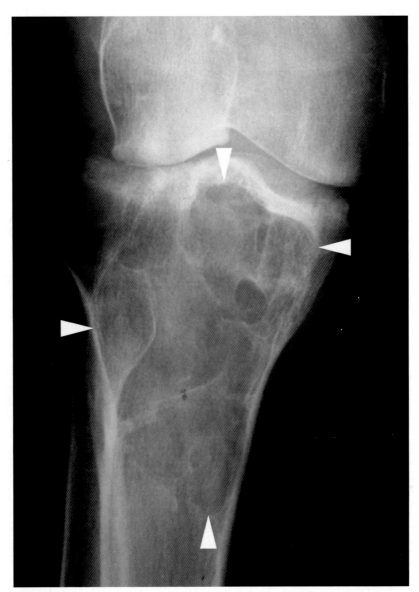

Fig B 6-28
PVNS. Large lucent lesion (arrowheads) in the proximal tibia extending to the
articular surface, mimicking a giant cell tumor.[14]

Moth-Eaten or Punched-Out Osteolytic Destructive Lesions of Bone

Condition	Imaging Findings	Comments
Osteolytic metastases (see Figs B 6-15 and B 6-16)	Single or multiple areas of bone destruction of variable size with irregular and poorly defined margins. Major sites of metastatic spread are bones containing red marrow, such as the spine, pelvis, ribs, skull, and the upper ends of the humerus and femur. Metastases distal to the knees and elbows are infrequent but do occur, especially with bronchogenic tumors. Periosteal reaction is rare.	Most common primary lesions causing osteolytic metastases are carcinomas of the breast, lung, kidney, and thyroid. Kidney and thyroid metastases typically produce a single large metastatic focus that may appear as an expansile trabeculated lesion (blowout metastasis). Elliptical lytic bone lesions suggest lymphoma. Metastatic neuroblastoma in children produces mottled bone destruction resembling leukemia. Spinal metastases typically destroy the pedicles, unlike multiple myeloma (in which the pedicles are infrequently involved). Because almost half the mineral content of a bone must be lost before it is detectable on plain radiographs, radionuclide bone scanning is far more sensitive for screening (false-negative bone scans occur with aggressively osteolytic lesions, especially multiple myeloma).
Multiple myeloma (Figs B 7-1 and B 7-2)	Multiple punched-out osteolytic lesions scattered throughout the skeletal system. Because bone destruction is due to proliferation of plasma cells distributed throughout the bone marrow, the flat bones containing red marrow (vertebrae, skull, ribs, pelvis) are primarily affected. The appearance may be indistinguishable from that of metastatic carcinoma, though the lytic defects in myeloma tend to be more discrete and uniform in size. Sharply circumscribed lytic lesions tend to eventually coalesce, destroying large segments of bone and often breaking through the cortex and periosteum to form a soft-tissue mass (especially involving a rib). Pathologic fractures are common, especially in the ribs, vertebrae, and long bones.	Disseminated malignancy of plasma cells that primarily affects persons between 40 and 70 years of age. Typical laboratory findings include an abnormal spike of monoclonal immunoglobulin and the presence of Bence Jones protein in the urine. Up to 20% of patients develop secondary amyloidosis. Extensive plasma cell proliferation in the bone marrow with no tendency to form discrete tumor masses may produce generalized skeletal deossification simulating postmenopausal osteoporosis. In the spine, there are often multiple vertebral compression fractures and usually sparing of the pedicles (lacking red marrow), which are frequently destroyed by metastatic disease. Because there is little or no stimulation of new bone formation, radionuclide bone scans may be normal even with extensive skeletal infiltration. Solitary or diffuse areas of sclerosis (simulating osteoblastic metastases) may rarely occur.
Ewing's sarcoma (Fig B 7-3; see Fig B 8-2)	Classic appearance (though seen in a majority of cases) is an ill-defined permeative area of bone destruction that involves a large central portion of the shaft of a long bone and is associated with a fusiform lamellated periosteal reaction parallel to the shaft. Other types of periosteal reactions include a thin periosteal elevation (Codman's triangle) or a sunburst pattern with horizontal spicules of bone extending into a soft-tissue mass.	Primary malignant tumor of children and young adults (peak incidence in the midteens) that arises in the bone marrow and most commonly involves the long bones of the extremities (especially the femur and tibia). Tends to metastasize early to the lungs and to other bones. Other appearances of Ewing's sarcoma include a purely lytic lesion or a mass of increased density (suggesting osteogenic sarcoma) in the metaphyseal region.

Condition	Imaging Findings	Comments
Reticulum cell sarcoma (Figs B 7-4 and B 7-5)	Moth-eaten pattern of permeative bone destruction that arises in the medullary cavity and then invades the cortex. There is often an amorphous or lamellated periosteal reaction. Most commonly involves a long bone (especially near the knee), but also can affect the pelvis, scapula, ribs, and vertebrae.	Primary malignant lesion of bone that is histologically similar to Ewing's sarcoma but tends to occur in older persons (average age, approximately 40 years). Unlike Ewing's sarcoma, reticulum cell sarcoma rarely causes systemic symptoms and the patient generally appears healthy even when local disease is extensive. The tumor tends to metastasize late to lymph nodes and the lungs and only rarely spreads to other bones.

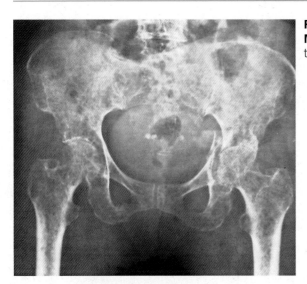

Fig B 7-1
Multiple myeloma. Diffuse, punched-out osteolytic lesions throughout the pelvis and proximal femurs.

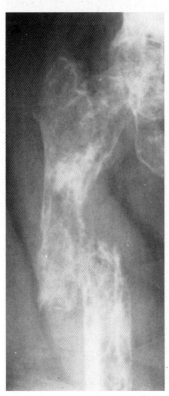

Fig B 7-2
Heavy chain disease. Diffuse, destructive bone lesions have led to a pathologic fracture of the midshaft of the femur.

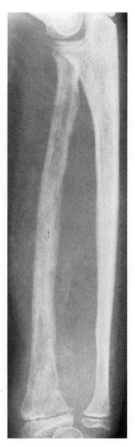

Fig B 7-3
Ewing's sarcoma. Diffuse permeative destruction involves virtually the entire radius.

Condition	Imaging Findings	Comments
Osteomyelitis (Figs B 7-6 and B 7-7)	In long bones, the earliest evidence of osteomyelitis is a localized, deep soft-tissue swelling adjacent to the metaphysis with displacement or obliteration of normal fat planes. Subtle areas of metaphyseal lucency reflecting resorption of necrotic bone are followed by more prominent bone destruction producing a ragged, moth-eaten appearance (the more virulent the organism, the larger the area of destruction). Subperiosteal spread of inflammation elevates the periosteum and stimulates the laying down of layers of new bone parallel to the shaft, producing a characteristic lamellated periosteal reaction. Eventually, a large amount of new bone surrounds the cortex in a thick, irregular bony sleeve (involucrum) and disruption of the cortical blood supply leads to bone necrosis and segments of avascular dead bone (sequestra). In vertebral osteomyelitis (see Figs SP 3-3 and SP 4-4), the earliest sign is subtle erosion of the subchondral bony plate with loss of the sharp cortical outline. This may progress to total destruction of the vertebral body associated with a paravertebral soft-tissue abscess. Unlike neoplastic processes, osteomyelitis usually affects the intervertebral disk space and often involves adjacent vertebrae.	Osteomyelitis is caused by a broad spectrum of infectious organisms that reach bone by hematogenous spread, by extension from a contiguous site of infection, or by direct introduction of organisms (trauma or surgery). Acute hematogenous osteomyelitis tends to involve bones with rich red marrow (metaphyses of long bones, especially the femur and tibia, in infants and children; vertebrae in adults). Because the earliest changes are usually not evident on plain radiographs until approximately 10 days after the onset of symptoms, radionuclide bone scanning is the most valuable imaging modality for early diagnosis (increased isotope uptake reflects the inflammatory process and increased blood flow). The radiographic findings, clinical history, and symptoms are generally sufficient to make the diagnosis of osteomyelitis, though at times aggressive bone destruction and bizarre periosteal reaction (especially in children) may suggest a malignant bone tumor and require biopsy. Chronic osteomyelitis results in a thick, irregular, sclerotic bone with central radiolucency, elevated periosteum, and often a chronic draining sinus.

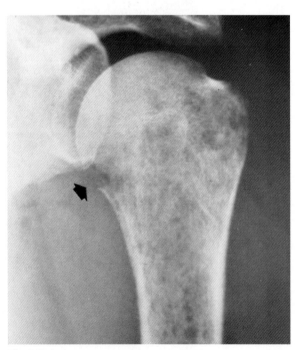

Fig B 7-4
Reticulum cell sarcoma. A moth-eaten pattern of bone destruction in the proximal humerus is associated with a pathologic fracture (arrow).

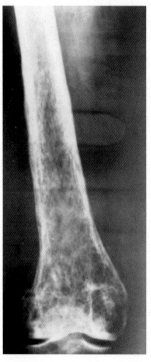

Fig B 7-5
Reticulum cell sarcoma. Diffuse permeative destruction with mild periosteal response involving the distal half of the femur.

Condition	Imaging Findings	Comments
Leukemia (Fig B 7-8)	Patchy lytic lesions produce a permeative moth-eaten appearance or diffuse destruction with cortical erosion. Reactive response to proliferating leukemic cells can cause patchy or uniform osteosclerosis, whereas subperiosteal proliferation of tumor cells incites periosteal new bone formation. In children, the knees, ankles, and wrists are most often affected; in adults, leukemic bone lesions most commonly involve the vertebrae, ribs, skull, and pelvis.	The earliest radiographic sign of disease in children is a transverse radiolucent band at the metaphyseal ends of long bones (most commonly the knees, ankles, and wrists). Though a nonspecific indication of severe illness younger than age 2, its presence after this age strongly suggests acute leukemia. Diffuse skeletal demineralization (especially in the spine where it leads to vertebral compression fractures) may result from both leukemic infiltration of the bone marrow and alteration of protein and mineral metabolism. Metastatic neuroblastoma may be indistinguishable from leukemia.
Lymphoma (see Fig B 4-3)	Hematogenous spread produces a mottled pattern of destruction and sclerosis that may simulate metastatic disease.	Other forms of skeletal involvement include dense vertebral sclerosis (ivory vertebra), discrete elliptical lytic lesions, and bone erosion (especially of the anterior surfaces of upper lumbar and lower thoracic vertebral bodies due to direct extension from adjacent nodes).
Fibrosarcoma (Fig B 7-9)	Initially, an irregular, destructive lesion arising in the medullary cavity that may cause thinning, expansion, and erosion of the cortex accompanied by periosteal proliferation. As the tumor develops, there may be massive invasion of the cortex and extension into the medullary canal.	Rare primary malignant tumor of fibroblastic tissue that most often involves tubular bones in young patients and flat bones in older ones. Tends to grow slowly and to have a somewhat better prognosis than osteogenic sarcoma. Unlike most primary bone tumors, fibrosarcomas tend to metastasize to lymph nodes.

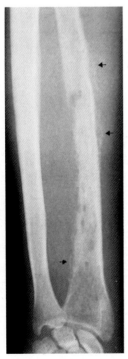

Fig B 7-6
Osteomyelitis. Patchy pattern of bone destruction involves much of the shaft of the radius. Note the early periosteal new bone formation (arrows).

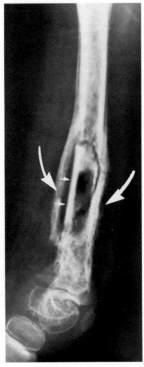

Fig B 7-7
Chronic osteomyelitis. The involucrum (curved arrows), a thick, irregular, bony sleeve, surrounds the sequestrum (straight arrows), a residual segment of avascular dead bone.

Condition	Imaging Findings	Comments
Osteogenic sarcoma (Fig B 7-10)	Purely lytic, destructive process is one manifestation.	More commonly a mixed form (combination of bone destruction and production) with an exuberant, irregular periosteal response.
Langerhans cell histiocytosis (see Fig B 6-18)	Initially, there is a small relatively well-defined lucent area that enlarges to produce endosteal scalloping, a multilocular appearance, and bone expansion with associated periosteal new bone formation. May produce more confluent areas of bone destruction simulating malignancy or osteomyelitis. Predominantly involves the skull, pelvis, spine, and ribs.	Bone lesions are most characteristic of Langerhans cell histiocytosis. A calvarial defect may demonstrate a bony density in its center (button sequestrum). Spinal involvement may lead to the collapse of a vertebral body, which assumes the shape of a thin flat disk (vertebra plana).
Massive osteolysis of Gorham	Initially, radiolucent foci in intramedullary or subcortical regions with slowly progressive atrophy, dissolution, fracture, fragmentation, and disappearance of a portion of the bone. The process spreads across joints and intervertebral spaces, leading to a dramatic pattern of regional destruction that generally increases relentlessly over a period of years (may eventually stabilize).	Rare disease of unknown etiology that usually is detected before age 40. May affect the axial or appendicular skeleton. One of the "primary osteolysis syndromes," many of which affect the hands and feet.
Diffuse lymphangiomatosis (Fig B 7-11)	Multiple cystic lesions throughout the skeleton causing erosions and progressive osteolytic defects in various bones.	Rare condition in children and adolescents that may be associated with widespread soft-tissue abnormalities and involvement of other organ systems.

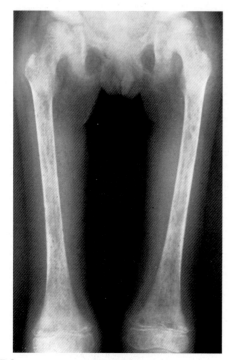

Fig B 7-8
Acute leukemia. Proliferation of neoplastic cells in the marrow has caused extensive destruction of bone in both femurs.

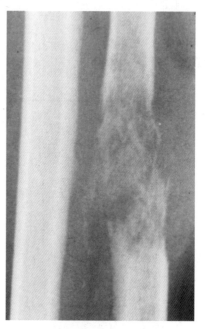

Fig B 7-9
Fibrosarcoma. Irregular destructive lesion of the shaft of the radius.

Condition	Imaging Findings	Comments
Intraosseous hemangiomatosis	Multiple widespread bone defects.	Rare condition without the characteristic appearance seen in other forms of the disease (no vertebral or skull hemangiomas).
Weber-Christian disease	Multiple punched-out or moth-eaten lesions involving the skull, pelvis, and medullary bone.	Rare disturbance of fat metabolism resulting in diffuse panniculitis, characteristic painful nodules in subcutaneous fat, and occasional bone lesions.
Membranous lipodystrophy	Multiple radiolucent cystic lesions symmetrically distributed in the carpal and tarsal bones and the ends of long bones.	Rare hereditary disease of unknown origin that usually affects young adults and is associated with presenile mental retardation.

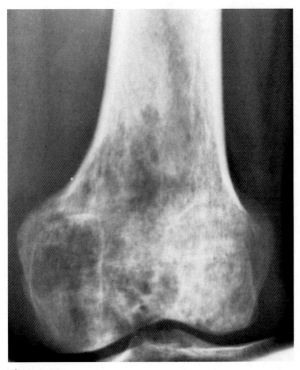

Fig B 7-10
Osteogenic sarcoma. Primarily a lytic, destructive process in the distal femur.

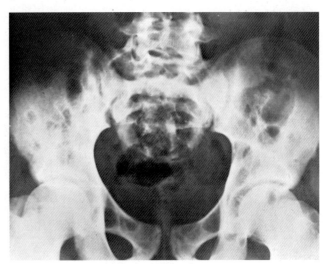

Fig B 7-11
Diffuse lymphangiomatosis. Multiple lytic lesions, some with thin sclerotic rims, diffusely involve the pelvis.

Localized Periosteal Reaction

Condition	Imaging Findings	Comments
Fracture	Localized periosteal reaction associated with traumatic or stress fracture.	May involve multiple bones in the battered child syndrome.
Primary malignant tumor of bone (Figs B 8-1 through B 8-3)	Localized periosteal reaction that may be solid, laminated, spiculated (perpendicular to the shaft), or amorphous. Codman's triangle may occur.	Most commonly, osteosarcoma and Ewing's sarcoma. Periosteal reaction is rare in other primary bone malignancies.

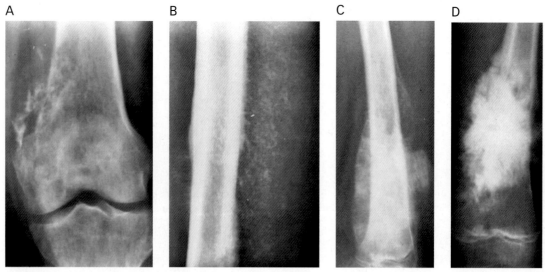

A   B   C   D

Fig B 8-1
Osteogenic sarcoma. (A to D) Four examples of osteogenic sarcoma of the femur illustrate the broad spectrum of radiographic changes. There are various amounts of exuberant, irregular periosteal response and ragged bone destruction.

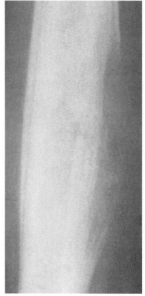

Fig B 8-2
Ewing's sarcoma. Laminated periosteal reaction on one side of the bone and thin periosteal elevation (Codman's triangle) on the other.

Condition	Imaging Findings	Comments
Secondary malignant tumor of bone (Fig B 8-4)	Multiple areas of localized solid or laminated periosteal reaction associated with an underlying destructive process. There may be perpendicular periosteal reaction in the skull.	Common manifestation in children with leukemia and metastases from neuroblastoma.
Benign bone tumor or cyst (Fig B 8-5)	Various patterns of periosteal reaction.	Solid periosteal reaction with expanding cysts or tumors, especially if there is an underlying pathologic fracture. Elliptical and dense periosteal reaction in osteoid osteoma (radiolucent intracortical nidus).
Osteomyelitis (Figs B 8-6 and B 8-7)	Solid or laminated periosteal reaction.	Subperiosteal spread of inflammation elevates the periosteum and stimulates the laying down of layers of new bone parallel to the shaft. Eventually, a large amount of new bone surrounds the cortex in a thick, irregular bony sleeve (involucrum). Disruption of the cortical blood supply leads to bone necrosis with dense segments of avascular dead bone (sequestra) remaining.
Subperiosteal hemorrhage	Solid or laminated periosteal reaction.	May result from trauma or hemophilia.

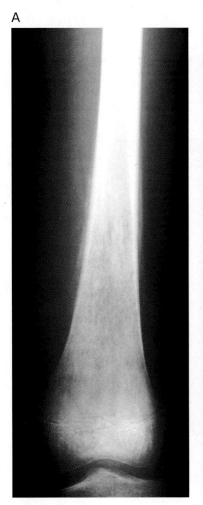
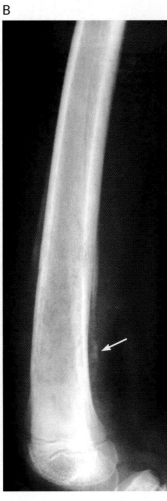

Fig B 8-3
Lymphoma. (A) Frontal radiograph of a child shows permeative changes of the distal femoral shaft with a dense periosteal reaction. (B) Lateral view clearly shows the laminated and interrupted periosteal reaction (arrow), a feature of round cell tumors including lymphoma and Ewing's sarcoma. [18]

Condition	Imaging Findings	Comments
Langerhans cell histiocytosis (see Fig B 6-18)	Solid or laminated periosteal reaction that may be localized or extensive.	Characteristic appearance of a sharply defined lucency with a peculiar beveled pattern and multiple undulating contours.
Arthritis	Solid or laminated periosteal reaction.	Most common in juvenile rheumatoid arthritis and reactive arthritis; rare in psoriatic arthritis.
Vascular stasis (Fig B 8-8)	Solid, often undulating, periosteal reaction primarily along the tibial and fibular shafts.	Chronic venous or lymphatic insufficiency or obstruction. Phleboliths often occur in varicose veins.

A
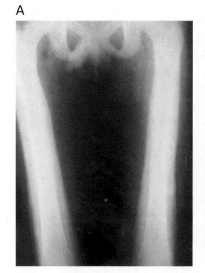

B
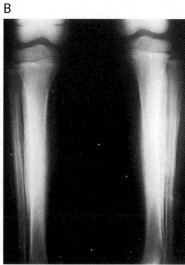

Fig B 8-4
Chronic leukemia. Pronounced periosteal new bone formation cloaking (A) the femurs and (B) the tibias and fibulas.

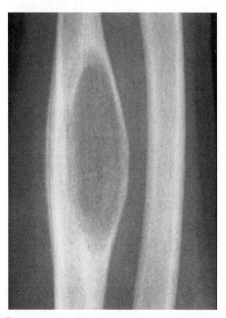

Fig B 8-5
Aneurysmal bone cyst of the radius. An expansile, eccentric, cyst-like lesion causes ballooning of the cortex and periosteal response.

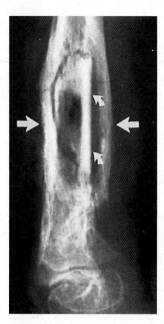

Fig B 8-6
Chronic osteomyelitis. The involucrum (straight arrows) surrounds the sequestrum (curved arrows).

Condition	Imaging Findings	Comments
Infantile cortical hyperostosis (Caffey's disease) (Fig B 8-9)	Laminated periosteal reaction in the healing phase. Primarily involves the mandible, scapula, clavicle, ulna, and ribs.	Now uncommon disease characterized by hyperirritability, soft-tissue swelling, periosteal new bone formation, and massive cortical thickening of underlying bones. Onset is almost always before 5 months of age.
Syphilis (acquired)/yaws (Figs B 8-10 and B 8-11)	Extensive, solid, often undulating, periosteal reaction occurring independently or in conjunction with gummas in the bone marrow.	Diffuse, widespread, and symmetric, periosteal reaction may reflect underlying infiltration by granulation tissue in congenital syphilis.

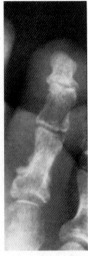

Fig B 8-7
Reiter's syndrome. Typical fluffy periosteal reaction about the proximal phalanx. There is also soft-tissue swelling of the toe.[19]

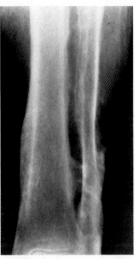

Fig B 8-8
Vascular stasis. Extensive periosteal changes about the tibial and fibular shafts.

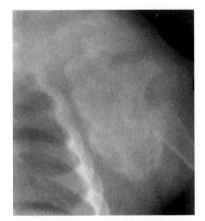

Fig B 8-9
Caffey's disease. Massive periosteal new bone formation about the left scapula.

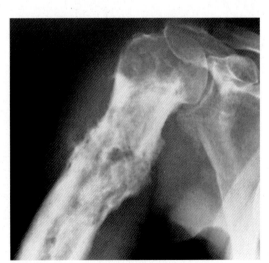

Fig B 8-10
Syphilis. Diffuse lytic destruction of the proximal humerus with reactive sclerosis and periosteal new bone formation.

Condition	Imaging Findings	Comments
Tropical ulcer (Fig B 8-12)	Fusiform periosteal reaction localized to the bone beneath the ulcer. Periosteal new bone blends with the cortex to produce the thickened, sclerotic cortex (often exceeding 1 cm) of a classic "ivory osteoma."	Extremely common disease throughout much of Africa that is caused by the Vincent types of fusiform bacilli and spirochetes. Chronic ulcers most often affect children and young adults and are usually located in the middle or lower leg.
Bone infarct	Solid periosteal response overlying the shaft of a large tubular bone (underlying patchy lucency and sclerosis of medullary bone).	Most common in sickle cell disease. Periosteal reaction may be radiographically indistinguishable from osteomyelitis.
Secondary osteomyelitis (spread from contiguous soft-tissue infection)	Solid periosteal reaction associated with bone destruction and sclerosis.	Most frequently occurs in patients with diabetes mellitus and vascular insufficiency and predominantly involves the hands and feet or the area adjacent to a decubitus ulcer.

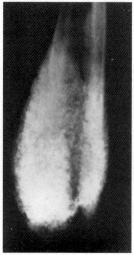

Fig B 8-11
Yaws. Massive patchy new bone formation affects both bones of the forearm. Strands of new bone extend in the line of the interosseous ligament.[8]

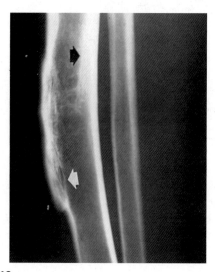

Fig B 8-12
Ivory osteoma of tropical ulcer. There is cortical thickening of the tibia on the side opposite the ulcer (black arrow), which had been present for 1 year. Medullary resorption is starting at the inner margin of the osteoma, and the solid cortex is beginning to show a trabecular pattern (white arrow).[20]

Widespread or Generalized Periosteal Reaction

Condition	Imaging Findings	Comments
Hypertrophic osteoarthropathy (Fig B 9-1)	Thick (initially thin), irregular, undulating periosteal reaction that eventually fuses with the cortex. Symmetrically involves the diaphyses of tubular bones (especially the long bones of the forearm and leg), sparing the ends. There is often associated soft-tissue swelling of the distal phalanges (clubbing) without changes in the underlying bone.	Most frequently arises in patients with primary intrathoracic neoplasms, especially bronchogenic carcinoma. Other common causes include tumors of the pleura and mediastinum, chronic suppurative lung lesions (lung abscess, bronchiectasis, empyema), and cystic fibrosis and pulmonary metastases in infants and children. Occasionally occurs in association with extrathoracic neoplasms and gastrointestinal diseases (biliary cirrhosis, ulcerative colitis, Crohn's disease).
Arthritis (see Fig B 8-6)	Generalized (or localized), solid or laminated periosteal reaction.	Juvenile rheumatoid arthritis (peripheral and axial skeleton, particularly at tendon and ligament insertions); reactive arthritis (calcaneus, short tubular bones of the foot, tibia, and fibula); psoriatic arthritis (infrequently).
Battered child syndrome (Fig B 9-2)	Exuberant solid or laminated periosteal reaction along the shafts of long bones (associated with multiple fractures).	Repeated traumatic injuries lead to multiple fractures in various stages of healing. There are often fractures of the corners of the metaphyses (with or without associated epiphyseal displacement) and one or more fractures at otherwise unusual sites (the ribs, scapula, sternum, spine, or lateral ends of the clavicles).

A
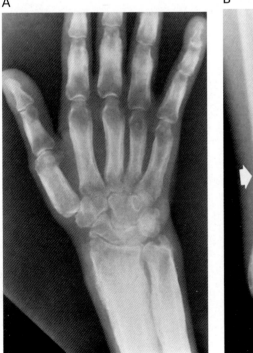

B
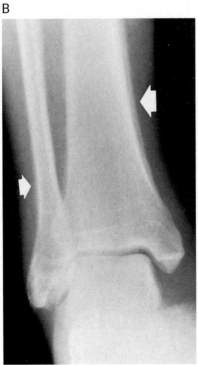

Fig B 9-1

Hypertrophic osteoarthropathy. Films of (A) the lower arm and hand and (B) the lower leg in patients with bronchogenic carcinoma and mesothelioma, respectively, demonstrate characteristic plaques of periosteal new bone (arrows). Note the irregular, undulating new bone formation affecting the distal radius and ulna. In the metacarpals, the periosteal reaction involves the diaphyses and spares the ends of these tubular bones. There is some periarticular demineralization about the metacarpophalangeal and metacarpocarpal joints but no evidence of bone erosion or cartilage destruction.

Condition	Imaging Findings	Comments
Physiologic periostitis of newborns	Generalized periosteal reaction along long bones of the extremities.	Occurs during the second and third months of life in up to 50% of infants (especially prematures). Generally considered to be a normal variation due to the exuberant bone growth at this age.
Idiopathic	Multiple and often symmetric solid periosteal reaction primarily involving tubular bones.	Most frequently occurs at tendon and ligament insertions into bone.
Venous or lymphatic stasis (Fig B 9-3)	Generalized (or localized) solid, thin or thick, often undulating periosteal reaction most commonly along the tibial and fibular shafts.	In venous stasis (eg, varicose veins), there may be development of phleboliths (calcified venous thrombi that appear as round densities and often contain lucent centers); there may also be plaque-like calcification in chronically congested subcutaneous tissues.
Thyroid acropachy (Fig B 9-4)	Generalized and symmetric spiculated periosteal reaction that primarily involves the midportions of the diaphyses of tubular bones of the hands and feet. Multiple small radiolucencies in the irregular periosteal new bone may produce a bubbly or lacy appearance.	Rare complication of hyperthyroid disease characterized by progressive exophthalmus, relatively asymptomatic swelling of the hands and feet, clubbing of the digits, and pretibial myxedema. Develops after thyroidectomy or radioactive iodine treatment of primary hyperthyroidism (most patients are euthyroid or hypothyroid when symptoms develop).

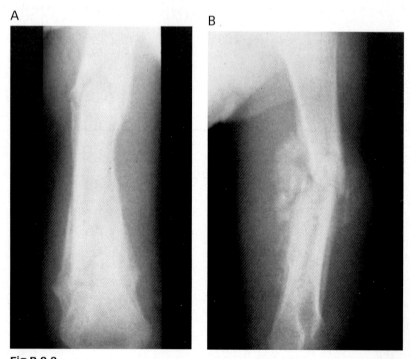

Fig B 9-2
Battered child. (A and B) Periosteal reaction about healing fractures of both humeri.

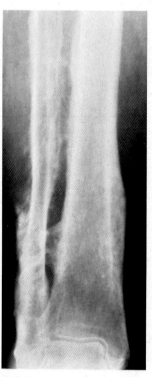

Fig B 9-3
Venous stasis. Periosteal new bone formation cloaking the tibia and fibula.

Condition	Imaging Findings	Comments
Pachydermoperiostosis (primary hypertrophic osteoarthropathy) (see Fig B 11-10)	Generalized and symmetric periosteal reaction that tends to blend with the cortex and primarily involves the distal ends of the radius, ulna, tibia, and fibula.	Inherited disorder characterized by marked thickening of the skin of the extremities, face, and scalp. Self-limited disease that most commonly affects adolescent males and progresses for several years before stabilizing.
Infantile cortical hyperostosis (Caffey's disease) (see Fig B 8-8)	Multiple areas of laminated periosteal reaction and massive cortical thickening in the healing phase. Primarily involves the mandible, scapula, clavicle, ulna, and ribs.	Now uncommon disease characterized by hyperirritability, soft-tissue swelling, periosteal new bone formation, and cortical thickening of underlying bones. Onset is almost always before 5 months of age. Scapular lesion (usually unilateral) may be mistaken for malignant tumor.
Hypervitaminosis A (Fig B 9-5)	Generalized solid or laminated periosteal reaction that is greatest near the center of the shaft and tapers toward the ends. Unlike Caffey's disease, periosteal thickening in hypervitaminosis A rarely involves the mandible.	Chronic excessive intake of vitamin A produces a syndrome characterized by bone and joint pain, hair loss, pruritus, anorexia, dryness and fissures of the lips, hepatosplenomegaly, and yellow tinting of the skin. The radiographic changes are most commonly seen between ages 1 and 3.
Fluorosis (see Fig B 18-16)	Generalized and symmetric periosteal reaction that primarily involves tubular bones (especially at sites of muscle and ligament attachments).	Fluorine poisoning causes dense skeletal sclerosis (most prominent in vertebrae and the pelvis) with calcification of ligaments (iliolumbar, sacrotuberous, and sacrospinous).
Gaucher's disease	Generalized periosteal reaction involving long tubular bones, the spine, and the pelvis.	Inborn error of lipid metabolism characterized by a ground-glass pattern, aseptic necrosis of the femoral head, and Erlenmeyer flask deformities.

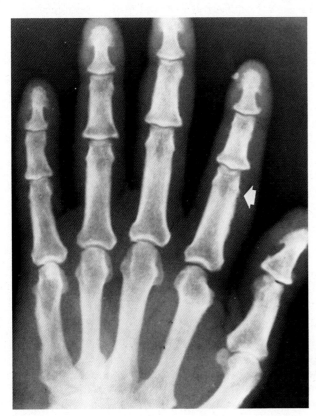

Fig B 9-4
Thyroid acropachy. Spiculated periosteal new bone formation, seen best on the radial aspect of the proximal phalanx of the second digit (arrow).

Condition	Imaging Findings	Comments
Congenital syphilis (see Fig B 21-1)	Diffuse, widespread, symmetric, and profound periosteal reaction primarily affecting long tubular bones.	Reflects underlying infiltration by syphilitic granulation tissue. Complete but slow resolution with treatment.
Tuberous sclerosis (see Fig B 31-6)	Diffuse undulating periosteal reaction or periosteal "nodules" involving tubular bones (especially metacarpals, metatarsals, and phalanges).	Rare inherited disorder presenting with clinical triad of convulsive seizures, mental deficiency, and adenoma sebaceum. There are often renal and intracranial hematomas and characteristic scattered intracerebral calcifications.
Thermal burns	Periosteal reaction in bones underlying areas of severe burns (represents local response to periosteal irritation).	Generally develops within several months after injury. In tubular bones, produces a radiographic appearance similar to that of hypertrophic osteoarthropathy.
Hand-foot syndrome (sickle cell anemia) (see Fig B 31-1)	Generalized periosteal reaction involving short tubular bones.	Follows infarctions in young children with sickle cell disease and produces a periosteal reaction indistinguishable from osteomyelitis.
Healing scurvy (Fig B 9-6)	Generalized massive periosteal reaction during the healing phase.	Findings in acute disease include characteristic "white line," Pelken's spur, Wimberger's sign, and demineralized epiphyseal ossification centers surrounded by dense sharply demarcated rings of calcification.
Healing rickets	Generalized solid or laminated periosteal new bone formation (represents remineralization of subperiosteal osteoid).	Thin stripes of density may develop along the outer cortical margins of long bones during acute disease. Although they resemble inflammatory periosteal reaction, these shadows represent zones of poorly calcified osteoid laid down by the periosteum.

A

B

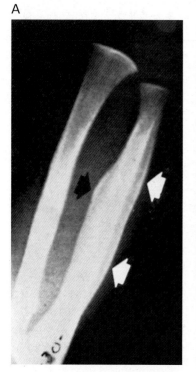
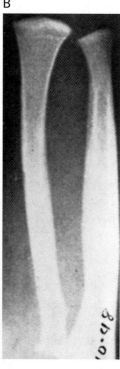

Fig B 9-5
Hypervitaminosis A. (A) Thin, wavy, shelf-like cortical thickening (arrows) during the active phase of poisoning. (B) Four months after stoppage of the vitamin concentrate, the hyperostosis is shrunken, smooth, and more sclerotic.[21]

Condition	Imaging Findings	Comments
Polyarteritis nodosa	Generalized symmetric periosteal reaction, most frequently involving the shafts of bones of the lower legs.	Pattern identical to that of hypertrophic osteoarthropathy.

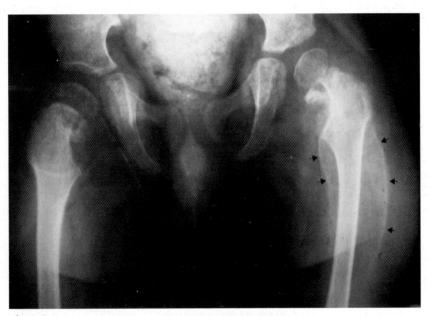

Fig B 9-6
Scurvy. Large, calcifying, subperiosteal hematoma of the femoral shaft (arrows).[16]

Arthritides

Condition	Joints Commonly Involved	Radiographic and Clinical Appearance
Osteoarthritis (degenerative joint disease) (Fig B 10-1)	Distal interphalangeal joints of the fingers; first carpometacarpal joint; hips; knees, first metatarsophalangeal joints; spine.	Bilateral, nonuniform joint space narrowing, subchondral sclerosis, and marginal osteophyte (spur) formation. Subchondral cysts are common, whereas osteoporosis is typically absent. Primary osteoarthritis most frequently affects postmenopausal women and is characterized by classic Heberden's nodes (enlargement of spurs to produce well-defined bony protuberances that appear clinically as palpable and visible knobby thickening). Osteoarthritis may also be secondary to trauma, ischemic necrosis, malalignment of bony structures, and other arthritides.
Erosive (inflammatory) osteoarthritis (Fig B 10-2)	Distal interphalangeal joints and first carpometacarpal joint.	Inflammatory process associated with proliferative and erosive abnormalities that predominantly involves middle-aged women. If proliferative changes (osteophytosis, sclerosis) predominate, the resulting radiographic appearance is identical to that of noninflammatory osteoarthritis. The erosions of inflammatory osteoarthritis frequently predominate in the central portion of the joint, unlike the marginal erosions of rheumatoid arthritis, psoriasis, gout, and multicentric reticulohistiocytosis.

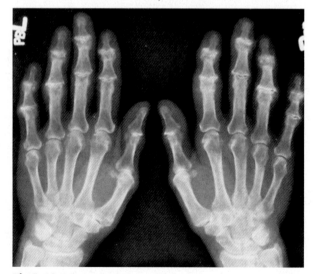

Fig B 10-1
Osteoarthritis of the fingers.

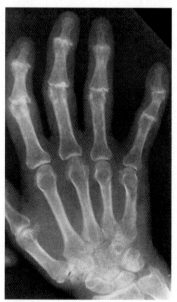

Fig B 10-2
Erosive osteoarthritis of the hand. Narrowing of the proximal and distal interphalangeal joints with erosions and spur formation.

Condition	Joints Commonly Involved	Radiographic and Clinical Appearance
Rheumatoid arthritis (Figs B 10-3 through B 10-6) (see Figs SP 13-1 and SP 17-6)	Bilateral, symmetric involvement of metacarpophalangeal, proximal interphalangeal, and carpal joints with similar involvement of the feet. Characteristic erosion of the ulnar styloid process. The condition often progresses toward the trunk until practically every joint in the body is involved. Atlantoaxial subluxation may develop due to weakening of the transverse ligaments from synovial inflammation.	Initially, fusiform periarticular soft-tissue swelling (due to joint effusion and hyperplastic synovitis) associated with periarticular osteoporosis (due to disuse and local hyperemia). Extension of pannus from synovial reflections onto the bones causes characteristic small foci of erosive destruction at the edges of the joint. Destruction of articular cartilage causes generalized joint space narrowing that is frequently associated with extensive bone resorption. Severe complications include opera-glass hand, solid bony ankylosis, and a variety of contractures and subluxations (boutonnière, swan neck, ulnar deviation). On MRI, pannus has a slightly higher signal than joint fluid on T1-weighted images, and this highly vascular tissue has been reported to demonstrate intense enhancement.

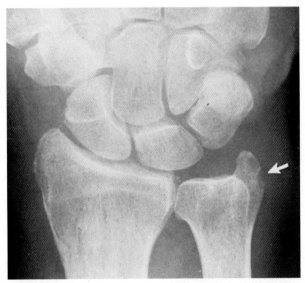

Fig B 10-3
Rheumatoid arthritis. Characteristic erosion of the ulnar styloid process (arrow) by an adjacent tenosynovitis of the extensor carpi ulnaris tendon. Note the associated soft-tissue swelling.

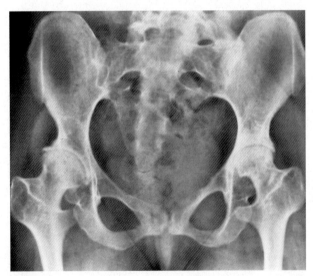

Fig B 10-4
Rheumatoid arthritis of the pelvis and hips. There is narrowing of the hip joints bilaterally with some reactive sclerosis. Note the relative preservation of the subchondral cortical margins. In contrast to degenerative disease, the joint space narrowing in rheumatoid arthritis is symmetric and not confined to weight-bearing surfaces. Note also the obliteration of both sacroiliac joints.

Condition	Joints Commonly Involved	Radiographic and Clinical Appearance
Juvenile rheumatoid arthritis (Fig B 10-7)	Rapidly growing joints (knees, ankles, wrists), unlike the peripheral distribution of involved joints in the adult form. Monarticular disease, especially in a knee, is more common in the juvenile type.	Initially, periarticular soft-tissue swelling and osteoporosis. Joint space narrowing and articular erosions are late findings. Periosteal calcification is much more common and severe than in the adult form, whereas synovial cysts infrequently occur. Ankylosis about the wrist and ankle is common. Variety of growth disturbances, including initial acceleration because of local hyperemia, then delay due to epiphyseal fusion or the administration of steroids. Overgrowth of the epiphysis of an affected joint may produce a characteristic balloon appearance. Other findings include apophyseal joint ankylosis and atlantoaxial subluxation in the cervical spine, erosion of the mandibular condyles and micrognathia, and erosion of the intercondylar notch of the femur (simulates hemophilia).

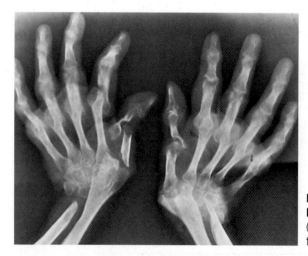

Fig B 10-5
Mutilating rheumatoid arthritis. Opera-glass hand (main en lorgnette deformity) due to extensive destruction and telescoping of bone ends.

A
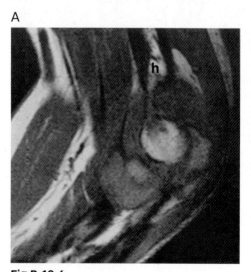

B
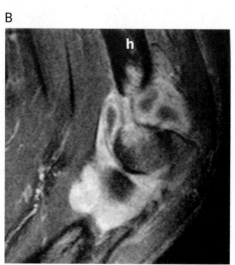

Fig B 10-6
Rheumatoid arthritis. (A) Sagittal T1-weighted image shows a distended joint as indicated by low signal surrounding the distal humerus (h). (B) T1-weighted, fat-suppressed image after contrast administration shows diffuse enhancement of the pannus.[22]

Condition	Joints Commonly Involved	Radiographic and Clinical Appearance
Psoriatic arthritis (Figs B 10-8 and B 10-9)	Bilateral, usually asymmetric, involvement of distal interphalangeal joints (may also affect proximal interphalangeal joints) of the hands and feet; sacroiliac joints; and spine.	Soft-tissue swelling, joint space narrowing, and periarticular erosions simulating rheumatoid arthritis (though psoriatic disease predominantly involves distal rather than proximal interphalangeal joints, is asymmetric, and causes little or no periarticular osteoporosis). Characteristic radiographic features include a tendency toward bony ankylosis of the interphalangeal joints, resorption of terminal tufts of the distal phalanges, fluffy periosteal reaction near joints and along shafts, and arthritis mutilans with "pencil-in-cup" deformity. Unilateral or bilateral sacroiliitis and asymmetric syndesmophytes in the thoracolumbar spine.
Reactive arthritis (arthritis, urethritis, conjunctivitis, mucocutaneous lesions) (Figs B 10-10 and B 10-11; see Fig B 8-6)	Sacroiliac joints; heels; toes.	Primarily affects young adults, mostly males (after certain types of venereal or enteric infections). Radiographic changes often mimic rheumatoid arthritis, though in reactive arthritis they tend to be asymmetric and primarily involve the feet. Typical manifestations include fluffy periostitis adjacent to the small joints of the foot, ankle, and calcaneus; inferior calcaneal spurs; asymmetric sacroiliitis; and asymmetric syndesmophytes in the thoracolumbar spine.

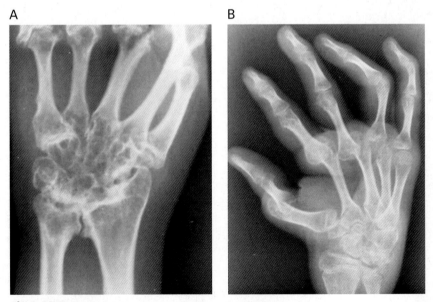

A   B

Fig B 10-7
Juvenile rheumatoid arthritis. (A) Severe deossification of the carpal bones with joint space narrowing and even obliteration. Note the virtual ankylosis between the distal radius and the proximal carpal row. (B) Multiple subluxations, especially involving the metacarpophalangeal joints. There is diffuse periarticular soft-tissue swelling with moderate osteoporosis.

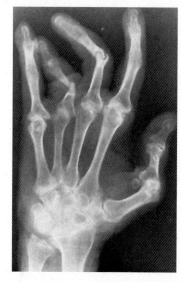

Fig B 10-8
Psoriatic arthritis. Bizarre pattern of asymmetric bone destruction, subluxation, and ankylosis. Note particularly the pencil-in-cup deformity of the third proximal interphalangeal joint and the bony ankylosis involving the wrist and the phalanges of the second and fifth digits.

A

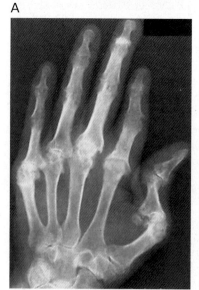

B

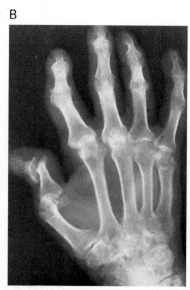

Fig B 10-9
Psoriatic arthritis. Views of both hands and wrists demonstrate ankylosis across many of the interphalangeal joints with scattered erosive changes involving several interphalangeal joints, most of the metacarpophalangeal joints, and the interphalangeal joint of the right thumb. Note the striking asymmetry of involvement of the carpal bones, an appearance unlike that expected in rheumatoid arthritis.

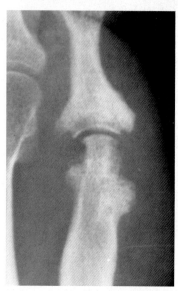

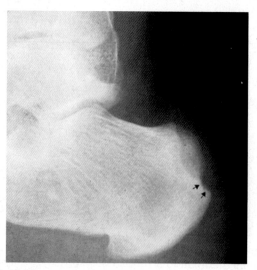

Fig B 10-10
Reactive arthritis. Erosive changes about the metatarso-phalangeal joint of the fifth digit. The erosions involve the juxtaarticular region, leaving the articular cortex intact.

Fig B 10-11
Reactive arthritis. Striking bony erosion (arrows) at the insertion of the Achilles tendon on the posterosuperior margin of the calcaneus.

Condition	Joints Commonly Involved	Radiographic and Clinical Appearance
Ankylosing spondylitis (Figs B 10-12 through B 10-14)	Sacroiliac joints; spine; hips; small joints of the hands and feet.	Almost always begins as bilateral, symmetric sacroiliitis that may lead to complete fibrous and bony ankylosis. In the lumbar spine, the disease tends initially to involve the lowermost levels and progress upward with characteristic squared vertebral bodies and bamboo spine (ossification in paravertebral tissues and longitudinal spinal ligaments combined with extensive lateral bony bridges [syndesmophytes] between vertebral bodies). Fractures often occur through a disk space (rather than a vertebral body) and continue through the posterior elements. Irregular proliferative new bone formation ("whiskering") often develops at sites of ligamentous or muscular attachments. Peripheral joint involvement (in up to half the patients) simulates psoriasis or Reiter's syndrome.
Jaccoud's arthritis (Fig B 10-15)	Multiple joints of the hands and, less frequently, the feet.	Rare occurrence after resolution of a severe attack of rheumatic fever. Usually there is only self-limited periarticular swelling, but it may rarely cause permanent deformities (ulnar deviation, flexion contractures) without joint space narrowing or bone erosion.
Arthritis associated with inflammatory bowel disease	Sacroiliac joints; spine; knees; elbows.	Spinal involvement identical to ankylosing spondylitis. Peripheral arthritis is usually limited to soft-tissue swelling and joint effusion, which tend to be migratory, usually follow the onset of colitis, generally flare up during exacerbations of colonic disease, and usually cause no residual damage. Some form of arthritis occurs in up to 25% of patients with ulcerative or Crohn's colitis.

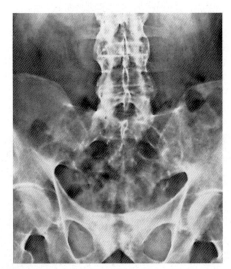

Fig B 10-12
Ankylosing spondylitis. Bilateral symmetric obliteration of the sacroiliac joints with prominent syndesmophytes in the lower lumbar spine.

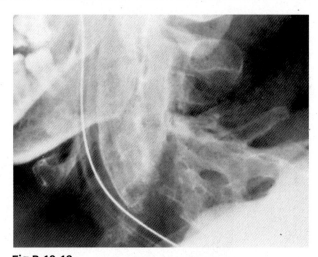

Fig B 10-13
Ankylosing spondylitis. Oblique fracture of the midcervical spine, with anterior dislocation of the superior segment, is seen in a patient who fell while dancing and struck his head. The fracture extends through the lateral mass and lamina. Because of loss of flexibility and osteoporosis, patients with ankylosing spondylitis can suffer a fracture with relatively slight trauma.

Condition	Joints Commonly Involved	Radiographic and Clinical Appearance
Gout (Figs B 10-16 through B 10-19)	First metatarsophalangeal joint; interphalangeal joints; elbows; knees.	Joint effusion, periarticular swelling, soft-tissue tophi, and characteristic "rat bite" erosions with sclerotic margins and overhanging edges adjacent to (but not involving) the articular surface. In advanced disease, severe destructive lesions are associated with joint space narrowing and even fibrous ankylosis. No osteoporosis (patients are symptom-free and without disability between acute attacks). There may be chondrocalcinosis and acro-osteolysis of terminal phalangeal tufts. On MRI, most tophi are isointense relative to muscle on T1-weighted images; on T2-weighted images, most have low to intermediate heterogeneous signal intensity, although lesions with high intensity have been reported. Homogeneous and intense contrast enhancement is frequently observed.

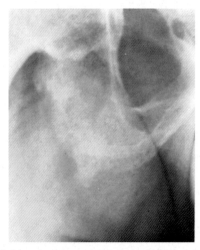

Fig B 10-14
Ankylosing spondylitis. Irregular proliferation of new bone (whiskering) along the inferior pubic ramus.

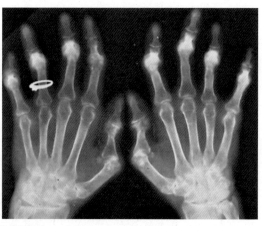

Fig B 10-15
Jaccoud's arthritis. Frontal views of the hands and wrists demonstrate mild ulnar deviation with pronounced flexion of the proximal interphalangeal joints. There is no evidence of joint space narrowing or bone erosion.

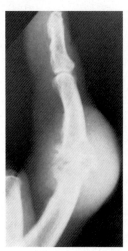

Fig B 10-16
Gout. Severe joint effusion and periarticular swelling about the proximal interphalangeal joint of a finger. Note the associated erosion of articular cartilage.

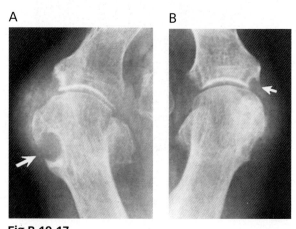

Fig B 10-17
Gout. Two examples of typical rat-bite erosions about the first metatarsophalangeal joint (arrows). The cyst-like lesions have thin sclerotic margins and characteristic overhanging edges.

Condition	Joints Commonly Involved	Radiographic and Clinical Appearance
Hemophilia (Figs B 10-20 through B 10-22)	Knees; elbows; ankles.	Recurrent bleeding into joints initially causes joint distention with cloudy increased density (deposition of iron pigment) in the periarticular soft tissues. In chronic disease, the hyperplastic synovium causes cartilage destruction and joint space narrowing with multiple subchondral cysts. Other characteristic findings include enlargement and premature ossification of epiphyseal centers, widening and deepening of the intercondylar notch of the femur, squaring of the inferior border of the patella, and destructive expansile bone lesions (pseudotumor of hemophilia) representing extensive intraosseous hemorrhage. On MRI, hypertrophied synovial membrane resulting from repetitive hemarthrosis has characteristic low signal in all pulse sequences, due to the magnetic susceptibility effect caused by hemosiderin.
CPPD disease (Fig B 10-23)	Knees; wrists; elbows; hips; shoulders.	Leads to the development of secondary osteoarthritis (subchondral cyst formation, hypertrophic spurring, joint space narrowing, and subchondral sclerosis). Frequent chondrocalcinosis.
Hydroxyapatite deposition disease	Shoulders; hips.	Amorphous calcifications in joints or bursae may cause inflammatory erosive changes.
Systemic lupus erythematosus (Fig B 10-24)	Hands.	Subluxations and malalignment of joints in the absence of erosions. Typical deformities include ulnar deviation at the metacarpophalangeal joints and hyperextension and hyperflexion deformities (boutonnière, swan neck) at the interphalangeal joints.

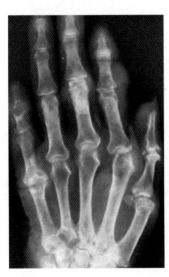

Fig B 10-18
Gout. Diffuse deposition of urate crystals in periarticular tissues of the hand produce multiple large, lumpy soft-tissue swellings representing gouty tophi. Note the erosive changes that typically involve the carpal bones and the distal interphalangeal and metacarpophalangeal joints of the fifth digits.

Condition	Joints Commonly Involved	Radiographic and Clinical Appearance
Scleroderma (see Fig B 19-1)	Hands and feet.	Soft-tissue swelling and periarticular osteoporosis along with characteristic terminal phalangeal resorption and soft-tissue calcifications. Erosive changes may represent coexistent rheumatoid arthritis.

A

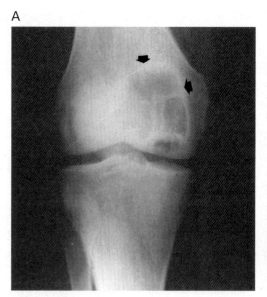

B

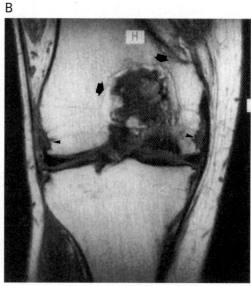

Fig B 10-19
Gout. (A) Frontal radiograph of the knee shows an osteolytic lesion involving the internal condyle and intercondylar area of the distal femur with a well-defined sclerotic margin (arrows). (B) Coronal T1-weighted MR image shows a well-defined lesion of heterogeneous signal intensity with a scalloped margin (arrows), which communicates with the joint space. Marrow surrounding the lesion shows normal intensity. The small erosions of the femoral condyles and adjacent soft-tissue masses (arrowheads) presumably represent juxta-articular tophi.[23]

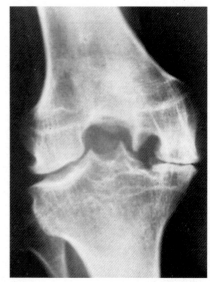

Fig B 10-20
Hemophilia. The intracondylar notch is markedly widened and there are coarsened trabeculae, narrowing of the joint space, and hypertrophic spurring.

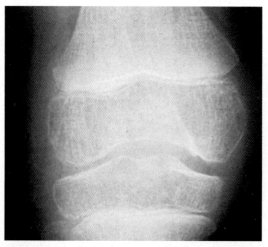

Fig B 10-21
Hemophilia of the knee in a child. There is demineralization and coarse trabeculation with overgrowth of the distal femoral and proximal tibial epiphyses. The intercondylar notch is moderately widened.

Condition	Joints Commonly Involved	Radiographic and Clinical Appearance
Sarcoidosis (see Fig B 31-5)	Hands.	In approximately 15% of patients, the disease presents as a transient acute polyarthritis with periarticular soft-tissue swelling. No significant osteoporosis or chronic radiographic deformities. The phalanges may show a coarsened trabecular pattern or sharply circumscribed, punched-out lucent areas.
Familial Mediterranean fever	Sacroiliac joints; large joints of the lower extremities.	Nonspecific transient soft-tissue swelling and osteoporosis with rare destructive changes. Bilateral, asymmetric involvement of sacroiliac joints.
Neuroarthropathies (see Section B 13)		See page 1053.
Multicentric reticulohistiocytosis (Fig B 10-25)	Bilateral, symmetric involvement of interphalangeal joints of the hands and feet. Atlantoaxial subluxation.	Well-circumscribed marginal erosions (simulating gout) due to the deposition of lipid-containing macrophages. May eventually cause dramatic resorption of phalanges, foreshortening of fingers, and end-stage arthritis mutilans. Characteristic development of multiple soft-tissue masses that produce a "lumpy-bumpy" appearance.
Ochronosis (homogentisic acid deposition) (see Fig SP 14-2)	Spine; shoulders; hips; knees.	Dense laminated calcification of multiple intervertebral disks (begins in the lumbar spine and may extend cephalad). Narrowing of intervertebral disk spaces and osteoporosis of vertebral bodies. Severe degenerative type of arthritis (joint space narrowing, marginal osteophytes, subchondral sclerosis) may develop in large peripheral joints at a young age.

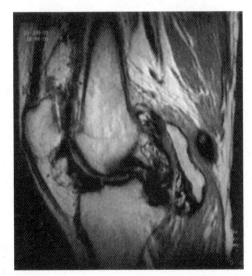

Fig B 10-22
Hemophilia. Sagittal T1-weighted MR image shows thickened synovial tissue with very low signal intensity due to hemosiderin deposits and to scar and fibrous tissue formation in this patient with chronic arthropathy.[23]

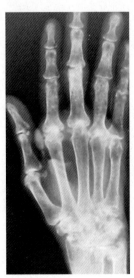

Fig B 10-23
CPPD arthropathy. Severe joint space narrowing, erosive changes, and sclerosis about the wrist. Less marked changes involve the metacarpophalangeal joints and the proximal interphalangeal joint of the third digit.

Condition	Joints Commonly Involved	Radiographic and Clinical Appearance
Hemochromatosis (synovial deposition of iron) (Fig B 10-26)	Metacarpophalangeal and interphalangeal joints of the hands.	Subarticular cysts and erosions, joint space narrowing, osteophytes, sclerosis, subluxation, and flattening and widening of the metacarpal heads (especially the second and third). May also produce osteoarthritic changes in large joints (knees, hips) and diffuse osteoporosis of the spine leading to vertebral collapse.

A
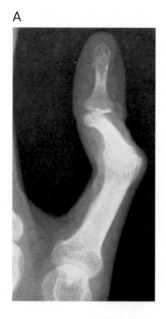

B
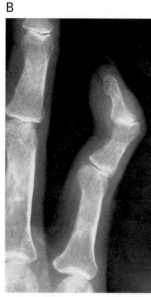

Fig B 10-24
Systemic lupus erythematosus. (A) Flexion of the proximal interphalangeal joint and hyperextension of the distal interphalangeal joint result in a boutonnière deformity. (B) Hyperextension of the proximal interphalangeal joint and flexion of the distal interphalangeal joint produce a swan-neck deformity.[19]

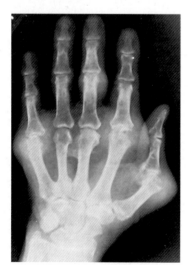

Fig B 10-25
Multicentric histiocytosis. Multiple soft-tissue masses produce a "lumpy-bumpy" appearance. The soft-tissue deposits of multinucleated giant cells have produced erosions of juxta-articular bone. Although at this stage most of the joint spaces are spared, extensive involvement of the second metacarpophalangeal joint has led to total joint destruction.[19]

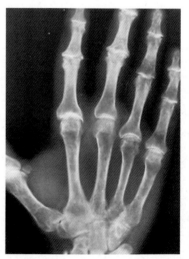

Fig B 10-26
Hemochromatosis. Diffuse joint space narrowing with scattered erosions, osteophytes, and articular sclerosis.

Condition	Joints Commonly Involved	Radiographic and Clinical Appearance
Acromegaly (excess growth hormone in adults) (Fig B 10-27)	Generalized cartilage overgrowth (especially metacarpophalangeal and hip joints).	Degenerative changes with prominent hypertrophic spurring develop at an early age, but, unlike typical osteoarthritis, acromegaly results in joint spaces that remain normal or are even widened. Associated findings include overgrowth of terminal phalangeal tufts, thickened heel pads, and micrognathia.
Pigmented villonodular synovitis (PVNS) (Figs B 10-28 and B 10-29)	Knees; ankles; hips.	Joint effusion with multiple nodular soft-tissue masses that never calcify but may appear dense because of hemosiderin deposits. Invasion of adjacent bone may cause subchondral cyst-like defects with sharp and sclerotic margins. Unlike rheumatoid or infectious arthritis, the joint space is usually preserved, and there is no osteoporosis as the disorder does not cause much disability. On MR, hemosiderin causes the synovial lesions to have low signal intensity (especially at the periphery) on T2-weighted images. On MRI, the diffuse or nodularly thickened synovium has low to intermediate signal intensity relative to that of muscle on T1-weighted images and low signal intensity on T2-weighted sequences (due to the magnetic susceptibility effect of hemosiderin and more manifest in the periphery of the lesions).

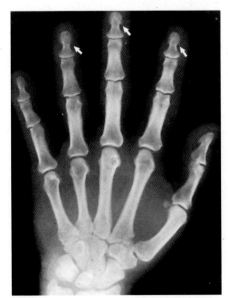

Fig B 10-27
Acromegaly. Widening of the metacarpophalangeal joints, thickening of the soft tissues of the fingers, and overgrowth of the tufts of the distal phalanges (arrows).

A 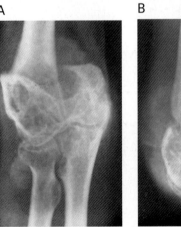 B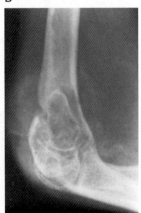

Fig B 10-28
Pigmented villonodular synovitis. (A) Frontal and (B) lateral views of the elbow demonstrate a joint effusion with nodular soft-tissue masses extending beyond the joint capsule. The soft-tissue mass appears dense because of deposits of hemosiderin in it. Large bone erosions reflect a combination of pressure effect and direct invasion by the synovial growth.

Condition	Joints Commonly Involved	Radiographic and Clinical Appearance

Infectious arthritis
  Pyogenic
  (Figs B 10-30 and B 10-31)
	Any joint (most commonly the knees, hips, shoulders, and spine).	Soft-tissue swelling followed by rapid destruction of cartilage (joint space narrowing) and bone that first appears on plain radiographs 8 to 10 days after the onset of symptoms. Severe, untreated infection causes extensive destruction and loss of the entire cortical outline. Complete destruction of articular cartilage leads to bony ankylosis. In the spine, pyogenic arthritis rapidly involves the intervertebral disks (unlike metastatic disease). On MRI, the joint effusion and synovitis are low signal intensity on T1-weighted images and have high signal on T2-weighted sequences.

A

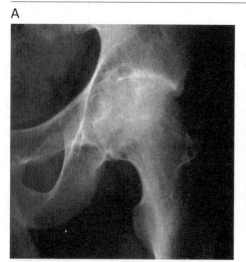

B

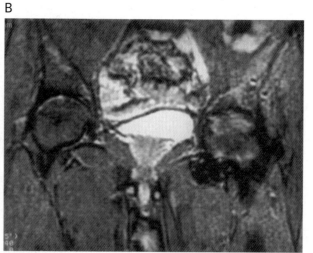

Fig B 10-29
Pigmented villonodular synovitis. (A) Frontal radiograph of the hip shows narrowing of the joint space and multiple subchondral lytic defects on both sides of the joint. (B) Coronal gradient-echo MR image shows tissue of very low signal intensity outlining the joint capsule. Note the prominent deposition of hemosiderin.[23]

A

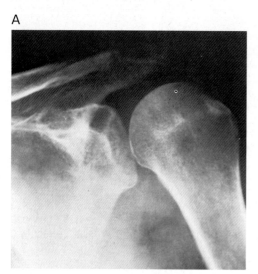

B

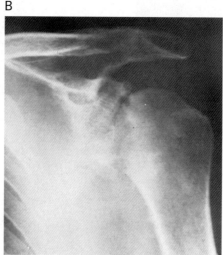

Fig B 10-30
Acute staphylococcal arthritis. (A) Several days after instrumentation of the shoulder for joint pain, there is separation of the humeral head from the glenoid fossa due to fluid in the joint space. (B) Six weeks later, there is marked cartilage and bone destruction, with sclerosis on both sides of the glenohumeral joint.

Condition	Joints Commonly Involved	Radiographic and Clinical Appearance
Tuberculous (Figs B 10-32 and B 10-33)	Spine; hips; knees.	Insidious onset and slowly progressive course characterized by extensive juxta-articular osteoporosis that precedes bone destruction (unlike pyogenic arthritis, in which osteoporosis is a relatively late finding). Cartilage and bone destruction occur relatively late and tend initially to involve the periphery of a joint, sparing the maximum-weight-bearing surfaces that are destroyed in pyogenic arthritis. In the spine, infection begins in the vertebral body (not the disk, as in pyogenic infection) and leads to vertebral collapse and often a characteristic sharp, angular kyphosis (gibbous deformity). Extension of the infection may produce a cold abscess (fusiform soft-tissue paraspinal mass).

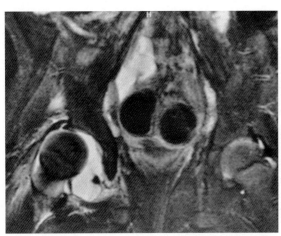

Fig B 10-31
Septic arthritis. Coronal STIR MR image in a child demonstrates a large, high-signal joint effusion in the right hip that causes the femoral head to sublux laterally from the acetabulum. No bone erosion or marrow edema is evident.[22]

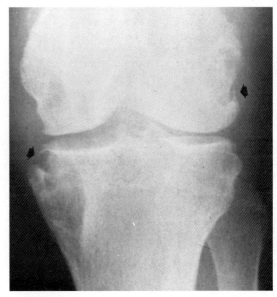

Fig B 10-32
Tuberculous arthritis of the knee. On both sides of the joint there are destructive bone lesions (arrows) involving the medial and lateral condyles and the medial aspect of the proximal tibia. Note the relative sparing of the articular cartilage and preservation of the joint space in view of the degree of bone destruction.

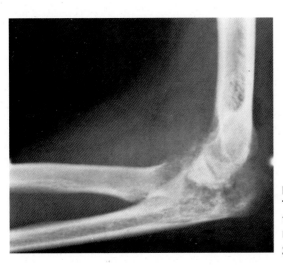

Fig B 10-33
Tuberculous arthritis of the elbow. Complete destruction of the joint space. The large antecubital mass reflects marked synovial hypertrophy resulting from chronic granulomatous infection.[19]

Condition	Joints Commonly Involved	Radiographic and Clinical Appearance
Fungal	Peripheral joints or the spine.	Variable radiographic manifestations requiring joint aspiration for diagnosis.
Viral	Small joints of the hands.	Transient joint effusion in rubella, mumps, or serum hepatitis, which usually subsides without bone lesions.
Transient arthritides	Variable pattern.	Episodes of arthritic symptoms that usually subside without residual joint damage may occur in such conditions as Behçet's syndrome. Sjögren's syndrome, polyarteritis, dermatomyositis, and relapsing polychondritis.
Amyloid (Fig B 10-34)	Axial (primarily cervical spine) or peripheral skeleton (especially shoulder).	In the glenohumeral and other large joints, amyloid arthropathy resembles inflammatory arthritis with juxta-articular soft-tissue swelling, mild periarticular osteoporosis, and subchondral cystic lesions, usually with sclerotic margins. On MRI, extensive amyloid deposition has low or intermediate signal on T1-weighted images and low to intermediate signal intensity of T2-weighted sequences.

A

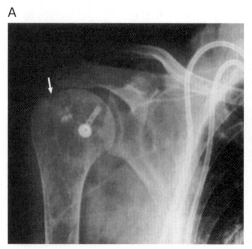

B

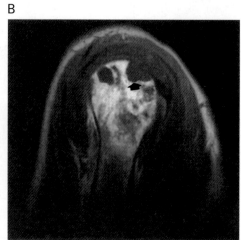

C

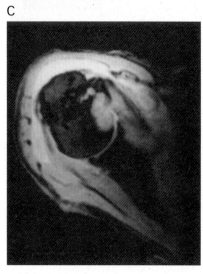

Fig B 10-34
Amyloid arthropathy. (A) Frontal radiograph shows diffuse soft-tissue swelling around the shoulder associated with small erosions in the humeral head (arrow). (B) Sagittal T1-weighted MR image shows extensive periarticular deposition of an abnormal soft tissue that is isointense relative to skeletal muscle and extends into subchondral defects (arrow). (C) Axial gradient-echo MR image shows distention of the subdeltoid bursa and an erosion of the anterior humeral head, which contains material of signal intensity less than that of fluid.[23]

Condition	Joints Commonly Involved	Radiographic and Clinical Appearance
Rapidly destructive articular disease (Fig B 10-35)	Hip (almost always unilateral).	Most frequently affects elderly women. Serial radiographs show progressive loss of joint space and loss of subchondral bone in the femoral head and acetabulum, resulting in marked flattening and deformity of the femoral head ("hatchet" deformity). Subchondral defects and mild sclerosis are common, though osteophytes are small or absent. Superolateral subluxation of the femoral head or intrusion deformity within the ilium can be observed.
Milwaukee shoulder (Fig B 10-36)	Shoulder.	Syndrome consisting of a complete tear of the rotator cuff, osteoarthritis changes, and noninflammatory joint effusion. Presents as joint space narrowing, subchondral sclerosis with cyst formation, capsular calcifications, and intra-articular loose bodies. MR shows a complete rotator cuff tear, large effusion, and thinning of cartilage with destruction of subchondral bone.

A   B

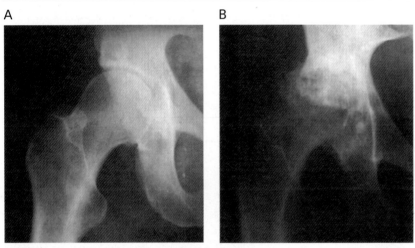

Fig B 10-35
Rapidly destructive articular disease. (A) Frontal radiograph of the hip obtained before the onset of symptoms shows mild osteoarthritic changes. (B) Radiograph obtained after 6 months of progressive pain shows flattening of the femoral head with superolateral subluxation, multiple subchondral defects, bone sclerosis, and narrowing of the articular space.[23]

A   B

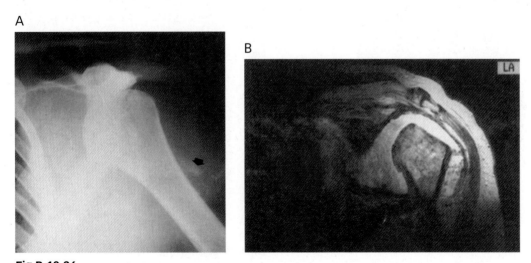

Fig B 10-36
Milwaukee shoulder. (A) Frontal radiograph shows soft-tissue swelling and irregular calcifications (arrow) around the shoulder. Note the anterior dislocation. (B) Coronal T2-weighted MR image shows a large joint effusion, resorption and deformity of the humeral head, and complete rupture of the rotator cuff.[23]

Erosion of Multiple Terminal Phalangeal Tufts (Acro-Osteolysis)

Condition	Comments
Scleroderma (Fig B 11-1)	Generalized resorption of the terminal phalanges of the hands or feet (or both), characterized by penciling of the tufts. A similar appearance may occur in other collagen vascular diseases (dermatomyositis, Raynaud's disease). Associated findings characteristic of scleroderma include skin atrophy and soft-tissue calcification.
Thermal injuries (burn, frostbite, electrical)	Resorption of the terminal tufts of the distal phalanges of the hand or foot probably reflects a combination of ischemic necrosis and secondary bacterial infection.
Diabetic gangrene (Fig B 11-2)	Diffuse destruction of terminal tufts (or more extensive involvement of the phalanges and metatarsals) associated with gas in the soft tissues of the foot reflects underlying vascular disease with diminished blood supply.

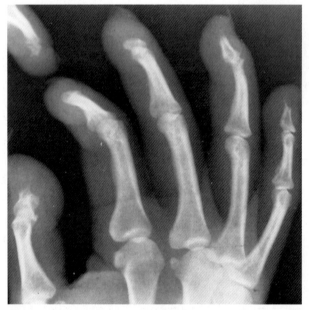

Fig B 11-1
Raynaud's disease. Severe trophic changes involve the distal phalanges with resorption of the terminal tufts.

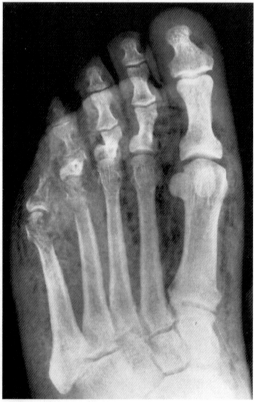

Fig B 11-2
Diabetic gangrene. Diffuse destruction of the phalanges and the metatarsal head of the fifth digit. Note the large amount of gas in the soft tissues of the foot.

Condition	Comments
Psoriatic arthritis (Fig B 11-3)	Resorption of the tufts of the distal phalanges of the hands and feet is a characteristic finding. Progressive osteolysis or "whittling" of bone may eventually lead to smoothly tapered or irregular destruction of most of the phalanx. Usually associated with skin lesions and an asymmetric arthritis that primarily involves the distal interphalangeal joints of the hands and feet.
Arteriosclerosis obliterans	Vascular insufficiency leads to resorption of distal phalanges and pencil-like deformities. A similar appearance may occur in Buerger's disease (thromboangiitis obliterans).
Neurotrophic disease (Fig B 11-4)	Resorption of terminal tufts occurs in such conditions as congenital indifference to pain, leprosy, diabetes mellitus, tabes dorsalis, syringomyelia, and meningomyelocele.

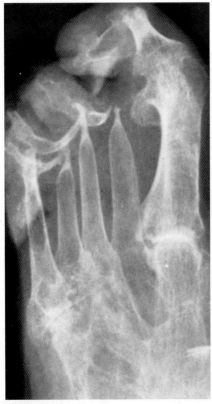

Fig B 11-3
Psoriatic arthritis. Arthritis mutilans of the foot and ankle. Severe pencil-like destruction of the metatarsals and phalanges with ankylosis of almost all the tarsal joints.

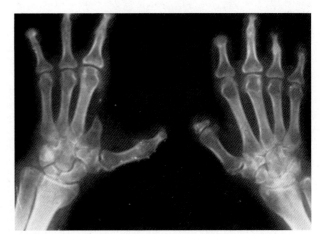

Fig B 11-4
Leprosy. Severe phalangeal resorption with evidence of typical pencil-like configurations.

Condition	Comments
Hyperparathyroidism (Fig B 11-5)	Tuft resorption is associated with characteristic subperiosteal resorption of the phalanges, metacarpals, and metatarsals.
Lesch-Nyhan syndrome (Fig B 11-6)	Rare inherited disorder of purine metabolism in which hyperuricemia is associated with mental and growth retardation and abnormal aggressive behavior. Characteristic self-mutilation by biting of the fingers and lips.
Epidermolysis bullosa (Fig B 11-7)	Rare hereditary disorder in which the skin blisters spontaneously or with injury. Severe scarring causes soft-tissue atrophy and the trophic changes of shortening and tapering of the distal phalanges.
Progeria (Fig B 11-8)	Nonhereditary congenital syndrome of dwarfism with premature aging and senility. There is typically shortening and abrupt tapering of the terminal phalanges of the hands and feet (and of the clavicles).

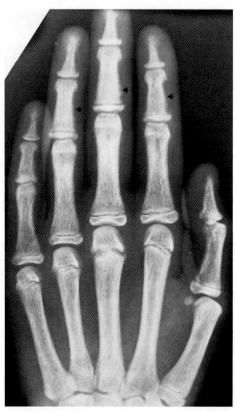

Fig B 11-5
Hyperparathyroidism. Tuft resorption associated with subperiosteal bone resorption that predominantly involves the radial margins of the middle phalanges of the second, third, and fourth digits (arrows).

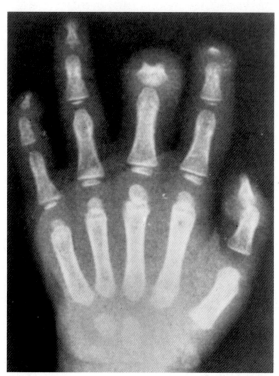

Fig B 11-6
Lesch-Nyhan syndrome. Amputation of the index and middle fingers from a self-inflicted bite. Although the child is 5 years old, the bone age is that of a 3-year-old.[24]

Condition	Comments
Familial acro-osteolysis (Fig B 11-9)	Diverse group of idiopathic disorders, several of which cause resorption of the terminal phalangeal tufts. This is often associated with band-like areas of lucency across the waists of the terminal phalanges.
Pachydermoperiostosis (primary hypertrophic osteoarthropathy) (Fig B 11-10)	Soft-tissue prominence of the distal digits may rarely be associated with bone resorption of the tufts that produces tapering, pointing, or disappearance of the terminal phalanges.
Pseudoxanthoma elasticum	Vascular occlusions lead to resorption of distal phalangeal tufts. Characteristic calcification of tendons, ligaments, and large peripheral arteries and veins.

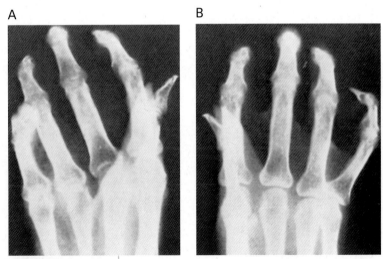

A B

Fig B 11-7
Epidermolysis bullosa. Diffuse trophic changes about the distal phalanges associated with bilateral contracture deformities resulting in a claw hand. Note the peculiar pointed, hook-like appearance of the terminal phalanges of the thumbs.[25]

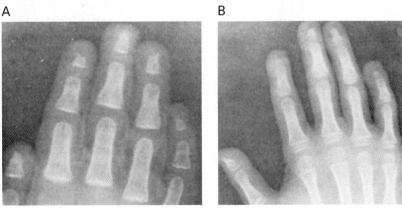

A B

Fig B 11-8
Progeria. Progressive absorption of the ungual tufts with preservation of soft tissues occurring over a 5-year period.[26]

Condition	Comments
Multicentric reticulohistiocytosis	Rare systemic disease of unknown cause in which severe inflammation of multiple joints progresses rapidly and leads to an incapacitating and deforming arthritis. The hands (especially the distal interphalangeal joints) are most often involved, and multiple soft-tissue masses typically produce a "lumpy-bumpy" appearance. Resorption of the distal phalangeal tufts frequently occurs.
Sjögren's syndrome	Classic triad of dry eyes (keratoconjunctivitis sicca), dry mouth (xerostomia), and a chronic polyarthritis that occurs in half the cases and is indistinguishable from ordinary rheumatoid arthritis. Bilateral parotid gland enlargement is common. May occasionally mimic psoriatic arthritis with distal interphalangeal joint involvement and resorption of terminal tufts.

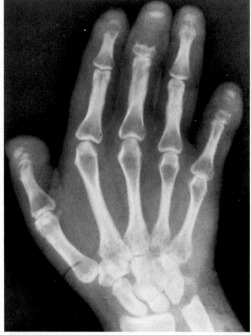

Fig B 11-9
Familial acro-osteolysis. Characteristic band-like areas of lucency crossing the waists of several phalanges.

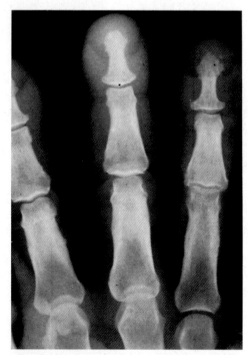

Fig B 11-10
Pachydermoperiostosis. Elephant-like thickening of the skin causes clubbing of the distal fingers and exaggerated knuckle pads in addition to a generalized increase in the bulk of the soft tissues surrounding the phalanges. Loss of the tufts accompanies the increase in the overlying soft tissues.[19]

Condition	Comments
Pyknodysostosis (see Fig B 5-6)	Rare hereditary dysplasia characterized by short stature; diffusely dense, sclerotic bones; and mandibular hypoplasia (loss of normal mandibular angle and craniofacial disproportion). Hypoplasia of the distal phalanges and absence of the terminal tufts cause the hands to be short and stubby.
Occupational acro-osteolysis	Primarily due to exposure to polyvinyl chloride (acro-osteolysis develops in 1% to 2% of workers involved in polymerization of vinyl chloride). Characteristic band-like radiolucent areas across the waist of one or more terminal phalanges (most commonly the thumb) may be combined with tuft resorption and beveling and osseous fragmentation.
Rothmund's syndrome	Rare hereditary ectodermal dysplasia associated with resorption of phalangeal tufts and dystrophic soft-tissue calcification.

Erosion, Destruction, or Defect of the Outer End of the Clavicle

Condition	Comments
Rheumatoid arthritis	Subchondral osteoporosis and erosions of the clavicle (and, to a lesser extent, the acromion) may progress to extensive osteolysis of the outer third of the clavicle, disruption of adjacent ligaments and capsular structures, and subluxation. The eroded end of the clavicle may be irregular or smoothly tapered.
Hyperparathyroidism (Fig B 12-1)	Subperiosteal bone resorption primarily involves the inferior aspect of the distal clavicle (the site of tendon and ligament attachment to the bone).
Neoplasm	Myeloma; metastases; lymphoma; Langerhans cell histiocytosis.
Cleidocranial dysostosis (Fig B 12-2)	Congenital hereditary disorder of membranous bone formation characterized by partial or total absence of the clavicles. Other major anomalies include multiple accessory bones along the sutures (wormian bones) and widening of the symphysis pubis.

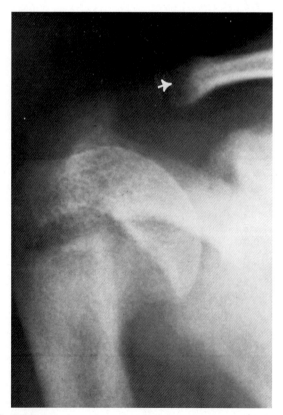

Fig B 12-1
Hyperparathyroidism. Characteristic erosion of the distal clavicle (arrow). Metaphyseal subperiosteal resorption beneath the proximal humeral head has led to a pathologic fracture with slippage of the humeral head.

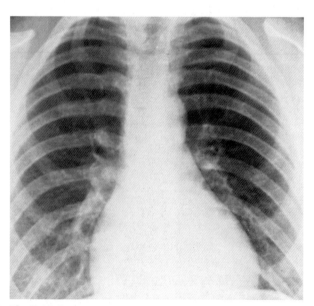

Fig B 12-2
Cleidocranial dysostosis. Total absence of both clavicles.

Condition	Comments
Scleroderma	Bone resorption of the distal clavicle (often with associated soft-tissue calcification) is an occasional finding. A far more frequent manifestation is resorption of the terminal tufts of the distal phalanges.
Gout	Erosion of the distal clavicle (occasionally with tophaceous calcification) is an uncommon appearance.
Osteomyelitis	Pyogenic or tuberculous infection can cause erosion or destruction of the distal clavicle.
Multicentric reticulohistiocytosis	Erosion of the distal clavicle is one manifestation of this rare systemic disease of unknown etiology that is characterized by severe inflammation of multiple joints and progresses rapidly to produce an incapacitating and deforming arthritis. The most common manifestations are resorption of the distal phalangeal tufts and development of multiple soft-tissue masses that typically produces a "lumpy-bumpy" appearance.
Hurler's syndrome	Shortening and thickening of the clavicles is a manifestation of this form of mucopolysaccharidosis. The most distinctive radiographic change in this condition is hypoplasia of L2 (causing accentuated kyphosis or gibbous deformity) with inferior beaking of the anterior margin of one or more vertebral bodies.
Post-traumatic osteolysis (Fig B 12-3)	Progressive resorption of the outer end of the clavicle may follow single or repeated episodes of local (often minor) trauma. The osteolytic process begins several weeks to several years after injury and is associated with erosion and cupping of the acromion, soft-tissue swelling, and dystrophic calcification. After the lytic phase stabilizes, reparative changes occur over several months until the subchondral bone becomes reconstituted (though the acromioclavicular joint can remain permanently widened).
Progeria (Fig B 12-4)	Shortening and abrupt tapering of the clavicles (and terminal phalanges of the hands and feet) is a common manifestation of this rare, nonhereditary congenital syndrome of dwarfism and premature aging and senility.
Pyknodysostosis	Hypoplasia of the lateral ends of the clavicles is a manifestation of this hereditary dysplasia that is characterized by short stature, diffusely dense sclerotic bones, and mandibular hypoplasia.

Condition	Comments
Holt-Oram syndrome	Hypoplasia of the clavicle (and radius of thumb) is among the upper extremity malformations associated with congenital heart disease (most often atrial septal defect) in this rare autosomal dominant condition.
Trisomy 13/trisomy 18	Tapering of the distal clavicles is one of multiple congenital anomalies associated with these rare syndromes.

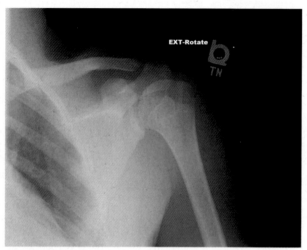

Fig B 12-3
Post-traumatic osteolysis. Resorption of the outer end of the clavicle in a young weightlifter with repetitive injury.

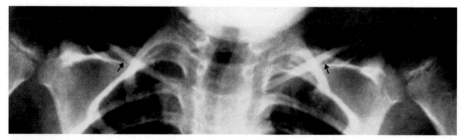

Fig B 12-4
Progeria. Thin and dense clavicles (arrows) with absence of the lateral thirds.[26]

Neuroarthropathy (Charcot Joint)

Condition	Comments
Tabes dorsalis (syphilis) (Fig B 13-1)	Primarily involves the weight-bearing joints of the lower extremities and lower lumbar spine. Approximately 5% to 10% of patients with tabes dorsalis have neuroarthropathy.
Syringomyelia (Fig B 13-2)	Primarily involves the upper extremity, especially the glenohumeral articulation, elbow, and wrist. Spinal changes are most common in the cervical region. Approximately 20% to 25% of patients with syringomyelia develop neuroarthropathy.
Diabetes mellitus (Fig B 13-3)	Primarily involves the metatarsophalangeal, tarsometatarsal, and intertarsal joints. Although the exact incidence of neuropathic joint disease in this condition is not clear, diabetes appears to be overtaking both syphilis and syringomyelia as the leading cause of neuroarthropathy.
Alcoholism	Primarily involves the metatarsophalangeal and interphalangeal joints. Probably an infrequent complication of the peripheral neuropathy seen in up to 30% of alcoholic patients.

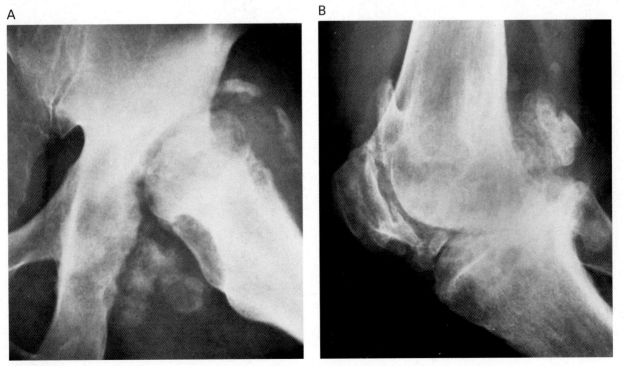

A   B

Fig B 13-1
Tabes dorsalis. Joint fragmentation, sclerosis, and calcific debris are seen about the hip (A) and the knee (B).

Condition	Comments
Congenital indifference to pain (Fig B 13-4)	Primarily involves the ankle and intertarsal joints. Neurologic deficit recognized in infancy or childhood in which pain sensation is decreased though there may be normal perception of touch and temperature and normal tendon reflexes. Identical skeletal abnormalities occur in familial dysautonomia (Riley-Day syndrome), which is characterized by autonomic dysfunction and sensory and motor disturbances.
Meningomyelocele/ spina bifida	Most frequent cause of neuroarthropathy in childhood. Primarily affects the ankle and inter-tarsal joints.
Leprosy (Fig B 13-5)	Chronic granulomatous mycobacterial infection that produces severe neuropathic changes in the hands and feet (due to insensitivity to pain that allows repeated trauma and infection to go untreated). Other radiographic findings include typical pencil-line tapering of the distal ends of the metatarsals and virtually pathognomonic calcification of nerves in the distal extremities.
Amyloidosis	Occasional manifestation in the knees or ankles that is probably related to vascular amyloid infil-tration in nerve tissue.

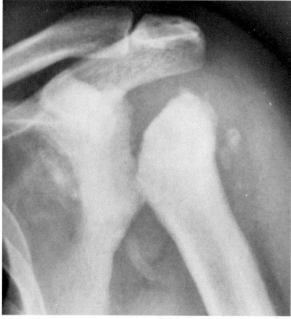

Fig B 13-2
Syringomyelia. Destruction with reactive sclerosis and calcific debris about the shoulder.

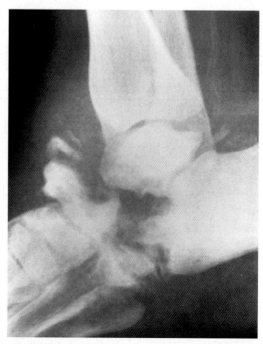

Fig B 13-3
Diabetes mellitus. Severe destructive changes with calcific debris about the intertarsal joints. Note the characteristic vascular calcification posterior to the ankle joint.

Condition	Comments
Steroid therapy	Systemically or locally administered steroid medication may produce a rapidly progressive, neuropathic-like joint disease characterized by severe osseous and cartilaginous destruction that most frequently involves the hips or knees.
Miscellaneous disorders	Spinal cord or peripheral nerve injury; myelopathy of pernicious anemia; inflammatory disease of the spinal cord (arachnoiditis, acute myelitis, poliomyelitis, and yaws).

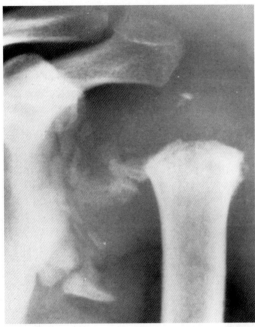

Fig B 13-4
Congenital indifference to pain. Virtually complete disappearance of the humeral head with reactive sclerosis and calcific debris.

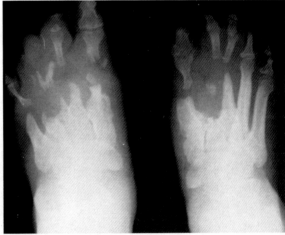

Fig B 13-5
Leprosy. Marked bone destruction and pencil-like resorption, most severe at the metatarsophalangeal joint.[25]

Loose Intra-Articular Bodies

Condition	Imaging Findings	Comments
Synovial osteochondromatosis (Fig B 14-1)	Multiple calcified or ossified bodies in a single joint. The calcifications vary in size, are usually irregular, and often have a laminated appearance. Most often involves the knees, with the hips next in frequency. Rarely affects the elbows, ankles, shoulders, or wrists.	Hypertrophic synovial membrane produces multiple metaplastic growths of cartilage that are most often intra-articular but may occasionally involve bursae and tendon sheaths. The cartilaginous masses frequently calcify or even ossify in part and often become detached and lie free in the joint cavity. Usually monarticular and tends to occur in young adults or the middle-aged. If not calcified (approximately one-third of cases), synovial chondromas cannot be detected on standard radiographs and arthrography is required to demonstrate these cartilaginous bodies.
Osteochondrial defect (Figs B 14-2 and B 14-3)	Small, round or oval necrotic segment of bone with its articular cartilage may separate to form a free joint body, leaving a residual pit in the articular surface. Primarily occurs about the knees, usually on the lateral aspect of the medial femoral condyle. Other common locations are the ankles, femoral heads, elbows, and shoulders.	Localized form of ischemic necrosis that most frequently affects young males and is probably caused by trauma. The necrotic segment of bone may remain attached and become denser and be separated from the surrounding bone by a crescentic lucent zone.
Trauma	Single or multiple joint bodies, usually associated with evidence of old trauma.	Secondary to avulsion of bone or cartilage (articular surface, meniscus). Uncalcified articular or meniscal cartilage may not be detected on plain radiographs.

A

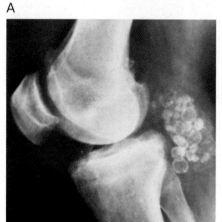

B

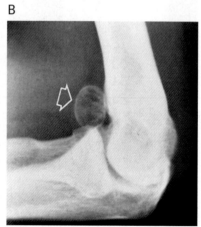

C

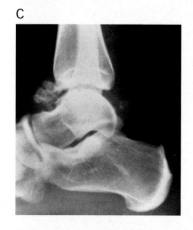

D

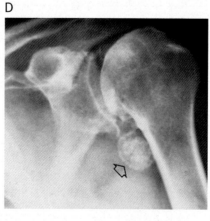

Fig B 14-1
Synovial osteochondromatosis. (A) Knee.
(B) Elbow. (C) Ankle. (D) Shoulder.

Condition	Imaging Findings	Comments
Neuroarthropathy (Charcot joint) (Fig B 14-4)	Calcified intra-articular bodies in one or more joints are associated with fracture, fragmentation, and sclerosis of articular surfaces, calcific and bony debris dissecting into soft tissues and extending about the joint and along muscle planes, and severe subluxations (due to laxity of periarticular soft-tissue structures).	Severe disorganization of a joint that develops in a variety of neurologic disorders in which loss of proprioception or deep pain sensation leads to repeated trauma to an unstable joint. Causes include diabetes, syphilis, syringomyelia, and leprosy. Degeneration of cartilage, recurrent fractures of subchondral bone, and marked proliferation of adjacent bone lead to total disorganization of the joint.
Degenerative joint disease	One or more detached hypertrophic spurs, primarily involving a weight-bearing joint.	Usually occurs in elderly patients and is associated with characteristic radiographic findings of osteophytosis, sclerosis, subchondral cysts, and joint space narrowing.
Intra-articular tumor calcification	Tumor may simulate a loose body. Predominantly involves the knees.	Rare appearance in synovial sarcoma or intracapsular chondroma. There is usually an associated soft-tissue mass.
Sequestrum (osteomyelitis)	Evidence of joint destruction or deformity.	Rare manifestation of tuberculous or pyogenic arthritis.

A
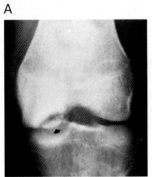
B
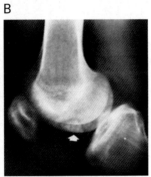

Fig B 14-2
Osteochondrial defect. (A) Frontal and (B) lateral views of the knee demonstrate the necrotic segment (arrows) separated from the femoral condyle by a crescentic lucent zone.

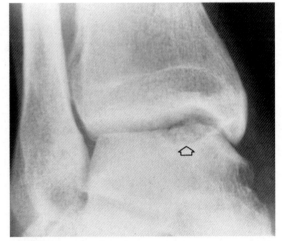

Fig B 14-3
Osteochondrial defect (arrow) at the ankle.

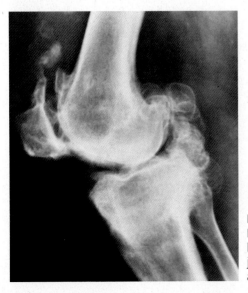

Fig B 14-4
Neuroarthropathy in syphilis. Multiple free joint bodies associated with disorganization of the knee joint, bone erosion, reactive sclerosis, and soft-tissue and ligamentous calcifications.

Chondrocalcinosis

Condition	Imaging Findings	Comments
CPPD disease (Figs B 15-1 and B 15-2)	Most commonly affects the knee joint with calcification in articular cartilage (fine linear densities parallel to subchondral bone surfaces) and menisci (dense linear deposits in the center of the knee joint). Other common sites include the triangular fibrocartilage of the wrists; vertical linear calcification of the symphysis pubis; articular cartilage in the shoulders, hips, elbows, and ankles; and the annulus fibrosus of intervertebral disks.	Inflammatory arthritis of older individuals caused by deposition of calcium pyrophosphate dihydrate crystals in the joints. May present as intermittent attacks of acute joint effusion and pain or as a progressive chronic arthritis. The acute arthritis of pseudogout may be clinically indistinguishable from gout or septic arthritis (diagnosis made by identification of calcium pyrophosphate crystals in synovial fluid). May produce a pattern of degenerative joint disease that primarily involves the radiocarpal, wrist, elbow, and shoulder joints (infrequently involved in osteoarthritis).
Degenerative joint disease/post-traumatic/ idiopathic	Calcification of cartilage in various areas.	Development of chondrocalcinosis without evidence of crystal arthropathy.
Gout (Fig B 15-3)	Calcification of fibrocartilage, most commonly involving the knees. The wrists, hips, and symphysis pubis may also be affected.	Increased serum urate concentration leads to deposition of uric acid crystals in joints, cartilage, and the kidneys. Chondrocalcinosis reported in 5% to 30% of patients.
Hemochromatosis	Calcification of cartilage that most often involves the knee. The shoulders, elbows, hips, symphysis pubis, and triangular cartilage of the wrist may also be affected.	Iron storage disorder that is either inherited or, more commonly, secondary to severe anemia with abnormal erythropoiesis (eg, thalassemia), liver disease in alcoholics, or chronic excessive iron ingestion. Chondrocalcinosis develops in approximately 50% of patients with arthropathy.

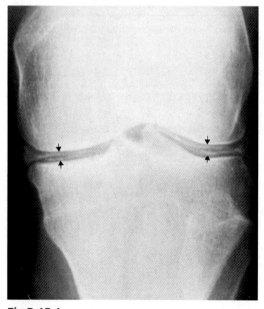

Fig B 15-1
CPPD disease. Calcification of both the medial and lateral menisci of the knee (arrows).

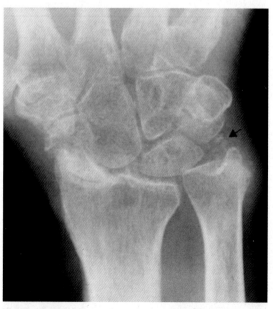

Fig B 15-2
CPPD disease. Characteristic calcifications in the triangular fibrocartilage of the wrist (arrow).

Condition	Imaging Findings	Comments
Hyperparathyroidism	Cartilage calcification most commonly involves the wrists, knees, hips, shoulders, and elbows.	Chondrocalcinosis reported in 20% to 40% of patients. Other common manifestations include subperiosteal bone resorption, rugger-jersey spine, brown tumors, erosion of the distal clavicles, and salt-and-pepper skull.
Ochronosis	Dense laminated calcification of multiple intervertebral disks. Cartilage calcification (with a severe type of degenerative arthritis) may develop in peripheral joints, especially the shoulders, hips, and knees.	Underlying condition is alkaptonuria, a rare enzyme deficiency that results in an abnormal accumulation of homogentisic acid in blood and urine (typically turns very dark on voiding or becomes black after standing or being alkalinized). Deposition of oxidized homogentisic acid in cartilage and other connective tissue produces a distinctive form of degenerative arthritis.
Wilson's disease (Fig B 15-4)	Cartilage calcification and arthropathy primarily involve the small joints of the hands and feet.	Rare familial disorder in which impaired hepatic excretion of copper results in toxic accumulation of the metal in the liver, brain, and other organs. Characteristic pigmentation of the cornea (Kayser-Fleischer ring). Skeletal changes occur in approximately half the patients.
Oxalosis	Deposition of calcium oxalate in cartilage.	Primary inborn error of metabolism or secondary to overabsorption of dietary oxalate (bacterial overgrowth syndromes, chronic disease of the pancreas and biliary tracts, decreased small bowel absorptive surface, Crohn's disease). Calcium oxalate is primarily deposited in the kidneys (nephrocalcinosis, nephrolithiasis), leading to recurrent urinary tract obstruction and infection, hypertension, and severe renal failure.
Acromegaly	Calcification of cartilage predominantly involving the knees.	Proliferation of articular cartilage leads to radiographically evident widening of joint spaces. Premature degenerative changes tend to develop.

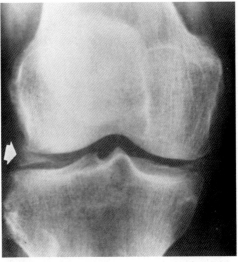

Fig B 15-3
Gout. Chondrocalcinosis about the knee (arrow) simulates CPPD disease.

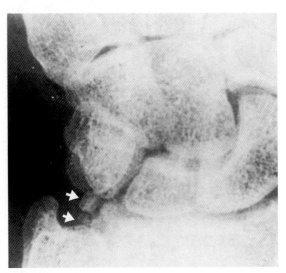

Fig B 15-4
Wilson's disease. Characteristic ossicles (arrows) in the region of the triangular fibrocartilage of the wrist.[28]

Periarticular Calcification

Condition	Comments
Calcific tendinitis and bursitis (Fig B 16-1)	Common cause of pain, limitation of motion, and disability about a joint. Although frequently associated with inflammation of an overlying bursa and often clinically termed "bursitis," the calcium deposits (primarily calcium hydroxyapatite) usually occur in the tendon and not in the overlying bursa (a mass of calcium may rupture into a bursa). Most commonly involves the shoulders, especially the supraspinatus tendon, in which the calcification is situated directly above the greater tuberosity of the humerus. Calcification is demonstrated radiographically in approximately half the patients with persistent pain and disability in this region. Other affected areas include the hips (calcification in gluteal insertions into the greater trochanter and surrounding bursae), elbows, knees, and wrists. Calcification in these areas usually appears as amorphous deposits that vary from thin curvilinear densities to large calcific masses.
CPPD disease	Accumulation of calcium pyrophosphate dihydrate crystals in tendinous structures. The calcification generally appears more diffuse and elongated than that associated with hydroxyapatite crystal deposition.

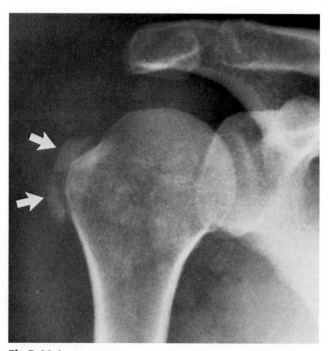

Fig B 16-1
Calcific tendinitis. Frontal view of the shoulder demonstrates amorphous calcium deposits (arrows) in the supraspinatus tendon.

Condition	Comments
Hyperparathyroidism (Fig B 16-2)	Calcific deposits (hydroxyapatite crystals) in joint capsules and periarticular tissues are common (especially in renal osteodystrophy), are often dense and massive, and may be observed in multiple (and often symmetric) locations. There is usually other radiographic evidence of hyperparathyroidism (subperiosteal bone resorption, rugger-jersey spine, salt-and-pepper demineralization of the skull, brown tumors).
Other disorders of calcium and phosphate metabolism	Metastatic calcification diffusely involving periarticular and other soft tissues may occur in such conditions as hypoparathyroidism, hypervitaminosis D, milk-alkali syndrome, and idiopathic hypercalcemia.
Collagen vascular disease (Fig B 16-3)	Widespread periarticular (and subcutaneous) calcification is common in scleroderma and dermatomyositis (there may be punctate, linear, or more massive "tumoral" calcification). Uncommon manifestation in rheumatoid arthritis, systemic lupus erythematosus, polyarteritis nodosa, and Raynaud's phenomenon.

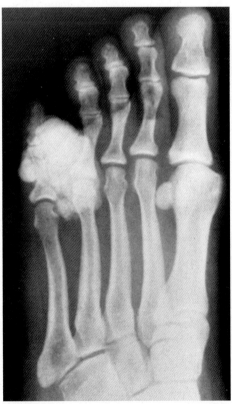

Fig B 16-2
Hyperparathyroidism. Dense mass of tumoral calcification in joint capsules and periarticular soft tissues of the lateral aspect of the foot in a patient with renal osteodystrophy.

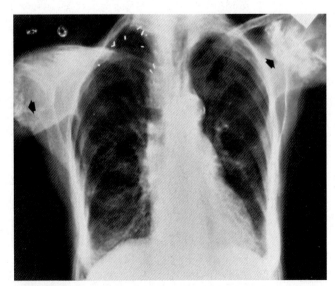

Fig B 16-3
Scleroderma. Clumps of calcification about the shoulder joints (arrows). Note the reticulonodular interstitial pattern at both lung bases. The surgical clips overlying the right apex are from a cervical sympathectomy for the treatment of associated Raynaud's phenomenon.

Condition	Comments
Tumoral calcinosis (Fig B 16-4)	Localized collections of calcium in periarticular soft tissues that may involve single or multiple joints and have a predilection for the hips, elbows, shoulders, ankles, and wrists. Primarily affects young and otherwise healthy individuals. Begins as small calcified nodules that enlarge to form solid, lobulated tumors that are extremely dense and have rough, irregular borders. Pathologically, the calcific masses reflect honeycomb-like clusters of cysts in a dense fibrous capsule. Because the cysts are filled with a granular, pasty, or liquid material, on upright views there may be sedimentation of calcium phosphate crystals with resulting fluid-calcium levels.
Calcinosis universalis (Fig B 16-5)	Rare disorder of unknown etiology affecting infants and children in which calcium is initially deposited subcutaneously and later in deep connective tissues throughout the body (similar to dermatomyositis). Periarticular tissues may also be involved.

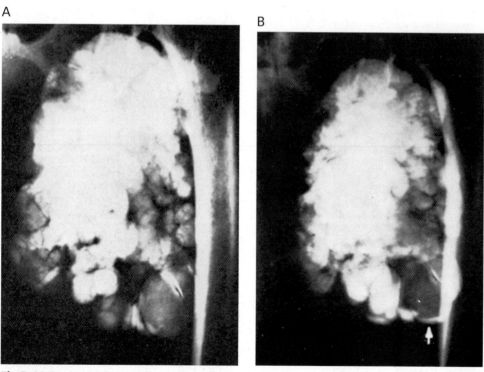

Fig B 16-4
Tumoral calcinosis. (A) Supine view demonstrates a large, irregular calcific mass with some relatively lucent areas in the proximal thigh. (B) Upright view shows sedimentation in the liquid-filled cysts (arrow), with absence of sedimentation in the more amorphous gritty deposits.[29]

Condition	Comments
Gout (Fig B 16-6)	Continued deposition of urate crystals in periarticular tissues causes the development of one or more characteristic large, lumpy soft-tissue swellings (gouty tophi) that may calcify. Classic sites include the first metatarsophalangeal joint, the insertion of the Achilles tendon, and the olecranon bursa (bilateral enlargement of the olecranon bursae, often with erosion or spur formation and calcified tophi, is virtually pathognomonic of gout).

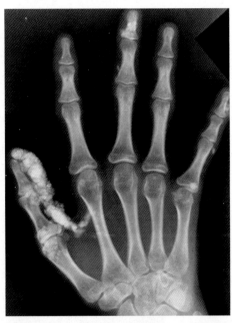

Fig B 16-5
Calcinosis universalis. Dense calcific deposits in the soft tissues on the ulnar aspect of the thumb.

A   B

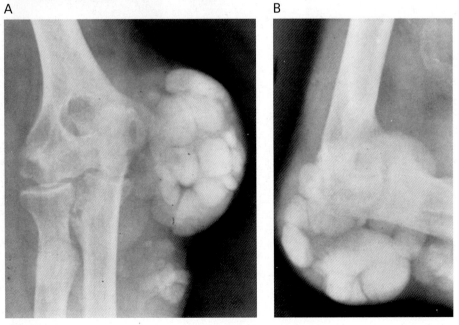

Fig B 16-6
Gout. (A) Frontal and (B) lateral views demonstrate massive deposition of calcium in a longstanding tophaceous lesion about the elbow.

Condition	Comments
Myositis ossificans (Fig B 16-7)	Osseous deposits in tendons and periarticular tissues (especially about the hips) develop in the paralyzed part in up to half of patients with paraplegia. In generalized (progressive) myositis ossificans, thick columns and plates of bone eventually replace tendons, fascia, and ligaments, causing such severe limitation of movement, contractures, and deformity that the patient becomes a virtual "stone person."
Sarcoidosis	Large periarticular soft-tissue masses, with or without calcification, are a rare manifestation.
Ochronosis	Tendinous calcification and ossification may involve the hips, knees, and shoulders. Characteristic ossification of intervertebral disks.
Trauma (Fig B 16-8)	Post-traumatic calcification may develop after capsular or ligamentous damage (eg, Pellegrini-Stieda calcification in the proximal attachment of the medial collateral ligament of the knee). Localized periarticular calcification also commonly develops around joint replacements.

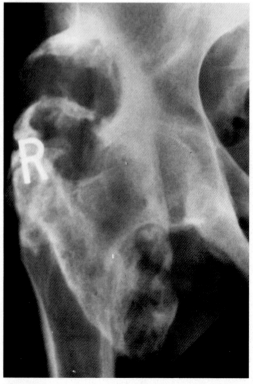

Fig B 16-7
Myositis ossificans. Marked heterotopic bone formation about the hip joint in a patient with paralysis.

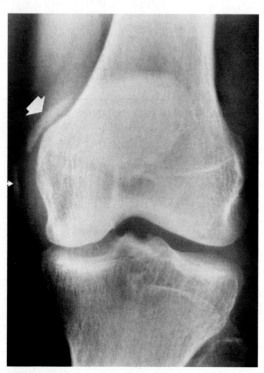

Fig B 16-8
Pellegrini-Stieda disease. Post-traumatic ossification (arrows) along the femoral condyle.

Condition	Comments
Synovial sarcoma (synovioma)	Malignant tumor that most frequently affects young adults and arises from a joint capsule, bursa, or tendon. The tumor usually develops from synovial tissue in the vicinity of a large joint (para-articular soft tissues just beyond the capsule), rather than in the synovial lining of the joint itself. Most often involves the knees, though the tumor may arise from a tendon sheath anywhere along a limb. Radiographically, a synovioma appears as a well-defined, round or lobulated soft-tissue mass adjacent to or near a joint. Amorphous punctate deposits or linear streaks of calcification frequently occur in the tumor (must be differentiated from pigmented villonodular synovitis, in which calcification does not occur though the mass may appear dense because of hemosiderin deposits).
Tuberculosis	Dystrophic calcification may follow tuberculous involvement of the synovial membranes of bursae and tendon sheaths. Primarily involves the hips and elbows.
Werner's syndrome	Rare condition characterized by symmetric growth retardation, premature aging, scleroderma-like skin changes, and cataracts. Soft-tissue calcification occurs in approximately one-third of cases, predominantly about bony protuberances (distal ends of the tibia and fibula) and the knees, feet, and hands. Other typical findings include patchy or generalized osteoporosis, extensive arterial calcifications, and premature osteoarthritis.

Localized Calcification or Ossification in Muscles and Subcutaneous Tissues

Condition	Comments
Idiopathic	Ligaments of the shoulder girdle and pelvis often calcify in normal individuals.
Myositis ossificans (post-traumatic) (Fig B 17-1)	Development of calcification or ossification in injured muscle that is usually related to acute or chronic trauma to the deep tissues of the extremities. Heterotopic calcification or ossification typically lies parallel to the shaft of a bone or the long axis of a muscle. Although the radiographic appearance may simulate that of parosteal sarcoma (Fig B 17-2), myositis ossificans is completely separated from the bone by a radiolucent zone, unlike the malignant tumor that is attached by a sessile base and has a discontinuous radiolucent zone.
Myositis ossificans associated with neurologic disorders (Fig B 17-3)	Up to half the patients with paraplegia demonstrate myositis ossificans in the paralyzed part. The osseous deposits occur in muscles, tendons, and ligaments. Heterotopic bone is most pronounced around large joints, especially the hips, and may proceed to complete periarticular osseous bridging.
Postinjection (Fig B 17-4)	Single or multiple irregular deposits of calcification may develop after the injection of bismuth, calcium gluconate, insulin, antibiotics, camphorated oil, or quinine. They also may occur after BCG vaccination or after the extravasation of an opaque substance.

A

B

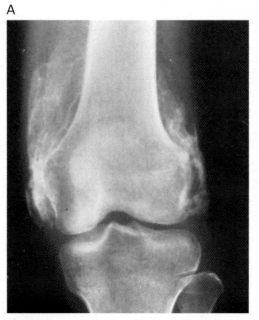
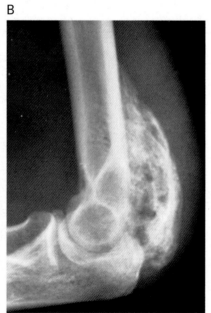

Fig B 17-1
Myositis ossificans. (A) Knee. (B) Elbow.

Condition	Comments
Thermal burn	Heterotopic calcification (most frequent in the periarticular region) not uncommonly becomes evident within several months.
Neoplasm (Figs B 17-5 through B 17-8)	Various patterns (from flecks of calcification to extensive ossification) can occur in benign neoplasms (chondroma, fibromyxoma, lipoma) and malignant neoplasms (soft-tissue osteosarcoma, chondrosarcoma, fibrosarcoma, liposarcoma, synovioma).

A B

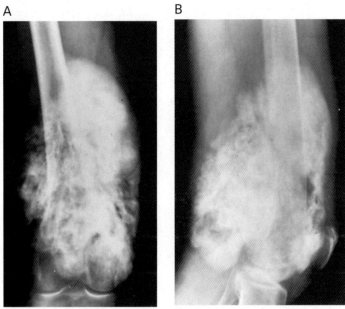

Fig B 17-2
Parosteal sarcoma. (A) Frontal and (B) lateral views of the leg demonstrate a broad-based, densely ossified mass extending outward from the distal femur. The characteristic radiolucent line separating the dense mass of tumor bone from the cortex is not seen in this huge lesion.

Fig B 17-3
Myositis ossificans associated with neurologic disorders. Diffuse osseous deposits in muscles, tendons, and ligaments about the hip in a patient with long-term paralysis.

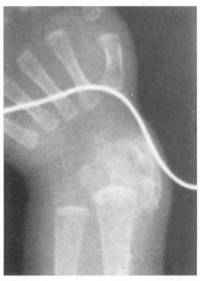

Fig B 17-4
Extravasation of a calcium gluconate injection. Soft-tissue opacification in a child.

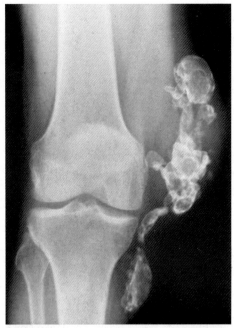

Fig B 17-5
Lipoma. Bizarre calcification in an extensive tumor about the knee.

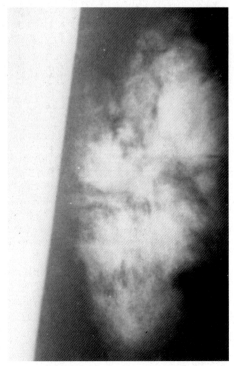

Fig B 17-7
Extraskeletal osteosarcoma of the posterolateral thigh.[30]

A

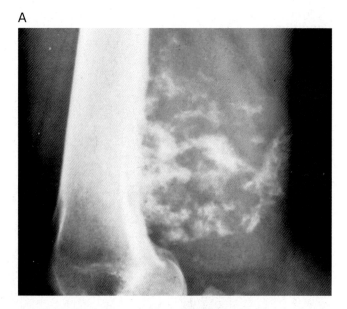

B

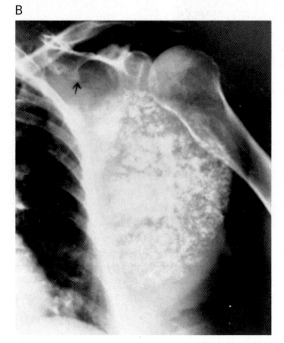

Fig B 17-6
Chondrosarcoma. (A) Prominent dense calcification in a large exostotic chondrosarcoma. (B) Extensive flocculent calcification in the cartilaginous matrix. The arrow points to a small osteochondroma in this patient with multiple hereditary exostoses.

Condition	Comments
Postsurgical scar (Fig B 17-9)	Calcification or ossification of an old surgical scar can produce linear densities on late postoperative radiographs.
Leprosy	Nerve abscesses produce soft-tissue masses that may calcify.
Healing infection or abscess	After pyogenic myositis or fibrositis.
Chronic venous stasis (Fig B 17-10)	A diffuse reticular ossification pattern may develop in an affected lower extremity. More commonly, single or multiple phleboliths and periosteal reaction occur about the distal tibia and fibula.

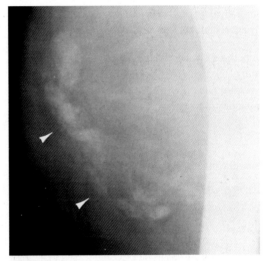

Fig B 17-8
Synovioma of the posteromedial thigh. Lateral view shows a large soft-tissue mass with extensive calcific deposits (arrowheads) in it.[30]

Fig B 17-9
Ossified surgical scar. Long, linear density on the anterior abdominal wall (arrows).

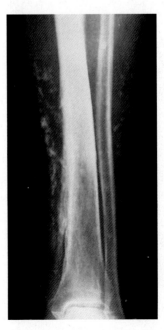

Fig B 17-10
Chronic venous stasis. Soft-tissue calcification associated with periosteal reaction about the distal tibia and numerous phleboliths.

Generalized Calcification or Ossification in Muscles and Subcutaneous Tissues

Condition	Comments
Dermatomyositis (Fig B 18-1)	Inflammatory disease of skeletal muscles in which a lymphocytic infiltration produces muscle fiber damage and degeneration. In adults, there is associated skin inflammation, a typical rash, and a relatively high incidence of underlying malignancy. Musculoskeletal changes are most severe in childhood dermatomyositis. A characteristic finding is extensive calcification in muscles and subcutaneous tissues underlying the skin lesions. The calcification may appear as superficial or deep masses, as linear deposits, or as a lacy, reticular, subcutaneous deposition of calcium encasing the torso.
Scleroderma (Fig B 18-2)	Multisystem disorder characterized by fibrosis that involves the skin and internal organs (especially the gastrointestinal tract, lungs, heart, and kidneys). Soft-tissue calcification often occurs in the hands and over pressure areas such as the elbows and ischial tuberosities. Other typical findings include soft-tissue atrophy in the fingertips with trophic osteolysis and resorption of terminal tufts and arthritic changes in the interphalangeal joints of the hands.
Calcinosis universalis (Fig B 18-3)	Disease of unknown etiology in which calcium is initially deposited subcutaneously and later in deep connective tissues throughout the body. Generally affects infants and children and is progressive.
Disorders of calcium and phosphorus metabolism (Figs B 18-4 through B 18-6)	Soft-tissue calcification in subcutaneous tissues, blood vessels, and periarticular regions may occur in hyperparathyroidism (especially in secondary renal osteodystrophy) as well as in other disorders of calcium and phosphorus metabolism such as hypervitaminosis D, milk-alkali syndrome, idiopathic hypercalcemia, hypercalcemia associated with bone destruction, hypoparathyroidism, and pseudohypoparathyroidism.
Vascular calcifications Arterial (Figs B 18-7 and B 18-8)	Arteriosclerosis; Mönckeberg's sclerosis; aneurysm; diabetes mellitus; hyperparathyroidism (hypercalcemia); Takayasu's arteritis.

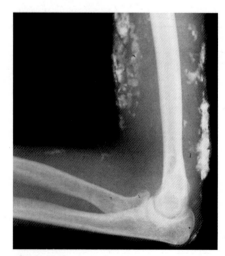

Fig B 18-1
Dermatomyositis. Extensive deposits of calcium in the soft tissues about the humerus and elbow and loss of the sharp demarcation between the muscles and the subcutaneous tissues.

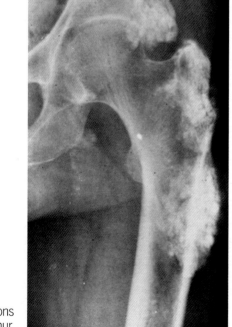

Fig B 18-2
Scleroderma. Extensive calcifications about the hip joint and proximal femur.

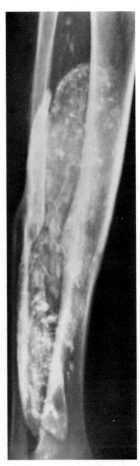

Fig B 18-3
Calcinosis universalis. Huge calcified mass in the subcutaneous and deep connective tissues of the lower leg.

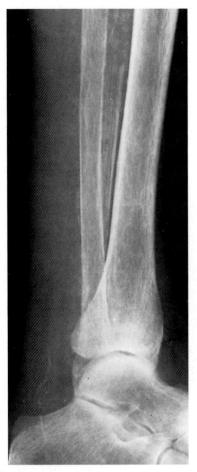

Fig B 18-4
Hypervitaminosis D. Diffuse calcification involving the interosseous ligament between the tibia and fibula as well as vascular structures.

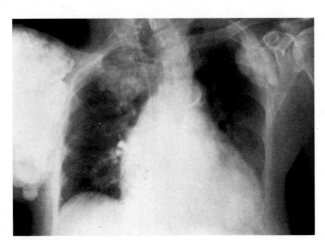

Fig B 18-5
Hypervitaminosis D. Huge masses of calcification near the shoulder joints bilaterally.

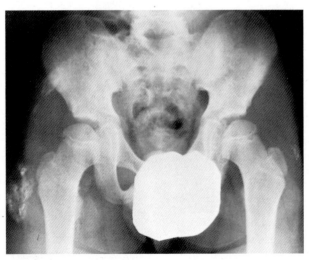

Fig B 18-6
Hypoparathyroidism. Soft-tissue calcifications lying in muscle bundles about both hip joints.

Condition	Comments
Venous (Figs B 18-9 through B 18-11)	Phleboliths may develop in association with varicose veins, hemangioma, Maffucci's syndrome (multiple enchondromatosis), and after irradiation.
Systemic lupus erythematosus (Fig B 18-12)	Calcification in the soft tissues is an occasional finding that most commonly involves the lower extremities and appears as diffuse, linear, streaky, or nodular calcification in subcutaneous and deeper tissues.

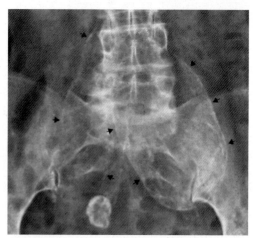

Fig B 18-7
Arteriosclerosis of the lower extremities. There are calcified plaques (arrows) in the walls of aneurysms of the lower abdominal aorta and both common iliac arteries.

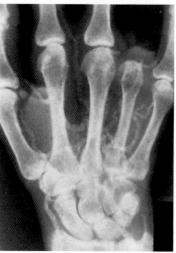

Fig B 18-8
Mönckeberg's sclerosis. Typical calcification of the media in moderate-sized vessels of a diabetic patient. Note the prior surgical resection of the phalanges of the fourth digit.

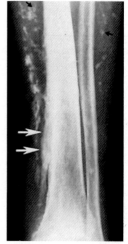

Fig B 18-9
Varicose veins. Multiple, round and oval calcifications in the soft tissues (phleboliths) representing calcified thrombi, some of which have characteristic lucent centers (black arrows). Extensive new bone formation along the medial aspect of the tibial shaft (white arrows) caused by long-standing vascular stasis.

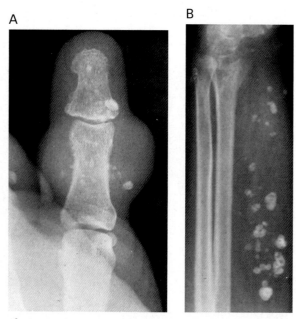

Fig B 18-10
Soft-tissue hemangiomas with phleboliths involving (A) the thumb and (B) the forearm.

Condition	Comments
Ehlers-Danlos syndrome	Generalized inherited disorder of connective tissue characterized by fragile and hyperextensible skin, easy bruising, and loose-jointedness. The most typical radiographic abnormality is calcification of fatty nodules in the subcutaneous tissues of the extremities. These nodules range from 2 to 10 mm and appear as central lucent zones with ring-like calcification, simulating phleboliths (must be differentiated from calcified subcutaneous parasites, which tend to be aligned along muscular and fascial planes rather than randomly distributed in the soft tissues). Other nonspecific musculoskeletal abnormalities include scoliosis, deformities of the thoracic cage, hypermobility of joints, and subluxations.
Pseudoxanthoma elasticum (Fig B 18-13)	Calcification typically occurs in the middle and deep layers of the dermis in this hereditary systemic disorder in which widespread degeneration of elastic fibers results in cutaneous, ocular, and vascular manifestations in children and young adults. Other sites of calcification include tendons, ligaments, and large peripheral arteries and veins.
Parasites	
Cysticercosis (*Taenia solium*) (Fig B 18-14)	Invasion of human tissue by the larval form of the pork tapeworm typically produces multiple linear or oval calcifications in the soft tissues. The calcified cysts often have a noncalcified central area and almost always have their long axes in the plane of the surrounding muscle bundle (unlike the random distribution of soft-tissue calcifications in Ehlers-Danlos syndrome). There may also be intracranial calcification (tiny central calcification representing the scolex surrounded by an area of radiolucency and rimmed by calcium deposition in the overlying cyst capsule).
Guinea worm (*Dracunculus medinensis*)	Serpiginous or curvilinear opacification (most often in the lower extremities) that is often coiled and may be several feet long. The calcification is frequently segmented and beaded because muscle movement breaks up the underlying necrotic worm.

B

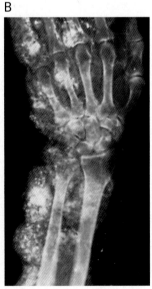

A

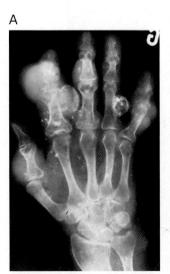

Fig B 18-11
Maffucci's syndrome. (A) Plain radiograph demonstrates multiple soft-tissue masses and calcified thrombi in association with expansile bony lesions. (B) Late film from an arteriogram shows contrast material filling many cavernous hemangiomas of the soft tissues.

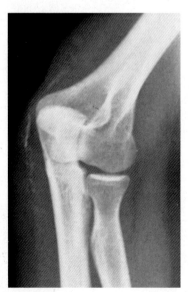

Fig B 18-12
Systemic lupus erythematosus. Lace-like calcification about the elbow.

Condition	Comments
Loa loa (*Filaria bancrofti*)	Calcified dead worm appears curled up into a coil or as a thin, cotton-like thread of density. The calcifications are often difficult to visualize and are best seen in the web spaces of the hands or feet.
Trichinosis (*Trichinella spiralis*)	Calcification of encysted larvae is common pathologically, though their small size (1 mm or less) makes them difficult to detect radiographically.
Hydatid disease (*Echinococcus*)	Infrequent calcification in cysts within muscles or subcutaneous tissue.
Myositis ossificans progressiva (Fig B 18-15)	Rare congenital dysplasia characterized by an interstitial myositis or fibrositis that undergoes cartilaginous and osseous transformation. Thick columns and plates of bone eventually replace tendons, fascia, and ligaments, causing severe limitation of motion, contractures, and deformity that the patient becomes a virtual "stone person" and death ensues. There are usually a variety of associated congenital anomalies, most frequently hypoplasia of the great toes or thumbs.
Fluorosis (Fig B 18-16)	Characteristic calcification of paraspinal, sacrotuberous, and iliolumbar ligaments as well as ligamentous calcification in the appendicular skeleton. Other skeletal findings include dense sclerosis (most prominent in the vertebrae and pelvis) and periosteal roughening and articular bone deposits arising at sites of muscular and ligamentous attachments.
Basal cell nevus syndrome	Soft-tissue calcification is occasionally seen in this inherited disorder characterized by multiple basal cell carcinomas, palmar pits, dentigerous cysts of the mandible, multiple rib and spinal anomalies, brachydactyly, and various neurologic and ophthalmologic abnormalities.

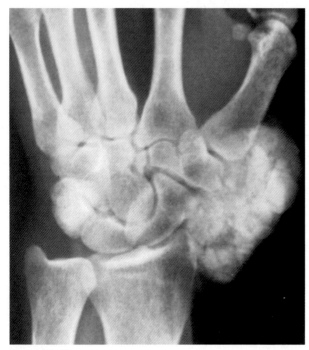

Fig B 18-13
Pseudoxanthoma elasticum. Extensive calcification in soft tissues on the radial side of the wrist.

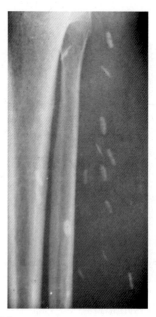

Fig B 18-14
Cysticercosis. Multiple, linear and oval calcifications along muscle bundles.

Condition	Comments
Werner's syndrome	Rare condition characterized by symmetric retardation of growth, premature aging, scleroderma-like skin changes, and cataracts. Soft-tissue calcification occurs in approximately one-third of cases, especially about bony protuberances (especially the distal ends of the tibia and fibula) and the knees, feet, and hands.

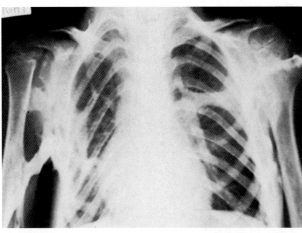

Fig B 18-15
Myositis ossificans progressiva. Frontal view of the chest demonstrates extensive new bone formation in the soft tissues, which severely limited arm motion. Note the exostosis of the left proximal humerus due to blending of the ossific foci with the cortex of the bone.[31]

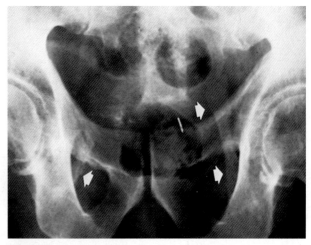

Fig B 18-16
Fluorosis. Calcification of the sacrotuberous ligaments (arrows).

Calcification About the Fingertips

Condition	Comments
Scleroderma (Fig B 19-1)	Digital calcification occurs in 10% to 20% of cases and may appear as small punctate deposits at the phalangeal tips or as more focal conglomerate calcific masses. Often associated with resorption of the terminal phalangeal tufts.
Raynauds disease	Discrete calcium deposits may develop in the fingertips in association with soft-tissue atrophy and resorption of terminal tufts. Cold sensitivity occurs almost exclusively in women and produces symptoms of peripheral arterial spasm (especially in the upper limbs). May be either an isolated finding or a symptom of a more severe underlying condition (eg, scleroderma or other collagen vascular disease).

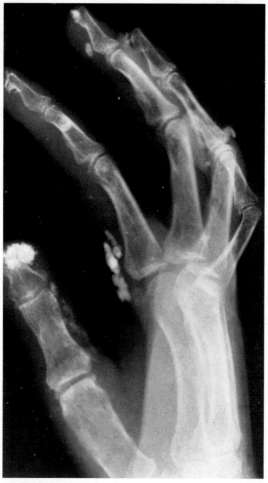

Fig B 19-1
Scleroderma. Amorphous clumps of calcium in the soft tissues of the fingers. Note the trophic changes about the terminal tufts.

Condition	Comments
Dermatomyositis (Fig B 19-2)	Calcification of the fingertips with associated terminal phalangeal erosion is one manifestation. More commonly, there is extensive calcification in muscles and subcutaneous tissue underlying the associated skin lesions.
Calcinosis universalis (Fig B 19-3)	Diffuse deposition of calcium in subcutaneous and later in deep connective tissues may involve the fingertips.
Systemic lupus erythematosus	Occasional manifestation (calcification more commonly involves the lower extremities).
Epidermolysis bullosa	Rare manifestation. Severe scarring causes soft-tissue atrophy and trophic changes involving the distal phalanges (may simulate scleroderma).
Rothmund syndrome	Rare hereditary type of ectodermal dysplasia associated with resorption of phalangeal tufts and dystrophic soft-tissue calcification.

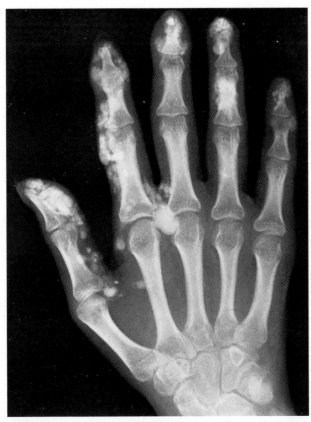

Fig B 19-2
Dermatomyositis. Irregular calcific deposits involve all the fingers.

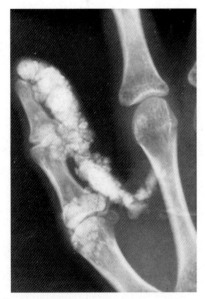

Fig B 19-3
Calcinosis universalis. Coned view of the thumb demonstrates dense calcific deposits in the soft tissues on the ulnar aspect. The distal phalangeal tufts are normal, which virtually excludes scleroderma as the underlying cause of the calcification.

Zones of Increased Density in the Metaphyses

Condition	Comments
Normal variant	Normal, active children younger than 3 years of age often have relative whiteness of the metaphyseal ends of tubular bones.
Lead poisoning (Fig B 20-1)	Dense transverse bands extending across the metaphyses of long bones and along the margins of flat bones such as the iliac crest. Predominantly involves the most rapidly growing portions of the skeleton (metaphyses at the distal ends of the femur and radius and both ends of the tibia). Lead lines can be observed in growing bones approximately 3 months after the inhalation of lead and 6 months after ingestion of the metal. Must be differentiated from the usual whiteness of the metaphyseal ends of tubular bones that is often seen in normal, active children younger than 3 years of age.
Other heavy metal or chemical absorption (Fig B 20-2)	Bismuth; arsenic; phosphorus; fluoride; mercury; lithium; radium. May also develop in children whose mothers received high doses of estrogen or heavy metal therapy during pregnancy.
Treated leukemia (Fig B 20-3)	Dense metaphyses (simulating lead poisoning) occur in a large percentage of patients with leukemia undergoing chemotherapy.
Transverse growth lines (growth arrest lines)	Fine, symmetric, opaque transverse lines (single or multiple, varying in thickness and number) paralleling the contour of the provisional zone of calcification may be related to such stresses as malnutrition or chronic disease. These dense zones probably result from overproduction of, and failure to destroy, calcified cartilage matrix.
Healing rickets (Fig B 20-4)	Represents mineralization of the zone of provisional calcification, which widens as healing progresses.
Hypervitaminosis D/ idiopathic hypercalcemia	Metaphyseal bands of increased density, reflecting heavy calcification of the matrix of proliferating cartilage, alternate with areas of increased lucency in the tubular bones of infants and children.
Cretinism	Dense transverse metaphyseal bands may occur in association with a typical delay in the appearance and subsequent growth of ossification centers, epiphyseal dysgenesis (fragmented epiphyses with multiple ossification foci), and retarded bone age.

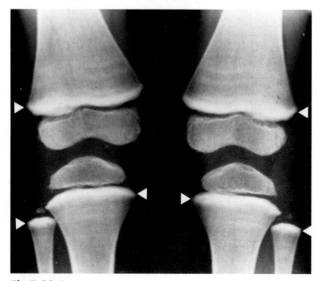

Fig B 20-1
Lead poisoning.

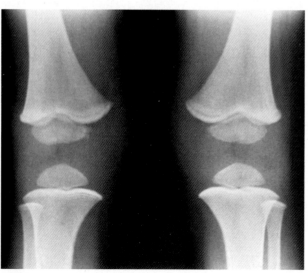

Fig B 20-2
Bismuth poisoning.

Condition	Comments
Healing scurvy	Increased density of the metaphyses may occur along with cortical thickening, increased density of the epiphyses, and massive subperiosteal bone formation.
Hypoparathyroidism	Zones of increased density in the metaphyseal regions of long bones may be associated with characteristic cerebral calcifications (primarily involving the basal ganglia, dentate nuclei of the cerebellum, and choroid plexus).
Osteopetrosis	Transverse radiodense metaphyseal bands often occur in the long bones and vertebrae. There may be alternating lucent transverse lines that probably reflect the intermittent nature of the pathologic process.
Congenital syphilis	Transverse metaphyseal stripes (sclerotic and lucent bands) may be an early finding. This pattern may also develop in other transplacental infections (rubella, toxoplasmosis, and cytomegalic inclusion disease).

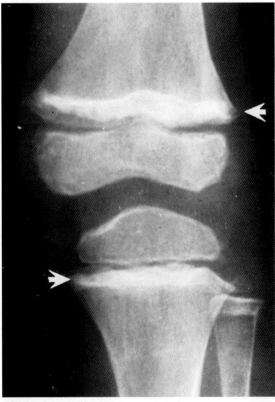

Fig B 20-3
Chronic leukemia. After therapy with methotrexate, dense, irregular sclerosis has developed about the metaphyses of the distal femur and proximal tibia (arrows).

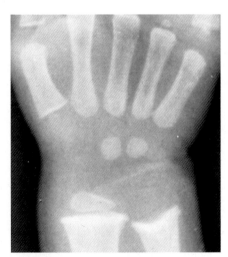

Fig B 20-4
Healed rickets. Increased sharpness of the metaphyseal lines after therapy with vitamin D.

Radiolucent Metaphyseal Bands

Condition	Comments
Normal variant	Striated appearance of the metaphyses is common in neonates.
Transplacental infection (Figs B 21-1 and B 21-2)	Rubella; syphilis; herpes; toxoplasmosis; cytomegalic inclusion disease. In rubella, there is a typical pattern of alternating dense and lucent longitudinal striations (celery stick sign).
Leukemia (Fig B 21-3)	Symmetric band-like lucent areas (not associated with actual leukemic cell infiltration) primarily affect sites of rapid bone growth (the distal femur, proximal tibia, proximal humerus, and distal radius). Nonspecific appearance that probably reflects a nutritional deficit that interferes with proper osteogenesis (after age 2, radiolucent metaphyseal bands strongly suggest leukemia).
Metastatic neuroblastoma	Lucent metaphyseal bands and other radiographic abnormalities (widespread osteolytic lesions, periosteal reaction) may be indistinguishable from leukemia. May be differentiated by the presence of vanillylmandelic acid (VMA) in the urine.

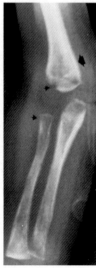

Fig B 21-1
Congenital syphilis. Transverse bands of increased density across the metaphyses (small arrows) associated with patchy areas of bone destruction in the diaphyses. There is solid periosteal new bone formation (large arrow), which is best seen about the distal humerus.

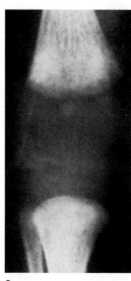

Fig B 21-2
Rubella. Radiograph of the knee in a 1-day-old girl with a maternal history of rubella demonstrates alternating lucent and sclerotic longitudinal striations extending perpendicular to the epiphyseal plate and parallel to the long axis of the bone (celery stick sign).[32]

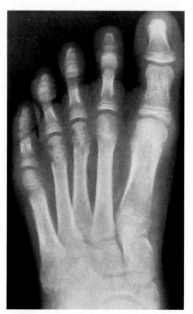

Fig B 21-3
Leukemia. In addition to radiolucent metaphyseal bands, there is frank bone destruction with cortical erosion involving many of the metatarsals and proximal phalanges.

Condition	Comments
Scurvy	Submetaphyseal band of lucency (Trümmerfeld zone) adjacent to the widened and increased density of the zone of provisional calcification (white line of scurvy). Other manifestations include Pelken's spur and Wimberger's sign.
Juvenile rheumatoid arthritis	Extensive deossification of an affected extremity may cause bands of metaphyseal lucency mimicking childhood leukemia. Primarily involves the areas of greatest bone growth (the knees, ankles, and wrists).
Craniometaphyseal dysplasia (Fig B 21-4)	Rare hereditary disorder in which failure of normal tubulation of bone is combined with hypertelorism, a broad flat nose, and defective dentition. Initial metaphyseal lucency and diaphyseal sclerosis progress to more normal mineralization and lack of modeling.
Systemic illness (Fig B 21-5)	Metaphyseal radiolucency is a nonspecific finding that may be encountered in various systemic illnesses of childhood (probably reflects a nutritional deficit interfering with proper osteogenesis).

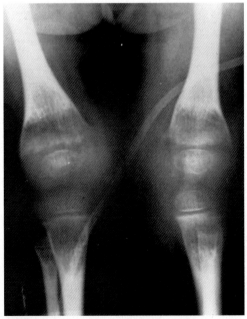

Fig B 21-4
Craniometaphyseal dysplasia. Severe metaphyseal lucency with diaphyseal sclerosis about the knees.

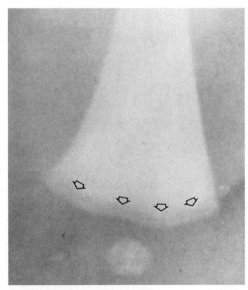

Fig B 21-5
Chronic systemic illness.

Underconstriction or Undertubulation (Wide Diametaphysis)

Condition	Comments

Lipid storage disease
  Gaucher's disease
  (Fig B 22-1)
	Inborn error of metabolism characterized by accumulation of abnormal quantities of complex lipids in the reticuloendothelial cells of the spleen, liver, and bone marrow. Skeletal infiltration causes a loss of bone density with expansion and cortical thinning of long bones, especially the femur. Marrow infiltration in the distal femur causes abnormal modeling and flaring and the characteristic Erlenmeyer flask deformity. Avascular necrosis (especially of the femoral heads) is a common complication. The spleen is usually markedly enlarged and hepatomegaly is common.

Niemann-Pick disease (Fig B 22-2)	Inborn error of lipid metabolism (abnormal deposition of sphingomyelin) that usually begins in infancy and is rapidly fatal. In patients with milder and more slowly progressive disease who survive until late adulthood or adolescence, the skeletal abnormalities are identical to those in Gaucher's disease. However, the early age of onset and the frequently associated nodular interstitial pulmonary infiltrates suggest Niemann-Pick disease.

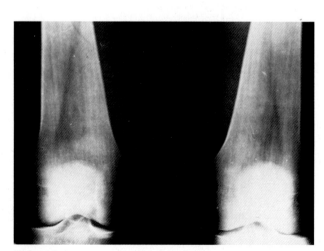

A 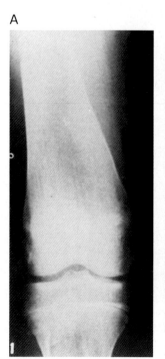 B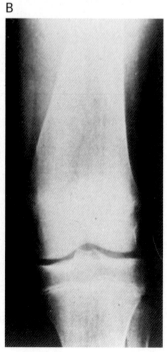

Fig B 22-1
Gaucher's disease. The distal ends of the femurs show typical underconstriction and cortical thinning (Erlenmeyer flask appearance).[33]

Fig B 22-2
Niemann-Pick disease. Thin cortices and a lack of normal modeling of the distal femurs simulate the pattern in Gaucher disease.[4]

Condition	Comments

Anemia
  Thalassemia
  (Fig B 22-3)
	Extensive marrow hyperplasia (due to ineffective erythropoiesis and rapid destruction of newly formed red blood cells) causes pronounced widening of the medullary spaces and thinning of the cortices. Normal modeling of long bones does not occur because the expanding marrow flattens or even bulges the normally concave surfaces of the shafts. Focal collections of hyperplastic marrow cause localized radiolucencies that have the appearance of multiple osteolytic lesions. Other characteristic findings include the "hair-on-end" appearance of the skull (vertical striations in a radial pattern) and paravertebral soft-tissue masses of extramedullary hematopoiesis.

Sickle cell anemia	Marrow hyperplasia in long bones causes widening of the medullary spaces, thinning of the cortices, and coarsening of the trabecular pattern. The expanding marrow prevents normal modeling, as in thalassemia. Other characteristic changes include "fish vertebrae," bone infarcts, osteomyelitis, and papillary necrosis.

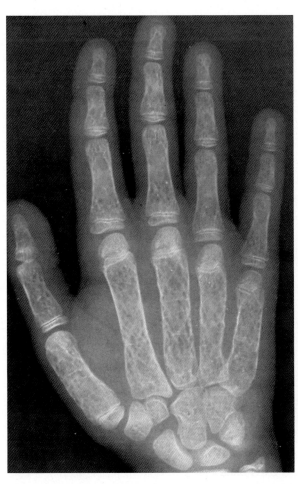

Fig B 22-3
Thalassemia. Pronounced widening of the medullary spaces with thinning of the cortices. Note the absence of normal modeling due to the pressure of the expanding marrow space. Localized radiolucencies simulating multiple osteolytic lesions represent tumorous collections of hyperplastic marrow.

Condition	Comments
Bone dysplasia Fibrous dysplasia (Fig B 22-4)	Proliferation of fibrous tissue in the medullary cavity produces a well-defined area that varies from completely lucent to a homogeneous ground-glass density (depending on the amount of fibrous or osseous tissue deposited in the medullary cavity). The bone is often locally expanded, most commonly at the metaphysis but sometimes extending to involve the entire shaft. Thinning of the cortices predisposes to pathologic fracture. In severe and long-standing disease, the affected bones may be bowed or deformed (eg, shepherd's crook deformity of the femur).
Multiple exostoses (diaphyseal aclasis) (Fig B 22-5)	Hereditary bone dysplasia in which multiple osteochondromas arise from the ends of the shafts of bones preformed in cartilage. Characteristic undertubulation and often bowing of long bones occurs with multiple osteochondromas in the metaphyseal regions. Frequently, there is deformity of the forearm due to shortening and bowing of the ulna.

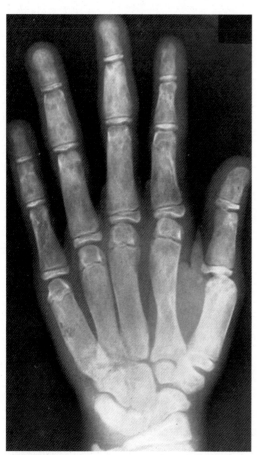

Fig B 22-4
Fibrous dysplasia. Smudgy, ground-glass appearance of the medullary cavities with failure of normal modeling.

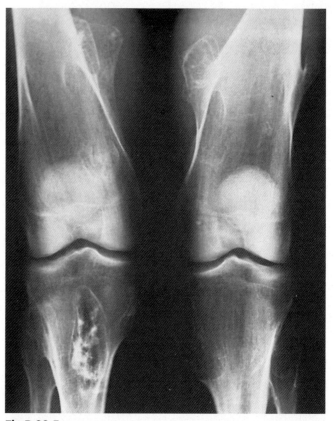

Fig B 22-5
Multiple exostoses. Bilateral involvement of the distal femurs and proximal tibias.

Condition	Comments
Craniometaphyseal dysplasia	Rare hereditary disorder in which failure of normal tubulation of bone is combined with hypertelorism, a broad, flat nose, and defective dentition. Additional findings include sclerosis of the base of the skull and calvarium, lack of aeration of the paranasal sinuses and mastoids, and thickening and sclerosis of the mandible.
Metaphyseal dysplasia (Pyle disease) (Fig B 22-6)	Rare hereditary disorder in which symmetric paddle-shaped enlargement of the metaphyses and adjacent diaphyses of long bones is associated with osteoporosis and cortical thinning. No evidence of skull abnormalities (unlike craniometaphyseal dysplasia).

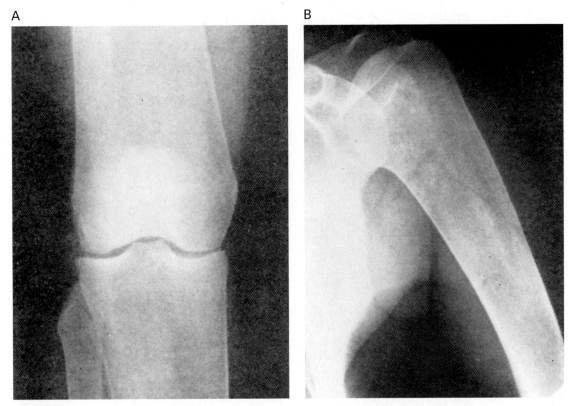

A

B

Fig B 22-6
Metaphyseal dysplasia. Frontal views of (A) the knee and (B) the proximal humerus show defective modeling leading to extreme widening of the metaphyseal areas of the visualized long bones. The cortices are markedly thin in the metaphyseal area.[34]

Condition	Comments
Multiple enchondromatosis (Olliers disease) (Fig B 22-7)	Bone dysplasia affecting the growth plate in which an excess of hypertrophic cartilage is not resorbed and ossified in a normal fashion. This causes proliferation of rounded masses or columns of decreased-density cartilage in the metaphyses and diaphyses of one or more tubular bones. The involvement is usually unilateral and the affected bones are invariably shortened and often deformed. In long bones, columns of radiolucent cartilage may be separated by bony septa, producing a striated appearance. In the hands and feet, the lesions are globular and expansile, often with stippled or mottled calcification.

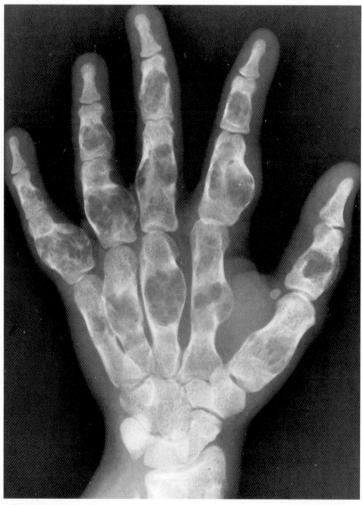

Fig B 22-7
Multiple enchondromatosis. Multiple globular and expansile lucent filling defects involving virtually all the metacarpals and the proximal and distal phalanges.

Condition	Comments
Progressive diaphyseal dysplasia (Camurati-Engelmann's disease) (Fig B 22-8)	Rare disorder in which symmetric cortical thickening in the midshafts of long bones is associated with a neuromuscular dystrophy that causes a wide-based waddling gait. A combination of endosteal and periosteal cortical thickening causes symmetric fusiform enlargement and undertubulation of long bones. Encroachment on the medullary canal may cause anemia and secondary hepatosplenomegaly. Amorphous increased density at the base of the skull may lead to impingement on the cranial nerves.

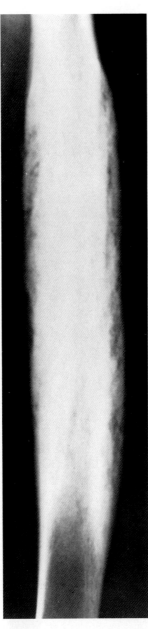

Fig B 22-8
Progressive diaphyseal dysplasia. Dense endosteal and periosteal cortical thickening causes fusiform enlargement of the midshaft of the femur.

Condition	Comments
Osteopetrosis (Fig B 22-9)	Rare hereditary bone dysplasia in which failure of the resorptive mechanism of calcified cartilage interferes with its normal replacement by mature bone. A dense, uniform, and symmetric increase in bone density is associated with undertubulation of long bones. Alternating dense and lucent transverse lines (probably reflecting the intermittent nature of the pathologic process) may develop in the metaphyses of long bones and vertebrae. Other characteristic findings include a miniature bone inset within each vertebral body (bone-within-a-bone appearance) and increased density at the end plates (sandwich vertebrae).

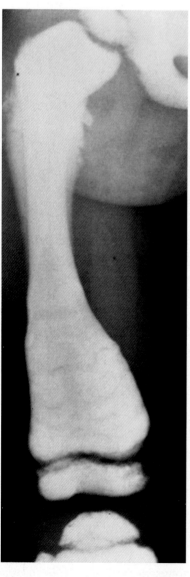

Fig B 22-9
Osteopetrosis. Dense, uniform, symmetric increase in the density of the femur with failure of proper modeling.

Condition	Comments
Hypophosphatasia	Mild form developing in adults is associated with lack of modeling of long bones, decreased stature, increased bone fragility, and various skeletal deformities.
Osteogenesis imperfecta	Inherited generalized disorder of connective tissue associated with blue sclerae, multiple fractures, and hypermobility of joints. The rarest "cystic" form is characterized by flared metaphyses that are hyperlucent and traversed by a honeycomb of coarse trabeculae. The shaft may be overconstricted and show severe bending deformities and healed fractures in addition to generalized osteopenia.
Metatropic dwarfism	Very rare short-limbed dwarfism in which the patient is normal at birth. Progressive kyphoscoliosis with characteristic trumpet-like expansion of multiple metaphyses, especially in the femurs and tibias.
Healing fracture/ metaphyseal injury	Common cause of localized undertubulation and deformity of a long bone. During the healing phase, an elevated solid periosteal reaction may simulate a "double cortex" (especially in infants and children), but disappears with further bone remodeling.
Biliary atresia	Most common cause of persistent neonatal jaundice; usually fatal within 2 years unless corrected surgically. Undertubulation of long bones is combined with signs of osteoporosis and rickets.

Metabolic and nutritional disorders
  Healing rickets and scurvy
  (Fig B 22-10)
	Widening of the diametaphyses with cortical thickening and undertubulation occurs in the healing phase of these diseases.

Mucopolysaccharidoses	Thickening and undertubulation of the shafts of long bones, often with irregular wavy contours, is common. Metaphyseal flaring may be seen in Morquio's disease, whereas tapering of the ends of long bones suggests Hurler's disease.
Homocystinuria	Inborn error of methionine metabolism in which there is usually widening of the metaphyses and enlargement of the ossification centers of long bones, most commonly at the knees. There is usually striking osteoporosis of the spine that is often associated with biconcave deformities of vertebral bodies. Long bones tend to be osteoporotic with cortical thickening.

Condition	Comments
Hypervitaminosis D/ idiopathic hypercalcemia	Undertubulation, especially in the distal femurs, may occur in association with generalized sclerosis, cortical thickening, and dense transverse metaphyseal bands. Prominent renal calcification and renal failure often develop.
Congenital rubella (see Fig B 21-2)	Undertubulation of long bones with radiolucent metaphyseal bands and characteristic alternating lucent and sclerotic longitudinal striations (celery stick pattern). Osseous changes regress in infants who grow normally, but may persist in those who fail to survive.
Bone cysts, tumors, and tumor-like conditions	Localized widening near the end of a long bone may be caused by a variety of benign expansile mass lesions (including Langerhans cell histiocytosis).
Lead poisoning	Wide sclerotic bands of lead deposited in the metaphyses can prevent normal bone remodeling and lead to residual deformity.

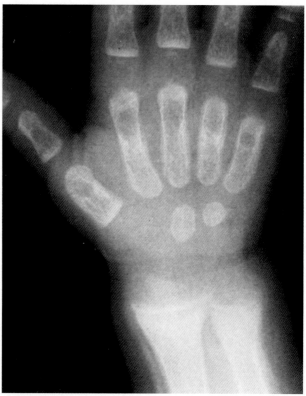

Fig B 22-10
Healing rickets. Widening of the metacarpals associated with diffuse periosteal reaction. There is still some bony demineralization and residual cupping and fraying of the distal radius and ulna.

Condition	Comments
Infantile cortical hyperostosis (Caffey disease)	Diffuse soft-tissue swelling, periosteal new bone formation, and massive cortical thickening cause generalized widening and undertubulation of affected bones. Primarily involves the mandible, scapula, clavicle, ulna, and ribs and almost always develops before the age of 5 months.
Chronic osteomyelitis	Sclerosis and solid periosteal new bone formation may produce marked thickening of the affected area.

Overconstriction or Overtubulation (Narrow Diametaphysis)

Condition	Comments
Disuse atrophy	Osteoporosis with cortical thinning and a decrease in the size and number of trabeculae in the spongiosa may develop after prolonged disuse. Concentric constriction of the shaft often occurs in children (rare in adults).
Paralysis (infancy and childhood) (Fig B 23-1)	Poliomyelitis, birth palsies, and congenital malformations of the spinal cord and brain result in decreased peripheral muscle tone and secondary bone atrophy. In addition to overconstriction of the shafts, there is generalized osteoporosis and cortical thinning.
Muscular disorders (Fig B 23-2)	Generalized overconstriction of the shafts of long bones (similar to that in paralysis) develops in such conditions as muscular dystrophy, arthrogryposis, amyotonia congenita, and infantile muscular atrophy (Werdnig-Hoffmann disease). Replacement of muscle by fat produces a characteristic finely striated or striped appearance. The fascial sheaths may appear as thin shadows of increased density surrounded by fat.

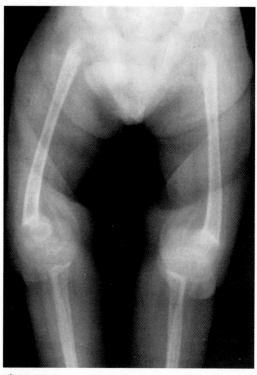

Fig B 23-1
Paralysis. Generalized narrowing of the bones of the leg with cortical thinning and diffuse osteoporosis.

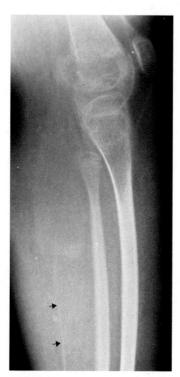

Fig B 23-2
Muscular dystrophy. Generalized thinning of the bones of the lower leg. The fascial sheaths appear as thin shadows of increased density (arrows) surrounded by fatty infiltration within muscle bundles.

Condition	Comments
Marfan's syndrome (Fig B 23-3)	Inherited generalized disorder of connective tissue in which there is elongation and thinning (without osteoporosis) of the tubular bones that is most pronounced in the hands and feet (arachnodactyly). Most patients are tall and appear emaciated because of a decrease in subcutaneous fat. Bilateral dislocation of the lens of the eye often occurs because of weakness and redundancy of its supporting structures. Laxity of ligaments elsewhere leads to loose-jointedness, double-jointedness, and recurrent dislocations. Dissecting aneurysm is the most serious cardiovascular complication.
Homocystinuria	Inborn error of methionine metabolism that produces a Marfan-like appearance of thin and elongated tubular bones. In contrast to Marfan's syndrome, the long tubular bones in homocystinuria have widened metaphyses and enlarged ossification centers and there is often striking osteoporosis (especially in the spine).
Osteogenesis imperfecta (Fig B 23-4)	Inherited generalized disorder of connective tissue in which long bones are slender and overconstricted. There is striking osteoporosis with thinning of the cortices and a marked susceptibility to fracture (from minimal trauma) that leads to bowing and other deformities.

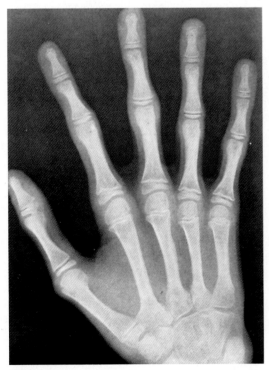

Fig B 23-3
Marfan's syndrome. The metacarpals and phalanges are unusually long and slender (arachnodactyly).

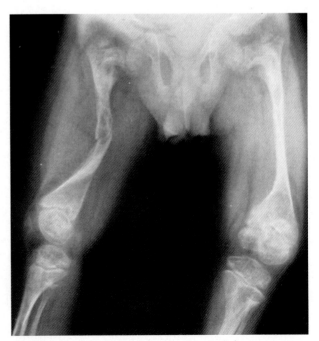

Fig B 23-4
Osteogenesis imperfecta. The bones of the lower extremity are thin and deformed with evidence of previous fracture.

Condition	Comments
Juvenile rheumatoid arthritis (Fig B 23-5)	Generalized connective tissue disease of children that most frequently affects the areas of greatest bone growth (the knees, ankles, and wrists). The long tubular bones may be overconstricted with generalized osteoporosis. Periosteal new bone formation is much more common and severe than in the adult form of the disease. Growth disturbances are common and include overgrowth of the epiphyses of an affected joint (balloon epiphysis), initially accelerated bone growth because of local hyperemia, and then delayed bone growth due to early epiphyseal fusion or the administration of steroids.
Neurofibromatosis (see Figs B 26-1, B 29-1, SK 13-2, and SK 24-14)	Overtubulation of bone may result in an extremely thin shaft that is usually associated with bowing deformities. Conversely, overgrowth of bone may produce elephantoid soft-tissue and bony thickening. Other major abnormalities include pseudoarthroses, "ribbon ribs," posterior vertebral scalloping, and orbital dysplasia.
Epidermolysis bullosa (see Fig B 11-7)	Thin, osteoporotic tubular bones may reflect chronic muscle atrophy in this rare hereditary disorder in which the skin blisters spontaneously or with injury. Flexion contractures and webbing between the fingers may produce a claw-like hand. Severe scarring causes soft-tissue atrophy and trophic changes of shortening and tapering of the distal phalanges. Healing of esophageal mucosal lesions may progress to stenotic webs.

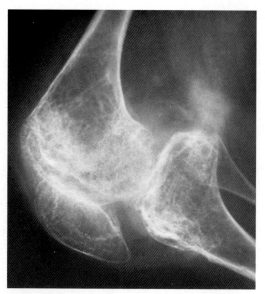

Fig B 23-5
Juvenile rheumatoid arthritis. Severe demineralization of bone with expansion of the epiphyseal and metaphyseal areas and relative constriction of the underdeveloped diaphyseal portions.

Condition	Comments

Dwarfism
  Progeria
  (Fig B 23-6)
	Nonhereditary congenital syndrome of dwarfism and premature aging and senility in which thin, osteoporotic long bones are associated with such findings as small facial bones and mandible; progressive resorption of terminal phalangeal tufts, clavicles, and occasionally ribs; thin calvarium with wormian bones; coxa valga; and coronary artery disease and hypertension that lead to prominent cardiomegaly.

Hypopituitarism	Proportional dwarfism that is often associated with narrowing of tubular bones and delayed epiphyseal closure. Hypogonadism and other endocrinologic disturbances commonly occur.
Tubular stenosis (Kenny-Caffey)	Proportional dwarfism characterized by overconstricted tubular bones that show symmetric internal thickening of the cortex and narrowing of the medullary cavity. Other manifestations include calvarial sclerosis and transient hypocalcemia with tetanic convulsions.

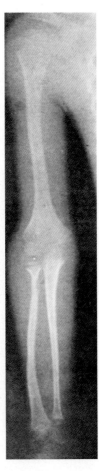

Fig B 23-6
Progeria. The ulna and radius are thin and osteoporotic.[26]

Avascular Necrosis of the Hip or Other Joints

Condition	Comments
Trauma	Disruption of the blood supply most commonly affects the hips and is secondary to an intracapsular femoral neck fracture, dislocation of the femoral head, or surgical correction of congenital hip dislocation or slipped femoral capital epiphysis. The carpal navicular is also frequently involved.
Sickle cell disease (Fig B 24-1)	Sludging of sickled erythrocytes in the sinusoidal vascular bed results in functional obstruction.
Steroid therapy/Cushing syndrome (Fig B 24-2)	Underlying pathophysiology is unclear. May be related to microscopic fat emboli in end-arteries of bone, steroid-induced osteoporosis with micro-fractures, or compression of the sinusoidal vascular bed by an increase in the marrow fat cell mass.
Occlusive vascular disease	Arteriosclerosis or thromboembolic disease disrupts the blood supply.

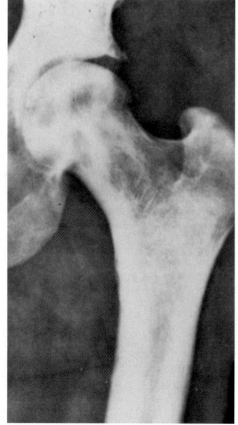

Fig B 24-1
Sickle cell disease. Avascular necrosis of the femoral head, with mottled areas of increased and decreased density reflecting osteonecrosis without collapse. The trabeculae in the neck and intertrochanteric region are thickened by apposition of new bone. A solid layer of new bone has been laid down in continuity with the inner aspect of the cortex of the femoral shaft, with consequent narrowing of the medullary canal.[30]

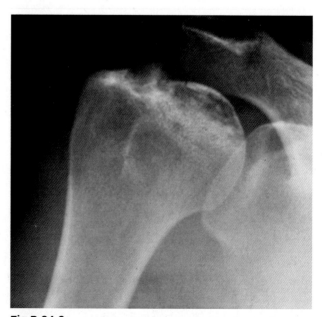

Fig B 24-2
Steroid therapy. Avascular necrosis of the head of the humerus in a transplant recipient.

Condition	Comments
Legg-Calvé-Perthes disease (Figs B 24-3 and B 24-4)	Osteochondritis of the femoral capital epiphyseal ossification center, most commonly occurring in boys between the ages of 5 and 9. There may be associated focal destructive lesions of the femoral neck (simulating an infectious or neoplastic process). Long-term complications include failure of the femoral neck to grow (with resultant shortening) and early development of degenerative arthritis.
Chronic alcoholism	Avascular necrosis, especially of the femoral head, is a fairly common complication. The underlying pathophysiologic mechanism is probably similar to that with steroid therapy. In alcoholic fatty liver disease, systemic fat emboli may lodge in bone and lead to necrosis.
Gaucher's disease (Fig B 24-5)	Inborn error of metabolism in which abnormal quantities of complex lipids may accumulate in the bone marrow, causing progressive obstruction of blood flow through the sinusoids and leading to infarction.
Chronic pancreatitis	The increased incidence of avascular necrosis probably represents a complication of underlying chronic alcoholism. Circulating lipases may produce areas of fat necrosis in the bones of patients with acute pancreatitis.

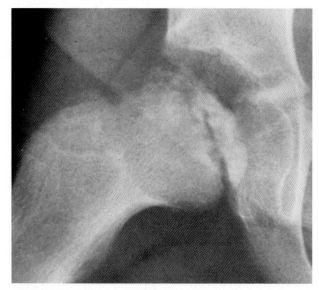

Fig B 24-3
Legg-Calvé-Perthes disease. Flattening of the femoral capital epiphyses along with fragmentation and sclerosis.

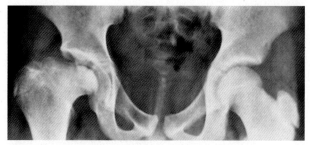

Fig B 24-4
Legg-Calvé-Perthes disease. In a teenager with chronic disease, there is severe flattening of the right femoral head with virtually complete failure of the ipsilateral femoral neck to grow. This led to shortening of the leg and a clinically obvious limp.

Condition	Comments
Gout	Infrequent, but important, cause of avascular necrosis that should be considered in the older age group when no other etiology is apparent. No definite pathophysiologic explanation (other than the frequent association of chronic alcoholism and gout).
Collagen disease	Systemic lupus erythematosus; rheumatoid arthritis; polyarteritis nodosa. Ischemic bone necrosis may be related to steroid therapy or vasculitis causing interruption of the arterial blood supply.
Radiation therapy/ radium poisoning (Fig B 24-6)	Direct cytotoxic effect (especially on the more sensitive hematopoietic marrow constituents) or damage to the arterial blood supply to bone.
Caisson disease (dysbaric disorders)	Result of air (nitrogen) embolization after rapid decompression. Because fat cells tend to absorb large quantities of dissolved nitrogen, rapid expansion of these cells in the marrow can cause increased intraosseous marrow pressure and vascular compromise.
Hemophilia	Hemarthrosis can occlude epiphyseal vessels and result in avascular necrosis. Most commonly involves the femoral and radial heads (both of which have a totally intracapsular epiphysis and are therefore especially vulnerable to deprivation of their vascular supply from compression by a tense joint effusion).

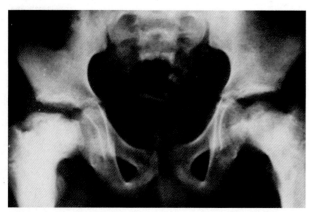

Fig B 24-5
Gaucher's disease. Bilateral avascular necrosis of the femoral heads.

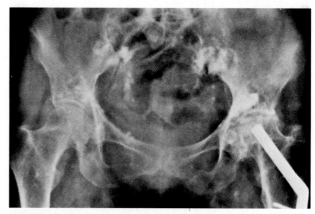

Fig B 24-6
Radiation therapy. After radiation therapy for carcinoma of the cervix, there has been flattening and sclerosis of the left femoral head (reflecting avascular necrosis) and patchy areas of dense sclerosis in the pelvis.

Condition	Comments
Osteomyelitis	Although no longer generally regarded in the context of osteonecrosis, the sequestrum of osteomyelitis is a manifestation of ischemic bone death occurring as a consequence of compressive and destructive suppuration that isolates a segment of bone from its blood supply.
Osteochondrial defect (Fig B 24-7)	Localized form of avascular necrosis that most frequently affects young males and is probably caused by trauma. Primarily involves the knees (usually the lateral aspect of the medial femoral condyle). Other common locations are the ankles, femoral heads, elbows, and shoulders. Radiographically, a small, round or oval, necrotic segment of bone with its articular cartilage detaches and lies in a depression in the joint surface. The necrotic segment is often denser than the surrounding bone and well demarcated by a crescentic lucent zone. Separation of the necrotic segment from the joint to form a free joint body leaves a residual pit in the articular surface.

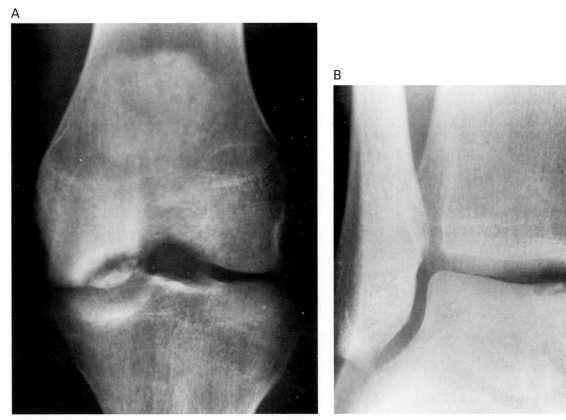

Fig B 24-7
Osteochondrial defect. (A) Knee. (B) Ankle.

Rib Notching

Condition	Comments
Arterial Coarctation of the aorta (Fig B 25-1)	By far the most common cause of rib notching. Usually involves the posterior fourth to eighth ribs and rarely develops before age 6. Aortic narrowing typically occurs at or just distal to the level of the ductus arteriosus. Characteristic double bulge in the region of the aortic knob (figure-3 sign on plain chest radiographs and reverse figure-3, or figure-E, sign on the barium-filled esophagus) represents prestenotic and poststenotic dilatation. Collateral flow bypassing the aortic constriction to reach the abdomen and lower extremities comes almost entirely from the two subclavian arteries via the thyrocervical, costocervical, and internal mammary arteries and their subdivisions to the posterior intercostals and then into the descending aorta. The large volume of blood traversing this route causes dilatation, tortuosity, and increased pulsation of the intercostal arteries, which result in gradual erosion of the adjacent bones. Unilateral rib notching in coarctation occasionally occurs on the left side when the constriction is located proximal to an anomalous right subclavian artery, and on the right side when the coarctation occurs proximal to the left subclavian artery (only the subclavian artery that arises proximal to the aortic obstruction transmits the collateral blood to the intercostals). Notching of the first two ribs does not occur because the first two intercostal arteries, arising from the supreme intercostals, do not convey blood directly to the postcoarctation segment of the aorta. The last three intercostal arteries conduct blood away from the postcoarctation aortic segment and thus do not greatly enlarge or cause rib notching.
Low aortic obstruction	Thrombosis of the lower thoracic or abdominal aorta causes collateral flow via the lower intercostal arteries to supply blood to the lower part of the body via anastomoses with arteries of the abdominal wall.
Subclavian artery obstruction	Unilateral rib notching commonly occurs secondary to interruption of a subclavian artery for the Blalock-Taussig subclavian artery–pulmonary artery anastomosis for congenital heart disease. The development of rib notching reflects increased blood flow through collateral vessels to the arm resulting from interruption of the subclavian and vertebral arteries on the involved side. Rib notching is also a rare complication of Takayasu arteritis ("pulseless disease") causing occlusion of one or both subclavian arteries.

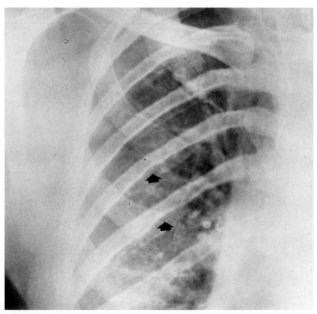

Fig B 25-1
Coarctation of the aorta. Notching of the posterior fourth through eighth ribs (arrows).[36]

Condition	Comments
Decreased pulmonary blood flow	The intercostal arteries may participate in the collateral circulation to the lungs whenever there is an obstruction to pulmonary blood flow. Nevertheless, despite abundant and well-developed collateral circulation, rib notching is uncommon in this situation. Conditions with decreased pulmonary blood flow in which rib notching has been reported include tetralogy of Fallot, unilateral absence of the pulmonary artery, Ebstein's anomaly, emphysema, pseudotruncus arteriosus, and pulmonary valvular stenosis or atresia.
Venous	Chronic obstruction of the superior vena cava (as in fibrosing mediastinitis) can produce rib notching. This is a very infrequent cause, as might be expected, as dilated intercostal veins do not erode the ribs as readily as do dilated, highly pulsatile intercostal arteries.
Arteriovenous	Pulmonary arteriovenous fistula (dilated intercostal arteries carrying a systemic supply to the fistula or contributing collateral circulation to that portion of the pulmonary vascular bed bypassed by the large flow through the fistula); arteriovenous fistula of the chest wall (intercostal artery–vein communication).
Neurogenic (Fig B 25-2)	Rib erosions due to multiple intercostal neurofibromas (in neurofibromatosis) or rare single intercostal nerve tumors (schwannoma or neurilemmoma). Rib deformities in neurofibromatosis frequently reflect the generalized bone dysplasia occurring in this condition.
Osseous	Periosteal irregularities mimicking rib notching rarely occur in hyperparathyroidism, tuberous sclerosis, and thalassemia. Poliomyelitis primarily causes irregularity of the superior surfaces of the ribs.
Idiopathic	Mild degrees of rib notching may develop in apparently healthy individuals with none of the underlying causes described above.

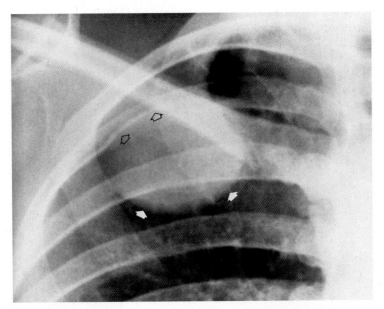

Fig B 25-2
Neurofibroma. Erosion of the inferior surface of the third rib (black arrows) associated with a large soft-tissue mass (white arrows).

Resorption or Notching of Superior Rib Margins

Condition	Comments
Disturbance of osteoblastic activity (decreased or deficient bone formation)	
Neurofibromatosis (Fig B 26-1)	Irregular, notched, scalloped, and twisted ribbon-like configuration of the ribs is a manifestation of dysplastic bone formation. Rib deformities also may be secondary to mechanical pressure caused by neighboring intercostal neurofibromas.
Collagen disease	Erosions of the superior margins of the posterior aspect of the upper ribs (third, fourth, fifth, and occasionally sixth). Most commonly occurs in rheumatoid arthritis and scleroderma, but may also develop in systemic lupus erythematosus and Sjögren's syndrome.
Paralytic poliomyelitis (Fig B 26-2)	Initially, a localized shallow indentation with progressive narrowing of the upper cortical margins of the ribs. As the condition progresses, the cortices of the ribs become increasingly thin, and there is localized osteoporosis. A similar, though slight, indentation may occasionally occur on the inferior cortical margin, producing an hourglass appearance. The underlying mechanism is most likely atrophy of the intercostal muscles (and their replacement by fat and fibrous tissue) at their attachment to the ribs, which decreases the normal "stress stimulus" required for osteoblastic bone production to replace the osteoid that has been lost by physiologic erosion. Another explanation is that the rib erosion is secondary to the continued pressure of the scapula against the posterior aspect of the ribs from prolonged use of a respirator. There may also be severe thinning of the humeri and usually pronounced scoliosis of the thoracic spine.
Localized pressure effect	May follow the use of rib retractors during surgery or intercostal chest drainage tubes. Also an underlying mechanism in patients with neurofibromatosis, thoracic neuroblastoma, and multiple hereditary exostoses. Severely tortuous intercostal arteries extending down from the lower border of a rib have been reported to erode the superior borders of the adjacent inferior rib.
Osteogenesis imperfecta	Systemic connective tissue disorder in which there is an inability to produce adequate amounts of osteoid to balance physiologic osteolysis. Produces a concave superior margin in multiple ribs associated with cortical thinning and abnormal rib rotation and curvature.

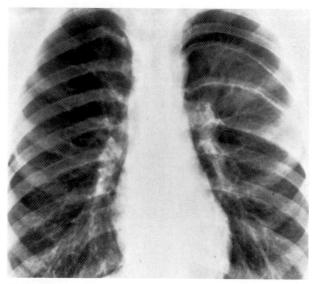

Fig B 26-1
Neurofibromatosis. Narrowing and irregularity of several upper ribs.

Condition	Comments
Marfan's syndrome (Fig B 26-3)	Narrow ribs with thin cortices reflect poor muscle tone rather than a primary alteration in the quality of osteoid bone formation. Both superior and inferior marginal defects may occur.
Radiation therapy	Rare delayed manifestation of radiation interference with normal osteoblastic activity.
Disturbance of osteoclastic activity (increased bone resorption)	
Hyperparathyroidism	Subperiosteal bone resorption commonly involves the superior margins of one or more ribs (most often unilateral).
Idiopathic	Rare cases of superior marginal rib defects have been reported in patients with no demonstrable underlying cause.

A   B

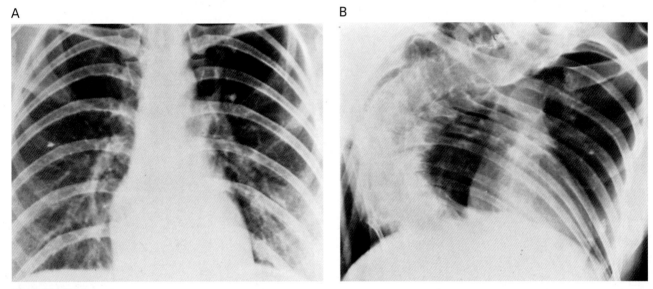

Fig B 26-2
Poliomyelitis. (A) Severe thinning of the humeri and ribs bilaterally. Note the bilateral shoulder dislocations. (B) In another patient, there is severe scoliosis of the thoracic spine producing an unusual configuration of the ribs.

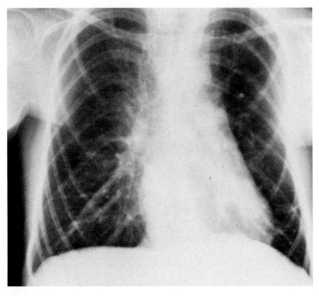

Fig B 26-3
Marfan's syndrome. Pronounced generalized narrowing of the ribs with thinning of the cortices.

Bone-within-a-Bone Appearance

Condition	Comments
Normal neonate (Fig B 27-1)	Not uncommon appearance in infants 1 to 2 months of age caused by loss of bone density at the periphery of vertebral bodies (but with retention of their sharp cortical outlines). The bone subsequently assumes a normal density; thus, this appearance probably reflects a normal stage in the transformation of the architecture of the neonatal vertebrae to that of later infancy.
Osteopetrosis (Fig B 27-2)	Miniature inset in each lumbar vertebral body is a typical manifestation of this rare hereditary bone abnormality characterized by a symmetric generalized increase in bone density and lack of tubulation.
Thorotrast administration (Fig B 27-3)	Radiographic densities of infantile vertebrae and pelvis (ghost vertebrae) in adult bones may be seen in adults who received intravenous Thorotrast during early childhood. The deposition of Thorotrast causes constant alpha radiation and temporary growth arrest so that the size of the ghost vertebrae corresponds to the vertebral size at the time of injection. Most patients also have reticular or dense opacification of the liver, spleen, and lymph nodes.

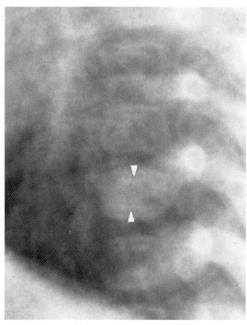

Fig B 27-1
Normal neonate. The arrowheads point to one example of the bone-within-a-bone appearance.

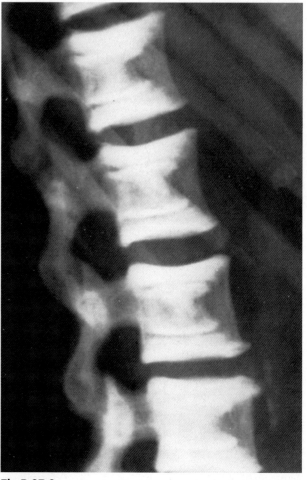

Fig B 27-2
Osteopetrosis. A miniature inset is seen in each lumbar vertebral body, giving it a bone-within-a-bone appearance. There is also sclerosis at the end plates.[31]

Condition	Comments
Transverse growth lines (growth arrest lines) (Fig B 27-4)	Opaque transverse lines paralleling the superior and inferior margins of vertebral bodies. Underlying causes include chronic childhood diseases, malnutrition, and chemotherapy.
Heavy metal poisoning	Radiodense lines paralleling the superior and inferior margins of multiple vertebral bodies are an infrequent manifestation of lead or phosphorus poisoning.
Gaucher's disease	Initial collapse of an entire vertebral body with subsequent growth recovery peripherally may be associated with horizontal and vertical sclerosis, giving the bone-within-a-bone appearance.
Paget's disease	May involve one or multiple vertebrae. More commonly produces enlarged, coarsened trabeculae with condensation of bone most prominent along the contours of a vertebral body (picture frame) or uniform increase in osseous density of an enlarged vertebral body (ivory vertebra).
Sickle cell anemia	Rare manifestation. More commonly generalized osteoporosis, localized step-like central depressions, and characteristic bioconcave indentations on both the superior and inferior margins of softened vertebral bodies (fish vertebrae).
Hypervitaminosis D	The margins of the vertebral bodies are outlined by dense bands of bone that are exaggerated by adjacent radiolucent zones. The central, normal-appearing bone may simulate the bone-within-a-bone appearance.

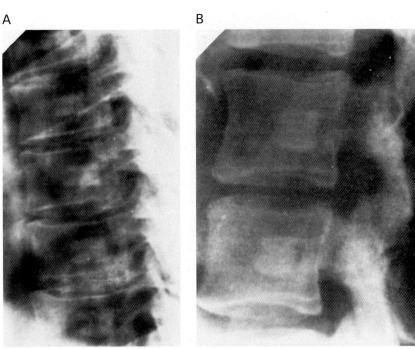

Fig B 27-3
Thorotrast. Two examples of persistence of radiographic densities of infantile vertebrae in adult bones of patients who received intravenous Thorotrast during early childhood.[37]

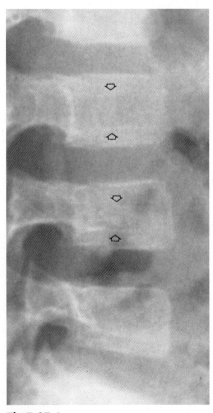

Fig B 27-4
Transverse growth lines. Opaque lines paralleling the superior and inferior margins of the vertebral body (arrows) in a child with severe chronic illness.

Heel Pad Thickening (>22 Millimeters)

Condition	Comments
Acromegaly (Fig B 28-1)	An excess of pituitary growth hormone causes generalized overgrowth of all body tissues. Other characteristic findings include joint space widening (especially metacarpophalangeal and hip joints) due to proliferation of cartilage, overgrowth of the tips of the distal phalanges producing thick bony tufts with pointed lateral margins (square, spade-shaped hand), thickening of the calvarium with frontal bossing and enlargement of the paranasal sinuses, prognathous jaw (lengthening of the mandible and increased mandibular angle), and scalloping of the posterior aspect of vertebral bodies.
Normal variant	Apparent thickening of the heel pad without any underlying cause may be a normal variant, especially in black males.
Obesity/high body weight	Although not directly proportional to body weight, heel pad thickening is common in people weighing more than 200 pounds.

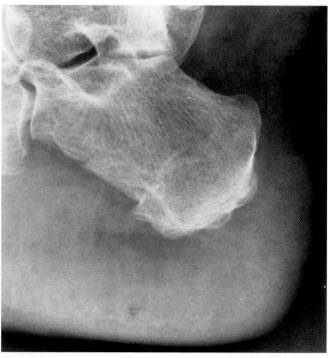

Fig B 28-1
Acromegaly. Prominent thickening of the heel pad, which measured 32 mm on the original radiograph.

Condition	Comments
Soft-tissue infection	Especially common in mycetoma (Madura foot), a chronic granulomatous fungal disease that affects the feet and is most prevalent in India. Pronounced soft-tissue swelling may be followed by bone destruction, deformity, and fistula formation.
Generalized edema	A manifestation of diffuse peripheral edema.
Myxedema/thyroid acropachy	Diffuse soft-tissue swelling of the hands and feet. In thyroid acropachy, a rare complication of hyperthyroid disease that develops after thyroidectomy or radioactive iodine treatment of primary hyperthyroidism. There is typically a generalized and symmetric spiculated periosteal reaction that primarily involves the midportion of the diaphyses of tubular bones of the hands and feet.
Dilantin therapy	The percentage of patients with abnormally thickened heel pads increases steadily with the length of treatment. Dilantin may also cause calvarial thickening that can be confused with acromegaly.
Trauma	Edema and bleeding in soft tissues. An associated fracture of the calcaneus may occur.

Pseudoarthrosis

Condition	Comments
Neurofibromatosis (Fig B 29-1)	Characteristic complication reflecting a fracture that failed to heal. Usually involves the junction of the middle and lower thirds of the tibia or fibula (or both) during the first year of life. Anterior bowing of the leg and severe disuse osteoporosis are typical findings. An abnormally formed, deficient, or gracile fibula is a frequent accompaniment of pseudoarthrosis of the tibia.
Nonunion of a fracture (Fig B 29-2)	A false joint may form at the fracture site, with one fragment presenting a convex surface that fits into the concave surface of the apposing fragment.

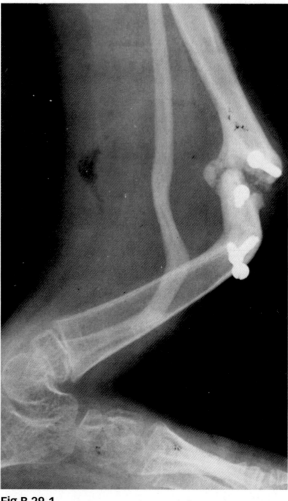

Fig B 29-1
Neurofibromatosis. A false joint of the midshaft of the tibia has developed after trauma. Note the severe disuse osteoporosis of the bones of the ankle and the ribbon-like shape of the lower fibula.

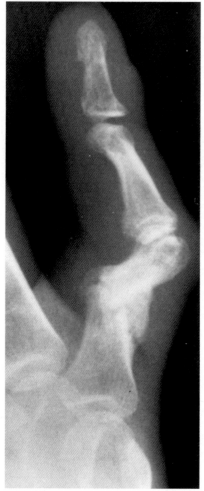

Fig B 29-2
Post-traumatic pseudoarthrosis. Nonunion about a fracture of the proximal phalanx of the fifth digit. Although there is extensive callus formation, the lucent fracture line can still be clearly seen.

Condition	Comments
Osteogenesis imperfecta (see Fig B 2-9)	Inherited generalized disorder of connective tissue that causes osteoporosis with abnormal fragility of the skeleton and an unusual tendency for fractures. Although fracture healing is often normal, exuberant callus formation and bizarre deformities (including pseudoarthrosis) may occur.
Fibrous dysplasia	Proliferation of fibrous tissue in the medullary cavity causes local expansion of bone and cortical erosion from within, predisposing to pathologic fractures that may lead to pseudoarthrosis. In severe and long-standing disease, affected bones may be bowed or deformed (eg, shepherd's crook deformity of the femur).
Congenital pseudoarthrosis	Rare condition that is generally unilateral, primarily involves the tibia, and develops during the first or second year of life. Initially, there is anterior bowing of the lower half of the tibia with sclerosis, narrowing of the medullary canal, and cystic abnormalities at the apex of the curve indicating impending fracture and pseudoarthrosis. Once the fracture appears, the margins of adjacent bone become increasingly tapered. After bone grafting, healing may be expected in approximately 30% of patients. Congenital pseudoarthrosis of the clavicle occurs almost exclusively on the right (bilateral in 10% of patients) and presents within the first few months of life as a painless lump over the medial third of the clavicle. Radiographs show the medial end of the clavicle superior to the lateral end, osseous discontinuity, and the absence of callus formation (absence of pain and visible callus permits differentiation from post-traumatic pseudoarthrosis).

Protrusio Acetabuli*

Condition	Comments
Normal variant	A normal phenomenon in children (4 to 12 years of age) that does not reflect any acetabular abnormality.
Rheumatoid arthritis	Common manifestation of severe rheumatoid hip disease. There is diffuse loss of the interosseous space and an eroded and often diminutive femoral head.
Rheumatoid variants	Ankylosing spondylitis; psoriatic arthritis; reactive arthritis syndrome; inflammatory bowel disease.
Acquired softening of bone	Paget's disease; osteomalacia or rickets; hyperparathyroidism. Rare manifestation of osteoporosis.
Osteoarthritis	Usually a mild degree of protrusion that is typically associated with medial migration of the femoral head. May be primary or secondary to hemophilia, pseudogout, hemochromatosis, or ochronosis.
Post-traumatic	May develop after an acetabular fracture with medial dislocation of the hip or after total hip replacement arthroplasty with marked thinning of the available acetabular roof.
Osteogenesis imperfecta	Caused by the osteoporotic and abnormally fragile bone in this inherited disorder of connective tissue.
Primary acetabular protrusion (Otto pelvis) (Fig B 30-2)	Usually bilateral and much more frequent in women. Associated loss of the joint space usually results in axial or medial migration of the femoral head with respect to the acetabulum. Although the etiology is unknown, postulated causes include failure of ossification or premature fusion of the Y cartilage or a direct consequence of normal stress on the Y cartilage (normally, the protrusion is reversible due to diminished stress after age 8; failure of correction of the protrusion resulting in its persistence into adult life may be due to premature fusion and coxa vara).
Miscellaneous causes	Destruction of the acetabulum resulting from septic arthritis, neoplasm, or radiation therapy.

*Pattern: Projection of the acetabular line (the medial wall of the acetabulum) medial to the ilioischial line (a portion of the quadrilateral surface) by 3 mm or more in adult men and by 6 mm or more in adult women (Fig B 30-1).

A

B

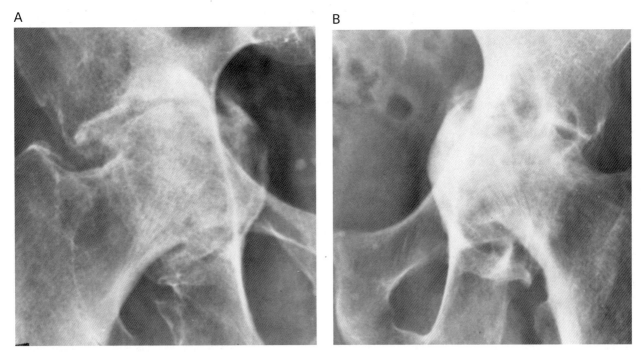

Fig B 30-1
Protrusio acetabuli. Two typical examples.

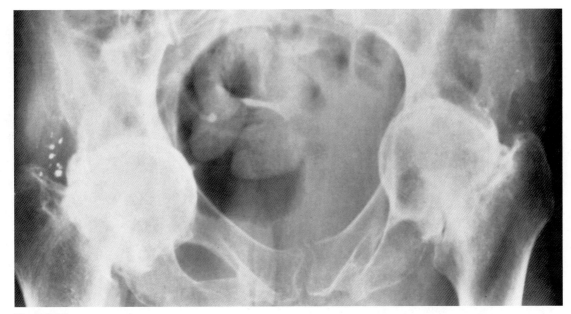

Fig B 30-2
Otto pelvis. Bilaterally symmetric protrusio acetabuli with superimposed degenerative changes.

Dactylitis*

Condition	Comments
Sickle cell anemia (hand-foot syndrome) (Fig B 31-1)	The small bones of the hands and feet are the most common sites of infarction in children. The peak incidence is between 6 and 24 months of age (children less than 6 months may still have the protection of their fetal hemoglobin). Differentiation from osteomyelitis is difficult both clinically and radiographically, though the lack of systemic symptoms and fever suggests infarction without osteomyelitis.
Pyogenic osteomyelitis	Most commonly represents *Salmonella* infection in a child with sickle cell anemia. Usually involves several bones in each hand. May be extremely difficult to differentiate from the hand-foot syndrome in this condition.
Tuberculosis ("spina ventosa") (Fig B 31-2)	Most often occurs in children, in whom it may be multiple. Sequestrum formation is uncommon, though it may be associated with small sinus tracts through which bony fragments may be extruded.

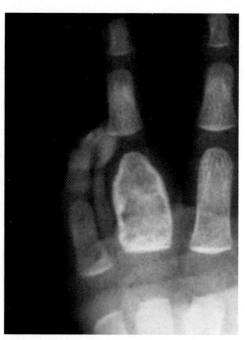

Fig B 31-2
Tuberculosis. Typical expansion of a phalanx along with irregular destruction of bone architecture. Note the absence of periosteal reaction, which differentiates the appearance from that of syphilitic dactylitis.[38]

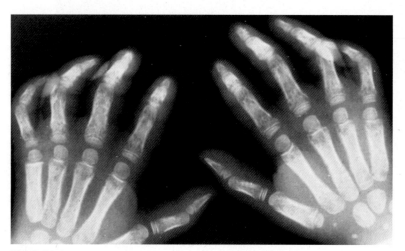

Fig B 31-1
Hand-foot syndrome in sickle cell anemia. Diffuse destruction of the shafts of multiple phalanges and metacarpals is due to infarction. There are reactive bone changes with sclerosis and periosteal thickening.

*Pattern: Soft-tissue swelling, periosteal reaction, and variable degrees of bone destruction and expansion involving one or multiple bones of the hands or feet or both.

Condition	Comments
Leprosy	Most frequently produces acro-osteolysis. More destructive lesions may lead to neuroarthropathy and a classic "licked candy stick" appearance and progress to a virtually fingerless hand.
Other infections (Figs B 31-3 and B 31-4)	Yaws, syphilis, smallpox, atypical mycobacteria, fungal disease.
Sarcoidosis (Fig B 31-5)	Approximately 15% of patients have bone involvement, predominantly in the middle and distal phalanges of the hand. Usually associated with characteristic hilar and paratracheal adenopathy, interstitial pulmonary disease, or both.
Leukemia	Leukemic changes are generally more diffuse than in osteomyelitis or sickle cell anemia, though the radiographic differentiation may be difficult.
Tuberous sclerosis (Fig B 31-6)	Characteristic abnormalities in the hands and feet are wavy periosteal new bone formation along the shafts of the metatarsals and metacarpals and cyst-like changes in the phalanges.
Pancreatic fat necrosis	Infrequent manifestation that probably results from elevated levels of lipase during the acute phase of the disease. In children, the lesions must be distinguished from those caused by infection or sickle cell dactylitis.

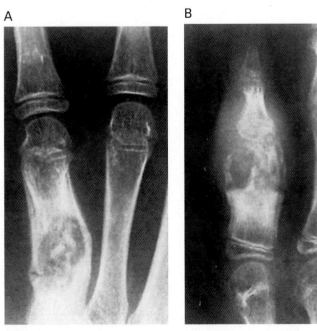

Fig B 31-3
Yaws. Examples of cortical and medullary granulomas along with intense periosteal new bone formation.[10]

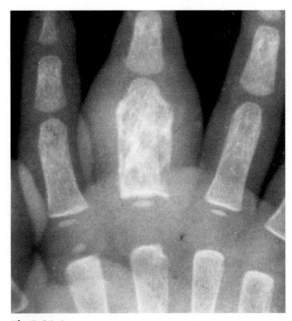

Fig B 31-4
Congenital syphilis. Typical destructive expansion of a phalanx with periosteal calcification forming a dense shell around the lesion.

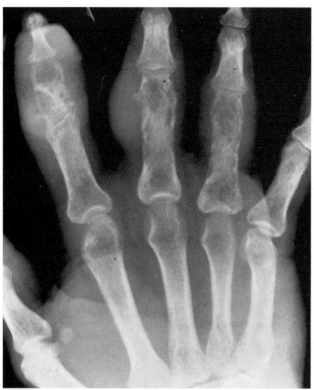

Fig B 31-5
Sarcoidosis. Destructive changes involving the middle phalanx of the second finger, with soft-tissue swelling about the third proximal interphalangeal joint and cortical thinning and a lace-like trabecular pattern affecting the proximal phalanges of the third and fourth digits.

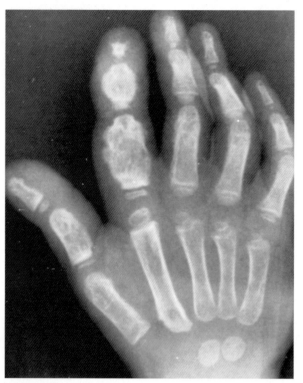

Fig B 31-6
Tuberous sclerosis. Cyst-like expansion and characteristic wavy periosteal new bone formation about the proximal and middle phalanges of the second digit. Periosteal new bone formation is also seen along the shaft of the second metacarpal.

Bony Whiskering (Proliferation of New Bone at Tendon and Ligament Insertions)

Condition	Comments
Diffuse idiopathic skeletal hyperostosis (DISH)	Common manifestation in this condition characterized by flowing calcification and ossification along the anterolateral aspect of at least four contiguous vertebral bodies with relative preservation of the intervertebral disk spaces and absence of the erosive and sclerotic changes seen in ankylosing spondylitis.
Ankylosing spondylitis (Fig B 32-1)	Characteristic bilateral erosion and sclerosis of the sacroiliac joints leading to complete fibrosis and bony ankylosis. Proliferation of new bone at tendon and ligament insertions also can occur in psoriatic arthritis, Reiter's syndrome, and inflammatory bowel disorders.
Fluorosis	In addition to periosteal roughening and bone deposits arising at sites of muscular and ligamentous attachments, typical skeletal findings include dense sclerosis (most prominent in the vertebrae and pelvis), vertebral osteophytosis (which can lead to encroachment on the spinal canal and intervertebral foramina), and calcification of paraspinal, sacrotuberous, and iliolumbar ligaments.
Hypoparathyroidism	Associated findings include generalized or localized osteosclerosis, band-like areas of increased opacity in the metaphyses of long bones, calvarial thickening, and cerebral calcification that especially involves the basal ganglia, dentate nuclei of the cerebellum, and the choroid plexus.
Familial vitamin D–resistant rickets	Hereditary disorder (also termed X-linked hypophosphatemia) secondary to renal tubular loss of phosphate, decreased intestinal absorption of calcium, and normal serum levels of calcium.
POEMS syndrome	Plasma cell dyscrasia characterized by chronic progressive polyneuropathy (P), hepatosplenomegaly (organomegaly [O]), endocrine disturbances including diabetes mellitus (E), abnormal myeloma-type proteins (M), and abnormal thickening and pigmentation of the skin (S). This condition of unknown cause is more frequent in men and has its onset at a young age.

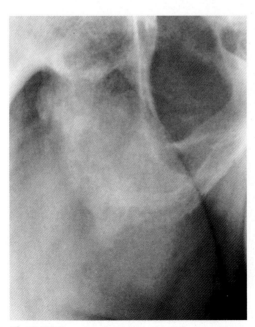

Fig B 32-1
Ankylosing spondylitis. Irregular proliferation of new bone ("whiskering") along the inferior pubic ramus.

Eponyms of Fractures

Condition	Imaging Findings	Comments
Upper extremity		
Mallet (baseball) finger (Fig B 33-1)	Avulsion from the dorsal aspect of the base of a distal phalanx at the insertion of the extensor tendon.	Occurs when a blow to the end of the finger forcibly flexes the distal phalanx while the extensor tendon is taut.
Bennett fracture (Fig B 33-2)	Oblique fracture of the base of the first metacarpal that transects the proximal articular surface.	Results from forcible abduction of the thumb and is associated with dorsal and radial subluxation or dislocation of the shaft of the first metacarpal. A triangular fragment consisting of the base of the bone remains in relation to the underlying greater multangular bone.
Rolando fracture (Fig B 33-3)	Y- or T-shaped, comminuted fracture of the base of the first metacarpal that extends into the articular surface.	Much less common though more serious than a Bennett fracture.
Gamekeeper thumb (Fig B 33-4)	Avulsion from the ulnar margin of the proximal phalanx at the site of insertion of the ulnar collateral ligament.	Valgus injury of the metacarpophalangeal joint resulting in a partial tear or disruption of the ulnar collateral ligament that may lead to decreased function of the thumb. In most cases, the radiographic examination is normal. A stress film may be required to demonstrate widening of the ulnar margin of the joint and radial subluxation of the proximal phalanx.

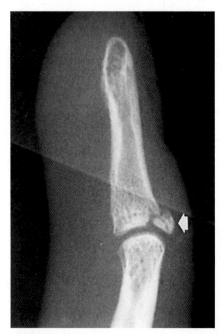

Fig B 33-1
Mallet (baseball) finger. The small triangular fragment (arrow) is proximally retracted by the action of the common extensor tendon. The flexion deformity results from the unopposed action of the flexor digiti profundus tendon.

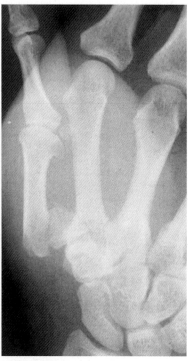

Fig B 33-2
Bennett fracture.

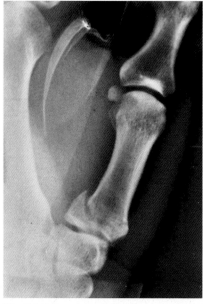

Fig B 33-3
Rolando fracture. In addition to the fracture of the ulnar margin, similar to that found in a Bennett fracture, there is a second fragment at the radial margin, which characterizes this as a Rolando fracture.[39]

Condition	Imaging Findings	Comments
Boxer fracture (Fig B 33-5)	Transverse fracture of the neck of the fifth and sometimes the fourth metacarpal with volar angulation of the distal fragment.	Characteristic injury resulting from a blow struck with the fist.
Colles' fracture (Fig B 33-6)	Transverse fracture of the distal radius with dorsal angulation and often overriding of the distal fracture fragment.	Caused by a fall on the outstretched hand. Associated fracture of the ulnar styloid process in more than half the cases.

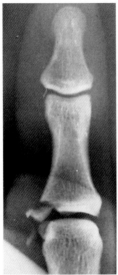

Fig B 33-4
Gamekeeper thumb with fracture.[39]

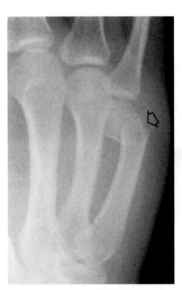

Fig B 33-5
Boxer fracture (arrow).

A   B

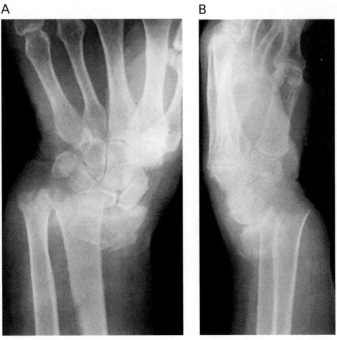

Fig B 33-6
Colles' fracture. (A) Frontal and (B) lateral projections show overriding and dorsal displacement of the distal fragment.

Condition	Imaging Findings	Comments
Smith fracture (Fig B 33-7)	Transverse fracture of the distal radius with volar angulation of the distal fragment.	Results from a fall on the back of the hand or a direct blow. Because Colles' and Smith fractures may have identical appearance on frontal views, a lateral projection is essential to show the direction of the displacement and angulation.
Chauffeur (Hutchinson) fracture (Fig B 33-8)	Avulsion of the radial styloid process.	Usually nondisplaced fracture occurring at the site of attachment of the radial collateral ligament.
Barton fracture (Fig B 33-9)	Fracture of the dorsal rim (Barton) or anterior rim (reverse Barton) of the distal radial joint surface with dislocation of the radiocarpal joint.	Typically occurs in younger persons as a result of motorcycle accidents or in the elderly following a fall on the outstretched hand. Fractures involving the anterior rim are more common.
Nightstick fracture (Fig B 33-10)	Isolated fracture of the distal shaft of the ulna.	Usually the result of a direct blow, as the forearm is raised to protect either the face or head from an assault by a club or other hard object.
Monteggia fracture (Fig B 33-11)	Combination of a fracture of the shaft of the ulna and anterior dislocation of the radius at the elbow.	The dislocation of the radial head can be missed clinically and cause aseptic necrosis with subsequent elbow dysfunction. Therefore, whenever the forearm is fractured, the elbow must be examined to exclude a dislocation.

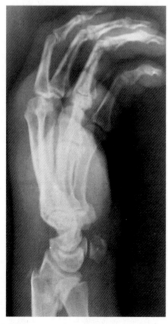

Fig B 33-7
Smith fracture. Lateral view shows volar angulation of the distal fragment, the reverse of that encountered in a Colles fracture.[39]

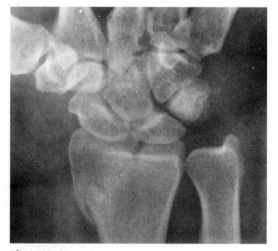

Fig B 33-8
Chauffeur fracture. Complete fracture extending diagonally across the base of the radial styloid.[39]

Condition	Imaging Findings	Comments
Galeazzi fracture (Fig B 33-12)	Combination of a fracture of the shaft of the radius and dorsal dislocation of the ulna at the wrist.	Much less common than a Monteggia fracture. The dislocated ulna is rarely missed clinically because the deformity at the wrist is usually obvious.

A

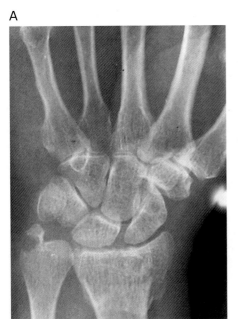

B

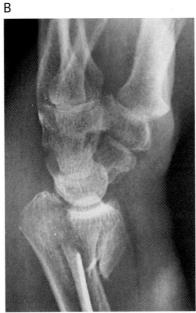

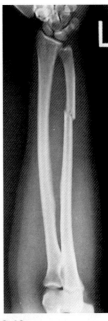

Fig B 33-9
Reverse Barton fracture. (A) Fracture of the distal radius with shortening of the radius and avulsion of the ulnar styloid. The appearance is similar to a Colles or a Smith fracture in this projection. (B) Lateral projection shows that the fracture of the distal radius creates a large fragment from the anterior rim of the distal radius. The posterior rim is intact. The anterior fragment includes approximately two-thirds of the joint surface.[39]

Fig B 33-10
Nightstick fracture. Minimally displaced oblique fracture of the ulna without associated fracture of the radius. (L, left.)[39]

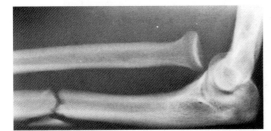

Fig B 33-11
Monteggia fracture. Displaced fracture of the ulnar shaft associated with anterior dislocation of the radial head.

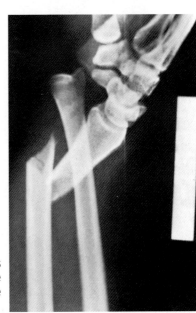

Fig B 33-12
Galeazzi fracture. A lateral projection shows the dorsally angulated distal radial fracture and the obvious disruption of the distal radioulnar joint. The ulna is intact.[39]

Condition	Imaging Findings	Comments
Greenstick fracture (Fig B 33-13)	Incomplete, angulated fracture of a long bone (usually in the forearm) that commonly occurs in young children.	Typically, the side opposite the bending force fractures completely, whereas the side under the force remains intact. As the name implies, the fracture resembles the break that results when a supple green branch of a tree is bent and breaks incompletely.
Little League elbow (Fig B 33-14)	Irregular lucent area in the capitellum, occasionally associated with loose bodies within the elbow joint.	Group of clinical disorders resulting from elbow overuse in children. In one common form, rarefaction and fragmentation of the capitellum occurs with repetitive motion of the arm. Continued valgus stress during the acceleration phase of pitching compresses the radial head on the capitellum and distracts the medial epicondyle apophysis. In some cases, this can lead to inflammation or avulsion of the medial epicondyle.
Hill-Sachs deformity (Fig B 33-15)	Large defect or groove in the posterolateral aspect of the head of the humerus.	The result of repeated anterior dislocations and best seen on internal rotation views, this indentation is probably caused by small compression fractures of this weakest point of the humeral head as it impinges against the anterior rim of the glenoid fossa.

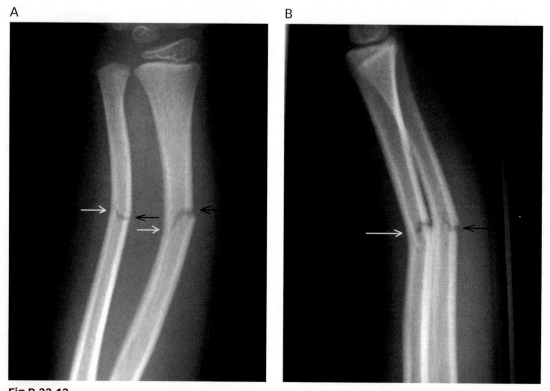

A B

Fig B 33-13

Greenstick fracture. Frontal image of a young child who fell off a bike shows incomplete fractures of the radius and ulna. The cortex is fully broken (black arrows) on one side of the bone and intact on the other side (white arrows).[40]

Condition	Imaging Findings	Comments
Bankhart fracture (Fig B 33-16)	Bony irregularity or fragmentation of the anterior margin of the glenoid fossa.	Complication of anterior dislocation of the humerus that results from the same mechanism as the Hill-Sachs deformity but is much less common.

A B

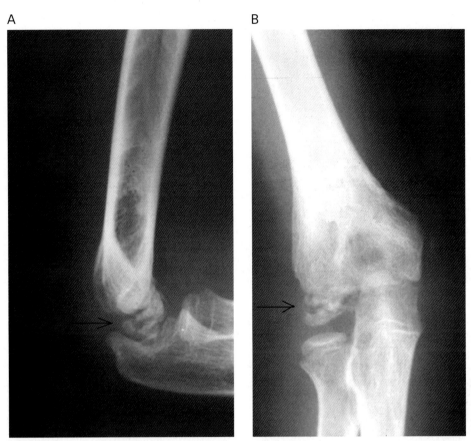

Fig B 33-14
Little League elbow. Frontal and lateral views of the elbow in an active pitcher shows rarefaction and fragmentation of the capitellum (arrow) from repetitive overuse of the elbow.[40]

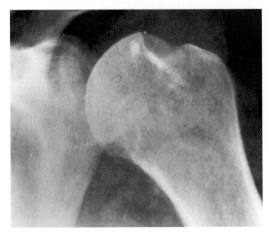

Fig B 33-15
Hill-Sachs deformity.

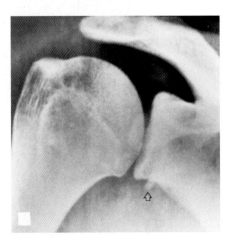

Fig B 33-16
Bankhart fracture. Fracture of the anterior rim of the glenoid (arrow) as a result of anterior dislocation of the shoulder.[39]

Condition	Imaging Findings	Comments
Lower extremity		
March fracture (Fig B 33-17)	Radiographs at the time of initial symptoms are normal. Early findings are mild periosteal change; later there is dense sclerosis about the fracture site.	Fatigue fracture of one of the metacarpals. Most commonly found in military recruits who frequently jump and march in their vigorous training
Jones (dancer's) fracture (Fig B 33-18)	Transverse fracture at the base of the fifth metatarsal.	Avulsion injury related to the peroneus brevis tendon. In children, this fracture must be differentiated from the longitudinally oriented apophysis found at the lateral margin of the base of the fifth metatarsal.
Lisfranc injury (Fig B 33-19)	Dislocation (usually lateral) of the second through fifth metatarsals (tarsometatarsal fracture dislocation). Medial displacement of the first metatarsal can occur.	Dorsal dislocation of the forefoot that may be produced by falling from a height, falling down a flight of stairs, or simply stepping off a curb. Disruption of the ligamentous attachments binding the cuneiform and cuboid bones to the bases of the metatarsals permits dorsal metatarsal dislocation. Associated fractures of the tarsal bones and the bases of the metatarsals may occur.
Chopart dislocation (Fig B 33-20)	Dislocation of the talonavicular and calcaneocuboid joints (midtarsal dislocation).	Disruption of the joint between the hindfoot and midfoot, named for the surgeon who described amputation of the foot at this level.

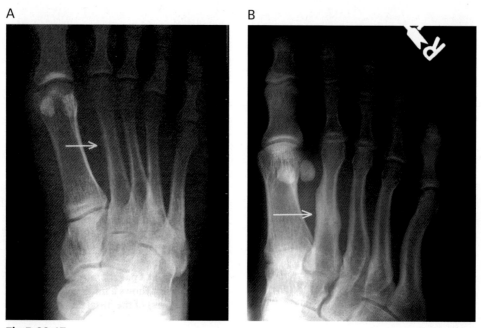

Fig B 33-17
March fracture. Frontal radiographs of the right foot of a college gymnast show the early (A) and late (B) findings of a fatigue fracture of the second metatarsal (arrow). The fracture completely healed with rest.[40]

Condition	Imaging Findings	Comments
Toddler fracture (Fig B 33-21)	Spiral hairline fracture in the distal shaft of the tibia that is seen in young children.	The fracture occurs when a child is running, or steps on something, and then loses his footing. The abrupt twisting of the tibia produces a fracture in a spiral pattern. As with other fractures in young children, these fractures tend to be incomplete or minimally displaced and therefore are sometimes difficult to recognize clinically or radiographically.

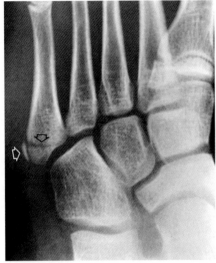

Fig B 33-18
Jones' fracture. Note that the fracture line is transverse (black arrow), whereas the normal apophysis in this child has a vertical orientation (white arrow).

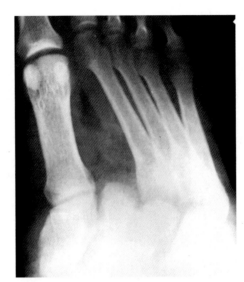

Fig B 33-19
Lisfranc injury. Gross lateral displacement of the second through fifth metatarsals.

A

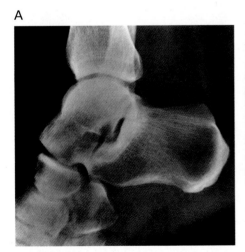

B

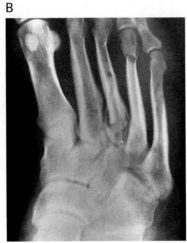

Fig B 33-20
Chopart dislocation. (A) Lateral and (B) frontal views. Lateral projection shows complete disruption of the calcaneocuboid joint. The cuboid bone is displaced plantarward, while the talonavicular joint is subluxed.[39]

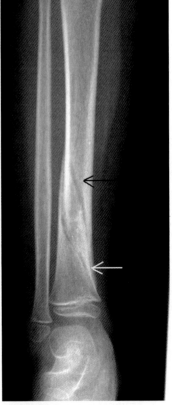

Fig B 33-21
Toddler fracture. Frontal radiograph of a young ambulatory infant, who fell and twisted his right lower leg, shows a spiral fracture (arrows) in the distal portion of the tibia.[40]

Condition	Imaging Findings	Comments
Maisonneuve fracture (Fig B 33-22)	Fracture of the posterior tibial tubercle (or rupture of the posterior inferior talofibular ligament), fracture of the medial malleolus (or rupture of the deltoid ligament), and fracture of the proximal part of the fibula.	Result of a pronation–external rotation injury. The importance of this fracture is that, whenever an apparent isolated fracture of the medial malleolus or the posterior lip of the tibia is seen without evidence of a fracture of the lateral malleolus or distal fibula, it is essential to obtain a view of the entire leg to identify the associated proximal fibular fracture.
Tillaux fracture	Avulsion from the anterior tubercle of the tibia.	Result of tension within the anterior inferior tibial-fibular ligament.
Wagstaffe–LeFort fracture	Avulsion fracture at the fibular attachment of the anterior tibial-fibular ligament.	Rare lesion that may occur in association with various fractures of the malleoli.
Spine and pelvis		
Jefferson fracture (Fig B 33-23)	Bilateral offset or spreading of the lateral articular masses of C1 in relation to the apposing articular surfaces of C2.	Comminuted fracture of the ring of the atlas that involves both the anterior and the posterior arches and causes centripetal displacement of the fragments.
Hangman's fracture (Fig B 33-24)	Fracture of the arch of C2 anterior to the inferior facet that is usually associated with anterior subluxation of C2 on C3.	Results from acute hyperextension of the head on the neck. Although originally described after hanging, this serious and unstable fracture is now usually the result of motor vehicle injury (hitting the head on a dashboard).

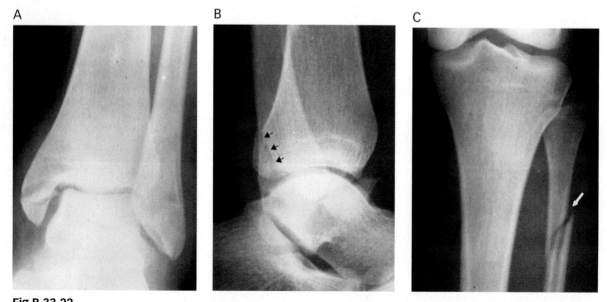

Fig B 33-22
Maisonneuve fracture. (A) Frontal and (B) lateral views of the ankle demonstrate an oblique fracture of the medial malleolus and a fracture of the posterior tibial tubercle (arrows). (C) A view of the proximal leg reveals the associated spiral fracture of the proximal shaft of the fibula (arrow).[41]

Condition	Imaging Findings	Comments
Clay shoveler fracture (Fig B 33-25)	Avulsion fracture of the C6 or C7 spinous process.	The result of rotation of the trunk relative to the head and neck. This fracture may be difficult to demonstrate on emergency cross-table lateral radiographs because the shoulders frequently obscure the lower cervical spine. On the frontal view, there may be a double shadow of the spinous processes due to caudad displacement of the avulsed fragment (unlike a bifid spinous process, which usually lies at a higher level and on a more horizontal plane).

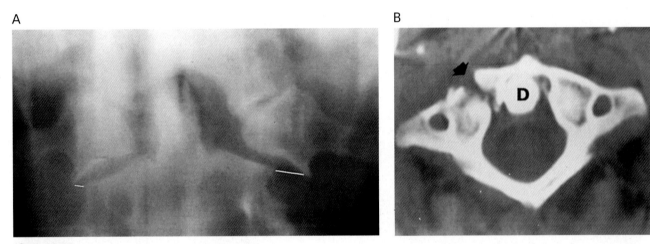

Fig B 33-23
Jefferson fracture. (A) On a frontal tomogram, there is lateral displacement of the lateral masses of C1 bilaterally (white lines). (B) A CT scan in another patient shows the unilateral break in the arch of C1 (arrow). (D, dens.)

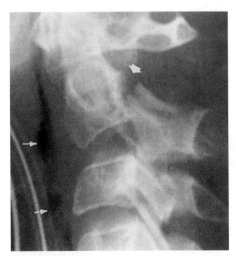

Fig B 33-24
Hangman fracture. Bilateral fracture of the neural arch of C2 (broad arrow). The abnormal air within the soft tissues (thin arrows) was due to an associated fracture of the larynx.

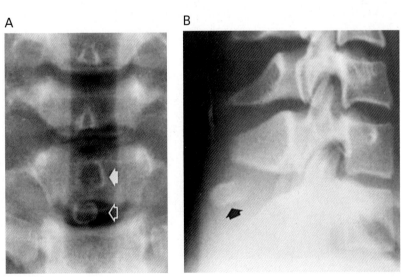

Fig B 33-25
Clay shoveler fracture. (A) Frontal view of the cervical spine shows the characteristic double–spinous-process sign resulting from the caudad displacement of the avulsed fragment (open arrow) with respect to the normal position of the major portion of the spinous process (closed arrow). (B) A lateral view clearly shows the avulsed fragment (arrow).

Condition	Imaging Findings	Comments
Chance fracture (Fig B 33-26)	Horizontal fracture of a lumbar vertebral body that extends to involve some or all of the posterior elements.	Often associated with significant visceral injuries in the "seat belt syndrome" (hyperflexion at the waist that occurs in a car accident when a person is restrained by a lap belt but no shoulder strap). On frontal views, separation and elevation of the posterior elements may produce an "empty" appearance of the involved vertebral body.
Malgaigne fracture (Figs B 33-27 and B 33-28)	Double vertical fractures and dislocations involving both the anterior and the posterior arches on the same side of the pelvis.	Unstable lesion that usually results from crush injuries in motor vehicle accidents or falls from a height. The most common combination is a fracture of both the superior and the inferior rami and a vertical fracture of the sacrum. Straddle fractures involve the inferior and posterior rami bilaterally; a combination of fractures of the superior and inferior rami on one side and the sacrum or ilium on the other is called a "bucket handle" fracture.

A

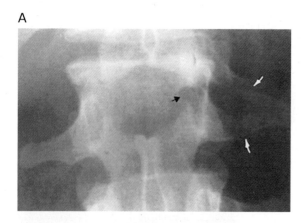

B

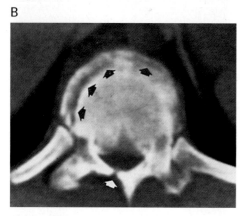

Fig B 33-26
Chance fracture. (A) A frontal view shows the characteristic empty appearance of the involved vertebral body due to fractures of the posterior elements. Note the fractures of the left pedicle (black arrow) and transverse process (white arrows). (B) CT scan in another patient shows a fracture of the lumbar vertebral body (black arrows) associated with a lamina fracture at the same level (white arrow).

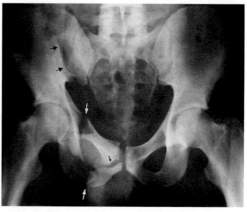

Fig B 33-27
Malgaigne fracture. There are fractures of the right superior and inferior pubic rami (white arrows) and wide separation of the ipsilateral sacroiliac joint (large black arrows). There is also some sacroiliac joint separation, an avulsion of the L5 transverse process on the left, and a fracture of the right pubic symphysis (small black arrow).

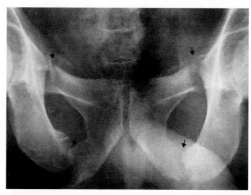

Fig B 33-28
Straddle fracture. Bilateral fractures (arrows) of the superior and inferior pubic rami.

Condition	Imaging Findings	Comments
LeFort fractures (Fig B 33-29)		Fractures of the facial bones along one or more planes of relative structural weakness in response to certain types of severe traumatic force.
LeFort I (transverse fracture)	Fracture line oriented transversely through the maxilla (above the line of dentition). It involves the nasal septum, the lower portions of the pterygoid processes, and the medial and lateral walls of the maxillary sinuses.	Secondary to a local impact sustained over the upper lip region (alveolar process), this injury results in a separated fracture segment (floating palate) composed of the lower portion of the maxillary sinus, the alveolar process, the entire palate, and the lower portions of the pterygoid plates.
LeFort II (pyramidal fracture)	Transverse fracture through the nasal bones that extends through the frontal processes of the maxillary bones and continues backward across the lacrimal bones before angling forward through the roofs of the maxillary sinuses to the anterior-inferior orbital rims. After descending through the anterior maxillary walls near the zygomaticomaxillary sutures, the fracture line extends through the posterior maxillary sinus walls and across the pterygomaxillary fissures, ending in the lower pterygoid processes.	Caused by a long, broad impact over the central facial area, in this injury the zygomatic bones remain attached to the cranium through the arch and the zygomaticofrontal process, giving rise to a "floating maxilla."
LeFort III (craniofacial dysjunction)	Fracture line that runs across the nasofrontal region, then backward across the frontal process of the maxilla, the lacrimal bones, and the ethmoid bones (upper medial orbital bones).	Caused by a strong, broad impact over the nasal area, orbital rims, and zygomas. After extending posteriorly across the orbital fissure, the fracture line extends in two different directions: upward across the lateral wall, ending near the zygomaticofrontal sutures; and backward into the sphenomaxillary fissures to the lower pterygoid processes.

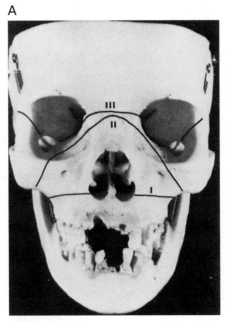
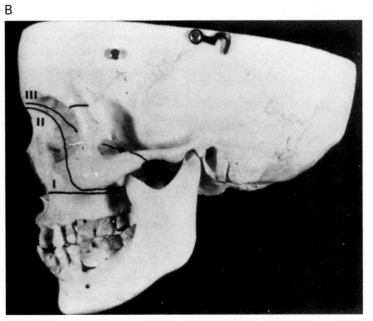

Fig B 33-29
LeFort planes of weakness. (A) Frontal view corresponding to a Caldwell projection. (B) Lateral view.[42]

Avulsion Injuries*

Condition	Imaging Findings	Comments
Pelvis		
Ischial tuberosity (Fig B 34-1)	Insertion of the hamstring muscle group. During the healing stage, the avulsion can have an aggressive appearance, including lysis and destruction. Chronic avulsions frequently result in prominent bone formation.	Most commonly, pelvic site. Usually occurs before closure of the apophysis secondary to extreme active hamstring contractions, as in sprinting by runners or sudden and excessive passive lengthening in cheerleaders or dancers. Patients typically present with pain in the buttock region, an antalgic gate, or inability to walk.
Anterior superior iliac spine (Fig B 34-2)	Attachment site for the sartorius muscle and the tensor muscle of the fascia lata.	Typically occurs in sprinters during forceful extension at the hip. Patients complain of pain just below the most anterior aspect of the iliac crest. Generally heals quickly without sequelae.
Anterior inferior iliac spine (Fig B 34-3)	Origin of the straight head of the rectus femoris muscle.	Results from forceful extension at the hip and heals within 5 to 6 weeks.
Symphysis pubis (Fig B 34-4)	Origin for the long adductor, short adductor, and gracilis muscles.	Virtually always due to chronic overuse, though occasionally arising acutely in athletes when there is forceful contraction against resistance (eg, two soccer players kicking the ball simultaneously). Pain is localized to the groin. Unlike other pelvic avulsions, discrete bone fragments are not seen. May lead to rarefaction or lysis and be confused with infection or tumor.

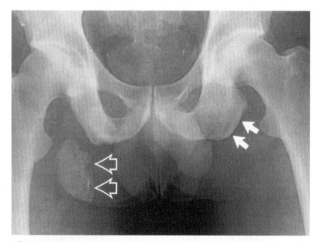

Fig B 34-1
Ischial tuberosity. Bilateral chronic avulsions. Note the protuberant bone (closed arrows) and a large, smooth fragment (open arrows).[43]

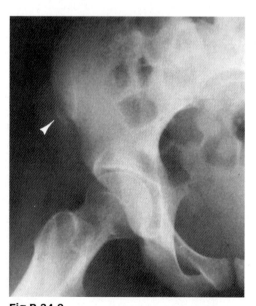

Fig B 34-2
Anterior superior iliac spine (arrowhead).[44]

---

*Acute avulsion injuries result from extreme, unbalanced, and often eccentric muscular contractions, produce severe pain and loss of function, and may be associated with avulsed bone fragments. Subacute injuries may include areas of mixed lysis and sclerosis. Chronic avulsions are the result of repetitive microtrauma or overuse, usually develop from organized sports activities, and may be associated with a protuberant mass of bone that simulates a neoplastic or infectious process.

Condition	Imaging Findings	Comments
Iliac crest	Insertion of the abdominal musculature.	Uncommon injury associated acutely with abrupt directional changes during motion or with repetitive microtrauma (as in long-distance runners). Radiographs may show asymmetry of the apophyses of the iliac crest.
Lesser trochanter (Fig B 34-5)	Insertion of the iliopsoas muscle.	Uncommon injury that predominantly affects young athletes, who complain of considerable pain and decreased function. In adults, this appearance virtually always is due to metastatic disease.
Greater trochanter (Fig B 34-6)	Attachment site for the hip rotators, including the middle and least gluteal, internal obturator, gemellus, and piriform muscles.	Results from a sudden directional change. The diagnosis may be difficult to make if there is only minimal displacement of the avulsed fragment (MR may show the lesion to better advantage).

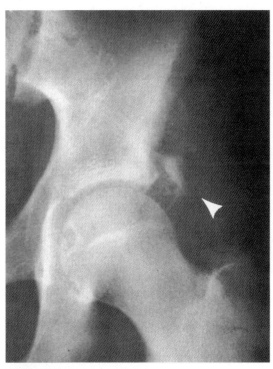

Fig B 34-3
Anterior inferior iliac spine (arrowhead).[44]

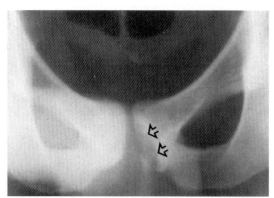

Fig B 34-4
Symphysis pubis (arrows).[43]

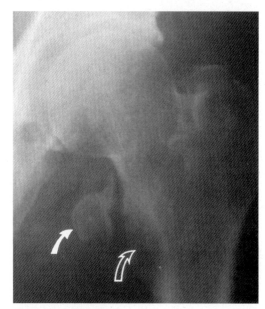

Fig B 34-5
Lesser trochanter (solid arrow). A lytic defect representing metastatic cancer is seen at the femur attachment site (open arrow).[43]

Condition	Imaging Findings	Comments
Knee		
Segond fracture (Fig B 34-7)	Involves the meniscotibial portion of the middle third of the lateral capsular ligament. The avulsed fragment lies immediately distal to the lateral tibial plateau and appears as an elliptical piece of bone parallel to the tibia.	Caused by forceful internal rotation and varus stress. Patients present with pain at the lateral joint line and anterolateral rotational instability (rotational subluxation). Often subtle, it is usually visible on AP or tunnel-view radiographs. MR is generally performed because the Segond fracture is frequently associated with other significant injuries, such as tears of the anterior cruciate ligament and menisci.
Fibular head (Fig B 34-8)	Attachment for the coronary, oblique popliteal, and lateral (fibular) collateral ligaments.	Results from force directed at the anteromedial tibia with the knee extended. Associated injuries include tears of the anterior cruciate ligament and damage to the peroneal nerve.

A

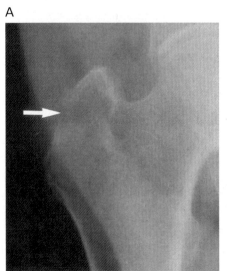

B

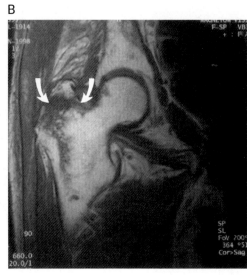

Fig B 34-6
Greater trochanter (arrows). (A) Plain film. (B) MRI.[43]

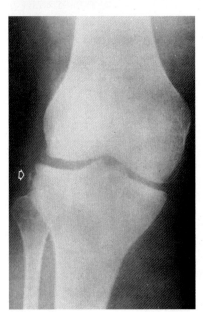

Fig B 34-7
Segond fracture (arrow).[44]

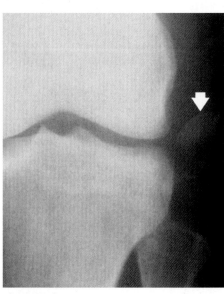

Fig B 34-8
Fibular head (arrow).[43]

Condition	Imaging Findings	Comments
Tibial eminence (Fig B 34-9)	Attachment site for the anterior cruciate ligament.	More common in children, in whom it results from forced flexion of the knee with internal rotation of the tibia. In adults, the injury is more often secondary to a motor vehicle injury in which the leg is hyperextended at impact (also more likely associated injuries, such as tear of the medial collateral ligament and focal bone contusions). Radiographic diagnosis can be difficult and often requires additional tunnel-view and oblique imaging (CT and MR generally show the avulsion to better advantage).
Posterior cruciate ligament (Fig B 34-10)	Posterior aspect of the tibial plateau.	Results from forceful displacement in a flexed knee or hyperextension. Findings are often subtle, especially if the fragment is not significantly displaced.
Tibial tuberosity (Fig B 34-11)	Attachment of the patellar tendon.	Results from violent extension of the knee or passive flexion against contracted quadriceps muscles in sports that require jumping, squatting, and kicking. Although an acute injury, it is most frequently seen in young adolescents with ongoing Osgood-Schlatter disease (bilateral in up to 50%).
Inferior pole of patella (Fig B 34-12)	Proximal insertion of the patellar tendon.	May reflect "jumper's knee" or "patella sleeve fracture." MR imaging may be required to demonstrate the patellar tendon and cartilage.
Ankle and foot Calcaneal insufficiency (Fig B 34-13)	Extra-articular fracture in the posterior third of the calcaneus that usually begins at the calcaneal tuberosity and extends superiorly, with the avulsed fragment displaced cephalad due to the pull of the Achilles tendon.	Seen almost exclusively in diabetic patients, this injury is probably related to osteopenia and superimposed neuropathic changes. May be differentiated from typical stress fractures in that the latter have normal bone density and do not become displaced.

A

B

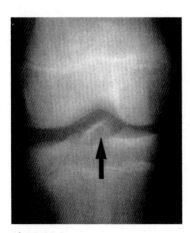

Fig B 34-9
Tibial eminence (arrow).[43]

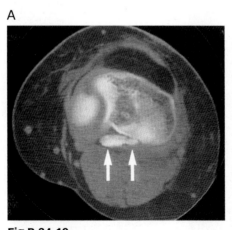
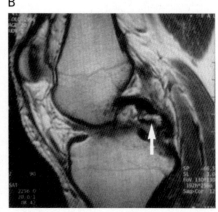

Fig B 34-10
Posterior cruciate ligament. (A) Axial CT shows minimal displacement of the avulsed fragment (arrows). (B) Sagittal proton-density-weighted MR image shows displacement of an avulsed fragment (arrow).[43]

Condition	Imaging Findings	Comments
Posterior capsule (Fig B 34-14)	Curvilinear calcification adjacent to the posterior aspect of the ankle joint, related to trauma to the distal tibia.	Rare injury that is presumably the result of forced dorsiflexion of the foot.
Anterior capsule (Fig B 34-15)	Protuberance of the anterior talus ("talar beak") at the insertion of the joint capsule.	Occurs in basketball players and represents a chronic injury caused by repetitive microtrauma.

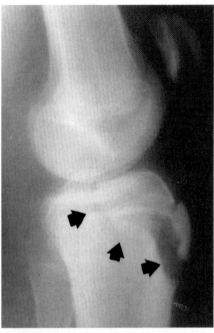

Fig B 34-11
Tibial tuberosity. There is displacement of the proximal base of the epiphysis and extension into the joint (arrows).[43]

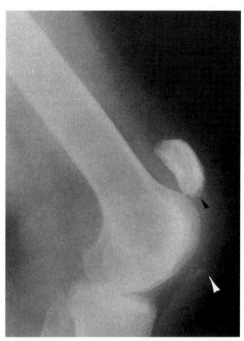

Fig B 34-12
Inferior pole of the patella (white arrowhead). The black arrowhead points to the site of the avulsion from the abnormally high patella.[44]

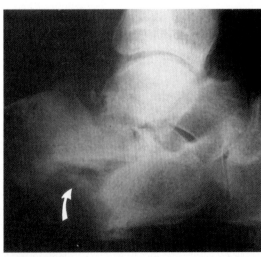

Fig B 34-13
Calcaneal insufficiency (arrow).[43]

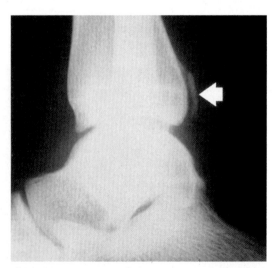

Fig B 34-14
Posterior capsule. Curvilinear calcification adjacent to the posterior tibial margin (arrow).[43]

Condition	Imaging Findings	Comments
Base of fifth metatarsal	Attachment of the peroneus brevis tendon.	Results from forceful contraction of the tendon against an inverted foot, as when stepping off a curb or tripping. In children, this horizontal fracture must be differentiated from the longitudinally oriented apophysis found at the lateral margin of the base of the fifth metatarsal.
Shoulder and elbow Greater tuberosity (Fig B 34-16)	Attachment site of the supraspinatus, infraspinatus, and teres minor tendons.	Patients present with a history of falling on an outstretched hand with the elbow extended (often with anterior dislocation). At radiography, the fracture may not be readily apparent and only seen on delayed images. Because the treatment of this isolated injury is different from the clinically similar rotator cuff tear, MR is often used to show the lesion to better advantage.

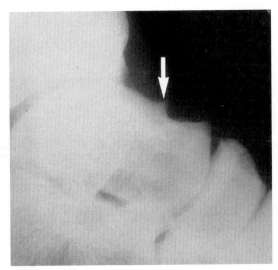

Fig B 34-15
Anterior capsule. Protuberance of the anterior talus (arrow) where the joint capsule is inserted, indicating a chronic avulsion.[43]

A
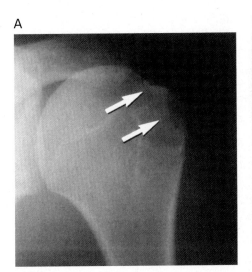

B
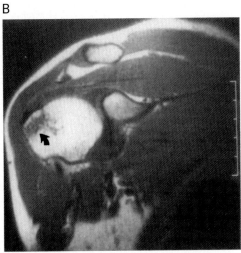

Fig B 34-16
Greater tuberosity. (A) Frontal radiograph shows the nondisplaced avulsion (arrows). (B) Coronal oblique T1-weighted MR image shows the fracture to greater advantage (arrow).[43]

Condition	Imaging Findings	Comments
Lesser tuberosity (Fig B 34-17)	Insertion of the subscapularis muscle. AP radiographs with the arm in internal rotation usually show a large fragment, but a small, minimally displaced fragment may be seen only on an axillary view.	Rare injury that occurs most commonly in strenuous sports (eg, wrestling) when the arm is abducted (60 to 90 degrees) and the subscapularis muscle forcefully contracts to resist further external rotation. The avulsed lesser tuberosity may retract and lie inferior and medial to the glenoid (may be misinterpreted as calcific tendonitis of the biceps or subscapularis tendon). May be associated with posterior glenohumeral or biceps tendon dislocation.
Medial epicondyle (Fig B 34-18)	If acute, separation of the medial epicondyle with soft-tissue swelling. In chronic injury, there may be fragmentation and roughening of the medial epicondyle.	Most commonly in adolescents and associated with recurrent contraction of the flexor pronator group of muscles during the acceleration phase of throwing ("Little League" elbow). An entrapped fragment may simulate the trochlear ossification center and, if not recognized and removed, lead to disabling degenerative osteoarthritis.

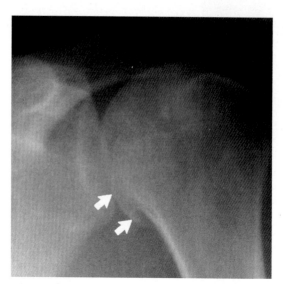

Fig B 34-17
Lesser tuberosity (arrows).[43]

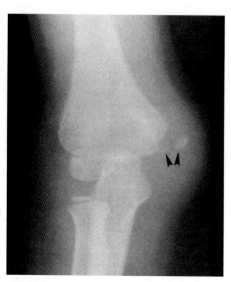

Fig B 34-18
Medial epicondyle (arrowheads).[44]

Benign Bone Tumors and Tumor-like Processes on Computed Tomography

Condition	Imaging Findings	Comments
Bone island	Single or multiple areas of dense sclerotic bone.	Typically an incidental finding on plain radiographs, on which the appearance is usually so characteristic that no additional imaging studies are required.
Simple bone cyst	Well-defined lesion of fluid attenuation with bony septations.	Most commonly involves the proximal humerus and femur. Asymptomatic unless pathologic fracture occurs.
Osteoid osteoma (Fig B 35-1)	Low-attenuation nidus within an area of thickened cortical bone.	Relatively common lesion with the characteristic clinical pattern of pain that is worse at night and often relieved by anti-inflammatory medications. Complete resection of the nidus is curative.
Osteoblastoma (Fig B 35-2)	Cortical expansion with ossified matrix.	Most commonly involves the posterior elements of the vertebrae. Bone expansion may simulate a malignant lesion.
Osteochondroma (Fig B 35-3)	Prominent cartilaginous cap (normally < 2 cm).	Common process that appears on plain radiographs as a bony projection with contiguous marrow and cortex from the bone of origin (best seen on CT).
Enchondroma (Fig B 35-4)	Well-defined lesion with cortical erosion and a central calcified matrix.	Most commonly an asymptomatic lesion involving the fingers. The presence of pain should suggest the possibility of a low-grade chondrosarcoma.

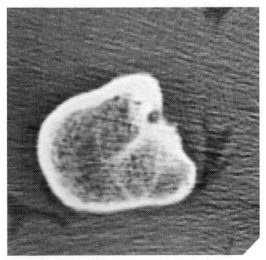

Fig B 35-1
Osteoid osteoma. Low-attenuation nidus within an area of thickened cortical bone in the lesser trochanter of the right femur.[45]

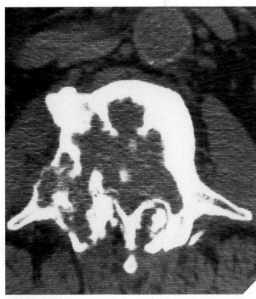

Fig B 35-2
Osteoblastoma. In this aggressive form, focal areas of bone formation within the lesion and invasion of the cortex simulate a malignant process. (Courtesy of Ibrahim F. Abdelwahab, MD, New York, NY.)[45]

Condition	Imaging Findings	Comments
Chondroblastoma (Fig B 35-5)	Well-defined epiphyseal lesion with sclerotic margins and often central calcification.	Most commonly occurs about the knee and generally presents as chronic local pain in a patient under age 25.
Chondromyxoid fibroma (Fig B 35-6)	Eccentric metaphyseal lesion with well-defined sclerotic margins.	Most commonly involves the knee and distal tibia. Calcifications of the chondroid matrix are best appreciated on CT.

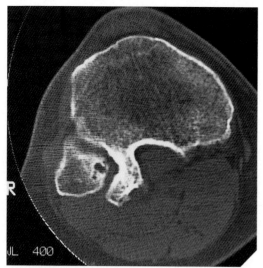

Fig B 35-3
Osteochondroma. There is continuity of the cortex, which extends without interruption from the osteochondroma into the tibia. Note also that the medullary portion of the lesion and the tibia communicate.[45]

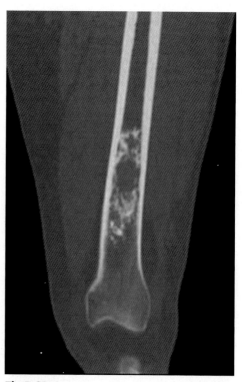

Fig B 35-4
Enchondroma. Characteristic calcifications within the lesion. The central area of lucency, devoid of calcifications, was worrisome for malignancy, but a biopsy demonstrated the benign nature of the lesion. (Courtesy of Jim Wu, MD, Boston)

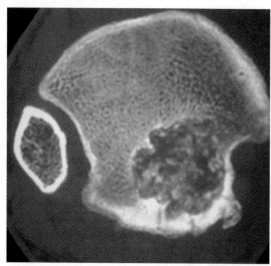

Fig B 35-5
Chondroblastoma. Well-defined lesion in the distal tibial epiphysis with calcifications.[46]

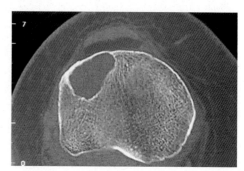

Fig B 35-6
Chondromyxoid fibroma. The lytic lesion has well-defined sclerotic margins with no matrix calcifications.[46]

Condition	Imaging Findings	Comments
Nonossifying fibroma (Fig B 35-7)	Well-defined eccentric metaphyseal lesion with scalloped sclerotic margins.	Also known as fibrous cortical defect, this lesion is typically discovered incidentally in the distal femur or distal tibia.
Aneursymal bone cyst (Fig B 35-8)	Well-defined expansile, eccentric lesion of fluid attenuation.	More than half occur in the long bones; up to 30% are found in the spine.
Fibrous dysplasia (Fig B 35-9)	Well-defined lesion with sclerotic margins. Lesions with greater fibrous content may show a low-attenuation matrix with an amorphous ground-glass texture.	Single lesion (monostotic) generally involve the femur, tibia, ribs, and skull base. Multiple lesions (polyostotic) usually affect one side of the skeleton. Abnormal bone growth may cause deformity.
Giant cell tumor (Fig B 35-10)	Metaphyseal lesion of low attenuation with no calcified matrix.	Typically occurs around the knee (distal femur or proximal tibia) in a subchondral location following epiphyseal closure.

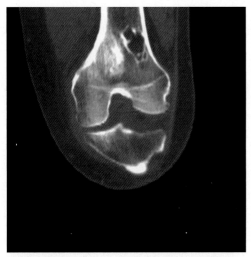

Fig B 35-7
Nonossifying fibroma. Well-defined eccentric metaphyseal lesion with scalloped sclerotic margins. (Courtesy of Jim Wu, MD, Boston)

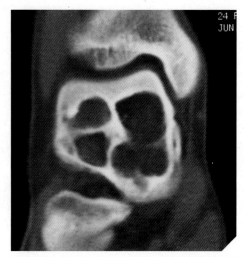

Fig B 35-8
Aneursymal bone cyst. Coronal image of the anterior portion of the talus demonstrates internal ridges within a well-defined expansile, eccentric lesion of fluid attenuation.[45]

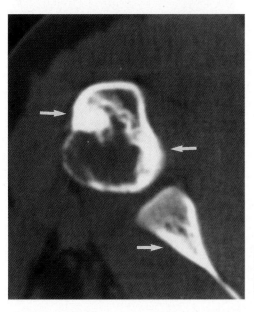

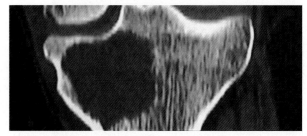

Fig B 35-10
Giant cell tumor. Coronal image shows a lytic lesion without sclerotic margins in the subchondral region of the proximal tibia.[46]

Fig B 35-9
Fibrous dysplasia. Image through the shoulder joint shows high-attenuation areas of sclerosis in the humeral head and scapula (arrows).[45]

Condition	Imaging Findings	Comments
Langerhans cell histiocytosis (Fig B 35-11)	Well-defined lesion typically with medullary expansion and periosteal response.	The cortical and periosteal changes are best seen on CT.
Adamantinoma	Eccentric, expansile lesion that occurs primarily in the tibia.	The cortical and soft-tissue involvement are best demonstrated on CT.
Bone infarct (Fig B 35-12)	Central coarse calcifications in medullary lesions, typically about the knee.	Unlike enchondroma, there is no evidence of endosteal scalloping.
Intraosseous ganglion (Fig B 35-13)	Area of low attenuation rimmed by a zone of reactive sclerosis.	Common finding with a predilection for the articular ends of long bones, usually the non-weight-bearing segment. The appearance is similar to that of a degenerative cyst, but in most cases there are no degenerative changes in the adjacent joint.

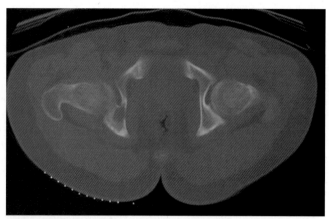

Fig B 35-11
Langerhans cell histiocytosis. Well-defined lucent lesion with medullary expansion in the acetabulum. (Courtesy of Jim Wu, MD, Boston)

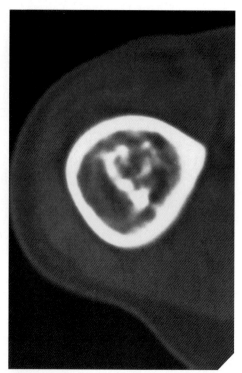

Fig B 35-12
Bone infarct. Distal femur lesion with central coarse calcification but no endosteal scalloping of the cortex.[45]

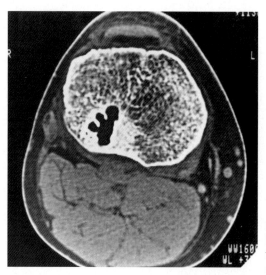

Fig B 35-13
Intraosseous ganglion. Eccentric oval lesion in the proximal tibia that has low attenuation and ramifications. Note the rim of reactive sclerosis.[45]

Condition	Imaging Findings	Comments
Brodie's abscess (Fig B 35-14)	Area of low attenuation that may contain a central sequestrum and often demonstrates a sinus tract extending through a thickening cortex.	Localized osseous infection that has a predilection for the metaphyses and the ends of long bones. Cortical lesions may be confused with osteoid osteoma.

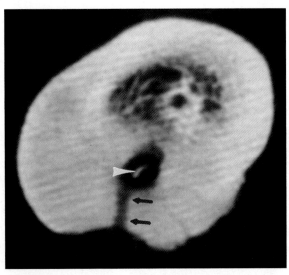

Fig B 35-14
Brodie's abscess. Area of low attenuation that contains a central sequestrum (arrowhead) and has a sinus tract extending through the thickening cortex.[46]

Benign Bone Tumors and Tumor-like Processes on Magnetic Resonance Imaging

Condition	Imaging Findings	Comments
Simple bone cyst (Fig B 36-1)	Uncomplicated fluid-filled cysts have low signal intensity on T1-weighted images and high signal intensity on T2-weighted images. Traumatic bleeding within the cyst produces heterogeneous signal intensities on both sequences.	Expansile lesion that is sharply demarcated from adjacent normal bone and may contain thin septa producing a multiloculated appearance. Typically has an oval configuration with its long axis parallel to that of the host bone.
Osteoid osteoma (Fig B 36-2)	Nidus appears as a round focus of low or intermediate signal intensity on T1-weighted images with variable signal intensity on T2-weighted images and variable contrast enhancement.	MRI may be misleading because of the often-misleading bone-marrow and soft-tissue changes that may mimic osteomyelitis, stress fracture, inflammatory arthritis, or a more aggressive bone tumor.

A

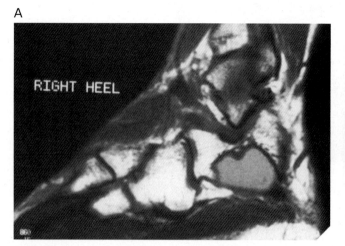

B

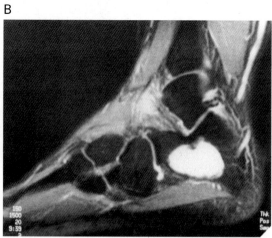

Fig B 36-1
Simple bone cyst. (A) Sagittal T1-weighted image shows homogeneous intermediate signal intensity within the lesion, which has a sclerotic margin that appears as low signal intensity. (B) On a T2-weighted image, the lesion has high signal intensity.[47]

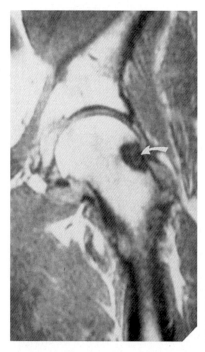

Fig B 36-2
Osteoid osteoma. Coronal T1-weighted image shows the low signal intensity lesion (curved arrow) in the lateral aspect of the neck of the left femur.[45]

Condition	Imaging Findings	Comments
Osteoblastoma (Fig B 36-3)	Low signal intensity of bone on all sequences.	Most commonly involves the posterior elements of the vertebrae. Radiographic features may be similar to a large osteoid osteoma. Bone expansion may simulate a malignant lesion.
Osteochondroma (Fig B 36-4)	Cartilaginous cap has low signal intensity on T1-weighted images and high signal intensity on T2-weighted sequences. Bone marrow is seen extending into the rest of the lesion.	Common process that appears on plain radiographs as a bony projection with contiguous marrow and cortex from the bone of origin. The cartilaginous cap is best seen on CT.
Enchondroma (Fig B 36-5)	Lobulated lesion with low signal intensity on T1-weighted images and high intensity on T2-weighted scans. Mineralized areas show decreased signal on all pulse sequences.	Most commonly an asymptomatic lesion involving the fingers. The presence of pain should suggest the possibility of a low-grade chondrosarcoma. Plain radiographs show single or multiple medullary lesions with sharp margins that often contain internal calcification of the chondroid matrix.
Chondroblastoma (Fig B 36-6)	Well-defined epiphyseal lesion with low signal intensity on T1-weighted images and variable intensity on T2-weighted sequences. Extensive surrounding edema is usually seen.	Generally presents as chronic local pain in a patient under age 25. On plain radiographs, the lesion has sharp margins and a sclerotic rim, with calcification seen in about half the cases.
Chondromyxoid fibroma (Fig B 36-7)	Well-defined lesion with uniform low intensity on T1-weighted images and high or intermediate intensity on T2-weighted sequences.	Most commonly involves the metaphyses of the knee and distal tibia. Plain radiographs show an eccentric lesion with sclerotic margins and often internal calcifications of the chondroid matrix.

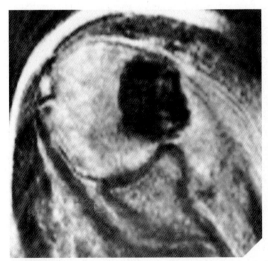

Fig B 36-3
Osteoblastoma. Axial T2-weighted image shows the low signal intensity of this proximal humeral lesion, indicating the bony matrix. The rim of high signal intensity adjacent to the posterolateral margin of the tumor reflects peritumoral edema.[45]

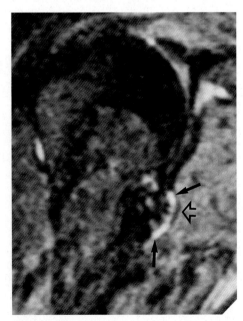

Fig B 36-4
Osteochondroma. T2-weighted image showing the thin cartilaginous cap as a band of high signal intensity (arrows), covered by a linear area of low signal representing perichondrium (open arrow).[45]

Condition	Imaging Findings	Comments
Nonossifying fibroma	Well-defined cortical lesion with low or intermediate intensity on both T1- and T2-weighted sequences.	Also known as fibrous cortical defect, this lesion is typically discovered incidentally in the distal femur or distal tibia. On plain radiographs, it appears as an eccentric metaphyseal lytic defect with scalloped sclerotic margins.
Aneursymal bone cyst (Fig B 36-8)	Well-defined lesion with high signal intensity on T2-weighted sequences. Fluid-fluid levels are common.	Plain radiographs show an eccentric lytic lesion with an expansile or ballooned bony contour. A sclerotic rim and periosteal response often occur.

A
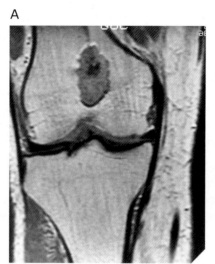

B
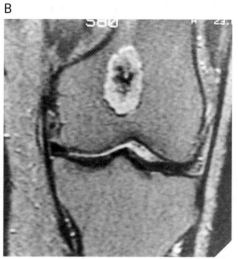

Fig B 36-5
Enchondroma. (A) Coronal T1-weighted image shows a well-circumscribed, lobulated lesion with intermediate signal intensity. The darker area in the center represents calcifications. (B) On the T2-weighted image, the lesion has a mixed-intensity signal, with the brighter areas representing cartilaginous tumor and the darker areas reflecting calcifications.[45]

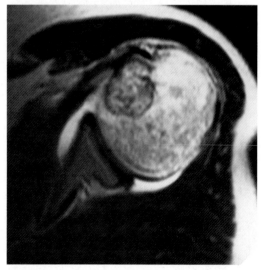

Fig B 36-6
Chondroblastoma. An axial T2-weighted image shows a sharply marginated lesion of the left humeral head that has a sclerotic border and central calcifications. Note the small amount of joint effusion and peritumoral edema.[45]

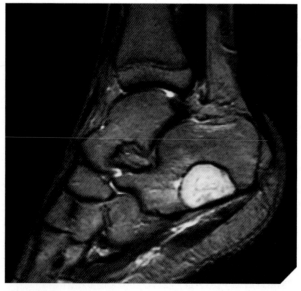

Fig B 36-7
Chondromyxoid fibroma. On this sagittal T2-weighted image, the lesion has uniform high signal intensity. The rim of low signal intensity represents the sclerotic border.[45]

Condition	Imaging Findings	Comments
Fibrous dysplasia (Fig B 36-9)	Well-defined lesion with low-intensity margins. The mass has low signal intensity on T1-weighted images and intermediate signal intensity on T2-weighted sequences.	Single lesion (monostotic) generally involves the femur, tibia, ribs, and skull base. Multiple lesions (polyostotic) usually affect one side of the skeleton. Abnormal bone growth may cause deformity.
Giant cell tumor (Fig B 36-10)	Low intensity lesion on T1-weighted images that has intermediate signal on T2-weighted sequences. Decreased signal intensity on T2-weighted images reflects hemosiderin deposition. Contrast enhancement is generally seen and there may be fluid-fluid-levels.	Typically occurs around the knee (distal femur or proximal tibia) in a subchondral location following epiphyseal closure. On plain radiographs, the lytic lesion has nonsclerotic margins.
Langerhans cell histiocystosis (Fig B 36-11)	Well-defined lesion with low signal intensity on T1-weighted images and high signal intensity on T2-weighted sequences. Marked contrast enhancement may be seen.	Increased signal intensity on T1-weighted images is due to xanthomatous histiocytes. Periosteal changes, best seen on CT, appears as low signal intensity on all images.

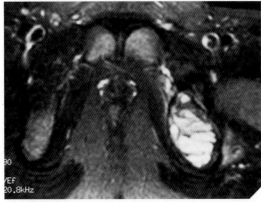

Fig B 36-8
Aneurysmal bone cyst. Axial T2-weighted image shows a lesion of the left inferior pubic ramus that has high signal intensity. Note the multiple fluid-fluid levels characteristic of an aneurysmal bone cyst.[45]

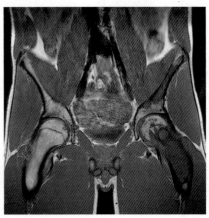

Fig B 36-9
Fibrous dysplasia. Coronal T1-weighted image demonstrates expansion of the left femoral neck and abnormal signal intensity in this area and the left ilium in a patient with polyostotic disease.[46]

A

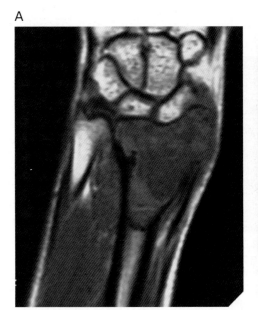

B

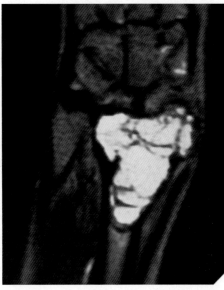

Fig B 36-10
Giant cell tumor. (A) Coronal T1-weighted image of the wrist shows the lesion to be of low signal intensity. (B) On a T2-weighted image, the tumor becomes bright, displaying low-signal septations.[45]

Condition	Imaging Findings	Comments
Adamantinoma (Fig B 36-12)	Variable pattern.	On plain radiographs, an eccentric lytic area with sclerosis that generally involves the tibia.
Brodie's abscess (Fig B 36-13)	Low intensity rim about a well-defined lesion that has low-to-intermediate signal on T1-weighted images and bright homogeneous signal on T2-weighted sequences.	This localized osseous infection demonstrates prominent contrast enhancement.
Bone island (Fig B 36-14)	Low signal intensity on both T1- and T2-weighted images.	Homogeneously dense, sclerotic focus in cancellous bone on conventional radiographs.

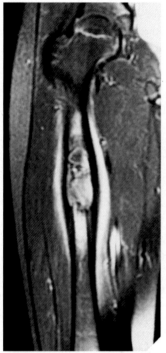

Fig B 36-11
Langerhans cell histiocytosis. This coronal contrast T1-weighted image shows marked enhancement of an expansile lesion of the right femur. Note the enhancement of the soft tissue adjacent to the thickened femoral cortex.[45]

A

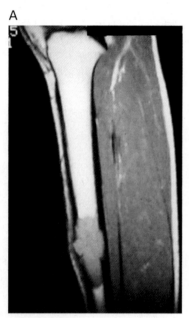

B

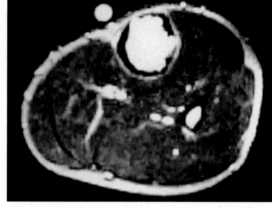

Fig B 36-12
Adamantinoma. This expansile lesion of the tibia has the signal intensity of muscle on a sagittal T1-weighted image (A) and high signal intensity on an axial T2-weighted sequence (B).[46]

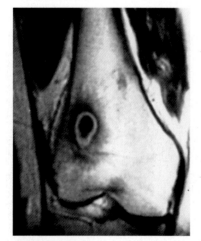

Fig B 36-13
Brodie's abscess. Coronal contrast T1-weighted image demonstrates rim enhancement about this lesion in the distal femur.[46]

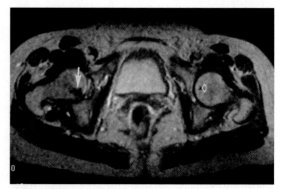

Fig B 36-14
Bone island. Axial T2-weighted image shows a low-intensity lesion with irregular margins (arrow) in the right femoral head. Note the tiny bone island in the opposite femoral head (open arrow).[46]

Malignant Bone Tumors on Magnetic Resonance Imaging

Condition	Imaging Findings	Comments
Osteosarcoma (Fig B 37-1)	Signal intensity varies with the matrix (decreased if blastic, increased with lytic) on T2-weighted sequences.	Metaphyseal lytic, blastic, or mixed lesions that most commonly involve the distal femur or proximal tibia. Staging of marrow and soft-tissue involvement is the primary indication for MR imaging.
Chondrosarcoma (Fig B 37-2)	Irregular mass with low signal intensity on T1-weighted images and intermediate-to-high signal intensity on T2-weighted scans. Calcification within the lesion appears as low signal intensity on all sequences.	May arise de novo in bone or develop secondarily in an osteochondroma or enchondroma. CT is superior for evaluating cortical destruction and matrix calcification, while MRI is better for showing soft-tissue extension.
Ewing's sarcoma (Fig B 37-3)	In lytic permeative lesions, low signal intensity on T1-weighted images and high signal intensity on T2-weighted scans. Variable pattern in mixed or sclerotic lesions.	Primarily affects children under age 20. In addition to local pain and swelling, there may be fever and increased white count suggesting infection. Most commonly involves the pelvis and sacrum or the femur and tibia.
Fibrosarcoma/Malignant fibrous histiocytoma (Fig B 37-4)	Low signal intensity on T1-weighted images and high signal intensity on T2-weighted scans. Areas of hemorrhage may demonstrate high signal intensity on T1-weighted images.	Uncommon malignancies that in almost a third of cases arise secondary to a preexisting lesion (irradiation, bone infarct, Paget's disease, chronic osteomyelitis). Best modality for demonstrating extent of marrow involvement and soft-tissue extension.

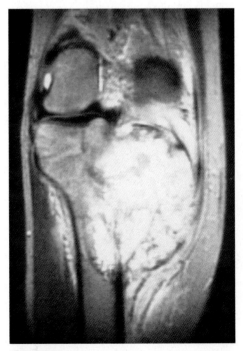

Fig B 37-1
Osteosarcoma. Coronal T1-weighted image shows extensive soft-tissue involvement of this large mass involving the proximal femur.[46]

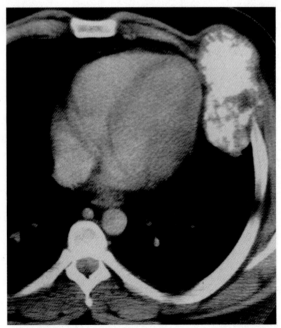

Fig B 37-2
Chondrosarcoma. Axial T2-weighted image of the chest demonstrates non-homogeneity of the rib lesion. Areas of low signal intensity represent calcified portions of the mass.[45]

Condition	Imaging Findings	Comments
Myeloma (Fig B 37-5)	Variable pattern, though generally low signal intensity of T1-weighted images and high signal intensity on T2-weighted scans.	Most common primary bone malignancy. Patients may present with local bone pain and constitutional symptoms of weakness and weight loss. Characteristic multiple small lytic foci on plain radiographs, though a single expansile process with soft-tissue mass may occur.

A

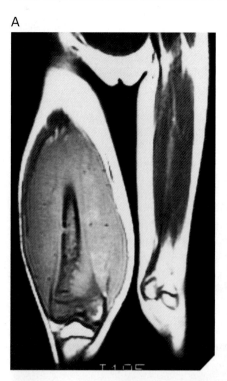

B

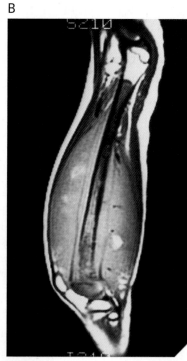

Fig B 37-3
Ewing's sarcoma. (A) Coronal and (B) sagittal T1-weighted images demonstrate the intraosseous and extraosseous extent of this tumor of the distal femur.[45]

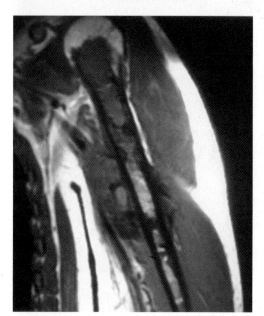

Fig B 37-4
Malignant fibrous histiocytoma. Coronal T1-weighted image shows the large humeral lesion with soft-tissue extension.[46]

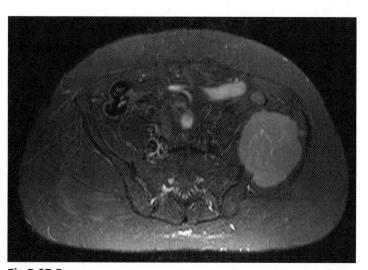

Fig B 37-5
Plasmacytoma. Axial contrast T1-weighted, fat-saturated image demonstrates an enhancing mass that arises from the left iliac bone and produces extensive bone destruction and a large soft-tissue mass. (Courtesy of Jim Wu, MD, Boston)

Condition	Imaging Findings	Comments
Lymphoma (Fig B 37-6)	Variable pattern.	MR imaging is primarily used in solitary lesions to define cortical destruction and soft-tissue extension (though this can be demonstrated by CT).
Paget's sarcoma (Fig B 37-7)	Low signal intensity on T1-weighted images in areas of lucency on plain radiographs suggests malignant degeneration.	Malignant degeneration (half osteosarcomas) occurs in up to 6% of patients and presents as increasing or new pain in the area of Paget's involvement.
Metastases (Fig B 37-8)	Variable pattern depending on the characteristics of the lesion. Sclerotic metastases have decreased signal intensity on all sequences. Lytic lesions have decreased signal intensity on T1-weighted images and increased signal intensity on T2-weighted sequences. Enhancement patterns vary.	Diffusion or chemical shift imaging may be of value in determining whether a compression fracture in the spine has a benign or malignant etiology.

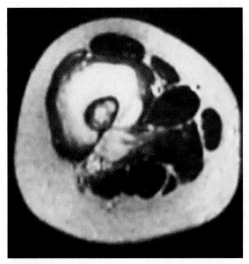

Fig B 37-6
Lymphoma. Axial T1-weighted image shows diffuse marrow changes and a large associated soft-tissue mass.[46]

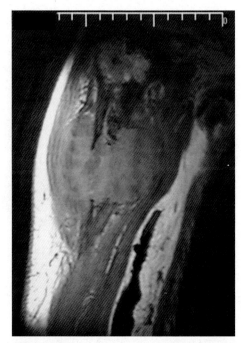

Fig B 37-7
Paget's sarcoma. Coronal T1-weighted image demonstrates both the bone destruction and the large soft-tissue mass.[46]

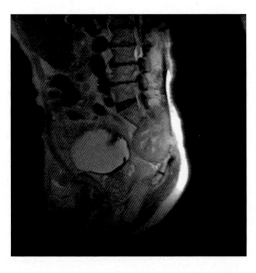

Fig B 37-8
Metastasis. Sagittal T2-weighted STIR image shows a mass arising in the sacrum that has a large soft-tissue component and causes extensive bone destruction. (Courtesy of Jim Wu, MD, Boston)

Benign Soft-Tissue Masses on Magnetic Resonance Imaging

Condition	Imaging Findings	Comments
Lipoma (Fig B 38-1)	Fat intensity on all pulse sequences. May have fibrous septa but no contrast enhancement.	This most common soft-tissue mass consists of mature adipose tissue.
Ganglion cyst (Fig B 38-2)	Well-defined mass with characteristics of a cyst (uniform low signal intensity on T1-weighted images and high signal intensity on T2-weighted sequences). The appearance varies if there is hemorrhage or thick proteinaceous debris within the lesion, and the wall shows contrast enhancement.	This juxta-articular lesion most commonly occurs in the wrist and hand.
Hemangioma (Fig B 38-3)	High signal intensity in characteristic serpiginous vessels on T2-weighted images.	Cavernous hemangiomas are larger than capillary hemangiomas and may have large amounts of fat and nonvascular tissue.

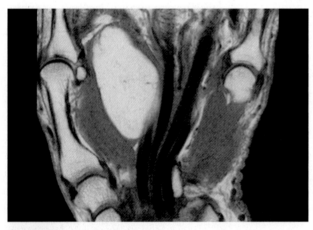

Fig B 38-1
Lipoma. Coronal T1-weighted image shows a well-defined mass of fat signal intensity along the flexor tendons of the hand.[46]

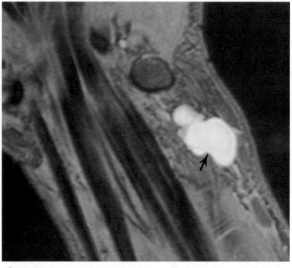

Fig B 38-2
Ganglion cyst. Coronal fat-suppressed T2-weighted image demonstrates a lobulated lesion of the wrist.[46]

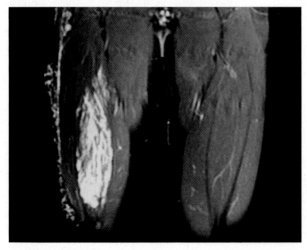

Fig B 38-3
Hemangioma. Coronal T2-weighted image shows deep and superficial hemangiomas in the distal thigh with markedly increased signal intensity in serpiginous vascular structures.[46]

Condition	Imaging Findings	Comments
Lymphangioma (Fig B 38-4)	Cyst-like low signal intensity on T1-weighted images and high signal intensity on T2-weighted scans.	Dilated serpiginous vessels are seen in the soft tissues.
Nerve sheath tumors (Fig B 38-5)	Low signal intensity on T1-weighted images and high signal intensity of T2-weighted scans.	Neurofibroma often has a target appearance on T2-weighted images, with a low-intensity center and peripheral higher intensity. Schwannoma has a similar appearance in almost half the cases.
Myxoma (Fig B 38-6)	Well-defined mass with low signal intensity on T1-weighted images and homogeneous high signal intensity on T2-weighted sequences.	Intramuscular mass that most commonly involves the thigh, upper arm and shoulder, and the gluteal region.
Desmoid (Fig B 38-7)	Low signal intensity (fibrous tissue) on all sequences that may involve parts of the mass or the entire lesion. More often, areas of intermediate signal intensity are seen on T2-weighted images.	Although benign lesions, desmoids may have an aggressive clinical behavior and are multiple in up to 15% of cases. Neurovascular and bone involvement may be identified on MRI.
Giant cell tumor of tendon sheath (Fig B 38-8)	Mass associated with a tendon that has low signal intensity (like muscle) on T1-weighted images and intermediate or low signal intensity on T2-weighted sequences. The lesion may show irregular contrast enhancement.	Most commonly a focal lesion involving the flexor tendons on the hand.

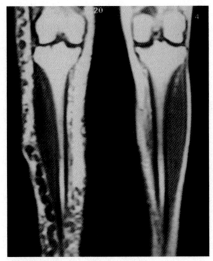

Fig B 38-4
Lymphangioma. Coronal T1-weighted images of the lower extremities demonstrate dilated lymphatic vessels of low signal intensity on the right.[46]

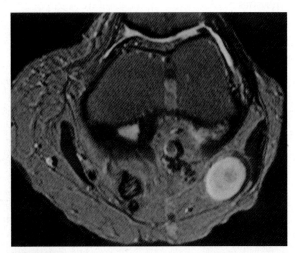

Fig B 38-5
Neurofibroma. Axial T2-weighted image shows a high-intensity lesion with central low intensity, the so-called "target appearance" that is characteristic of this tumor.[46]

Condition	Imaging Findings	Comments
Hematoma (Fig B 38-9)	Signal intensity varies depending on the age of the lesion. Subacute or chronic hematomas have increased signal intensity on all sequences, often with a low-intensity fibrous rim. Acute hematomas have muscle intensity on T1-weighted images and a variable pattern on T2-weighted sequences.	Patients present with a history of trauma or a painful mass.

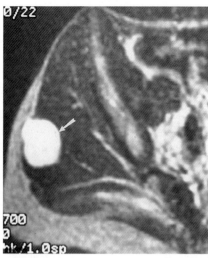

Fig B 38-6
Myxoma. T2-weighted axial image shows homogeneous high signal intensity in this gluteal lesion.[46]

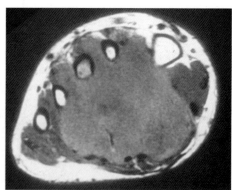

Fig B 38-7
Desmoid. Axial T1-weighted image shows a poorly defined foot mass that contains areas of low signal intensity characteristic of a fibrous lesion.[46]

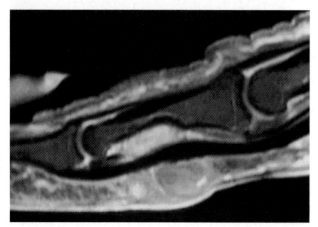

Fig B 38-8
Giant cell tumor of tendon sheath. Sagittal T2-weighted contrast image shows irregular enhancement of this soft-tissue mass, which has produced a broad erosion of the underlying middle phalanx of the finger.[46]

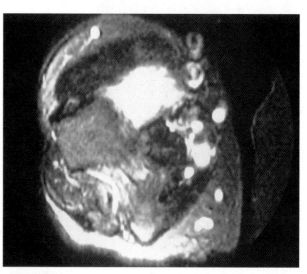

Fig B 38-9
Hematoma. T2-weighted image shows a high signal intensity mass.[46]

Condition	Imaging Findings	Comments
Myositis ossificans (Fig B 38-10)	Signal intensity varies with age of the process. In early stages, it has low signal intensity on T1-weighted images and high signal intensity on T2-weighted sequences. As the process develops, there is a peripheral rim of low signal intensity on all sequences. Irregular areas of increased signal intensity may be seen on T2-weighted images, and there may be fluid-fluid levels. In the late stage, there is central signal intensity similar to fat on all sequences, or areas of low intensity caused by ossification or fibrosis.	A history of trauma may not be given. Common clinical findings include pain, tenderness, and a soft-tissue mass. Plain radiographs show characteristic calcification or ossification within the mass, which typically has a long axis parallel to the adjacent bone.
Abscess (Fig B 38-11)	Soft-tissue mass, often with bone erosions, that generally has low signal intensity on T1-weighted images and high signal intensity on T2-weighted sequences.	Various infectious organisms may produce this nonspecific appearance, for which the correct diagnosis requires clinical correlation.

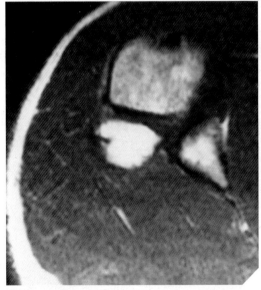

Fig B 38-10
Myositis ossificans. On this axial T1-weighted image, the center of the lesion demonstrates high signal intensity, while the periphery exhibits low-to-intermediate signal.[45]

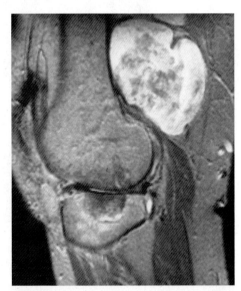

Fig B 38-11
Abscess. Sagittal T2-weighted image shows a large, inhomogeneous posterior soft-tissue abscess with bone erosion due to *Mycobacterium tuberculosis*.[46]

Malignant Soft-Tissue Masses on Magnetic Resonance Imaging

Condition	Imaging Findings	Comments
Liposarcoma (Fig B 39-1)	Fat-intensity mass with thickened septa and areas of inhomogeneity (decreased signal intensity on T1-weighted images; increased signal intensity on T2-weighted scans).	Second most common soft-tissue sarcoma in adults. High-grade tumors have variable signal intensity (little fat intensity) and irregular contrast enhancement).
Malignant fibrous histiocytoma (Fig B 39-2)	Irregular mass with low signal intensity on T1-weighted images and inhomogeneous high signal intensity on T2-weighted scans. Various enhancement patterns.	Most common soft-tissue sarcoma in adults over age 45. Typically presents as a painless enlarging mass involving the lower extremity.

A
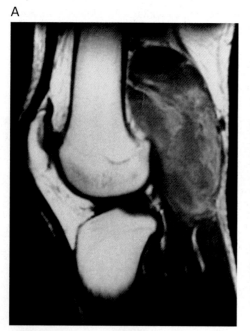
B
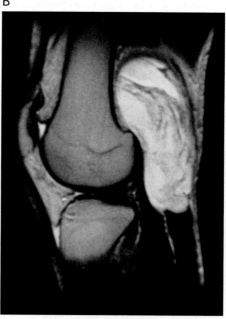

Fig B 39-1
Liposarcoma. (A) Sagittal T1-weighted image shows little fat signal in this intermediate-grade lesion. (B) On the T2-weighted image, the tumor has high signal intensity.[46]

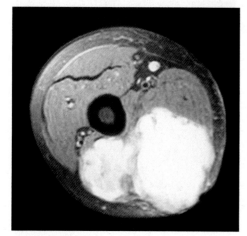

Fig B 39-2
Malignant fibrous histiocytoma. Axial T2-weighted image shows the lesion to have generally high signal intensity with some areas of inhomogeneity.[46]

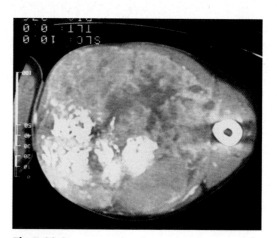

Fig B 39-3
Synovial sarcoma. T2-weighted coronal image shows a large inhomogeneous mass. Calcifications appear as low-intensity regions in the medial aspect of the mass, while hemorrhage is seen inferiorly.[46]

Condition	Imaging Findings	Comments
Synovial sarcoma (Fig B 39-3)	Inhomogeneous signal intensity on T2-weighted images. Calcifications appear as areas of low signal intensity on all sequences. There may be a cystic appearance with fluid-fluid levels.	Common soft-tissue tumor that typically appears as a slow-growing, often-painful mass near a joint. Metastases are present in about 25% of patients at the time of diagnosis.
Rhabomyosarcoma (Fig B 39-4)	Mass that often has poorly defined margins and low signal intensity on T1-weighted images and high signal intensity (may be inhomogeneous) on T2-weighted scans.	Most common soft-tissue mass in children under age 15, but also frequently occurs in adolescents and young adults. Metastases are present in about 20% at the time of diagnosis. Most common locations (in decreasing order of frequency) are the head, neck, genitourinary tract, retroperitoneum, and extremities.
Peripheral nerve tumors (Fig B 39-5)	Irregular mass with signal inhomogeneity on T2-weighted images.	About half occur in patients with neurofibromatosis. Irregular bone destruction may be seen.

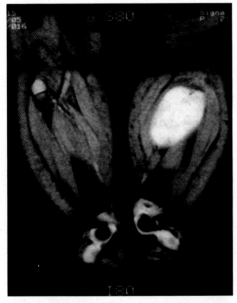

Fig B 39-4
Rhabomyosarcoma. Coronal gradient echo image demonstrates the high signal intensity of this muscle mass.[46]

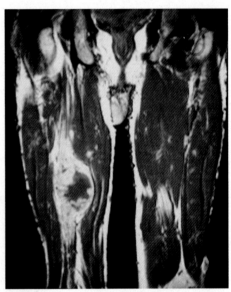

Fig B 39-5
Malignant nerve sheath tumor. T1-weighted contrast image shows peripheral enhancement of the large tumor and adjacent nerve.[46]

Intra-Articular Masses on Magnetic Resonance Imaging

Condition	Imaging Findings	Comments
Noninfectious synovial proliferative processes		
Lipoma arborescens (Fig B 40-1)	Lobulated mass with the signal intensity of fat on all sequences.	Rare intra-articular lesion in which replacement of subsynovial tissue by mature fat cells leads to a villous synovial proliferation. Usually monoarticular, it most frequently affects the knee, especially the suprapatellar pouch. Ultrasound demonstrates a hyperechoic, frond-like mass that bends and waves in real time during manipulation of the joint.
Synovial osteo-chondromatosis (Figs B 40-2 and B 40-3)	Variable appearance depending on the relative proportion of synovial proliferation and calcified nodule formation. Nonmineralized lesions form an intra-articular conglomerate mass that is isointense relative to muscle on T1-weighted images and hyperintense on T2-weighted images. Nodules containing calcification have low signal intensity on all pulse sequences. On T1-weighted images, intra-articular bodies with mature bone and fatty marrow display the low signal intensity of cortical bone peripherally and the high signal intensity of bone marrow centrally.	Proliferation and metaplastic transformation of the synovium with formation of multiple cartilaginous nodules. The knee is the most commonly affected joint, followed by the elbow, hip, and shoulder. In the late stage, the nodules may break off into the joint space.

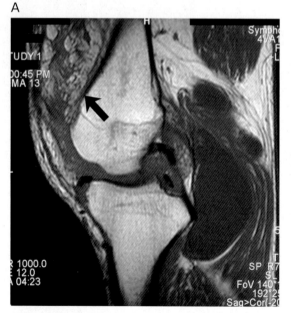
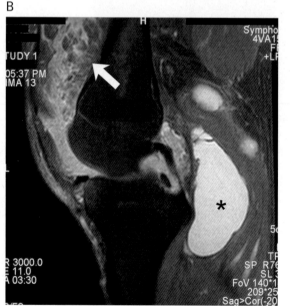

Fig B 40-1
Lipoma arborescens. (A) Sagittal proton density-weighted image shows a lobulated mass in the suprapatellar bursa (arrow) with signal intensity equivalent to that of fat. (B) A fat-saturation sequence shows loss of signal of the synovial proliferation (arrow) surrounded by a large joint effusion extending into the popliteal bursa (*).[48]

Condition	Imaging Findings	Comments
Pigmented villonodular synovitis (PVNS) (Figs B 40-4 and B 40-5)	The mass-like proliferative synovium has a lobulated margin. It may be extensive in diffuse disease or limited to a single nodule in the focal form. Bleeding is common, resulting in hemosiderin deposition and a characteristic low signal intensity on all pulse sequences. Areas of high signal intensity on T2-weighted images are likely caused by inflamed synovium or joint effusions.	Benign proliferative disorder of the synovium that may affect joints, bursae, or tendon sheaths. Diffuse or, less commonly, a focal process, it most frequently involves the knee, followed by the hip, ankle, and shoulder.
Rheumatoid arthritis (Fig B 40-6)	Pannus appears as intermediate-to-low signal intensity on both T1- and T2-weighted images of affected joints. Synovial rice bodies may be seen.	Chronic systemic disorder that predominantly affects women. Most commonly involving the hands, wrists, and feet, it is characterized by an inflammatory response that results in a proliferative, hyperplastic, and hypervascular synovium (pannus).
Infectious granulomatous diseases Tuberculous arthritis (Fig B 40-7)	Joint effusion with proliferative synovium, bone erosions, and periarticular abscesses that may mimic neoplastic involvement. Synovial rice bodies may be seen.	Most commonly involving the hip and knee, tuberculous arthritis usually results from hematogenous spread of an active pulmonary or lymphatic focus of disease to the synovium. Synovial rice bodies, which represent detached synovial villi lying within the joint cavity that resemble grains of rice, may also be seen with rheumatoid and coccidiodomycosis arthritis.

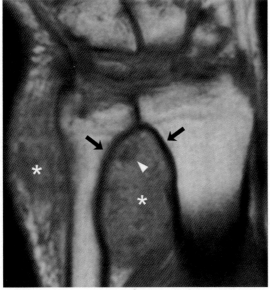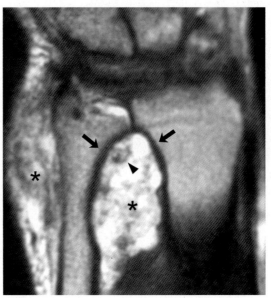

Fig B 40-2
Synovial osteochondromatosis. (A) Coronal proton density-weighted image demonstrates an intermediate-signal-intensity mass (*) in the radioulnar joint. (B) Coronal T2-weighted image shows that the mass (*) is hyperintense. On both MR images, note the multiple low-signal-intensity areas (arrowhead) representing regions of calcification that were evident on plain radiographs.[48]

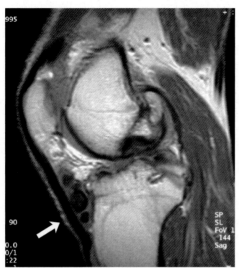

Fig B 40-3
Synovial osteochondromatosis. Sagittal proton density-weighted image demonstrates calcified nodules as masses of low signal intensity (arrow) in the deep infrapatellar bursa.[48]

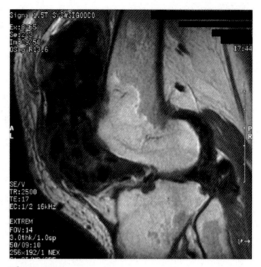

Fig B 40-4
Diffuse PVNS. Sagittal proton density-weighted image shows lobulated, mass-like synovial proliferation with characteristic low signal intensity. Note the tibial articular erosions.[48]

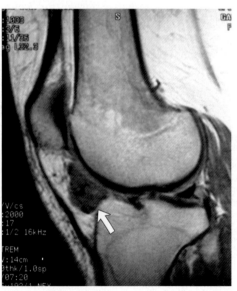

Fig B 40-5
Focal PVNS. Sagittal proton density-weighted image shows a low-signal-intensity mass (arrow) in the anterior joint space.[48]

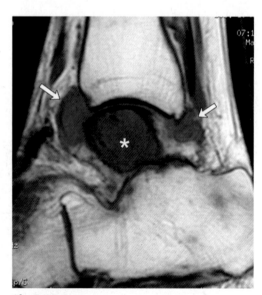

Fig B 40-6
Rheumatoid arthritis. A sagittal T1-weighted image shows a low-signal-intensity lesion (*) in the talus, with low-signal-intensity pannus (arrows) in the joint space.[48]

Condition	Imaging Findings	Comments
Coccidiodomycosis arthritis (Fig B 40-8)	Joint effusion with marginal erosions. Synovial rice bodies may be seen.	A fungal infection that is endemic in areas of Mexico, South America, and the southwestern United States, coccidioidomycosis arthritis primarily involves the ankle and knee. Articular infections usually result from direct extension of a focus of osteomyelitis, though direct hematogenous spread to a joint can rarely occur.
Deposition diseases Gout (Fig B 40-9)	Well-defined erosions with overhanging edges and preservation of the joint space. The gouty tophus has intermediate signal intensity on T1-weighted images and intermediate-to-low signal intensity on T2-weighted images.	Metabolic disorder in which hyperuricemia results from either an increased production or decreased excretion of uric acid. The deposition of local aggregates of urate crystals and proteinaceous material surrounded by an intense inflammatory reaction (tophus) most commonly involves the joints of the hands and feet.
Amyloid	Amyloid deposits have low-to-intermediate signal intensity on all pulse sequences.	Accumulation of amyloid in and around joints, most frequently the shoulders, hips, knees, and wrists. Usually bilateral, amyloid arthropathy most frequently develops in patients undergoing chronic hemodialysis or with plasma cell dyscrasia.

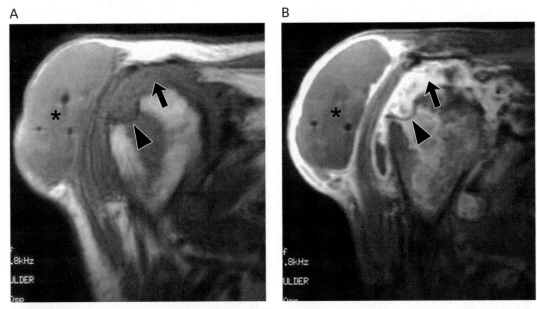

Fig B 40-7
Tuberculous arthritis. (A) Coronal T1-weighted image of the right shoulder demonstrates an erosion of the humeral head (arrowhead) and a distended joint space with proliferative synovium (arrow). Note the adjacent large mass (*). (B) On a T1-weighted contrast study with fat saturation, the mass (*) appears as a fluid-filled collection with an enhancing periphery rather than a solid tumor. Note the enhancement of the synovium within the joint (arrow) and the marginal erosion (arrowhead). The combination of a destructive inflammatory arthritis decompressing into the adjacent subdeltoid bursa to form a cold abscess is typical of tuberculous arthritis.[48]

Condition	Imaging Findings	Comments
Vascular malformations Arteriovenous malformations	Soft-tissue mass containing serpiginous areas of low-signal intensity on all sequences.	Shunting of arterial blood to the venous system in a central confluence of tortuous vessels. Although arteriovenous malformations are congenital, they are often not discovered until later in life. Involvement of the extremities is relatively common and may be manifest as single or multifocal lesions or even as a diffuse process affecting the entire extremity and adjacent trunk.
Klippel-Trenaunay-Weber syndrome (Fig B 40-10)	Joint effusion, arteriovenous malformation of intermediate signal intensity with a prominent flow void represent a large feeding artery, and superficial dilated veins.	Rare congenital abnormality consisting of cutaneous hemangiomas (nevus flammeus), hypertrophy of bone and soft tissue, varicose veins, and arteriovenous malformations, all usually affecting a single limb.
Synovial hemangioma (Figs B 40-11 and B 40-12)	Lobulated intra-articular mass with intermediate signal intensity on T1-weighted images and striking hyperintensity on T2-weighted images (probably related to pooling of blood within vascular spaces). Low-signal-intensity linear structures traversing the lesion on T2-weighted images likely represent fibrous septa or vascular channels.	Rare benign vascular malformation that occurs predominantly in the knee and usually affects children and young adults.

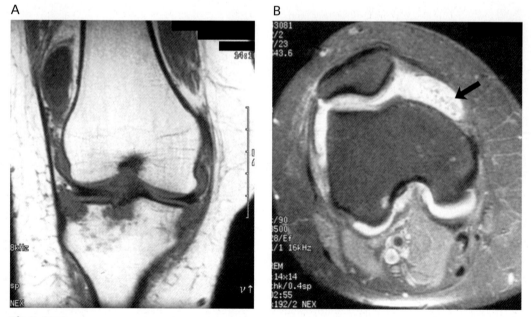

Fig B 40-8
Coccidiodomycosis. (A) Coronal T1-weighted image demonstrates a joint effusion and marginal erosions of the proximal tibia with preservation of the joint spaces. (B) Axial proton density-weighted image with fat saturation demonstrates multiple rice bodies (arrow) within a joint effusion.[48]

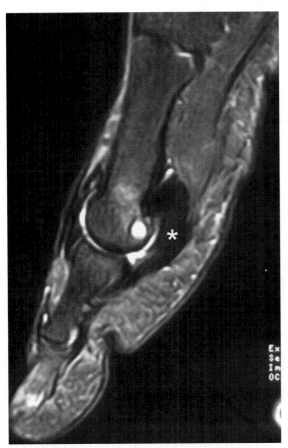

Fig B 40-9
Gout. Sagittal STIR image demonstrates low signal intensity of the gouty tophus (*). There is erosion with an overhanging edge at the distal head of the first metatarsal and preservation of the joint space.[48]

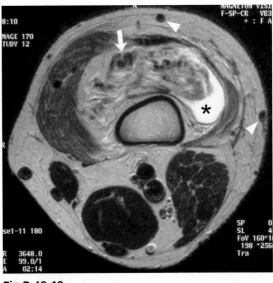

Fig B 40-10
Klippel-Trenaunay-Weber syndrome. An axial T2-weighted image demonstrates a joint effusion (*) and an intermediate-signal-intensity AVM in the suprapatellar bursa with a prominent serpentine signal void (arrow) from a large feeding artery. Note the large, dilated superficial veins (arrowheads).[48]

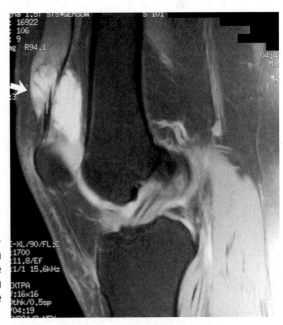

Fig B 40-11
Synovial hemangioma. Sagittal proton density-weighted image with fat saturation demonstrates a mass in the suprapatellar bursa that invades the musculature anteriorly (arrow). The markedly high signal of the mass reflects pooling of blood within the vascular spaces of this synovial hemangioma.[48]

Condition	Imaging Findings	Comments
Malignancies		
Synovial sarcoma (Fig B 40-13)	Mass of low signal intensity on T1-weighted images and high signal intensity on T2-weighted scans. There are often cystic areas of hemorrhage and fluid-fluid levels. Foci of persistent low signal intensity on all sequences are consistent with areas of calcification. Contrast enhancement is seen.	Accounting for 10% of primary soft-tissue malignant tumors, most synovial sarcomas are located in the extremities, especially around the knee. Despite its name, synovial sarcoma does not arise from the synovial membrane but rather from primitive mesenchymal cells in the extra-articular soft tissues. Fewer than 5% of synovial sarcomas arise within the joint space.
Synovial chondrosarcoma (Fig B 40-14)	Often-lobulated mass that is isointense on T1-weighted images and hyperintense on T2-weighted sequences. Calcification within the cartilaginous nodules appear as small areas of low signal intensity on all pulse sequences. Bone erosion also can be seen, and there is heterogeneous contrast enhancement.	Metastatic transformation of the synovium with the formation of multiple cartilaginous nodules that can calcify and ossify. It most commonly involves the knee and hip; distant metastases usually appear in the lungs.

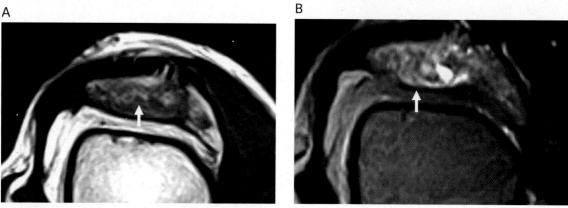

A   B

Fig B 40-12
Synovial hemangioma. (A) Axial T1-weighted image shows an intermediate-signal-intensity lesion in the suprapatellar pouch (arrow) containing areas of high signal intensity. (B) Corresponding fat-suppressed T2-weighted image shows a characteristic circular-linear pattern (arrow) that probably represents fibrous septa or vascular channels traversing the lesion.[49]

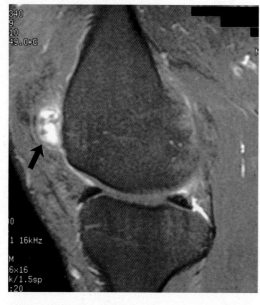

Fig B 40-13
Synovial sarcoma. Sagittal contrast T1-weighted image with fat saturation demonstrates enhancement of a mass (arrow) in the anterior joint space of the knee. Note the foci of low signal intensity, which persisted on all pulse sequences, consistent with areas of calcification.[48]

Condition	Imaging Findings	Comments
Synovial metastases	Variable appearance.	Despite the highly vascular nature of the synovium, it rarely is the site of metastatic spread. Lung cancer is the most common primary tumor that metastasizes to the synovium.
Cyclops lesion (Fig B 40-15)	Anterior or anterolateral soft-tissue mass in the intercondylar notch near the tibial insertion of the reconstructed anterior cruciate ligament. It has intermediate-to-low signal intensity on all pulse sequences due to its fibrous content.	Central granulation tissue surrounded by dense fibrous tissue, which occurs in up to 10% of patients following anterior cruciate ligament reconstruction. The lesion was named for the bulbous appearance and characteristic focal areas of reddish blue discoloration (from venous channels) that resembles an eye at arthroscopy.

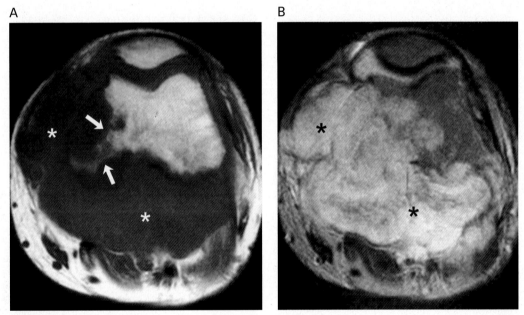

Fig B 40-14
Synovial chondrosarcoma. (A) Axial T1-weighted image demonstrates a large, lobulated, low-signal-intensity mass (*) distending the knee joint space, with erosions and invasion of the femoral condyles (arrows). (B) Axial T2-weighted image obtained more distally demonstrates high signal intensity (*) within the mass.[48]

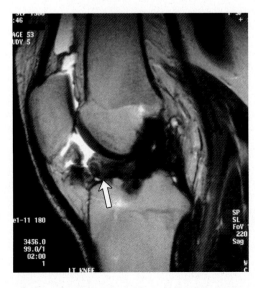

Fig B 40-15
Cyclops lesion. Sagittal T2-weighted image following anterior cruciate ligament reconstruction demonstrates a mass anteriorly in the joint space of the knee. Note the characteristic low signal intensity of this fibrous mass (arrow).[48]

Sources

1. Reprinted with permission from "Bone Changes Following Electrical Injury" by LB Brinn and JE Moseley, *American Journal of Roentgenology* (1966;97:682–686), Copyright ©1966, American Roentgen Ray Society.

2. Smith SS, Murphey MD, Kambiz M, et al. Radiologic spectrum of paget disease of bone and its complications with pathologic correlation. *RadioGraphics* 2002;22:1191–2012.

3. Reprinted with permission from "Radiologic Diagnosis of Metabolic Bone Disease" by WA Reynolds and JJ Karo, *Orthopedic Clinics of North America* (1972;3:521–532), Copyright ©1972, WB Saunders Company.

4. Reprinted with permission from "Radiologic Findings in Niemann-Pick Disease" by R Lachman et al, *Radiology* (1973;108:659–664), Copyright ©1973, Radiological Society of North America Inc.

5. Reprinted with permission from "The Radiologic Assessment of Short Stature" by JP Dorst, CI Scott, and JG Hall, *Radiologic Clinics of North America* (1972;10:393–414), Copyright ©1972, WB Saunders Company.

6. Reprinted with permission from "Skeletal Changes in Wilson's Disease" by R Mindelzun et al, *Radiology* (1970;94:127–132), Copyright ©1970, Radiological Society of North America Inc.

7. Reprinted with permission from "Brodie's Abscess: Reappraisal" by WB Miller, WA Murphy, and LA Gilula, *Radiology* (1979;132:15–23), Copyright ©1979, Radiological Society of North America Inc.

8. Reprinted with permission from "Tumoural Gummatous Yaws" by WP Cockshott and AGM Davies, *Journal of Bone and Joint Surgery* (1960;42B:785–791), Copyright ©1960, Journal of Bone and Joint Surgery Inc.

9. Ejindu VC, Hine, AL, Mashayekhi M, et al. Musculoskeletal manifestations of sickle cell disease. *RadioGraphics* 2007;27:1005–1021.

10. Reprinted from *Clinical Radiology in the Tropics* by WP Cockshott and H Middlemiss (Eds) with permission of Churchill Livingstone Inc, ©1979.

11. Reprinted with permission from "The Many Facets of Multiple Myeloma" by WT Meszaros, *Seminars in Roentgenology* (1974;9:219–228), Copyright ©1974, Grune & Stratton Inc.

12. Reprinted with permission from "The 'Fallen Fragment Sign' in the Diagnosis of Unicameral Bone Cysts" by J Reynolds, *Radiology* (1969;92:949–953), Copyright ©1969, Radiological Society of North America Inc.

13. Reprinted from *Roentgen Diagnosis of Diseases of Bone* by J Edeiken with permission of Williams & Wilkins Company, ©1981.

14. Stacy GS, Peabody TD, Dixon LB. Mimics on radiography of giant cell tumor of bone. *AJR Am J Roentgenol* 2003;182:1583–1589.

15. Reprinted with permission from "Classic and Contemporary Imaging of Coccidioidomycosis" by JP McGahan et al, *American Journal of Roentgenology* (1981;136:393–404), Copyright ©1981, American Roentgen Ray Society.

16. Reprinted with permission from "Skeletal Changes in Hemophilia and Other Bleeding Disorders" by DJ Stoker and RO Murray, *Seminars in Roentgenology* (1974;9:185–193), Copyright ©1974, Grune & Stratton Inc.

17. Boyse TD, Jacobson JA. Case 45: Cystic angiomatosis. *Radiology* 2002;223:164–167.

18. Krishnan A, Ahirkhoda A, Tehranzadeh J, et al. Primary bone lymphoma: Radiographic-MR imaging correlation. *RadioGraphics* 2003;23:1371–1387.

19. Reprinted from *The Radiology of Joint Disease* by DM Forrester, JC Brown, and JW Nesson with permission of WB Saunders Company, ©1978.

20. Reprinted with permission from "Ulcer Osteoma: Bone Response to Tropical Ulcer" by TM Kolawole and SP Bohrer, *American Journal of Roentgenology* (1970;109:611–618), Copyright ©1970, American Roentgen Ray Society.

21. Reprinted with permission from "Chronic Poisoning Due to Excess of Vitamin A" by J Caffey, *Pediatrics* (1950;5:672–688), Copyright ©1950, American Academy of Pediatrics.

22. Reprinted with permission from *Musculoskeletal MRI* by PA Kaplan, CA Helms, et al. Philadelphia: W.B. Saunders, 2001.

23. Reprinted with permission from "Nonseptic Monoarthritis: Imaging Features with Clinical and Histopathologic Correlation" by J Llauger, J Palmer, N Roson, et al., *RadioGraphics* (2000;20:S263278).

24. Reprinted with permission from "Congenital Hyperurecosuria" by MH Becker and JK Wallin, *Radiologic Clinics of North America* (1968;6:239–243), Copyright ©1968, WB Saunders Company.

25. Reprinted with permission from "Epidermolysis Bullosa with Characteristic Hand Deformities" by LB Brinn and MT Khilnani, *Radiology* (1967;89:272–277), Copyright ©1967, Radiological Society of North America Inc.

26. Reprinted with permission from "Progeria" by FR Margolin and HL Steinbach, *American Journal of Roentgenology* (1968;103:173–178), Copyright ©1968, American Roentgen Ray Society.

27. Reprinted from *Diagnostic Imaging in Internal Medicine* by RL Eisenberg with permission of McGraw-Hill Book Company, ©1985. Courtesy of Robert R Jacobson, Pearl Mills, and Tanya Thomassie.

28. Reprinted with permission from "Calcium Deposition Diseases" by MK Dalinka, AJ Reginato, and DA Golden, *Seminars in Roentgenology* (1982;17:39–48), Copyright ©1982, Grune & Stratton Inc.

29. Reprinted with permission from "Tumoral Calcinosis with Sedimentation Sign" by I Hug and J Guncaga, *British Journal of Radiology* (1974;47:734–736), Copyright ©1974, British Institute of Radiology.

30. Reprinted with permission from "Tumors of the Soft Tissues of the Extremities" by RC Cavanagh, *Seminars in Roentgenology* (1973;8:83–89), Copyright ©1973, Grune & Stratton Inc.

31. Reprinted from *Radiology of Bone Diseases* by GB Greenfield, JB Lippincott Company, with permission of the author, ©1986.

32. Reprinted with permission from "The Roentgenographic Manifestations of the Rubella Syndrome in Newborn Infants" by EB Singleton et al, *American Journal of Roentgenology* (1966;97:82–91), Copyright ©1966, American Roentgen Ray Society.

33. Reprinted with permission from "Gaucher's Disease" by B Levin, *American Journal of Roentgenology* (1961;85:685–696), Copyright ©1961, American Roentgen Ray Society.

34. Reprinted with permission from "Familial Metaphyseal Dysplasia" by MG Hermel, J Gershon-Cohen, and DT Jones, *American Journal of Roentgenology* (1953;70:413–421), Copyright ©1953, American Roentgen Ray Society.

35. Reprinted with permission from "Skeletal Changes in the Anemias" by JE Moseley, *Seminars in Roentgenology* (1974;9:169–184), Copyright ©1974, Grune & Stratton Inc.

36. Reprinted from *Plain Film Interpretation in Congenital Heart Disease* by LE Swischuk with permission of Williams & Wilkins Company, ©1979.

37. Reprinted with permission from "Ghost Infantile Vertebrae and Hemipelves within Adult Skeletons from Thorotrast Administration in Childhood" by JG Teplick et al, *Radiology* (1978;129:657–660), Copyright ©1978, Radiological Society of North America Inc.

38. Reprinted with permission from "Tuberculosis of the Bones and Joints" by M Chapman, RO Murray, and BJ Stoker, *Seminars in*

Roentgenology (1979;14:266–282), Copyright ©1979, Grune & Stratton Inc.

39. Reprinted from *Radiology of Skeletal Trauma* by LF Rogers with permission of Churchill Livingstone Inc., ©1982.

40. Lee P, Hunter TB, Taljanovic. Musculoskeletal Cooloquialisms: How Did We Come Up with These Names? *RadioGraphics* 2004;24:1009–1027.

41. Reprinted with permission from "Maison Neuve Fracture of the Fibula" by AM Pankovich, *Journal of Bone and Joint Surgery* (1976; 58:337–339), Copyright ©1976, Journal of Bone and Joint Surgery Inc.

42. Reprinted with permission from "The Radiology of Facial Fractures" by K Dolan, C Jacob, and W Smoker, *Radiographics* (1984;4:576–663), Copyright ©1984, Radiological Society of North America Inc.

43. Stevens MA, El-Khoury GY, Kathol MH, et al. Imaging features of avulsion injuries. *RadioGraphics* 1999;19:655.

44. Tehranzadeh J. The spectrum of avulsion and avulsion-like injuries of the musculoskeletal system. *RadioGraphics* 1987;7:945.

45. Greenspan A. *Orthopedic Imaging, 4th edition*. Philadelphia: Lippincott Williams & Wilkins, 2004.

46. Berquist TH. *Musculoskeletal Imaging Companion, 2nd edition*. Philadelphia: Lippincott Williams & Wilkins, 2007.

47. Greenfield GB and Arrington JA. *Imaging of Bone tumors*. Philadelphia, Lippincott, 1995.

48. Sheldon PJ, Forrester DM, Learch TJ. Imaging of intraarticular masses. *RadioGraphics* 2005;25:105–119.

49. Vilanova JC, Barcelo J, Smirniotopoulos JG, et al. Hemangioma from Head to Toe: MR imaging with pathologic correlation. *RadioGraphics* 2004;24:367–385.

6

Spine Patterns

Generalized Vertebral Osteoporosis

Condition	Comments
Osteoporosis of aging (senile or postmenopausal osteoporosis) (Fig SP 1-1)	Most common form of generalized osteoporosis. As a person ages, the bones lose density and become more brittle, fracturing more easily and healing more slowly. Many elderly persons are also less active and have poor diets that are deficient in protein. Females are affected more often and more severely than males, as postmenopausal women have deficient gonadal hormone levels and decreased osteoblastic activity.
Drug-induced osteoporosis (Fig SP 1-2)	Patients receiving large doses of steroids over several months often develop generalized osteoporosis. Patients treated with 15,000 to 30,000 U of heparin for 6 months or longer also may develop generalized osteoporosis (possibly due to a direct local stimulating effect of heparin on bone resorption).
Deficiency states Protein deficiency (or abnormal protein metabolism)	Inability to produce adequate bone matrix in such conditions as malnutrition, nephrosis, diabetes mellitus, Cushing's syndrome, and hyperparathyroidism. Also patients with severe liver disease (hepatocellular degeneration, large or multiple liver cysts or tumors, biliary atresia). Pure dietary protein deficiency is rare in developed countries.

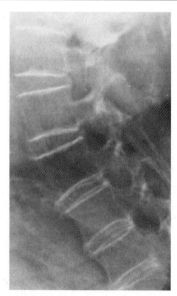

Fig SP 1-1
Osteoporosis of aging. Generalized demineralization of the spine in a postmenopausal woman. The cortex appears as a thin line that is relatively dense and prominent (picture-frame pattern).

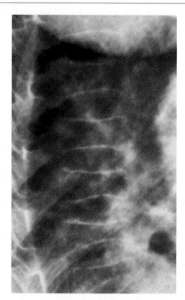

Fig SP 1-2
Steroid-induced osteoporosis. Lateral view of the thoracic spine in a patient on high-dose steroid therapy for dermatomyositis demonstrates severe osteoporosis with thinning of cortical margins and biconcave deformities of vertebral bodies.

Condition	Comments
Vitamin C deficiency (scurvy)	Scurvy is now rarely seen in adults, though it can develop in severely malnourished individuals, especially elderly persons. There must be a prolonged period of vitamin C deficiency before symptoms become manifest. Osteoporosis is prominent in the axial skeleton, especially the spine. Biconcave deformities of vertebral bodies, condensation of bone at the superior and inferior vertebral margins, and centralized osteopenia are identical to the changes of osteoporosis in other disorders.
Intestinal malabsorption	Underlying mechanism in such conditions as sprue, scleroderma, pancreatic disease (insufficiency, chronic pancreatitis, mucoviscidosis), Crohn's disease, decreased absorptive surface of the small bowel (resection, bypass procedure), infiltrative disorders of the small bowel (eosinophilic enteritis, lactase deficiency, lymphoma, Whipple's disease), and idiopathic steatorrhea.
Endocrine disorders (Fig SP 1-3)	Hypogonadism (especially Turner's syndrome and menopause); adrenocortical abnormality (Cushing's syndrome, Addison's disease); nonendocrine steroid-producing tumor (eg, oat cell carcinoma); diabetes mellitus; pituitary abnormality (acromegaly, hypopituitarism); thyroid abnormality (hyperthyroidism and hypothyroidism).

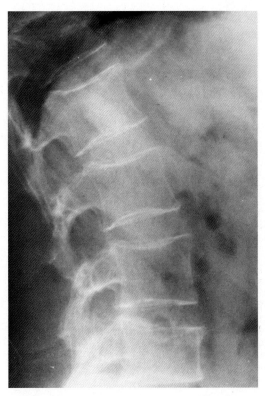

Fig SP 1-3
Cushing's syndrome due to adrenal hyperplasia. Marked demineralization and an almost complete loss of trabeculae in the lumbar spine. The vertebral end plates are mildly concave and the intervertebral disk spaces are slightly widened. Note the compression of the superior end plate of L4.[1]

Condition	Comments
Neoplastic disorders (Fig SP 1-4)	Diffuse cellular proliferation in the bone marrow with no tendency to form discrete tumor masses may produce generalized skeletal deossification simulating postmenopausal osteoporosis in adults with multiple myeloma or diffuse skeletal metastases and in children with acute leukemia. Pressure atrophy produces cortical thinning and trabecular resorption.
Anemia (Fig SP 1-5)	Extensive marrow hyperplasia within the vertebral bodies produces a decrease in the number of trabeculae, thinning of the subchondral bone plates, accentuation of vertical trabeculation, and biconcave or central squared-off vertebral depressions. This appearance can be seen with thalassemia and sickle cell disease, as well as in severe iron deficiency anemia.
Ankylosing spondylitis	In long-standing disease, osteoporosis of the vertebral bodies becomes apparent and may be severe. Biconcave deformities of the vertebral bodies may develop.

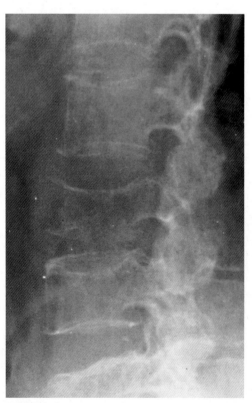

Fig SP 1-4
Multiple myeloma. Diffuse myelomatous infiltration causes generalized demineralization of the vertebral bodies and a compression fracture of L2.

Condition	Comments
Osteogenesis imperfecta (Fig SP 1-6)	Inherited generalized disorder of connective tissue with multiple fractures, hypermobility of joints, blue sclerae, poor teeth, deafness, and cardiovascular disorders such as mitral valve prolapse or aortic regurgitation. In the spine, osteoporosis, ligamentous laxity, and post-traumatic deformities may result in severe kyphoscoliosis. Vertebral bodies are flattened and may be biconvex or wedge shaped anteriorly.
Neuromuscular diseases and dystrophies	Decreased muscular tone leading to osteoporosis, bone atrophy with cortical thinning, scoliosis, and joint contractures occurs in congenital disorders and such acquired conditions as spinal cord disease and immobilization for chronic disease or major fracture. Lack of the stress stimulus of weight bearing is the underlying cause of the generalized disuse atrophy termed *space flight osteoporosis*.
Homocystinuria (Fig SP 1-7)	Inborn error of methionine metabolism that causes a defect in the structure of collagen or elastin and a radiographic appearance similar to that of Marfan's syndrome. Striking osteoporosis of the spine and long bones (extremely rare in Marfan's syndrome).

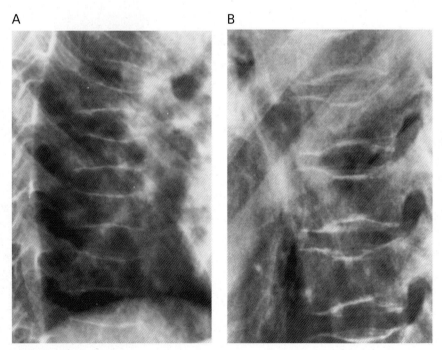

A   B

Fig SP 1-5
Sickle cell anemia. (A) Biconcave indentations on both the superior and inferior margins of the soft vertebral bodies produce the characteristic fish vertebrae. (B) Localized step-like central depressions of multiple vertebral end plates.

Condition	Comments
Lipid storage diseases	Gaucher's disease and Niemann-Pick disease. Accumulation of abnormal quantities of complex lipids in the bone marrow produces a generalized loss of bone density and cortical thinning.
Hemochromatosis	Iron-storage disorder often associated with diffuse osteoporosis of the spine and vertebral collapse. Approximately half the patients have a characteristic arthropathy that most frequently involves the small joints of the hand. Hepatosplenomegaly and portal hypertension are common.
Idiopathic juvenile osteoporosis (Fig SP 1-8)	Rare condition characterized by the abrupt onset of generalized or focal bone pain in children 8 to 12 years of age. Osteoporosis of the spine, particularly in the thoracic and lumbar regions, may be combined with vertebral collapse. The disease is usually self-limited with spontaneous clinical and radiologic improvement.

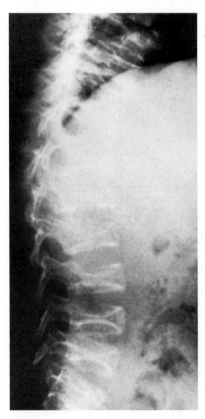

Fig SP 1-6
Osteogenesis imperfecta. In addition to generalized osteoporosis, some vertebrae show biconcave deformities, whereas others demonstrate anterior wedging.[2]

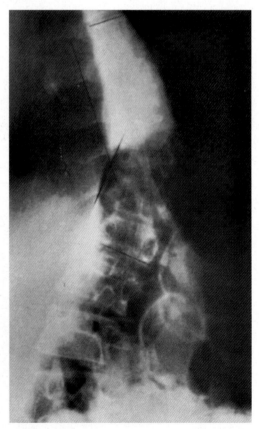

Fig SP 1-7
Homocystinuria. Scoliosis and osteoporosis.[2]

A B

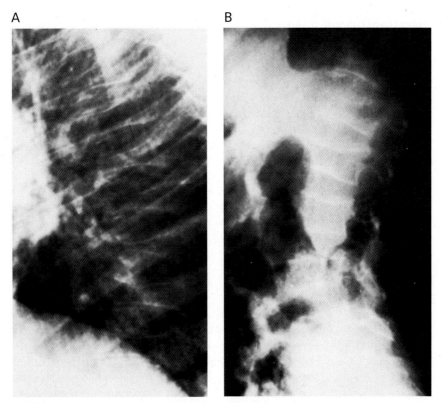

Fig SP 1-8
Idiopathic juvenile osteoporosis. Lateral radiographs of (A) thoracic and (B) lumbar regions of the spine show striking osteoporotic lucency associated with severe compression and collapse of multiple vertebral bodies. Note the ballooning of several disk spaces.[2]

Lytic Lesion of a Vertebral Body or Posterior Elements

Condition	Imaging Findings	Comments
Osteoblastoma (Figs SP 2-1 and SP 2-2)	Expansile lucent (or opaque) lesion that grows rapidly, readily breaking through the cortex and producing a sharply defined soft-tissue component that is often circumscribed by a thin calcific shell.	Rare bone neoplasm that involves the vertebral column (most frequently the neural arches and spinous processes) in approximately half of patients. Most frequently occurs in the second decade of life and produces a dull aching pain, tenderness, and soft-tissue swelling. May contain some internal calcification.
Hemangioma (Fig SP 2-3)	Demineralized and occasionally expanded vertebral body with characteristic multiple, coarse linear striations running vertically.	Benign, slow-growing tumor composed of vascular channels. Usually asymptomatic and identified in middle-aged patients. The coarse vertical trabecular pattern may extend into the pedicles and laminae. Soft-tissue and intraspinal extension of the tumor or secondary hemorrhage can produce a paraspinal mass.
Aneurysmal bone cyst (Fig SP 2-4)	Expansile, trabeculated, lucent lesion that primarily involves the posterior elements. There may be extension into or primary involvement of a vertebral body.	Consists of numerous blood-filled arteriovenous communications, rather than being a true neoplasm. Most frequently occurs in children and young adults and presents as mild pain of several months' duration, swelling, and restriction of movement. May cross a vertebral interspace and involve adjacent vertebrae.
Giant cell tumor (Fig SP 2-5)	Slow-growing lucent lesion that often has ill-defined margins and may progress to vertebral collapse.	Most giant cell tumors of the spine occur in the sacrum, where the tumor has an expansile appearance.

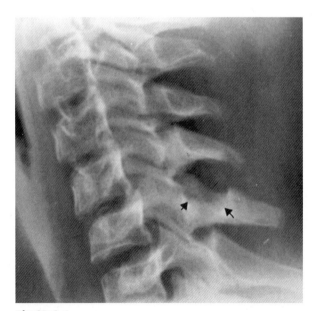

Fig SP 2-1
Osteoblastoma of the cervical spine. Sharply defined, erosive lesion (arrows) involves the superior margin of a lower cervical spinous process

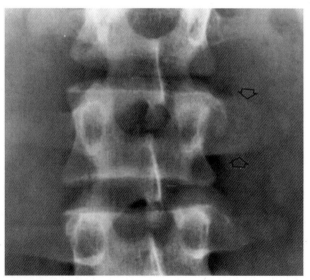

Fig SP 2-2
Osteoblastoma of the lumbar spine. Well-circumscribed, expansile lesion (arrows) involves the left transverse process of a midlumbar vertebra.

Condition	Imaging Findings	Comments
Chordoma (see Figs SK 7-6 and SK 8-7)	Bulky mass causing ill-defined bone destruction or cortical expansion. Flocculent calcifications may develop in a large soft-tissue mass.	Arises from remnants of the notochord and primarily involves the sacrococcygeal region (50%) and clivus (30%). The remainder of the tumors occurs elsewhere in the spine. Locally invasive, but does not metastasize.
Langerhans cell histiocytosis (see Fig SP 6-7)	Bubbly, lytic, expansile lesions of both vertebral bodies and posterior elements can occur without significant collapse.	Most common manifestation is the characteristic collapse of a vertebral body (vertebra plana). A paraspinal mass can simulate a soft-tissue abscess related to vertebral osteomyelitis.

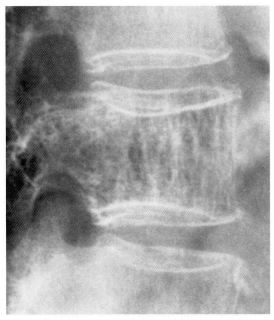

Fig SP 2-3
Hemangioma of a vertebral body. Multiple coarse, linear striations run vertically in the demineralized vertebral body.

A

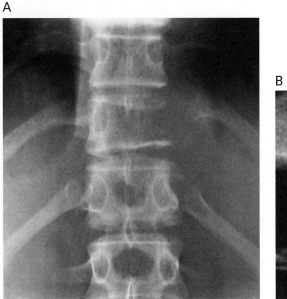

B

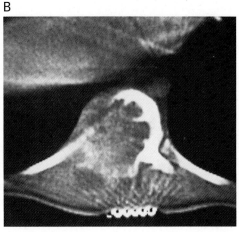

Fig SP 2-4
Aneurysmal bone cyst of a thoracic vertebral body. (A) Destruction of the body and posterior elements. No peripheral shell of bone can be recognized. (B) CT scan shows irregular destruction suggesting a malignant process.[3]

Condition	Imaging Findings	Comments
Fibrous dysplasia	Expansile lesion with a ground-glass or purely lytic appearance.	Infrequent manifestation. Vertebral collapse or a posteriorly expanding fibrous-tissue mass can result in cord compression.
Hydatid (echinococcal) cyst (Fig SP 2-6)	Single or multiple expansile lytic lesions containing trabeculae. May be associated with cortical erosion and a soft-tissue mass.	Bone involvement occurs in approximately 1% of patients and most commonly affects the vertebral bodies, pelvis, and sacrum. Infiltration of daughter cysts into the bone produces a multiloculated appearance that resembles a bunch of grapes. Rupture into the spinal canal may produce neurologic abnormalities, including paraplegia.
Metastases (Fig SP 2-7)	Single or multiple areas of bone destruction of variable size with irregular and poorly defined margins.	Spinal metastases typically destroy the pedicles (unlike multiple myeloma, in which the pedicles are infrequently destroyed). Because almost half the mineral content of a bone must be lost before it is detectable on plain radiographs, radionuclide bone scanning is far more sensitive for screening.
Plasmacytoma	Multicystic expansile lesion with thickened trabeculae. Primarily involves the vertebral body.	Involved vertebral body may collapse and disappear completely, or the lesion may extend across the intervertebral disk to invade the adjacent vertebral body (simulating infection). Multiple myeloma causes generalized decreased bone density and destructive changes involving multiple vertebral bodies and often results in multiple vertebral compression fractures (see Fig SP 6-2).

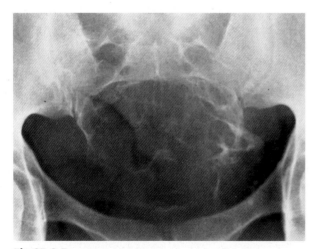

Fig SP 2-5
Giant cell tumor of the sacrum. Huge expansile lesion.

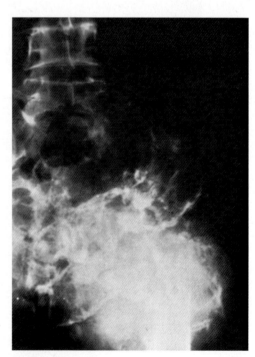

Fig SP 2-6
Echinococcosis. Expansile, bubbly, lytic lesions of the pelvis, sacrum, and proximal femur associated with deformity, osseous fragmentation, and soft-tissue swelling.[2]

Condition	Imaging Findings	Comments
Lymphoma (Fig SP 2-8)	Patchy osteolysis, with or without associated osteosclerosis.	Single or multiple lesions may have well- or ill-defined margins. Vertebral compression fractures may occur.
Osteomyelitis (see Figs SP 6-3 and SP 6-4)	Earliest sign is subtle erosion of the subchondral bony plate with loss of the sharp cortical outline. This may progress to total destruction of the vertebral body associated with a paravertebral soft-tissue abscess. Unlike neoplastic processes, osteomyelitis usually affects the intervertebral disk space and often involves adjacent vertebrae.	Osteomyelitis is caused by a broad spectrum of infectious organisms that reach bone by hematogenous spread, extension from a contiguous site of infection, or direct introduction (trauma or surgery). Because the earliest changes are usually not evident on plain radiographs until at least 10 days after the onset of symptoms, radionuclide bone scanning is the most valuable imaging modality for early diagnosis (increased isotope activity reflects the inflammatory process and increased blood flow).

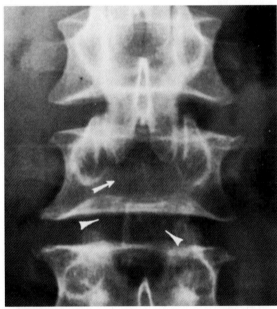

Fig SP 2-7
Metastasis. Osseous destruction (arrowheads) of a portion of the pedicles, the entire lamina, the inferior articulating processes, and the spinal process produces the appearance of an empty vertebral body (arrow).[2]

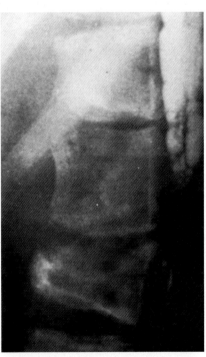

Fig SP 2-8
Lymphoma. Lateral radiograph of the thoracolumbar junction shows lucency of multiple vertebral bodies with destruction and collapse. There is some patchy sclerosis and evidence of a previous myelogram.[2]

Osteosclerotic Vertebral Lesions

Condition	Imaging Findings	Comments
Bone island (enostosis/endosteoma)	Circular or triangular areas of dense compact bone in the vertebral body (occasionally the posterior elements) that are usually homogeneous with a well-defined margin but infrequently show radiating spicules.	Asymptomatic, completely benign, and detected in approximately 1% of individuals. May present a diagnostic dilemma when seen in a patient with a known malignancy and possible metastases. Typically shows no activity on radionuclide bone scans (unlike metastases), though some bone islands may demonstrate isotope uptake.
Osteoblastic metastases (Fig SP 3-1)	Single or multiple ill-defined areas of increased density that may progress to complete loss of normal bony architecture. Vary from a small, isolated round focus of sclerotic density to a diffuse sclerosis involving most or all of a bone (eg, ivory vertebral body).	Osteoblastic metastases are most commonly secondary to lymphoma and carcinomas of the breast and prostate. Other primary tumors include carcinomas of the gastrointestinal tract, lung, and urinary bladder. Osteoblastic metastases are generally considered to be evidence of slow growth in a neoplasm that has allowed time for reactive bone proliferation.
Paget's disease (Fig SP 3-2)	In the reparative stage, there is a mixed lytic and sclerotic pattern with cortical thickening and enlargement of affected bone. In the sclerotic stage, there may be a uniform increased density (eg, ivory vertebra).	The purely sclerotic phase is less common than the combined destructive and reparative stages. An ivory vertebra may simulate osteoblastic metastases or Hodgkin's disease, though in Paget's disease the vertebra is also expanded.

A   B

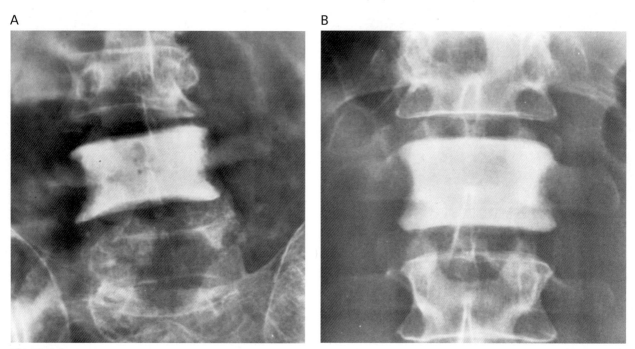

Fig SP 3-1
Osteoblastic metastases (ivory vertebrae). (A) Carcinoma of the prostate. (B) Lymphoma.

Condition	Imaging Findings	Comments
Osteomyelitis (chronic or healed) (Fig SP 3-3)	Thickening and sclerosis of bone with an irregular outer margin surrounding a central ill-defined area of lucency.	After a variable period (10 to 12 weeks), regenerative changes appear in the bone with sclerosis or eburnation. The severity of osteosclerotic response is variable. Although extensive sclerosis has been described as typical of pyogenic rather than tuberculous infection, this appearance may also be evident in tuberculosis, particularly in black patients. With early and proper treatment of pyogenic infection, a completely radiodense (ivory) vertebra may be produced.
Osteoid osteoma (Fig SP 3-4)	Small, round or oval lucent nidus surrounded by a large, dense sclerotic zone of cortical thickening. The nidus may only be detectable on tomography.	Benign bone tumor that usually develops in young men. Classic clinical symptom is local pain that is worse at night and is dramatically relieved by aspirin. In the spine, osteoid osteomas most commonly arise in the posterior elements and are often associated with scoliosis. Surgical excision of the nidus is essential for cure. (It is not necessary to remove the reactive calcification.)
Osteochondroma (exostosis)	Cartilage-covered osseous excrescence that arises from the surface of a bone. Typically, there is a blending of the cortex of an osteochondroma with that of normal bone.	Although the spine is affected infrequently, lesions developing in the vertebral column or ribs can cause spinal cord compression. Vertebral osteochondromas primarily involve the posterior elements, especially the spinous processes, and tend to arise in the lumbar and cervical regions. Rapid growth or the development of localized pain suggests malignant degeneration to chondrosarcoma.

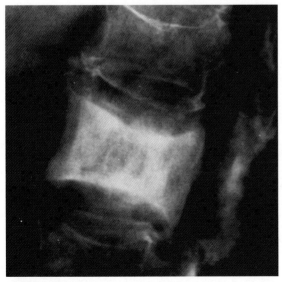

Fig SP 3-2
Paget's disease. Sclerotic vertebral body with associated enlargement and cortical thickening.[4]

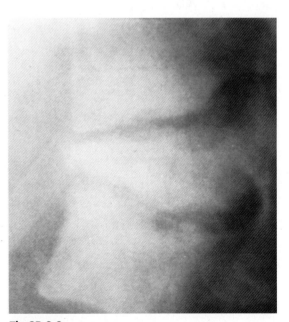

Fig SP 3-3
Chronic osteomyelitis. There is destruction and collapse of bone with reactive sclerosis and narrowing of two intervertebral disk spaces. Note the poorly defined or fuzzy diskovertebral junctions associated with this pyogenic infection.[2]

Condition	Imaging Findings	Comments
Multiple myeloma	Generalized patchy or uniform bone sclerosis.	Very rare manifestation. Scattered, slow-growing osteoblastic lesions with dense plasmacytic infiltrates and normal laboratory findings may be termed *plasma-cell granuloma*.
Mastocytosis (Fig SP 3-5)	Scattered sclerotic foci (simulating metastases) or uniform ivory vertebra.	Caused by diffuse deposits of mast cells in the bone marrow. Episodic release of histamine from mast cells causes typical symptoms of pruritus, flushing, tachycardia, asthma, and headaches, as well as an increased incidence of peptic ulcers. There often is hepatosplenomegaly, lymphadenopathy, and pancytopenia.

A

B

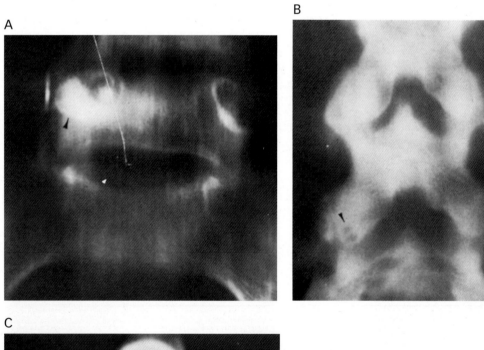

C

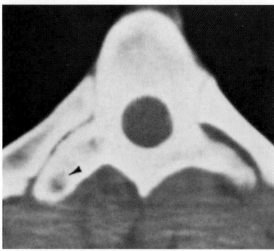

Fig SP 3-4
Osteoid osteoma. (A) Sclerotic lesion of a pedicle (arrowhead).
(B) Radiolucent nidus (arrowhead) in an inferior articular process.
(C) Axial CT scan clearly shows the radiolucent nidus (arrowhead) in
a transverse process.[2]

Condition	Imaging Findings	Comments
Osteopoikilosis (Fig SP 3-6)	Multiple sclerotic foci (2 mm to 2 cm) producing a typical speckled appearance.	Rare asymptomatic hereditary condition that infrequently involves the spine but tends to affect the small bones of the hands and feet, the pelvis, and the epiphyses and metaphyses of long bones.
Melorheostosis (Fig SP 3-7)	Irregular sclerotic thickening of the cortex, usually confined to one side of a single bone or to multiple bones of one extremity.	Rare disorder. Axial involvement may be accompanied by fibrolipomatous lesions in the spinal canal. In the extremities, sclerosis typically begins at the proximal end of the bone and extends distally, resembling wax flowing down a burning candle.
Congenital stippled epiphyses (chondrodysplasia punctata) (Fig SP 3-8)	Multiple punctate calcifications occurring in epiphyses before the normal time for appearance of ossification centers.	Rare condition that most commonly involves the hips, knees, shoulders, and wrists. Affected bones may be shortened, or the process may regress and leave no deformity. Abnormalities of vertebral end plates may cause the vertebral bodies to have an irregular shape and lead to the development of kyphoscoliosis.

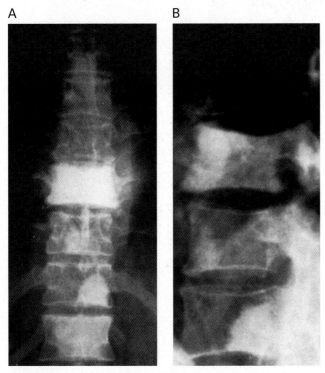

Fig SP 3-5
Mastocytosis. (A) Frontal and (B) lateral radiographs of the thoracic region of the spine show focal osteosclerotic lesions associated with paravertebral swelling.[2]

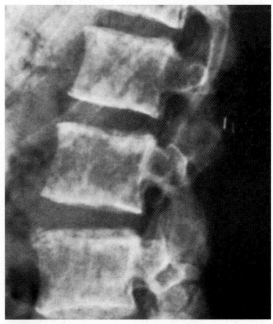

Fig SP 3-6
Osteopoikilosis. Multiple sclerotic foci in the margins of the vertebral bodies and posterior elements.[2]

Condition	Imaging Findings	Comments
Tuberous sclerosis (Fig SP 3-9)	Dense sclerotic foci that may be discrete and round, ovoid, or flame-shaped. In the spine, the pedicles and posterior portions of the vertebral bodies are most often involved.	Rare inherited disorder presenting with the clinical triad of convulsive seizures, mental deficiency, and adenoma sebaceum. Associated with renal and intracranial hamartomas and characteristic scattered intracerebral calcifications.

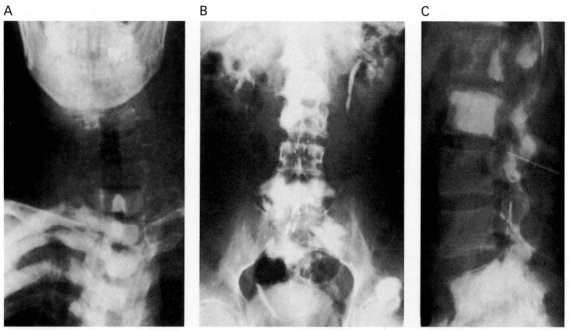

A B C

Fig SP 3-7
Melorheostosis. (A, B, and C) Three radiographs of the axial skeleton show hyperostosis and enostoses involving the upper right ribs, the thoracic and lumbar vertebrae, the sacrum, and the ilium. Quadriparesis developed in this 21-year-old man because of a diffuse intramedullary lipoma in the spinal cord.[2]

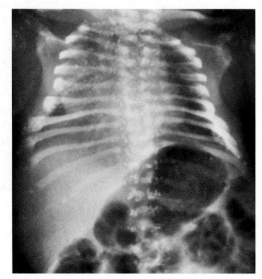

Fig SP 3-8
Congenital stippled epiphyses. Multiple, small punctate calcifications of various sizes involve virtually all the epiphyses in this view of the chest and upper abdomen.

Condition	Imaging Findings	Comments
Callus formation	Localized increase in bone density about a healed or healing fracture.	History of trauma is helpful in making this diagnosis.

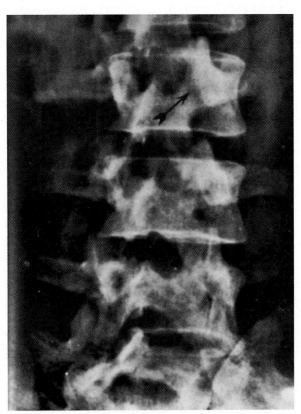

Fig SP 3-9
Tuberous sclerosis. Left oblique view shows a homogeneously dense left pedicle and superior articular facet (arrow). This was an incidental finding on excretory urography.[2]

Generalized Vertebral Osteosclerosis

Condition	Imaging Findings	Comments
Myelofibrosis (myelosclerosis, myeloid metaplasia) (Fig SP 4-1)	Approximately half the patients have a widespread, diffuse increase in bone density (ground-glass appearance) that primarily affects the spine, ribs, and pelvis. Increased radiodensity or condensation of bone at the inferior and superior margins of the vertebral body can produce a "sandwich" appearance.	Hematologic disorder in which gradual replacement of marrow by fibrosis produces a varying degree of anemia and a leukemoid blood picture. Most commonly idiopathic, though a large percentage of patients have antecedent polycythemia vera. Extramedullary hematopoiesis causes massive splenomegaly, often hepatomegaly, and sometimes tumor-like masses in the posterior mediastinum. Uniform obliteration of fine trabecular margins of the ribs results in sclerosis simulating jail bars crossing the thorax.
Osteoblastic metastases (Fig SP 4-2)	Generalized diffuse osteosclerosis.	Primarily lymphoma and carcinomas of the prostate and breast.
Paget's disease (Fig SP 4-3)	Diffuse osteosclerosis may develop in advanced stages of polyostotic disease.	Although the radiographic appearance may simulate that of osteoblastic metastases, characteristic cortical thickening and coarse trabeculation should suggest Paget's disease.
Sickle cell anemia	Diffuse sclerosis with coarsening of the trabecular pattern may be a late manifestation reflecting medullary infarction.	Initially, generalized osteoporosis due to marrow hyperplasia. Common findings include typical "fish vertebrae," a high incidence of acute osteomyelitis in the extremities (often caused by *Salmonella* infection), splenomegaly, and extramedullary hematopoiesis.

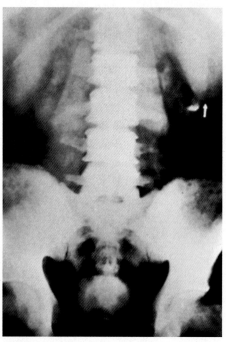

Fig SP 4-1
Myelofibrosis. Uniform sclerosis of the spine and pelvis seen on a film from an excretory urogram. The renal function is obviously diminished, and the spleen is enlarged (arrow).[2]

Condition	Imaging Findings	Comments
Osteopetrosis (Albers-Schönberg disease, marble bones) (Fig SP 4-4)	Symmetric, generalized increase in bone density involving the entire skeleton. Typical patterns in the spine are a "bone-within-a-bone" appearance (a miniature bone inset in each vertebral body) and "sandwich" vertebrae (increased density at the end plates). In the extremities, lack of modeling causes widening of the metaphyseal ends of tubular bones.	Rare hereditary bone dysplasia in which failure of the resorptive mechanism of calcified cartilage interferes with its normal replacement by mature bone. Varies in severity and age of clinical presentation from a fulminant, often fatal condition at birth to an essentially asymptomatic form that is an incidental radiographic finding. Although radiographically dense, the involved bones are brittle, and fractures are common even with trivial trauma. Extensive extramedullary hematopoiesis (hepatosplenomegaly and lymphadenopathy).

A

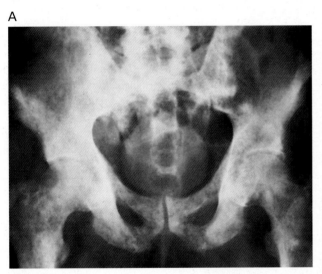

B

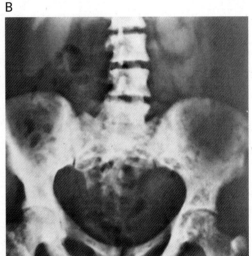

Fig SP 4-2
Osteoblastic metastases. (A) Carcinoma of the prostate. (B) Carcinoma of the breast.

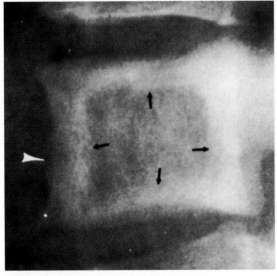

Fig SP 4-3
Paget's disease. Picture-frame vertebral body with condensation of bone along its peripheral margins (arrows). There is straightening of the anterior surface of the bone (arrowhead) and involvement of the pedicles.[2]

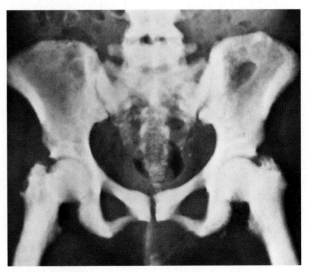

Fig SP 4-4
Osteopetrosis. Generalized sclerosis of the lower spine, pelvis, and hips in a 74-year-old woman with the tarda form of this condition.

Condition	Imaging Findings	Comments
Pyknodysostosis	Diffuse dense, sclerotic bones. Characteristically there is mandibular hypoplasia with loss of the normal mandibular angle and craniofacial disproportion.	Rare hereditary bone dysplasia. Patients have short stature, but hepatosplenomegaly is infrequent. Numerous wormian bones may simulate cleidocranial dysostosis. Unlike osteopetrosis, in the long bones the medullary cavities are preserved, and there is no metaphyseal widening.
Fluorosis (Fig SP 4-5)	Dense skeletal sclerosis most prominent in the vertebrae and pelvis. Obliteration of individual trabeculae may cause affected bones to appear chalky white. There is often calcification of interosseous membranes and ligaments (paraspinal, iliolumbar, sacrotuberous, and sacrospinous). Vertebral osteophytosis can lead to encroachment of the spinal canal and neural foramina.	Fluorine poisoning may result from drinking water with a high concentration of fluorides, industrial exposure (mining, smelting), or excessive therapeutic intake of fluoride (treatment of myeloma or Paget's disease). Periosteal roughening, hyperostosis, and bony excrescences often develop at sites of muscular and ligamentous attachments at the iliac crests, ischial tuberosities, and long bones.
Mastocytosis (see Fig SP 3-5)	Diffuse sclerosis; single ivory vertebra; or scattered, well-defined sclerotic foci simulating metastases.	Caused by diffuse deposits of mast cells in the bone marrow. Episodic release of histamine from mast cells causes typical symptoms of pruritus, flushing, tachycardia, asthma, and headaches, as well as an increased incidence of peptic ulcers. There often is hepatosplenomegaly, lymphadenopathy, and pancytopenia.

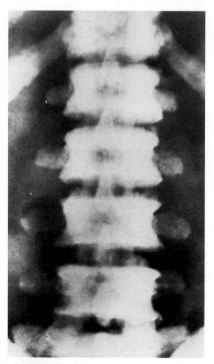

Fig SP 4-5
Fluorosis. Diffuse vertebral sclerosis with obliteration of individual trabeculae.[5]

Condition	Imaging Findings	Comments
Renal osteodystrophy (Fig SP 4-6)	Thick bands of increased density adjacent to the superior and inferior margins of vertebral bodies producing the characteristic "rugger jersey" spine.	Other findings include generalized demineralization of vertebral bodies producing arch-like contour defects of the end plates (simulating osteoporosis) and herniation of disk material into the vertebral bodies because of weakening of the diskovertebral junction related to subchondral resorption.
Multiple myeloma	Uniform sclerosis of bone.	Very rare manifestation.

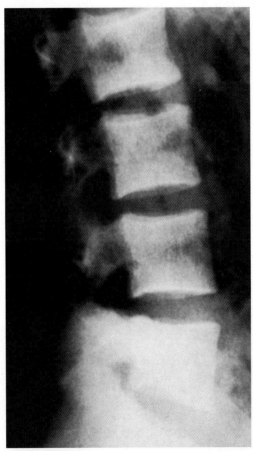

Fig SP 4-6
Renal osteodystrophy. Areas of increased sclerosis subjacent to the cartilaginous plates produce the characteristic "rugger jersey" spine in this patient with chronic renal failure.[2]

Increase in Size of One or More Vertebrae

Condition	Comments
Acromegaly (Fig SP 5-1)	Appositional bone growth results in a generalized increase in the size of the vertebral bodies. Hypertrophy of cartilage widens the intervertebral disk spaces, whereas hypertrophy of soft tissue may lead to an increased concavity (scalloping) of the posterior aspects of the vertebral bodies.
Paget's disease (Fig SP 5-2)	Generalized enlargement of affected vertebral bodies. Increased trabeculation, which is most prominent at the periphery of the bone, produces a rim of thickened cortex and a picture-frame appearance. Dense sclerosis of one or more vertebral bodies (ivory vertebrae) may present a pattern simulating osteoblastic metastases or Hodgkin's disease, though in Paget's disease the vertebrae are also enlarged.
Congenital (Fig SP 5-3)	Fusion or partial fusion of two or more vertebral bodies (block vertebra) is a frequent occurrence. The underlying bone is otherwise normal. Congenital fusion can usually be differentiated from that resulting from disease because the total height of the combined fused bodies is equal to the normal height of two vertebrae less the intervertebral disk space.

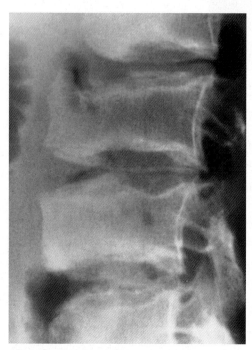

Fig SP 5-1
Acromegaly. Enlargement of all vertebral bodies, especially in the anteroposterior direction. Note the mild posterior scalloping.

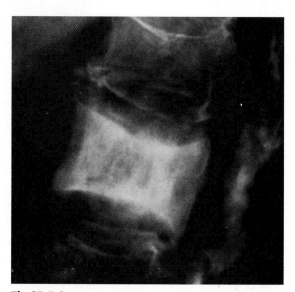

Fig SP 5-2
Paget's disease. Enlargement and cortical thickening of a vertebral body, producing an ivory vertebra.[4]

Condition	Comments
Neuromuscular deficit	Increased height of the vertebral bodies related to the absence of normal vertical stress may develop in patients who cannot bear weight (eg, paralysis, Down's syndrome, rubella syndrome).
Benign bone tumor	Expansion of a vertebral body may result from hemangioma, aneurysmal bone cyst, osteoblastoma, or giant cell tumor.
Fibrous dysplasia	Proliferation of fibrous tissue in the medullary cavity may infrequently involve the spine and cause one or more vertebral bodies to expand. Complications include vertebral collapse and spinal cord compression.

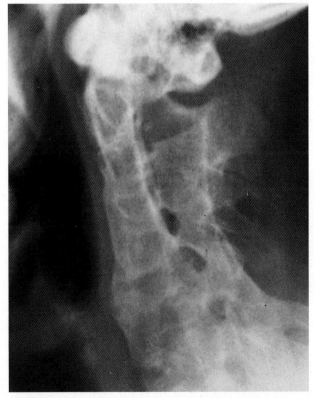

Fig SP 5-3
Block vertebrae. Essentially complete fusion of the cervical spine into a solid mass in a patient with Klippel-Feil deformity.

Loss of Height of One or More Vertebral Bodies

Condition	Imaging Findings	Comments
Osteoporosis (Fig SP 6-1)	Smooth, arch-like indentations of the vertebral end plates that are most marked centrally in the region of the nucleus pulposus. Primarily involves the lumbar and lower thoracic spine (where weight-bearing stress is directed toward the axes of the vertebral bodies).	Regardless of the cause (most commonly senile or postmenopausal osteoporosis, steroid therapy), as the bone density of the vertebral body decreases the cortex appears as a thin line that is relatively dense and prominent, producing a picture-frame pattern. In addition to the typical "fish vertebrae" appearance, osteoporotic vertebral bodies may demonstrate anterior wedging and compression fractures. The characteristic concave contours of the superior and inferior disk surfaces result from expansion of the nucleus pulposus into the weakened vertebral bodies.
Hyperparathyroidism	Generalized demineralization of the vertebral bodies produces arch-like contour defects of the superior and inferior vertebral surfaces, simulating osteoporosis.	Subchondral resorption at the diskovertebral junctions produces areas of structural weakening that allow herniation of disk material into the vertebral body (cartilaginous or Schmorl's nodes). In patients with hyperparathyroidism secondary to renal failure, thick bands of increased density adjacent to the superior and inferior margins of vertebral bodies produce the characteristic "rugger jersey" spine.

A   B

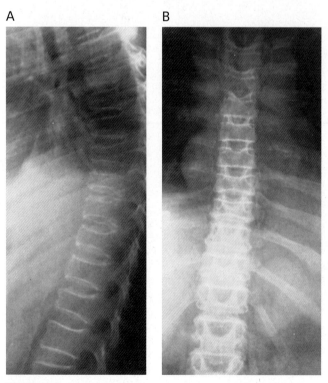

Fig SP 6-1
Severe osteoporosis. (A) Lateral and (B) frontal views of the thoracolumbar spine show striking demineralization and compression of multiple vertebral bodies in a 14½-year-old girl treated with steroids for 5 years for chronic glomerulonephritis. The height age of the girl was only 9 years at this time.[6]

Condition	Imaging Findings	Comments
Osteomalacia	Arch-like contour defects of the superior and inferior surfaces of multiple vertebral bodies, simulating osteoporosis.	Insufficient mineralization of the vertebral bodies. In osteomalacia secondary to renal tubular disorders, hyperostosis may be more prominent than deossification. This results in a striking thickening of the cortices and increased trabeculation of spongy bone. Nevertheless, the bony architecture is abnormal and is prone to fracture with relatively minimal trauma.
Multiple myeloma (Fig SP 6-2)	Generalized skeletal deossification simulating osteoporosis or destructive changes mimicking metastases. Severe loss of bone substance in the spine often results in multiple vertebral compression fractures.	Decreased bone density and destructive changes are usually limited to the vertebral bodies, sparing the pedicles (lacking red marrow) that are frequently destroyed by metastatic disease. Because multiple myeloma causes little or no stimulation of new bone formation, radionuclide bone scans may be normal even with extensive skeletal infiltration.
Metastases	Destructive process involving not only the vertebral bodies but also the pedicles and neural arches. Pathologic collapse of vertebral bodies frequently occurs in advanced disease.	Destruction of one or more pedicles may be the earliest sign of metastatic disease and aids in differentiating this process from multiple myeloma (pedicles are much less often involved). Because cartilage is resistant to invasion by metastases, preservation of the intervertebral disk space may help to distinguish metastases from an inflammatory process.
Osteomyelitis Pyogenic	Various radiographic patterns, including disk space narrowing, loss of the normally sharp adjacent subchondral plates, areas of cortical demineralization, vertebral body destruction and even collapse, and sclerotic new bone formation.	Rapid involvement of the intervertebral disks (loss of disk spaces and destruction of adjacent end plates), in contrast to the vertebral body involvement and preservation of disk spaces in metastatic disease.

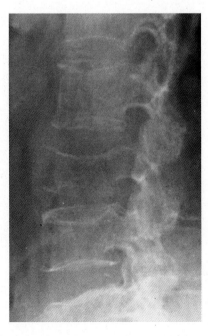

Fig SP 6-2
Multiple myeloma. The diffuse myelomatous infiltration causes generalized demineralization of the vertebral bodies and a compression fracture of L2.

Condition	Imaging Findings	Comments
Tuberculous (Fig SP 6-3)	Irregular, poorly marginated bone destruction in a vertebral body, with narrowing of the adjacent intervertebral disk and extension of infection and bone destruction across the disk to involve the contiguous vertebral body.	Most commonly involves the anterior part of vertebral bodies in the thoracic and lumbar region. Often associated with a paravertebral abscess, an accumulation of purulent material that produces a soft-tissue mass about the vertebra. Unlike pyogenic infection, tuberculous osteomyelitis is rarely associated with periosteal reaction or bone sclerosis. In the untreated patient, progressive vertebral collapse and anterior wedging lead to the development of a characteristic sharp kyphotic angulation and gibbous deformity. Healed lesions may demonstrate mottled calcific deposits in a paravertebral abscess and moderate recalcification and sclerosis of the affected bones.
Brucellosis (Fig SP 6-4)	In the less common central type of vertebral lesion, lytic destruction of the vertebral body leads to vertebral collapse with various degrees of wedging and often the development of a paraspinal abscess (overall pattern closely simulates that of tuberculous infection).	Primarily a disease of animals (cattle, swine, goats, sheep) that is transmitted to humans by the ingestion of infected dairy products or meat or through direct contact with animals, their carcasses, or their excreta. In the more common peripheral form, loss of cortical definition or frank erosions of the anterior and superior margins of the vertebral bodies and disk space narrowing is followed by reactive sclerosis and hypertrophic spur formation.
Fungal infections	Generally produce spinal involvement mimicking tuberculosis.	Infrequent manifestation of actinomycosis, blastomycosis, coccidioidomycosis, cryptococcosis, or aspergillosis. The diagnosis depends on biopsy and culture of the organism.

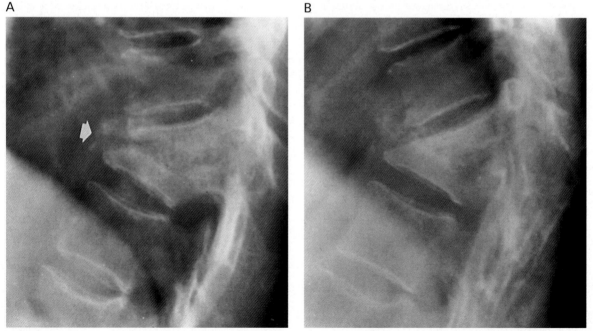

Fig SP 6-3
Tuberculous osteomyelitis of the thoracic spine. (A) Initial film demonstrates vertebral collapse and anterior wedging of adjacent midthoracic vertebrae (arrow). The residual intervertebral disk space can barely be seen. (B) Several months later, there is virtual fusion of the collapsed vertebral bodies, producing a characteristic sharp kyphotic angulation (gibbous deformity).

Condition	Imaging Findings	Comments
Fractures (Fig SP 6-5)	Primarily anterior wedging of the superior end plate of a vertebral body. Severe compressive forces may drive the nucleus pulposus into the vertebral body, resulting in a burst fracture with the posterosuperior fragment often driven into the spinal canal. In patients who have jumped from great heights, compression fractures of the thoracolumbar junction are frequently associated with a fracture of the calcaneus.	Primarily involve the T11 to L4 region. In older patients, it may be difficult to distinguish an acute spinal fracture from the vertebral compression that is frequently associated with osteoporosis. In acute trauma, there is often evidence of cortical disruption, a paraspinal soft-tissue mass, or an ill-defined increase in density beneath the end plate of an involved vertebra, indicating bone impaction. In osteoporosis, vertebral compression is often associated with osteophytic spurs arising from the apposing margins of the involved and adjacent vertebral bodies. An acute spinal fracture may be difficult to distinguish from a pathologic fracture caused by metastases or multiple myeloma. (The presence of bone destruction, especially involving the cortex, indicates a pathologic fracture.)
Scheuermann's disease (vertebral epiphysitis) (Fig SP 6-6)	Irregularity and loss of the sharp outline of the ring-like epiphyses along the upper and lower margins of vertebral bodies that are followed by fragmentation and sclerosis, causing the adjacent border of the vertebral body to become irregular. The affected vertebrae tend to become wedge shaped (they decrease in height anteriorly).	Occurs in both sexes between the ages of 12 and 17. Although the cause of this familial condition is unclear, possible contributing factors include circulatory disturbances, early disk degeneration, and faulty ossification. Wedging of vertebral bodies produces a dorsal kyphosis, which persists even after the disease has healed.
Langerhans cell histiocytosis (Fig SP 6-7)	Spotty destruction in a vertebral body that proceeds to collapse. The vertebra assumes the shape of a thin flat disk (vertebra plana).	Most commonly occurs in children younger than age 10. The intervertebral disk spaces are preserved.

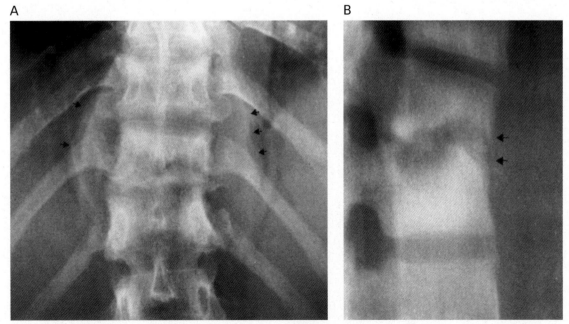

Fig SP 6-4
Brucellosis. (A) Frontal plain film of the lower thoracic spine demonstrates loss of height of the T11 and T12 vertebral bodies with destruction of the end plates and swelling of the paravertebral soft tissues (arrows). (B) A lateral tomogram of the lower thoracic spine demonstrates cortical destruction with sclerosis of the inferior end plate of T11 and the superior end plate of T12 (arrows). There is a mild degree of anterior wedging. The overall radiographic appearance is indistinguishable from that of tuberculous spondylitis.

Condition	Imaging Findings	Comments
Morquio syndrome (Fig SP 6-8)	Universal flattening of vertebral bodies (vertebrae planae).	Characteristic central anterior beaking in this form of mucopolysaccharidosis.

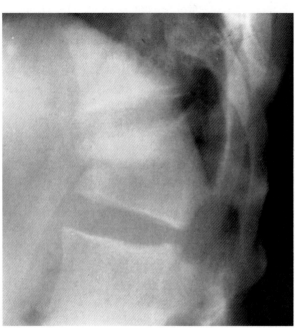

Fig SP 6-5
Fracture. Characteristic anterior wedging of the superior end plate of the L1 vertebral body.

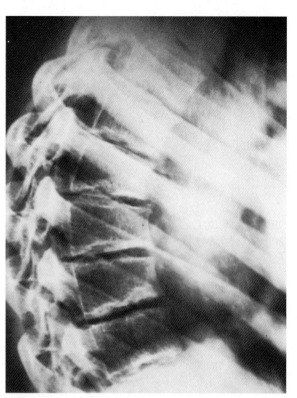

Fig SP 6-6
Scheuermann's disease. Irregularity of the vertebral end plates and wedging of the vertebral bodies, which causes an arcuate kyphosis.[7]

A

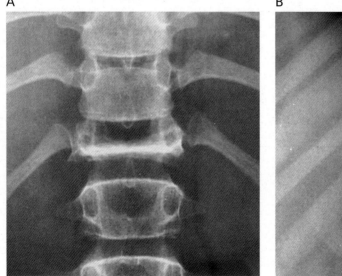

B

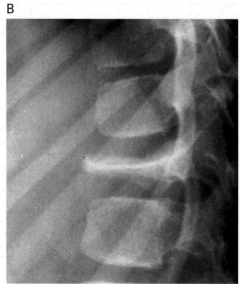

Fig SP 6-7
Langerhans cell histiocytosis. (A) Frontal and (B) lateral views of the spine show complete collapse with flattening of the T12 vertebral body (vertebra plana).

Condition	Imaging Findings	Comments
Spondyloepiphyseal dysplasia (Fig SP 6-9)	Generalized flattening of lumbar vertebral bodies, often with a distinctive hump-shaped mound of bone on their superior and inferior surfaces.	Rare hereditary dwarfism that affects both the extremities and the vertebrae. Characteristic findings include flattening of the femoral capital epiphyses with early degenerative changes, a small pelvis, and a general delay in ossification of the skeleton.
Paget's disease	Arch-like contour defects of the superior and inferior vertebral surfaces or a pathologic fracture.	Although there is typically enlargement of the vertebral body with increased trabeculation that is most prominent at the periphery, the weakened bone permits expansion of the nucleus pulposus and results in an increased incidence of pathologic fracture.
Sickle cell anemia (Fig SP 6-10)	Localized step-like central depression of multiple vertebral end plates. There may also be biconcave indentations on the superior and inferior margins of the softened vertebral bodies due to expansile pressure of the adjacent intervertebral disks.	Probably caused by circulatory stasis and ischemia, which retard growth in the central portion of the vertebral cartilaginous growth plate while the periphery of the growth plate (with a different blood supply) continues to grow at a more normal rate.
Gaucher's disease	Localized step-like central depression of multiple vertebral end plates.	Probably caused by circulatory stasis and ischemia, which retard growth in the central portion of the vertebral cartilaginous growth plate while the periphery of the growth plate (with a different blood supply) continues to grow at a more normal rate. This inborn error of metabolism is characterized by the accumulation of abnormal quantities of complex lipids in the reticuloendothelial cells of the spleen, liver, and bone marrow.

B

A

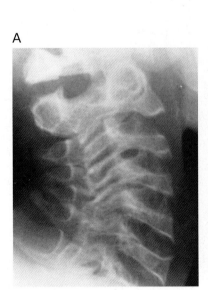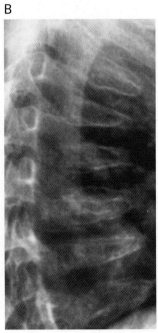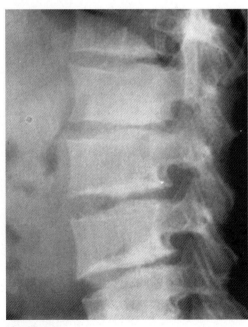

Fig SP 6-8
Morquio syndrome. Generalized flattening of the vertebral bodies in the (A) cervical and (B) lumbar regions.

Fig SP 6-9
Spondyloepiphyseal dysplasia. Generalized flattening of the vertebral bodies (platyspondyly).

Condition	Imaging Findings	Comments
Primary bone neoplasm	Various patterns of bone destruction and patho-logic fracture.	Benign tumor (hemangioma, giant cell tumor, aneurysmal bone cyst); lymphoma; sarcoma; chordoma (sacrum).
Osteogenesis imperfecta (Fig SP 6-11)	Flattening of vertebral bodies, which are either biconcave or wedge shaped anteriorly.	Inherited generalized disorder of connective tissue causing thin, brittle bones. Severe kyphoscoliosis results from a combination of ligamentous laxity, osteoporosis, and post-traumatic deformities.
Convulsions (Fig SP 6-12)	Multiple compression fractures, primarily invol-ving the midthoracic vertebrae.	Tetanus (*Clostridium tetani*); tetany; hypoglycemia; shock therapy. Although the degree of compression may be substantial, the fractures infrequently cause pain and usually do not lead to neurologic sequelae.
Vanishing bone disease	Diffuse destruction of multiple vertebral bodies.	Rare condition that most often involves the pelvis, ribs, spine, and long bones. No sclerotic or periosteal reaction.
Amyloidosis	Loss of bone density and collapse of one or more vertebral bodies.	Rare manifestation caused by diffuse infiltration of the bone marrow by the amorphous protein. Generalized demineralization with collapse of vertebral bodies is usually a manifestation of underlying multiple myeloma.
Hydatid (echinococcal) cyst	Expanding lytic lesion causing a pathologic fracture.	Bone involvement occurs in approximately 1% of patients and most commonly affects the vertebral bodies, pelvis, and sacrum.

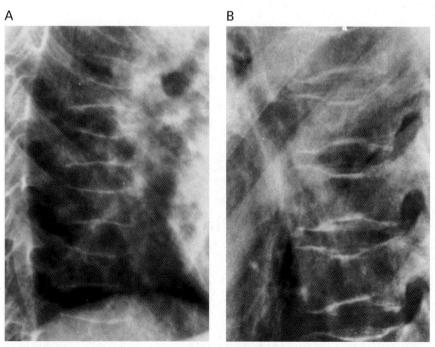

A   B

Fig SP 6-10
Sickle cell anemia. (A) Biconcave indentations on both the superior and inferior margins of the soft vertebral bodies produce the characteristic "fish vertebrae." (B) Localized step-like central depressions of multiple vertebral end plates.

Condition	Imaging Findings	Comments
Traumatic ischemic necrosis (Kümmell's spondylitis)	Delayed post-traumatic reaction characterized by rarefaction of the vertebral body, intravertebral vacuum cleft, and vertebral collapse.	The existence of this condition is controversial. Most authorities believe that significant trauma to the spine occurred at the time of the initial injury in instances of alleged Kümmell's spondylitis.
Thanatophoric dwarfism	Extreme flattening of hypoplastic vertebral bodies.	An H or U configuration of the vertebral bodies can be seen on frontal projections.

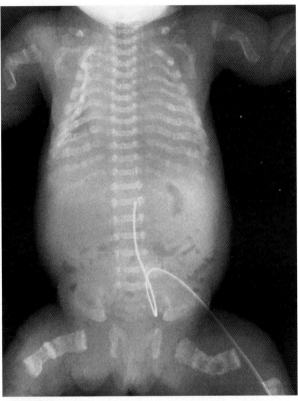

Fig SP 6-11
Osteogenesis imperfecta. Generalized flattening of vertebral bodies associated with fractures of multiple ribs and long bones in an infant.

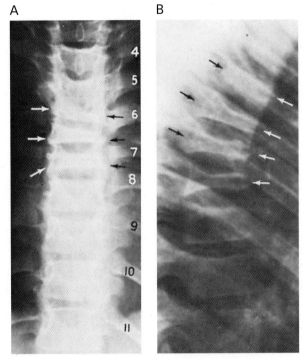

Fig SP 6-12
Tetanus. (A) Frontal and (B) lateral projections show residual fractures and compression deformities of vertebral bodies (arrows).[8]

Narrowing of the Intervertebral Disk Space and Adjacent Sclerosis

Condition	Imaging Findings	Comments
Intervertebral osteochondrosis (degenerative disk disease) (Fig SP 7-1)	Well-defined sclerosis of vertebral margins and characteristic "vacuum" phenomenon.	Degeneration of the nucleus pulposus and the cartilaginous end plate.
Infection (Figs SP 7-2 through SP 7-4)	Ill-defined vertebral margins and often a soft-tissue mass. Reactive sclerosis is common with pyogenic inflammation but infrequent with tuberculosis.	Depending on the site of disease, anterior extension of vertebral osteomyelitis may cause retropharyngeal abscess, mediastinitis, pericarditis, subdiaphragmatic abscess, psoas muscle abscess, or peritonitis. Posterior extension of inflammatory tissue can compress the spinal cord or produce meningitis if the infection penetrates the dura to enter the subarachnoid space.
Trauma	Well-defined sclerotic vertebral margins, soft-tissue mass, and evidence of fracture.	Disk injury and degeneration is the underlying mechanism.
Neuroarthropathy (Fig SP 7-5)	Extensive sclerosis of the vertebrae associated with osteophytosis, fragmentation, and malalignment.	Caused by repetitive trauma in patients with loss of sensation and proprioception due to such conditions as diabetes, syphilis, syringomyelia, leprosy, and congenital insensitivity to pain.
Calcium pyrophosphate dihydrate deposition (CPPD) disease	Ill- or well-defined sclerotic vertebral margins associated with fragmentation, subluxation, and calcification.	Degenerative process secondary to the deposition of calcium pyrophosphate dihydrate crystals in cartilaginous end plates and intervertebral disks.
Ochronosis (see Fig SP 14-2)	Well-defined sclerotic vertebral margins with "vacuum" phenomena and pathognomonic diskal calcification.	Degenerative change resulting from the deposition of the black pigment of oxidized homogentisic acid in cartilaginous end plates and intervertebral disks.

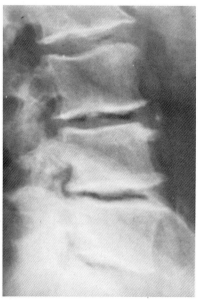

Fig SP 7-1
Degenerative disk disease. Hypertrophic spurring, intervertebral disk space narrowing, and reactive sclerosis. Note the linear lucent collections (vacuum phenomenon) overlying several of the intervertebral disks.

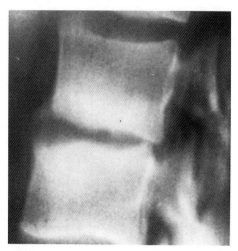

Fig SP 7-2
Pyogenic vertebral osteomyelitis. Narrowing of the intervertebral disk space with irregularity of the end plates and reactive sclerosis.

Condition	Imaging Findings	Comments
Rheumatoid arthritis	Ill- or well-defined sclerotic vertebral margins associated with subluxations and apophyseal joint abnormalities.	Loss of the intervertebral disk space (usually in the cervical region) may reflect apophyseal joint instability with recurrent diskovertebral trauma or extension of inflammatory tissue from neighboring articulations.

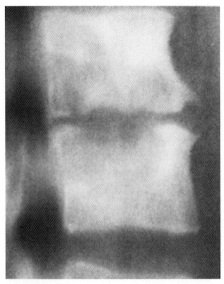

Fig SP 7-3
Pseudomonas osteomyelitis. Tomogram shows the destructive process in L2 and L3, irregular narrowing of the intervertebral disk space, and reactive sclerosis.

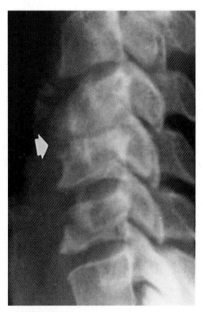

Fig SP 7-4
Tuberculous osteomyelitis of the cervical spine. Narrowing of the intervertebral disk space (arrow) is accompanied by diffuse bone destruction involving the adjacent vertebrae. Note the lack of sclerotic reaction.

A   B

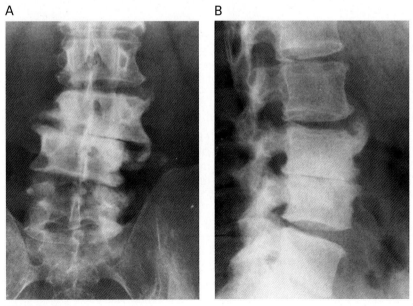

Fig SP 7-5
Neuroarthropathy. (A) Frontal and (B) lateral views of the lumbosacral spine in a patient with tabes dorsalis show marked hypertrophic spurring with virtual obliteration of the intervertebral disk space between L3 and L4. Note the reactive sclerosis of the apposing end plates and the subluxation of the vertebral bodies seen on the frontal view.

Localized Widening of the Interpedicular Distance

Condition	Comments
Intramedullary neoplasm of spinal cord	Large tumors can cause localized thinning and remolding of the pedicles, most commonly at the L1 to L3 level. The most common cause is an ependymoma of the cord, especially of the conus or filum terminale. Also may occur with astrocytoma, oligodendroglioma, glioblastoma multiforme, and medulloblastoma.
Meningocele/ myelomeningocele (Fig SP 8-1)	Large posterior spinal defect through which there is herniation of the meninges (meningocele) or of the meninges and a portion of the spinal cord or nerve roots (myelomeningocele). The posterior defect is marked by absence of the spinous processes and laminae and widening of the interpedicular distance, as well as a soft-tissue mass representing the herniation itself.
Diastematomyelia (Fig SP 8-2)	Fusiform widening of the spinal canal with an increase in the interpedicular distance that extends over several segments is a characteristic finding in this rare malformation in which the spinal cord is split by a midline bony, cartilaginous, or fibrous spur extending posteriorly from a vertebral body. If the septum dividing the cord is ossified, it may appear on frontal views as a pathognomonic thin vertical bony plate lying in the middle of the neural canal. The condition most commonly occurs in the lower thoracic and upper lumbar regions and is often associated with a variety of skeletal and central nervous system anomalies.

A
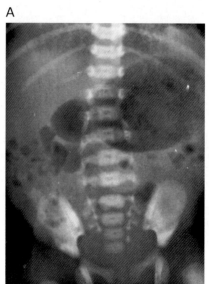
B
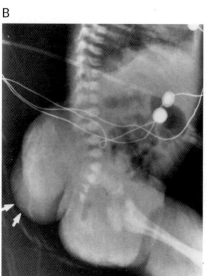

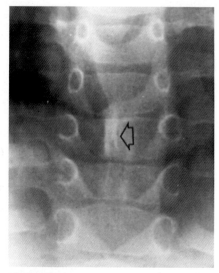

Fig SP 8-1
Meningomyelocele. (A) Frontal view of the abdomen shows the markedly increased interpedicular distance of the lumbar vertebrae. (B) In another patient, a lateral view demonstrates the large soft-tissue mass (arrows) situated posterior to the spine. Note the absence of the posterior elements in the lower lumbar and sacral regions.

Fig SP 8-2
Diastematomyelia. Note the pathognomonic ossified septum (arrow) lying in the midline of the neural canal.

Anterior Scalloping of a Vertebral Body

Condition	Comments
Lymphoma/chronic leukemia	Erosion of the anterior surfaces of upper lumbar and lower thoracic vertebral bodies is caused by direct neoplastic extension from adjacent lymph nodes. Other skeletal abnormalities include paravertebral soft-tissue masses, dense vertebral sclerosis (ivory vertebrae), and a mottled pattern of destruction and sclerosis with hematogenous spread that may simulate metastatic disease.
Other causes of lymphadenopathy	Metastases or inflammatory processes (especially tuberculosis).
Aortic aneurysm	Continuous pulsatile pressure can rarely cause erosions of the anterior aspect of one or more vertebral bodies. The concomitant demonstration of the calcified wall of the bulging aneurysm is virtually pathognomonic.

Posterior Scalloping of a Vertebral Body

Condition	Comments
Normal variant (physiologic scalloping)	Minimal to moderate posterior scalloping limited to the lumbar spine can be demonstrated in approximately half of normal adults. The appearance is identical to that of a mild degree of pathologic scalloping, but there is no associated pedicle abnormality or widening of the interpedicular distance.
Increased intraspinal pressure	Posterior scalloping most commonly occurs with local expanding lesions that are situated in the more caudal portion of the spinal canal, are relatively large and slow growing, and originate during the period of active growth and bone modeling. Generally reflects an intraspinal neoplasm (ependymoma, dermoid, lipoma, or neurofibroma). Intraspinal meningiomas rarely produce even minor bone changes because they are situated above the level of the conus and tend to produce cord symptoms while still relatively small. Other rare underlying causes include spinal cysts, syringomyelia and hydromyelia, and severe, generalized communicating hydrocephalus.
Achondroplasia (Fig SP 10-1)	Decreased endochondral bone formation causes the pedicles to be short and the interpedicular spaces to narrow progressively from above downward (opposite of normal), thus reducing the volume of the spinal canal. This is postulated to limit the normal posterior enlargement of the vertebral canal during the early growth period, with the result that the growing subarachnoid space must gain room for expansion through scalloping of the posterior aspects of the vertebral bodies.
Neurofibromatosis (Fig SP 10-2)	Posterior scalloping may reflect an osseous dysplasia, weakness of the dura (permitting transmission of cerebrospinal fluid pulsations to the bone), or an associated thoracic meningocele.
Hereditary connective tissue disorders (dural ectasia)	Posterior scalloping is secondary to loss of the normal protection afforded the posterior surfaces of the vertebral bodies by an intact, strong dura. The underlying mesodermal dysplasia causes dural ectasia or weakness that permits transmission of cerebrospinal fluid pulsations to the bone. Occurs in such congenital syndromes as Ehlers-Danlos, Marfan's, and osteogenesis imperfecta tarda.
Mucopolysaccharidoses (Fig SP 10-3)	Inborn disorders of mucopolysaccharide metabolism in Hurler's and Morquio's syndromes may produce abnormal vertebral bodies that are unable to resist the normal cerebrospinal fluid pulsations over their posterior surfaces (even though the dura is normal).

A

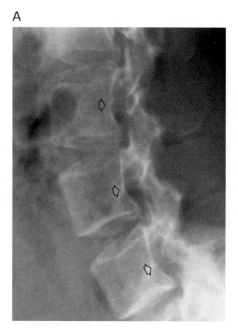

B

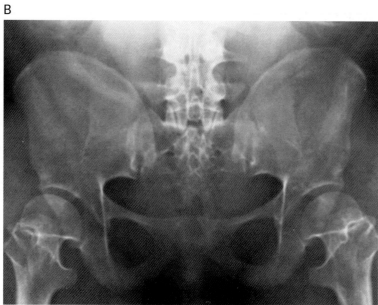

Fig SP 10-1
Achondroplasia. (A) Posterior scalloping of multiple vertebral bodies (arrows). (B) Characteristic short, broad pelvis with small sacrosciatic notch.

Condition	Comments
Acromegaly (Fig SP 10-4)	Hypertrophy of soft tissue may produce posterior scalloping.

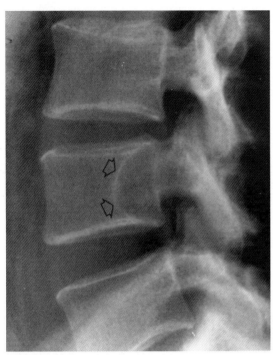

Fig SP 10-2
Neurofibromatosis (arrows).

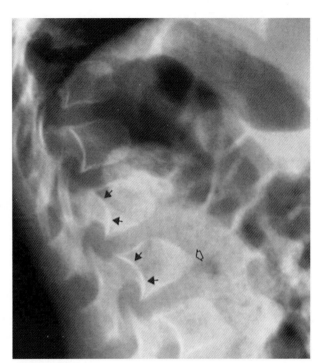

Fig SP 10-3
Hurler's syndrome. In addition to the posterior scalloping (closed arrows), there is typical inferior breaking (open arrow) of the anterior margin of the vertebral body.

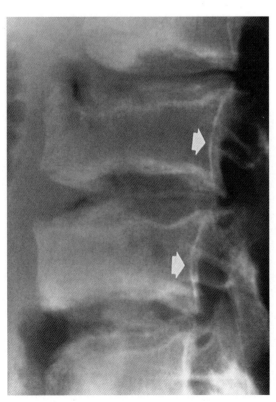

Fig SP 10-4
Acromegaly. Posterior scalloping (arrows) associated with enlargement of vertebral bodies (especially in the anteroposterior dimension).

Squaring of One or More Vertebral Bodies

Condition	Comments
Ankylosing spondylitis (Fig SP 11-1)	Erosive osteitis of the corners of the vertebral bodies produces a loss of the normal anterior concavity and a characteristic squared vertebral body. Spinal involvement initially involves the lower lumbar area and progresses upward to the dorsal and cervical regions. Characteristic bilateral and symmetric sacroiliitis and a "bamboo" spine (ossification in paravertebral tissues and longitudinal spinal ligaments combined with extensive lateral bony bridges, or syndesmophytes).
Paget's disease	Enlargement of affected vertebral bodies with increased trabeculation that is most prominent at the periphery of the bone and produces a rim of thickened cortex and a squared, picture-frame appearance. Dense sclerosis may produce an ivory vertebra.
Rheumatoid variants	Uncommon manifestation of rheumatoid arthritis, psoriatic arthritis, or Reiter's syndrome.
Down's syndrome (mongolism)	Manifestations include a decrease in the acetabular and iliac angles with hypoplasia and marked lateral flaring of the iliac wings, multiple manubrial ossification centers, the presence of 11 ribs, and shortening of the middle phalanx of the fifth finger.

A

B

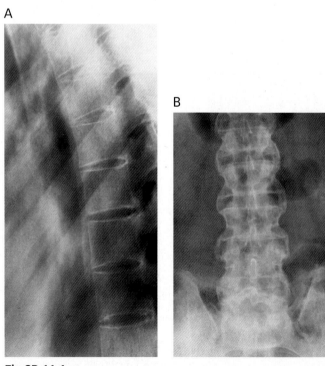

Fig SP 11-1
Ankylosing spondylitis. (A) Characteristic squaring of thoracic vertebral bodies. (B) Extensive lateral bony bridges (syndesmophytes) connect all the lumbar vertebral bodies to produce a bamboo spine.

Enlarged Cervical Intervertebral Foramen

Condition	Comments
Neurofibroma (Fig SP 12-1)	The most common cause of an enlarged cervical intervertebral foramen is the "dumbbell" type of neurofibroma (intradural and extradural components) that erodes the superior or inferior margins of the pedicles. Enlargement of an intervertebral foramen may also develop because of protrusion of a lateral intrathoracic meningocele in a patient with generalized neurofibromatosis.
Other spinal tumors	Rare manifestation of dermoid, lipoma, lymphoma, meningioma, and neuroblastoma.
Congenital absence of pedicle	Produces the radiographic appearance of an enlarged cervical intervertebral foramen.
Vertebral artery aneurysm or tortuosity (Fig SP 12-2)	Erosion is caused by pulsatile flow as the vertebral artery passes through the foramina transversaria of the upper six cervical vertebrae between its origin from the subclavian artery and its entrance into the cranial vault through the foramen magnum.
Traumatic avulsion of nerve root (Fig SP 12-3)	On myelography, a brachial root avulsion produces a pouch-like appearance of the root sleeve, which is blunted and distorted and extends for a variable distance into the intervertebral foramen. Nerve root avulsions can be readily differentiated from diverticula of the subarachnoid space, which have smooth, delicately rounded contours and exhibit the normal radiolucent outlines of intact nerve roots within the opaque, contrast-filled pocket.

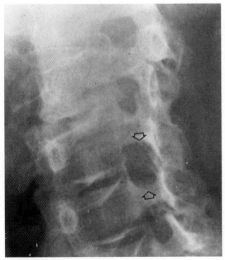

Fig SP 12-1
Neurofibroma. Smooth widening (arrows) due to the contiguous mass, without evidence of bone destruction.

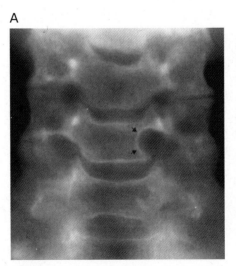
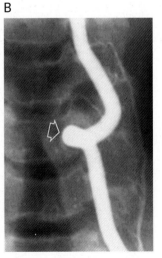

Fig SP 12-2
Tortuous vertebral artery. (A) Frontal tomogram shows the enlarged foramen (arrows). (B) Arteriogram shows the tortuous vertebral artery (arrow) entering the enlarged foramen.

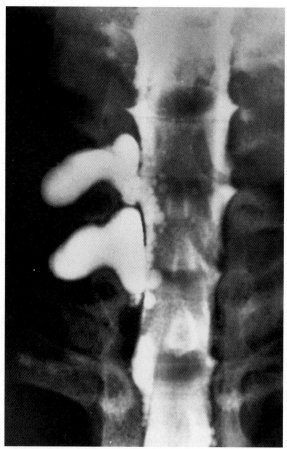

Fig SP 12-3
Traumatic avulsion of nerve roots. Note the pouch-like appearance of the blunted nerve roots that extend into the cervical foramina.

Atlantoaxial Subluxation

Condition	Comments
Rheumatoid arthritis (Fig SP 13-1)	Synovial inflammation causes weakening of the transverse ligaments. The odontoid process is often eroded, and the dens may be completely destroyed. Upward displacement of C2 may permit the dens to impinge on the upper cervical cord or medulla, producing acute neurologic symptoms requiring immediate traction or decompression. Atlantoaxial subluxation also occurs in juvenile rheumatoid arthritis.
Rheumatoid variants	Ankylosing spondylitis; psoriatic arthritis. Inflammatory changes of the synovial and adjacent ligamentous structures can lead to erosion of the dens.
Trauma	Almost always accompanied by a fracture of the odontoid process resulting from hyperflexion (dens and atlas displaced anteriorly) or hyperextension (posterior displacement). Isolated atlantoaxial subluxation (without fracture) indicates tearing of the transverse ligaments.
Congenital cervicobasilar anomaly	Absent anterior arch of the atlas; absent or separate odontoid process; atlanto-occipital fusion.
Retropharyngeal abscess (child)	Presumably causes laxity of the transverse ligaments due to the hyperemia associated with the inflammatory process.
Down's syndrome	Results from laxity of the spinal ligaments and has been reported in up to 20% of cases. Although usually mild and asymptomatic, a few patients develop symptoms ranging from discomfort in the neck to quadriparesis.
Morquio syndrome	Hypoplasia of the dens in this condition predisposes to atlantoaxial subluxation with consequent damage to the spinal cord. This risk is so high that some recommend early prophylactic posterior cervical fusion for patients with this disease.

A

B

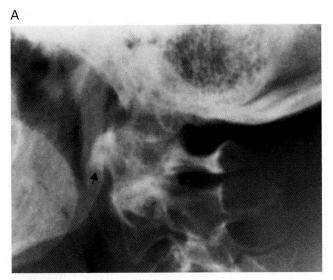
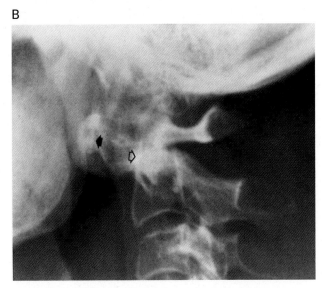

Fig SP 13-1
Rheumatoid arthritis. (A) Routine lateral film of the cervical spine shows a normal relation between the anterior border of the odontoid process and the superior portion of the anterior arch of the atlas (arrow). (B) With flexion, there is wide separation between the anterior arch of the atlas (closed arrow) and the odontoid (open arrow).

Calcification of Intervertebral Disks

Condition	Comments
Degenerative disk disease (Fig SP 14-1)	Radiographic manifestations include osteophytosis, narrowing of intervertebral disk spaces with marginal sclerosis, and the vacuum phenomenon (linear lucent collection overlying one or more intervertebral disks).
Transient calcification in children	Unlike most other causes of intervertebral disk calcification, in children the cervical region is most commonly involved, and there is a high frequency of associated clinical signs and symptoms. A self-limited condition requiring only conservative symptomatic treatment.
Post-traumatic	Associated findings of previous spinal injury.
Ochronosis (Fig SP 14-2)	Dense laminated calcification of multiple intervertebral disks (beginning in the lumbar spine and extending to the dorsal and cervical regions) is virtually pathognomonic of this rare inborn error of metabolism in which deposition of the black pigment of oxidized homogentisic acid in cartilage and other connective tissue produces a distinctive form of degenerative arthritis. The intervertebral disk spaces are narrowed, the vertebral bodies are osteoporotic, and limitation of motion is common. Severe degenerative arthritis may develop in peripheral joints, especially the shoulders, hips, and knees (an infrequent manifestation of osteoarthritis, especially in young patients).
Ankylosing spondylitis (Fig SP 14-3)	Central or eccentric, circular or linear calcific collections may appear in the intervertebral disks at single or multiple sites along the spinal column. Usually associated with apophyseal joint ankylosis at the same vertebral levels and adjacent syndesmophytes. The development of similar calcific deposits in other conditions affecting the vertebral column that are characterized by ankylosis (diffuse idiopathic skeletal hyperostosis, juvenile rheumatoid arthritis) suggests that immobilization of a segment of the spine may interfere with diskal nutrition and lead to degeneration and calcification.
Calcium pyrophosphate dihydrate deposition (CPPD) disease	Calcification frequently affects the intervertebral disks and may be associated with back pain. The deposits involve the annulus fibrosis (not the nucleus pulposus, as in ochronosis). Disk space narrowing often occurs.

Condition	Comments
Hemochromatosis	Deposition of calcium pyrophosphate dihydrate crystals occurs in the outer fibers of the annulus fibrosis, as in CPPD. Other radiographic manifestations include diffuse osteoporosis of the spine associated with vertebral collapse and a peripheral arthropathy that most commonly involves the small joints of the hands (especially the second and third metacarpophalangeal joints).
Hypervitaminosis D	Calcification of the annulus fibrosis is an uncommon finding. More often causes generalized osteoporosis with extensive masses of soft-tissue calcification.

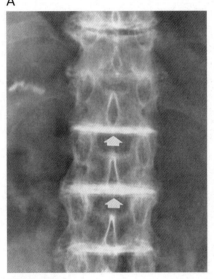

Fig SP 14-2
Ochronosis. (A) Frontal and (B) lateral views of the lumbar spine in two different patients show dense laminated calcification of multiple intervertebral disks (arrows).

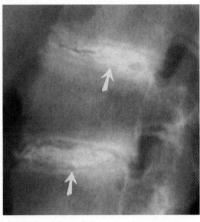

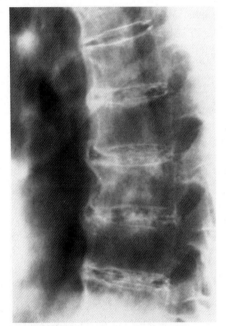

Fig SP 14-1
Degenerative disk disease. Note the anterior osteophytes, narrowing of intervertebral disk spaces, and calcification in the anterior longitudinal ligament.

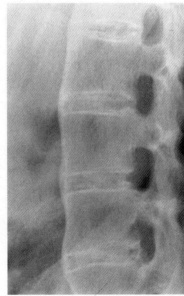

Fig SP 14-3
Ankylosing spondylitis. Calcification of intervertebral disks is associated with squaring of vertebral bodies and dense calcification of the anterior longitudinal ligament.

Bone-Within-A-Bone Appearance

Condition	Comments
Normal neonate (Fig SP 15-1)	Not uncommon appearance in infants 1 to 2 months of age caused by loss of bone density at the periphery of vertebral bodies (but with retention of their sharp cortical outlines). The bone subsequently assumes a normal density; thus, this appearance probably reflects a normal stage in the transformation of the architecture of the neonatal vertebrae to that of later infancy.
Osteopetrosis (Fig SP 15-2)	Miniature inset in each lumbar vertebral body is a typical manifestation of this rare hereditary bone abnormality characterized by a symmetric, generalized increase in bone density and lack of tubulation.
Thorotrast administration (Fig SP 15-3)	Radiographic densities of infantile vertebrae and pelvis (ghost vertebrae) in adult bones may be seen in adults who received intravenous Thorotrast during early childhood. The deposition of Thorotrast causes constant alpha radiation and temporary growth arrest, so that the size of the ghost vertebrae corresponds to the vertebral size at the time of injection. Most patients also have reticular or dense opacification of the liver, spleen, and lymph nodes.
Transverse growth lines (growth arrest lines) (Fig SP 15-4)	Opaque transverse lines paralleling the superior and inferior margins of vertebral bodies. Underlying causes include chronic childhood diseases, malnutrition, and chemotherapy.

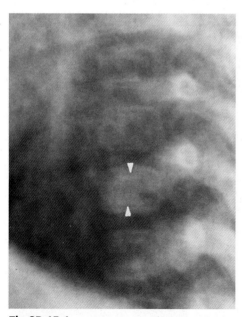

Fig SP 15-1
Normal neonate. The arrowheads point to one example of the bone-within-a-bone appearance.

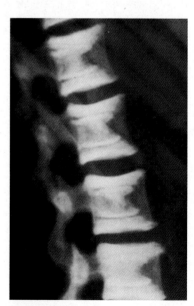

Fig SP 15-2
Osteopetrosis. A miniature inset is seen in each lumbar vertebral body, giving it a bone-within-a-bone appearance. There is also sclerosis at the end plates.[7]

Condition	Comments
Heavy metal poisoning	Radiodense lines paralleling the superior and inferior margins of multiple vertebral bodies are an infrequent manifestation of lead or phosphorus poisoning.
Gaucher's disease	Initial collapse of an entire vertebral body with subsequent growth recovery peripherally may be associated with horizontal and vertical sclerosis, giving the bone-within-a-bone appearance.
Paget's disease	May involve one or multiple vertebrae. More commonly produces enlarged, coarsened trabeculae with condensation of bone most prominent along the contours of a vertebral body (picture frame) or uniform increase in osseous density of an enlarged vertebral body (ivory vertebra).
Sickle cell anemia	Rare manifestation. More commonly generalized osteoporosis, localized step-like central depressions, and characteristic biconcave indentations on both the superior and inferior margins of softened vertebral bodies (fish vertebrae).
Hypervitaminosis D	The margins of the vertebral bodies are outlined by dense bands of bone that are exaggerated by adjacent radiolucent zones. The central, normal-appearing bone may simulate the bone-within-a-bone appearance.

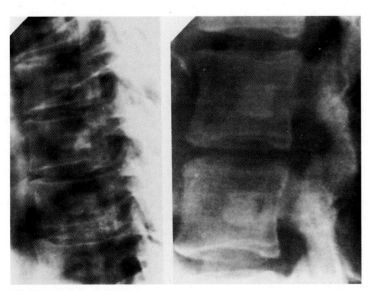

Fig SP 15-3
Thorotrast. Two examples of persistence of radiographic densities of infantile vertebrae in adult bones of patients who received intravenous Thorotrast during early childhood.[9]

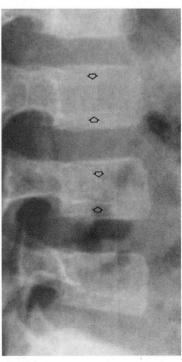

Fig SP 15-4
Transverse growth lines. Opaque lines paralleling the superior and inferior margins of the vertebral body (arrows) in a child with severe chronic illness.

Beaked, Notched, or Hooked Vertebrae in a Child

Condition	Imaging Findings	Comments
Normal variant	Variable pattern of vertebral notching.	Vertebral notching can be seen in infants who are presumably normal. This incidental finding is probably secondary to subclinical hyperflexion trauma or to the exaggerated thoracolumbar kyphosis that is seen in all young infants who are unable to remain erect in the sitting position because of normal muscular immaturity.
Mucopolysaccharidoses		Genetically determined disorders of mucopolysaccharide metabolism that result in a broad spectrum of skeletal, visceral, and mental abnormalities.
Hurler syndrome (gargoylism) (Fig SP 16-1)	Inferior beaking. The centrum of the second lumbar vertebra is usually hypoplastic and displaced posteriorly, giving rise to an accentuated kyphosis, or gibbous, deformity.	Other radiographic manifestations include swelling of the central portions of long bones (due to cortical thickening or widening of the medullary canal), "canoe-paddle" ribs, and J-shaped sella (shallow, elongated sella with a long anterior recess extending under the anterior clinoid processes).
Morquio syndrome (Fig SP 16-2)	Generalized flattening of the vertebral bodies with central anterior beaking. There is often hypoplasia and posterior displacement of L1 or L2, resulting in a sharp, angular kyphosis.	Other radiographic manifestations include tapering of long bones (less marked than in Hurler syndrome) and flaring, fragmentation, and flattening of the femoral heads combined with irregular deformity of the acetabula (often results in subluxations at the hip).
Cretinism (hypothyroidism)	Inferior or central beaking.	Radiographic manifestations include delay in appearance and subsequent growth of ossification centers, epiphyseal dysgenesis (fragmented epiphyses with multiple foci of ossification), retarded bone age, increased thickness of the cranial vault, and widened sutures with delayed closure.
Achondroplasia (Fig SP 16-3)	Central anterior wedging of vertebral bodies. Progressive narrowing of the interpedicular distances from above downward (opposite of normal) and scalloping of the posterior aspects of the vertebral bodies.	Radiographic manifestations include symmetric shortening of all long bones, ball-and-socket epiphyses, trident hand, and a characteristic short, broad pelvis with short and square ilia and decreased acetabular angles.
Down's syndrome (mongolism)	Variable pattern of vertebral notching.	Radiographic manifestations include a decrease in the acetabular and iliac angles with hypoplasia and marked lateral flaring of the iliac wings, squaring of vertebral bodies, multiple manubrial ossification centers, the presence of only 11 ribs, and shortening of the middle phalanx of the fifth finger.
Neuromuscular disease with generalized hypotonia	Variable pattern of vertebral notching.	Niemann-Pick disease, phenylketonuria, Werdnig-Hoffmann disease, mental retardation. Probably related to an exaggerated kyphotic curvature of the thoracic spine.

Condition	Imaging Findings	Comments
Trauma	Variable pattern of vertebral notching.	Hyperflexion-compression spinal injuries. Repeated hyperflexion of the spine is postulated to be the underlying cause of vertebral notching in battered children.

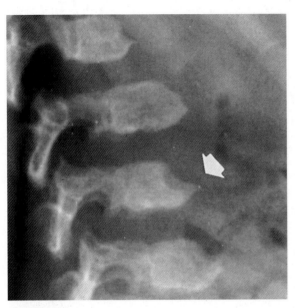

Fig SP 16-1
Hurler syndrome. Typical inferior beaking (arrow) of the anterior margin of a vertebral body.

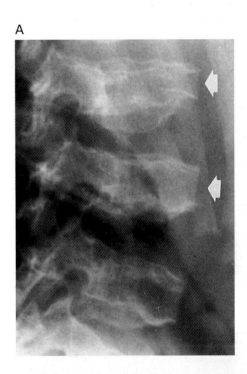

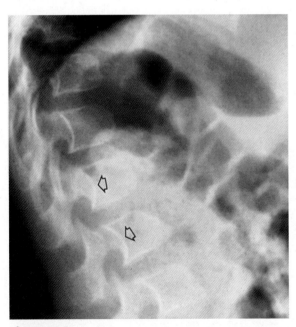

Fig SP 16-3
Achondroplasia. Central anterior wedging of several vertebral bodies. Note the characteristic posterior scalloping (arrows).

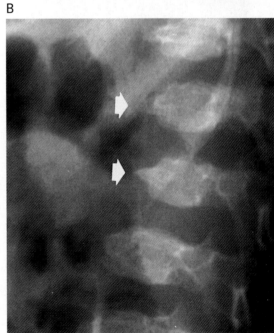

Fig SP 16-2
Morquio syndrome. (A and B) Two examples of universal flattening of the vertebral bodies with central anterior beaking (arrows).

Sacroiliac Joint Abnormality

Condition	Comments
Bilateral symmetric distribution Ankylosing spondylitis (Fig SP 17-1)	Sacroiliac joints are the initial site of involvement. Early findings include blurring of articular margins, irregular widening of the joints, and patchy sclerosis. This generally progresses to narrowing of the joint spaces and may lead to complete fibrosis and bony ankylosis. Dense reactive sclerosis often occurs, though it may become less prominent as the joint spaces become obliterated.
Inflammatory bowel disease (Fig SP 17-2)	Appearance identical in all respects to that of classic ankylosing spondylitis. Underlying conditions include ulcerative colitis, Crohn's disease, and Whipple's disease.
Hyperparathyroidism/ renal osteodystrophy	Subchondral resorption of bone (predominantly in the ilia) leads to irregularity of the osseous surface, adjacent sclerosis, and widening of the interosseous joint space. Articular space narrowing and bony fusion do not occur.
Osteitis condensans ilii (Fig SP 17-3)	Triangular zone of dense sclerosis along the inferior aspect of the ilia. The surfaces are well defined, the sacrum is normal, and the sacroiliac joint spaces are preserved. The condition probably represents a reaction to the increased stress to which the sacroiliac region is subjected during pregnancy and delivery (a similar type of sclerotic reaction, osteitis pubis, may occur in the pubic bones adjacent to the symphysis in women who have borne children).

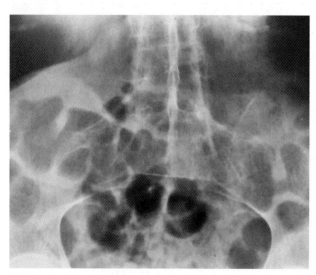

Fig SP 17-1
Ankylosing spondylitis. Bilateral, symmetric obliteration of the sacroiliac joints.

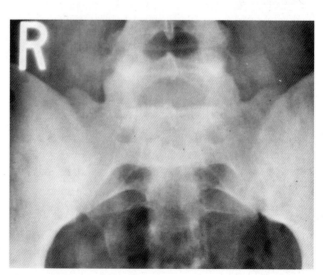

Fig SP 17-2
Inflammatory bowel disease. Bilateral, symmetric involvement of the sacroiliac joints in a patient with ulcerative colitis.

Condition	Comments
Osteoarthritis	After age 40, most patients have some narrowing of the sacroiliac joint spaces, which may involve the entire articulations or appear as focal areas of abnormality at the inferior aspect of the joints. In comparison with ankylosing spondylitis, sacroiliac joint disease in osteoarthritis occurs in older patients, is often associated with prominent osteophytosis (especially at the anterosuperior and anteroinferior limits of the articular cavity) and prominent subchondral sclerosis, does not show erosions, and rarely demonstrates intra-articular bony ankylosis (though periarticular bridging osteophytes are common). Degenerative joint disease also may have a bilateral and asymmetric or a unilateral distribution.
Gout	Irregularity and sclerosis of articular margins are common (may reflect osteoarthritis in older patients). Large cystic areas of erosion in the subchondral bone of the ilia and sacrum are uncommon. Sacroiliac joint changes occur more frequently with early-onset disease and tend to have a left-sided predominance. As with degenerative joint disease, sacroiliac joint involvement in gouty arthritis may be bilateral and asymmetric or unilateral.
Multicentric reticulohistiocytosis	Erosions and joint space narrowing leading to bony ankylosis, but no subchondral sclerosis.

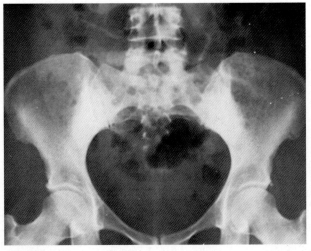

Fig SP 17-3
Osteitis condensans ilii. Sharply demarcated sclerosis of the ilia adjacent to the sacroiliac joints. The sacrum is not affected, and the margins of the sacroiliac joints are sharp and without destruction. The sclerosis that overlies the sacral wing is actually in the ilium, where it curves posteriorly behind the sacrum.[4]

Condition	Comments
Bilateral asymmetric distribution	
Psoriatic arthritis (Fig SP 17-4)	Bilateral, asymmetric distribution is probably most common, though bilateral, symmetric abnormalities are frequent and even unilateral involvement may occur. The radiographic changes include erosions and sclerosis, predominantly affecting the ilium, and widening of the articular space. Although joint space narrowing and bony ankylosis can occur, this is much less frequent than in classic ankylosing spondylitis. A prominent finding may be blurring and eburnation of apposing sacral and iliac surfaces above the true joint in the region of the interosseous ligament.
Reactive arthritis (Fig SP 17-5)	Bilateral, asymmetric distribution is probably most common, though bilateral, symmetric abnormalities are frequent and unilateral sacroiliac joint abnormalities may infrequently occur (especially early in the disease process). Sacroiliac joint changes are common in reactive arthritis, eventually developing in approximately 50% of patients. Osseous erosions primarily involve the iliac surface, and adjacent sclerosis varies from mild to severe. Early joint space widening may later be replaced by narrowing. Although intra-articular bony ankylosis may eventually appear, it occurs much less frequently than in ankylosing spondylitis. A prominent finding may be blurring and eburnation of apposing sacral and iliac surfaces above the true joint in the region of the interosseous ligament.
Rheumatoid arthritis (Fig SP 17-6)	Relatively uncommon manifestation that usually produces minor subchondral erosions, mild or absent sclerosis, and either no or only focal intra-articular bony ankylosis. Infrequently has a unilateral distribution.

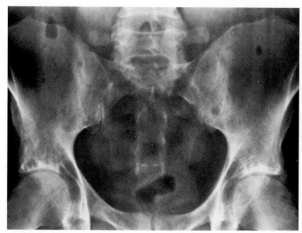

Fig SP 17-4
Psoriatic arthritis. Bilateral, though somewhat asymmetric, narrowing of the sacroiliac joints.

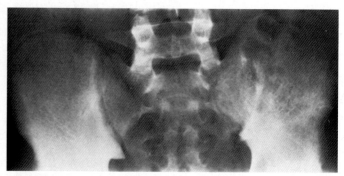

Fig SP 17-5
Reactive arthritis. Bilateral, though asymmetric, sclerosis and narrowing of the sacroiliac joints with reactive sclerosis.

Condition	Comments
Familial Mediterranean fever (Fig SP 17-7)	Initially, widening of the articular space with loss of normal cortical definition primarily involving the ilium. Eventually, sclerosis with or without erosions and even bony ankylosis. Involvement may also be bilateral and symmetric or even unilateral.
Relapsing polychondritis	Joint space narrowing, erosion, and eburnation. Involvement may also be bilateral and symmetric or even unilateral.
Unilateral distribution	
Infection (Fig SP 17-8)	By far the most common cause of unilateral sacroiliac involvement. May be related to bacterial, mycobacterial, or fungal agents and is relatively common in drug abusers.
Paralysis	Cartilage atrophy accompanying paralysis or disuse produces diffuse joint space narrowing with surrounding osteoporosis and may even lead to intra-articular osseous fusion (perhaps related to chronic low-grade inflammation).
Osteoarthritis	May occur in conjunction with degenerative joint disease involving the contralateral hip.

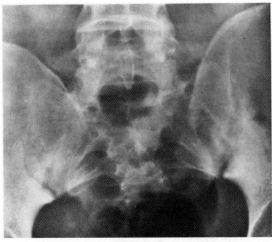

Fig SP 17-6
Rheumatoid arthritis. Bilateral, though asymmetric, sclerosis and narrowing of the sacroiliac joints.

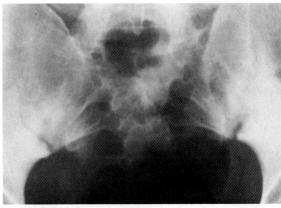

Fig SP 17-7
Familial Mediterranean fever. Bilateral, though asymmetric, narrowing, erosive changes, and reactive sclerosis about the sacroiliac joints.

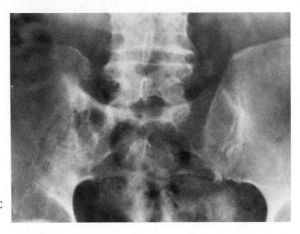

Fig SP 17-8
Healed tuberculosis. Obliteration of the right sacroiliac joint. The left sacroiliac joint remains intact.

Spinal Cord Tumors on Magnetic Resonance Imaging

Condition	Imaging Findings	Comments
Intramedullary Ependymoma (Fig SP 18-1)	Isointense or hypointense fusiform widening of the spinal cord on T1-weighted images. Increased signal, often with a multinodular appearance, on T2-weighted images. Generally intense, homogeneous, and sharply marginated focal contrast enhancement.	Most common primary tumor of the spinal cord. Predominantly occurs in the lower spinal cord, conus medullaris, and filum terminale. Boundaries of the tumor are difficult to define on T1-weighted images unless they are outlined by syrinx cavities capping the upper and lower poles of the tumor. On T2-weighted images, it is difficult to distinguish the tumor from surrounding edema. Often evidence of prior hemorrhage.
Astrocytoma (Fig SP 18-2)	Widening of the spinal cord that is isointense on T1-weighted images and hyperintense on T2-weighted images. Tendency to more patchy and irregular contrast enhancement consistent with a more diffusely infiltrating tumor.	Second most common primary spinal cord tumor. Typically involves the cervicothoracic region. Although different patterns of contrast enhancement have been reported in some ependymomas and astrocytomas, they cannot be reliably differentiated by MRI.
Hemangioblastoma (Fig SP 18-3)	Irregular and diffuse widening of the cord with cystic components and heterogeneous signal intensity. Intense enhancement of the highly vascular tumor nidus.	Dilated posterior pial venous plexus draining the tumor nodule may produce serpentine flow voids (simulating an arteriovenous malformation) on the dorsal aspect of the cord. The association of a strongly enhancing tumor nodule within a cystic intramedullary mass is very suggestive of hemangioblastoma.

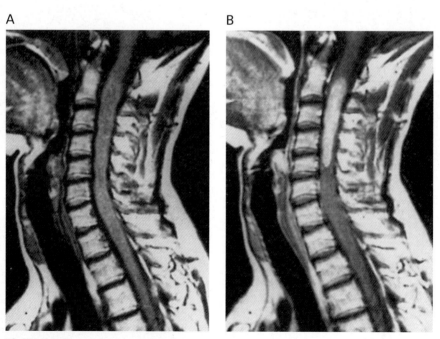

A   B

Fig SP 18-1
Ependymoma. (A) Nonenhanced sagittal T1-weighted image shows widening of the cervical cord from C1 to T2, suggesting intramedullary tumor. (B) Postcontrast scan shows a well-defined oval area of enhancement extending from C2 to C5.[10]

Condition	Imaging Findings	Comments
Metastasis (Fig SP 18-4)	Single or multiple masses producing fusiform or irregular widening of the cord (or no cord enlargement at all) that is hypointense on T1-weighted images and hyperintense on T2-weighted images. Generally marked contrast enhancement.	May develop from primary CNS neoplasms via CSF pathways or hematogenous spread from non-CNS primary tumors. After contrast injection, the enhancing tumor nodule (often smaller than the area of cord enlargement) can be distinguished from surrounding edema.
Intradural extramedullary Meningioma (Fig SP 18-5)	Generally isointense on T1-weighted images and only slightly hyperintense on T2-weighted images. Immediate and uniform contrast enhancement.	Typically occurs in the thoracic region (80%) in middle-aged or elderly women. Like meningiomas in the head, spinal tumors tend to maintain signal intensity similar to that of cord parenchyma.

A
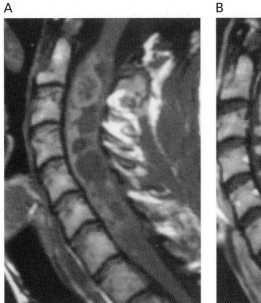
B
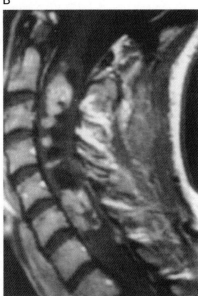

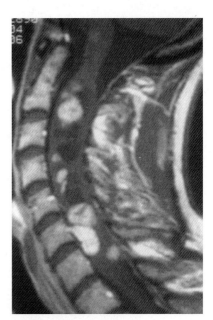

Fig SP 18-2
Astrocytoma. (A) Noncontrast midsagittal T1-weighted image shows a nonhomogeneous lesion involving the spinal cord from C2 to T1. (B) Corresponding postcontrast image shows enhancement of several tumor nodules. (Courtesy M. Smith, M.D., Nashville, TN.)[11]

Fig SP 18-3
Hemangioblastoma. A midsagittal post-contrast T1-weighted image shows multiple solid and cystic lesions in the cervical spinal cord in this patient with von Hippel-Lindau disease.[11]

A
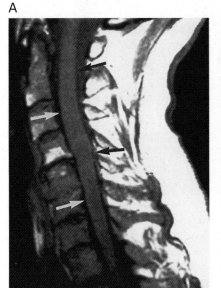
B
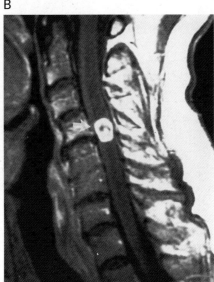

Fig SP 18-4
Metastasis. (A) Nonenhanced sagittal T1-weighted image shows nonspecific intramedullary expansion of a long segment of the cervical spinal cord (arrows). (B) Postcontrast scan shows intense enhancement of a partially necrotic mass at the C4 level (arrow). The intramedullary expansion of the cord above and below this level was attributed to cord edema.[12]

Condition	Imaging Findings	Comments
Neurofibroma (Fig SP 18-6)	Smooth, sharply marginated mass that tends to be relatively isointense to the spinal cord on all sequences. Variable pattern of contrast enhancement depending on internal architecture of the tumor.	In contrast to meningiomas, neurofibromas have no sex predilection and are more evenly distributed along the course of the spinal canal. They may have a characteristic extradural component that extends through the neural foramen into the paraspinal tissues (dumbbell tumor). Neurofibromas have a more variable MR appearance than meningiomas because of their propensity to undergo cystic degeneration and central necrosis, which makes them hypointense on T1-weighted images and hyperintense on T2-weighted images.
Metastasis ("seeding") (Fig SP 18-7)	Multiple focal nodular masses that show intense contrast enhancement.	Unless large, these tumor deposits generally are not visualized on noncontrast scans. Other patterns include enhancement of a thin leptomeningeal veil that diffusely coats the spinal cord or nerve roots and a homogeneous increase in signal within the subarachnoid space.
Lipoma (Fig SP 18-8)	Well-circumscribed mass that has the characteristic signal intensity of fat (homogeneous high signal on T1-weighted images and decreasing intensity on progressively more T2-weighted images); parallels the signal intensity of subcutaneous fat.	Uncommon lesion that can occur anywhere in the spinal canal and has no age or sex predilection. The characteristic bright signal on T1-weighted images can be confused with contrast enhancement if only post-contrast studies are obtained, thus leading to the erroneous diagnosis of meningioma or neurofibroma. In the lumbar area, before making the diagnosis of intradural lipoma, it is important to note that fat may be present in the distal conus medullaris and filum terminale in approximately 5% of normal individuals.

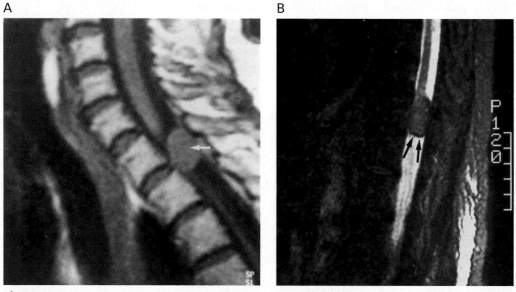

A   B

Fig SP 18-5
Meningioma. (A) Sagittal T1-weighted scan demonstrates an isointense intradural soft-tissue mass (arrow) in the dorsal aspect of the upper thoracic canal. Note the displacement of the spinal cord.[13] (B) Sagittal T2-weighted image in another patient shows a well-circumscribed intradural mass at the T10 level. The linear area of signal loss at the periphery of the mass (arrows) represents calcifications.[12]

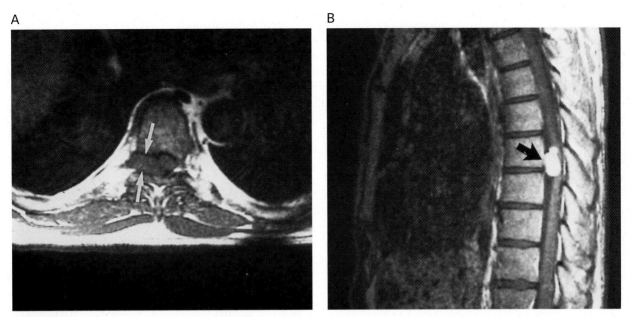

Fig SP 18-6
Neurofibroma. (A) Axial T1-weighted image demonstrates an oval, right-sided intraspinal mass that extends through an expanded T8 neural foramen (arrows). (B) Postcontrast midline sagittal scan in another patient shows a slightly loculated, homogeneously enhancing intradural extramedullary mass (arrow).[12]

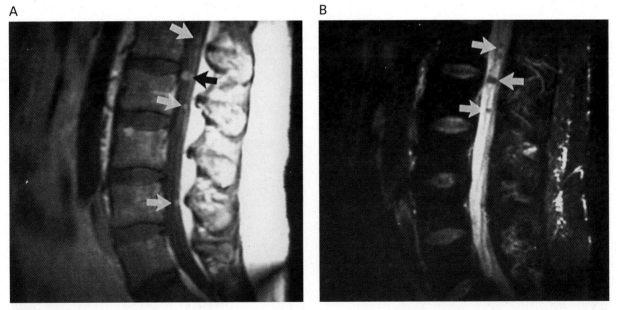

Fig SP 18-7
Metastatic seeding. (A) Sagittal T1-weighted image shows multiple high-intensity nodules (arrows) involving the nerve roots of the cauda equina in this patient with metastatic melanoma. The high intensity could represent either contrast enhancement or the paramagnetic effect of melanin. (B) The nodules also can be identified on a T2-weighted scan (arrows).[12]

Condition	Imaging Findings	Comments
Epidermoid/dermoid/ teratoma (Fig SP 18-9)	Variable appearance depending on the nature of the tissues (fat, solid keratin or cholesterol, fibrous tissue, muscle, bone) comprising the mass.	Epidermoids are ectodermal in origin; dermoids arise from both extoderm and mesoderm; teratomas are composed of tissue from all three germ layers. Epidermoids usually contain a significant fluid component that is isointense to CSF on all pulse sequences, whereas dermoids often mimic the signal intensity of fat.
Extradural Metastasis (Fig SP 18-10)	Mass that is hypointense on T1-weighted images and of increased signal intensity on T2-weighted images.	The most common primary tumors to metastasize to the spine are lung and breast carcinoma, followed by prostate carcinoma. Epidural metastases almost always occur in association with osseous metastases, in which the bright signal of marrow in the vertebral body is replaced by low-signal tumor on T1-weighted images. Contrast studies may mask metastases by increasing the signal of osseous metastases, so that they appear isointense to normal marrow on T1-weighted scans.
Lymphoma	Mass that is hypointense on T1-weighted images and of increased signal intensity on T2-weighted images.	Bulky soft-tissue mass insinuating itself into foramina, extending over multiple segments, and producing less skeletal involvement than expected for lesion size.
Vertebral neoplasm with intraspinal extension	Mass that is hypointense on T1-weighted images and of increased signal intensity on T2-weighted images.	Myeloma; chordoma; sarcoma.

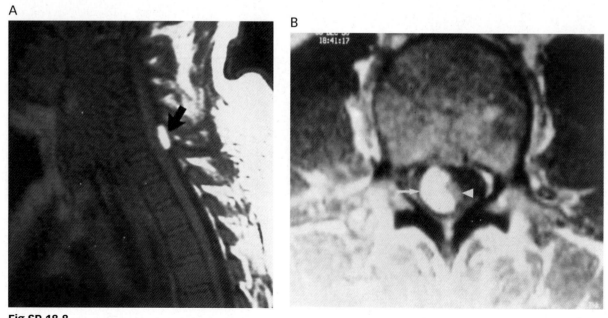

Fig SP 18-8
Lipoma. (A) Sagittal[12] and (B) axial[13] T1-weighted scans in two different patients show a homogeneously hyperintense intradural mass. Note how the intensity of the lesions is similar to that of paraspinal and subcutaneous fat.

Condition	Imaging Findings	Comments
Hemangioma	Lesion within the vertebral body that tends to be of high signal intensity on both T1- and T2-weighted images.	Although usually an incidental finding of little clinical significance, hemangiomas occasionally expand and break through the cortex to cause a myelopathic or radiculopathic syndrome. Hemangiomas can be differentiated from relatively common interosseous islands of fat because they maintain their high signal intensity on T2-weighted images.

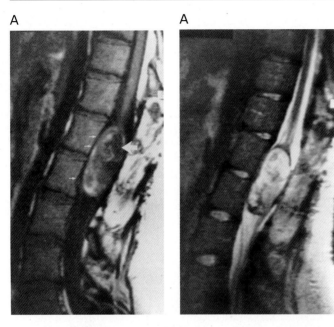

Fig SP 18-9
Epidermoid. (A) Sagittal T1-weighted image shows an ovoid, well-circumscribed, heterogeneous intradural mass (large arrow) inferior to the conus. Note the widening of the spinal canal with posterior scalloping of adjacent vertebral bodies (small arrows). (B) Sagittal T2-weighted scan shows the mass to be heterogeneously hyperintense.[13]

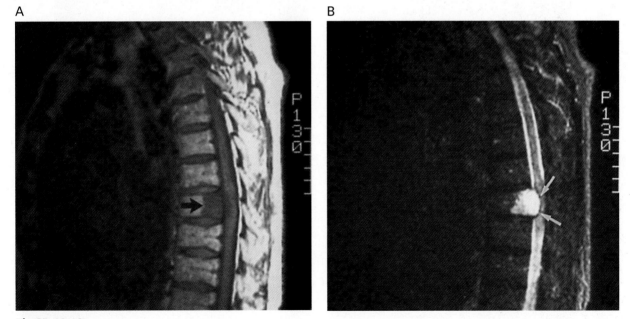

Fig SP 18-10
Metastasis. (A) A T9 bony metastasis from known cranial chordoma is seen as a loss of the normal marrow fat on this T1-weighted scan in a patient with a thoracic myelopathy (arrow). (B) An associated epidural soft-tissue component is seen to better advantage with T2 weighting (arrows), resulting in spinal canal narrowing and compression of the thoracic spinal cord.[13]

Nonneoplastic Lesions of Vertebral Bodies on Magnetic Resonance Imaging

Condition	Imaging Findings	Comments
Degenerative disk disease		Marrow signal intensity abnormalities have been reported in up to 50% of intervertebral levels showing degenerative disk changes.
Type I (Fig SP 19-1)	Decreased signal intensity on T1-weighted images and increased signal intensity on T2-weighted images.	Associated with local replacement of normal cellular marrow with vascularized fibrous tissue. Tends to convert to type II lesions over time.
Type II (Fig SP 19-2)	Increased signal intensity on T1-weighted images and slightly increased signal intensity on T2-weighted images.	Associated with local fatty replacement of marrow. Type I and II changes are thought to represent a continuum in the response of adjacent marrow to degenerative disk disease.
Type III (Fig SP 19-3)	Decreased signal intensity on both T1- and T2-weighted images.	Least common pattern that probably represents bone sclerosis or fibrosis adjacent to the end plate.
Schmorl's node (Fig SP 19-4)	Continuous with the disk and of identical signal intensity.	Superior or inferior displacement of disk material through a cartilaginous and osseous end plate. Large lesions must be differentiated from metastases or infection based on their sharp margins, low intensity of their rims, and association with narrowed disk spaces.

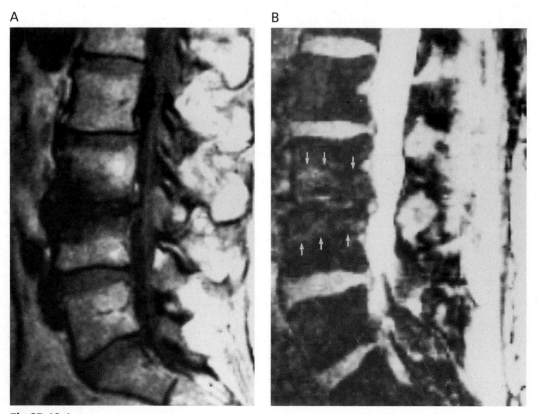

A   B

Fig SP 19-1
Degenerative disk disease (type I changes). (A) Sagittal T1-weighted image shows a broad area of decreased signal intensity adjacent to the L3-4 disk. (B) Gradient echo image shows mildly increased signal intensity (arrows) in the corresponding area.[11]

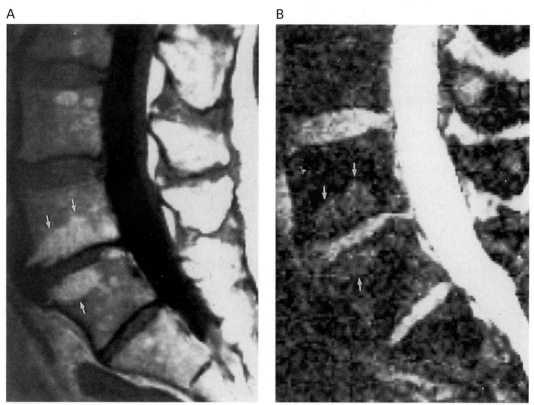

Fig SP 19-2
Degenerative disk disease (type II changes). (A) Sagittal T1-weighted image shows a sharply marginated area of increased signal intensity (arrows) adjacent to a narrowed disk space. (B) On the T2-weighted image, this area has a slightly increased signal intensity.[14]

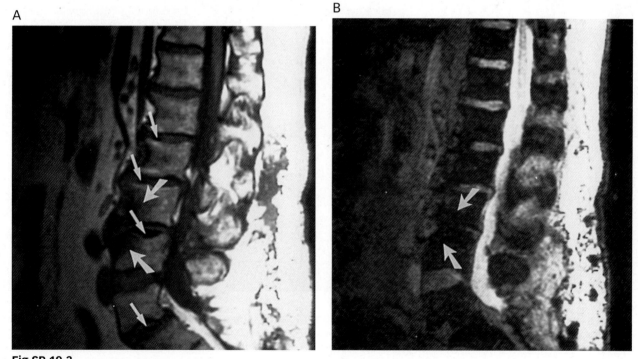

Fig SP 19-3
Degenerative disk disease (type III changes). (A) Sagittal T1-weighted image shows ill-defined zones of decreased signal intensity within the end plates adjacent to the L3-4 intervertebral disk (thick arrows). (Thin arrows indicate lumbar interspaces.) (B) On the T2-weighted image, these end plates become isointense with normal marrow (arrows).[12]

Condition	Imaging Findings	Comments
Compression fracture Subacute (Fig SP 19-5)	Decreased signal intensity on T1-weighted images and increased signal intensity on T2-weighted images.	Cannot reliably differentiate between simple osteoporotic and pathologic fractures on the basis of signal intensity alone. Findings that suggest neoplasm include a large soft-tissue mass, destruction of bone cortex, and involvement of multiple levels. One clear indication of metastases is the presence of another lesion with similar signal characteristics at a nonfractured vertebral level.
Chronic (healed) (Fig SP 19-5)	Signal intensity varies with the underlying cause.	In simple osteoporotic disease, the signal intensity of the marrow generally returns to normal on all sequences. Pathologic fractures secondary to metastatic disease usually are hypointense to marrow on T1-weighted images and hyperintense on T2-weighted images.
Infection (Fig SP 19-6)	Involved marrow shows decreased signal intensity on T1-weighted images and increased signal intensity on T2-weighted images.	Generally associated with a narrowed disk that on T2-weighted images has increased signal intensity, unlike the decreased signal intensity seen with disk degeneration.
Radiation therapy (Fig SP 19-7)	On T1-weighted images, characteristic high signal intensity involving multiple contiguous vertebral bodies.	Areas of abnormal signal intensity reflect progressive fatty degeneration of bone marrow in a region corresponding to the radiation port.

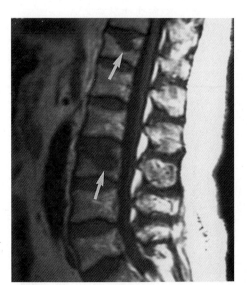

A
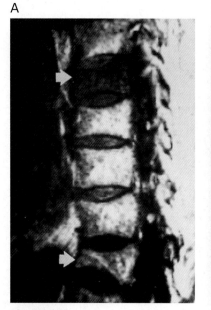

B
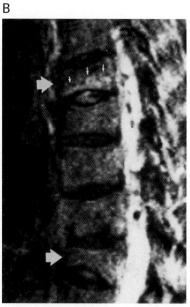

Fig SP 19-4
Schmorl's nodes. Central herniation of disk material through the superior end plates of T12 and L3 (arrows).[12]

Fig SP 19-5
Compression fractures (subacute and chronic). Sagittal (A) T1-weighted and (B) T2-weighted images show anterior compression deformities (wedging) of the T7 and T11 vertebral bodies (large arrows). The signal intensity of the marrow is normal at T11, indicating a healed chronic compression fracture. At T7, the signal intensity of the marrow is decreased on the T1-weighted image and slightly increased on the T2-weighted image in a linear, heterogeneous fashion (small arrows, B), consistent with a subacute compression fracture.[14]

Condition	Imaging Findings	Comments
Focal fatty infiltration	Focal area or areas of increased signal intensity on T1-weighted images. On T2-weighted images, the area(s) have signal intensity equal to or slightly higher than normal bone marrow (but substantially less than CSF).	Common phenomenon in both sexes after age 30. Must not be confused with metastases.
Paget's disease (Fig SP 19-8)	In the initial osteolytic phase, fibrous conversion of marrow, which contains multiple enlarged vessels (these changes disappear in the mixed phase). In the final osteosclerotic phase, the marrow returns to normal, and the bony cortices are thickened.	Single or multiple lesions affect approximately 3% of the population older than age 40. Multiple sites include primarily the spine (75%), skull (65%), and pelvis (40%). New onset of pain in a bone involved in Paget's disease should raise the possibility of sarcomatous degeneration.

A
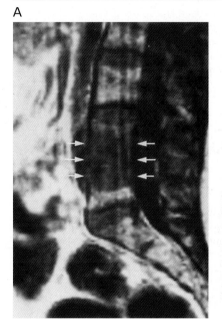

B
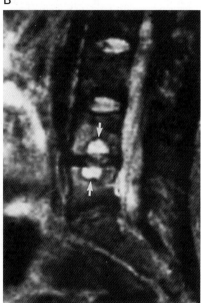

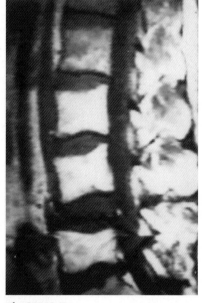

Fig SP 19-6
Infection. (A) Sagittal T1-weighted image shows a large area of decreased signal intensity involving both sides of the L4-5 disk space. The boundaries between the disks and the end plates are obliterated (arrows). (B) T2-weighted image shows sharply marginated areas of increased signal intensity (arrows) adjacent to the disk, which shows mottled, irregular signal characteristics.[14]

Fig SP 19-7
Radiation therapy. Axial T1-weighted image in a patient after radiation therapy for a plasmacytoma of L4 shows the typically increased signal intensity from L2, L3, L4, and the inferior aspect of L1, consistent with fatty replacement of bone marrow in a distribution corresponding to the radiation therapy port.[14]

A
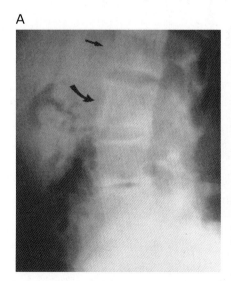

B
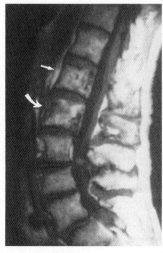

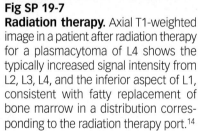

Fig SP 19-8
Paget's disease. (A) Lateral radiograph showing involvement of L3 (curved arrow) and L2 (straight arrow). (B) Midsagittal T1-weighted MR image shows mottled signal intensity in L3 (curved arrow) and T2 (straight arrow). The affected vertebrae appear slightly enlarged.[11]

Neoplastic Lesions of Vertebrae on Magnetic Resonance Imaging

Condition	Imaging Findings	Comments
Hemangioma (Fig SP 20-1)	Increased signal intensity on both T1- and T2-weighted images.	Benign vascular tumor that is usually an incidental finding. MRI can show paravertebral and epidural extension of tumor, which lacks adipose tissue and thus appears isointense on T1-weighted images.
Osteochondroma	Heterogeneous appearance with the cartilaginous components of increased signal intensity on T2-weighted images, whereas the osteoid or calcified portions have low signal intensity.	Primarily involves the posterior elements, especially the spinous processes. Rapid growth is an ominous sign. Factors favoring a benign lesion include cortical margins that are contiguous with the adjacent bone, well-defined lobular surfaces, lack of adjacent bone involvement, and a thin cartilaginous cap (usually less than 1 cm).
Osteoid osteoma	Heterogeneous appearance with the calcification within the nidus and the surrounding bony sclerosis having low signal intensity on all sequences, whereas the noncalcified portion of the nidus itself has increased signal intensity on T2-weighted images.	Intense enhancement of the highly vascular nidus, which not only helps to localize the nidus but also aids in differentiating the lesion from a nonenhancing process such as a Brodie's abscess.
Osteoblastoma (Fig SP 20-2)	High signal intensity on T2-weighted images. Intense contrast enhancement.	May have an inhomogeneous appearance if there is hemorrhage or calcification.
Aneurysmal bone cyst (Fig SP 20-3)	Expansile lesion of the posterior elements, often with internal septations and lobulations, that frequently has a thin, well-defined rim of low signal intensity.	A characteristic appearance is multiple fluid-fluid levels that can have varying signal intensities based on hemorrhage of different ages within the large anastomosing blood-filled cavernous spaces of the lesion.

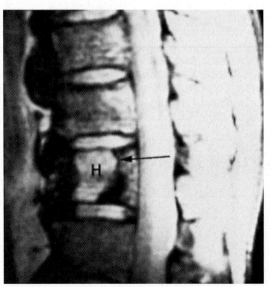

Fig SP 20-1
Hemangioma. Sagittal proton-density image shows a high-signal lesion (H) within a lower thoracic vertebral body. The lesion is well defined, and a discrete cortical margin is evident posteriorly (arrow).[15]

Condition	Imaging Findings	Comments
Giant cell tumor (Fig SP 20-4)	Expansile lesion of low signal intensity on T1-weighted images and increased signal intensity on T2-weighted images.	Unenhanced scans show tumor displacing normal bright marrow fat, whereas contrast enhancement can separate tumor from adjacent normal structures.
Sacrococcygeal teratoma (Fig SP 20-5)	Pelvic mass adjacent to the coccyx that often contains cystic components and has variable intensity patterns. After injection of contrast material, solid portions of the tumor enhance.	Rare childhood tumor arising from multipotential cells of Hensen's node that migrate to lie within the coccyx. Cystic components generally have low signal intensity on T1-weighted images and are of increased signal intensity on T2-weighted images, though they may have different intensities if they contain hemorrhage.

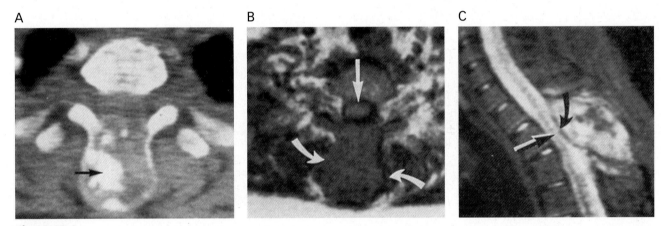

Fig SP 20-2
Osteoblastoma. (A) Axial CT scan shows an expanded spinous process of T2 with internal amorphous calcifications (arrow). The anterior extent of the tumor and its relationship with the cord cannot be established. (B) Axial T1-weighted and (C) midline sagittal T2-weighted images show the cord (straight arrows) and its relationship with the tumor (curved arrows in B). Note the partial obliteration of the posterior subarachnoid space (curved arrow in C) on the sagittal image.[16]

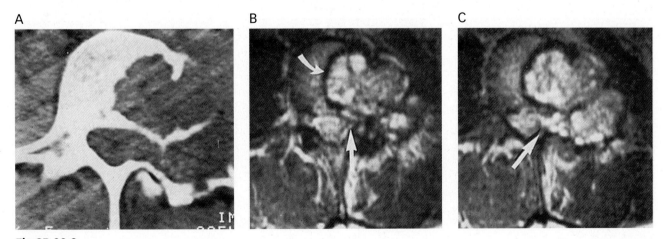

Fig SP 20-3
Aneurysmal bone cyst. (A) Axial CT scan shows osseous extension of the tumor but cannot evaluate possible spinal canal invasion. (B) Axial T2-weighted image shows the relationship between the tumor and the thecal sac (straight arrows). Note the bubbly appearance of the tumor, with small cysts of different signal intensity. (C) Left parasagittal proton-density image shows the superior extension of the tumor into the spinal canal (straight arrows). Note the band of decreased signal intensity (curved arrow in B) between the tumor and vertebral body, representing the rim of sclerosis.[16]

Condition	Imaging Findings	Comments
Langerhans cell histiocytosis (Fig SP 20-6)	Lytic process, frequently with vertebral collapse, that has decreased signal intensity on T1-weighted images and increased signal intensity on T2-weighted images.	MRI can well delineate any spinal cord compression resulting from vertebral collapse or an associated epidural hematoma. The lesion may be difficult to differentiate from metastatic disease.
Chordoma (Fig SP 20-7)	Isointense or hypointense to spinal cord on T1-weighted images. High signal intensity on T2-weighted images.	Frequently has internal septations and a surrounding capsule of low signal intensity. May contain areas of hemorrhage and cystic change. Although CT is superior for showing bone destruction or calcification, MRI better shows any epidural disease.
Primary malignant tumors (Fig SP 20-8)	Destructive lesions that have decreased signal intensity on T1-weighted images and increased signal intensity on T2-weighted images.	Osteosarcoma, chondrosarcoma, Ewing's sarcoma. Leukemia and lymphoma can present an identical appearance, as can metastatic carcinoma.

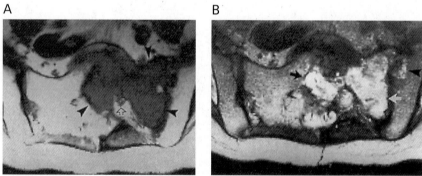

Fig SP 20-4
Giant cell tumor. (A) Axial T1-weighted image shows tumor (arrowheads) replacing normal marrow fat in the left sacral ala and body of S1. Tumor surrounds the neural canal containing the first left ventral sacral nerve root (arrow). (B) On the T2-weighted image, the tumor (arrows) is inhomogeneous and of intermediate signal intensity. Note the tumor extension (arrowhead) across the left sacroiliac joint.[17]

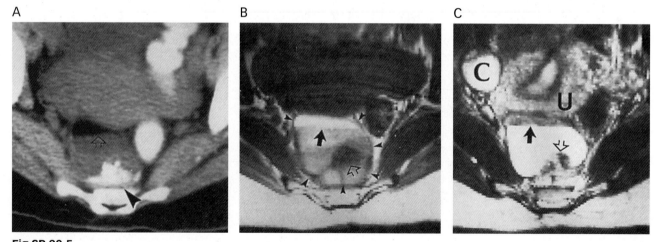

Fig SP 20-5
Sacral teratoma. (A) CT scan shows a presacral mass without evidence of sacral erosion. Note the posterior calcification (arrowhead) and fat-fluid level (arrow) in the lesion. (B) Axial T1-weighted MR scan shows the presacral mass (arrowheads). The high-intensity fat (solid arrow) is layering on the lower intensity fluid in the lesion. The low-intensity area posteriorly (open arrow) represents calcification. (C) On the T2-weighted image, the signal intensities have reversed at the fat-fluid interface (solid arrow). The posterior calcification (open arrow) remains of low intensity. (C, ovarian cyst; U, uterus.)[17]

Condition	Imaging Findings	Comments
Metastases (Fig SP 20-9)	Low-intensity lesions on T1-weighted images. On contrast scans, most vertebral metastases become isointense to normal marrow and difficult to visualize (may require fat suppression).	Vertebral metastases occur in 5% to 10% of patients with cancer, especially those with primary tumors of the breast, prostate, uterus, or lung. They are multiple in approximately 90% of patients and primarily involve the thoracic spine.

A

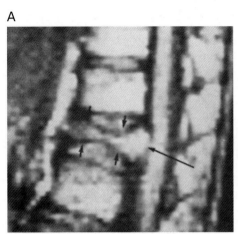

B

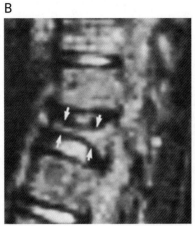

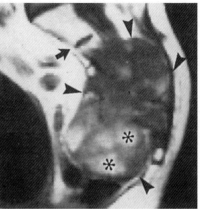

Fig SP 20-6
Langerhans cell histiocytosis. (A) T1-weighted and (B) proton-density sagittal images demonstrate compression deformity (vertebra plana) of the T11 vertebral body (short arrows). Soft tissue (long arrow) also projects posteriorly into the ventral epidural space. The intervertebral disks are not involved.[15]

Fig SP 20-7
Chordoma. Sagittal T1-weighted scan shows an extensive neoplasm (arrowheads) with obliteration of the sacral canal and presacral and postsacral extension. Note preservation of the S1-S2 disk (arrow), which indicates potential for radical resection. High-intensity areas in the neoplasm (asterisks) represent areas of hemorrhage.[17]

A

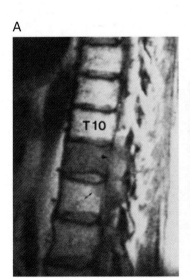

B

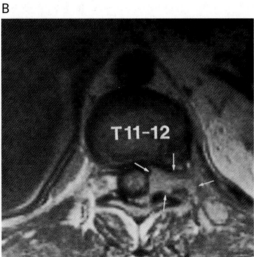

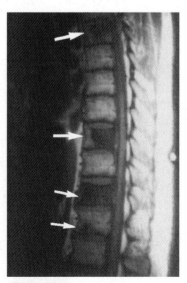

Fig SP 20-8
Lymphoma. (A) Parasagittal T1-weighted image shows tumor replacement of much of the normal marrow of the T11 vertebral body. The tumor has broken through the cortex posteriorly (arrowhead) and displaces the high-signal epidural fat. Note that the posterosuperior portion of T12 has decreased signal intensity consistent with tumor involvement (small arrow). (B) Axial T1-weighted scan through the T11-T12 foramen shows tumor infiltration (arrows) into the left epidural space, compressing the left side of the thecal sac and filling the left neural foramen.[15]

Fig SP 20-9
Metastases. A noncontrast midsagittal T1-weighted image shows areas of low signal intensity (arrows) in multiple vertebrae representing metastases from breast cancer.[11]

Postoperative Lumbar Region of Spine on Magnetic Resonance Imaging

Condition	Imaging Findings	Comments
Herniated disk (Fig SP 21-1)	Hypointense or isointense to disk (on T1-weighted images) and contiguous with it. No contrast enhancement.	May show some delayed enhancement 30 to 60 minutes after injection, though not to the same degree as a scar. The perimeter of a disk may enhance because of the development of vascular granulation tissue surrounding it.
Epidural fibrosis (scar) (Fig SP 21-2)	Hypointense or isointense to disk on T1-weighted images. Often linear and extending above or below level of disk. Conforms to epidural space, and tends to retract thecal sac. Intense contrast enhancement.	Enhancing scar occasionally may obscure tiny disk fragments or cause underestimation of disk size. Must not be confused with normal epidural venous plexus and dorsal root ganglia that also show contrast enhancement. Distinction of postoperative scar from recurrent herniated disk is critical because second operation of scar generally leads to a poor surgical result, as opposed to removal of a reherniated disk.
Arachnoiditis (Fig SP 21-3)	Centrally clumped (intradural pseudomass) or peripheral adherent nerve roots (empty thecal sac). Mild contrast enhancement.	Best detected on T2-weighted images because of high contrast between hyperintense CSF and low-intensity signal of the nerves. Extensive clumping of nerves may make it difficult to determine where the spinal cord ends and the cauda equina begins.
Infection	Mass that is hypointense on T1-weighted images and of increased signal intensity on T2-weighted images.	Because of its high soft-tissue sensitivity, MRI can detect changes in the disk, adjacent end plates, and bone marrow, whereas plain radiographs and radionuclide scans are still negative.
Hematoma	Usually an epidural mass containing material that has varying signal characteristics depending on the stage of its hemorrhagic contents.	Patient generally presents with a neurologic deficit in the immediate postoperative period.

A   B

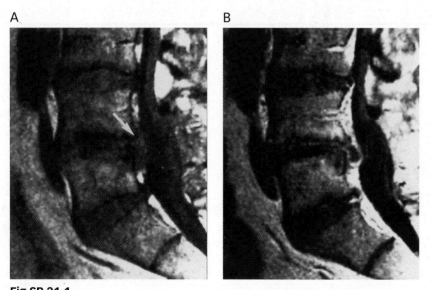

Fig SP 21-1
Herniated disk. (A) Sagittal T1-weighted precontrast image shows a very ill-defined anterior epidural soft-tissue mass at the L4-L5 level (arrow), with slight mass effect on the anterior thecal sac. Differentiation of scar from disk is not possible. (B) Repeat scan after intravenous injection of contrast material clearly defines the central nonenhancing herniation surrounded by enhancing scar tissue.

Condition	Imaging Findings	Comments
Pseudomeningocele	Well-circumscribed mass posterior to the thecal sac that is of CSF density (hypointense on T1-weighted images and hyperintense on T2-weighted images).	Usually does not produce symptoms until weeks or months after surgery. Caused by a small dural tear at the time of surgery that allows progressive herniation of the arachnoid membrane or produces a CSF leak into adjacent soft tissues.

A

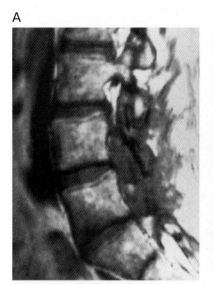

B

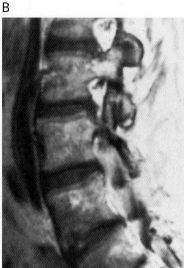

Fig SP 21-2
Epidural scar. (A) Sagittal T1-weighted precontrast image shows a large amount of abnormal tissue within the epidural space at the L4-L5 through L5-S1 levels. (B) Repeat scan after intravenous injection of contrast material demonstrates diffuse and intense enhancement throughout the epidural tissue, consistent with scar.[18]

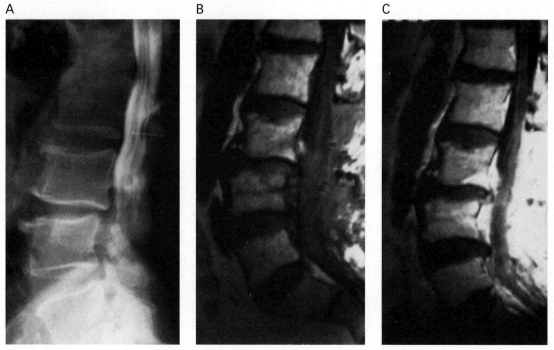

Fig SP 21-3
Arachnoiditis. (A) Lateral view of a lumbar myelogram shows irregular collection of contrast within the most distally filled aspect of the thecal sac, thickened nerve roots, and a block at L3-L4. Sagittal precontrast (B) and postcontrast (C) T1-weighted images were performed. After contrast infusion, there is inhomogeneous, amorphous enhancement of the contents of the thecal sac. Note also the marked enhancement of the postoperative scar posterior to the thecal sac at the site of previous laminectomy and enhancement of the epidural venous plexus or postoperative scar (or both) posterior to the L3 and L4 vertebral bodies.[19]

Demyelinating and Inflammatory Disease of the Spinal Cord on Magnetic Resonance Imaging

Condition	Imaging Findings	Comments
Multiple sclerosis (Figs SP 22-1 and SP 22-2)	Areas of increased signal on T2-weighted images. In acute stage, there may be associated swelling of the spinal cord, which can mimic an intramedullary neoplasm. In late disease, the cord may become atrophic.	Most plaques are peripherally located, are less than two vertebral segments in length, and occupy less than half the cross-sectional area of the cord. Enhancement of spinal cord lesions appears to correlate with active disease. In approximately one-third of patients with multiple sclerosis who present clinically with myelopathy, no associated periventricular lesions can be detected on MR scans of the brain.

A

B

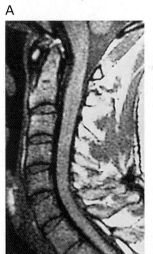
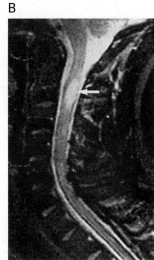

Fig SP 22-1
Multiple sclerosis. (A) T1-weighted and (B) T2-weighted sagittal images show focal enlargement of the cord at the C2 level that demonstrates high signal intensity (arrow, B).[20]

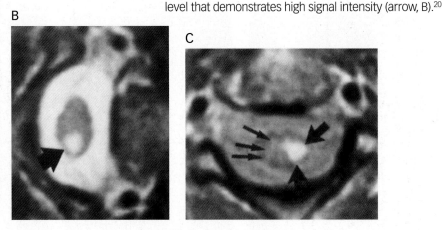
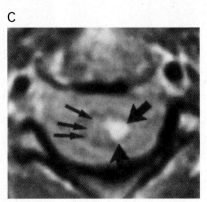

Fig SP 22-2
Multiple sclerosis. (A) Sagittal T2-weighted image shows focal increased signal posteriorly (arrows) at the level of C3 in a normal-sized spinal cord. The plaque is approximately half a vertebral segment in length and is longer than it is wide. (B) Axial T2-weighted scan through the plaque shows the typical peripheral posterolateral location in cross section (arrow). Note that the plaque involves less than half the cross-sectional area of the cord. (C) Axial proton-density image at the same level shows clear involvement of the left dorsal and lateral horns of the central gray matter (large arrows) compared with the appearance of the normal right dorsal and lateral horns (small arrows).[21]

Condition	Imaging Findings	Comments
Transverse myelitis (Figs SP 22-3 and SP 22-4)	Increased intramedullary signal on T2-weighted images in a cord that may be of normal or slightly expanded caliber. The abnormal signal may extend above the level of clinical deficit. A diffuse, peripheral, punctate, or speckled pattern of enhancement may occur.	Rapidly progressing myelopathy that occurs in the absence of any known neurologic disease. It has been associated with viral illness, vasculitides (such as lupus), vaccinations, and multiple sclerosis. In patients who recover, follow-up MR scans may demonstrate resolution of the abnormal signal and return of the cord to a normal caliber.
AIDS–related myelopathy (Fig SP 22-5)	Various patterns may occur. The study may be normal or show areas of increased signal on T2-weighted images that are indistinguishable from transverse myelitis due to other causes. Some contrast enhancement may occur.	In addition to other cerebral neurologic complications, persons with AIDS may experience a vacuolar myelopathy that is probably related to direct injury to the neurons by the HIV virus. Demyelination of the posterior and lateral columns resembling subacute combined degeneration also occurs.
Postradiation myelitis (Fig SP 22-6)	Depending on the time elapsed since radiation, the cord may appear normal, atrophic, or enlarged. Lesions may have increased signal intensity on T2-weighted images and may show contrast enhancement.	The effects of radiation for the treatment of an intramedullary neoplasm may be difficult to differentiate from tumor. Radiation also produces fatty replacement of vertebral body marrow that results in a characteristic high signal intensity on T1-weighted images.

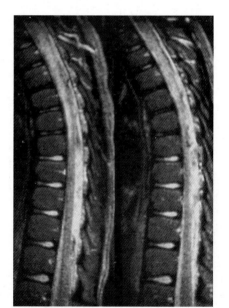

Fig SP 22-3
Transverse myelitis. T2-weighted sagittal images in a young boy with rapid onset of back pain and paraplegia 3 weeks after a viral illness show diffuse, increased signal intensity in the cord, consistent with edema.[20]

A

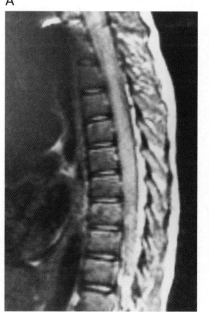

B

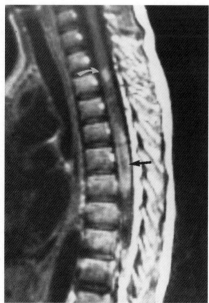

Fig SP 22-4
Inflammatory myelitis. (A) Initial parasagittal proton-density image shows diffuse enlargement of the thoracic cord, which has a heterogeneously high signal. (B) After contrast administration, there are several areas of abnormal enhancement within the enlarged thoracic cord. The largest of these areas demonstrates a peripheral, diffuse pattern of enhancement (arrow). A separate area of enhancement is noted superiorly (curved arrow). (Courtesy of Linda L. Coleman, M.D.)[22]

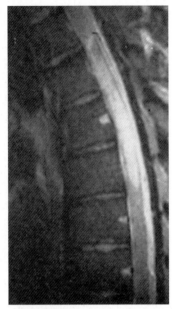

Fig SP 22-5
AIDS-related myelopathy. T2-weighted sagittal image demonstrates high intramedullary signal in a somewhat swollen area of the thoracic cord.[20]

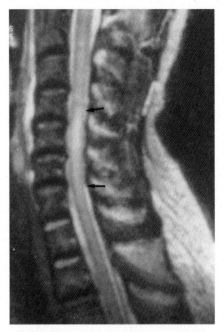

Fig SP 22-6
Postradiation myelitis. T2-weighted image after radiation therapy for laryngeal cancer shows increased signal intensity (arrows) in the spinal cord from C4-C7.[11]

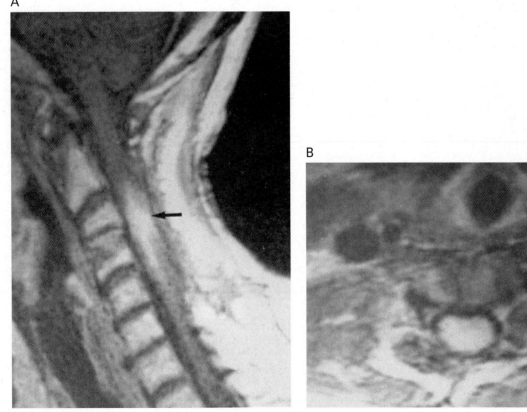

Fig SP 22-7
Intramedullary sarcoidosis. (A) Sagittal and (B) axial T1-weighted images after injection of contrast material show an enhancing intramedullary mass (arrow, A) indistinguishable from a glioma.[20]

Condition	Imaging Findings	Comments
Sarcoidosis (Figs SP 22-7 and SP 22-8)	Enhancing intramedullary or pial lesion that is usually not evident on standard spin echo scans.	Although clinical involvement of the CNS occurs in 5% of patients with sarcoidosis, primary involvement is very rare. The involvement may be intramedullary or extramedullary (or both). Pial enhancement is not pathognomonic because it can be seen with tuberculous, toxoplasmic, or HIV-related meningitis; leptomeningeal metastases; and post-shunting meningeal fibrosis.

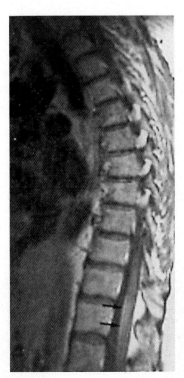

Fig SP 22-8
Pial sarcoidosis. T1-weighted axial image of the thoracic region of the spine after injection of contrast material demonstrates pial enhancement along the conus (arrows). The patient's bilateral lower extremity numbness resolved after steroid therapy.[20]

Congenital Anomalies of the Spine on Magnetic Resonance Imaging

Condition	Imaging Findings	Comments
Tethered cord syndrome (Fig SP 23-1)	Caudal displacement of the conus below the L2-L3 level in neonates and young children or below the middle of L2 after age 12.	Clinically presents with motor and sensory dysfunction of the lower extremities (unrelated to myotomal or dermatomal pattern), muscle atrophy, decreased or hyperactive reflexes, urinary incontinence, spastic gait, scoliosis, or foot deformities. Causes include lipomatous lesions (intramedullary lipomas, lipomyelomeningoceles, lipoma of the filum terminale); myelomeningocele; diastematomyelia; and a short, thickened filum terminale (>2 mm).
Syringomyelia/ hydromyelia (Fig SP 23-2)	Fusiform widening of the spinal cord, which contains a dilated central cavity filled with CSF-intensity material.	Usually associated with the Chiari I malformation. In adults without this malformation, syringomyelia/hydromyelia suggests the presence of a spinal cord tumor.
Failure of fusion of posterior elements (Fig SP 23-3)	Various patterns of posterior protrusion of meninges, neural elements, and fat through a midline bony defect.	Meningocele; myelomeningocele (usually with Chiari II malformation); lipomyelomeningocele.
Diastematomyelia (Fig SP 23-4)	Longitudinal splitting of the spinal cord.	Often occurs in association with a bony or fibrous spur (best seen on plain films or CT) that divides the cord and may cause tethering.

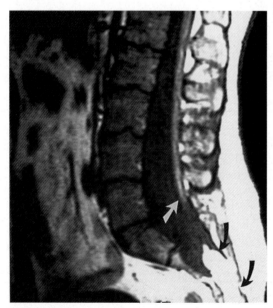

Fig SP 23-1
Tethered cord syndrome. Sagittal T1-weighted image in a patient who had undergone a myelomeningocele repair at birth shows that the cord ends at the L5 level (straight arrow). Note the absence of the posterior elements of the sacrum, as well as the presence of a high-signal-intensity mass (lipoma) within the sacral spinal canal (curved arrows).[12]

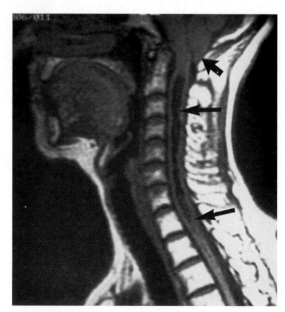

Fig SP 23-2
Syringomyelia in Chiari I malformation. Sagittal T1-weighted image of the cervical region of the spine shows the characteristic low position of the cerebellar tonsils (short arrow). The intramedullary cord syrinx extends from C2 to T2 (long arrows).[12]

Condition	Imaging Findings	Comments
Dorsal dermal sinus	Single or double low-intensity line extending downward and inward from the skin through the subcutaneous tissue. If present, the dermoid/epidermoid lesion can be clearly delineated.	Epithelial tract connecting the spinal canal with the skin of the back (most commonly the sacrococcygeal or lumbar region). Approximately half terminate in an epidermoid or dermoid lesion (about 25% of dermoids are associated with dermal sinuses). Clinically, the sinus most frequently appears as a pinpoint hole or a small atrophic zone in the skin. A tuft of short, small, wiry hairs may emerge from the ostium.

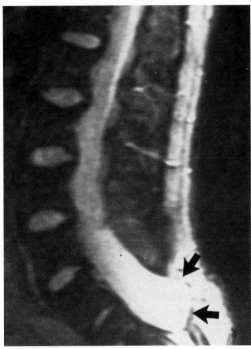

Fig SP 23-3
Meningocele. Sagittal T2-weighted image shows extension of the meninges and subarachnoid space through a bony defect in the upper sacrum (arrows).[12]

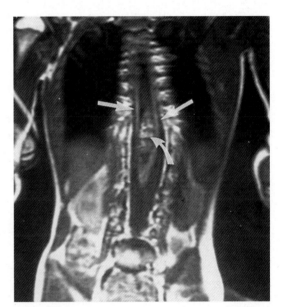

Fig SP 23-4
Diastematomyelia. Coronal MR scan shows the two hemicords (straight arrows) separated by a bony spur that contains marrow (curved arrow). The hemicords unite inferior to the bony spur.[12]

Sources

1. Reprinted with permission from "Radiologic Diagnosis of Metabolic Bone Disease" by WA Reynolds and JJ Karo, *Orthopedic Clinics of North America* (1972;3:521–532), Copyright ©1972, WB Saunders Company.

2. Reprinted from *Diagnosis of Bone and Joint Disorders*, ed 2, by DL Resnick and G Niwayama, with permission of WB Saunders Company, ©1988.

3. Reprinted with permission from "Benign Tumors" by JW Beabout, RA McLeod, and DC Dahlin, *Seminars in Roentgenology* (1979;14:33–43), Copyright ©1979, Grune & Stratton Inc.

4. Reprinted from *Roentgen Diagnosis of Disease of Bone*, ed 3, by J Edeiken with permission of Williams & Wilkins Company, ©1981.

5. Reprinted from *Clinical Radiology in the Tropics* by WP Cockshott and H Middlemiss (Eds) with permission of Churchill Livingstone Inc, ©1979.

6. Reprinted with permission from "The Radiologic Assessment of Short Stature" by JP Dorst, CI Scott, and JG Hall, *Radiologic Clinics of North America* (1972;10:393–414), Copyright ©1972, WB Saunders Company.

7. Reprinted from *Radiology of Bone Diseases* by GB Greenfield, JB Lippincott Company, with permission of the author, ©1986.

8. Reprinted from *Caffey's Pediatric X-Ray Diagnosis*, ed 8, by FN Silverman with permission of Year Book Medical Publishers Inc, ©1985.

9. Reprinted with permission from "Ghost Infantile Vertebrae and Hemipelves within Adult Skeletons from Thorotrast Administration in Childhood" by JG Teplick et al, *Radiology* (1978;120:657–660), Copyright ©1978, Radiological Society of North America Inc.

10. Reprinted with permission from "Gd-DTPA-Enhanced MR Imaging of Spinal Tumors" by BD Parizel et al, *AJR Am J Roentgenol* (1989;152:1087–2020), Copyright ©1989, Williams & Wilkins Company.

11. Reprinted with permission from *Neuroradiology Companion*, by M Castillo, Lippincott-Raven, with permission of the author.

12. Reprinted from *MRI of the Musculoskeletal System*, ed 2, by TH Berquist (Ed) with permission of Mayo Foundation, ©1990.

13. Reprinted with permission from "Magnetic Resonance Imaging of Extramedullary-Intradural Spinal Masses" by JL Port, JS Ross, *The Radiologist* (1995;2:163–171).

14. Reprinted with permission from "Non-neoplastic Lesions of Vertebral Bodies: Findings in Magnetic Resonance Imaging" by CW Hayes, ME Jensen, and WF Conway, *Radiographics* (1989;9:883–903), Copyright ©1989, Radiological Society of North America Inc.

15. Reprinted with permission from *Clinical Magnetic Resonance Imaging*, RR Edelman, JR Hesselink (Eds), Copyright ©1990, WB Saunders Company.

16. Reprinted with permission from "Tumors of the osseous spine: staging with MR imaging versus CT" by J Beltran, AM Noto, DW Chakeres et al, *Radiology* (1987;162:565–569).

17. Reprinted with permission from "MR Imaging of Sacral and Presacral Lesions" by LH Wetzel, E Levine, *AJR Am J Roentgenol* (1990;154:771–775).

18. Reprinted with permission from "MR Imaging of the Postoperative Lumbar Spine: Assessment with Gadopentetate Dimeglumine" by JS Ross, TJ Masaryk, M Schrader et al, *American Journal of Roentgenology* (1990;155:867–872), Copyright ©1990, American Roentgen Ray Society.

19. Reprinted with permission from "Benign Lumbar Arachnoiditis: MR Imaging with Gadopentetate Dimeglumine" by CE Johnson and G Sze, *AJR Am J Roentgenol* (1990;155:873–880), Copyright ©1990, American Roentgen Ray Society.

20. Reprinted with permission from "MRI of Infectious and Inflammatory Diseases of the Spine" by AS Mark, *MRI Decisions* (1991;5:12–26), Copyright ©1991, PW Communications, International. All rights reserved.

21. Reprinted with permission from "Multiple Sclerosis in the Spinal Cord: MR Appearance and Correlation with Clinical Parameters" by LM Tartaglino, DP Friedman, AE Flanders et al, *Radiology* (1995;195:725–732).

22. Reprinted with permission from "Intramedullary Cord Lesions: MR Evaluation" by AJ Johnson, *The Radiologist* (1994;1:131–139).

7 Skull Patterns

Dilated Cerebral Ventricles

Condition	Imaging Findings	Comments
Noncommunicating (obstructive) hydrocephalus	Symmetric distention of the ventricular system proximal to the obstruction and a ventricular system of normal or less than normal size distal to the obstruction.	Possible site of obstruction should be examined in detail with thin CT slices and, if necessary, overlapping cuts to establish the pathogenesis of the obstruction.
Level of foramen of Monro (Fig SK 1-1)	Enlargement of the lateral ventricles with normal-sized third and fourth ventricles.	Colloid cyst; suprasellar tumors (especially craniopharyngioma); intraventricular tumors; arachnoid cysts of the suprasellar cistern; intraventricular hemorrhage (trauma, arteriovenous malformation, hemophilia). Unilateral tumors, such as those arising in the hypothalamus, basal ganglia, or cerebral parenchyma, may obstruct only one side and cause dilatation of the opposite ventricle and mass compression of the ipsilateral ventricle.
Level of aqueduct (Fig SK 1-2)	Enlargement of the lateral and third ventricles with a normal-sized fourth ventricle.	Most common causes are congenital aqueduct stenosis or occlusion (most commonly associated with the Arnold-Chiari malformation) and neoplasm (pinealoma, teratoma). Other underlying conditions include cyst of the quadrigeminal cistern, brainstem edema, aneurysmal dilatation of the vein of Galen, hemorrhage, and acute infection.
Level of outlet of fourth ventricle (Fig SK 1-3)	Enlargement of the entire ventricular system (with the fourth ventricle often dilated out of proportion).	Atresia of fourth ventricle foramina (Dandy-Walker cyst); Arnold-Chiari malformation; basilar arachnoiditis (eg, tuberculous meningitis); tonsillar herniation; neoplasm (medulloblastoma, ependymoma); basilar impression (eg, Paget's disease); arachnoid cyst.

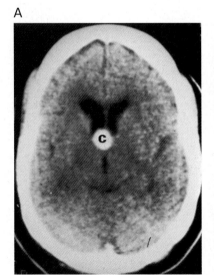 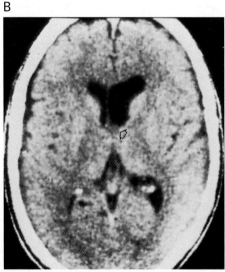

Fig SK 1-1
Level of the foramen of Monro. (A) Bilateral enlargement of the frontal horns with a normal-sized third ventricle in a patient with a hyperdense colloid cyst (c). (B) Unilateral enlargement of the left frontal horn caused by a tiny hypodense unilateral tumor (arrow).

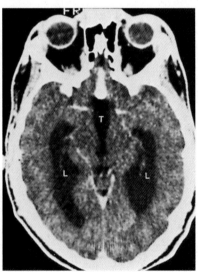

Fig SK 1-2
Level of the aqueduct. Dilatation of the lateral (L) and third (T) ventricles in a patient with congenital hydrocephalus. The symptoms of headache and papilledema were resolved after ventricular shunting.

Condition	Imaging Findings	Comments
Communicating hydrocephalus (Fig SK 1-4)	Generalized ventricular enlargement with normal or absent sulci.	Obstruction of the normal cerebrospinal fluid pathway distal to the fourth ventricle (usually involves the subarachnoid space at the basal cisterns, cerebral convexity, or foramen magnum). Causes include infection (meningitis, empyema), subarachnoid or subdural hemorrhage, congenital anomalies, neoplasm, and dural venous thrombosis. A similar pattern is seen in "normal-pressure" hydrocephalus, a syndrome of gait ataxia, urinary incontinence, and dementia associated with ventricular dilatation and relatively normal cerebrospinal fluid pressure.
Overproduction of cerebrospinal fluid (Fig SK 1-5)	Generalized enlargement of the ventricular system.	Choroid plexus papilloma or carcinoma that causes overproduction of cerebrospinal fluid. This rare tumor usually occurs in the fourth ventricle in adults and the lateral ventricle in children. Differentiation from other intraventricular masses is made by the CT demonstration of its choroid location and the typical choroidal pattern of contrast enhancement.
Atrophy (atrophic hydrocephalus) (Figs SK 1-6 through SK 1-8)	Diffuse dilatation of the lateral and third ventricles as well as the cisterns. The sulci over the surfaces of the cerebral hemispheres are prominent and appear as wide linear lucent stripes.	Multiple causes, including normal aging, degenerative diseases (Alzheimer's, Pick's, Jakob-Creutzfeldt, Binswanger's), Huntington's disease, congenital inflammatory disease (eg, toxoplasmosis, torulosis, cytomegalic inclusion disease), vascular disease (multifocal infarct, arteriovenous malformation).

A

B

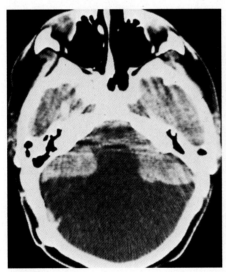

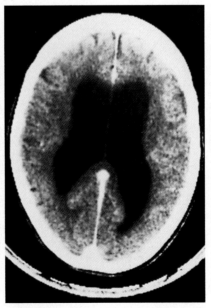

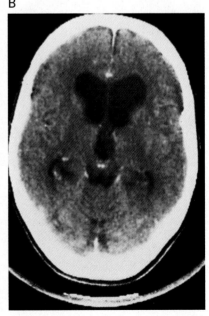

Fig SK 1-3
Dandy-Walker cyst. Huge low-density cyst that occupies most of the enlarged posterior fossa and represents an extension of the dilated fourth ventricle.

Fig SK 1-4
Communicating hydrocephalus. Generalized ventricular enlargement in a 69-year-old patient with ataxia, dementia, and incontinence. Note the absence of the dilated sulci in the obstructive hydrocephalus.[1]

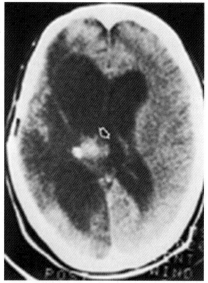

Fig SK 1-5
Choroid plexus papilloma. Enhancing ventricular mass (arrow) causing pronounced generalized enlargement of the ventricular system.

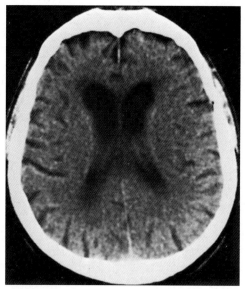

Fig SK 1-6
Normal aging. CT scan of a 70-year-old man shows generalized ventricular dilatation with prominence of the sulci over the surfaces of the cerebral hemispheres.

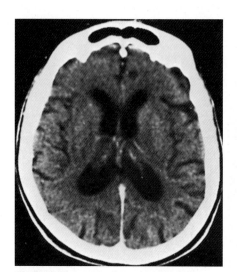

Fig SK 1-7
Alzheimer's disease. Noncontrast scan of a 56-year-old woman with progressive dementia shows generalized enlargement of the ventricular system and sulci.

A

B

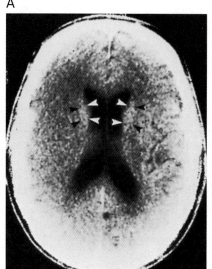

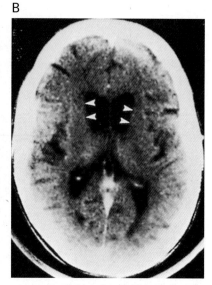

Fig SK 1-8
Huntington's disease. (A) CT scan in a normal patient shows the heads of the caudate nucleus (black arrowheads) producing a normal concavity of the frontal horns (white arrowheads). (B) In a patient with Huntington's disease, atrophy of the caudate nucleus causes a characteristic loss of the normal concavity (white arrowheads) of the frontal horns.

Condition	Imaging Findings	Comments
Atrophy of one cerebral hemisphere (Fig SK 1-9)	Enlargement of the ipsilateral lateral ventricle and sulci and a shift of midline structures to the affected side.	Usually the result of complete occlusion of the ipsilateral middle cerebral artery. If the occlusion occurs in early childhood, the affected half of the skull is underdeveloped.
Localized atrophy (Fig SK 1-10)	Focal enlargement of a part of one ventricle or a group of sulci.	Usually a late residual of previous insult to the brain (eg, infarct, hematoma, severe contusion, abscess).

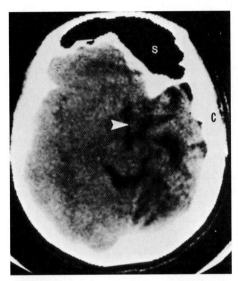

Fig SK 1-9
Cerebral hemiatrophy (Davidoff-Dyke syndrome). CT scan of a 5-year-old boy who had intrauterine difficulties demonstrates extensive loss of brain volume in the left hemisphere. There is also enlargement of the left hemicalvarium (C), enlargement of the left frontal sinus (S), and a shift of midline structures such as the third ventricle (arrowhead) from right to left. The low density in the remainder of the hemisphere represents encephalomalacia.

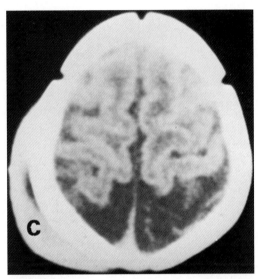

Fig SK 1-10
Localized atrophy. Contrast-enhanced scan of an infant with intrauterine infection shows bilateral occipital atrophy. Note the cephalhematoma (C) on the right.

Ring-Enhancing Lesions

Condition	Comments
Glioblastoma multiforme (Figs SK 2-1 and SK 2-2; see Figs SK 4-2 and SK 6-2)	Thick, irregular ring enhancement in a solitary lesion that tends to be situated in a deep hemispheric location and associated with surrounding low-attenuation edema and glial cell infiltration. May occasionally have a relatively uniform rim of enhancement that mimics the capsule of an abscess.
Metastasis (Fig SK 2-3)	Irregular rim enhancement with a relatively lucent center due to tumor necrosis. Typically located at the gray matter–white matter junction and usually associated with surrounding low-density edema that tends to be relatively concentric and uniform in the adjacent white matter (unlike glial cell infiltration with glioblastoma multiforme, which is usually eccentric and irregular in both gray and white matter).
Lymphoma (Fig SK 2-4)	Single or multiple ring-enhancing lesions that primarily affect transplant recipients (high incidence of central nervous system lymphoma in these patients).

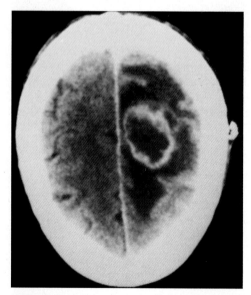

Fig SK 2-1
Glioblastoma multiforme. Thick irregular ring-enhancing lesion associated with a large amount of surrounding low-attenuation edema.

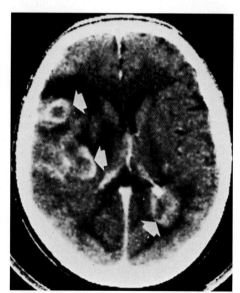

Fig SK 2-2
Multicentric glioblastoma multiforme. Bilateral, irregular enhancing masses (arrows) with surrounding low-density edema.

Condition

Abscess
(Figs SK 2-5 through SK 2-8)

Comments

Usually a relatively thin, uniform ring of enhancement associated with considerable reactive edema and a strongly suggestive clinical picture of fever, leukocytosis, obtundation, extracranial infection, or a previous operation. Some pyogenic or fungal abscesses may develop a relatively thick capsule, which resembles the periphery of a high-grade glioma or metastasis. The relatively poor inflammatory response of deep hemispheric white matter may cause the capsule of an abscess to be less developed along the medial wall than along the lateral margin, a feature that may aid in distinguishing an abscess from a neoplasm.

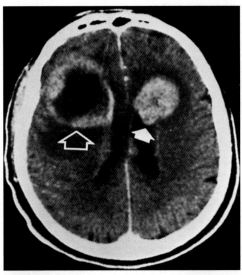

Fig SK 2-3
Metastases. Enhancing metastases from squamous cell carcinoma of the lung that are both ring-enhancing (open arrow) and solid (solid arrow).

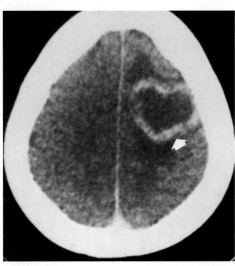

Fig SK 2-4
Lymphoma developing after renal transplantation. Heart-shaped, peripherally enhancing, central lucent lesion (arrow) situated in the frontoparietal region. There is moderate surrounding edema.[2]

A

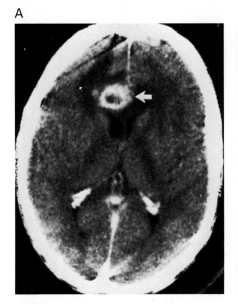

B

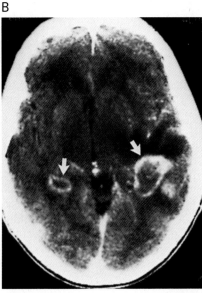

Fig SK 2-5
Brain abscess in acquired immunodeficiency syndrome. (A) Candidal abscess appears as a cystic lesion with a thick zone of enhancement (arrow) near the genu of the corpus callosum. (B) In another patient, multiple toxoplasmic brain abscesses appear as lucent lesions with rings of enhancement (arrows).[3]

Condition	Comments
Infection following transplantation (Fig SK 2-9)	Infection by one of a broad spectrum of organisms is the most common complication of transplantation and may be the cause of a rim-enhancing lesion. Epstein-Barr virus causes focal infarcts that produce a rim-enhancing pattern.

A   B

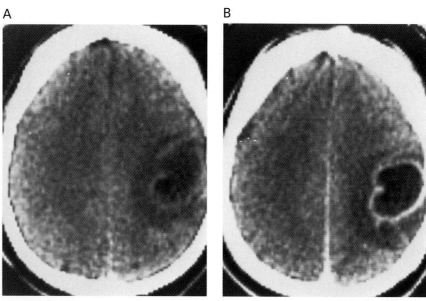

Fig SK 2-6
Cysticercosis. (A) Precontrast CT scan shows a primarily low-density area in the right frontoparietal region. The ring of increased density around the lesion is vaguely evident initially, but becomes readily apparent after contrast enhancement (B).[4]

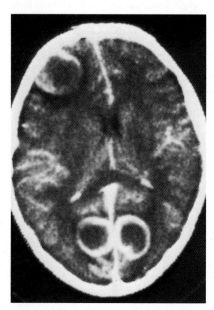

Fig SK 2-7
Pyogenic brain abscesses. One frontal and two occipital lesions with relatively thin, uniform rings of enhancement.

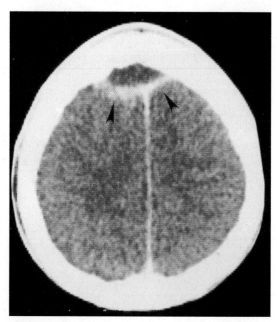

Fig SK 2-8
Epidural abscess. Biconvex hypodense lesion with contrast-enhanced dural margin (arrowheads) that crosses the falx and displaces the falx away from the inner table of the skull.[5]

Condition	Comments
Resolving intracerebral hematoma (3–6 weeks old) (Fig SK 2-10)	Thin, uniform ring of contrast enhancement that initially represents perivascular inflammation and defects in the tight capillary junctions and eventually reflects the collagenous capsule. Causes of intracerebral hematoma include trauma, surgery, hypertensive vascular disease, vascular malformation, mycotic aneurysm, and berry aneurysm.
Nonacute subdural hematoma	Occasionally produces a pattern of thick rim enhancement with loculation, reflecting its richly vascular surrounding membrane.
Atypical meningioma (Fig SK 2-11)	A few meningiomas contain low-attenuation, nonenhancing areas (necrosis, old hemorrhage, cyst formation, or fat in the meningioma tissue) that produce a thick, often irregular, rim. This pattern, especially if associated with prominent edema, may mimic a malignant glioma or metastasis. Coronal scans demonstrating that the mass arises from a dural base suggest the diagnosis of meningioma, though superficial gliomas may invade the dura and dural-based metastases may occur.

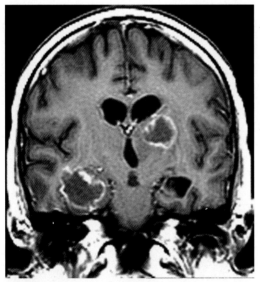

Fig SK 2-9
Epstein-Barr virus infection. Contrast MR image shows rim enhancement of lesions in the deep gray matter on the left and the temporal lobe on the right. The signal hyperintensity in the periventricular white matter is related to treatment. This infection developed following bone marrow transplantation for acute lymphoblastic leukemia.[6]

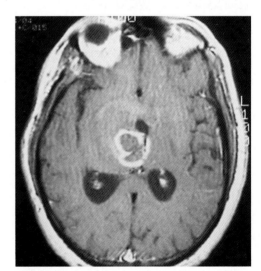

Fig SK 2-10
Resolving intracerebral hematoma. Five weeks after the initial episode of bleeding, there is peripheral contrast enhancement of the thalamic lesion.

Condition	Comments
Radiation necrosis (Fig SK 2-12)	Occasional manifestation. Develops in the tumor bed 9 to 24 months after radiation therapy and may be impossible to differentiate from recurrent or residual tumor.
Radiation complications (Fig SK 12-13)	Radiation necrosis occasionally develops in the tumor bed 9 to 24 months after radiation therapy and may be impossible to differentiate from recurrent or residual tumor. Radiation-induced cerebral malignancies, such as glioblastoma multiforme, are well documented.

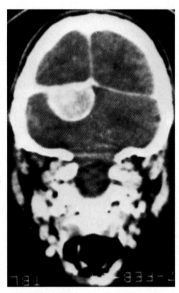

Fig SK 2-11
Atypical meningioma. The contrast enhancement is predominantly peripheral, with the area of central necrosis remaining relatively nonenhanced. The correct diagnosis is indicated by the origin of the tumor from the thickened tentorium.

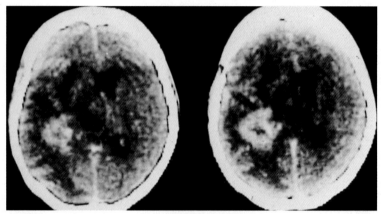

Fig SK 2-12
Radiation necrosis. Lesion with ring enhancement and surrounding edema that could represent a primary or metastatic tumor. At autopsy, the mass was found to represent postradiation necrosis with sarcomatous changes in a patient who had undergone surgery for a solitary metastasis.[5]

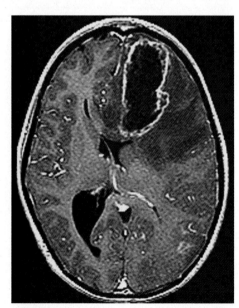

Fig SK 2-13
Radiation-induced malignancy. Contrast scan shows a lesion with rim enhancement in the left frontal lobe.[6]

Multiple Enhancing Cerebral and Cerebellar Nodules

Condition	Comments
Metastases (Figs SK 3-1 and SK 3-2)	Round, well-marginated, homogeneously enhancing nodules that are typically located at the gray matter–white matter junction and are often associated with some peritumoral edema. The major malignant tumors causing intracranial metastases are, in decreasing order of frequency, lung, breast, skin (melanoma), colon, rectum, and kidney.
Primary lymphoma (Fig SK 3-3)	Homogeneously and often intensely enhancing masses that most commonly occur in the basal ganglia, corpus callosum, or periventricular region. Peritumoral edema is usually slight. Primary lymphoma of the brain is rare in otherwise healthy individuals and is much more common in patients who are immunosuppressed (especially organ transplant recipients).

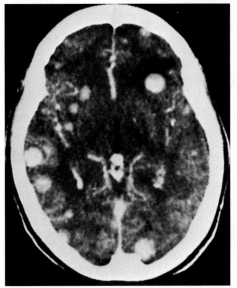

Fig SK 3-1
Metastatic carcinoma. Multiple enhancing masses of various shapes and sizes representing hematogenous metastases from carcinoma of the breast.

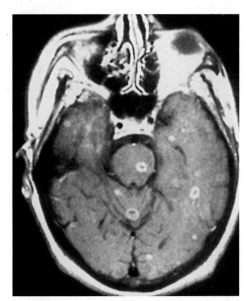

Fig SK 3-2
Metastatic carcinoma. Multiple enhancing masses representing hematogenous metastases from carcinoma of the lung.

Condition	Comments
Multiple sclerosis (Figs SK 3-4 and SK 3-5)	Contrast enhancement in plaques of demyelination is unusual except in rapidly evolving ones with surrounding inflammatory changes. The plaques in multiple sclerosis usually have a more central or periventricular location, unlike the more peripheral position of metastases near the gray matter–white matter junction.

A   B

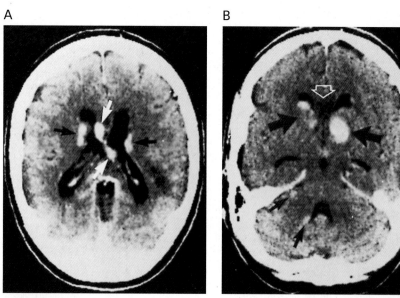

Fig SK 3-3
Primary lymphoma. (A) Homogeneous enhancement of multiple periventricular nodules (arrows). (B) Another section shows additional enhancing lymphomatous nodules in the basal ganglia (large arrows) and posterior fossa (small arrows). Note the cystic cavum septum pellucidi (open arrow).[1]

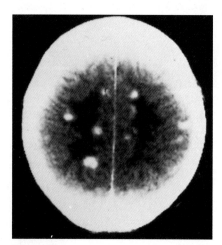

Fig SK 3-4
Multiple sclerosis simulating metastases. Nodular enhancement in periventricular and subcortical white matter resulting from demyelination.[1]

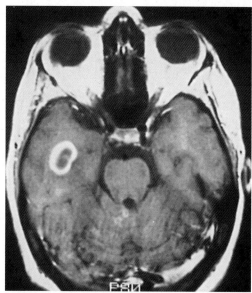

Fig SK 3-5
Multiple sclerosis. Single large ring-enhancing lesion.

Condition	Comments

Disseminated infection
  Cysticercosis
  (Figs SK 3-6 and SK 3-7)
	Multiple, small, homogeneously enhancing nodules may develop after infection by the larvae of the pork tapeworm (*Taenia solium*). Usually associated with much more extensive edema than are metastases. May demonstrate multiple enhancing rings, some of which contain focal calcification representing the scolices of degenerated larvae.

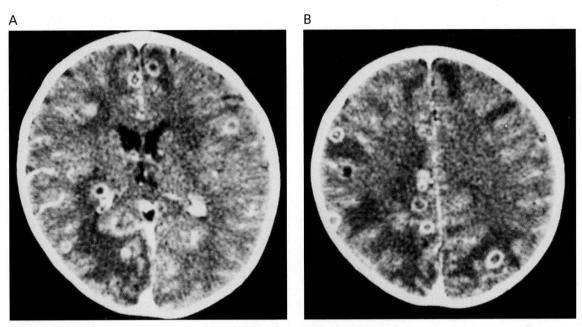

Fig SK 3-6
Cysticercosis. Multiple, enhancing nodules or rings, some of which contain focal calcification representing the scolices of erupted larvae. Note the zones of surrounding edema.[1]

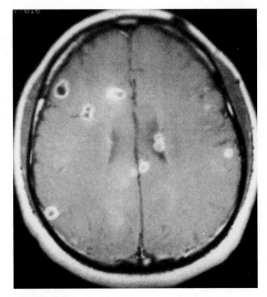

Fig SK 3-7
Cysticercosis. Multiple enhancing nodules.

Condition	Comments
Tuberculosis	Homogeneously enhancing nodules or small rings with central punctate lucencies representing foci of cavitation surrounded by a rim of inflammatory cells.
Histoplasmosis	Pattern identical to that of multiple tuberculous abscesses.
Toxoplasmosis	Multiple, densely enhancing nodules (or ring-enhancing lesions) that occur at both the gray matter–white matter junction and in a periventricular location.

Subacute, multifocal infarction
   Arterial
   (Fig SK 3-8)
	Small focal enhancing lesions distributed along vascular watersheds. Underlying causes include hypoperfusion, multiple emboli, cerebral vasculitis (eg, systemic lupus erythematosus), and meningitis.

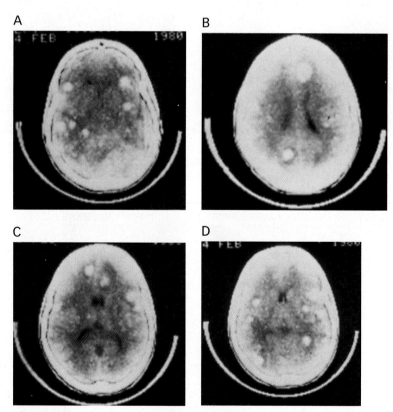

Fig SK 3-8
Subacute, multifocal infarction. Multiple enhancing nodules producing a pattern mimicking metastases.

Condition	Comments
Venous	Parasagittal hemorrhages due to cortical venous infarction are a highly specific secondary finding in superior sagittal sinus thrombosis.
Sarcoidosis (Fig SK 3-9)	Homogeneous enhancement of the noncaseating granulomas (more often affects the meninges than the brain).

A
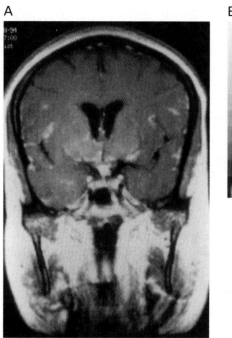

B
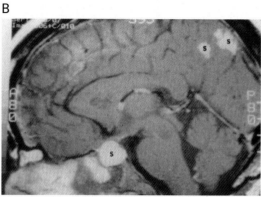

C
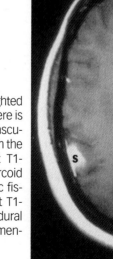

Fig SK 3-9
Sarcoidosis. (A) Coronal postcontrast T1-weighted image shows abnormal pial enhancement. There is also abnormal enhancement along the perivascular spaces for the lenticulostriate arteries and in the pituitary stalk. (B) Midsagittal postcontrast T1-weighted image (different patient) shows sarcoid deposits (s) in the posterior interhemispheric fissure and in the sella. (C) Axial postcontrast T1-weighted image of a different patient shows dural and mass-like (s) sarcoid deposits simulating meningiomas (avascular at angiography).[7]

Hypodense Supratentorial Masses on Computed Tomography

Condition	Imaging Findings	Comments
Astrocytoma (Fig SK 4-1)	Hypodense lesion with little contrast enhancement or peritumoral edema. Calcification frequently occurs.	Slowly growing tumor that has an infiltrative character and can form large cavities or pseudocysts.
Glioblastoma multiforme (Fig SK 4-2)	Large, inhomogeneous mass with irregular, poorly defined margins and central hypodense zones. Contrast enhancement is usually intense and inhomogeneous, and a ring with thickened irregular walls or nodules of enhancement is common.	Highly malignant lesion that is predominantly cerebral in location. Typically has low-attenuation tissue consisting of edema and malignant glial cells surrounding the enhancing portion of the tumor.
Oligodendroglioma (Fig SK 4-3)	Large, irregular, inhomogeneous mass containing calcification and hypodense zones. Variable peritumoral edema and contrast enhancement.	Slow-growing tumor that originates from oligodendrocytes in the central white matter (especially the anterior half of the cerebrum). Calcification (peripheral or central, nodular or shell-like) occurs in approximately 90% of tumors.
Metastasis (Fig SK 4-4)	Hypodense mass surrounded by edema (which usually exceeds tumor volume). Variable contrast enhancement depending on the size and type of tumor.	The density of a metastasis depends on its cellularity and neovascularity and the presence of central necrosis or hemorrhage. Epithelial tumors are typically hypodense; melanoma, choriocarcinoma, and osteosarcoma are usually hyperdense.
Ganglioglioma/ ganglioneuroma	Small, well-defined hypodense or ill-defined isodense mass. Calcified and cystic areas are frequent, and most tumors show homogeneous contrast enhancement.	Rare, relatively benign, slow-growing tumors containing mature ganglion cells and stromal elements derived from glial tissue. Typically occur in adolescents and young adults in the temporal and frontal lobes, basal ganglia, and anterior third ventricle.

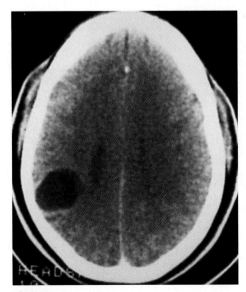

Fig SK 4-1
Cystic astrocytoma. Hypodense mass with a thin rim of contrast enhancement.

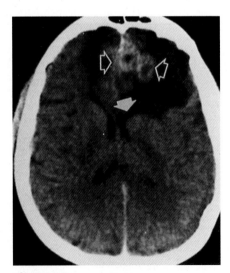

Fig SK 4-2
Glioblastoma multiforme. Irregular enhancing lesion (open arrows). The substantial mass effect of the tumor distorts the frontal horns (closed arrow).

Condition	Imaging Findings	Comments
Epidermoid (primary cholesteatoma) (Fig SK 4-5)	Round, sharply marginated, nearly homogeneous hypodense mass. May have extremely low attenuation due to a high fat content. No contrast enhancement.	The result of inclusion of ectodermal germ layer elements in the neural tube during its closure between the third and fifth weeks of gestation. Ectodermal inclusion early in this period produces a midline tumor, whereas later inclusion produces an eccentrically located lesion. More common in the cerebellopontine angle and suprasellar region.

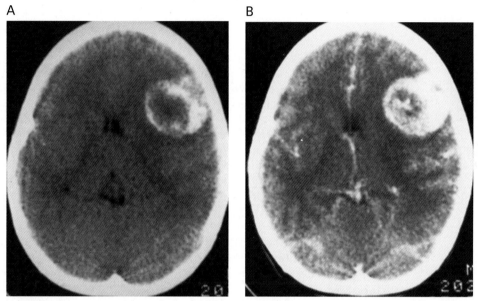

Fig SK 4-3
Oligodendroglioma. (A) Nonenhanced scan showing a hypodense mass containing amorphous areas of calcification. (B) After the intravenous injection of contrast material, there is marked contrast enhancement.

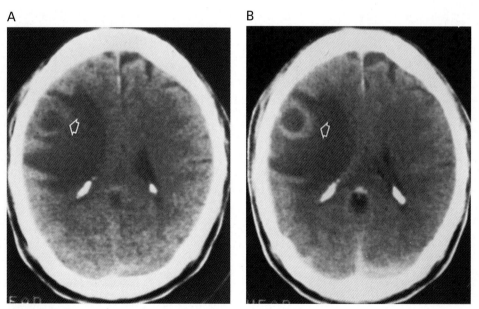

Fig SK 4-4
Metastasis. (A) Nonenhanced scan shows a small hypodense mass with an isodense rim (arrow) surrounded by extensive edema. (B) After the intravenous injection of contrast material, there is prominent ring enhancement (arrow) about the metastasis.

Condition	Imaging Findings	Comments
Dermoid	Inhomogeneous midline mass that often contains focal areas of fat, mural or central calcification, or bone. No contrast enhancement.	Congenital inclusion of both ectodermal and mesodermal germ layer elements at the time of neural tube closure. Contains hair follicles and sebaceous and apocrine glands (derived from mesoderm) that produce a thick, buttery mixture of sweat and sebum.
Lipoma (Fig SK 4-6)	Well-defined, homogeneously hypodense fatty mass that occurs in the midline. No contrast enhancement.	Uncommon congenital tumor resulting from inclusion of mesodermal adipose tissue at the time of neural tube closure. Most commonly involves the corpus callosum (often with dense, curvilinear mural calcification).
Radiation necrosis (see Fig SK 6-11)	Deep, focal, hypodense mass that is usually in or near the irradiated tumor bed. May show an irregular ring of contrast enhancement.	Develops 9 to 24 months after radiation therapy and may be impossible to differentiate from recurrent or residual tumor.
Cerebral infarction (Figs SK 4-7 through SK 4-10)	Triangular or wedge-shaped area of hypodensity involving the cortex and the underlying white matter down to the ventricular surface.	Unlike a hypodense glioma, an infarct has a distinctive shape that corresponds to the distribution of a specific vessel or vessels and has a characteristic pattern of peripheral, rarely central, enhancement. The clinical diagnosis is usually obvious because of the abrupt onset of symptoms.
Pyogenic abscess (Fig SK 4-11)	Central hypodense zone (pus, necrotic tissue) surrounded by a thin, isodense ring (fibrous capsule) and peripheral low-density tissue (reactive edema).	Unlike intermediate-grade and highly aggressive gliomas, in which enhancement is often ring-like but irregular in thickness, a cerebral abscess is characterized by a thin uniform ring of enhancement. There also is usually a strongly suggestive clinical picture of fever, leukocytosis, obtundation, extracranial infection, or a previous operation.

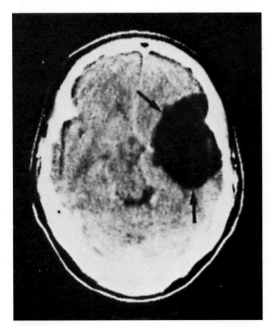

Fig SK 4-5
Epidermoid. Enhanced scan shows a large, sharply marginated, low-attenuation, extra-axial sylvian mass (arrows).[1]

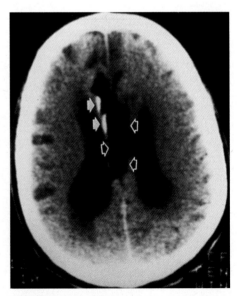

Fig SK 4-6
Lipoma of the corpus callosum. Extremely low-density mass (open arrows) involving much of the corpus callosum. Note the peripheral calcifications (closed arrows).

Condition	Imaging Findings	Comments
Hydatid (echinococcal) cyst (Fig SK 4-12)	Round, sharply marginated, smooth-walled hypodense mass.	Rare manifestation of this parasitic infection. The parenchymal cysts tend to be large and multiple, with no reactive edema or contrast enhancement.
Herpes simplex encephalitis (Fig SK 4-13)	Poorly defined, frequently bilateral areas of decreased attenuation, especially involving the temporal and parietal lobes.	Most common cause of nonepidemic fatal encephalitis in the United States. The putamen, which is spared by this infection, often forms the sharply defined, slightly concave or straight medial border of the low-density zone. Various patterns of contrast enhancement develop in approximately half the patients.

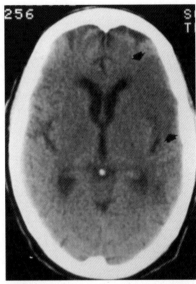

Fig SK 4-7
Acute left middle cerebral artery infarct. Scan obtained 20 hours after the onset of acute hemiparesis and aphasia shows obliteration of the normal sulci (arrows) in the involved hemisphere. There is low density of the gray and white matter in the distribution of the left middle cerebral artery.

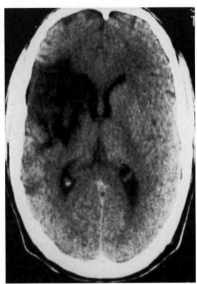

Fig SK 4-8
Chronic right middle cerebral artery infarct. Low-attenuation region with sharply defined borders and some dilatation of the adjacent ventricle.

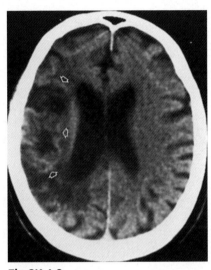

Fig SK 4-9
Old infarct in the distribution of the right middle cerebral artery. There is a thin peripheral rim of contrast enhancement (arrows) about the hypodense region. Note the enlargement of the right lateral ventricle.

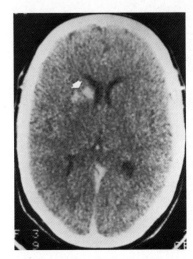

Fig SK 4-10
Basal ganglia infarction. Hypodense region (arrow) involving the right head of the caudate and putamen and passing through the anterior limb of the internal capsule. This distribution reflects a lesion of the artery of Heubner. After the intravenous injection of contrast material, there is contrast enhancement of the area of infarction (arrow).

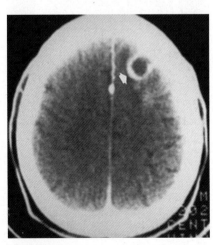

Fig SK 4-11
Pyogenic abscess. Hypodense lesion surrounded by a uniform ring of contrast enhancement (arrow).

Condition	Imaging Findings	Comments
Cerebritis	Irregular, poorly marginated hypodense area (representing edema) in the white matter or basal ganglia that may behave as a mass and result in effacement of the adjacent sulci or ventricle. Unlike most cerebral abscesses, there is no discrete ring-like capsule on unenhanced scans in patients with cerebritis.	Focal inflammatory process in the brain, usually resulting from bacteria or fungi, which may progress to abscess formation (requires approximately 10 to 14 days). After administration of contrast material, may show a well-defined ring that tends to increase in thickness on serial scans.
Resolving intracerebral hematoma (3 to 6 weeks old) (see Fig SK 6-9)	Hypodense region with a thin uniform ring of enhancement that mimics a neoplasm.	There is usually a history of previous intracerebral hematoma.
Resolving subdural hematoma (Figs SK 4-14 and SK 4-15)	Well-defined, hypodense, crescentic mass adjacent to the inner table of the skull.	After the injection of contrast material there is characteristic enhancement of the richly vascular membrane that forms around a subdural hematoma 1 to 4 weeks after injury. Occasionally, contrast material seeps into the hematoma and produces a fluid-fluid level.
Subdural empyema (Fig SK 4-16)	Crescentic or lentiform, extra-axial hypodense collection (representing pus) adjacent to the inner border of the skull. After administration of contrast material, a narrow zone of enhancement of relatively uniform thickness separates the hypodense extracerebral collection from the brain surface.	Suppurative process in the cranial subdural space that is most commonly the result of the spread of infection from the frontal or ethmoid sinuses. Less frequent causes include mastoiditis, middle ear infection, purulent meningitis, penetrating wounds to the skull, craniectomy, or osteomyelitis of the skull. Often bilateral and associated with a high mortality rate, even if properly treated.

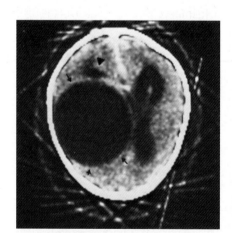

Fig SK 4-12
Echinococcal cyst. Huge right supratentorial hypodense mass (arrows). The right ventricle is partially visible posterior and medial to the cyst (arrowhead), and the left ventricle is enlarged.[8]

A

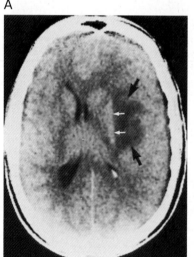

B

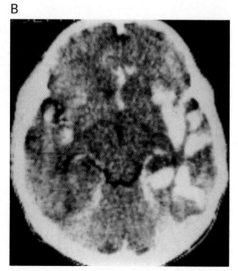

Fig SK 4-13
Herpes simplex encephalitis. (A) Nonenhanced scan demonstrates a hypodense area deep in the left frontotemporal region (large black arrows) and a shift of midline structures. The putamen, with its well-defined lateral border (small white arrows), is not affected by infection. (B) In another patient, there is dramatic gyral contrast enhancement that is most prominent on the left.[1]

SK 4 / HYPODENSE SUPRATENTORIAL MASSES ON CT

1263

Condition	Imaging Findings	Comments
Epidural abscess (see Fig SK 6-8)	Poorly defined area of low density adjacent to the inner table of the skull. There may be an adjacent area of bone destruction or evidence of paranasal sinus or mastoid infection. After the intravenous injection of contrast material, the inflamed dural membrane appears as a thickened zone of enhancement on the convex inner side of the lesion.	Almost invariably associated with cranial bone osteomyelitis originating from an infection in the ear or paranasal sinuses. The infectious process is localized outside the dural membrane and beneath the inner table of the skull. The frontal region is most frequently affected because of its close relation to the frontal sinuses and the ease with which the dura can be stripped from the bone.
Multiple sclerosis (Fig SK 4-17)	Multifocal, nonconfluent, low-attenuation regions with distinct margins near the atria of the lateral ventricles.	Contrast enhancement in the plaques is unusual except in rapidly evolving ones with surrounding inflammatory changes.
Necrosis of the globus pallidus	Bilaterally symmetric areas of low attenuation in the basal ganglia.	Causes include carbon monoxide poisoning, barbiturate intoxication, cyanide or hydrogen sulfide poisoning, hypoglycemia, hypoxia, hypotension, and Wilson's disease.

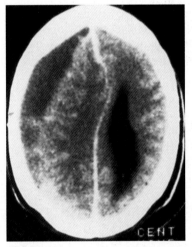

Fig SK 4-14
Right subdural hematoma. Crescent-shaped, low-density region in the right frontoparietal area. Note the marginal contrast enhancement, dilated left ventricle, and evidence of subfalcine and transtentorial herniation.

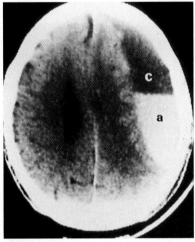

Fig SK 4-15
Mixed acute and chronic left subdural hematoma. The high-density acute hemorrhage (a) is layered in the dependent portion of the hematoma, with the lower density chronic collection (c) situated anteriorly.

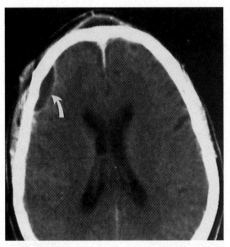

Fig SK 4-16
Subdural empyema. Lens-shaped extra-axial hypodense collection (arrow) that complicated a severe sinus infection. Note the thin rim of peripheral contrast enhancement.

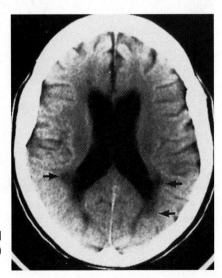

Fig SK 4-17
Multiple sclerosis. Multiple, discrete, homogeneous, and slightly irregular regions of diminished attenuation (arrows) adjacent to the slightly enlarged ventricles.[1]

High-Attenuation Masses in a Cerebral Hemisphere on Computed Tomography

Condition	Imaging Findings	Comments
Meningioma (Figs SK 5-1 and SK 5-2)	Rounded, sharply delineated hyperdense mass in a juxtadural location. Often contains calcification and usually shows intense homogeneous contrast enhancement.	Benign tumor that arises from arachnoid lining cells and is attached to the dura. The hyperdense matrix of a meningioma is the result of diminished water content, tumor hypervascularity, and microscopic psammomatous calcification. The detection of hyperostosis is virtually pathognomonic.
Metastasis (Fig SK 5-3)	Some dense metastases mimic meningiomas because of their superficial location and well-defined margins, though they are entirely intraparenchymal.	Metastatic colon carcinoma, which has a very dense cellular structure, and metastatic osteosarcoma, which contains osteoid and calcification, tend to be extremely dense. Melanoma and choriocarcinoma also tend to be hyperdense.
Primary lymphoma (Fig SK 5-4)	Slightly hyperdense mass that enhances homogeneously and often intensely.	Rare malignant neoplasm derived from microglial cells (histologically similar to lymphocytes) that is often multifocal and has a markedly increased incidence in organ transplant recipients.
Acute intracerebral hemorrhage (Fig SK 5-5)	Homogeneously dense, well-defined lesion with a round to oval configuration.	Causes include head trauma, surgery, hypertensive vascular disease, or rupture of a vascular malformation, mycotic aneurysm, or berry aneurysm.
Acute epidural hematoma (Figs SK 5-6 and SK 5-7)	Biconvex (lens-shaped), peripheral high-density lesion.	Caused by acute arterial bleeding; most commonly develops over the parietotemporal convexity.
Acute subdural hematoma (Fig SK 5-8)	Peripheral zone of increased density that follows the surface of the brain and has a crescentic shape adjacent to the inner table of the skull.	Caused by venous bleeding, most commonly from ruptured veins between the dura and leptomeninges. Serial scans demonstrate a gradual decrease in the attenuation of a subdural lesion over several weeks.

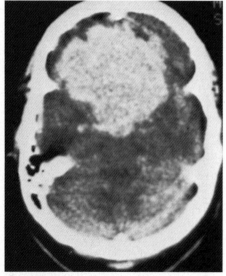

Fig SK 5-1
Meningioma. Huge hyperdense mass in the frontal lobe.

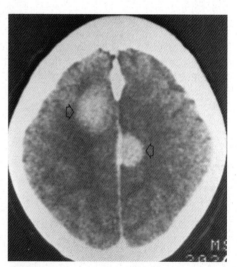

Fig SK 5-2
Meningioma. Bilateral hyperdense masses (arrows) in juxtadural locations.

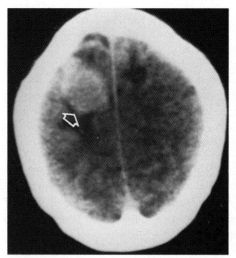

Fig SK 5-3
Metastasis. Nonenhanced scan shows a hyperdense mass (arrow) in the right frontal region representing a metastasis from carcinoma of the lung.

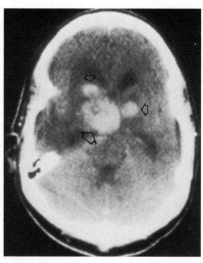

Fig SK 5-4
Primary lymphoma. Multifocal hyperdense masses (arrows).

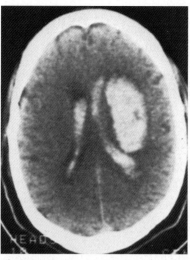

Fig SK 5-5
Intracerebral hematoma. Large, homogeneous high-density area with extensive acute bleeding into the lateral ventricles.

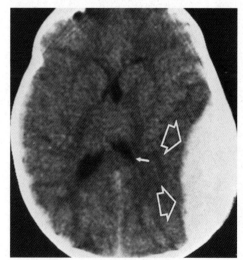

Fig SK 5-6
Acute epidural hematoma. CT scan of a 4-year-old child involved in a motor vehicle accident shows a characteristic lens-shaped epidural hematoma (open arrows). The substantial mass effect associated with the hematoma distorts the lateral ventricle (closed arrow).

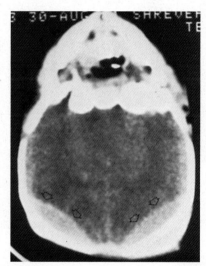

Fig SK 5-7
Epidural hematoma. Bilaterally symmetric posterior high-density areas (arrows) with lens-shaped configurations.

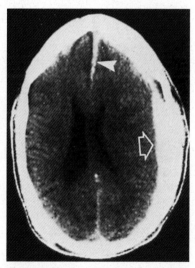

Fig SK 5-8
Acute subdural hematoma. High-density, crescent-shaped lesion (open arrow) adjacent to the inner table of the skull. The hematoma extends into the interhemispheric fissure (closed arrowhead).

Supratentorial Masses on Magnetic Resonance Imaging

Condition	Imaging Findings	Comments
Astrocytoma (Fig SK 6-1)	Hypointense lesion on T1-weighted images. High-intensity signal on proton-density and T2-weighted images.	Low-grade tumors tend to be homogeneous and lack central necrosis. They may contain large cystic components that have smooth walls and contain uniform-signal fluid, unlike the heterogeneous appearance of necrosis.
Glioblastoma multiforme (Figs SK 6-2 and SK 6-3)	Hypointense lesion on T1-weighted images. Hyperintense signal on proton-density and T2-weighted images.	These high-grade gliomas appear heterogeneous as a result of central necrosis with cellular debris, fluid, and hemorrhage. These tumors infiltrate along white matter fiber tracts. Deeper lesions frequently extend across the corpus callosum into the opposite hemisphere.

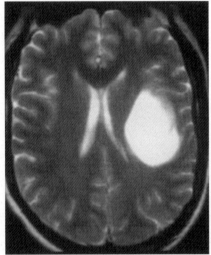

Fig SK 6-1
Low-grade astrocytoma. T2-weighted image shows a high-signal-intensity lesion with well-defined margins, no surrounding edema, and little mass effect.[7]

A   B

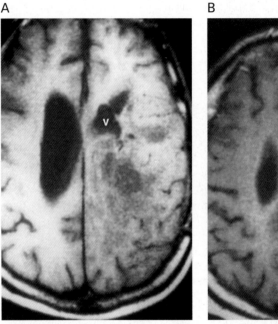

Fig SK 6-2
Glioblastoma multiforme. (A) Axial T1-weighted image shows a large mass of inhomogeneous low-intensity signal compressing the left lateral ventricle (v). (B) After the injection of gadolinium, there is striking enhancement of this complex necrotic mass.

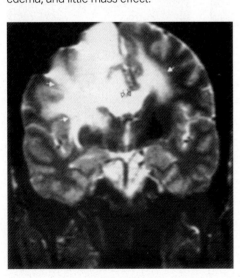

Fig SK 6-3
Glioblastoma crossing the corpus callosum. Coronal T2-weighted scan shows high intensity in the left and right centrum semiovale (white arrows) and extension of tumor across the corpus callosum (open arrows).[9]

Condition	Imaging Findings	Comments
Oligodendroglioma (Fig SK 6-4)	Hypointense lesion on T1-weighted images. Hyperintense signal on proton-density and T2-weighted images.	Although conventional spin-echo MRI is insensitive to the frequent calcification in these slow-growing tumors, it can demonstrate a heterogeneous appearance caused by cystic and hemorrhagic regions in the mass.
Metastasis (Fig SK 6-5)	Generally hypointense on T1-weighted images and of increased signal intensity on proton-density and T2-weighted images. Peritumoral edema is usually prominent, but unlike infiltrative gliomas, the edema accompanying a metastasis usually does not cross the corpus callosum or involve the cortex.	Areas of nonhemorrhagic cystic necrosis appear as irregular regions of intensity similar to that of cerebrospinal fluid (CSF) surrounded by the nonnecrotic portion of the lesion. Intratumoral hemorrhage occurs in approximately 15% to 20% of metastases, especially melanoma, choriocarcinoma, and renal cell, thyroid, and bronchogenic carcinoma. Melanotic melanoma metastases without hemorrhage typically are of high intensity on T1-weighted images and are isointense or hypointense to cortex on T2-weighted sequences.
Lymphoma (Fig SK 6-6)	Hypointense or isointense mass on T1-weighted images. Typically a homogeneous, slightly high-signal to isointense mass deep in the brain on T2-weighted images.	The mild T2 prolongation is probably related to dense cell packing in the tumor, leaving relatively little interstitial space for the accumulation of water. Like glioblastoma, lymphoma tends to extend across the corpus callosum into the opposite hemisphere. Central necrosis is uncommon, however, and there is usually only a mild or moderate amount of peritumoral edema.

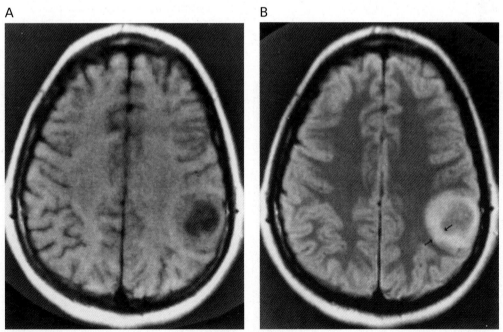

A   B

Fig SK 6-4
Oligodendroglioma. (A) T1-weighted and (B) proton-density images show a well-differentiated left parietal lobe mass containing a central cystic component. The arrows (B) point to the thickened wall of the enhancing lesion.[10]

Condition	Imaging Findings	Comments
Meningioma (Fig SK 6-7)	Usually hypointense to white matter on T1-weighted images. At 1.5 T, the lesion is hyperintense to white matter on T2-weighted images.	At lower field strength, approximately half of meningiomas are isointense to cortex on T1- and T2-weighted images. The tumor usually has a mottled pattern resulting from a combination of flow void from vascularity, focal calcification, small cystic foci, and entrapped CSF spaces. An interface is often seen between the brain and the lesion, representing a CSF cleft, a vascular rim, or a dural margin.

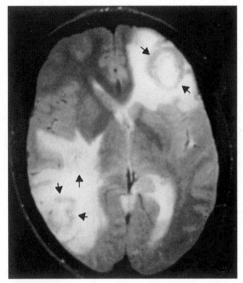

Fig SK 6-5
Metastases. Axial T2-weighted scan demonstrates three large masses (arrows) surrounded by extensive high-signal edema.

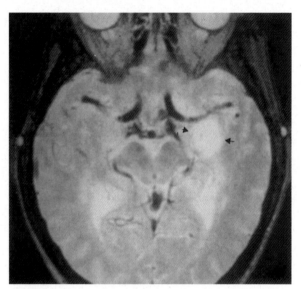

Fig SK 6-6
Lymphoma. Homogeneous mass of increased signal intensity (arrows) extending to involve the uncus.

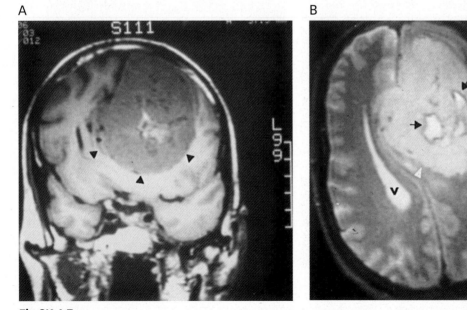

Fig SK 6-7
Meningioma. Huge mass (black and white arrowheads) that appears hypointense on a T1-weighted coronal scan (A) and hyperintense on a T2-weighted image (B). Note the dramatic shift of the ventricle (v) caused by the mass effect of the tumor. The arrows point to areas of hemorrhage in the neoplasm.

Condition	Imaging Findings	Comments
Epidermoid (see Fig SK 14-4)	Heterogeneous texture and variable signal intensity. Most epidermoids are of slightly higher signal than CSF on both T1- and T2-weighted images.	Some epidermoids appear bright on T1-weighted images. The heterogeneous signal pattern is probably related to various concentrations of keratin, cholesterol, and water in the cyst as well as the proportion of cholesterol and keratin in crystalline form.
Dermoid	Heterogeneous texture as a result of the multiple cell types in it.	Fatty components are common and produce high signal on T1-weighted images. A characteristic fat-fluid level may be seen.
Lipoma (see Fig SK 24-8B)	High signal intensity on T1-weighted images. Isointense or mildly hyperintense on proton-density images. Low intensity on T2-weighted sequences.	Typically a midline lesion that is often associated with partial or complete agenesis of the corpus callosum.
Choroid plexus papilloma (Fig SK 6-8)	Mildly hyperintense on T2-weighted images.	Relatively homogeneous, although hypervascularity can result in areas of flow void. Intense, homogeneous contrast enhancement.
Colloid cyst (Fig SK 6-9; see also Fig SK 20-2)	Smoothly marginated spherical mass with two signal patterns: low density on CT, isointense on T1-weighted MR images, and hyperintense on T2-weighted MR images; and isodense or slightly hyperdense on CT with a high-signal capsule and a hypointense center on T2-weighted MR images.	The first pattern corresponds to a fluid composition similar to CSF. In the second pattern, the hypointense center on MRI has been attributed to high concentrations of metal ions (sodium, calcium, magnesium, copper, and iron) or a high cholesterol content of the cystic fluid.

A   B

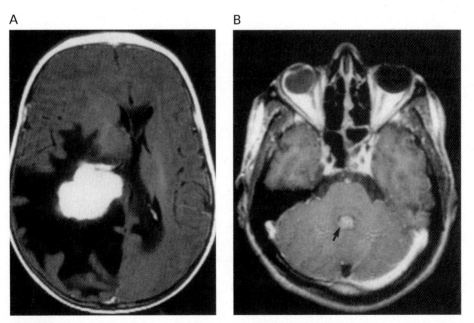

Fig SK 6-8
Choroid plexus papilloma. (A) Axial postcontrast T1-weighted image shows a large enhancing mass in the trigone of the right lateral ventricle with extensive surrounding edema. (B) Scan at a lower level shows a small papilloma (arrow) in the fourth ventricle.[7]

Condition	Imaging Findings	Comments
Cerebral abscess (Fig SK 6-10)	Hypointense mass with isointense capsule surrounded by low-signal edema on T1-weighted images. Hyperintense mass surrounded by a hypointense capsule and high-signal edema on T2-weighted images.	In the cerebritis stage, there is high signal intensity on T2-weighted images both centrally from inflammation and peripherally from edema. Areas of low signal are variably imaged on T1-weighted scans. As this process develops into a discrete abscess, the capsule becomes highlighted as a relatively isointense structure containing and surrounded by low signal on T1-weighted images and high signal on T2-weighted images.
Herpes simplex encephalitis	Ill-defined areas of high signal intensity on T2-weighted images. This process usually begins unilaterally but progresses to become bilateral.	MRI can demonstrate positive findings more quickly (as soon as 2 days) and more definitively than CT.
Intraparenchymal hematoma (Fig SK 6-11)		Well-defined, although somewhat variable, progression of signal intensity changes primarily related to the paramagnetic effects of the breakdown products of hemoglobin.
Very acute (0 to 3 hours)	Isointense to slightly hyperintense on T1-weighted images. Isointense to bright signal on T2-weighted images.	Immediately after an intracerebral bleed, the liquefied mass in the brain substance contains oxyhemoglobin but no paramagnetic substances. Therefore, it looks like any other proteinaceous fluid collection.
Acute (3 hours to 3 days)	Isointense to slightly hyperintense on T1-weighted images. Isointense to bright signal on T2-weighted images.	Reduction in oxygen tension in the hematoma results in the formation of intracellular deoxyhemoglobin and methemoglobin in intact red cells. These substances have a paramagnetic effect that produces T2 shortening. A thin rim of increased signal surrounding the hematoma on T2-weighted images represents edema.
Subacute (3 days to 3 weeks)	Bright rim of hyperintense signal on T1-weighted images that extends inward to fill the entire lesion. Increased signal on T2-weighted images, although to a lesser extent.	As red blood cells lyse, redistribution of methemoglobin into the extracellular space changes the effect of this paramagnetic substance to one of predominantly T1 shortening. The longer T2 results from a combination of (1) red blood cell lysis (T2 shortening disappears), (2) osmotic effects that draw fluid into the hematoma, and (3) the repetition times (TR) that are in general use for T2-weighted sequences, which are not sufficiently long to eliminate T1 contrast effects in the image.
Chronic (3 weeks to 3 months or more)	Variable appearance on T1-weighted images. Pronounced hypointense rim or completely low-signal lesion on T2-weighted images.	Phagocytic cells invade the hemorrhage (starting at the outer rim and working inward), metabolizing the hemoglobin breakdown products and storing the iron as superparamagnetic hemosiderin and ferritin.

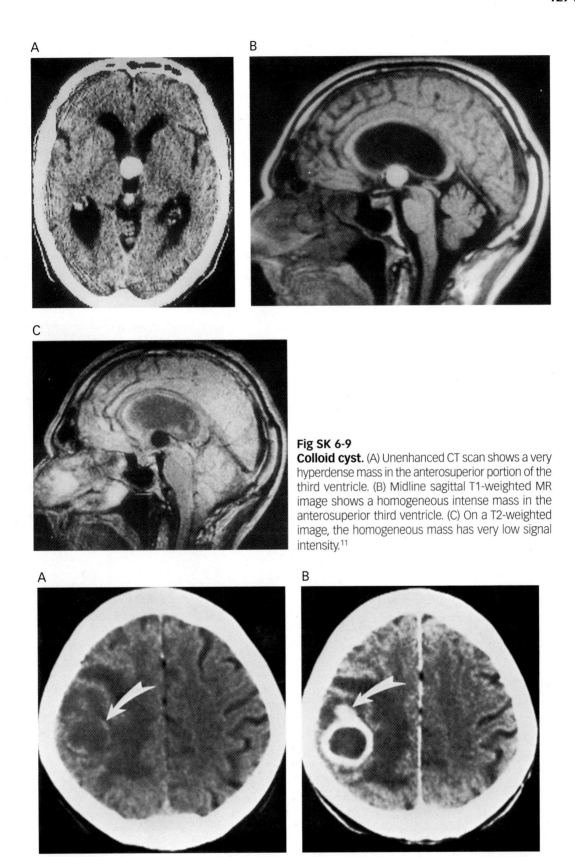

Fig SK 6-9
Colloid cyst. (A) Unenhanced CT scan shows a very hyperdense mass in the anterosuperior portion of the third ventricle. (B) Midline sagittal T1-weighted MR image shows a homogeneous intense mass in the anterosuperior third ventricle. (C) On a T2-weighted image, the homogeneous mass has very low signal intensity.[11]

Fig SK 6-10
Brain abscess. (A) Nonenhanced CT scan shows vasogenic edema in the right anterior parietal white matter. The isodense ring of the abscess capsule can be seen (white arrow). (B) Contrast-enhanced study shows a thick but uniformly enhancing capsule with the beginnings of a daughter abscess anteriorly (arrow). The enhancement of an abscess is typically circular and nearly uniform except along the medial surface.[12]

Condition	Imaging Findings	Comments
Vascular diseases Infarction (Fig SK 6-12)	Hypointense on T1-weighted images. Hyperintense on proton-density and T2-weighted images. Old infarcts may have a more complex signal pattern that is related both to hemorrhagic components and to the evolution of infarcts, the latter resulting in areas of microcystic and macrocystic encephalomalacia and gliosis.	Classic pattern of cerebral infarction is a wedge-shaped abnormality that involves both the cortex and a variable amount of the subcortical tissue, in either a major vascular territory or a watershed area. Because MRI is extremely sensitive to edema, experimental infarcts have been detected as soon as 2–4 hours after vessel occlusion, at a time when CT has shown no abnormality.
Arteriovenous malformation (AVM) (Fig SK 6-13)	Cluster of serpiginous flow voids (representing rapid blood flow) and areas of high signal (slow flow in draining veins).	The use of partial flip-angle techniques can distinguish hemosiderin or calcification associated with the lesion from vessels containing rapidly flowing blood.

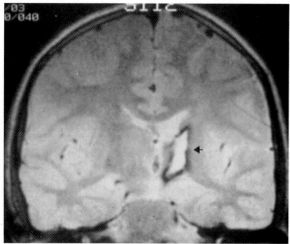

Fig SK 6-11
Intraparenchymal hematoma. Coronal T2-weighted scan shows a large hematoma in the left thalamic region (arrow). The hematoma consists of two portions: a central area of increased signal intensity representing methemoglobin, and a surrounding area of low signal intensity representing hemosiderin.

Fig SK 6-12
Infarction. Axial T2-weighted image shows a wedge-shaped area of increased signal intensity involving both cortex and subcortical tissue in the right occipital lobe.

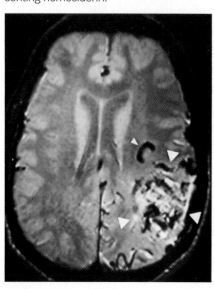

Fig SK 6-13
Arteriovenous malformation (AVM). Axial proton-density scan shows a large left parietal mass (large arrowheads) consisting of vascular structures of various intensities, depending on whether there is rapid flow (black) or slow flow (white). Note the markedly dilated vessel (small arrowhead) that feeds the malformation.

Condition	Imaging Findings	Comments
"Cryptic" AVM (Fig SK 6-14)	On T2-weighted images, an island of bright signal (methemoglobin) is surrounded by an extensive region of very low signal (hemosiderin).	This lesion may be responsible for spontaneous hemorrhage but is angiographically occult.
Venous malformation (Fig SK-15)	Solitary or stellate collection of flow voids (draining vein) that may be associated with increased signal in the body of the angioma.	Radiating or spoke-like pattern of tributaries draining into a single large vein that courses perpendicular to the surface of the brain to enter a major vein or dural sinus.
Aneurysm (Fig SK 6-16)	Flow void that may be surrounded by a heterogeneous signal intensity pattern representing turbulence or thrombus.	MRI may be unable to distinguish small aneurysms from normal vessels. Partial flip-angle imaging produces fairly consistent flow-related enhancement in the lumen and more clearly differentiates this from surrounding clot.

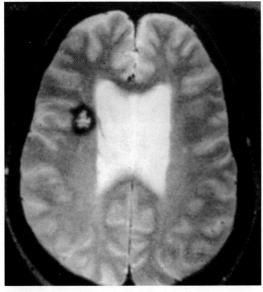

Fig SK 6-14
Cryptic AVM. Axial T2-weighted scan shows the characteristic appearance of an island of bright signal (methemoglobin) surrounded by an extensive region of very low signal (hemosiderin).

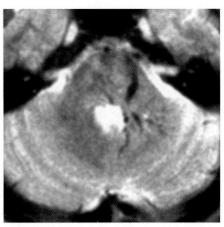

Fig SK 6-15
Venous malformation. Axial T2-weighted image shows a tubular flow void with a radiating "crown of voids" in the left side of the pons.[13]

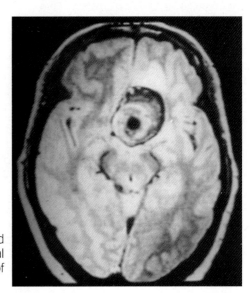

Fig SK 6-16
Aneurysm of the supraclinoid portion of the internal carotid artery. The low-signal flow void representing the residual patent lumen is surrounded by a heterogeneous region of increased signal representing lamellar thrombus.

Sellar and Juxtasellar Masses on Computed Tomography

Condition	Imaging Findings	Comments
Pituitary adenoma (Figs SK 7-1 and SK 7-2)	Typically a well-circumscribed tumor of slightly greater than brain density that shows homogeneous contrast enhancement. Regions of necrosis or cyst formation in the tumor produce internal areas of low density. Microadenomas (<10 mm) are usually less dense than the normal pituitary gland.	CT can demonstrate adjacent bone erosion, extension of the tumor beyond the confines of the sella, and impression of nearby structures such as the third ventricle, optic nerves, or optic chiasm.
Craniopharyngioma (Fig SK 7-3)	Typically a mixed-density lesion containing cystic and solid areas and dense globular or, less commonly, rim calcification. Variable contrast enhancement of the solid portion of the tumor.	Benign, congenital, or rest-cell, tumor with cystic and solid components that usually originates above the sella turcica, depressing the optic chiasm and extending up into the third ventricle. Less commonly, a craniopharyngioma lies in the sella, where it compresses the pituitary gland and may erode adjacent bony walls.
Meningioma (Fig SK 7-4)	Hyperdense mass that enhances intensely and homogeneously after intravenous administration of contrast material. May have associated hyperostosis of adjacent bone.	Suprasellar meningiomas arise from the tuberculum sellae, clinoid processes, optic nerve sheath, cerebellopontine angle cistern, cavernous sinus, or medial sphenoidal ridge.
Glioma Optic chiasm (Fig SK 7-5)	Suprasellar mass that is isodense on nonenhanced scans and shows moderate and variable enhancement after administration of contrast material.	Benign globular mass occupying the anterior aspect of the suprasellar cistern that most often occurs in adolescent girls, gradually produces bilateral visual abnormalities and optic atrophy, and is often associated with neurofibromatosis.

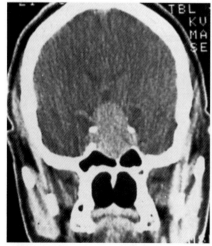

Fig SK 7-1
Pituitary adenoma. Coronal scan shows an enhancing mass filling and extending out from the pituitary fossa. Note the remodeling of the base of the sella.

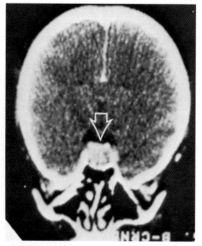

Fig SK 7-2
Nelson's syndrome. Hyperdense tumor filling the enlarged sella (arrow) in a patient whose pituitary adenoma developed after adrenal surgery.

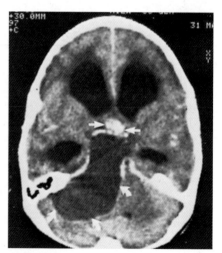

Fig SK 7-3
Craniopharyngioma. A rim-enhancing tumor containing dense calcification (straight arrows) and a large cystic component (curved arrows) that extends into the posterior fossa. Note the associated hydrocephalus.[1]

Condition	Imaging Findings	Comments
Hypothalamus	Usually a large, well-defined, irregularly contoured mass that is inhomogeneous with low-density and markedly enhancing regions.	Slow-growing astrocytoma that usually occurs in children and young adults. In infants, it typically produces a syndrome of failure to thrive despite adequate caloric intake, unusual alertness, and hyperactivity.
Chordoma (Fig SK 7-6)	Well-defined mass with variable enhancement and homogeneity. Usually associated with destruction of the clivus and retrosellar calcification.	Locally invasive tumor that arises from remnants of the fetal notochord and most commonly occurs in patients 50 to 70 years of age.
Metastasis (Fig SK 7-7)	Smooth or irregular mass that usually enhances homogeneously and is associated with bone destruction.	Most metastases to the sellar and juxtasellar region originate from tumors of the lung, breast, kidney, or gastrointestinal tract or are due to direct spread from carcinomas of the nasopharynx or sphenoid sinus.
Germ cell tumor (germinoma/teratoma) (Fig SK 7-8)	Various patterns of density and enhancement.	Occasionally involve the suprasellar region and frequently calcify (especially teratomas). May spread via cerebrospinal fluid pathways.
Epidermoid/dermoid (Fig SK 7-9)	Smooth or lobulated suprasellar masses of low attenuation (usually of less than cerebrospinal fluid density). Usually nonenhancing (may have a thin peripheral rim of contrast enhancement).	Epidermoids are lined with squamous epithelium, whereas dermoids typically contain hair, dermal elements, calcification, and fat. Intrathecal contrast material may be required to find the margins of these lesions.
Neuroma	Inhomogeneously enhancing mass. A trigeminal tumor typically erodes the base of the skull (especially the foramen ovale and apex of the petrous pyramid).	Arises from cranial nerves III to VI. Gasserian ganglion neuroma appears as a large filling defect in the enhanced cavernous sinus.

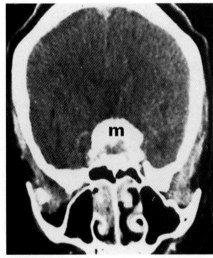

Fig SK 7-4
Meningioma. Coronal reconstruction demonstrates shows the large calcified mass (m) and associated bone destruction.

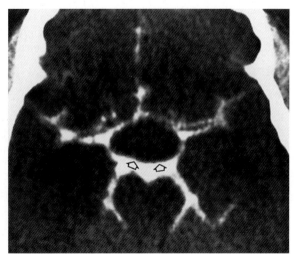

Fig SK 7-5
Optic chiasm glioma. Axial suprasellar metrizamide cisternogram demonstrates a tumor filling the suprasellar cistern (arrows). Only faint enhancement was present on the standard contrast-enhanced CT scan.[14]

Condition	Imaging Findings	Comments
Hamartoma of the tuber cinereum (Fig SK 7-10)	Small, smooth, isodense and nonenhancing mass attached to the posterior aspect of the hypothalamus between the tuber cinereum and the pons.	Rare lesion of early childhood that usually presents with precocious puberty, seizures, and mental changes (behavioral disorders and intellectual deterioration).
Aneurysm Intracavernous	Well-defined, oval or teardrop-shaped, eccentric mass that is slightly denser than cerebral tissue on unenhanced scans and markedly and homogeneously enhanced after intravenous administration of contrast material.	Intracavernous internal carotid aneurysms are saccular, occasionally have an intrasellar component, and are bilateral in approximately 25% of cases. They may have rim calcification and contain a low-density area representing a thrombus. An aneurysm can erode bone and compress the cavernous sinus (causing cranial nerve palsy) or rupture and produce a carotid-cavernous fistula.

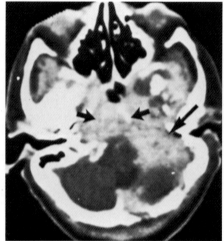

Fig SK 7-6
Chordoma. Enlarging mass with destruction of the entire clivus (short arrows) and only small bone fragments remaining. The left petrous pyramid is also destroyed (long arrow).[5]

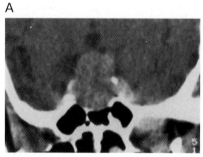

Fig SK 7-7
Metastasis (oat cell carcinoma of the lung). (A) Noncontrast coronal scan shows a somewhat hyperdense mass filling the pituitary fossa and extending into the suprasellar region. (B) After intravenous injection of contrast material, there is dense enhancement of the metastasis.

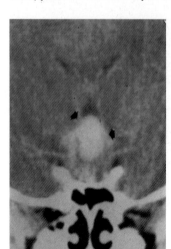

Fig SK 7-8
Ectopic pinealoma. Enhancing suprasellar mass (arrows).

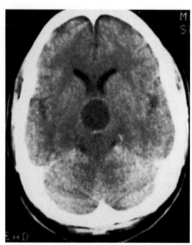

Fig SK 7-9
Epidermoid. Smooth, low-attenuation suprasellar mass with a thin rim of contrast enhancement.

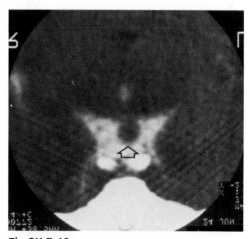

Fig SK 7-10
Hamartoma of the tuber cinereum. Intrathecally enhanced coronal scan shows a small mass (arrow) that was isodense and nonenhancing on initial CT scans.

Condition	Imaging Findings	Comments
Suprasellar (Fig SK 7-11)	Slightly hyperdense mass that enhances intensely and homogeneously. May have rim calcification and contain a low-density thrombus.	Usually most common in the fourth to sixth decades, congenital (berry aneurysm), and the result of maldevelopment of the media (especially at points of arterial bifurcation). The sudden onset of headache or neck stiffness suggests aneurysmal leakage or rupture.
Carotid-cavernous fistula	Focal or diffuse enlargement of one or both enhancing cavernous sinuses (most prominent on the side of the fistula) and enlargement of the superior ophthalmic vein (especially on the side of the fistula) and edematous extraocular muscles.	Arises from traumatic rupture of the internal carotid artery or spontaneous rupture of a carotid aneurysm. May occasionally produce a normal CT scan for a few days after head trauma because the fistula develops slowly or after a delay.
Arachnoid cyst (Fig SK 7-12)	Well-defined, nonenhancing mass of cerebrospinal fluid density. Sharp, noncalcified margin.	A suprasellar cyst often causes hydrocephalus (most common in infancy), visual impairment, and endocrine dysfunction.
Inflammatory lesion	Various patterns.	Infrequent manifestation of sarcoidosis, tuberculosis, sphenoid mucocele, pituitary abscess, or lymphoid hypophysitis (an autoimmune disorder in which lymphocytes infiltrate the pituitary gland).
Langerhans cell histiocytosis	Irregularly marginated, relatively well-defined enhancing suprasellar mass.	Involvement of the hypothalamus and sella turcica, which is most common in children, is usually associated with multiple destructive skeletal lesions.

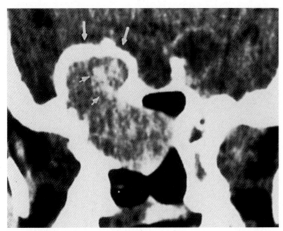

Fig SK 7-11
Giant parasellar aneurysm. There is a rim of calcification (long arrows) along the superior margin of the aneurysm. Areas of enhancement in the aneurysm (short arrows) represent the patent lumen; the rest of the aneurysm is filled with nonenhancing thrombus.

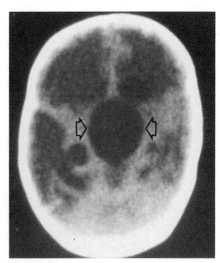

Fig SK 7-12
Arachnoid cyst. Large, well-defined suprasellar mass of cerebrospinal fluid density (arrows). Note the prominent associated hydrocephalus.

Sellar and Juxtasellar Masses on Magnetic Resonance Imaging

Condition	Imaging Findings	Comments
Pituitary adenoma Microadenoma (Fig SK 8-1)	Usually hypointense compared with the normal gland on T1-weighted images. After contrast injection, the tumor typically does not enhance to the same extent as the normal pituitary gland and thus stands out as an area of relative hypointensity.	Important secondary signs of microadenoma include asymmetric upward convexity of the gland surface, deviation of the infundibulum, and focal erosion of the sellar floor. The preferred imaging planes are coronal and sagittal.
Macroadenoma (Fig SK 8-2)	Generally isointense to the normal gland and brain parenchyma unless there are cystic and hemorrhagic components. Homogeneous contrast enhancement permits clear demarcation of the tumor from normal suprasellar structures.	Adenoma larger than 10 mm. It may be hormone secreting (especially prolactin producing) and associated with amenorrhea and galactorrhea. MRI is ideal for demonstrating extension of tumor to involve the cavernous sinus, optic chiasm, inferior recesses of the third ventricle, and hypothalamus.
Craniopharyngioma (Fig SK 8-3)	Variable appearance depending on the solid or cystic nature of the mass and the specific cyst contents. Solid lesions are hypointense on T1-weighted images and hyperintense on T2-weighted images. Cysts also have a long T2 but show high signal intensity on T1-weighted images if they have a high cholesterol content or methemoglobin.	The solid and wall portions of a craniopharyngioma show contrast enhancement. Truncation of the dorsum sellae and upward growth into the third ventricle may be seen. Calcification (seen well on CT) is not reliably detected by MRI.
Rathke's cleft cyst (Fig SK 8-4)	Either a mass with CSF intensity on both T1- and T2-weighted images or a lesion that is markedly hyperintense on both sequences.	Remnant of an embryologic invagination cephalad up out of the pharynx that gives rise to the anterior and intermediate pituitary lobes. Bright signal on T1-weighted images appears to reflect the high protein or starch content of the mucoid material in the cyst.

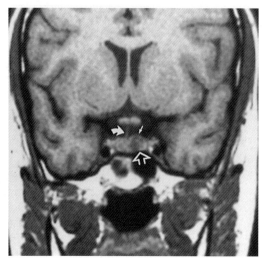

Fig SK 8-1
Pituitary microadenoma. Coronal T1-weighted image demonstrates a prolactin-secreting microadenoma (open arrow) as a focal area of decreased signal in the pituitary gland. Associated findings include displacement of the pituitary stalk contralaterally (curved arrow) and elevation of the upper border of the gland (straight solid arrow).[15]

A
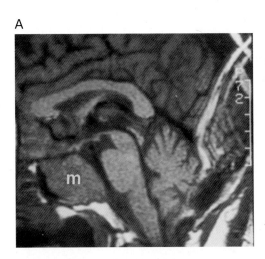

B
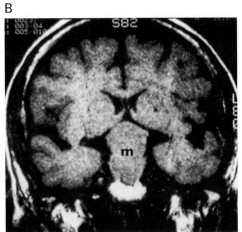

C
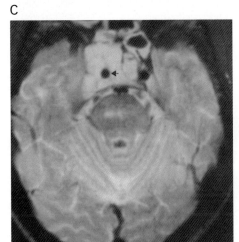

Fig SK 8-2
Pituitary macroadenoma. (A) Sagittal and (B) coronal MR scans demonstrate a large mass (m) that arises from the sella turcica and extends upward to fill the suprasellar cistern. (C) In another patient, an axial scan shows tumor involvement of the right cavernous sinus with encasement of the ipsilateral carotid artery (arrow).

A
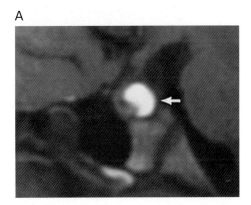

B
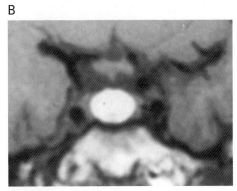

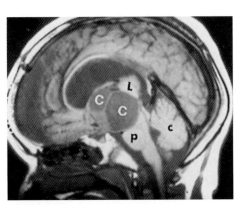

Fig SK 8-3
Craniopharyngioma. Sagittal MR image demonstrates a large, multiloculated, suprasellar mass with cystic (C) and lipid (L) components. (c, cerebellum; p, pons.)

Fig SK 8-4
Rathke's cleft cyst. (A) Sagittal and (B) coronal T1-weighted images show an ovoid lesion of high intensity (arrow) in the middle to posterior portion of the pituitary fossa.[16]

Condition	Imaging Findings	Comments
Meningioma (Fig SK 8-5)	Isointense to hypointense mass on T1-weighted images. Isointense or slightly hyperintense mass on T2-weighted images. Marked homogeneous contrast enhancement.	Sagittal and coronal planes show the anatomic location of the mass as well as whether the internal carotid artery and its branches are encased by tumor and whether there is involvement of the optic nerve and chiasm. Unlike a pituitary adenoma, a suprasellar meningioma usually does not project into the intrasellar space.
Glioma Optic chiasm (Fig SK 8-6)	Isointense or slightly hypointense on T1-weighted images. Hyperintense on T2-weighted images.	Posterior extension to the lateral geniculate body and beyond into the optic radiations and appears as areas of increased signal on axial T2-weighted images.

A

B

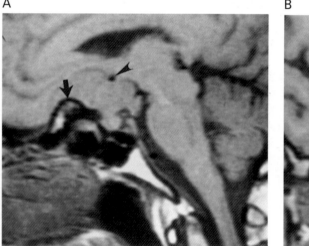 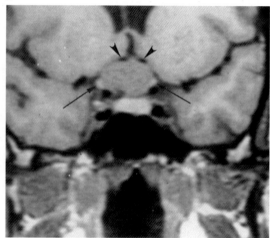

Fig SK 8-5
Planum sphenoidale meningioma growing over the diaphragma sellae. (A) Sagittal T1-weighted scan shows a soft-tissue mass isointense to brain that elevates the anterior cerebral artery (arrowhead) and produces hyperostosis of the planum sphenoidale (arrow). (B) Coronal T1-weighted image shows a mass in the suprasellar space sitting on the diaphragma sellae, lying above the pituitary gland, elevating the two anterior cerebral arteries (arrowheads), and displacing both optic nerves (arrows).[16]

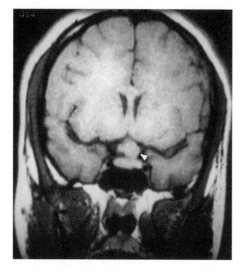

Fig SK 8-6
Optic chiasm glioma. A suprasellar mass is seen on the left (arrowhead).

Condition	Imaging Findings	Comments
Hypothalamus	Isointense or slightly hypointense on T1-weighted images. Hyperintense on T2-weighted images.	Subtle deformity of the inferior recesses of the third ventricle can be visualized on coronal views. As with chiasmatic glioma, the tumor tends to have moderate contrast enhancement.
Chordoma (Fig SK 8-7)	Hypointense on T1-weighted images. Hyperintense signal on T2-weighted images.	Alteration of the normal high-signal fat in the clivus on T1-weighted images is a sensitive indicator of disease.
Metastasis (Fig SK 8-8)	Hypointense lesion on T1-weighted images. Hyperintense signal on T2-weighted images.	Most metastases to the sellar and juxtasellar region originate from tumors of the lung, breast, kidney, or gastrointestinal tract or result from direct spread from carcinomas of the nasopharynx or sphenoid sinus.
Germ cell tumor (germinoma/teratoma)	Isointense to hypointense on T1-weighted images. Slightly to moderately increased signal on T2-weighted images.	Detection of a suprasellar germ cell tumor mandates close inspection of the pineal region because it may represent a forward extension of a pineal tumor or a multifocal process.
Epidermoid (Fig SK 8-9)	Heterogeneous texture and variable signal intensity. Most are of slightly higher signal than CSF on both T1- and T2-weighted images.	Some epidermoids appear bright on T1-weighted images.
Dermoid	Heterogeneous texture as a result of the multiple cell types in it.	Fatty components are common and produce high signal on T1-weighted images.
Neuroma (Fig SK 8-10)	Isointense or hypointense lesion on T1-weighted images. Isointense to hyperintense lesion on T2-weighted images.	Prominent homogeneous contrast enhancement. Coronal scans may show extension of a mandibular (V_3) neuroma downward through the foramen ovale.

A   B

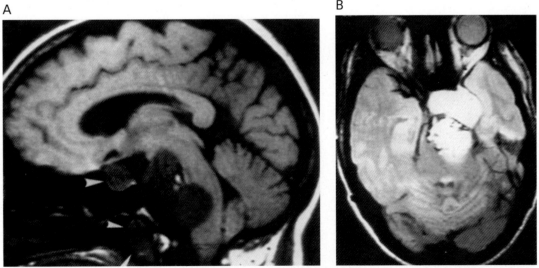

Fig SK 8-7
Clival chordoma. (A) Sagittal MR scan shows a low-intensity multilobulated mass deforming and displacing the brainstem, destroying the clivus, and extending into the sella turcica (upper arrowhead) and nasopharynx (lower two arrowheads). (B) Axial T2-weighted scan shows that the hyperintense mass with peripheral vessels invaginates into the brainstem and also occupies the region of the sella turcica and left cavernous sinus.[17]

Condition	Imaging Findings	Comments
Aneurysm (Fig SK 8-11)	Flow void that may be surrounded by a pattern of heterogeneous signal intensity representing turbulence or thrombus.	Aneurysms in the suprasellar, intrasellar, and parasellar spaces can mimic a neoplasm by producing a mass lesion.
Arachnoid cyst	Smoothly marginated and homogeneous mass containing cyst fluid that is isointense to CSF on all pulse sequences.	The presence of mass effect and the lack of adjacent brain reaction are usually sufficient to differentiate an arachnoid cyst from atrophic encephalomalacia.

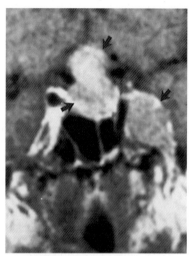

Fig SK 8-8
Metastasis. Coronal T1-weighted image shows an enhanced mass (arrows) in the sella, suprasellar space, and left parasellar cavernous sinus.[16]

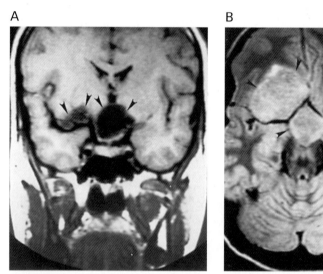

Fig SK 8-9
Epidermoid tumor. (A) Coronal T1-weighted image shows a hypointense suprasellar mass (arrowheads) that extends into the fissure of the right middle cerebral artery. (B) Axial proton-density image shows the suprasellar mass to have slightly increased signal intensity (arrowheads) and to extend into the inferior right frontal region.[16]

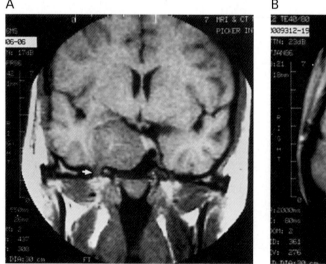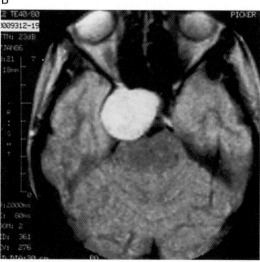

Fig SK 8-10
Trigeminal schwannoma of the right gasserian ganglion. (A) T1-weighted coronal image shows the mass to be of relatively low signal intensity and to involve the mandibular division (arrow). (B) On the T2-weighted scan, the lesion has high homogeneous signal intensity.[18]

Condition	Imaging Findings	Comments
Ectopia of the posterior pituitary lobe (Fig SK 8-12)	Posterior pituitary bright spot located cephalad in the median eminence of the hypothalamus rather than in its usual location.	Occurs most commonly in pituitary dwarfism (short stature), although it has been reported as being a normal variant. It also can be an acquired abnormality with traumatic stalk transection and compression or destruction of the neurohypophysis.
Lesion of the infundibular stalk	Various appearances.	True primary neoplasms (choristoma or pituicytoma) are extremely rare. More common neoplasms of the infundibulum are germinoma, lymphoma, leukemia, and other metastatic tumors. Nonneoplastic causes of infundibular enlargement include histiocytosis and sarcoidosis.

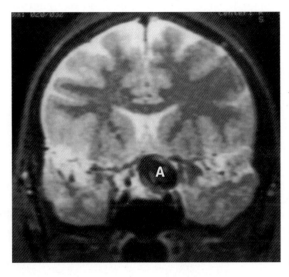

Fig SK 8-11
Distal left carotid artery aneurysm. On this coronal T2-weighted scan, the predominantly flow-void mass (A) extends into the suprasellar cistern and displaces the pituitary stalk.[15]

B

A

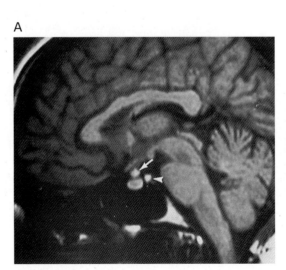
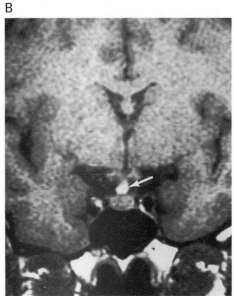

Fig SK 8-12
Ectopia of the posterior pituitary lobe. (A) Sagittal and (B) coronal T1-weighted images in a patient with diabetes insipidus that developed after an automobile accident. Hyperintensity in the region of the tuber cinereum (arrows) indicates transection of the pituitary stalk. Note the separate hyperintense area of fat in the dorsum sellae (arrowhead, A).[19]

Masses in the Pineal Region

Condition	Imaging Findings	Comments
Pineal tumors		
Germinoma ("atypical teratoma") (Figs SK 9-1 and SK 9-2)	On CT, an isodense or hyperdense mass in the posterior third ventricle adjacent to or surrounding the pineal gland. Usually shows intense, homogeneous contrast enhancement. On MRI, usually isointense to brain on both T1- and T2-weighted images. A few lesions have long T1 and T2, which may correlate with embryonal cell elements.	Malignant primitive germ cell neoplasm that occurs almost exclusively in males, is usually radiosensitive, and is the most common tumor of the pineal region. May occur in association with a suprasellar germinoma. Because of their proximity to the aqueduct, these tumors frequently cause hydrocephalus. May produce ependymal or cisternal seeding.
Teratoma (Figs SK 9-3 and SK 9-4)	On CT, an inhomogeneous mass containing regions of low and high attenuation representing fat and calcification, respectively. On MRI, teratomas are of mixed signal intensity and often contain cystic components and fat.	Rare benign tumor that has a marked predominance in males and contains elements of all three germ layers. Usually shows minimal contrast enhancement (intense enhancement suggests malignant degeneration).
Teratocarcinoma (Fig SK 9-5)	Irregularly marginated mass that varies in density and typically shows intense homogeneous contrast enhancement.	Malignant tumors (embryonal cell carcinoma; choriocarcinoma) that arise from primitive germ cells and are characterized by intratumoral hemorrhage, invasion of adjacent structures, and seeding via cerebrospinal fluid pathways.

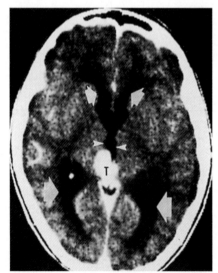

Fig SK 9-1
Germinoma. Enhancing tumor (T) in the pineal region of a young girl with paralysis of upward gaze, headaches, and nausea (Parinaud's syndrome). The minimal dilatation of the third ventricle (arrowheads) and lateral ventricles (arrows) indicates mild hydrocephalus, which developed because of obstruction of the posterior portion of the third ventricle by the tumor.

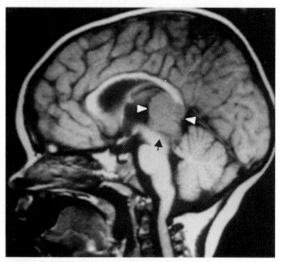

Fig SK 9-2
Germinoma. Sagittal T1-weighted MR image shows a large isointense mass (arrowheads) that compresses the midbrain (arrow) and elevates the splenium of the corpus callosum.

Condition	Imaging Findings	Comments
Pineocytoma (Fig SK 9-6)	On CT, a slightly hyperdense mass that often contains dense, focal calcification. Variable contrast enhancement. On MRI, a hypointense mass on T1-weighted images that becomes hyperintense on T2-weighted images.	Slow-growing tumor composed of mature pineal parenchymal cells and usually confined to the posterior third ventricle. Indistinct tumor margins suggest infiltration of adjacent structures. May spread via cerebrospinal fluid pathways.
Pineoblastoma (Fig SK 9-7)	Poorly marginated isodense or slightly hyperdense mass typically containing dense calcification. Homogeneous and intense contrast enhancement.	Highly malignant tumor of primitive pineal parenchymal cells that frequently spreads via cerebrospinal fluid pathways.

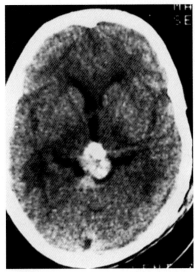

Fig SK 9-3
Teratoma. Nonenhanced scan shows an inhomogeneous mass containing a large amount of calcification.

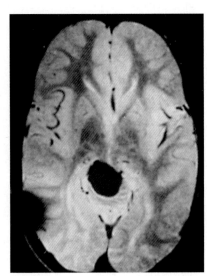

Fig SK 9-4
Teratoma. Axial T2-weighted MR image shows a pineal mass that is markedly hypointense because of high fat content and extensive calcification.

A
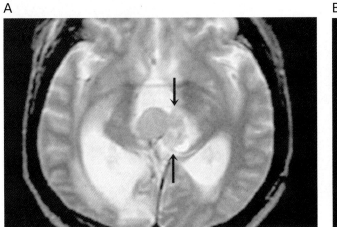

B
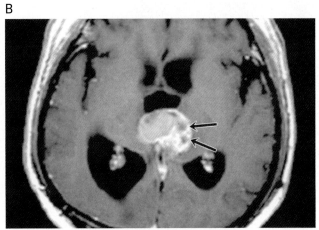

Fig SK 9-5
Embryonal cell carcinoma. (A) Axial T2-weighted MR image shows a tumor with heterogeneous signal intensity in the pineal gland (arrows). (B) Contrast T1-weighted image shows some enhancing foci within the tumor (arrows).[20]

Condition	Imaging Findings	Comments
Metastasis (Fig SK 9-8)	Indistinct hypodense or isodense mass that shows homogeneous enhancement. Occasionally hyperdense.	Infrequent manifestation that must be considered in older adults with known malignant disease.
Glioma of nonpineal origin	Low-density mass with poorly defined margins, minimal or moderate enhancement, and no calcification. May displace the normal calcified pineal gland.	Tumors arising from the thalamus, posterior hypothalamus, tectal plate of the mesencephalon, or splenium that extend into the quadrigeminal cistern. Usually occur in older patients.

B

A

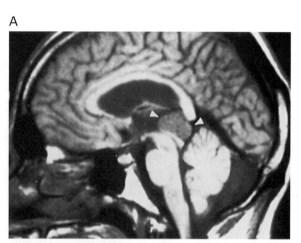
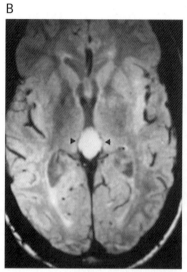

Fig SK 9-6
Pineocytoma. Pineal mass that is hypointense (arrowheads) on a sagittal T1-weighted image (A) and hyperintense (arrows) on an axial T2-weighted image (B).

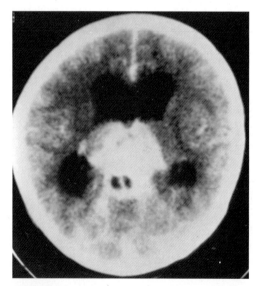

Fig SK 9-7
Pineoblastoma. Huge densely calcified mass in the pineal region causing obstructive hydrocephalus.

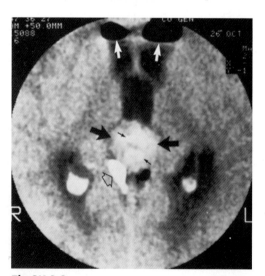

Fig SK 9-8
Metastasis. In this patient with lung carcinoma, an unenhanced scan shows a well-circumscribed, hyperdense pineal mass (large arrows) containing dense punctate calcification (small arrows). Air in the frontal horns (white arrows) resulted from a recent ventricular shunting procedure. Note the tentorial calcification (open arrow) adjacent to the metastasis.[1]

Condition	Imaging Findings	Comments
Meningioma (Fig SK 9-9)	On CT, a round, sharply delineated isodense or hyperdense mass that is often calcified and shows intense homogeneous contrast enhancement. On MRI, generally a relatively isointense mass with intense enhancement.	Midline tumors arising from the edge of the tentorium may be difficult to distinguish from pineal tumors. However, they are usually eccentrically located and often have a flat border along the tentorium close to the dural margin.
Vein of Galen aneurysm (Fig SK 9-10)	Mass of uniform density and intense contrast enhancement that mimics a pineal tumor.	Arteriovenous malformation that often presents in childhood, produces high blood flow, and is an important cause of neonatal heart failure.
Pineal cyst (Fig SK 9-11)	Sharply circumscribed mass that is best seen as a round area of high signal intensity on T2-weighted images.	Benign lesion seen in 4% of normal patients in one series. They are not associated with hydrocephalus or a pineal mass and are of no clinical significance.

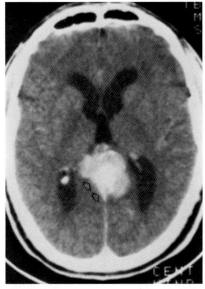

Fig SK 9-9
Meningioma. Densely enhancing mass in the pineal region that arises from the incisura of the tentorium. Note the characteristic flat border (arrows) along the tentorium.

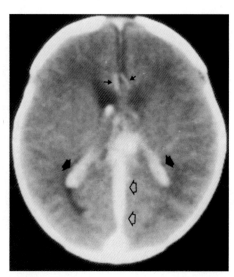

Fig SK 9-10
Vein of Galen aneurysm. A contrast-enhanced scan shows dilatation of the vein of Galen and straight sinus (open arrows). Note the prominent feeding vessels of the choroid plexus (closed arrows) and the anterior cerebral arteries (thin arrows).

A

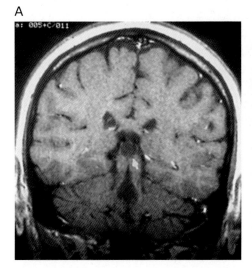

B

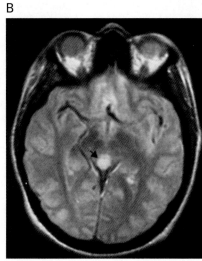

Fig SK 9-11
Pineal cyst. Round pineal mass (arrows) that is markedly hypointense on a coronal T1-weighted image (A) and hyperintense on an axial T2-weighted image (B).

Hypothalamic Lesions on Magnetic Resonance Imaging

Condition	Imaging Findings	Comments
Glioma (Fig SK 10-1)	Suprasellar mass that is isointense or hypointense on T1-weighted images and hyperintense on T2-weighted images. Inhomogeneous contrast enhancement.	Hypothalamic gliomas frequently invade the optic chiasm and vice versa, so that the primary site of origin may be difficult to determine. The tumor is slow growing and usually occurs in children and young adults.
Germinoma (Fig SK 10-2)	Usually mildly hypointense on T1-weighted images and hyperintense on T2-weighted images, though it may be isointense on both pulse sequences.	Second most frequent site (most common in the pineal region). Hypothalamic germinomas affect men and women equally, unlike the strong male predominance in pineal lesions. These low-grade malignant tumors are radiosensitive and may spread via CSF pathways.

A
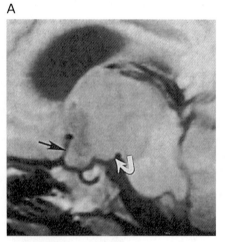

B
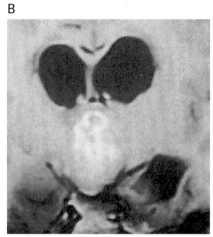

Fig SK 10-1
Glioma. (A) Sagittal T1-weighted image in a 2-year-old emaciated and hyperactive girl shows a large midline mass involving the optic chiasm (straight arrow) and hypothalamus (curved arrow). (B) Coronal contrast-enhanced T1-weighted image shows nonuniform enhancement of the tumor, which extends superiorly to the foramen of Monro and causes obstructive hydrocephalus.[21]

A
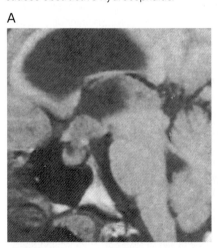

B
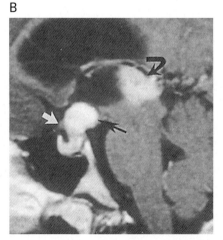

Fig SK 10-2
Germinoma. Sagittal T1-weighted scans before (A) and after (B) administration of contrast material in an 18-year-old man with diabetes insipidus show enhancing masses in the floor of the anterior third ventricle (straight black arrow) and pineal region (curved arrow). The optic chiasm (white arrow) is not involved.[21]

Condition	Imaging Findings	Comments
Primary lymphoma (Fig SK 10-3)	Slightly hypointense on T1-weighted images. Variable appearance on T2-weighted images. Usually shows contrast enhancement.	Prevalence of primary CNS lymphoma is increased in AIDS patients and other immunosuppressed individuals. Most common presentation is solitary or multicentric, well-defined enhancing masses in the deep gray nuclei, periventricular white matter, or corpus callosum.
Hamartoma (Fig SK 10-4)	Mass in the region of the tuber cinereum that is isointense on T1-weighted images and isointense or mildly hyperintense on T2-weighted images. The lesion is stable over time and typically does not show contrast enhancement.	Rare lesion of early childhood that usually presents with precocious puberty, seizures, and mental changes (behavioral disorders and intellectual deterioration). It may be found incidentally in adults and mimic low-grade gliomas.

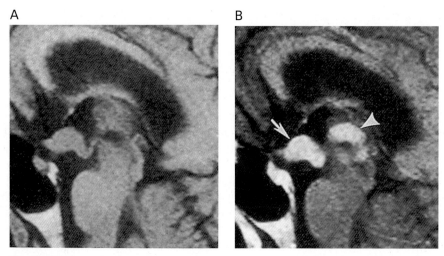

Fig SK 10-3
Primary CNS lymphoma. (A) Sagittal and (B) axial T1-weighted images after injection of contrast material show enhancing mass lesions in the hypothalamus (arrow) and left thalamus (arrowhead).[21]

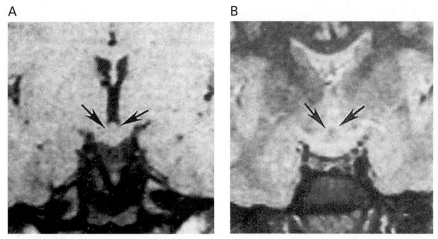

Fig SK 10-4
Hamartoma. Coronal (A) T1-weighted and (B) T2-weighted scans in a 5-year-old girl with precocious puberty show a midline hypothalamic mass (arrows) bulging into the inferior floor of the third ventricle. The lesion is isointense on both images and is centered in the region of the tuber cinereum.[21]

Condition	Imaging Findings	Comments
Langerhans cell histiocytosis (Fig SK 10-5)	Suprasellar mass involving the infundibulum and hypothalamus that is hypointense on T1-weighted images and hyperintense on T2-weighted images. The lesion enhances homogeneously with contrast material.	Multisystem disorder associated with proliferation of macrophages. Hypothalamic involvement, most common in children, is usually associated with multiple destructive skeletal lesions. Dramatic response to low-dose radiation, strongly favors the diagnosis of histiocytosis over hypothalamic glioma.
Metastasis (Fig SK 10-6)	Typically intense contrast enhancement with extensive bone destruction without marked sellar enlargement.	Metastatic involvement of the hypothalamus is unusual, most commonly due to breast cancer in women and lung cancer in men.
Hemangioblatoma (Fig SK 10-7)	Complex cystic mass, often with an intensely enhancing mural nodule.	This benign vascular neoplasm rarely occurs in the hypothalamic-pituitary axis, and its discovery in this location should raise a strong suspicion for von Hippel-Lindau disease.
Choristoma (Fig SK 10-8)	Variable appearance with the solid parts of the tumor being isointense to brain on both T1- and T2-weighted images. Inhomogeneous enhancement may be seen.	Low-grade glioma arising along the distribution of the neurohypophysis. This rare tumor is essentially benign and has minimal tendency for invasion or recurrence.
Craniopharyngioma (Fig SK 10-9)	Variable appearance depending on the solid or cystic nature of the mass and the specific cyst contents. The lesion is generally hypointense on T1-weighted images and hyperintense on T2-weighted images. High signal intensity on T1-weighted images can reflect high cholesterol content or methemoglobin within a cystic mass.	The solid and wall portions of a craniopharyngioma show contrast enhancement. The lesion may arise anywhere along the infundibular stalk from the floor of the third ventricle to the pituitary gland. Craniopharyngiomas have two peaks of prevalence, one between 10 and 14 years of age and the other in the fourth to sixth decades of life.

A   B

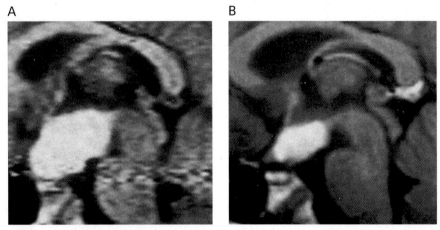

Fig SK 10-5
Langerhans cell histiocytosis. (A) Initial sagittal T1-weighted image after injection of contrast material in a 9-year-old boy with diabetes insipidus shows a large enhancing hypothalamus mass splaying the cerebral peduncles. (B) Corresponding image 3 weeks after low-dose radiation treatment shows a significant decrease in size of the lesion.[21]

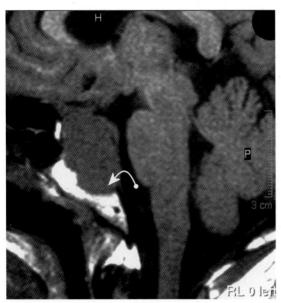

Fig SK 10-6
Metastasis. Sagittal T1-weighted contrast image demonstrates a large clival mass with destruction of the sella and invasion of the suprasellar region. Note the small enhancing hypothalamic mass (arrow) representing metastasis from breast cancer.[22]

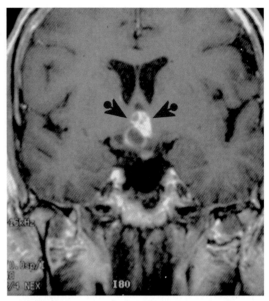

Fig SK 10-7
Hemangioblastoma. Coronal T1-weighted contrast image indicates that the complex mass contains cystic components with marginal enhancement (short arrow) and an intensely enhancing mural nodule (long arrow).[22]

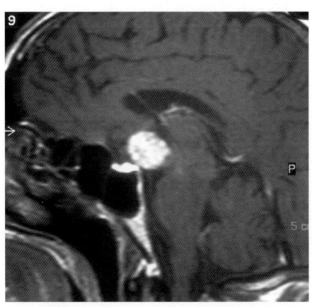

Fig SK 10-8
Choristoma. Sagittal T1-weighted contrast image shows a well-defined suprasellar mass (arrow). Initially isointense relative to brain, the mass shows inhomogeneous enhancement.[22]

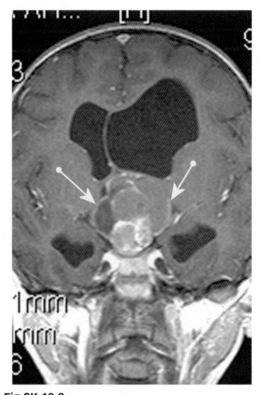

Fig SK 10-9
Craniopharyngioma. Coronal T1-weighted contrast image shows a lobulated suprasella tumor with intrasellar extension. The tumor is formed predominantly of multiple cysts with varying signal intensities that show thin mural enhancement (arrows). Note the associated asymmetric dilatation of the lateral ventricle.[22] (Courtesy of Yasser Regab, M.D., Cairo, Egypt.)

Condition	Imaging Findings	Comments
Dermoid cyst (Fig SK 10-10)	Heterogeneous texture due to the multiple cell types within it.	Fatty components are common and produce high signal on T1-weighted images. Dermoid cysts with low fat content may demonstrate signal intensity similar to that of CSF.
Rathke's cleft cyst (Fig SK 10-11)	Either a mass with CSF intensity on both T1- and T2-weighted images or a lesion that is markedly hyperintense on both sequences.	Bright signal on T1-weighted images appears to reflect the high protein content or starch content of the mucoid material in the cyst.
Colloid cyst (Fig SK 10-12)	Although a highly variable appearance, most commonly hyperintense on T1-weighted images and iso- to hypointense on T2-weighted sequences. No contrast enhancement or calcification.	Slow-growing mass usually located in the antero-superior third ventricle close to the foramen of Monro.
Encephalitis (Fig SK 10-13)	Extensive edema appears hyperintense on T2-weighted images.	Most commonly due to viral infection. MR imaging shows the extent of the inflammation and helps differentiate encephalitis from other hypothalamic conditions that produce discrete masses.
Sarcoidosis (Fig SK 10-14)	Leptomeningeal form, involving the infundibulum and hypothalamus, typically is isointense on T1-weighted images and mildly hyperintense on T2-weighted images. It shows homogeneous contrast enhancement.	Systemic noncaseating granulomatous disease that involves the central nervous system in approximately 5% of individuals. It is common in blacks and usually occurs in the third to fourth decades of life. There is usually a positive response to steroid therapy.

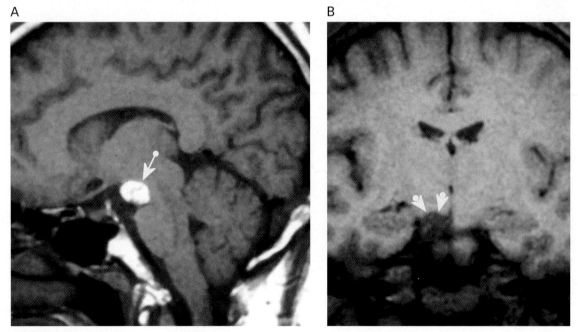

A   B

Fig SK 10-10
Dermoid cyst. (A) Sagittal T1-weighted image shows a well-defined hyperintense lesion (arrow) at the floor of the hypothalamus, posterior to the infundibular stalk. (B) On a coronal fat-suppressed T1-weighted image, the lesion (arrowheads) exhibits suppressed signal intensity, a finding that indicates fat deposition.[22]

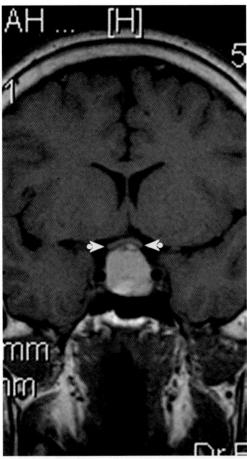

Fig SK 10-11
Rathke's cleft cyst. Coronal T1-weighted image shows a well-defined intra- and suprasellar lesion that displaces the optic chiasm upward (arrowheads). The high signal intensity reflects the high concentration of mucopolysaccharides within the mass.[22] (Courtesy of Yasser Regab, M.D., Cairo, Egypt.)

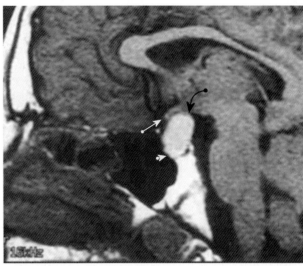

Fig SK 10-12
Colloid cyst. Sagittal T1-weighted image shows a well-defined, homogeneously hyperintense suprasellar cyst (curved arrow) that displaces the optic chiasm upward (straight arrow). Intrasellar extension compresses the pituitary gland (arrowhead).[22]

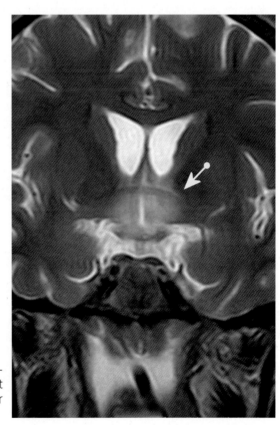

Fig SK 10-13
Encephalitis. Coronal T2-weighted image shows a hyperintense area in the thalamic-hypothalamic region (arrow) that corresponds to edematous changes.[22] (Courtesy of Yasser Regab, M.D., Cairo, Egypt.)

Condition	Imaging Findings	Comments
Ectopic posterior pituitary gland (Fig SK 10-15)	Small midline mass within the tuber cinereum–infundibular region that has homogeneous high signal intensity on T1-weighted images and is isointense on T2-weighted images. Characteristic absence of normal infundibulum and high-signal-intensity tissue within the posterior sella on T1-weighted images.	May be caused by trauma or an adjacent mass or be of congenital origin. Often associated with dwarfism, though many patients are asymptomatic. Transection, compression, or absence of the infundibulum and its neurohypophyseal tract results in the proximal build-up of neurosecretory granules within liposome vesicles before the point of interruption. The bright signal associated with the phospholipid membranes of these hormone-carrying vesicles is thus displaced proximally and cannot be seen in its normal location in the posterior lobe of the pituitary gland at the back of the sella.
Wernicke's encephalopathy (Fig SK 10-16)	Nearly complete absence of the mamillary bodies, best seen on T1-weighted images.	Atrophy of the mamillary bodies is a characteristic feature of this disorder. The disease is caused by thiamine deficiency and is most commonly seen in alcoholics. It is associated with the classic triad of oculomotor dysfunction, ataxia, and encephalopathy.

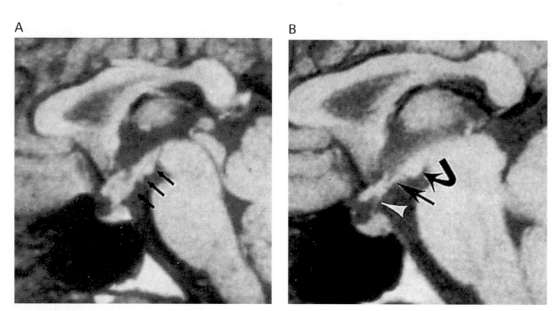

Fig SK 10-14
Sarcoidosis. (A) Sagittal T1-weighted image in a black woman with recent onset of visual difficulties shows abnormal thickening in the hypothalamic region (arrows) involving the tuber cinereum, mamillary bodies, and infundibulum. (B) After a 3-week course of steroids, a repeat sagittal scan shows dramatic resolution with a return to normal of hypothalamic region anatomy. Note the mamillary bodies (curved arrow), tuber cinereum (straight arrow), and infundibulum (arrowhead).[21]

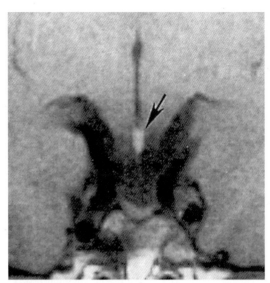

Fig SK 10-15
Ectopic posterior pituitary gland. Coronal T1-weighted image in a young boy with short stature shows a hyperintense, oblong nodule (arrow) in the inferior portion of the tuber cinereum. Pituitary tissue within the sella does not show high signal in its posterior portion, and there is no evidence of an infundibulum connecting the pituitary gland to the hypothalamus.[21]

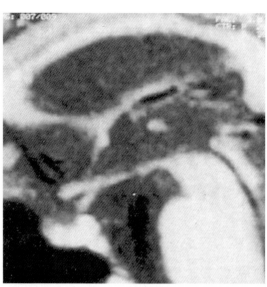

Fig SK 10-16
Wernicke's encephalopathy. Sagittal T1-weighted image in an elderly alcoholic man shows striking atrophy of the mamillary bodies.[21]

Hyperintense Basal Ganglia on T1-Weighted Magnetic Resonance Imaging

Condition	Comments
Paramagnetic substances	
Methemoglobin (subacute intracranial hemorrhage or hemorrhagic infarct) (Figs SK 11-1 and SK 11-2)	In the late subacute stage, hemolysis brings about the release of methemoglobin contained in red blood cells, which results in an area of hyperintensity on both T1- and T2-weighted images.
Manganese (parenteral nutrition) (Fig SK 11-3)	Symmetric increase in signal intensity on T1-weighted images in the globus pallidus and subthalamic nucleus, without corresponding abnormalities on T2-weighted images or CT. Cessation of parenteral nutrition usually results in regression of the abnormal signal intensity.
Calcification (Fig SK 11-4)	Although usually isointense or hypointense on both T1- and T2-weighted images, calcification occasionally may appear hyperintense on T1-weighted scans. This is believed to relate to the varying crystalline structure of the calcification, with those calcium particles with greater surface area showing greater T1-relaxation.

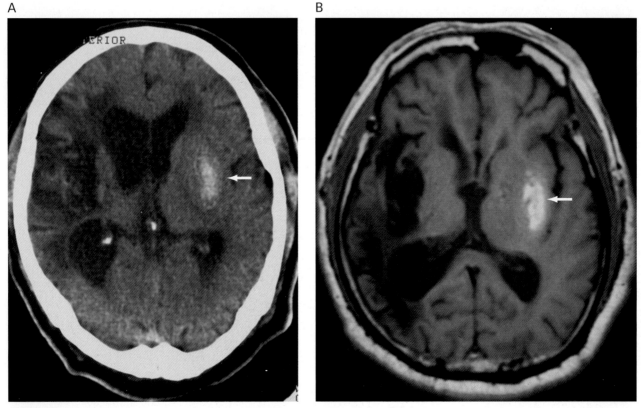

A   B

Fig SK 11-1
Intracranial hemorrhage. (A) Increased signal in the left basal ganglion. (B) Unenhanced CT shows slightly increased attenuation in the same region.[23]

Condition	Comments
Neurofibromatosis (type 1) (Fig SK 11-5)	In this, the most common of the phakomatoses, abnormal increased signal in the basal ganglia on T1-weighted images usually occurs in the globus pallidus and internal capsule. Small foci of hyperintensity may affect the brainstem, cerebellar white matter, dentate nucleus, basal ganglia, and periventricular white matter on T2-weighed images. These lesions typically resolve by adulthood and do not exhibit mass effect, edema, or contrast enhancement.
Hypoxic ischemic encephalopathy (Fig SK 11-6)	Global, rather than focal, brain injury due to perfusion or oxygenation disturbance most frequently involves the basal ganglia and parasagittal cortical areas. The hyperintensity in the basal ganglia on T1-weighted images may represent minor hemorrhage related to reperfusion in the subacute stage. Cortical laminar hyperintensity in the subacute stage represents depositions of lipid-laden macrophages of laminar necrosis.

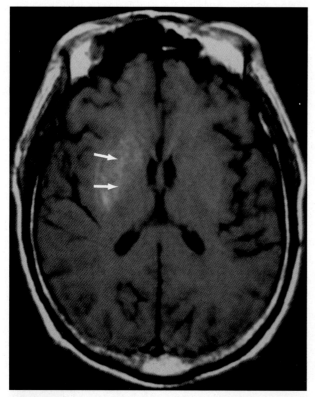

Fig SK 11-2
Petechial hemorrhagic infarct. Increased signal in the right basal ganglion (straight arrows) and temporal area (curved arrows).[23]

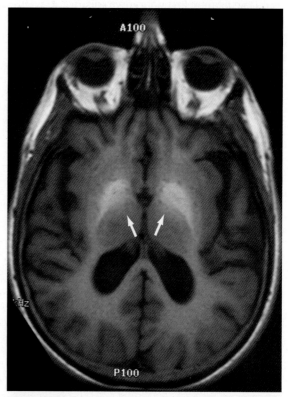

Fig SK 11-3
Parenteral nutrition. Increased signal intensity in the globus pallidus (arrows).[23]

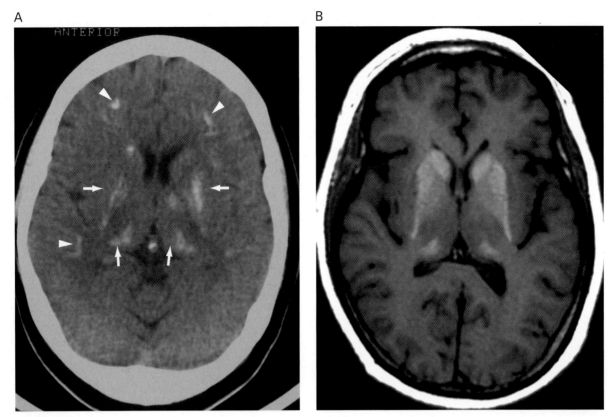

Fig SK 11-4
Calcification (hypoparathyroidism). (A) Unenhanced CT scan shows extensive calcification in the basal ganglia (arrows) and subcortical white matter (arrowheads) bilaterally. (B) T1-weighted MR image shows increased signal intensity in the basal ganglia.[23]

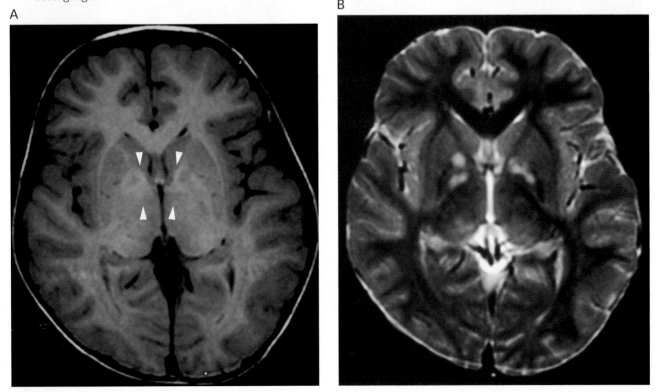

Fig SK 11-5
Neurofibromatosis. (A) T1-weighted image shows hyperintensity involving the globus pallidus and internal capsule (arrowheads) bilaterally. (B) On the corresponding T2-weighted image, there are small nodular foci of increased intensity in the globus pallidus and internal capsule bilaterally, but the extent and morphology of the signal abnormality differ from those on the T1-weighted image.[23]

Condition	Comments
Chronic hepatic failure (Fig SK 11-7)	Acquired hepatocerebral degeneration is an irreversible neurologic syndrome occurring in patients who have chronic liver disease and a portocaval shunt. There is symmetric hyperintensity of the globus pallidus that shows no enhancement and is not present on T2-weighted images or CT.
Diabetic hyperglycemia (Fig SK 11-8)	Hyperintensity of the putamen and/or caudate nucleus on T1-weighted images with no significant T2 signal alteration, mass effect, or contrast enhancement. Acute chorea-ballism with hyperglycemia usually has a benign clinical course, though some patients may have persistent or recurrent symptoms.
Japanese encephalitis (Fig SK 11-9)	Epidemic throughout Asia during the rainy season, the characteristic MR finding is bilateral hemorrhagic lesions in the thalami and basal ganglia that may produce hyperintensity on T1-weighted images.

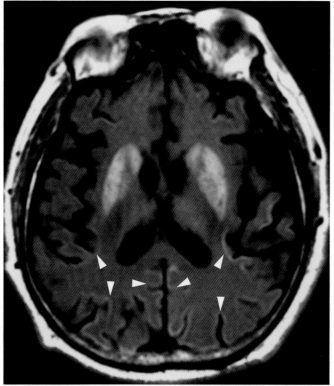

Fig SK 11-6
Hypoxic ischemic encephalopathy. Hyperintense foci in the basal ganglia bilaterally and laminar hyperintensity along the cerebral cortex (arrows) that is more prominent in the parieto-occipital region.[23]

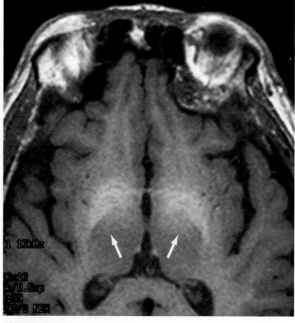

Fig SK 11-7
Chronic hepatic failure. Increased signal intensity in the globus pallidus (arrows).[23]

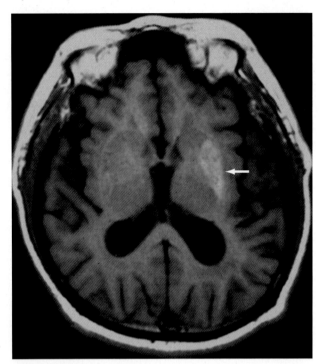

Fig SK 11-8
Diabetic hyperglycemia. Increased signal intensity in the left putamen (arrow). The patient had an abrupt onset of involuntary movements involving the right limbs.[23]

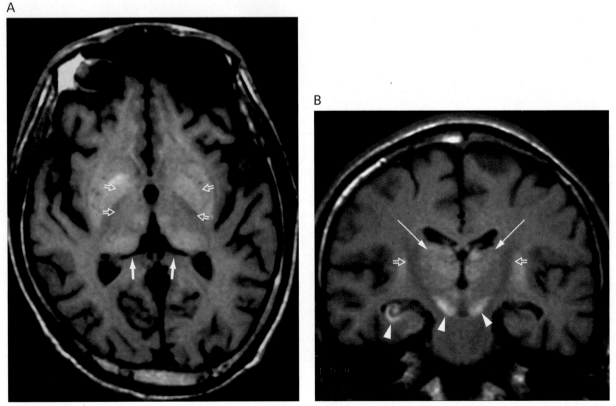

Fig SK 11-9
Japanese encephalitis. (A) Axial T1-weighted image shows increased signal intensity suggestive of subacute hemorrhage in the thalamus (solid arrows) and corpus striatum (open arrows) bilaterally. (B) On a coronal T1-weighted image, there is increased signal intensity in the corpus striatum (open arrows), thalamus (short arrows), and cerebral peduncle (long arrows) bilaterally, as well as in the right hippocampus (arrowhead).[23]

Cerebellar Masses on Computed Tomography

Condition	Imaging Findings	Comments
Astrocytoma (Fig SK 12-1)	Cystic or hypodense solid mass. Variable contrast enhancement (cystic astrocytomas may display an enhancing rim of tissue surrounding the circumference of the cyst or an enhancing localized mural nodule along nonenhancing cyst margins).	Occurs more commonly in children (first or second most frequent tumor of the posterior fossa) than in adults. Affects the cerebellar hemispheres more commonly than the vermis, tonsils, or brainstem. Approximately 20% of the tumors calcify. Malignant astrocytomas show edema and necrosis in addition to enhancement after the administration of contrast material.
Medulloblastoma (Fig SK 12-2)	Sharply marginated, spherical midline mass that is hyperdense and shows uniform and intense contrast enhancement.	Embryonal tumor consisting of primitive and poorly differentiated cells that originate immediately above the fourth ventricle and migrate during gestation toward the surface of the cerebellum. One of the two most common posterior fossa tumors in children. May occur in the cerebellar hemispheres in older patients. Metastasizes along the cerebrospinal fluid pathways in approximately 10% of cases (abnormal contrast enhancement or irregular thickening of the lining of the subarachnoid spaces).
Ependymoma	Isodense or slightly hyperdense midline mass. Unlike medulloblastomas, ependymomas are often inhomogeneous with cystic or hemorrhagic areas and frequently calcify. The tumor margins are often irregular and poorly defined, and the enhancement pattern is usually less homogeneous and intense than in medulloblastoma.	Fourth ventricular tumor that is more common in children than in adults. A characteristic finding is a thin, well-defined, low-attenuation halo that represents the distended and usually effaced fourth ventricle surrounding the tumor. The lesion frequently extends through the foramina of Luschka into the cerebellopontine angle or through the foramen of Magendie into the cisterna magna and typically causes hydrocephalus.

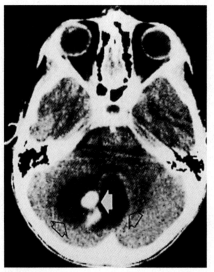

Fig SK 12-1
Cystic astrocytoma. The cystic posterior fossa lesion (open arrows) contains a central nodular area of enhancement (closed arrow).

Condition	Imaging Findings	Comments
Hemangioblastoma (Fig SK 12-3)	Most commonly a cystic hemispheric mass, typically with one or more small intensely enhancing mural nodules. May appear as a solid mass. Calcification is extremely rare.	Relatively uncommon tumor of the posterior fossa and spinal cord that is usually seen in adults. Hemangioblastomas tend to be smaller than hemispheric astrocytomas and almost never calcify. Characteristic intense tumor stain on angiography (more sensitive and specific than CT for this type of tumor).

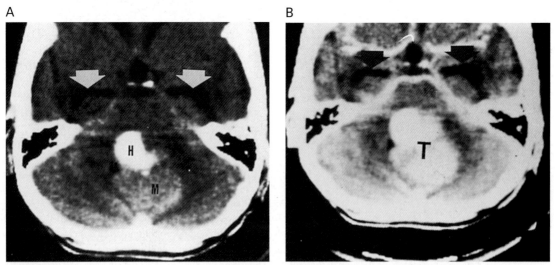

Fig SK 12-2
Medulloblastoma. (A) Noncontrast scan in an 8-year-old girl shows the tumor as a mixed high-density (H) and medium-density (M) mass in the posterior fossa. (B) After the intravenous injection of contrast material, there was marked enhancement of the tumor (T). The arrows point to the dilated temporal horns representing hydrocephalus.

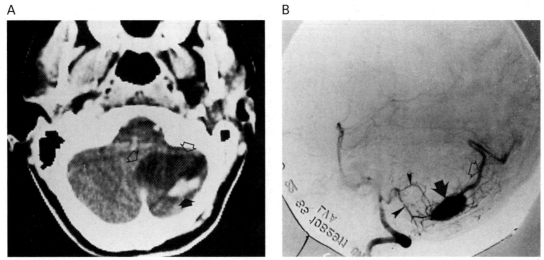

Fig SK 12-3
Hemangioblastoma in von Hippel-Lindau syndrome. (A) CT scan shows a cystic lesion (open arrows) with an enhancing nodule (closed arrow) in the left cerebellar hemisphere. (B) Vertebral arteriogram shows the vascular nodule (solid arrow) of the tumor with multiple feeding arteries (black arrowheads) and a large draining vein (open arrow).

Condition	Imaging Findings	Comments
Cerebellar sarcoma (lateral medulloblastoma) (Fig SK 12-4)	Large, solid, lobulated mass that is hyperdense or heterogeneous.	Probably represents a variety of desmoplastic peripheral medulloblastoma that is never calcified or predominantly cystic (as may be a central medulloblastoma).
Metastasis (Fig SK 12-5)	Various appearances (densely enhancing nodules surrounded by edema; large, inhomogeneous, poorly enhancing mass; ring enhancement in tumors with central necrosis).	Most common cerebellar tumors of older patients. There is usually a history of an extracerebral tumor and evidence of other cerebral metastases.

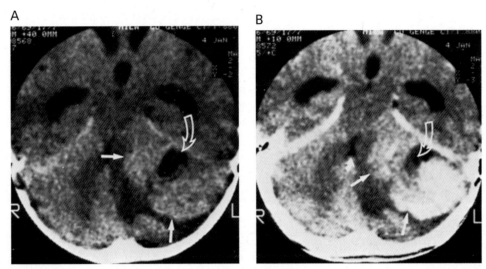

Fig SK 12-4
Cerebellar sarcoma. (A) Noncontrast scan shows dense tumor (straight arrows) in the left cerebellar hemisphere. Note the cystic region (open curved arrow) within it. (B) After intravenous contrast infusion, the tumor is notably enhanced (straight arrows). The fourth ventricle is displaced severely from left to right (open curved arrow), causing noncommunicating hydrocephalus.[1]

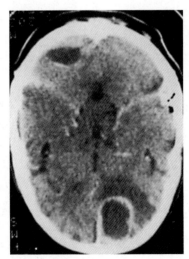

Fig SK 12-5
Metastasis. Ring-enhancing lesion with surrounding edema.

Condition	Imaging Findings	Comments
Lymphoma	Solid, hyperdense, densely enhancing mass that is located near the fourth ventricle or cerebellar surface and is usually associated with little or no edema.	Often multicentric with infiltration into adjoining tissue and across the midline (no respect for normal anatomic boundaries). Tumor margins are invariably poorly defined and irregular, probably because of the characteristic perivascular and vascular infiltration pattern of the tumor cells.
Epidermoid	Sharply marginated, nearly homogeneous, hypodense mass that may have an extremely low attenuation due to a high fat content.	Result of inclusion of ectodermal germ layer elements in the neural tube during its closure between the third and fifth weeks of gestation. Most commonly occurs in the cerebellopontine angle and suprasellar region, though it may develop in the fourth ventricle. Rupture into the ventricular system may produce a characteristic fat–cerebrospinal fluid level.
Choroid plexus papilloma	Homogeneous isodense or hyperdense intraventricular mass with smooth, well-defined, frequently lobulated margins. Intense homogeneous contrast enhancement.	Most commonly occurs in the first decade of life, usually in infancy. Typically develops in the lateral ventricles, though the fourth ventricle may be involved. In choroid plexus carcinoma, there are low-attenuation zones in the adjacent brain (representing edema or tumor invasion) and massive hydrocephalus.
Infarct (Fig SK 12-6)	Well-defined, low-attenuation region in a cerebellar hemisphere.	Contrast enhancement in a subacute infarction may simulate a cerebellar tumor.
Hemorrhage (Fig SK 12-7)	High-attenuation process that may appear round or irregular in shape and compress the fourth ventricle to cause hydrocephalus.	Hemorrhage into the cisterns usually produces a thin layer of high-density tissue adjacent to the tentorium or in the pontine cistern.

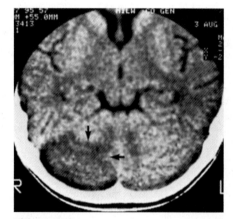

Fig SK 12-6
Right cerebellar infarction. The low-attenuation process (arrows) has well-defined margins consistent with chronic infarction.[1]

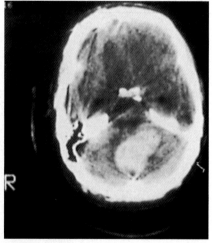

Fig SK 12-7
Cerebellar hemorrhage. There is a well-circumscribed, high-attenuation mass.

Condition	Imaging Findings	Comments
Arteriovenous malformation (Fig SK 12-8)	Large, tortuous, high-attenuation structures (representing serpiginous dilated vessels) that are seen after contrast enhancement.	An unruptured arteriovenous malformation may appear normal or only subtly abnormal on unenhanced CT studies, since the abnormal vessels are usually only slightly hyperdense with respect to the brain and are therefore difficult to identify. In some cases, calcification in the malformation or a low-density cyst or damaged cerebral tissue from previous hemorrhage suggests the presence of a malformation.
Abscess	Various patterns.	Pyogenic; tuberculous; fungal; parasitic.

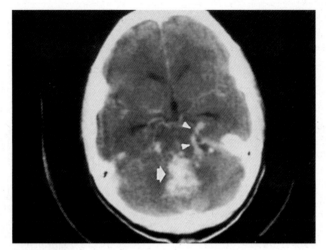

Fig SK 12-8
Arteriovenous malformation. Irregular mass of increased attenuation in the vermis (arrow). Note the dilated vein (arrowheads) draining the lesion.

Cerebellar Masses on Magnetic Resonance Imaging

Condition	Imaging Findings	Comments
Astrocytoma (Fig SK 13-1)	Hypointense on T1-weighted images. Increased signal intensity on T2-weighted images.	More than 50% of these tumors are cystic with smooth margins and a relatively homogeneous appearance.
Medulloblastoma (Fig SK 13-2)	Hypointense on T1-weighted images. Increased signal intensity on T2-weighted images.	Necrosis, hemorrhage, and cavitation are common and may produce a heterogeneous appearance (although to a lesser degree than with ependymoma). Dense cell packing with relatively little extracellular water may cause the tumor to appear only mildly hyperintense relative to brain on T2-weighted images.
Ependymoma (Fig SK 13-3)	Hypointense on T1-weighted images. Increased signal intensity on T2-weighted images.	Typically heterogeneous appearance because of frequent calcification and cystic and necrotic areas.
Hemangioblastoma (Figs SK 13-4 and SK 13-5)	Cystic portion is hypointense on T1-weighted images. The solid tumor nodules are isointense to or of slightly lower intensity than gray matter. Generalized increased signal intensity on T2-weighted images.	Classic MR appearance is a cystic mass with a brightly enhancing nodule. The hypervascular tumor often shows areas of signal void, representing enlarged tumor vessels either in the mass or on its periphery.
Metastasis (Fig SK 13-6)	Hypointense on T1-weighted images. Increased signal intensity on T2-weighted images.	Contrast-enhanced MRI is the most sensitive technique for the evaluation of posterior fossa metastasis. Hemorrhagic tumors (eg, melanoma, choriocarcinoma, and lung, thyroid, and renal carcinoma) produce various patterns depending on the chronicity of the bleeding.

B

A

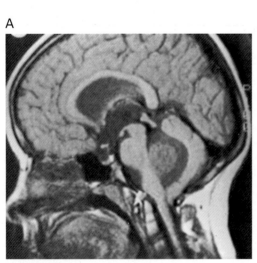
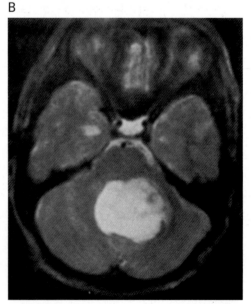

Fig SK 13-1
Cystic astrocytoma. (A) Sagittal T1-weighted image shows a large cerebellar vermian cyst containing fluid that is more intense than the dilated third ventricle. There is a central nodule of decreased intensity relative to the cerebellum. (B) On the axial T2-weighted image, the cyst fluid is markedly hyperintense. The central nodule has a somewhat lesser signal intensity.[24]

Condition	Imaging Findings	Comments
Lymphoma	Hypointense or isointense mass on T1-weighted images. Typically homogeneous, slightly high-signal to isointense mass on T2-weighted images.	The mild T2 prolongation is probably related to dense cell packing in the tumor, leaving relatively little interstitial space for the accumulation of water. The mass may be multicentric and exhibit infiltration into adjoining tissue and across the midline (no respect for normal anatomic boundaries).
Epidermoid	Heterogeneous texture and variable signal intensity. Most are of slightly higher signal than CSF on both T1- and T2-weighted images.	Some epidermoids appear bright on T1-weighted images because of their high fat content.

B

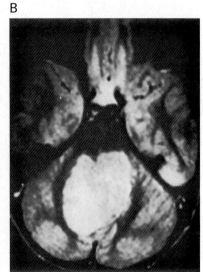

A

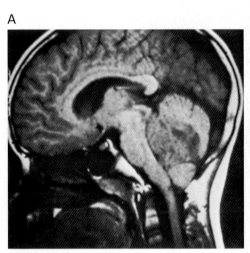

Fig SK 13-2
Cystic medulloblastoma. (A) Sagittal T1-weighted image demonstrates a mottled but predominantly hypointense cerebellar vermian lesion compressing the roof of the fourth ventricle. (B) Axial T2-weighted image shows the solid portion of the tumor to be hyperintense, whereas the cystic-necrotic component has an even more marked hyperintensity.[24]

B

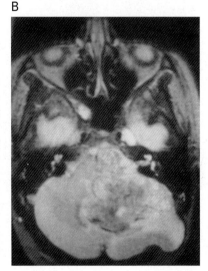

A

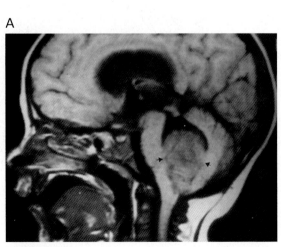

Fig SK 13-3
Ependymoma. (A) Sagittal T1-weighted image shows a large hypointense mass (arrows) in an expanded fourth ventricle. (B) Axial T2-weighted image shows the markedly heterogeneous quality of the mass. Note the extension of peritumoral edema into the adjacent cerebellar hemisphere.

Condition	Imaging Findings	Comments
Infarct (Figs SK 13-7 and SK 13-8)	Well-defined lesion that is hypointense on T1-weighted images and hyperintense on T2-weighted images. Old infarcts may have a more complex signal pattern that is related both to hemorrhagic components and to the evolution of infarcts, the latter resulting in areas of microcystic and macrocystic encephalomalacia and gliosis.	Involvement of both the cortex and a variable amount of subcortical tissue in a defined vascular territory. Contrast enhancement in a subacute infarction may simulate the appearance of a cerebellar tumor.

A

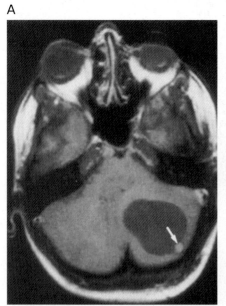

B

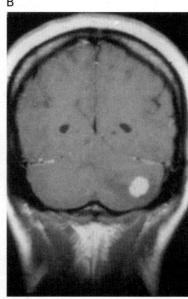

Fig SK 13-4
Hemangioblastoma. (A) Axial postcontrast T1-weighted image shows a mostly cystic left cerebellar lesion with a small nodule (arrow) of enhancement. (B) In another patient, a coronal scan shows a solid and enhancing hemangioblastoma in the left cerebellum.[6]

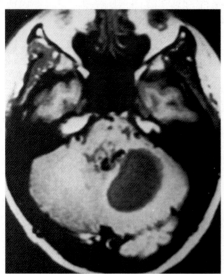

Fig SK 13-5
Cystic hemangioblastoma. Axial T1-weighted scan demonstrates a large cystic mass within the left cerebellar hemisphere. The cyst is markedly hypointense and well marginated and has a nodular component along its medial aspect. Note the virtually pathognomonic appearance of large arteries feeding the solid component of this cystic lesion.[24]

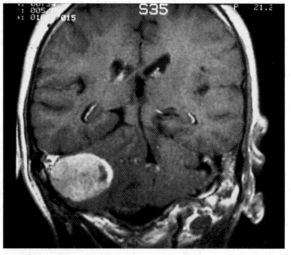

Fig SK 13-6
Metastasis. Coronal MR scan after gadolinium administration shows an enhancing right cerebellar lesion with a pronounced mass effect on midline structures.

Condition	Imaging Findings	Comments
Hemorrhage (Fig SK 13-9)	Variable pattern of signal intensity depending on the chronicity of the process.	The lesion may appear round or irregular in shape and may compress the fourth ventricle to cause hydrocephalus.
Arteriovenous malformation	Cluster of serpiginous flow voids (representing rapid blood flow) and areas of high signal (slow flow in draining veins).	The use of partial flip-angle techniques can distinguish hemosiderin or calcification associated with the lesion from vessels containing rapidly flowing blood.
Abscess	Hypointense mass with an isointense capsule surrounded by low-signal edema on T1-weighted images. Hyperintense mass surrounded by a hypointense capsule and high-signal edema on T2-weighted images.	Pyogenic; tuberculous; fungal; parasitic.

A

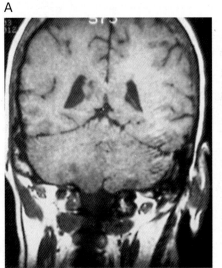

B

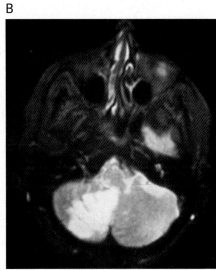

Fig SK 13-7
Infarction in the territory of the right posterior inferior cerebellar artery. The well-defined lesion is hypointense on the coronal T1-weighted image (A) and hyperintense on the axial T2-weighted scan (B).

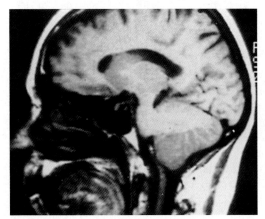

Fig SK 13-8
Infarction in the territory of the left posterior inferior cerebellar artery. Parasagittal T1-weighted image shows hypointensity of the entire lower half of the cerebellar hemisphere on that side.

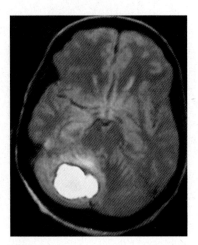

Fig SK 13-9
Resolving hemorrhage. The right cerebellar mass consists of hyperintense methemoglobin surrounded by a thin, hypointense rim of hemosiderin.

Cerebellopontine Angle Masses on Computed Tomography

Condition	Imaging Findings	Comments
Acoustic neuroma (Figs SK 14-1 through SK 14-3)	Well-defined, uniformly enhancing tumor with smooth, rounded margins. Typically there are enlargement and erosion of the internal auditory canal. May contain low-attenuation cystic areas and simulate an epidermoid. Bilateral acoustic neuromas suggest neurofibromatosis.	Represents approximately 10% of primary intracranial tumors and accounts for most masses in the cerebellopontine angle. Small intracanalicular tumors confined to the internal auditory canal may cause bony changes or clinical findings suggesting an acoustic neuroma in the absence of CT evidence of a discrete mass. In such cases (if MRI not available), repeat CT examination is required after the intrathecal administration of contrast material (metrizamide or air).
Meningioma (Fig SK 14-4)	Hyperdense mass on noncontrast scans that shows dense enhancement after the intravenous injection of contrast material. Unlike acoustic neuromas, meningiomas commonly show calcification and cystic changes. Typically, they are larger and more broadly based along the petrous bone than neuromas.	Second most common cerebellopontine angle mass. Usually centered above or below the internal auditory meatus and infrequently associated with widening of the internal auditory canal (or hearing loss).
Epidermoid (Fig SK 14-5)	Low-density mass on both pre- and post-contrast scans (though occasional high-density and enhancing lesions have been recorded). Infrequently has a calcified margin.	Most common location for this fat-containing tumor. Because the tumor tends not to stretch or distort the brainstem or cranial nerves but to surround them, an extensive neoplasm may be present before symptoms occur.

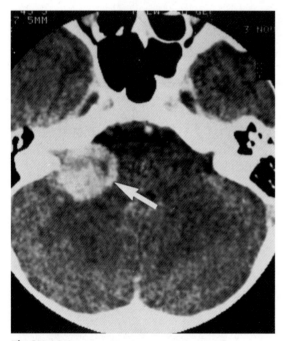

Fig SK 14-1
Acoustic neuroma. Contrast-enhancing mass (arrow) in the right internal auditory canal and cerebellopontine angle cistern.[1]

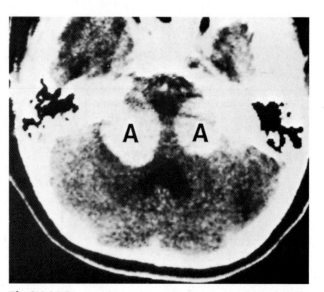

Fig SK 14-2
Neurofibromatosis. Bilateral acoustic neuromas (A) in a young girl with progressive bilateral sensorineural hearing loss.

Condition	Imaging Findings	Comments
Metastasis (Fig SK 14-6)	Enhancing mass with bone erosion (often without distinct margins) and sometimes edema in the adjacent cerebellum.	Usually a history of a primary neoplasm elsewhere.

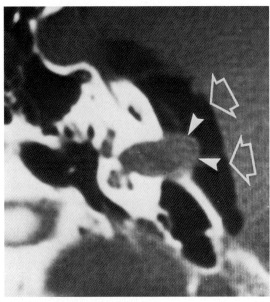

Fig SK 14-3
Intracanalicular acoustic neuroma. Air injected into the subarachnoid space shows the cerebellopontine angle cistern (open arrows) and outlines the small tumor (arrowheads).

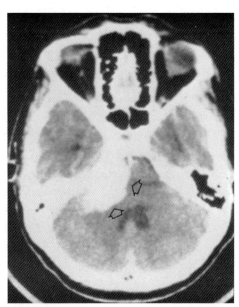

Fig SK 14-4
Meningioma. Dense enhancing lesion (arrows) that is more broadly based along the petrous bone than a typical acoustic neuroma.

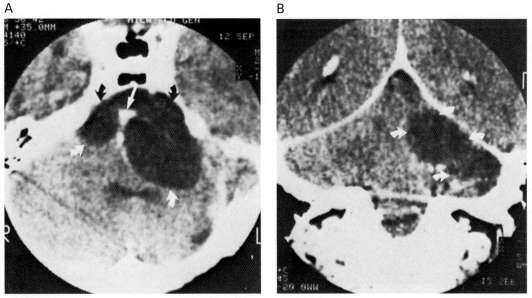

Fig SK 14-5
Epidermoid. Irregularly shaped, low-density mass (curved arrows) in front of the basilar artery (arrow) and brainstem on (A) axial and (B) coronal images.[1]

Condition	Imaging Findings	Comments
Arachnoid cyst (Fig SK 14-7)	Cystic structure with a density equal to that of cerebrospinal fluid. With positive contrast cisternography, there is enhancement of the adjacent cisterns without enhancement of the cyst (some intrathecal contrast eventually penetrates the cyst).	Typically displaces adjacent brainstem and cerebellar structures to a much greater degree than a cystic epidermoid tumor. Arachnoid cysts do not calcify, unlike epidermoids.
Aneurysm of basilar or vertebral artery (Fig SK 14-8)	Usually has greater than brain density on pre-contrast scans.	The amount of contrast enhancement depends on the degree of luminal thrombosis. A characteristic appearance is concentric or eccentric circles representing the enhanced lumen, the less dense thrombus, and the dense wall of the aneurysm.
Arterial ectasia	Curvilinear, homogeneously enhancing structure that may simulate a cerebellopontine angle tumor.	Elongation and ectasia of the vertebral, basilar, or inferior cerebellar artery. Digital or conventional arteriography or dynamic CT can show the true nature of the process.
Glomus jugulare tumor (Fig SK 14-9)	Lobulated, uniformly dense, and densely enhancing mass. Although the highly vascular mass may simulate other enhancing extra-axial lesions at this site, associated erosion of the jugular foramen usually permits the diagnosis.	The tumor arises in the middle ear and produces a blue or red polypoid mass, which can be visualized otoscopically, or a mass in the jugular foramen. Although most of these tumors are histologically benign, they may be locally invasive and cause irregular and poorly defined bone erosion suggesting malignancy.
Extension of adjacent tumor	Various patterns.	May be secondary to brainstem or cerebellar glioma, chordoma, pituitary adenoma, craniopharyngioma, fourth ventricular tumor, choroid plexus papilloma, or neuroma of one of the lowest four cranial nerves.

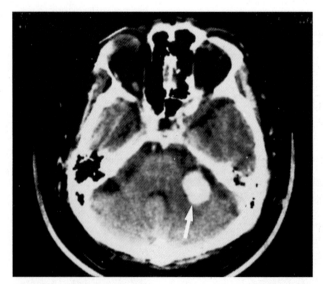

Fig SK 14-6
Metastasis to left flocculus. Contrast-enhancing nodule (arrow) displaces the brainstem. It is distinguished from an acoustic neuroma by its location posterior and medial to the porus acousticus.[1]

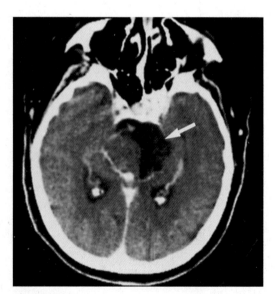

Fig SK 14-7
Arachnoid cyst. Slightly irregular cystic mass (arrow) of cerebrospinal fluid density that displaces the brainstem and basilar artery to the right.[1]

Condition	Imaging Findings	Comments
Normal flocculus	Nodule along the lateral surface of the cerebellum near the internal auditory canal.	The flocculus is located posterior to the internal auditory canal, does not enhance as prominently as the usual acoustic neuroma, and is not associated with widening of the internal auditory canal.

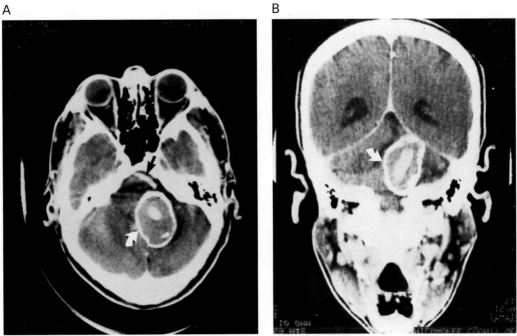

Fig SK 14-8
Giant aneurysm with thrombus simulating meningioma. (A) Axial and (B) coronal images show the mass (arrow) with calcific rim and high density within it displacing the pons and cerebellum. The aneurysm fails to enhance as densely as the basilar artery (arrow).[1]

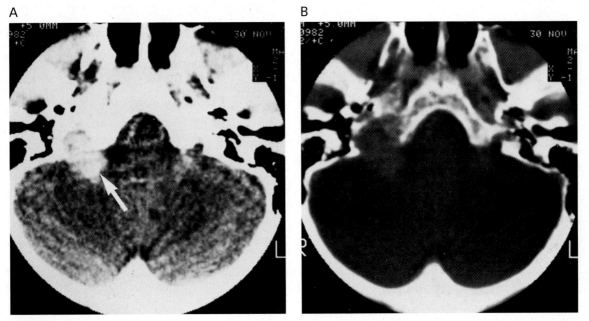

Fig SK 14-9
Glomus jugulare tumor. Densely enhancing mass (arrow) that has eroded the osseous margins adjacent to the right jugular foramen.[1]

Cerebellopontine Angle Masses on Magnetic Resonance Imaging

Condition	Imaging Findings	Comments
Acoustic neuroma (Figs SK 15-1 and SK 15-2)	Isointense or slightly hypointense lesion on T1-weighted images. Hyperintense signal on T2-weighted images.	Prominent contrast enhancement permits demonstration of even small intracanalicular masses on coronal or axial images.
Meningioma (Fig SK 15-3)	Usually hypointense to white matter on T1-weighted images. At 1.5 T, the lesion is hyperintense to white matter on T2-weighted images.	Prominent and homogeneous contrast enhancement. Typically larger and more broadly based along the petrous bone than an acoustic neuroma.
Epidermoid (Fig SK 15-4)	Heterogeneous texture and variable signal intensity. Most are of slightly higher signal than CSF on both T1- and T2-weighted images.	Some epidermoids appear bright on T1-weighted images.

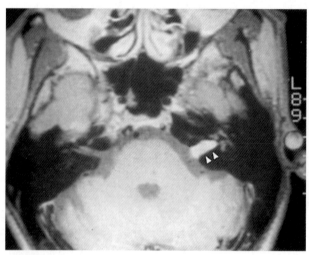

Fig SK 15-1
Acoustic neuroma. Marked contrast enhancement of the left-sided lesion (arrowheads). Note the normal neural structures on the right.

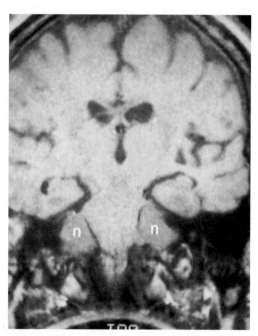

Fig SK 15-2
Acoustic neuroma. Bilateral tumors (n) are seen in this coronal scan of a patient with neurofibromatosis.

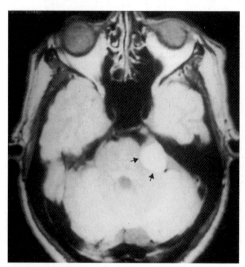

Fig SK 15-3
Meningioma. Note that the mass (arrows) has a relatively broad base along the petrous bone.

Condition	Imaging Findings	Comments
Lipoma (Fig SK 15-5)	Homogeneous high signal of T1-weighted images, which decreases on fat-suppressed images.	No enhancement after contrast material administration.
Metastasis (Fig SK 15-6)	Generally hypointense on T1-weighted images and of increased signal intensity on T2-weighted images.	Intratumoral hemorrhage and cystic necrosis may occur. There is usually a history of a primary neoplasm elsewhere.
Arachnoid cyst (Fig SK 15-7)	Smoothly marginated and homogeneous lesion containing cyst fluid that is isointense to CSF on all pulse sequences.	Typically displaces adjacent brainstem and cerebellar structures to a much greater degree than a cystic epidermoid tumor.

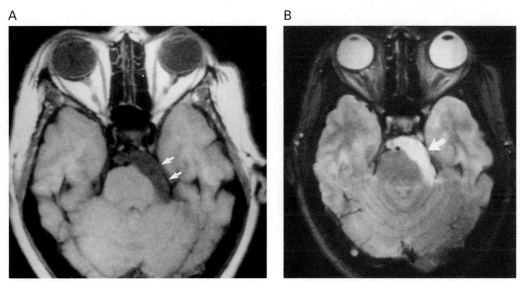

Fig SK 15-4
Epidermoid. (A) Axial T1-weighted and (B) axial T2-weighted scans show an oblong mass (arrows) of slightly higher signal than CSF enveloping the basilar artery and extending around the pons.

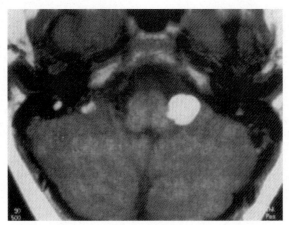

Fig SK 15-5
Lipoma. Axial T1-weighted image shows that the lesion has signal intensity similar to that of subcutaneous fat.[25]

Condition	Imaging Findings	Comments
Aneurysm of posterior fossa artery (Figs SK 15-8 and SK 15-9)	Flow void that may be surrounded by a pattern of heterogeneous signal intensity representing turbulence or thrombus.	Partial flip-angle imaging produces fairly consistent flow-related enhancement in the lumen and more clearly differentiates it from surrounding clot.
Arterial ectasia	Curvilinear flow void that may simulate a cerebellopontine angle tumor.	Elongation and ectasia of the vertebral, basilar, or superior cerebellar artery.

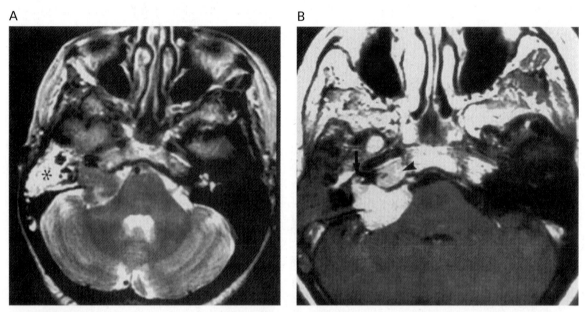

Fig SK 15-6
Metastasis. (A) Axial T2-weighted image shows a metastasis of the right cerebellopontine angle (from lung carcinoma) that mimics an acoustic neuroma but is associated with unusual middle ear retention (*). (B) Contrast-enhanced axial T1-weighted scan shows intense enhancement of the lesion, which extends into the cochlea (arrow). Note the presence of another enhancing lesion at the tip of the right petrous bone (arrowhead).[25]

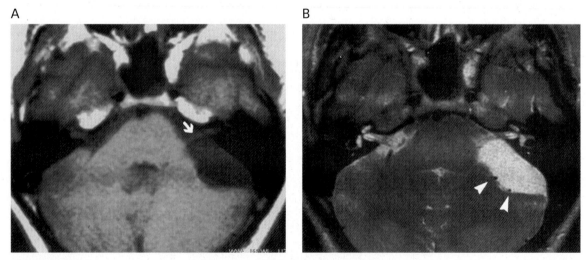

Fig SK 15-7
Arachnoid cyst. (A) Axial T1-weighted image shows the CSF-intensity cyst stretching the left 7th and 8th cranial nerve complex (arrow). (B) Axial T2-weighted scan shows the cyst displacing the vascular structures of the cerebellopontine angle (arrowheads).[25]

Condition	Imaging Findings	Comments
Glomus jugulare tumor (Fig SK 15-10)	Isointense lesion on T1-weighted images. Hyperintense signal on T2-weighted images.	This highly vascular tumor contains multiple signal voids representing enlarged vessels. There is marked contrast enhancement.

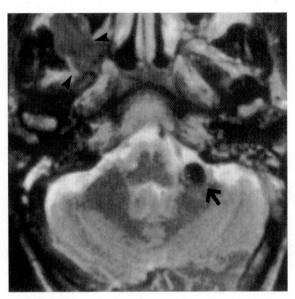

Fig SK 15-8
Aneurysm of the left posterior inferior cerebellar artery. Axial T2-weighted image shows the typical lack of signal (arrow) within the aneurysm. Note the lymphoma in the right pterygopalatine fossa (arrowheads), which explained the patient's neuralgia.[25]

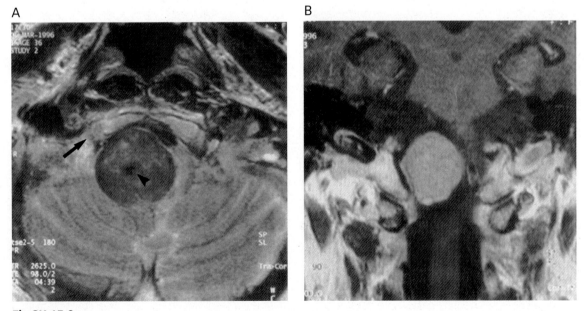

Fig SK 15-9
Thrombosed aneurysm of the right posterior inferior cerebellar artery. (A) Axial T2-weighted image shows a focal area of calcification (arrowhead). Note the normal right hypoglossal canal (arrow), a finding inconsistent with an acoustic neuroma. (B) Contrast coronal T1-weighted scan shows homogeneous enhancement of the organized thrombus, which completely fills the aneurysm.[25]

Condition	Imaging Findings	Comments
Extension of adjacent tumor (Figs SK 15-11 through SK 15-15)	Generally a hypointense lesion on T1-weighted images. Hyperintense signal on T2-weighted images.	May be secondary to brainstem or cerebellar glioma, chordoma, pituitary adenoma, craniopharyngioma, fourth ventricular tumor, choroid plexus papilloma, chondrosarcoma, or neuroma of the 5th or 9th through 12th cranial nerves.

A
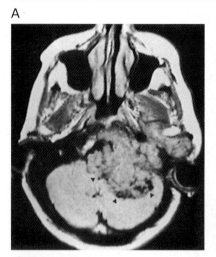

B
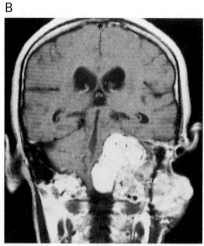

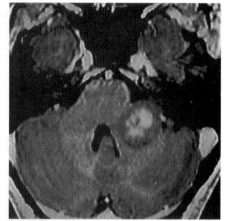

Fig SK 15-10
Glomus jugulare tumor with intracranial involvement and bony erosion. (A) Axial T1-weighted image shows the mass (arrowheads) in the left temporal bone and posterior fossa extending across the midline. Note the large veins on the surface of the tumor. (B) Coronal contrast-enhanced image shows displacement of the brainstem, bony erosion from the large enhanced mass, and parotid involvement.[26]

Fig SK 15-11
Brainstem glioma. A contrast axial T1-weighted image shows central enhancement in an unusual round grade III glioma located in front of the porus.[25]

A
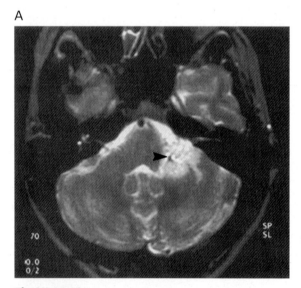

B
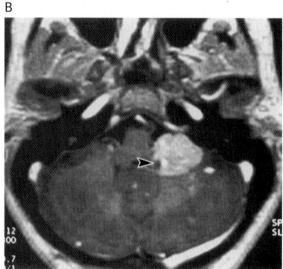

Fig SK 15-12
Hemangioblastoma. (A) Axial T2-weighted image in a patient with von Hippel-Lindau disease shows a solid tumor in the left cerebellopontine angle. Note the vascular pedicle (arrowhead), which appears as a flow void with all sequences. (B) Contrast T1-weighted axial image shows homogeneous enhancement of the tumor (arrowhead).[25]

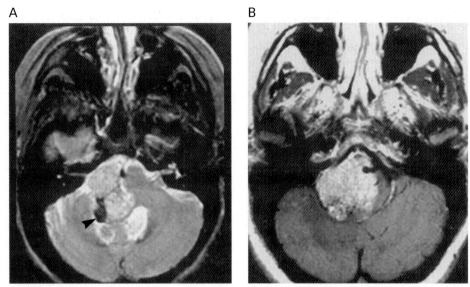

Fig SK 15-13
Choroid plexus papilloma. (A) Axial T2-weighted image shows a right cerebellopontine angle papilloma extending through the foramen of Luschka. The tumor contains massive hypointense calcification (arrowhead). (B) Contrast T1-weighted axial scan shows intense enhancement of the hypervascularized tumor. Note the normal choroid plexus in the left foramen of Luschka.[25]

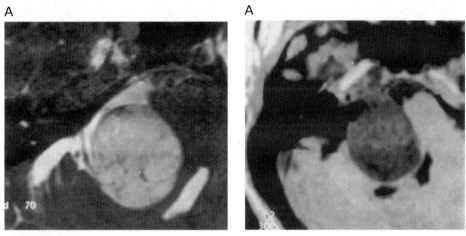

Fig SK 15-14
Chondrosarcoma. (A) Axial T1-weighted image shows the large tumor with its skull base pedicle. (B) Contrast T1-weighted coronal scan shows punctate enhancement, which could suggest a chondromatous lesion.[20]

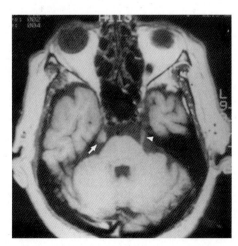

Fig SK 15-15
Trigeminal neuroma. Isointense mass on the right (arrow). Note the normal 5th cranial nerve on the left (arrowhead).

Low-Density Mass in the Brainstem on Computed Tomography

Condition	Imaging Findings	Comments
Glioma (Fig SK 16-1)	Typically a low-attenuation area with indistinct margins in an asymmetrically expanded brainstem. The tumor may be relatively isodense (and be difficult to detect) or occasionally show increased attenuation or even gross calcification.	The mass effect depends on tumor size and may be generalized or focal. Contrast enhancement may be obvious, minimal, or absent. Cysts may occur, allowing palliative decompression.
Metastasis (Fig SK 16-2)	Mass of inhomogeneous density with expansion of the brainstem and variable contrast enhancement (typically better defined than with gliomas).	More likely than primary glioma in a patient older than 50 years of age with progressive brainstem signs. Usually there is evidence of other intracranial lesions (isolated metastasis to the brainstem is unusual).
Other tumors	Various patterns.	Hamartoma, teratoma, epidermoid, lymphoma.
Infarction (Fig SK 16-3)	Combination of low attenuation, mass effect, and vague contrast enhancement may resemble a tumor.	Clinical information or follow-up scans can usually establish the diagnosis.
Multiple sclerosis	Combination of low attenuation, mass effect, and vague contrast enhancement may resemble a tumor.	Clinical information or follow-up scans can usually establish the diagnosis.
Central pontine myelinolysis (Fig SK 16-4)	Central region of diminished attenuation in the pons and medulla without marked contrast enhancement.	Although initial reports were largely confined to chronic alcoholics, the condition is also seen in patients with electrolyte disturbances (particularly hyponatremia) that have been corrected rapidly.
Syringobulbia (Fig SK 16-5)	Central mass of cerebrospinal fluid density within and usually enlarging the medulla. Sharply defined margins. Does not show contrast enhancement (unlike cyst neoplasm).	Cystic process in the medulla that is most frequently found in conjunction with syringomyelia (an Arnold-Chiari malformation) and less often with a tumor or degeneration in the brain.
Granuloma/abscess	Appearance mimicking that of a neoplasm.	Rare manifestation of tuberculosis, sarcoidosis, or infection. Diagnosis may require biopsy.

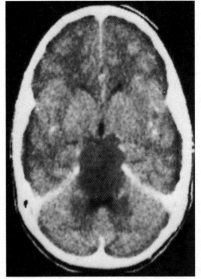

Fig SK 16-1
Glioma. Poorly defined low-attenuation mass causing irregular expansion of the brainstem and compression of the fourth ventricle.

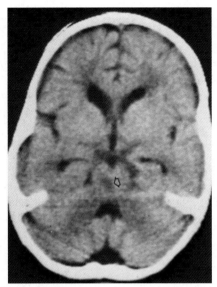

Fig SK 16-2
Metastasis. Subtle, ill-defined area of low density (arrow).

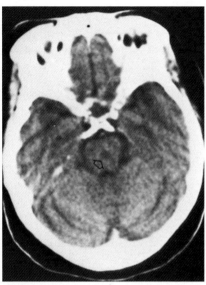

Fig SK 16-3
Infarction. Central low-attenuation region (arrow).

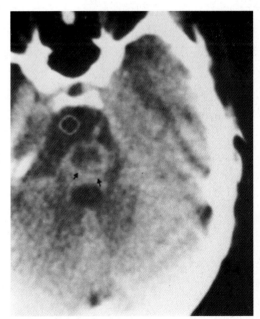

Fig SK 16-4
Central pontine myelinolysis. Low-attenuation region (arrows) in the center of the pons in a comatose alcoholic patient. Note the widening of the prepontine subarachnoid space, indicating loss of brainstem volume due to atrophy.

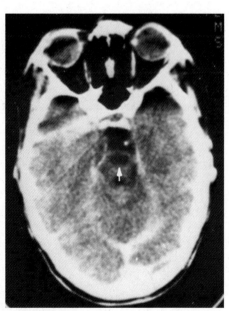

Fig SK 16-5
Syringobulbia. Well-demarcated mass of cerebrospinal fluid density (arrow) in the center of the brainstem.

Brainstem Lesions on Magnetic Resonance Imaging

Condition	Imaging Findings	Comments
Glioma (Fig SK 17-1)	Hypointense mass on T1-weighted images. High-intensity signal on proton-density and T2-weighted images.	The mass effect depends on tumor size and may be generalized or focal. Low-grade tumors tend to be homogeneous; high-grade gliomas may be heterogeneous as a result of central necrosis with cellular debris, fluid, and hemorrhage.
Metastasis (Fig SK 17-2)	Generally hypointense on T1-weighted images and of increased signal intensity on proton-density and T2-weighted images.	More likely than primary glioma to be seen in a patient older than 50 years of age with progressive brainstem signs. Usually there is evidence of other intracranial lesions (isolated metastasis to the brainstem is unusual).

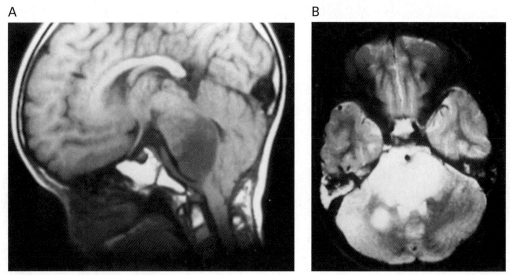

Fig SK 17-1
Brainstem glioma. (A) Sagittal scan shows a huge low-intensity mass involving most of the pons and medulla and compressing the fourth ventricle. (B) On an axial scan, the mass is hyperintense, encases the basilar artery, and extends to affect the cerebellar peduncles and right cerebellar hemisphere.

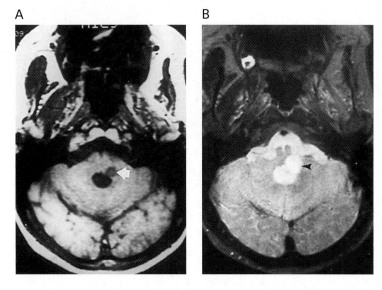

Fig SK 17-2
Metastasis. Pontine mass (arrow and arrowhead) that appears hypointense on a T1-weighted image (A) and hyperintense on a T2-weighted scan (B).

Condition	Imaging Findings	Comments
Other tumors	Various patterns.	Hamartoma; teratoma; epidermoid; lymphoma.
Infarction	Hypointense on T1-weighted images. Hyperintense on proton-density and T2-weighted images.	Associated mass effect and vague contrast enhancement may resemble features of a neoplasm.
Multiple sclerosis	Hypointense on T1-weighted images. Hyperintense on proton-density and T2-weighted images.	Usually associated with similar areas of demyelination elsewhere in the brain.
Central pontine myelinolysis (Fig SK 17-3)	Central region of hypointensity on T1-weighted images and hyperintensity on T2-weighted images in the pons and medulla.	Although initially reported in chronic alcoholics, this condition also presents in patients with electrolyte disturbances (especially hyponatremia) that have been corrected rapidly. In extreme cases, there may be extension to the tegmentum, midbrain, thalamus, internal capsule, and cerebral cortex.
Syringobulbia	Central mass of CSF density (hypointense on T1-weighted images; hyperintense on T2-weighted images) lying in and usually enlarging the medulla. Sharply defined margins, and no contrast enhancement (unlike cystic neoplasm).	Cystic process in the medulla that is more frequently found in conjunction with syringomyelia and less often with a tumor or degenerative process.
Granuloma/abscess	Appearance mimicking that of a neoplasm.	Rare manifestation of tuberculosis, sarcoidosis, or infection. Diagnosis may require biopsy.

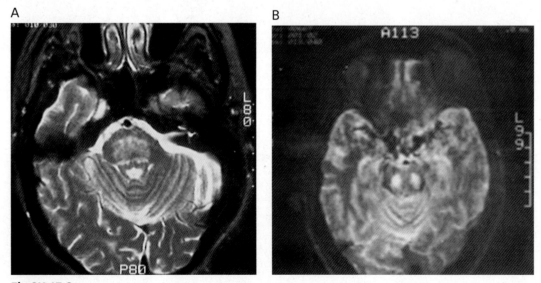

Fig SK 17-3
Central pontine myelinolysis. (A) T1-weighted axial image shows a hyperintense lesion in the central portion of the midpons. (B) More rostral scan shows symmetric lesions in the cerebral peduncles.

Masses Involving the Jugular Foramen on Magnetic Resonance Imaging

Condition	Imaging Findings	Comments
Glomus jugulare tumor (Fig SK 18-1)	Large, irregular mass that obscures the contents of the jugular foramen. It is nearly isointense with the brainstem on T1-weighted images and usually has high signal intensity on T2-weighted images. Intense contrast enhancement.	A characteristic finding is the appearance of prominent blood vessels within the mass. These vessels show negligible signal on T1-weighted images and high-signal intensity on gradient echo images. CT better shows the ill-defined osseous erosion at the margins of a glomus tumor.
Neurofibroma/schwannoma (Fig SK 18-2)	Smooth or irregular mass that is nearly isointense with the brainstem on T1-weighted images and generally shows high signal intensity on T2-weighted images. Intense contrast enhancement.	Typically no prominent vessels can be identified within the tumor. CT better shows adjacent bony erosion.

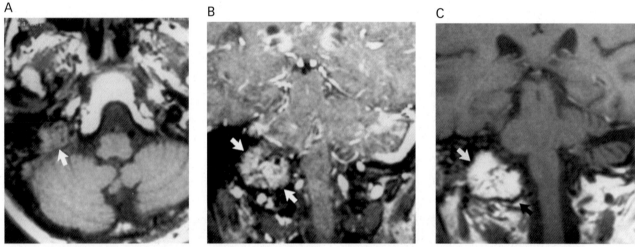

Fig SK 18-1
Glomus jugulare tumor. T1-weighted (A) axial, (B) coronal, and (C) contrast-enhanced coronal images show the tumor (arrows). The tumor contains small blood vessels, which demonstrate negligible signal intensity in A and C and high signal intensity in B. The tumor occludes the ipsilateral jugular bulb.[27]

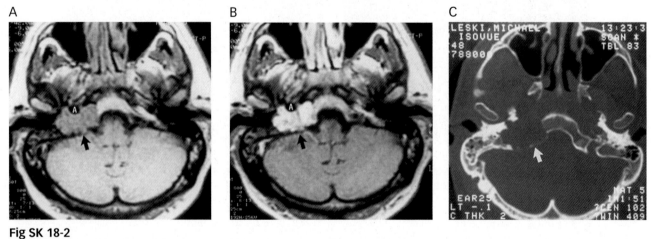

Fig SK 18-2
Schwannoma of 10th cranial nerve. (A) Initial and (B) post-contrast T1-weighted axial images show intense enhancement of the tumor (arrows). Note the anterior displacement of the internal carotid artery (A). (C) Axial CT scan with bone-window technique shows irregular erosion of the right jugular foramen area by the tumor (arrow).[27]

Condition	Imaging Findings	Comments
Meningioma (Fig SK 18-3)	Mass with a signal intensity that is usually the same as the brainstem on T1-weighted images and variable on T2-weighted images. Intense contrast enhancement.	Extension of tumor along the posteromedial edge of the petrous bone into a jugular foramen can be demonstrated by MRI even when no bony erosion can be detected by CT. Calcification may produce areas of low signal intensity within the tumor. No prominent vessels are typically seen within the lesion.
Other tumors (Fig SK 18-4)	Various patterns. Some tumors may contain areas of hemorrhage that produce high signal intensity on both T1- and T2-weighted images. Prominent blood vessels may sometimes be demonstrated.	Rare aggressive tumors (carcinoma, metastases, non-Hodgkin's lymphoma, childhood rhabdomyosarcoma, minor salivary gland malignancy, chondrosarcoma) may be difficult to differentiate from the more common lesions.

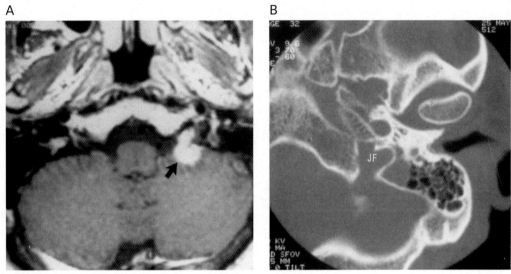

Fig SK 18-3
Meningioma. (A) Axial T1-weighted scan after administration of contrast material shows the enhancing tumor (arrow) extending into the jugular foramen. (B) Axial CT scan with bone-window technique demonstrates that the tumor has not eroded the margins of the jugular foramen (JF).[27]

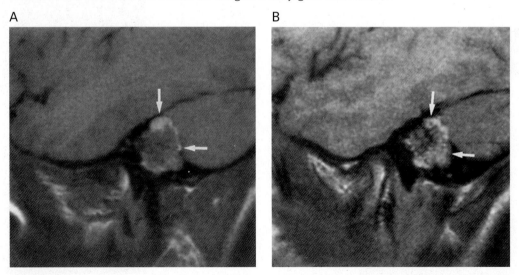

Fig SK 18-4
Adenocarcinoma. (A) T1-weighted and (B) T2-weighted parasagittal images of the tumor (arrows) in the jugular foramen. Note regions of high signal intensity from chronic hemorrhage, and small blood vessels with negligible signal.[27]

Periventricular White Matter Abnormalities on Magnetic Resonance Imaging

Condition	Imaging Findings	Comments
Virchow-Robin spaces (Fig SK 19-1)	CSF spaces that appear as punctate (1 to 2 mm) areas of high signal intensity on T2-weighted images but isointense or of low intensity on proton-density images.	Small subarachnoid spaces that follow the pia mater that is carried along with nutrient vessels as they penetrate the brain substance. Commonly seen in superficial white matter on higher axial sections through the cerebral hemispheres, where nutrient arteries for the deep white matter enter the brain. Other common locations include the lower basal ganglia and the lateral aspects of the anterior commissure, where the lenticulostriate arteries enter the anterior perforated substance.
Deep white matter ischemia (Fig SK 19-2)	Multiple high-intensity foci on both T2-weighted and proton-density images. Individual lesions have well-defined but irregular margins, tend to become confluent, and are usually relatively symmetric. No contrast enhancement is seen unless there is superimposed subacute infarction.	Most frequently detected in patients with ischemic cerebrovascular disease, hypertension, and aging, although in general there is poor correlation between the MR findings and neurologic function. The most common locations are the periventricular white matter, optic radiations, basal ganglia, centrum semiovale, and brainstem, in decreasing order of frequency.
Multiple sclerosis (Fig SK 19-3)	Periventricular high-intensity foci best shown on proton-density scans (high-signal plaques may be obscured by CSF on T2-weighted images). Typically found in a periventricular distribution, particularly along the lateral aspects of the atria and occipital horns. Usually there are discrete foci with well-defined margins. Contrast enhancement can be detected for up to 8 weeks after acute demyelination.	Chronic inflammatory disease of myelin that produces a relapsing and remitting course and is characterized by disseminated lesions in central nervous system white matter. In addition to involving periventricular sites, multiple sclerosis commonly involves the corona radiata, internal capsule, centrum semiovale, brainstem, and spinal cord. In contrast to deep white matter ischemia, multiple sclerosis is a disease of young adults and frequently involves the subcortical U fibers and the corpus callosum, where plaques often have a characteristic horizontal orientation.

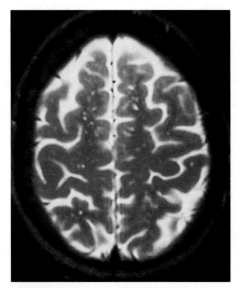

Fig SK 19-1
Prominent Virchow-Robin spaces.

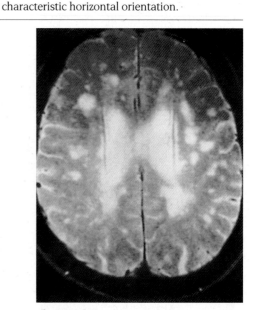

Fig SK 19-2
Deep white matter ischemia. Multiple areas of increased signal intensity around the ventricles and in the deep white matter.

Condition	Imaging Findings	Comments
Radiation injury (Fig SK 19-4)	Symmetric high-signal foci in the periventricular white matter on both T2-weighted and proton-density images. As the process extends outward to involve the peripheral arcuate fibers of the white matter, the margins become scalloped.	Effects of radiation injury to the brain are first detected on imaging studies approximately 6–8 months after the initial therapy. Imaging findings may continue to progress for 2 years or more after radiation therapy. With high-dose therapy, radiation necrosis may lead to profound edema, focal mass effect, and contrast enhancement. In such cases, it may be extremely difficult if not impossible to distinguish radiation change from recurrent tumor.
Hydrocephalus with transependymal CSF flow	Smooth high-signal halo of relatively even thickness along the lateral ventricles, which are dilated out of proportion to the cortical sulci.	Must be distinguished from the normal appearance on axial T2-weighted images of a cap of high signal around the frontal horns of the lateral ventricles ("ependymitis granularis"), which represents a normal accumulation of fluid in this subependymal area containing a loose network of axons with low myelin content.
Leukodystrophy (Fig SK 19-5)	Symmetric, diffuse, and confluent pattern of involvement.	Genetic disorders of children (adrenoleukodystrophy, metachromatic leukodystrophy, globoid cell leukodystrophy, Canavan's disease, Krabbe's disease, Alexander's disease, Pelizaeus-Merzbacher disease) that result in abnormal accumulation of specific metabolites in brain tissue and lead to progressive visual failure, mental deterioration, and spastic paralysis early in life.

B

A

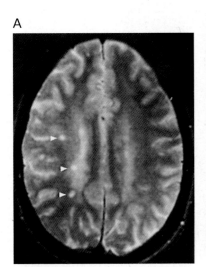
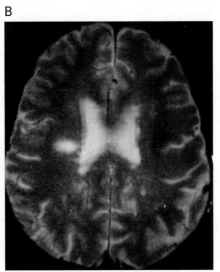
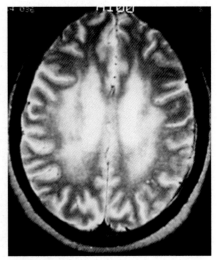

Fig SK 19-3
Multiple sclerosis. (A) Characteristic areas of increased signal intensity (arrow-heads) in the deep white matter of this 35-year-old woman. (B) In another patient, note the characteristic horizontal orientation of the right periventricular plaque.

Fig SK 19-4
Radiation injury. Symmetric foci of high signal intensity in the periventricular white matter on this T2-weighted image.

Condition	Imaging Findings	Comments
Subacute white matter encephalitis (Fig SK 19-6)	Bilateral, diffuse, patchy to confluent areas of increased signal intensity with poorly defined margins.	Inflammatory process involving the white matter of the cerebrum, cerebellum, and brainstem. It is occurring with increasing frequency in patients with acquired immunodeficiency syndrome (AIDS) secondary to human immunodeficiency virus (HIV) or cytomegalovirus infection.
Progressive multifocal leukoencephalopathy (PML) (see Fig SK 26-7)	Patchy, round or oval foci of increased signal intensity that eventually become large and confluent. The process is often distinctly asymmetric and initially involves the peripheral white matter, following the contours of the gray matter–white matter interface to give outer scalloped margins. Although PML is not primarily a periventricular process, the deeper white matter is also affected as the disease progresses.	Demyelinating disease resulting from reactivation of latent papovavirus in an immunocompromised individual. In the past, most cases occurred in patients with Hodgkin's disease or chronic lymphocytic leukemia or in those treated with steroids or immunosuppressive drugs. PML is occurring with increasing frequency in persons with AIDS.
Vasculitis	Multifocal, periventricular high-intensity foci.	Seen in systemic lupus erythematosus and Behçet's disease. These conditions occur in young adults and can produce a neurologic picture similar to that of multiple sclerosis. Factors suggesting vasculitis include associated systemic features and the presence of cortical infarcts in addition to the periventricular lesions.

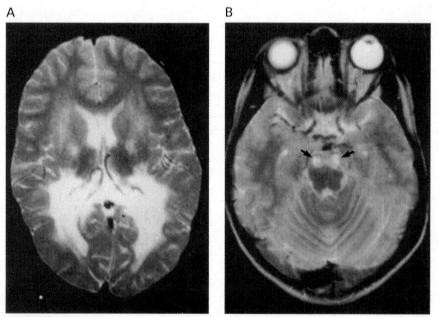

Fig SK 19-5
Adrenoleukodystrophy. (A) Axial T2-weighted image shows abnormal high signal intensity in the occipital lobes, splenium of the corpus callosum, and genu of the internal capsules. (B) In this child, the only abnormality is increased signal intensity in the corticospinal tracts (arrows) as they course in the midbrain.[6]

Condition	Imaging Findings	Comments
Migraine (Fig SK 19-7)	Periventricular hyperintense foci.	Lesions resembling those of multiple sclerosis and deep white matter ischemia have been reported in approximately half the patients with migraine. The classic pattern of headaches should suggest the correct diagnosis.
Mucopolysaccharidoses	Multifocal, periventricular high-intensity foci. Dural thickening and hydrocephalus may be noted.	Group of inherited metabolic diseases in which an enzyme deficiency leads to the deposition of mucopolysaccharides in various body tissues. Punctate white matter lesions reflect perivascular involvement with the disease, in which there is a large accumulation of vacuolated cells distended with mucopolysaccharide. As the disease progresses, the lesions become more widespread and larger, reflecting the development of infarcts and demyelination.

A   B

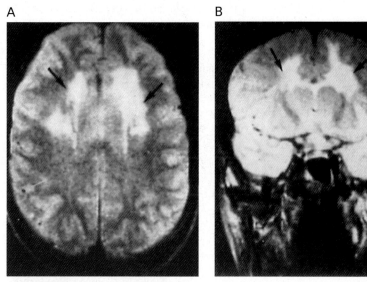

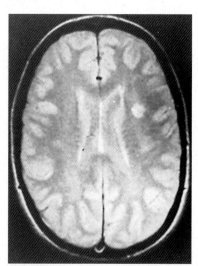

Fig SK 19-6
HIV encephalitis. (A) Axial and (B) coronal T2-weighted images show extensive white matter lesions (arrows) around the ventricles and in the centrum semiovale without evidence of mass effect.[28]

Fig SK 19-7
Migraine. Focal area of hyperintensity in the left frontal white matter in a woman with classic migraine headaches.[29]

Degenerative and Metabolic Disorders of the Brain on Magnetic Resonance Imaging

Condition	Imaging Findings	Comments
Degenerative disorders Parkinsonism (Fig SK 20-1)	Generalized atrophy with prominent sulci and arachnoid spaces. Described findings include (1) areas of hypointensity (correlating with sites of iron deposition) in the putamen, (2) return to normal signal intensity rather than the usual low signal of the dorsolateral aspect of the substantia nigra; and (3) narrowing of the pars compacta, a band of relatively increased signal between the hypointense red nucleus and the pars reticularis of the substantia nigra.	Extrapyramidal disorder that characteristically presents with slowness of movement, poverty of facial expression, flexed posture, immobility, and resting tremor. Pathologically, there is a loss of pigmented cells in the pars compacta of the substantia nigra.
Parkinsonism-plus syndromes	Various patterns in addition to generalized atrophy and enlarged cortical sulci and arachnoid spaces.	A term that refers to the approximately 25% of patients with Parkinsonian features who have more severe symptoms and respond poorly to dopamine replacement therapy.
Striatonigral degeneration (Fig SK 20-2)	Striking hypointensity of the putamen, particularly along its posterolateral margin, on T2-weighted images.	Degree of hypointense putaminal signal (representing pigment accumulation) has a significant correlation with the severity of rigidity.
Shy-Drager syndrome	Various patterns, depending on associated degenerative processes.	Pontocerebellar atrophy and neuronal degeneration in the sympathetic and vegetative nuclei causing orthostatic hypotension, urinary incontinence, and an inability to sweat.

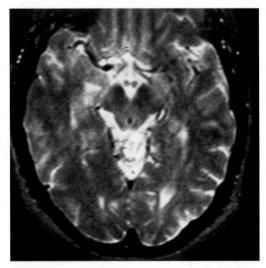

Fig SK 20-1
Parkinson's disease. Complete loss bilaterally of the normal hyperintense band between the red nuclei and the pars reticularis of the substantia nigra.[30]

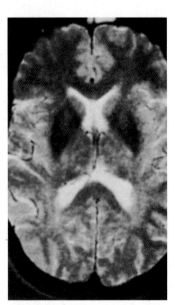

Fig SK 20-2
Striatonigral degeneration. Axial T2-weighted image shows striking hypointensity in the putamen.[24]

Condition	Imaging Findings	Comments
Olivopontocerebellar atrophy (Fig SK 20-3)	Atrophy and abnormal signal in the pons, middle cerebellar peduncles, cerebellum (hemispheric greater than vermian), and inferior olives.	Atrophic changes with prominent demyelination. Degenerative neuronal abnormalities in the substantia nigra, putamen, globus pallidus, dentate nuclei, and subthalamic nucleus of Luys.
Progressive supranuclear palsy (Fig SK 20-4)	Focal atrophy or signal changes (or both) of midbrain structures.	In addition to the neuronal degeneration and gliosis in the areas noted above, there are symptoms of supranuclear ocular palsies, nuchal dystonia, generalized hypotonia, and disturbances of wakefulness.
Alzheimer's disease (Fig SK 20-5)	In addition to generalized cortical and central atrophy, there is typical focal enlargement of the temporal horns (correlating with hippocampal atrophy) best seen on coronal scans.	Characterized by disorders of memory followed by language disturbances and visuospatial disorientation. Although there are few specific findings, the absence of white matter abnormality, hydrocephalus, mass lesion, or metabolic disorder in a demented patient strongly indicates Alzheimer's (or Parkinson's) disease.

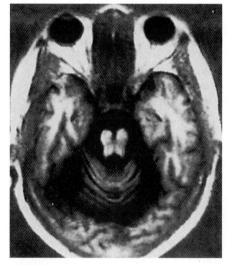

Fig SK 20-3
Olivopontocerebellar atrophy.[31]

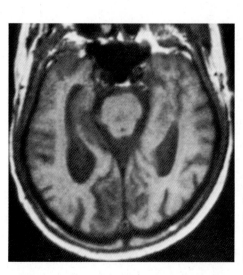

Fig SK 20-5
Alzheimer's disease. Axial T1-weighted scan shows bilateral temporal horn dilatation, more marked on the right, and a prominent area of decreased signal intensity in the right hippocampal region.[24]

Fig SK 20-4
Progressive supranuclear palsy. Axial T2-weighted scan shows atrophy of the midbrain with prominence of the perimesencephalic cisterns.[32]

Condition	Imaging Findings	Comments
Pick's disease (Fig SK 20-6)	Striking focal atrophy of both gray and white matter, typically involving the inferior frontal and temporal lobes, with severe reduction of affected gyri to a paper-thin edge ("knife-blade atrophy").	Much less common disorder in which the symptoms are largely indistinguishable from those of Alzheimer's disease, although abnormal behavior and difficulty with language occur more frequently than memory disturbances.
Huntington's chorea (Fig SK 20-7)	Atrophy of the head of the caudate nucleus and putamen bilaterally and moderate fronto-temporal atrophy.	Inherited disorder (autosomal dominant) characterized by dementia and choreoathetosis that progresses relentlessly.
Creutzfeldt-Jakob disease (spongiform encephalopathy) (Fig SK 20-8)	Rapid progression of central and peripheral atrophy. On T2-weighted images, there is increased signal intensity of gray matter affecting the corpus striatum, thalamus, and cerebral cortex.	Caused by a virus-like infectious agent with a long incubation period of up to several years. Unremitting and fatal course characterized by severe dementia, ataxia, visual disturbances, and myoclonus. Relatively few white matter abnormalities, unlike dementia related to vascular disorders.
Wernicke's encephalopathy	Atrophic changes in the superior vermis and mamillary bodies with generalized sulcal enlargement. On T2-weighted images, there may be increased signal in multiple subcortical areas.	Disorder due to alcoholism or nutritional deficiency (or both) that is associated with confusion, apathy, truncal ataxia, and ophthalmoparesis.
Metabolic disorders Central pontine myelinolysis (see Fig SK 16-3)	Central region in the pons and medulla that is hypointense on T1-weighted images and hyperintense on T2-weighted images.	Although initially reported in chronic alcoholics, this condition also presents in patients with electrolyte disturbances (especially hyponatremia) that have been corrected rapidly. In extreme cases, there may be extension to the tegmentum, midbrain, thalamus, internal capsule, and cerebral cortex.

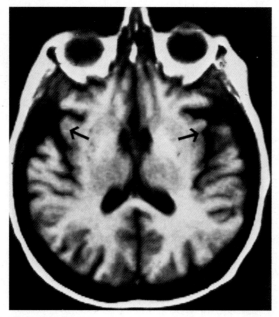

Fig SK 20-6
Pick's disease.[12]

Condition	Imaging Findings	Comments
Leigh's disease (Fig SK 20-9)	On T2-weighted images, there are symmetric areas of increased signal intensity in the basal ganglia, thalamus, brainstem, and cerebellum (seen as low attenuation on CT).	Fatal familial disorder (autosomal recessive) that may be due to an abnormality in pyruvate metabolism and produces bilaterally symmetric foci of necrosis and degeneration leading to multiple neurologic defects.

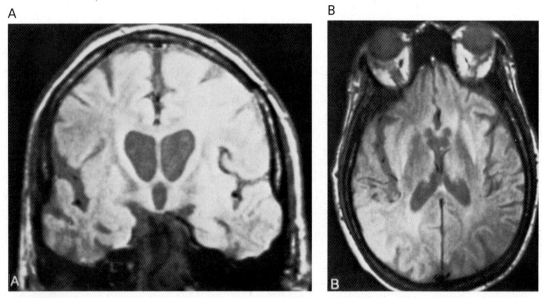

Fig SK 20-7
Huntington's chorea. (A) Coronal proton-density scan demonstrates atrophy of the caudate nuclei, associated with dilatation of the frontal horns of the lateral ventricles. (B) On an axial scan, the putamen is also small and atrophic bilaterally.[32]

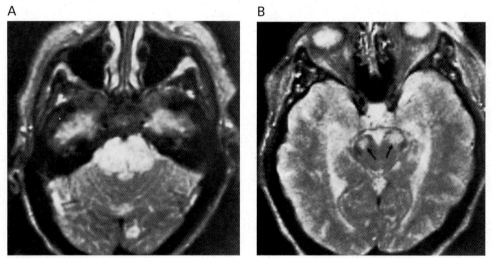

Fig SK 20-8
Central pontine myelinolysis. Axial T2-weighted images show (A) extensive increased signal intensity at the level of the midpons (with sparing of a thin band of tissue in the pontine tegmentum) and (B) symmetric hyperintense lesions in the cerebral peduncles (arrows).[27]

Condition	Imaging Findings	Comments
Wilson's disease (Fig SK 20-10)	On T2-weighted images, areas of increased signal intensity most commonly in the putamen and caudate, but also in the thalamus, dentate nuclei, midbrain, and subcortical white matter. Generalized cortical and central atrophy usually occurs.	Also termed hepatolenticular degeneration, this autosomal recessive disorder of copper metabolism produces the classic syndrome of dysphagia, slowness and rigidity of movements, dysarthria, and tremor that usually occurs during the second or third decade of life. Pathologically, there is softening and atrophy or frank cavitation in the lentiform nuclei.
Hallervorden-Spatz disease (Fig SK 20-11)	Decreased signal in the lentiform nuclei and perilentiform white matter (due to excess iron deposition) on T2-weighted images. There may be areas of increased signal in the periventricular white matter (disordered myelination) and disproportionate atrophy of the brainstem and cerebellum.	Progressive inherited (autosomal recessive) disorder of movement that arises in late childhood or early adolescence and is characterized by abnormal iron deposition in the globus pallidus, reticular zone of the substantia nigra, and red nucleus.
Adrenoleukodystrophy (Fig SK 20-12)	Large, usually symmetric and confluent areas of increased signal intensity on T2-weighted images that tend to involve the white matter of the occipital, posterior parietal, and temporal lobes.	Metabolic encephalopathy typically affecting boys between ages 4 and 8 years in which there is myelin degeneration involving various parts of the cerebrum, brainstem, and optic nerves, as well as the spinal cord. The neurologic findings of behavioral problems, intellectual impairment, and long tract signs can appear before or after adrenal gland insufficiency.
Mucopolysaccharidoses (see Fig SK 18-9)	In severe disease, multiple scattered small areas of increased signal on T2-weighted images in the periventricular white matter. Central atrophy with dilated ventricles usually occurs.	

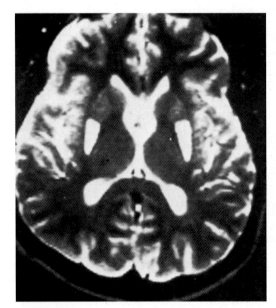

Fig SK 20-9
Leigh's disease. Axial T2-weighted scan shows characteristic prominent hyperintense signal in the putamen.[24]

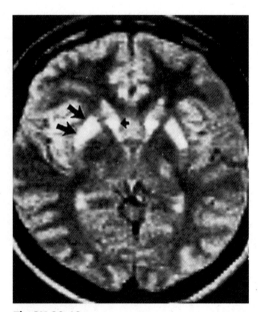

Fig SK 20-10
Wilson's disease. Axial T2-weighted image shows increased signal intensity in the lenticular nuclei (large arrows) and the posterior aspects of the heads of the caudate nuclei (small arrow).[33]

Condition	Imaging Findings	Comments
Nonketotic hyperglycemia	Severe atrophy of the cerebrum and cerebellum. Decreased or absent myelination in supratentorial white matter tracts with sparing of the brainstem and cerebellum.	Inherited disorder of amino acid metabolism in which large quantities of glycine accumulate in body fluids, plasma, urine, and cerebrospinal fluid. Affected persons present in infancy with seizures, abnormal muscle tone, and severe developmental delay.
Phenylketonuria	Widening of sulci and ventricles that may progress to frank atrophy of the cerebrum and cerebellum with confluent widespread white matter lesions on T2-weighted images.	Accumulation of phenylalanine in the brain, which leads to severe developmental delay and mental retardation.

A B

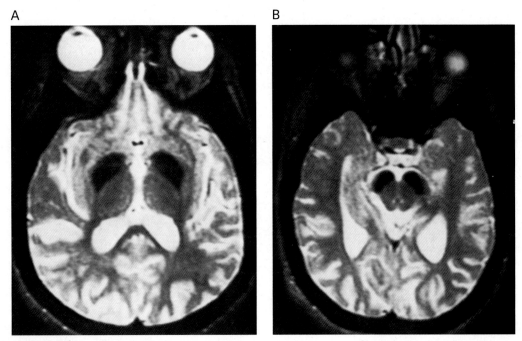

Fig SK 20-11
Hallervorden-Spatz disease. Axial T2-weighted images in a 16-year-old show striking hypointense signal in the globus pallidus (A) and substantia nigra (B) bilaterally.[24]

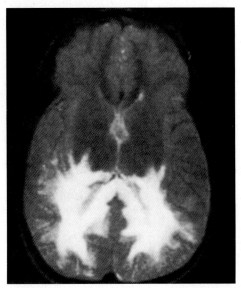

Fig SK 20-12
Adrenoleukodystrophy. Axial T2-weighted scan demonstrates bilaterally symmetric hyperintense signal in the white matter of the occipital and parietal lobes. The posterior temporal lobe is also involved and the abnormality extends into the splenium of the corpus callosum.[32]

Enhancing Ventricular Margins on Computed Tomography

Condition	Comments
Meningeal carcinomatosis (Fig SK 21-1)	Most commonly secondary to oat cell carcinoma of the lung, melanoma, or breast carcinoma. Unlike meningitis, leukemia, or lymphoma, meningeal metastases usually occur in patients with a disseminated malignancy and are seldom associated with fever, leukocytosis, or meningismus.
Leukemia	Meningeal infiltration occurs in up to 10% of patients with acute leukemia. Although systemic chemotherapy, which penetrates the blood-brain barrier ineffectively, fails to prevent cerebral leukemia, the combination of intrathecal methotrexate and whole-brain irradiation effectively eradicates leukemic cells in the central nervous system (except for subarachnoid deposits isolated by adhesions).
Lymphoma (Fig SK 21-2)	Most common form of intracranial lymphoma, which typically occurs in patients with diffuse histiocytic or undifferentiated lymphoma and poorly differentiated Hodgkin's disease.
Subependymal spread of primary brain tumor (Fig SK 21-3)	Periventricular "cast" of tumor may reflect the ependymal seeding or subependymal spread of gliomas or other intracranial neoplasms (eg, medulloblastoma, germinoma).
Inflammatory ventriculitis (Figs SK 21-4 and SK 21-5)	May be secondary to bacterial, fungal, viral, or parasitic infections or to noninfectious inflammatory disease (eg, sarcoidosis).

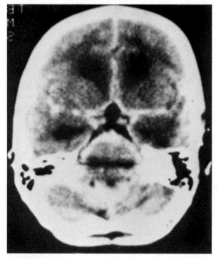

Fig SK 21-1
Meningeal carcinomatosis. Generalized enhancement of the meninges with obstructive hydrocephalus.

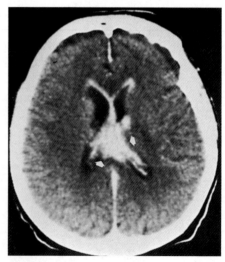

Fig SK 21-2
Histiocytic lymphoma. Homogeneously enhancing lesions (arrows) deep in the brain associated with enhancement of ventricular margins.

A

B

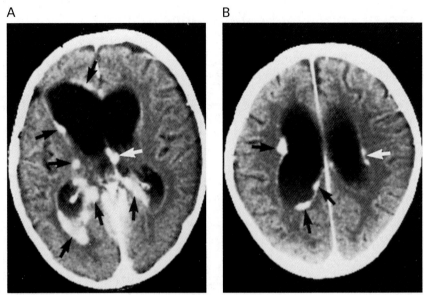

Fig SK 21-3
Subependymal metastases. Multiple enhancing ependymal nodules (arrows) in a patient with posterior fossa ependymoblastoma and hydrocephalus.[1]

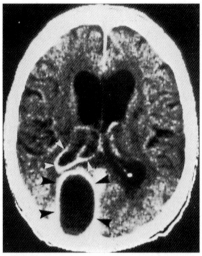

Fig SK 21-4
Brain abscess with ventriculitis. CT scan following the intravenous injection of contrast material in a drug addict with lethargy and confusion demonstrates enhancement of the ventricular system (white arrowheads) due to extensive spread of infection. Note the ring-enhancing abscess (black arrowheads) in the right occipital lobe.

A

B

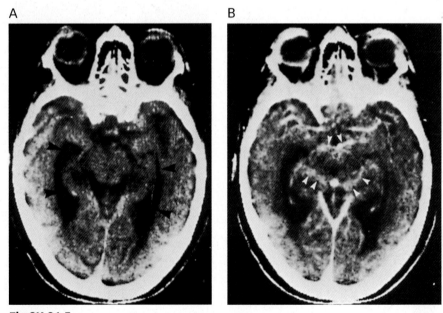

Fig SK 21-5
Pneumococcal meningitis. (A) Noncontrast scan shows dilatation of the temporal horns of the lateral ventricles (arrowheads). (B) After the intravenous injection of contrast material, there is enhancement of the meninges in the basal cisterns (arrowheads), reflecting the underlying inflammation due to meningitis. The hydrocephalus in meningitis is due to blockage of the normal flow of cerebrospinal fluid by inflammatory exudate at the level of the aqueduct and the basal cisterns.

Meningeal Enhancement on Magnetic Resonance Imaging

Condition	Comments
Infectious meningitis (Figs SK 22-1 and SK 22-2)	May be secondary to bacterial, fungal, viral, or parasitic infections. MRI is of special value in detecting meningeal inflammation in patients with AIDS.
Meningeal carcinomatosis (Fig SK 22-3)	Most commonly secondary to oat cell carcinoma of the lung, melanoma, or breast carcinoma. Neoplastic involvement of the leptomeningeal membranes, however, may occur as a complication of any neoplasm arising in the central nervous system or as a metastatic process originating from a distant primary tumor.
Lymphoma (Fig SK 22-4)	The dramatic increase in the incidence of central nervous system lymphoma in recent years has been attributed to AIDS.
Neurosarcoidosis (Fig SK 22-5)	Clinically apparent involvement of the central nervous system occurs in 2% to 5% of patients.
Dural venous sinus thrombosis	Associated with oral contraceptive use, craniotomy, infection, and, in children, dehydration. In a significant percentage of cases, no etiology can be determined.

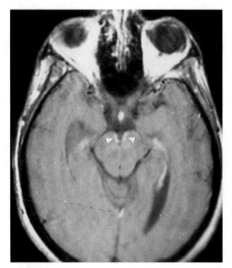

Fig SK 22-1
Cryptococcal meningitis in AIDS. Meningeal enhancement along the cerebral peduncles (arrowheads).

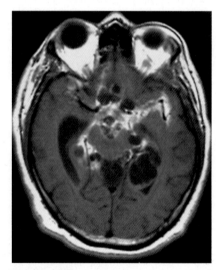

Fig SK 22-2
Cysticercosis. Subarachnoid enhancement in the basal cisterns and left sylvian fissure.[38]

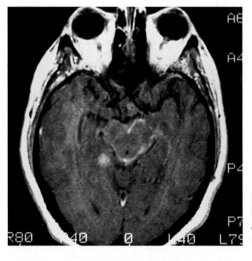

Fig SK 22-3
Meningeal carcinomatosis. Enhancement around the midbrain and cerebral peduncles represents pial spread of tumor.[38]

A

B

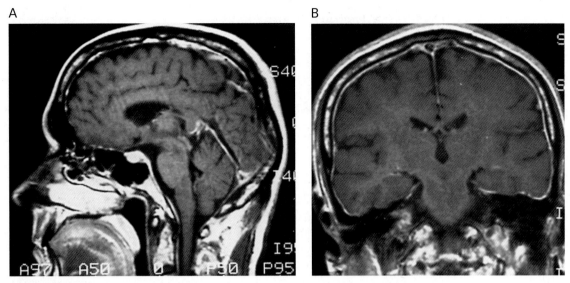

Fig SK 22-4
Lymphoma. (A) Sagittal and (B) coronal scans show enhancement of the falx cerebri as well as about the convexity and at the base of the temporal lobes.[38]

A

B

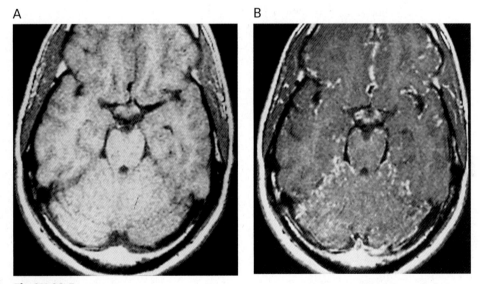

Fig SK 22-5
Neurosarcoidosis. (A) Unenhanced image reveals no parenchymal or meningeal abnormalities. (B) An enhanced scan shows diffuse leptomeningeal involvement.[38]

Intraventricular Masses

Condition	Imaging Findings	Comments
Choroid plexus papilloma (Fig SK 23-1)	Well-defined intraventricular mass, often with lobulated margins, that is hyperdense on CT and only mildly hyperintense on T2-weighted MR images. Intense homogeneous contrast enhancement.	Uncommon tumor that primarily occurs in children younger than 5 years of age. It most frequently occurs in the lateral ventricles in children and in the fourth ventricle in adults. Calcifications are common. Overproduction of CSF or obstruction of CSF pathways causes hydrocephalus. Parenchymal invasion suggests malignant degeneration to choroid plexus carcinoma.
Colloid cyst (Fig SK 23-2)	Smooth, spherical or ovoid mass in the anterior part of the third ventricle that usually has homogeneously high density on CT. Minimal if any contrast enhancement.	Papillomatous lesion containing mucinous fluid with variable amounts of proteinaceous debris, fluid components, and desquamated cells. Classic symptoms are positional headaches related to intermittent obstruction of the foramen of Monro. Most present during adult life, are relatively small (less than 2 cm), and cause dilatation of the lateral ventricles.
Meningioma (Fig SK 23-3)	Smoothly marginated mass that is hyperdense on CT and shows marked homogeneous contrast enhancement. On MRI, variable signal intensity and intense contrast enhancement.	Only 1% of meningiomas are intraventricular. They are found most commonly in the atrium, more often on the left than on the right. As with other meningiomas, they most frequently occur in middle-aged or older women.

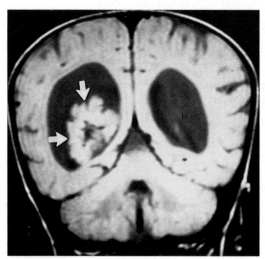

Fig SK 23-1
Choroid plexus papilloma. T1-weighted coronal image shows a lobulated isointense mass (arrows) in a markedly dilated right lateral ventricle.

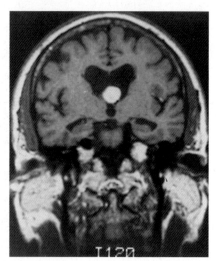

Fig SK 23-2
Colloid cyst. T1-weighted coronal MR scan shows a hyperintense mass in the third ventricle just posterior to the foramen of Monro. There is ventricular dilatation in this elderly man with a history of recurrent headache.[27]

Condition	Imaging Findings	Comments
Ependymoma (Fig SK 23-4)	Well-defined mass that typically arises in the floor of the fourth ventricle. It is hyperdense and shows homogeneous enhancement on CT. On MRI, the tumor has a heterogeneous internal texture as a result of the frequent occurrence of calcification, cysts, and necrotic areas in the lesion.	Rare lesion of the first and second decades that affects boys twice as often as girls. Ependymomas are slow-growing but malignant tumors that may expand and infiltrate into the ventricle or adjacent brain substance. They frequently extend through the foramina of Luschka and Magendie into the basal cisterns and cause ventricular and subarachnoid seeding.
Giant cell astrocytoma (Fig SK 23-5)	Often lobulated or calcified intraventricular mass that may arise from a subependymal nodule. Uniform contrast enhancement.	This malignant transformation of a hamartoma occurs in approximately 10% of patients with tuberous sclerosis. It is usually situated in the region of the foramen of Monro. The presence of other subependymal or parenchymal hamartomas strongly suggests this diagnosis.

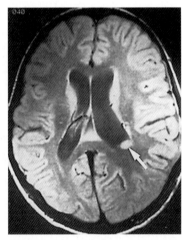

Fig SK 23-3
Intraventricular meningioma. Well-circumscribed mass (arrow) in the posterior aspect of the left lateral ventricle in a patient with neurofibromatosis.

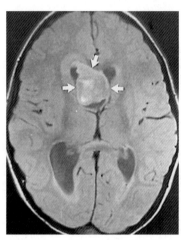

Fig SK 23-4
Ependymoma. Large intraventricular mass (arrows) located in the third ventricle and anterior horns of both lateral ventricles; there is associated hydrocephalus. Areas of greatest hyperintensity in the tumor represent subacute hemorrhage.[34]

A

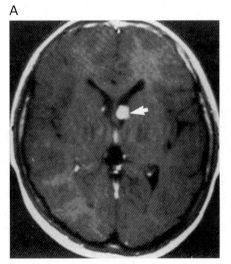

B

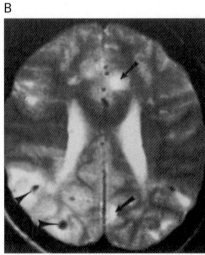

Fig SK 23-5
Giant cell astrocytoma. (A) Contrast-enhanced T1-weighted MR image shows a markedly hyperintense intraventricular mass (arrowhead) in this young boy with clinical stigmata of tuberous sclerosis. (B) T2-weighted image at another level shows characteristic high-signal cortical hamartomas (arrows) as well as dense calcifications (arrowheads).[35]

Condition	Imaging Findings	Comments
Dermoid/epidermoid (Figs SK 23-6 and SK 23-7)	Intraventricular mass.	MR can identify material within the cyst that has a signal intensity of fat or cerebrospinal fluid, respectively.
Primitive neuroectodermal tumor (Fig SK 23-8)	Well-circumscribed mass with intense and homogeneous enhancement.	Cyst formation may occur, especially in infratentorial tumors, and account for the large size of the neoplasm.
Teratoma (Fig SK 23-9)	Various epidermal components (fat and calcification) can be identified easily on CT or MRI.	Typically occurs in children younger than 1 year old. An elevated serum α-fetoprotein level suggests that the lesion is malignant.
Lymphoma	Variable signal intensity, though most lymphomas are isointense or slightly hyperintense on T2-weighted images. On CT, the tumor has mildly increased attenuation and shows intense contrast enhancement.	More commonly presents as mass(es) adjacent to the lateral ventricles (often crossing the corpus callosum to the opposite side) or as diffuse infiltration of the parenchyma.

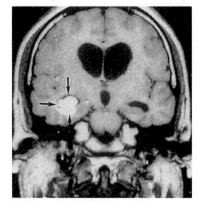

Fig SK 23-6
Dermoid cyst. Coronal T1-weighted MR image shows a hyperintense mass (arrows) filling the dilated right temporal horn. The lateral and third ventricles are enlarged.[36]

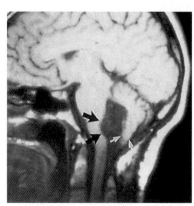

Fig SK 23-7
Epidermoid tumor. Sagittal T-weighted MR image shows a large mass filling the fourth ventricle. The mass has a slightly higher signal intensity than CSF. It depresses the brainstem (black arrows) and elevates the tonsil and inferior vermis (white arrows).[36]

A

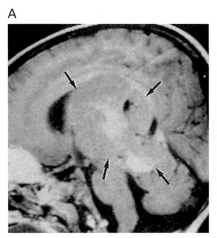

B

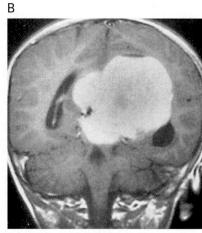

Fig SK 23-8
Primitive neuroectodermal tumor. (A) Sagittal T1-weighted MR image shows a large, inhomogeneously isointense mass (arrows) filling the entire body of the left lateral ventricle and compressing the third ventricle, midbrain, and upper vermis of the cerebellum. (B) Coronal T1-weighted scan demonstrates intense enhancement of the lesion.[36]

Condition	Imaging Findings	Comments
Oligodendroglioma (Fig SK 23-10)	Intraventricular mass that may contain calcification.	Adult neoplasm that usually arises in the fronto-temporal region.
Neurocytoma (neuroblastoma) (Fig SK 23-11)	Intraventricular mass that is mainly isointense relative to cortical gray matter on both T1- and T2-weighted images. Often contains areas of heterogeneous intensity reflecting tumor calcification (best seen on CT), cystic spaces, and vascular flow voids within the tumor.	Benign primary neoplasm of young adults that tends to occur in the lateral and third ventricles and has a characteristic attachment to the septum pellucidum. On light microscopy it appears identical to oligodendroglioma.
Metastasis (Fig SK 23-12)	Intraventricular mass.	Most commonly from melanoma and carcinomas of the lung and breast.

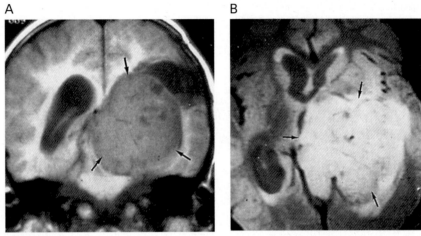

Fig SK 23-9
Malignant teratoma. (A) Coronal T1-weighted MR image shows a large, irregular, lobulated mass (arrows) of inhomogeneous hypointensity in the body and occipital horn of the left lateral ventricle. (B) On the axial proton-density-weighted image, the mass is hyperintense (arrows).[36]

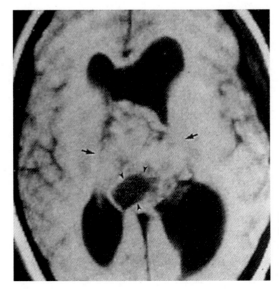

Fig SK 23-10
Oligodendroglioma. Axial T1-weighted MR image shows a large lobulated isointense mass (arrows) with cystic components (arrowheads) involving the septum pellucidum and bodies of the lateral ventricles.[36]

A

B

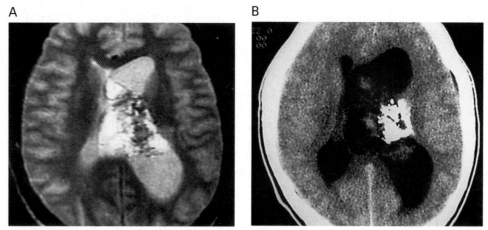

Fig SK 23-11
Neurocytoma. (A) Axial T2-weighted MR image shows the heterogeneous appearance of the lesion, reflecting the presence of cystic spaces and calcifications. (B) CT scan shows coarse, conglomerate calcification and large cystic areas within the intraventricular tumor.[37]

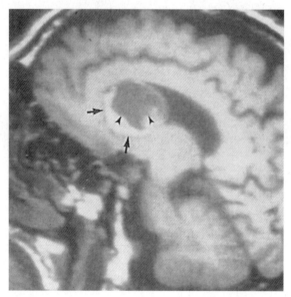

Fig SK 23-12
Hemorrhagic metastatic melanoma. Sagittal T1-weighted MR image shows a round mass filling the left frontal horn near the foramen of Monro. The mass has a hyperintense rim (arrows), most likely representing methemoglobin, and a hypointense center (arrowheads).[36]

Periventricular Calcification in a Child on Computed Tomography

Condition	Comments
Tuberous sclerosis (Fig SK 24-1)	Small, round, calcified nodules along the lateral wall of the frontal horn and anterior third ventricle are a hallmark of this inherited neurocutaneous syndrome, which is manifested by the clinical triad of convulsive seizures, mental deficiency, and adenoma sebaceum.
Intrauterine infection (Fig SK 24-2)	Diffuse calcifications and ventricular enlargement associated with substantial cerebral atrophy and microcephaly typically develop in patients with congenital infections due to cytomegalovirus or toxoplasmosis.

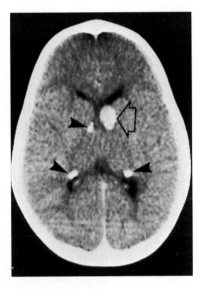

Fig SK 24-1
Tuberous sclerosis. Multiple calcified hamartomas (solid black arrowheads) lying along the ependymal surface of the ventricles. The open arrow points to a giant cell astrocytoma at the foramen of Monro.

A   B

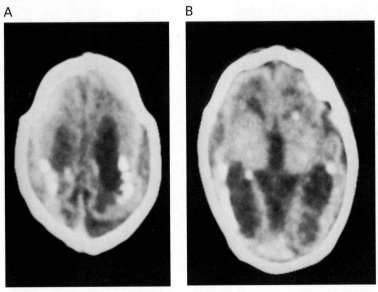

Fig SK 24-2
Cytomegalovirus infection. Two scans of an infant show multiple periventricular calcifications and dilatation of the ventricular system.

Common Congenital Malformations of the Brain on Computed Tomography and Magnetic Resonance Imaging

Condition	Imaging Findings	Comments
Disorders of neural tube closure (encephalocele/ meningocele) (Fig SK 25-1)	Herniation of brain, meninges, or both through a variably sized skull defect that is smooth and well defined and tends to have slightly sclerotic margins.	Most frequently involves the occipital bone (70%). Other sites (approximately 9% each) are the parietal, frontal, and nasal regions.
Disorders of neuronal migration		Congenital malformations of the cerebral wall and cortex that result from deranged migration of neuroblasts and abnormal formation of gyri and sulci. They are believed to arise during weeks 6 to 15 of gestation when successive waves of neuroblasts normally migrate from the subependymal germinal matrix to the surface of the brain to form the standard six-layered cortex.
Lissencephaly (Fig SK 25-2)	Abnormal cerebral surface that may be completely smooth and agyric (rare), almost agyric with a few areas of pachygyria (too broad, flattened gyri), or nearly equally agyric and pachygyric.	The cerebrum has an hourglass or figure-of-8 contour because the brain fails to develop opercula. The insulae are exposed, and the middle cerebral arteries course superficially along shallow sylvian grooves. No sylvian triangle is present. The cortical gray matter is thickened (despite a reduced number of cell layers). The white matter is deficient, and there is a thin subcortical layer, hypoplasia of the centrum semiovale, and reduced to absent digitations of white matter into the cortex.

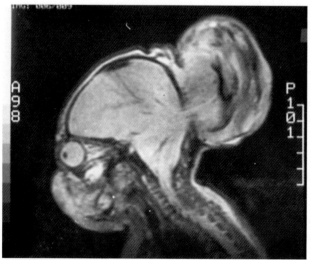

Fig SK 25-1
Occipital encephalocele. Parasagittal MR image shows brain parenchyma that has herniated through a posterior calvarial defect. Although the protrusion contains a large vessel, represented by a linear signal void, it is difficult to identify possible ventricular structures because of distortion.[39]

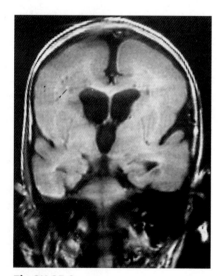

Fig SK 25-2
Agyria.[40]

Condition	Imaging Findings	Comments
Pachygyria (Fig SK 25-3)	Abnormally thickened cortical gray matter with coarse, broadened gyri separated by shallow sulci. All or only a part of the brain may be involved.	Pachygyria with no associated agyria is a distinct migrational disorder in which patients live longer than those with lissencephaly, sometimes surviving into later childhood. Nevertheless, they have developmental delay, severe retardation, and seizures. The interface between gray and white matter is abnormally smooth and has incomplete or absent white matter digitations.
Polymicrogyria	Too many gyri of small size separated by wandering sulci.	Because the sulci may not reach the surface of the brain, areas of polymicrogyria may resemble pachygyria on imaging studies and on gross inspection.
Heterotopia (Fig SK 25-4)	Single or multiple masses of gray matter of various size and shape in the subependymal or subcortical white matter. These masses maintain the same signal intensity as cortical gray matter on all MR pulse sequences.	Heterotopic rests of gray matter result from arrest of neuronal migration along their paths to the cortex. Heterotopia can be an isolated entity, part of more diffuse migrational disorders, or associated with other malformations.
Schizencephaly (Fig SK 25-5)	A pattern varying from unilateral or bilateral slit-like clefts to large, bilateral, fan-shaped defects that extend from the lateral ventricles to the pial surface of the brain.	Full-thickness, transcerebral columns of gray matter that extend in continuity from the subependymal layer of the ventricle to the cortex. Gray matter lines the thin slits (or fan-shaped defects), which are filled with CSF.
Other disorders of organogenesis		
Holoprosencephaly (Fig SK 25-6)	Spectrum of complex patterns that, in the most severe form, includes a single ventricle and an array of facial deformities.	Complex developmental abnormality of the brain arising from failure of cleavage of the forebrain.
Septo-optic dysplasia (Fig SK 25-7)	Absence of the septum pellucidum in 50% to 75% of patients. Other findings include flattening of the roof of the frontal horns, pointing of the floors of the lateral ventricles in coronal section, dilatation of the suprasellar cistern and anterior third ventricle, small optic nerves, and small optic chiasm.	Heterogeneous syndrome of optic nerve hypoplasia associated with pituitary-hypothalamic insufficiency (and other endocrine abnormalities) and often with an abnormal corpus callosum, fornix, and infundibulum.

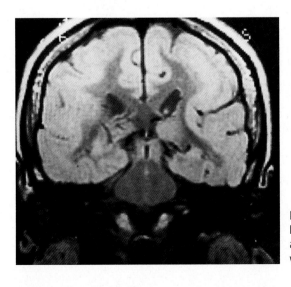

Fig SK 25-3
Pachygyria. Coronal MR scan shows broad gyri, an abnormally thick cortex, and poor arborization of white matter.[40]

Condition	Imaging Findings	Comments
Complete agenesis of the corpus callosum (Fig SK 25-8)	Increased separation of the lateral ventricles, enlargement of the occipital horns and atria, and upward displacement of the third ventricle.	Although occasionally seen as an isolated lesion agenesis of the corpus callosum, frequently is associated with various other central nervous system malformations and syndromes. Partial agenesis of the corpus callosum may occur.

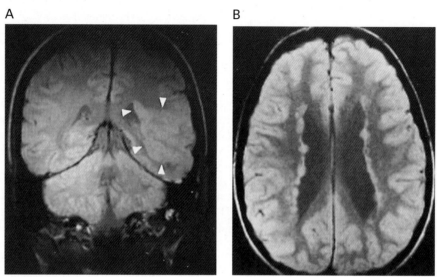

A   B

Fig SK 25-4
Heterotopia. (A) Coronal scan shows hemiatrophy and a gray matter mass bridging from ventricular to cortical surfaces (arrowheads). The intensity of the abnormal bridge of tissue was the same as that of gray matter on all pulse sequences.[39] (B) Gray matter collections lining the subependymal regions of both lateral ventricles.[41]

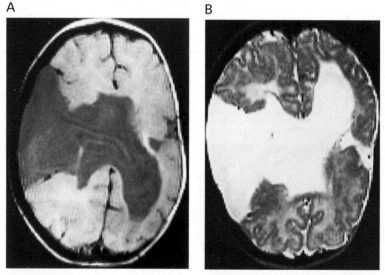

A   B

Fig SK 25-5
Schizencephaly. (A) Proton-density and (B) T2-weighted MR scans show bilateral full-thickness clefts (more marked on the right) that are lined by gray matter. Note the absence of the septum pellucidum.[40]

Condition	Imaging Findings	Comments
Lipoma of the corpus callosum (see Fig SK 25-8)	Focal, midline, nearly symmetric mass of fat in the interhemispheric fissure, usually near the genu of the corpus callosum.	Although asymptomatic in approximately 10% of cases, most lipomas of the corpus callosum are associated with seizures, mental disturbance, paralysis, or headache. About half the patients have callosal agenesis.
Dandy-Walker malformation (Fig SK 25-9)	Cystic mass in the posterior fossa associated with a defect in or agenesis of the vermis and separation of the cerebellar hemispheres.	Spectrum of disorders characterized by abnormal development of the cerebellum and fourth ventricle. Commonly associated with hydrocephalus.

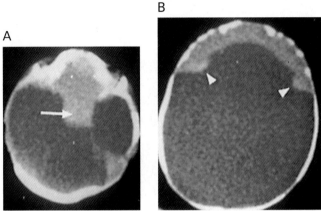

Fig SK 25-6
Holoprosencephaly. Nonsequential transverse CT scans show a monoventricle with anteriorly fused thalami (arrow). There is absence of the interhemispheric fissure, third ventricle, and corpus callosum. A crescent-shaped anterior cerebral mantle represents the undivided prosencephalon, the posterior margin of which cannot be identified on the CT scan. The monoventricle is distorted by a large compression dorsal cyst, the anterior border of which is approximated by the hippocampal fornix (arrowheads).[39]

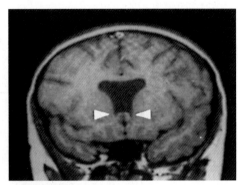

Fig SK 25-7
Septo-optic dysplasia. Coronal T1-weighted image shows absence of the septum pellucidum and squared-off frontal horns that have inferior points (arrowheads).[39]

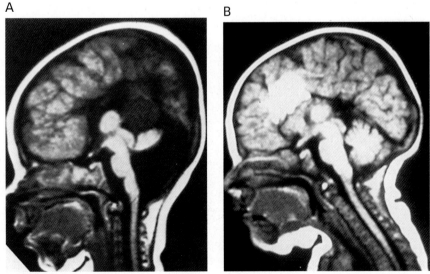

Fig SK 25-8
Agenesis of the corpus callosum. (A) Associated findings include a posterior interhemispheric cyst and a Dandy-Walker cyst of the posterior fossa. (B) In this patient, there is a lipoma involving the anterior aspect of the interhemispheric region.[41]

Condition	Imaging Findings	Comments
Cerebellar aplasia/ hypoplasia (Fig SK 25-10)	Partial absence of the vermis (usually the inferior lobules) and/or small size or partial absence of one or both cerebellar hemispheres.	Associated findings include absence or decreased size of the cerebellar peduncles (especially the brachium pontis), small size of the brainstem (especially the pons), and enlargement of the surrounding CSF spaces (fourth ventricle, vallecula, cisterna magna, and cerebellopontine angle cisterns).
Chiari malformations Chiari I (Fig SK 25-11)	Causal displacement of the cerebellar tonsils through the foramen magnum into the cervical spinal canal.	May be associated with hydromyelia (60% to 70%), hydrocephalus (20% to 25%), and basilar impression (25%). No association with myelomeningocele.

A   B

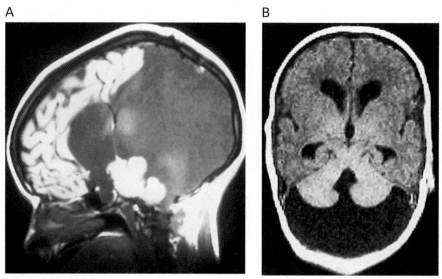

Fig SK 25-9
Dandy-Walker malformation. (A) Sagittal and (B) axial[40] MR scans in two different patients show large posterior fossa cystic masses associated with agenesis of the vermis and separation of the cerebellar hemispheres.

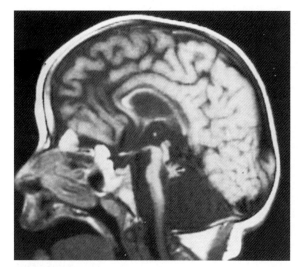

Fig SK 25-10
Cerebellar hypoplasia. Sagittal MR scan shows almost total absence of the cerebellum except for a small portion of the superior vermis.[41]

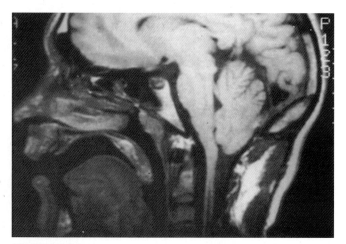

Fig SK 25-11
Chiari I malformation. Caudal displacement of the cerebellar tonsils 15 mm below the foramen magnum. Note the associated hydromyelia.

Condition	Imaging Findings	Comments
Chiari II (Fig SK 25-12)	Common findings include protrusion of the brainstem downward through the foramen magnum into the upper cervical spinal canal, with the upper spinal cord being driven inferiorly and compacted along its long axis; kinking at the cervicomedullary junction; marked elongation of the fourth ventricle, which descends into the spinal canal along the posterior surface of the medulla; beaked tectum; and hydromyelia.	Complex anomaly affecting the calvarium, spinal column, dura, and hindbrain that is nearly always associated with myelomeningocele. Because of the low position of the medulla and upper spinal cord, the upper cervical nerve roots course upward to their exit foramina, and the lower cranial nerves arise from the medulla in the cervical spinal canal and ascend through the foramen magnum before turning downward to exit their normal foramina.
Chiari III (Fig SK 25-13)	Herniation of brain contents through a bony defect involving the inferior occiput, foramen magnum, and posterior elements of the upper cervical vertebrae.	Cervico-occipital encephalocele containing nearly all the cerebellum. Variable amounts of brainstem, upper cervical cord, and meninges may be found in the posterior hernia sac.
Phakomatoses (neurocutaneous syndromes)		Hereditary developmental anomalies characterized by disordered histogenesis with abnormal cell proliferation in the nervous system and skin.
Neurofibromatosis (Fig SK 25-14)	Cranial nerve schwannomas (especially acoustic neuromas) that are often bilateral; meningiomas, frequently bilateral; optochiasmal gliomas (may be bilateral and affect the entire length of the visual apparatus); and cerebral hamartomas.	Autosomal dominant disorder characterized by dysplasia of neural ectodermal and mesodermal tissue. Other cerebral manifestations include orbital dysplasia, in which unilateral absence of a large part of the greater wing of the sphenoid and hypoplasia and elevation of the lesser wing result in a markedly widened superior orbital fissure; brainstem and supratentorial gliomas; arachnoid cysts; and vascular dysplasia with multiple infarctions.

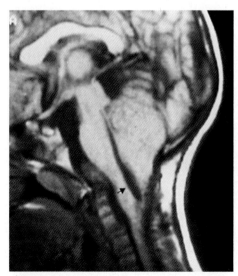

Fig SK 25-12
Chiari II malformation. Markedly elongated and inferiorly displaced fourth ventricle (arrow).[41]

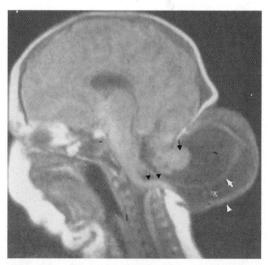

Fig SK 25-13
Chiari III malformation with cervico-occipital encephalocele. Sagittal MR scan shows the bony defect involving the inferior occiput, foramen magnum, and posterior elements of C1 and C2 with herniation of the cerebellum (black arrow), dilated posterior aspect of the fourth ventricle (white arrow), brainstem, upper cervical cord (black arrowheads), and meninges (white arrowhead) into the posterior sac.[41]

Condition	Imaging Findings	Comments
Tuberous sclerosis (Bourneville's disease) (Fig SK 25-15)	Cortical, subcortical, white matter, and subependymal tubers; small, round, calcified nodules along the lateral wall of the frontal horn and anterior third ventricle.	Inherited disorder in which the brain is typically involved with hyperplastic nodules of malformed glial-neuroglial tissue. Classic clinical triad of convulsive seizures, mental deficiency, and adenoma sebaceum. Giant cell astrocytoma develops in approximately 10% of patients; renal angiomyolipomas occur in about half. Large tumors or tubers may obstruct the aqueduct or ventricular foramina and produce hydrocephalus.

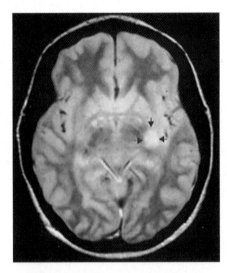

Fig SK 25-14
Neurofibromatosis with hamartoma (arrows).

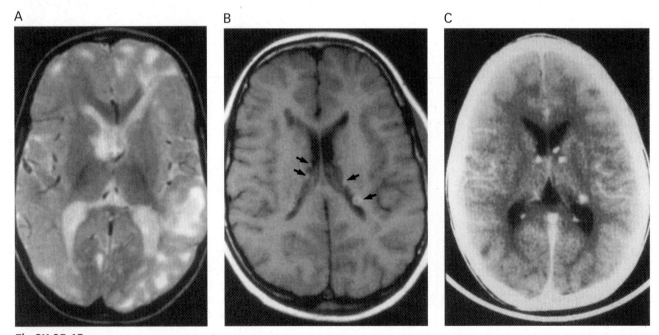

Fig SK 25-15
Tuberous sclerosis. (A) Axial T2-weighted MR image shows multiple subcortical and periventricular bright hamartomas. (B) Noncontrast axial T1-weighted MR image of a different patient shows slightly bright periventricular hamartomas (arrows). (C) CT scan of a different patient shows multiple calcified periventricular hamartomas.[6]

Condition	Imaging Findings	Comments
Sturge-Weber syndrome (encephalotrigeminal angiomatosis) (Fig SK 25-16)	Undulating parallel plaques of calcification in the brain cortex that appear to follow the cerebral convolutions and most often develop in the parieto-occipital area.	Congenital vascular anomaly in which a localized meningeal venous angioma occurs in conjunction with an ipsilateral facial angioma (port-wine nevus). Clinical findings include mental retardation, seizure disorders, and hemiatrophy and hemiparesis. Hemiatrophy leads to elevation of the base of the skull and enlargement and increased aeration of the ipsilateral mastoid air cells.
von Hippel-Lindau disease (Fig SK 25-17)	Single or multiple hemangioblastomas. Most are cystic, often with a mural enhancing nodule.	Autosomal dominant disorder in which vascular malformations of the retina (usually multiple capillary angiomas) are combined with one or more slow-growing hemangioblastomas of the cerebellum or spinal cord. There also may be angiomas in the liver, pancreas, and kidneys; renal tumors; and pheochromocytomas.
Congenital aqueductal stenosis (Fig SK 25-18)	Enlargement of the lateral and third ventricles with a normal-sized fourth ventricle. Causes deformity of the tectum, which may appear thick (but never bulbous) and has normal signal intensity on T2-weighted sequences (unlike a tectal tumor, which would be bright).	Congenital aqueductal stenosis accounts for 20% of instances of hydrocephalus. It generally presents in infancy, but may manifest itself at any time during life. May be associated with Chiari I and II malformations. Endocrine dysfunction, seen in up to 20% of patients, is probably caused by compression of the hypothalamus-pituitary axis from the enlarged third ventricle.

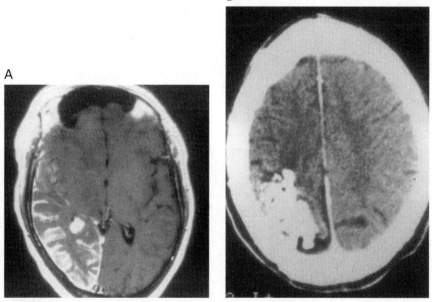

Fig SK 25-16
Sturge-Weber syndrome. (A) Postcontrast T1-weighted MR image shows extensive enhancement of the leptomeningeal angioma in the right occipital lobe and a prominent glomus of the right choroids plexus, which served for collateral venous drainage. (B) Axial CT scan in a different patient shows the classic parenchymal calcification in the right parietal lobe.[6]

Condition	Imaging Findings	Comments
Arachoid cyst (Fig SK 25-19)	Fluid-filled mass between the cerebellum and the occipital or petrous bones. At times, it may appear anterior to the cerebellum or in the cerebellopontine angle.	Congenital lesion of the arachnoid membrane that expands with cerebrospinal fluid. About 25% occur in the posterior fossa in a retrocerebellar location. Less commonly, they develop within the fourth ventricle or cerebellopontine cistern. Other congenital nervous system abnormalities are rarely associated with arachnoid cysts.
Vein of Galen malformation (Fig SK 25-20)	Large cystic-appearing, midline, mass-like structure located superior to the cerebellum that communicates through a persistent falcine sinus into a prominent torcular.	Venous ectasis secondary to a midline embryonic arteriovenous shunt, which drains directly into the vein of Galen or into a tributary. It may manifest with high-output congestive heart failure, hydrocephalus, or seizures in a neonate and as hemorrhage in older children.

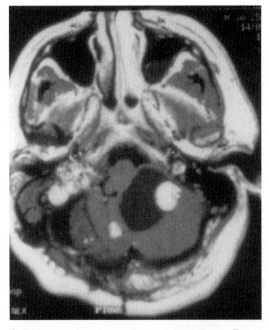

Fig SK 25-17
von Hippel-Lindau disease. Axial postcontrast T1-weighted MR image shows a left-sided cystic hemangioblastoma with an enhancing nodule and multiple small enhancing solid lesions in the right cerebellar hemisphere.[6]

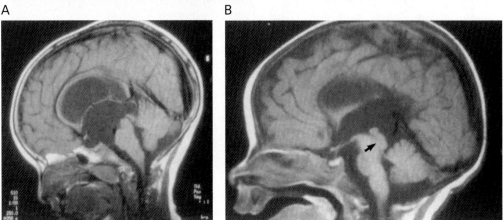

A   B

Fig SK 25-18
Congenital aqueductal stenosis. (A) Midsagittal T1-weighted MR image shows marked dilatation of the lateral and third ventricles with a normal-sized fourth ventricle. (B) Midsagittal T1-weighted image in another patients shows absence of the lumen in the aqueduct (arrow). The tectum is deformed but was of normal signal intensity on a T2-weighted scan (not shown). The lateral and third ventricles are large, for the fourth ventricle is normal in size.[6]

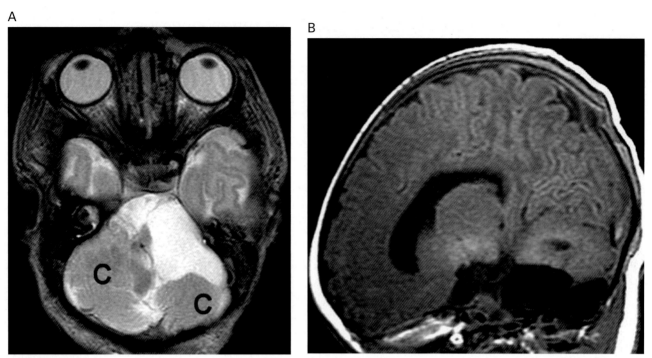

Fig SK 25-19
Arachnoid cyst. Axial T2-weighted MR image demonstrates a collection of cerebrospinal fluid anterior to the cerebellum in the cerebellopontine angle region. Note the small cerebellum (C) on the left. (B) Left parasagittal T1-weighted MR image shows the low-signal-intensity fluid lesion.[42]

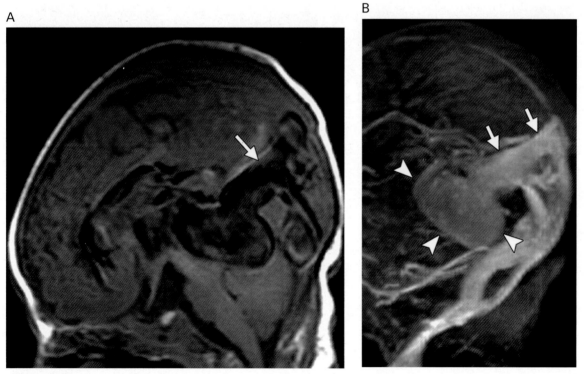

Fig SK 25-20
Vein of Galen malformation. (A) Sagittal T1-weighted MR image shows an apparent cystic mass in a supracerebellar location. The dilated vein of Galen communicates with a persistent falcine sinus (arrow). Note the extensive phase artifact due to the malformation. (B) Lateral MR venogram shows numerous dilated arteries and drainage of the large vein of Galen malformation (arrowheads) into a prominent torcular through a persistent falcine sinus (arrows).[42]

Midline Congenital Anomalies on Ultrasonography

Condition	Imaging Findings	Comments
Vein of Galen malformation (Fig SK 26-1)	Large, fluid-filled structure that lies between the lateral ventricles and can be followed posteriorly into the straight sinus and the torcular Herophili.	Arteriovenous malformation resulting from failure of the normal embryonic arteriovenous shunts to be replaced by capillaries. Doppler studies can confirm the markedly increased flow in the lesion and permit differentiation of this dilated vessel from a cyst.
Chiari II malformation (Fig SK 26-2)	Caudal displacement of the cerebellum and a narrowed and elongated fourth ventricle. Enlarged massa intermedia and often dilatation of the third and lateral ventricles.	Complex anomaly affecting the calvarium, spinal column, dura, and hindbrain that is nearly always associated with myelomeningocele. Hydromyelia commonly occurs.
Dandy-Walker syndrome (Fig SK 26-3)	Posterior fossa cyst (representing the ballooned fourth ventricle) and partial or complete absence of the vermis with separation of the cerebellar hemispheres.	Occasionally, an arachnoid cyst or an elongated cisterna magna may mimic the Dandy-Walker syndrome, but in these former conditions the vermis and cerebellum are normal. Hydrocephalus may be apparent at birth or develop later.

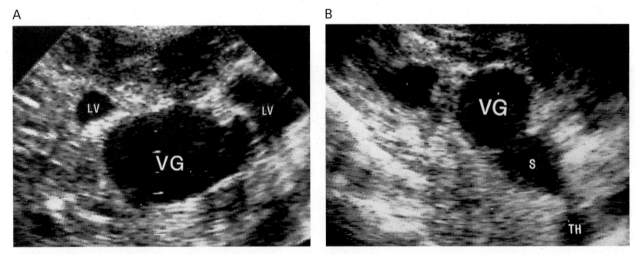

A   B

Fig SK 26-1
Vein of Galen malformation. (A) Coronal sonogram shows the large vein of Galen (VG) lying between the dilated lateral ventricles (LV). Note the parenchymal atrophy, seen as hypoechoic areas above the vein of Galen. (B) On the sagittal image, the dilated vein of Galen can be followed posteriorly into the straight sinus (S) and the torcular Herophili (TH).[43]

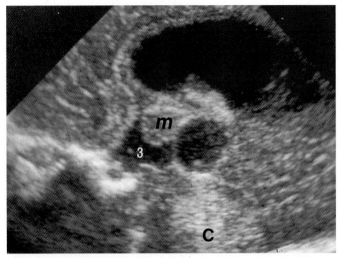

Fig SK 26-2
Chiari II malformation. Sagittal sonogram shows the cerebellum (C) and fourth ventricle situated low in the posterior fossa and obliteration of the cisterna magna. An enlarged massa intermedia (M) partially fills the third ventricle (3).[43]

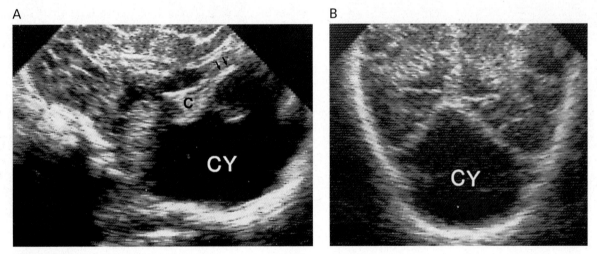

Fig SK 26-3
Dandy-Walker syndrome. (A) Sagittal sonogram demonstrates such characteristic features as a posterior fossa cyst (CY) representing the ballooned fourth ventricle and partial or complete absence of the vermis. The often huge cyst displaces the cerebellum (C) and tentorium (arrows) superiorly. (B) Posterior coronal image shows the large cyst (CY) filling the posterior fossa.[4,3]

Condition	Imaging Findings	Comments
Dandy-Walker variant (Fig SK 26-4)	Large posterior fossa cyst connected to a partially formed fourth ventricle by a narrow vallecula. The inferior vermis is absent, and the cerebellum is often hypoplastic.	When the separation between the cerebellar hemispheres is very narrow (slitlike), a CT, MR, or ultrasound scan through the posterior fossa is required to establish the communication of the cyst with the fourth ventricle.
Agenesis of the corpus callosum (Fig SK 26-5)	Increased separation of the lateral ventricles. Enlargement of the occipital horns and atria. Upward displacement of the third ventricle.	Although occasionally seen as an isolated lesion, agenesis of the corpus callosum is frequently associated with various other central nervous system malformations and syndromes.
Lipoma of the corpus callosum (Fig SK 26-6)	Focal echogenic mass of fat in the inter-hemispheric fissure, usually near the genu.	Approximately half the patients with lipomas have absence of the corpus callosum, with the echogenic mass lying just above an elevated third ventricle.

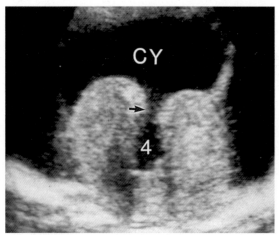

Fig SK 26-4
Dandy-Walker variant. Sonogram through the posterior fontanelle demonstrates a large cyst (CY) and fourth ventricle (4), connected by a narrow vallecula (arrow).[43]

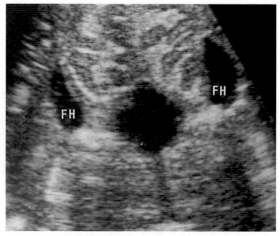

Fig SK 26-5
Agenesis of corpus callosum. Coronal sonogram shows separation of the frontal horns (FH), which have concave medial borders.[43]

Condition	Imaging Findings	Comments
Holoprosencephaly (Fig SK 26-7)	Spectrum of complex patterns that, in the most severe form (alobar), includes a single ventricle and an array of facial deformities.	Complex developmental abnormality of the brain resulting from failure of cleavage of the forebrain into cerebral hemispheres and lateral ventricles.

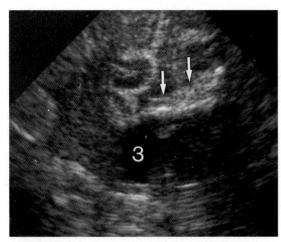

Fig SK 26-6
Intracerebral lipoma with absent corpus callo-sum. Coronal sonogram shows an echogenic area (arrows) superior and to the left of the elevated third ventricle (3).[43]

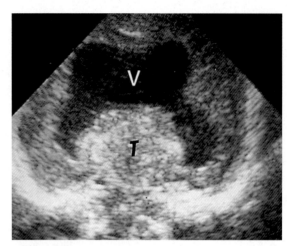

Fig SK 26-7
Alobar holoprosencephaly. Posterior coronal sonogram demonstrates the single ventricle (V) and the fused thalami (T).[43]

Central Nervous System Changes in Acquired Immunodeficiency Syndrome

Condition	Imaging Findings	Comments
Focal lesions		
Toxoplasmosis (Figs SK 27-1 and SK 27-2)	Single or multiple ring-enhancing lesions. Most commonly located at the corticomedullary junction and in the basal ganglia and white matter. Variable amount of peripheral edema.	This protozoan is the most common opportunistic infection in AIDS patients. Early in their development, the lesions may show more homogeneous enhancement with little mass effect or edema.
Cryptococcosis (Figs SK 27-3 and SK 27-4)	Initially, imaging studies may be negative or show only mild ventricular dilatation. Chronic relapsing infection can result in a parenchymal abscess and meningeal enhancement.	Most common fungal infection of the central nervous system in AIDS. Pathologically, a granulomatous meningitis is the most common manifestation.
Other infections (Fig SK 27-5)	Single or multiple enhancing lesions.	Herpes simplex encephalitis, tuberculosis, candidiasis, aspergillosis, and bacterial infections.
Lymphoma (Fig SK 27-6)	Single or multiple masses that often show central necrosis and ring enhancement. Favored sites include the deep white matter of the frontal and parietal lobes, basal ganglia, and hypothalamus.	Lymphoma in AIDS patients has a higher incidence of multiplicity and aggressive behavior. The lesions are frequently found close to the corpus callosum and tend to cross the midline into the opposite hemisphere, a feature that mimics glioblastoma. Unlike gliomastoma and metastases, lymphomas often are associated with only a relatively mild amount of peritumoral edema and mass effect.
Kaposi's sarcoma	Nonspecific enhancing lesion(s).	Rare direct involvement of the brain cannot be distinguished from other masses. Almost all AIDS patients with Kaposi's sarcoma have visible skin lesions.

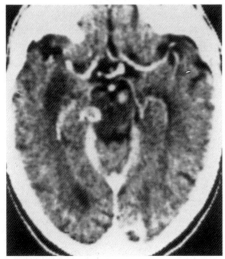

Fig SK 27-1
Toxoplasmosis. Contrast-enhanced CT scan shows multiple small areas of ring and solid enhancement in the region of the cerebral peduncles and pons. A small round area of enhancement is seen in the left occipital lobe.[44]

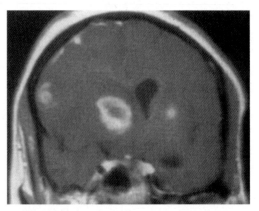

Fig SK 27-2
Toxoplasmosis. Postcontrast T1-weighted MR image shows at least three enhancing lesions.[6]

Condition	Imaging Findings	Comments
Diffuse atrophy or white matter disease		
Progressive multifocal leukoencephalopathy (PML) (Fig SK 27-7)	Round or oval lesions that become larger and more confluent and are often asymmetric. No enhancement or mass effect.	Reactivation of latent papovavirus in an immuno-compromised host that initially tends to involve the subcortical white matter and later spreads to the deeper white matter. The high signal on T2-weighted MR scans is related to both demyelination and edema.

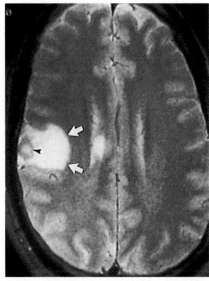

Fig SK 27-3
Cryptococcosis. Axial T2-weighted MR scan shows a relatively isointense peripheral mass (black arrowhead) with prominent surrounding edema (white arrows).

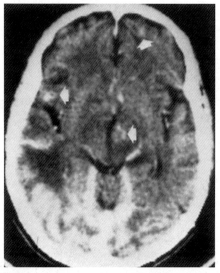

Fig SK 27-4
Cryptococcal meningitis. Contrast-enhanced CT scan demonstrates dense enhancement of the free edge of the tentorium and prominent enhancement of meninges in the right temporal and both occipital regions. Scattered focal intracerebral areas of enhancement (arrows) were thought to be caused by cryptococcal granulomas.[44]

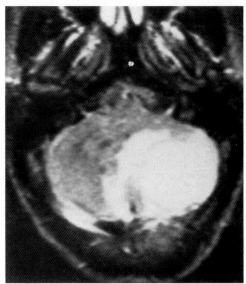

Fig SK 27-5
Streptococcal abscess. T2-weighted MR scan shows a well-defined, slightly lobulated mass in the left cerebellum. The margin of the abscess has a rim of decreased signal intensity, and there is moderate surrounding edema.[44]

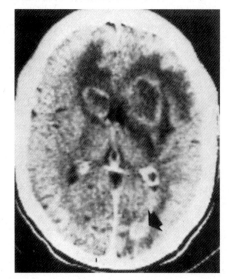

Fig SK 27-6
Lymphoma. Contrast-enhanced CT scan shows large, bilateral areas of enhancement with surrounding edema in the basal ganglia bilaterally. Another lesion is seen in the left occipital pole (arrow).[44]

Condition	Imaging Findings	Comments
HIV infection (Fig SK 27-8)	Ill-defined, diffuse or confluent patches of abnormal signal intensity without mass effect in the deep white matter of the cerebral hemispheres.	HIV encephalopathy is a progressive subcortical dementia attributed to direct infection of the central nervous system with the virus rather than to an opportunistic infection. Developing in up to 60% of AIDS cases, it typically produces bilateral but not always symmetric lesions that characteristically do not involve the gray matter.
Cytomegalovirus (Figs SK 27-9 and SK 27-10)	Abnormal signal intensity in the ependymal and subependymal regions. There is often peripheral contrast enhancement of periventricular lesions and generally evidence of volume loss (rather than mass effect).	The periventricular changes are better demonstrated on T1-weighted and proton-density images because on T2-weighted images the abnormal areas of increased signal intensity may not be clearly differentiated from the normal signal of CSF.

A   B

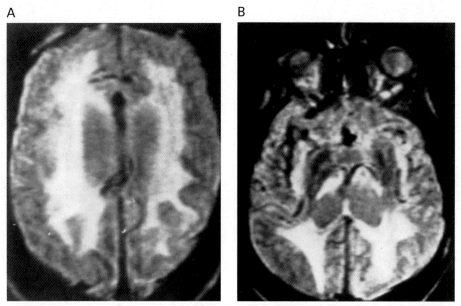

Fig SK 27-7
Progressive multifocal leukoencephalopathy. (A) Initial T2-weighted MR scan shows irregularly marginated areas of increased signal intensity in the region of the centrum semiovale bilaterally. There is no mass effect, but severe atrophy is seen. (B) Repeat study 3 months later shows progression of the white matter abnormalities, especially in the occipital region.[45]

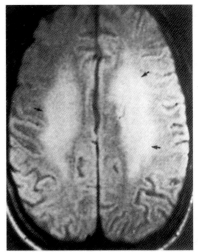

Fig SK 27-8
HIV encephalitis. Axial proton-density MR image shows symmetric regions of abnormally increased signal intensity without mass effect in the centrum semiovale bilaterally (arrows).[45]

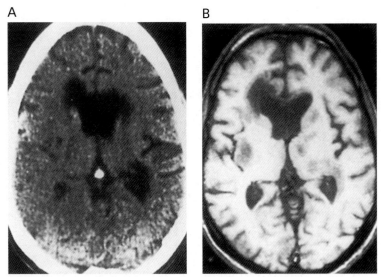

Fig SK 27-9
Cytomegalovirus ventriculitis. (A) Nonenhanced CT scan and (B) T1-weighted MR scan show bilateral periventricular areas of decreased attenuation/signal intensity, which is most marked near the right frontal horn. Note additional bilateral lesions in the basal ganglia.[45]

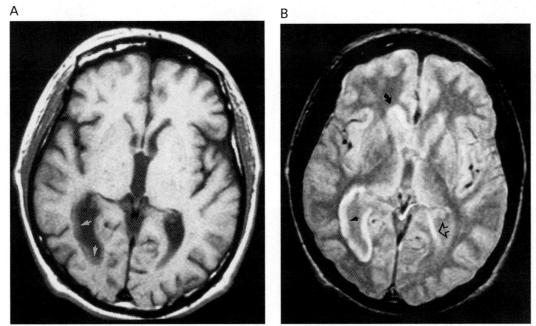

Fig SK 27-10
Cytomegalovirus. (A) Axial T1-weighted MR image demonstrates an irregular low-signal halo (arrows) surrounding the right occipital horn. There is no evidence of mass effect. (B) Axial proton-density image shows corresponding high signal in the right periatrial white matter (straight arrow). There are similar high-signal foci in the periventricular white matter adjacent to the right frontal horn (curved arrow) and the medial left atrium (open arrow).[46]

Thickening of the Optic Nerve

Condition	Comments
Optic nerve glioma (Figs SK 28-1 and SK 28-2)	Most common cause of optic nerve enlargement. Typically causes uniform thickening of the nerve with mild undulation or lobulation. In children (especially pre-adolescent girls), optic nerve gliomas are usually hamartomas that spontaneously stop enlarging and require no treatment. In older patients, however, these gliomas may have a progressive malignant course despite surgical or radiation therapy. Optic nerve gliomas are a common manifestation of neurofibromatosis (typically low-grade lesions that act more like hyperplasia than neoplasms).
Optic nerve sheath meningioma (Fig SK 28-3)	Most commonly occurs in middle-aged women and typically has a greater density, greater enhancement, and less homogeneous appearance than optic nerve gliomas. Other CT features include sphenoid bone hyperostosis and calcification, either eccentric when the tumor is polypoid or on both sides of the optic nerve with a tramline appearance when the tumor circumferentially surrounds the nerve.
Cyst of optic nerve sheath (Fig SK 28-4)	Cystic dilatation of the optic nerve sheath produces a mass that is less dense than a meningioma. May develop after irradiation of an optic nerve glioma.

A   B

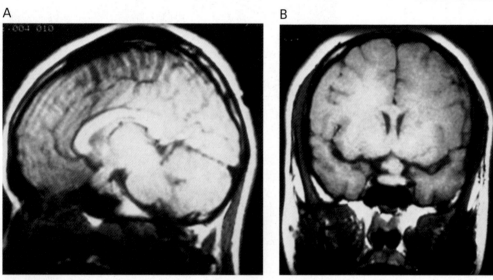

Fig SK 28-1
Optic nerve glioma. (A) Sagittal and (B) coronal T1-weighted MR scans show involvement of the chiasm and left optic nerve.

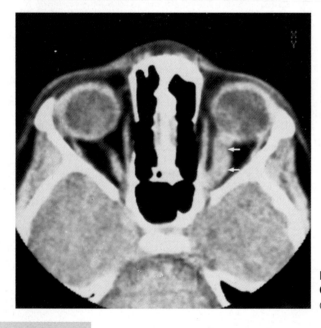

Fig SK 28-2
Optic nerve glioma. Diffuse enlargement of the left optic nerve (arrows) in an 8-year-old girl.[1]

Condition	Comments
Optic neuritis (Fig SK 28-5)	General term referring to thickening of the optic nerve developing from such non-neoplastic processes as multiple sclerosis, infection, ischemia (occlusion of vessels at the anterior portion of the optic nerve associated with temporal arteritis), and degenerative changes resulting from toxic, metabolic, or nutritional factors. After steroid therapy, enlargement of the optic nerve usually resolves.

A
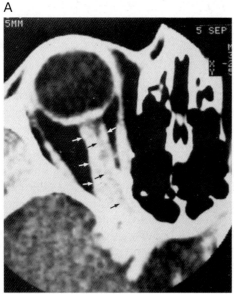
B
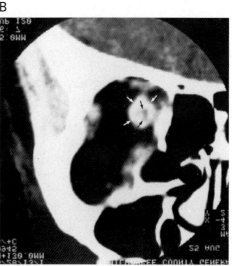

Fig SK 28-3
Optic nerve sheath meningioma. (A) Axial scan shows the enhancing tumor (white arrows) along the entire length of the intraorbital optic nerve (black arrows). Note the intracranial portion of the tumor. (B) Coronal scan demonstrates the meningioma (white arrows) surrounding the optic nerve.[1]

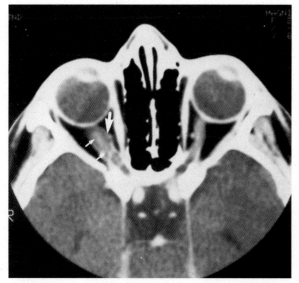

Fig SK 28-4
Cyst of optic nerve sheath. Large, smoothly marginated retrobulbar mass (arrows) that produced proptosis in this 43-year-old man.[1]

A
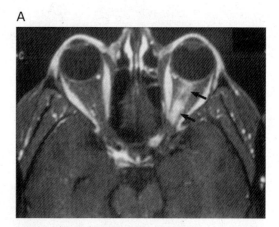
B
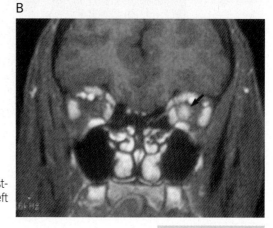

Fig SK 28-5
Optic neuritis. (A) Axial fat-suppressed and (B) coronal post-contrast T1-weighted images show a swollen and enhancing left optic nerve (arrows) secondary to multiple sclerosis.[6]

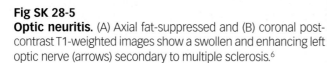

Orbital Masses Not Involving the Optic Nerve

Condition	Imaging Findings	Comments
Predominantly intraconal masses		
Cavernous hemangioma (Figs SK 29-1 and SK 29-2)	Well-defined intraconal mass that typically occurs lateral to the optic nerve. On CT, the mass is of high density and shows homogeneous contrast enhancement. Calcifications commonly occur, and the lesion may expand bone.	Most common benign orbital neoplasm in adults. They frequently occur in childhood, may cause proptosis, and may be associated with skin or conjunctival lesions. An identical imaging pattern can be seen with the less common lymphangiomas.
Retinoblastoma (Fig SK 29-3)	Fusiform or globular mass that often occurs near the orbital apex. On MRI, high flow usually results in signal void on all imaging sequences, although heterogeneous or even high signal intensity may be seen on T2-weighted images as a result of turbulent or slow flow, respectively.	Classic history of intermittent exophthalmos associated with crying or coughing. These lesions may be extremely difficult to diagnose because the varix may expand intermittently and not be obvious unless the venous pressure is increased during a Valsalva maneuver.

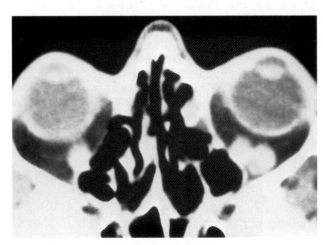

Fig SK 29-1
Cavernous hemangioma. Contrast-enhanced CT scan shows a typical homogeneous enhancing intraconal mass.[47]

A

B

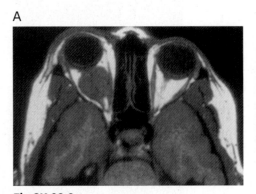 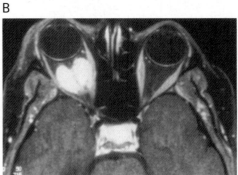

Fig SK 29-2
Cavernous hemangioma. (A) Precontrast axial T1-weighted MR image shows a focal intraconal mass surrounding the right optic nerve. There is mild proptosis. This condition did not alter the patient's visual acuity. (B) Corresponding postcontrast fat-suppressed T1-weighted image shows that the lesion becomes intensely enhanced.[6]

Condition	Imaging Findings	Comments
Melanoma (Fig SK 29-4)	Most commonly, proptosis with no intraorbital abnormality other than a slight increase in fat density. The next most common appearance on CT is diffuse, irregular increased density of the orbital soft tissues with variable contrast enhancement. This nonfocal process tends to involve both intraconal and extraconal regions and obliterates the usual soft-tissue density differences between muscle and fat. Least frequently, there may be a more sharply margi-nated focal mass that cannot be differentiated from a true neoplasm.	Nonspecific inflammation of orbital tissues that accounts for approximately 25% of all cases of unilateral exophthalmos. The condition can be remitting or chronic and progressive and may regress spontaneously or respond to steroids. The infiltrative process predominantly involves the tissues immediately behind the globe. On MRI, this chronic inflammatory process usually has low signal on both T1- and T2-weighted images, unlike the high signal on T2-weighted images seen with most other orbital lesions.
Orbital varix (Fig SK 29-5)	Intraocular calcified mass.	Childhood tumor (average age at diagnosis, 13 months; most found before age 5) that is hereditary in 40% of cases. Approximately 25% are bilateral.

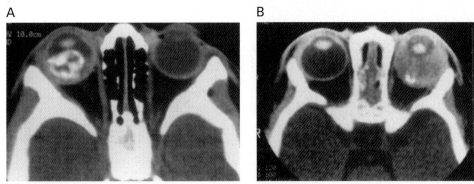

Fig SK 29-3
Retinoblastoma. (A) Axial CT scan shows a large calcified mass in the right eye. The posterior sclera is thick, implying invasion by tumor. (B) Axial noncontrast scan of a different patient shows the hyperdense tumor that fills most of the vitreous chamber and contains a small focus of calcification. The eye is enlarged. In both cases, there is no tumor extension outside of the globe.[6]

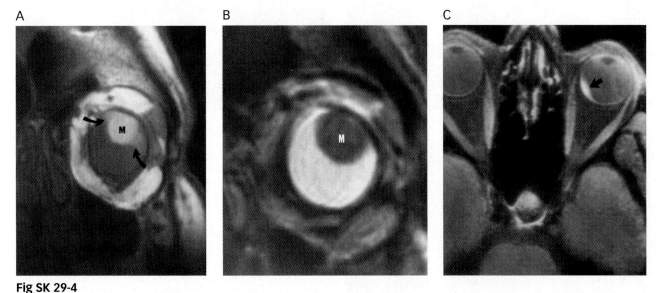

Fig SK 29-4
Melanoma. (A) Coronal (surface coil) noncontrast T1-weighted image shows the bright melanoma (M) with retinal effusions (arrows). (B) Coronal T2-weighted scan shows the tumor (M) to be dark. The effusions blend with the bright vitreous. (C) Axial postcontrast T1-weighted image with fat suppression shows the enhancing melanoma (arrow).[6]

Condition	Imaging Findings	Comments
Orbital pseudotumor (Fig SK 29-6)	Hyperdense, moderately enhancing mass on CT. On MR, classically bright on T1-weighted images, dark on T2-weighted sequences, and demonstrating contrast enhancement.	The most common ocular tumor among adults, melanoma arises from the choroids and occurs almost exclusively among white persons. Associated effusions are well visualized and are slightly bright on both T1-weighted MR images (because of the presence of protein and blood) and T2-weighted scans.

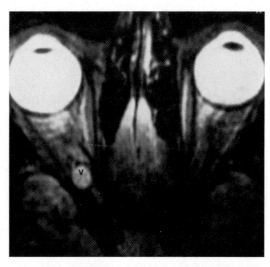

Fig SK 29-5
Orbital varix. T2-weighted MRI scan shows round, hyperintense mass compatible with surgically proved orbital varix (V).[48]

A
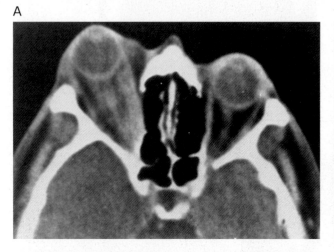

B
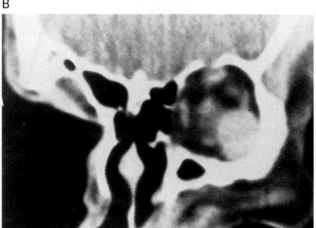

C
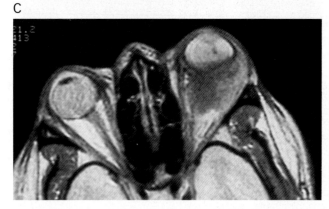

Fig SK 29-6
Orbital pseudotumor. (A) Axial enhanced CT scan shows a typical poorly defined intraconal mass on the right with marked proptosis.[48] (B) Less common appearance of a focal pseudotumor, predominantly extraconal, in the inferolateral aspect of the right orbit associated with mild proptosis.[48] (C) Proton-density MR scan shows an ill-defined region of relatively low signal intensity behind the globe.

Condition	Imaging Findings	Comments
Predominantly extraconal masses		
Extension from adjacent structures		
Orbital cellulitis/ abscess (Fig SK 29-7)	Preseptal cellulitis produces a soft-tissue mass with swelling of the anterior orbital tissues and obliteration of the fat planes. Extension of infection across the fibrous orbital septum into the posterior compartment of the orbit causes edema of the orbital fat and subsequent development of a more discrete mass as the infectious process proceeds.	Acute bacterial infection most often extending from the paranasal sinuses or eyelid. The orbits are predisposed to infections because (1) they are surrounded by the paranasal sinuses that are commonly infected, (2) the thin lamina papyracea offers little resistance to an aggressive process in the ethmoid sinuses, and (3) the veins of the face have no valves and thus serve as another pathway for extension of inflammation into the orbit. In most cases, the cellulitis is confined to the extraconal space; if left untreated, however, it can enter the muscle cone and the intraconal space.
Mucocele (Fig SK 29-8)	Paranasal sinus mass that may break through bone and extend into the orbit. On MRI, a mucocele typically has high signal on both T1- and T2-weighted images.	Complication of inflammatory disease that probably reflects obstruction of the ostium of the sinus and the accumulation of mucous secretions. Primarily involves the frontal sinuses (65%). Approximately 25% affect the ethmoid sinuses and 10% the maxillary sinuses.
Direct extension of neoplasm (Figs SK 29-9 and SK 29-10)	Extraorbital mass with extension into the orbit. MRI and CT can define the degree of soft-tissue extension into the orbit; the latter can demonstrate bony destruction.	Neoplasms include carcinomas of the sinuses and nasal cavity, angiofibromas of the pterygopalatine fossa, meningiomas of the floor of the anterior or middle cranial fossa, basal cell carcinomas of the skin, and primary and secondary tumors of the bony orbital wall.

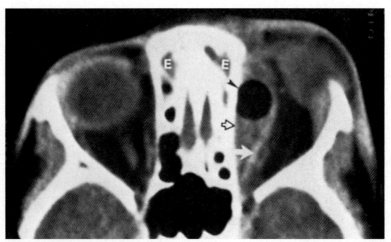

Fig SK 29-7
Orbital subperiosteal abscess. CT scan shows proptosis of left eye with subperiosteal abscess (open arrow). Note air bubble (arrowhead) within abscess and swollen left medial rectus muscle (white arrow).[48]

A

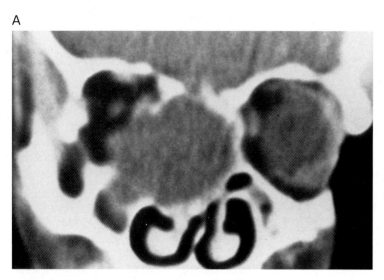

B

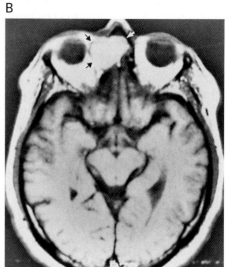

C

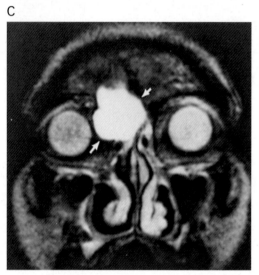

Fig SK 29-8
Mucocele. (A) CT scan shows benign expansion of bone by a sharply marginated, lucent, nonenhanced ethmoid mass that has extended into the medial aspect of the right orbit by eroding the lamina papyracea.[48] (B) In another patient, a T1-weighted MR image shows an expansile, hyperintense abnormality of the anterior ethmoids bilaterally that is greater on the right (arrows).[49] (C) T2-weighted MR image shows greater signal hyperintensity in the mucocele (arrows) and involvement of the lower right frontal sinus.[49]

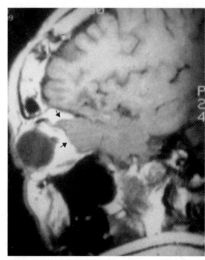

Fig SK 29-9
Meningioma. MR image shows a large mass virtually isointense to brain that arose from the planum sphenoidale and extended into the posterior aspect of the orbit (arrows).

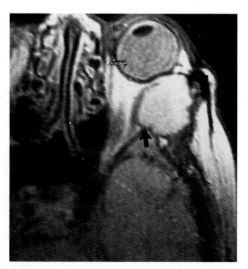

Fig SK 29-10
Adenoid cystic carcinoma. MR scan shows an ill-defined mass (arrow) invading the lateral rectus muscle and breaking through the lateral wall of the orbit.[47]

Condition	Imaging Findings	Comments
Hematogenous metastases (Fig SK 29-11)	Well- or ill-defined masses that are most frequently extraconal, although they may extend into the intraconal region.	Orbital metastases occur in approximately 10% of patients with generalized malignancy. Primary tumors that most frequently metastasize to the orbit are lung and breast cancers; in children, orbital metastases are seen in 50% of patients with neuroblastoma.
Benign bone lesions	Typically have low signal on all MR sequences.	Osteoma (especially in patients with Gardner's syndrome) and fibrous dysplasia (frequently involves the superolateral aspect of the orbit).
Lacrimal gland tumors (Fig SK 29-12)	Soft-tissue mass in the superolateral aspect of the orbit with proptosis and downward displacement of the globe.	Approximately half of primary lacrimal gland masses are of epithelial origin, being equally divided between benign mixed adenomas and carcinomas (most frequently adenoid cystic carcinomas). The remaining 50% include lymphoid lesions, such as dacryoadenitis and pseudotumors. Malignant lacrimal gland lesions generally are more poorly defined and demonstrate invasion of surrounding tissues.
Dacryocystitis	Well-defined, homogeneous mass of fluid intensity in the inferomedial part of the orbit.	Dilatation of the nasolacrimal sac as a result of obstruction or inflammation.
Dermoid cyst (Fig SK 29-13)	Well-circumscribed mass that may displace but not infiltrate adjacent structures. Characteristic fat-fluid level is often seen on MRI. May appear as homogeneous high signal on both T1- and T2-weighted images.	Congenital lesion arising from epithelial rests that typically presents as painless proptosis and a palpable mass in the upper orbit. The presence of fat excludes most other orbital neoplasms; the dependent fluid excludes lipoma.
Epidermoid cyst	Sharply marginated mass.	Like other extraconal masses, an epidermoid cyst typically has low signal on T1-weighted images and high signal on T2-weighted images.

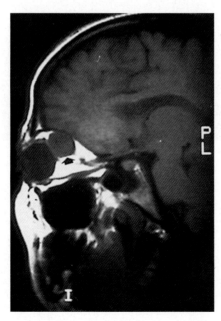

Fig SK 29-11
Hematogenous metastasis. Well-circumscribed retrobulbar mass (arrow).

Condition	Imaging Findings	Comments
Lymphoma (Fig SK 29-14)	Intraconal or extraconal mass that usually has ill-defined margins and may show invasion of surrounding structures.	As with most orbital lesions, lymphomas typically have low signal on T1-weighted images and high signal on T2-weighted images.

A

B

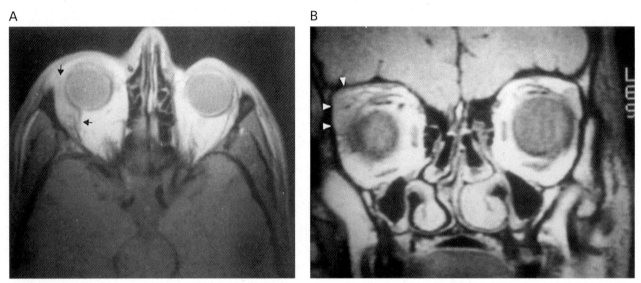

Fig SK 29-12
Lacrimal gland tumor. (A) Coronal and (B) axial MR scans show the mass in the superolateral aspect of the right orbit (arrows).

A

B

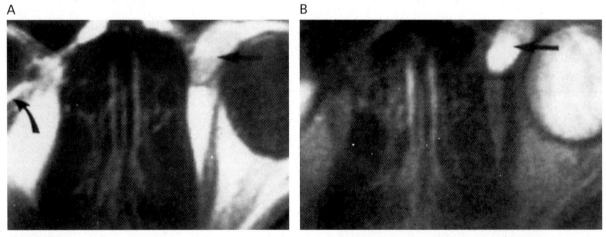

Fig SK 29-13
Dermoid cyst. A fat-fluid level (arrows) is seen in this well-defined extraconal lesion on (A) T1-weighted and (B) T2-weighted MR images. The artifact in the right orbit (curved arrow) is due to cosmetics.[47]

A

B

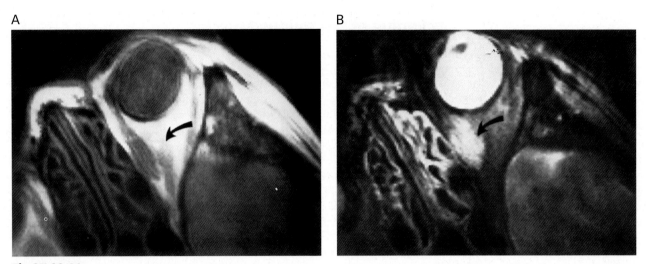

Fig SK 29-14
Lymphoma. Ill-defined enlargement of the medial rectus muscle (arrow) that typically has low signal on T1-weighted images (A) and high signal on T2-weighted images (B).[47]

Thickening of the Rectus Muscles

Condition	Comments
Thyroid ophthalmopathy (Graves' disease) (Fig SK 30-1)	Hypersecretion by fibroblasts of mucopolysaccharides, collagen, and glycoproteins causes binding of water and increased intraorbital pressure, leading to ischemia, edema, and sometimes fibrosis of extraocular muscles. The medial and inferior rectus muscles are usually affected before and to a greater degree than the lateral rectus or superior muscle group. The two eyes may be involved symmetrically or asymmetrically.
Rhabdomyosarcoma (Fig SK 30-2)	Uncommon, highly malignant orbital tumor arising from extraocular muscle that typically presents with rapidly progressive exophthalmos in boys younger than 10 years of age. Appears as a large, noncalcified, enhancing retrobulbar mass, often with adjacent bone destruction. The identification of a displaced, but otherwise normal, optic nerve helps to exclude an optic nerve tumor.
Metastasis	Unusual manifestation of infiltration by such neoplasms as lymphoma, leukemia, and neuroblastoma. An orbital neurofibroma may rarely produce a mass thickening the contour of a rectus muscle.
Orbital myositis	Inflammatory process that usually affects multiple muscles in children and a single muscle in adults and presents with rapid onset of proptosis, erythema of the lids, and injection of the conjunctiva. In most cases, steroid therapy causes the enlarged muscles to return to a normal appearance.
Orbital pseudotumor (Fig SK 30-3)	Inflammatory process that can affect virtually all the intraorbital soft-tissue structures. The variable appearances of this condition include enlargement of one or more extraocular muscles, a discrete or poorly defined intraconal or extraconal mass that may obliterate the muscle-fat planes, enlargement of the lacrimal gland, and scleral thickening. There is generally improvement after steroid therapy.

A

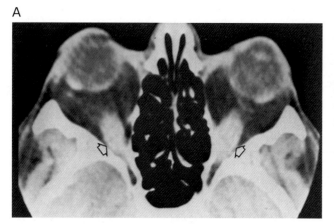

B

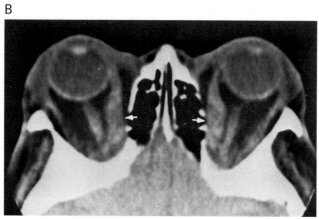

C

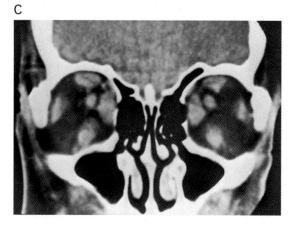

Fig SK 30-1
Thyroid ophthalmopathy. (A) Axial view shows bilateral thickening of the inferior rectus muscles (arrows). (B) At a higher level, there is thickening of the medial rectus muscles bilaterally (arrows). (C) Coronal view shows thickening of virtually all the rectus muscles on both sides.

Condition	Comments
Infiltrative processes	Orbital cellulitis, Wegener's granulomatosis, lethal midline granuloma, sarcoidosis, foreign body reaction.
Carotid-cavernous fistula Fig SK 30-4)	Dilatation of the cavernous sinus may cause enlargement of the extraocular muscles due to venous congestion. Typical findings consist of unilateral proptosis and enlargement of the superior ophthalmic vein.

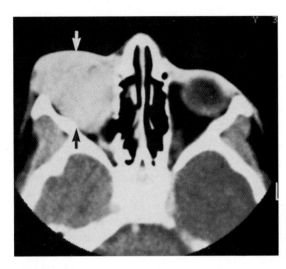

Fig SK 30-2
Rhabdomyosarcoma. Enhancing tumor (arrows) fills virtually the entire right orbit in a 6-year-old child with rapidly progressing proptosis.[1]

A

B

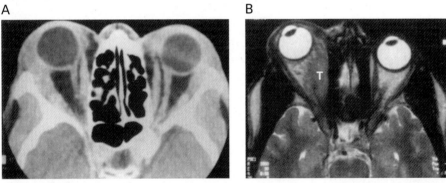

Fig SK 30-3
Orbital pseudotumor. (A) Axial CT scan shows that both lateral rectus muscles are thick (including their insertions). There is bilateral proptosis. (B) Axial T2-weighted MR image of a different patient shows the tumefactive type of pseudotumor (T), which involves the right medial rectus muscle, extends into the retro-ocular fat, and is of low signal intensity.[6]

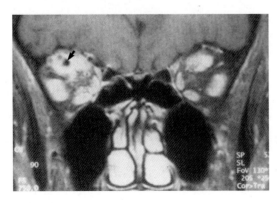

Fig SK 30-4
Carotid-cavernous fistula. Coronal postcontrast fat-suppressed T1-weighted image shows enlargement of the extraocular muscles in both orbits. Note the prominent right superior ophthalmic vein (arrow).[6]

Aneurysms and Vascular Malformations

Condition	Comments
Anterior communicating artery aneurysm (Fig SK 31-1)	Approximately 30% to 35% of intracranial aneurysms. Rupture results in hemorrhage in the gyri recti, anterior interhemispheric fissure, septum pellucidum, and frontal horns of the lateral ventricles.
Posterior communicating artery aneurysm (Fig SK 31-2)	Approximately 30% to 35% of intracranial aneurysms. Rupture tends to result in diffuse subarachnoid hemorrhage, but bleeding may be concentrated in the basilar cisterns.
Middle cerebral artery bifurcation aneurysm (Fig SK 31-3)	Approximately 20% of intracranial aneurysms. Rupture results in hemorrhage in the sylvian fissures, frontal opercula, and basilar cisterns.
Basilar artery tip aneurysm (Fig SK 31-4)	Approximately 5% of intracranial aneurysms. Rupture results in hemorrhage in the basilar cisterns and posterior portion of the third ventricle.
Posterior inferior cerebellar artery aneurysm (Fig SK 31-5)	Approximately 1% to 3% of intracranial aneurysms. Rupture may produce hemorrhage isolated to the posterior fossa or fourth ventricle.
Post-traumatic aneurysm (Fig SK 31-6)	Less than 1% of intracranial aneurysms. Common sites include the intracavernous portion of the internal carotid artery, the distal part of the anterior cerebral artery, and distal branches of the middle cerebral artery.

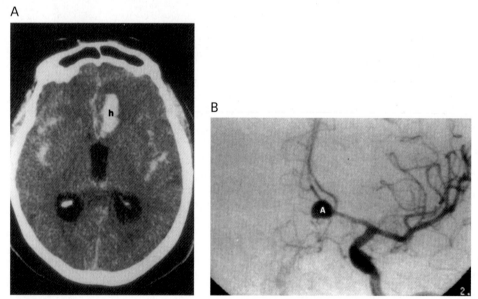

Fig SK 31-1
Anterior communicating artery aneurysm. (A) Axial CT scan shows clot (h) in the left gyrus rectus. There is blood in the anterior interhemispheric fissure and sylvian fissures. Note the hydrocephalus. (B) Oblique view from a catheter angiogram shows an aneurysm in the anterior communicating artery (A).[6]

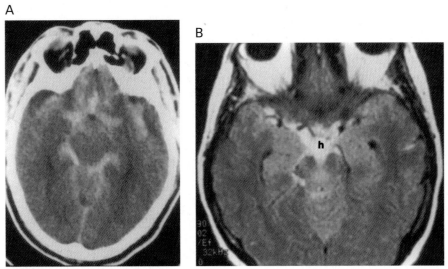

Fig SK 31-2
Posterior communicating artery aneurysm. (A) Axial CT and (B) MR images show subarachnoid hemorrhage (h) in the basilar cisterns.[6]

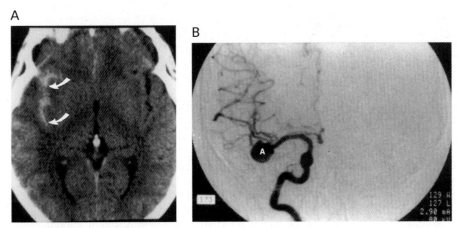

Fig SK 31-3
Middle cerebral artery bifurcation aneurysm. (A) Axial CT scan shows subarachnoid hemorrhage confined mostly to the right sylvian fissure (arrows). (B) Frontal view from a catheter angiogram shows an aneurysm (A) at the bifurcation of the right middle cerebral artery.[6]

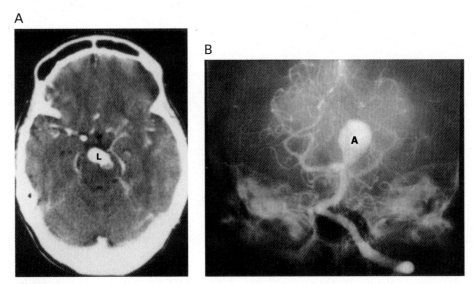

Fig SK 31-4
Basilar artery tip aneurysm. (A) Contrast-enhanced CT scan shows a large aneurysm (L) at the level of the basilar artery tip. (B) Frontal projection from a catheter angiogram shows a giant aneurysm (A) arising from the tip of the basilar artery.[6]

Condition	Comments
Giant aneurysm (Fig SK 31-7)	Aneurysms measuring more than 2.5 cm in diameter tend to occur in middle-aged women, with the most common sites being the bifurcation and intracavernous portion of the internal carotid artery, and the tip of the basilar artery. Probably caused by intramural hemorrhage, these aneurysms grow slowly and produce symptoms primarily due to their mass effect (seizures, headaches, focal neurologic deficits, and cranial nerve palsies, especially if located within the cavernous sinus). MRI may reveal complex concentric layers of clot along the wall.

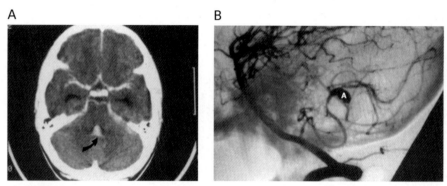

Fig SK 31-5
Posterior inferior cerebellar artery aneurysm. (A) Axial CT scan shows hemorrhage (arrow) in the fourth ventricle. (B) Lateral projection of a posterior fossa catheter angiogram shows an aneurysm (A) arising in the supratonsillar segment of a posterior inferior cerebellar artery.[6]

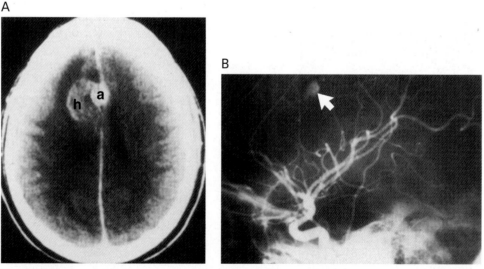

Fig SK 31-6
Post-traumatic aneurysm. (A) CT scan obtained 2 weeks after head injury shows a hematoma (h) as well as a central enhancing abnormality (a), which was shown at angiography (B) to represent a post-traumatic aneurysm (arrow) in the pericallosal artery.[6]

Condition	Comments
Arteriovenous malformation (AVM) (see Fig SK 6-13)	Approximately 25% of intracranial vascular malformations. Although congenital, they generally present during middle age (65% in patients older than age 40). More than 80% are supratentorial (especially parietal), and a similar number are solitary (multiple AVMs are seen in Osler-Weber-Rendu disease). CT demonstrates calcification in about 30% of intracranial AVMs. On MR, a cluster of serpiginous flow voids (representing rapid blood flow) and areas of high signal (slow flow in draining veins).
Cavernous angioma (see Fig SK 6-14)	Approximately 10% of intracranial vascular malformations. Slow-flow, low-pressure malformation with no normal intervening parenchyma. About 80% are supratentorial and 15% are multiple (often a familial component). When bleeding occurs, it tends to be self-limited and of no clinical significance. CT shows a slightly hyperdense, enhancing focal lesion with calcifications. On T2-weighted MR images, the lesion appears as an island of bright signal (methemoglobin) surrounded by an extensive region of very low signal (hemosiderin). Cavernous angiomas are often termed *cryptic* or *occult* because they generally are not visible on conventional angiograms.

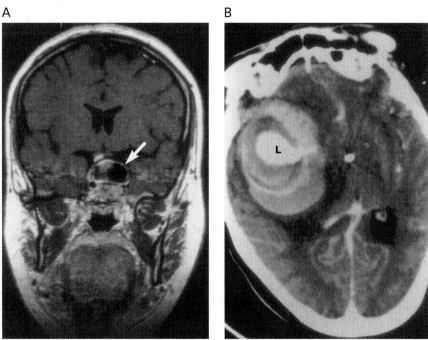

A B

Fig SK 31-7
Giant aneurysm. (A) Coronal T1-weighted MR image shows a large intrasellar aneurysm (arrow). (B) Axial postcontrast CT scan in another patient shows opacification of the lumen (L) of a giant aneurysm arising in the bifurcation of the right middle cerebral artery. Note the concentric and hyperdense layers of clot along the walls of this aneurysm.[6]

Condition	Comments
Developmental venous anomaly (Fig SK 31-8)	This most common cerebrovascular malformation is generally asymptomatic and an incidental finding. More than 65% are supratentorial, especially in the frontal lobe, and most are solitary.
Capillary telangiectasia (Fig SK 31-9)	Most common in the pons, these generally are asymptomatic lesions that are usually found incidentally at MRI. They typically enhance after contrast administration, are of low signal intensity on gradient echo imaging (probably because of magnetic susceptibility effects caused by oxyhemoglobin), and show no abnormality on precontrast T1-weighted and conventional or fast spin echo T2-weighted images.
Dural arteriovenous malformation and fistula	Generally asymptomatic, most occur in the cavernous sinuses and the posterior fossa (near the transverse and sigmoid sinuses). They are probably secondary to occlusion of a venous sinus.
Carotid artery-cavernous sinus fistula (see Fig SK 30-4)	More common high-flow type usually occurs in young men and constitutes almost 10% of intracranial vascular malformations. They develop secondary to traumatic tear of the internal carotid artery or rupture of an intracavernous internal carotid artery aneurysm. They usually drain into the superior ophthalmic vein and present with pulsatile exophthalmus, bruit, conjunctival chemosis, and cranial nerve palsies. The less common low-flow type, which typically occurs spontaneously among middle-aged women, is caused by communication of multiple dural branches from the external or internal cerebral artery with the cavernous sinus.

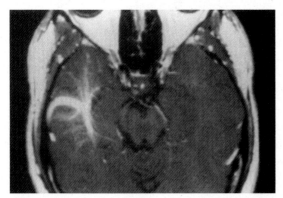

Fig SK 31-8
Developmental venous anomaly. Postcontrast axial T1-weighted MR image shows a venous angioma in the right temporal lobe. Slow flow results in enhancement of the lesion.[6]

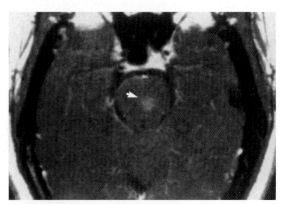

Fig SK 31-9
Capillary telangiectasia. Postcontrast T1-weighted MR image shows enhancement in this pontine lesion (arrow). The non-contrast images showed no abnormality.[6]

Condition	Comments
Vein of Galen aneurysm (Fig SK 31-10)	Arteriovenous malformation that often presents in childhood, produces high blood flow, and is an important cause of neonatal heart failure.

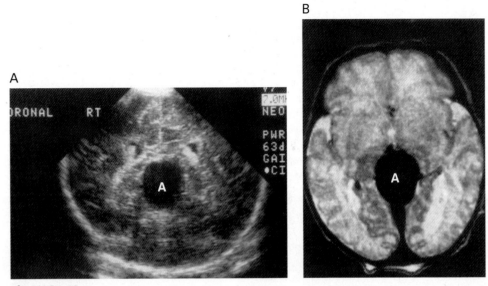

Fig SK 31-10
Vein of Galen aneurysm. (A) Coronal sonogram shows a hypoechoic and dilated vein of Galen. (B) T2-weighted MR image confirms the aneurysmal dilatation of the vein of Galen (A).[6]

Mandible Lesions on Computed Tomography

Condition	Comments
Cystic lesions	
Periapical (radicular) cyst (Fig SK 32-1)	The most common odontogenic cyst, it results from inflammation secondary to caries or other entities. Infection typically spreads to the apex (root) of the tooth, leading to secondary apical peridontitis, granuloma, or abscess, and eventually to cyst formation.
Follicular (dentigerous) cyst (Fig SK 32-2)	Most common developmental odontogenic cyst. The lesion forms around the crown of an unerupted tooth (commonly the third molar). Unlike radicular cysts, a follicular cyst may become extremely large, distorting the roots of adjacent teeth and remodeling the mandible, though the cortical bone is usually preserved.
Odontogenic keratocyst (Fig SK 32-3)	Most frequently located in the body or ramus of the mandible, these multiloculated lesions possess destructive potential and have a high recurrence rate after resection. Unlike follicular cysts, they can expand cortical bone and erode the cortex, though they rarely exhibit malignant transformation. Multiple lesions in a young patient are suggestive of basal cell nevus syndrome.

A

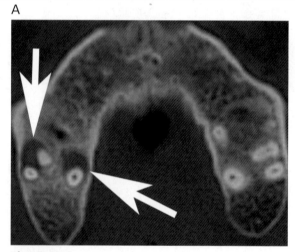

B

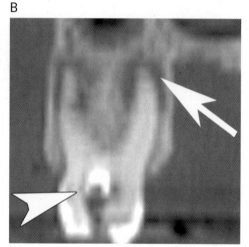

Fig SK 32-1
Periapical cyst. (A) Axial scan and (B) reformatted image demonstrate a radiolucent lesion (arrows) surrounding the apex of a molar. A defect with dental filling (arrowhead) is present within the crown of the tooth.[50]

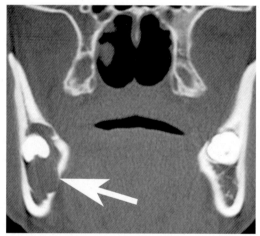

Fig SK 32-2
Follicular cyst. Coronal reformatted image reveals a cystic lesion with an unerupted tooth in the right molar region (arrow). The crown of the tooth is contained within the lesion. Note the presence of bone remodeling rather than expansion.[50]

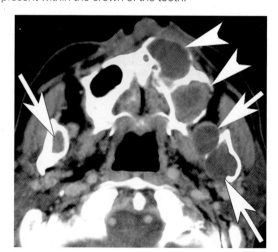

Fig SK 32-3
Odontogenic keratocyst. In this patient with the basal cell nevus syndrome, there are multiple cysts (arrows) in the mandible. Cystic lesions (arrowheads) are also identified within the maxilla.[50]

Condition	Comments
Solitary bone cyst (Fig SK 32-4)	Pseudocyst resulting from trauma, which leads to intramedullary hemorrhage and subsequent resorption. Most commonly located in the posterior marrow space of the mandible, they appear slightly irregular with poorly defined borders. A characteristic scalloped superior margin extends between the roots of adjacent teeth. Osseous expansion may thin the mandibular cortex.
Solid benign lesions Odontoma	The most common odontogenic tumor of the mandible, it consists of various tooth components, including dentin and enamel, which have developed abnormally to form a "hamartomatous" lesion. About half are associated with an impacted tooth. Forming between the roots of teeth, the tumor is initially radiolucent, then develops small calcifications, and eventually forms a radiopaque mass with a lucent rim.
Ameloblastoma (Figs SK 32-5 and SK 32-6)	Slow-growing tumor that arises from enamel-forming cells that failed to regress during embryonic development. Most commonly found in the posterior mandible, this expansile, radiolucent tumor can be unilocular or multilocular and contain cystic areas of low attenuation and scattered isoattenuating regions. The lesion may cause significant expansion of the mandible and even erode through the cortex, with extension into the surrounding oral mucosa. Erosion of the roots of adjacent teeth is pathognomonic and indicates aggressive behavior of the tumor.
Ossifying fibroma (Fig SK 32-7)	Tumor that contains fibrous tissue with varying amounts of bony trabeculae and usually occurs in the posterior mandible. An encapsulated, well-circumscribed lesion, it can appear radiolucent, radiopaque, or with mixed opacity depending on the degree of calcification.
Solid malignant lesions Ameloblastic carcinoma (Fig SK 32-8)	Although rare, malignant transformation of an ameloblastoma does occur. Aggressive features suggesting this diagnosis include cortical destruction, extraosseous extension, and extensive solid components. Most carcinomatous involvement of the mandible is secondary to invasion from the surrounding mucosa.

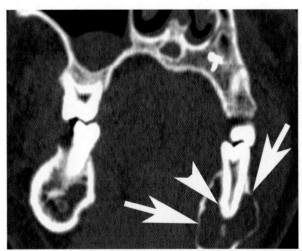

Fig SK 32-4
Solitary bone cyst. Coronal reformatted image demonstrates a cystic lesion (arrows) within the body of the mandible. The mandibular cortex is thinned. Note the normal tooth (arrowhead) within the lesion, a finding that helps distinguish the cyst from radicular or other odontogenic cysts.[50]

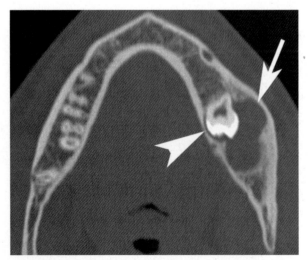

Fig SK 32-5
Ameloblastoma. Multiloculated cystic lesion (arrow) within the left mandible. The crown of an impacted tooth (arrowhead) within the lesion is a clue to the diagnosis.[50]

Condition	Comments
Sarcoma (Fig SK 32-9)	Osteosarcoma, chondrosarcoma, fibrosarcoma, and leiomyosarcoma can cause both osteolytic and osteoblastic lesions.
Metastasis (Fig SK 32-10)	Metastatic disease often involves the mandible, especially the posterior body and angle that have increased marrow vascularity. Although most are radiolucent with ill-defined borders, blastic lesions may occur in carcinoma of the prostate. The most common primary sites for mandibular metastasis are kidney, lung, and breast.

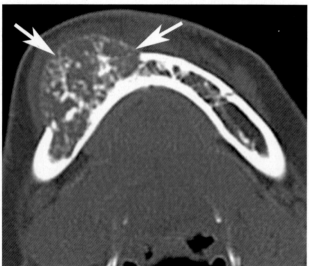

Fig SK 32-6
Aggressive ameloblastoma. Expansile enhancing lesion within the right mandibular body (arrows) that causes significant buccal cortical destruction. (Courtesy of Akifumi Fujita, M.D., Jichi Medical University, Shimotsuke, Japan.).[50]

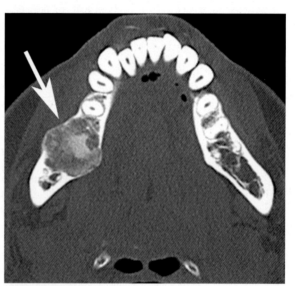

Fig SK 32-7
Ossifying fibroma. A circular, partially calcified lesion (arrow) within the mandible. Note the internal ground-glass calcifications.[50]

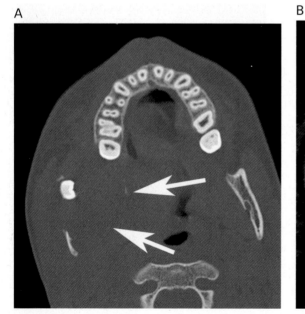

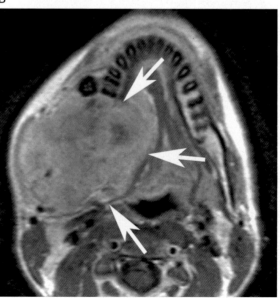

Fig SK 32-8
Ameloblastic carcinoma. (A) Contrast CT scan with bone windowing shows an enhancing multiloculated soft-tissue mass (arrows) with adjacent bone destruction. (B) Contrast T1-weighted MR image demonstrates the enhancing soft-tissue mass.[50]

Condition	Comments
Infectious lesions	
Apical periodontitis (Fig SK 32-11)	Generalized term for the spectrum of periapical cysts, granulomas, and abscesses, most of which are caused by dental caries. An apical abscess demonstrates an enhancing rim.
Osteomyelitis (Figs SK 32-12 and SK-13)	Rare in healthy individuals due to the early administration of antibiotics. There often are no imaging abnormalities in the acute suppurative stage. Chronic lesions demonstrate a variety of bone reactions, including focal radiolucent and radiopaque areas. Low-grade infections can cause sclerosing osteomyelitis, in which bone is deposited along the osseous cortex and trabeculae.
Vascular and neurogenic lesions	
Central giant cell granuloma (Giant cell reparative cyst) (Fig SK 32-14)	Most often found in the anterior mandible of girls or young women, this lesion is believed to be within the spectrum of altered vascular and reactive responses within bone. It initially appears as a small, unilocular radiolucent lesion that can mimic an ontogenic cyst. As it develops, it becomes multilocular with bone septa traversing the lesion and producing a honeycomb appearance. There may be expansion of the lesion, root resorption, and erosion or modeling of the cortex, and the lesion may cross the midline.
Arteriovenous malformation (Fig SK 32-15)	Although uncommon in the jaw, it may occur in the ramus and posterior body of the mandible. Contrast enhanced scans demonstrate dilated and tortuous vessels within the multiloculated lesion. Identification of an AVM is critical because of the potential for fatal hemorrhage after tooth extraction.
Others	Central hemangioma, neurofibroma, and schwannoma appear as well-defined soft-tissue structures with well-corticated margins.
Metabolic abnormalities (Fig SK 32-16)	Systemic disorders such as osteoporosis, osteomalacia, renal osteodystrophy, and hyperparathyroidism may cause lesions in the mandible that appear similar to those occurring elsewhere in the body.

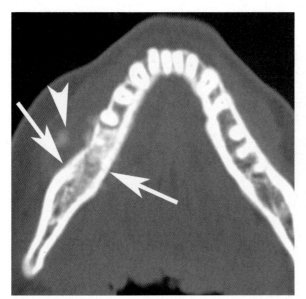

Fig SK 32-9
Osteosarcoma. Osteoblastic changes (arrows) are seen with the right mandibular body. Note the abnormal soft-tissue ossification (arrowhead).[50]

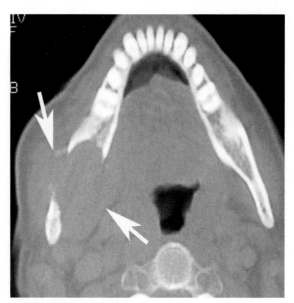

Fig SK 32-10
Metastasis. Expansile, osteolytic mass (arrows) within the right mandibular body, which represents a metastasis from hepatocellular carcinoma.[50]

Condition	Comments
Tumor-like conditions (Figs SK 32-17 and SK 32-18)	Torus mandibularis produces exostoses in the mandible. Multiple osteomas may develop in Gardner's syndrome, associated with impacted and supernumerary teeth. Fibrous dyplasia and Paget's disease appear the same in the mandible as they do in other parts of the body. Osteonecrosis from radiation therapy can demonstrate both sclerotic and lytic components with poorly defined borders and enlarged trabecular spaces.

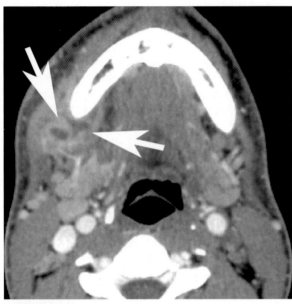

Fig SK 32-11
Apical peridontitis. Rim-enhancing fluid collection (arrows) within the perimandibular soft tissues.[50]

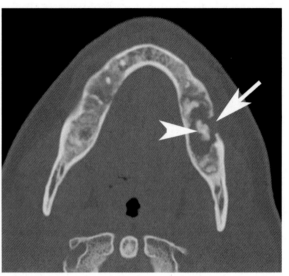

Fig SK 32-12
Chronic osteomyelitis. Osteolytic lesion (arrow), containing a bony sequestrum (arrowhead) within the left mandibular body.[50]

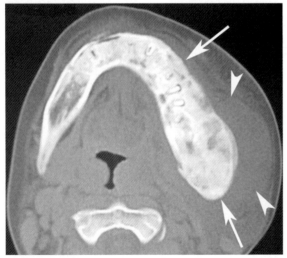

Fig SK 32-13
Sclerosing osteomyelitis. Diffuse sclerotic changes with expansion of the left mandibular body (arrows). Note the diffuse soft-tissue swelling (arrowheads).[50]

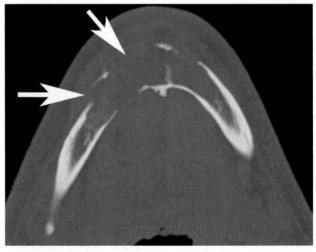

Fig SK 32-14
Central giant cell granuloma. Cystic lesion (arrows) within the mandible with erosion of the mandibular cortex.[50]

A

B

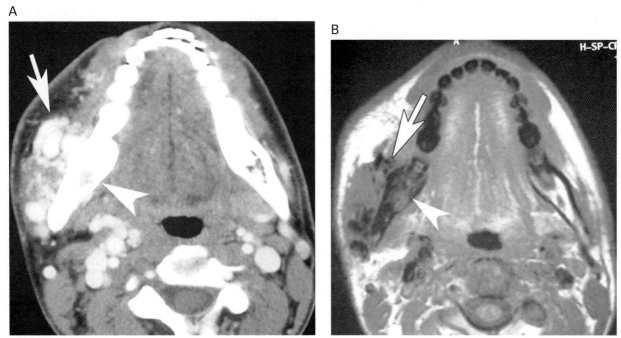

Fig SK 32-15
Arteriovenous malformation. (A) Contrast CT scan reveals multiple dilated and tortuous vessels (arrow) within the right masseter muscle. Note the abnormal enhancement (arrowhead) within the marrow of the mandible. (B) T1-weighted MR image demonstrates a slightly expansile lesion (arrow) within the right mandibular angle and body. Multiple flow voids are present within the right masseter muscle. Note the loss of normal fatty marrow (arrowhead) within the mandible.[50]

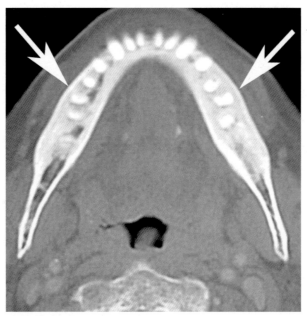

Fig SK 32-16
Renal osteodystrophy. Diffuse sclerotic changes (arrows) throughout the entire mandible.[50]

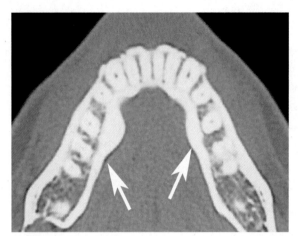

Fig SK 32-17
Torus mandibularis. Bilateral exostoses (arrows) in the lingual aspects of the mandible.[50]

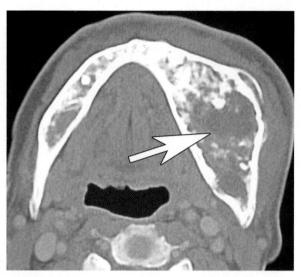

Fig SK 32-18
Fibrous dysplasia. Expansile lesion containing numerous unorganized bone trabeculae (arrow) within the left mandibular body.[50]

Sources

1. Reprinted from *Cranial Computed Tomography* by AL Williams and VM Haughton with permission of The CV Mosby Company, St Louis, ©1985.

2. Reprinted with permission from "Lymphoma after Organ Transplantation: Radiological Manifestations in the Central Nervous System, Thorax, and Abdomen" by DE Tubman, MP Frick, and DW Hanto, *Radiology* (1984;149:625–631), Copyright ©1984, Radiological Society of North America Inc.

3. Reprinted with permission from "Acquired Immunodeficiency Syndrome: Neuroradiologic Findings" by WM Kelly and MB Brant-Zawadzki, *Radiology* (1983;149:485–491), Copyright ©1983, Radiological Society of North America Inc.

4. Reprinted with permission from "Unusual Neuroradiological Features of Intracranial Cysticercosis" by CS Zee et al, *Radiology* (1980;137:397–407), Copyright ©1980, Radiological Society of North America Inc.

5. Reprinted from *Cranial Computed Tomography* by SH Lee and HCVG Rao (Eds) with permission of McGraw-Hill Book Company, ©1983.

6. Levine DS, Navarro OM, Chaudry G, et al. Imaging the complications of bone marrow transplantation in children. *RadioGraphics* 2007;27:307–324.

7. Reprinted with permission from *Neuroradiology Companion* by M Castillo, Lippincott-Raven, © 1999.

8. Reprinted with permission from "CT in Hydatid Cyst of the Brain" by K Abbassioun et al, *Journal of Neurosurgery* (1978;49:408–411), Copyright ©1978, American Association of Neurological Surgeons.

9. Reprinted with permission from "Adult Supratentorial Tumors" by SW Atlas, *Seminars in Roentgenology* (1990;25:130–154), Copyright ©1990, Grune & Stratton Inc.

10. Reprinted with permission from "Intracranial Oligodendrogliomas" by YY Lee and P Van Tassel, *American Journal of Roentgenology* (1989;152:361–369), Copyright ©1989, American Roentgen Ray Society.

11. Reprinted with permission from "Colloid Cysts of the Third Ventricle" by PP Maeder et al, *American Journal of Roentgenology* (1990; 155:135–141), Copyright ©1990, American Roentgen Ray Society.

12. Reprinted from *Essentials in Neuroimaging* by B Kirkwood, with permission of Churchill Livingstone, Copyright ©1991.

13. Vilanova JC, Barcelo J, Smirniotopoulos JG, et al. Hemangioma from Head to Toe: MR Imaging with Pathologic Correlation. *RadioGraphics* 2004;24:367–385.

14. Reprinted with permission from "The Radiology of Pituitary Adenoma" by SM Wolpert, *Seminars in Roentgenology* (1984;19:53–69), Copyright ©1984, Grune & Stratton Inc.

15. Reprinted with permission from "Amenorrhea and Galactorrhea: A Role for MRI" by LP Mark and WM Haughton, *MRI Decisions* (Jan-Feb 1989:26–32), Copyright ©1989, PW Communications, International. All rights reserved.

16. Reprinted with permission from "Imaging of Intrasellar, Suprasellar, and Parasellar Tumors" by RA Zimmerman, *Seminars in Roentgenology* (1990;25:174–197), Copyright ©1990, Grune & Stratton Inc.

17. Reprinted with permission from "Adult Infratentorial Tumors" by LT Bilaniuk, *Seminars in Roentgenology* (1990;25:155–173), Copyright ©1990, Grune & Stratton Inc.

18. Reprinted with permission from "MR Imaging of Primary Tumors of Trigeminal Nerve and Meckel's Cave" by WTC Yuh et al, *American Journal of Neuroradiology* (1988;9:665–670), Copyright ©1988, Williams & Wilkins Company.

19. Reprinted with permission from "MRI of the Pituitary Gland: Adenomas" by SC Patel and WP Sanders, *MRI Decisions* (1990; 4:12–20), Copyright ©1990, PW Communications, Int'l. All rights reserved.

20. Ueno T, Tanaka YO, Nagata M, et al. Spectrum of Germ Cell Tumors: From Head to Toe. *RadioGraphics* 2004;24:387–404.

21. Reprinted with permission from "MR Anatomy and Pathology of the Hypothalamus" by DJ Loes, TJ Barloon, WTC Yuh, et al, *American Journal of Roentgenology* (1991;156:579–585), Copyright ©1991, American Roentgen Ray Society.

22. Saleem SN, Said A-H M, Lee DH. Lesions of the hypothalamus: MR imaging diagnostic features. *RadioGraphics* 2007;27:1087–1108.

23. Lai PH, Chen C, Liang HL, Pan HB. Hyperintense Basal Ganglia on T1-Weighted MR Imaging. *AJR Am J Roentgenol* 1999;172:1109–1115.

24. Reprinted from *MR and CT Imaging of the Head, Neck and Spine* (2nd ed.), by RE Latchaw (Ed), with permission of CV Mosby Company, Copyright ©1991.

25. Reprinted with permission from "Unusual Lesions of the Cerebellopontine Angle: A Segmental Approach" by F Bonneville et al, *Radiographics* (2001;21:419).

26. Reprinted with permission from "Paragangliomas of the Jugular Bulb and Carotid Body" by T Vogl et al, *American Journal of Roentgenology* (1989;153:583–587), Copyright ©1989, American Roentgen Ray Society.

27. Reprinted with permission from "MRI of the Jugular Foramen" by DL Daniel and LP Mark, *MRI Decisions* (1991;5:2–11), Copyright ©1991, PW Communications, Int'l. All rights reserved.

28. Reprinted with permission from "CT, MR, and Pathology in HIV Encephalitis and Meningitis" by MJD Post et al, *AJR Am J Roentgenol* (1988;151:373–380), Copyright ©1988, American Roentgen Ray Society.

29. Reprinted with permission from "Imaging Decisions in the Evaluation of Headache" by CE Johnson and RD Zimmerman, *MRI Decisions* (1989;3:2–16), Copyright ©1989, PW Communications, International. All rights reserved.

30. Courtesy of Bruce H. Braffman, MD.

31. Reprinted with permission from "Multiple System Atrophy (Shy-Drager Syndrome): MR Imaging" by B Pastakia, R Polinsky, G DiChiro, et al, *Radiology* (1986;159:499–502), Copyright ©1986, Radiological Society of North America.

32. Reprinted from *Clinical Magnetic Resonance Imaging* by RR Edelman and JR Hesselink (Eds) with permission of WB Saunders Company, ©1990.

33. Reprinted with permission from "Wilson's Disease of the Brain, MR Imaging" by AM Aisen, W Martel, TO Grabielsen, et al, *Radiology* (1985;157:137–141), Copyright ©1985, Radiological Society of North America.

34. Reprinted with permission from "Intracranial Ependymoma and Subependymoma: MR Manifestations" by GP Spoto et al, *American Journal of Neuroradiology* (1990;11:83–91), Copyright ©1990, American Society of Neuroradiology.

35. Reprinted with permission from "Gd-DTPA-Enhanced Cranial MR Imaging in Children: Initial Clinical Experience and Recommendations for Its Use" by AD Elster and GD Rieser, *American Journal of Neuroradiology* (1989;10:1027–1030), Copyright ©1989, American Society of Neuroradiology.

36. Reprinted with permission from "Intraventricular Mass Lesions of the Brain: CT and MR Findings" by RD Tien, *AJR Am J Roentgenol* (1991;157:1283–1290), Copyright ©1991, American Roentgen Ray Society.

37. Reprinted with permission from "Intraventricular Neurocytoma: Radiological Features and Review of the Literature" by SK Goergen, MF Gonzales, and CA McLean, *Radiology* (1992;182:787–792), Copyright ©1992, Radiological Society of North America.

38. Reprinted with permission from "Intracranial Meningeal Pathology: Use of Enhanced MRI" by MR Ross, DO Davis, AS Mark, *MRI Decisions*

(1990;4:24–33), Copyright ©1990, PW Communications, International. All rights reserved.

39. Reprinted with permission from "Congenital Central Nervous System Anomalies" by LB Poe, LL Coleman, F Mahmud, *Radiographics* (1989;9:801–826), Copyright ©1989, Radiological Society of North America Inc.

40. Reprinted with permission from "Magnetic Resonance Imaging of Disturbances in Neuronal Migration: Illustration of an Embryologic Process" by AS Smith et al, *Radiographics* (1989;9:509–522), Copyright ©1989, Radiological Society of North America Inc.

41. Reprinted with permission from "Common Congenital Brain Anomalies" by SE Byrd and TP Naidich, *Radiologic Clinics of North America* (1988;26:755–772), Copyright ©1988, WB Saunders Company.

42. Epelman M, Daneman A, Blaser SI, et al. Differential diagnosis of intracranial cystic lesions at head US: Correlation with CT and MR imaging. *RadioGraphics* 2006;26:173–196.

43. Reprinted with permission from "Sonography of Congenital Midline Brain Malformations" by KC Funk and MJ Siegel, *Radiographics* (1988;8:11–25), Copyright ©1988, Radiological Society of North America, Inc.

44. Reprinted with permission from "CNS Complications of AIDS: CT and MR Findings" by RG Ramsey and GK Geremia, *AJR Am J Roentgenol* (1988;151:449–454), Copyright ©1988, American Roentgen Ray Society.

45. Reprinted with permission from "Encephalitis Caused by Human Immunodeficiency Virus: CT and MR Imaging Manifestations with Clinical and Pathologic Correlation" by HS Chrysikopoulos et al, *Radiology* (1990;175:184–191), Copyright ©1990, Radiological Society of North America Inc.

46. Reprinted with permission from "Intracranial Manifestations of Acquired Immunodeficiency Syndrome" by WW Woodruff, *The Radiologist* (1994;1:357–365).

47. Reprinted with permission from "Surface-Coil MR Imaging of Orbital Neoplasms" by JA Sullivan and SE Harms, *Am J Neuroradiol* (1986;7:29–34), Copyright ©1986, Williams & Wilkins Company.

48. Reprinted from *Head and Neck Imaging* by RT Bergeron, AG Osborn, and PM Som (Eds) with permission of The CV Mosby Company, St Louis, ©1990.

49. Reprinted with permission from "Mucoceles of the Paranasal Sinuses: MR Imaging with CT Correlation" by P Van Tassel et al, *AJR Am J Roentgenol* (1989;153:407–412), Copyright ©1989, American Roentgen Ray Society.

50. Dunfee BL, Sakai O, Pistey R, Gohel A. Radiologic and pathologic characteristics of benign and malignant lesions of the mandible. *RadioGraphics* 2006;26:1751–1768.

8

Breast Disease and Mammography

Well-Circumscribed Breast Masses*

Condition	Imaging Findings	Comments
Cyst (Fig MA 1-1)	Round or ovoid mass with density equal to or slightly greater than that of the breast parenchyma and oriented along the path of the ducts. A halo sign is often present.	Most commonly seen in women from 30 to 50 years old. May be associated with pain and tenderness, with symptoms occurring just before and with the menstrual cycle. May be multilocular or multiple and associated with other findings of fibrocystic disease. When multiple masses are present, it is essential that each be evaluated individually so that a well-defined carcinoma is not missed.
Fibroadenoma (Fig MA 1-2; see Fig MA 3-2)	Round, ovoid, or smoothly lobulated mass of medium density. Often contains calcification varying from punctate peripheral deposits to characteristic coarse, popcorn-like densities.	Common benign, estrogen-sensitive tumor that usually appears in adolescents and young women before age 30. Tumor growth may be enhanced by pregnancy or lactation. After menopause, the tumors undergo mucoid degeneration, hyalinize, and become calcified. Occasionally, myxoid degeneration in the mass can cause retraction of surrounding tissue and irregular, poorly circumscribed margins that simulate malignancy.

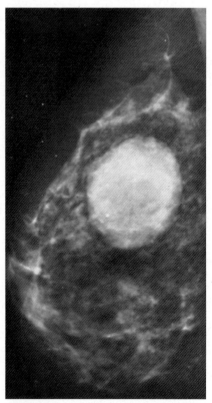

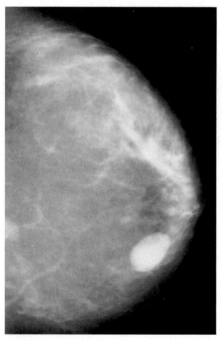

Fig MA 1-2
Fibroadenoma. Smooth, round mass with clearly defined margins.[2]

Fig MA 1-1
Benign cyst. Large homogeneous mass partially surrounded by a lucent halo.[1]

*High-density lesions are more dense than surrounding parenchyma. Structures such as veins, trabeculae, and the like cannot be seen "through" the lesion. Medium-density lesions have density similar to that of surrounding parenchymal structures (veins, trabeculae, and so forth), which can be seen "through" the lesion. Low-density lesions are less dense than surrounding breast parenchyma. Lucent lesions are of fat density

Condition	Imaging Findings	Comments
Carcinoma Medullary (Fig MA 1-3)	Medium- to high-density mass without calcification.	Represents approximately 4% of all malignant tumors of the breast. Because they are well demarcated and have a soft consistency, they can be mistaken for benign tumors both radiographically and clinically. They are typically located either deep in the breast or in the areolar or subcutaneous areas. Irregular margins can suggest underlying malignancy, although the border can be sharp, and there can even be a halo sign.
Mucinous (mucoid; colloid) (Fig MA 1-4)	Low-density mass because of the presence of mucin.	Represents approximately 3% of all breast malignancies. As with medullary carcinomas, mucoid carcinoma tends to be peripherally located and may mimic a benign process when its margins are well circumscribed and there is an associated halo sign.
Papillary (Fig MA 1-5)	Low-density mass.	Slow-growing tumors (intraductal, intracystic, and invasive types) that may mimic benign lesions on mammography. Calcification may develop in the wall of an intracystic papillary carcinoma.

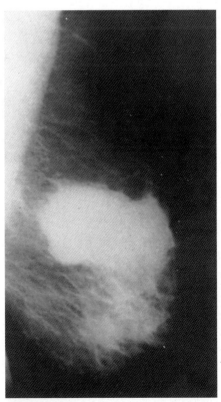

Fig MA 1-3
Medullary carcinoma. Large, lobulated, high-density mass.[3]

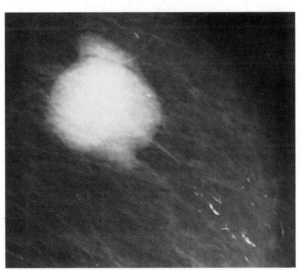

Fig MA 1-4
Mucinous carcinoma. Enlargement from a mediolateral view in an elderly woman with a palpable mass shows a large, lobulated mass of low density partially surrounded by a halo. Note the secretory calcifications.[1]

Condition	Imaging Findings	Comments
Papilloma (Fig MA 1-6)	Low- to medium-density mass. Crescent, rosette, or eggshell calcification can occur.	Most common cause of bloody or serious nipple discharge. Solitary papillomas usually develop in the retroareolar ducts; multiple papillomas generally occur in the peripheral ducts. Most papillomas are not detectable on mammography; intraductal papillomas may be shown on galactography. Intracystic papillomas may be visualized on pneumocystography.
Hematoma (Fig MA 1-7)	Medium- to high-density mass, often having slightly irregular margins. Overlying skin edema is usually present in the acute stage if the hematoma is secondary to trauma.	Most commonly caused by blunt or surgical trauma, although hematomas may develop in patients who are anticoagulated or have clotting abnormalities. The combination of hemorrhage and edema more commonly results in an ill-defined mass or a diffuse area of increased density. Although the mammographic findings simulate carcinoma, a history of trauma suggests a conservative approach. Follow-up examinations show gradual decrease in size or even disappearance of the lesion. An organized hematoma may occasionally persist as a more sharply defined mass.

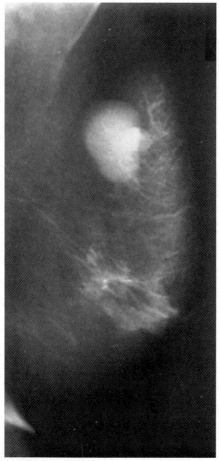

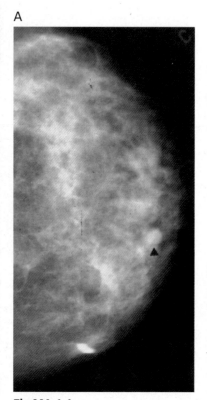

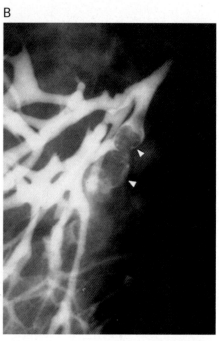

Fig MA 1-5
Papillary carcinoma. Large, low-density, lobulated mass with distinct margins.[1]

Fig MA 1-6
Papilloma. (A) Plain mammogram shows a possible nodule (arrowhead) on the craniocaudal projection that could not be confirmed on the mediolateral view. (B) Film obtained during galactography shows contrast material outlining a lobulated mass (arrowheads) in the region of the nodule.[4]

Condition	Imaging Findings	Comments
Lipoma (Fig MA 1-8)	Lucent mass with a thin surrounding capsule.	Common slow-growing benign tumor that usually presents in older women. More easily detected in a dense, fibroglandular breast than in the fatty replaced breast. Uncommon infarction may result in coarse or plaque-like calcifications. Lipomas can be mimicked by fatty lobules, which are partially surrounded by trabeculae and Cooper's ligaments.
Oil cyst (Fig MA 1-9)	Lucent mass surrounded by ring-like calcification.	Form of post-traumatic fat necrosis that may occur after breast surgery or trauma.
Galactocele (Fig MA 1-10)	Lucent or mixed-density mass that may demonstrate a characteristic fat-fluid level when imaged with a horizontal beam.	Milk-containing cyst caused by obstruction of a duct by inspissated milk in a woman who has abruptly stopped breast-feeding. The lucency reflects the lipid content of milk. Typically multiple, with individual lesions measuring less than 3 cm in diameter.
Fibroadenolipoma (hamartoma) (Fig MA 1-11)	Varies from a relatively lucent to a relatively dense mass, depending on the amount of fat compared to parenchymal tissue. Sharply demarcated capsule.	Uncommon benign tumor composed of normal or dysplastic mammary tissue, including adipose and fibrous tissues and ducts and lobules in variable amounts. Loss of normal architecture with lack of orientation of glandular elements toward the nipple results in an appearance resembling a slice of sausage.

A B

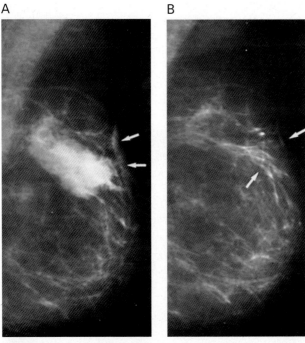

Fig MA 1-7
Hematoma. (A) Mammogram of a firm, palpable mass that arose at a recent biopsy site shows a dense lesion associated with skin thickening (arrows). (B) Three months later, there has been almost complete resolution of the hematoma with only minimal residual architectural distortion (arrows).[1]

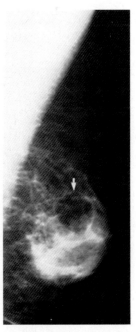

Fig MA 1-8
Lipoma. Well-delineated, 3-cm area of lucency with a surrounding capsule (arrow).[1]

Condition	Imaging Findings	Comments
Cystosarcoma phyllodes (Fig MA 1-12)	Solitary, large, rounded mass of medium to high density, or a conglomeration of smaller individual masses.	Rare fibroepithelial tumor. Approximately 80% are benign, although they can have tentacle-like projections extending out into the breast parenchyma that lead to recurrence after surgery. An indistinct portion of the margin of the tumor may indicate invasion into adjacent fibroglandular tissue. Coarse calcification in the mass suggests that it probably represents a large fibroadenoma.

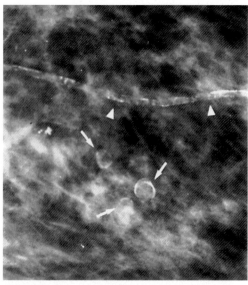

Fig MA 1-9
Oil cysts. Multiple, partially calcified cysts (arrows). Note the vascular calcification (arrowheads).[1]

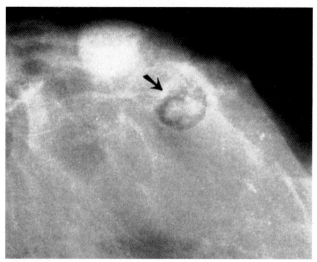

Fig MA 1-10
Galactocele. Sharply defined lesion (arrow) containing both lucent and opaque components in a young woman who noted a lump in her breast during nursing.[3]

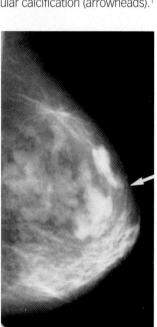

Fig MA 1-11
Fibroadenolipoma. Large, well-defined mass of mixed density in the upper central portion of the right breast. The mass contains fat as well as ovoid soft-tissue masses and is surrounded by a thin capsule (arrow).[2]

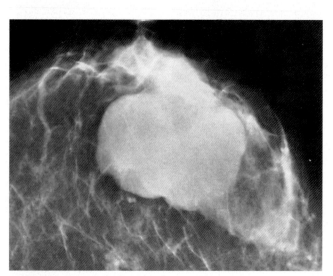

Fig MA 1-12
Cystosarcoma phyllodes. Huge, sharply outlined, radiopaque tumor that is mammographically benign.[5]

Condition	Imaging Findings	Comments
Metastasis (Fig MA 1-13)	Most commonly a solitary mass of medium density in a peripheral location (especially the superolateral quadrant). May present as multiple masses or as diffuse involvement of the breast.	Most frequently from a contralateral breast carcinoma, although a second primary breast carcinoma is far more common than a contralateral metastasis. Most frequent primary tumors that metastasize on the breast are melanoma, carcinoma of the lung, sarcoma, ovarian carcinoma, and lymphoma.
Skin lesions/ normal variants (Fig MA 1-14)	Medium-density lesion that is extremely well defined (as a result of air trapped around the lesion as it is compressed against the breast). Crenulated margin if the surface is irregular.	Epidermoid inclusion cyst, subcutaneous cyst, neurofibroma, mole, keratoses, retracted nipple. If the breast is turned with the lesion in tangent, the mass disappears or projects at the skin surface.
Nipple out of profile	Medium- to high-density appearance.	Different appearance of the "mass" on an orthogonal projection.
Intramammary lymph node (Fig MA 1-15)	Medium- to low-density lesion with a fatty notch or center. Often bilateral and multiple, and almost always located in the superolateral quadrant.	A node may increase in size and still be benign, although if it does not have a definable lucent hilum and measures 1 cm or more a biopsy may be necessary to exclude malignancy. Benign conditions associated with intramammary (as well as axillary) nodes include rheumatoid arthritis, sarcoidosis, psoriatic arthritis, and systemic lupus erythematosus.

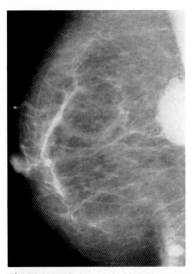

Fig MA 1-13
Metastasis from melanoma. Mediolateral oblique projection shows two circumscribed tumors near the chest wall.[5]

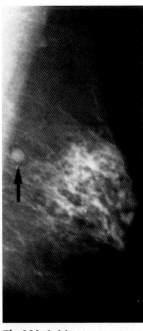

Fig MA 1-14
Mole on the skin surface. The broad rim of lucency surrounding the mass (arrow) indicates that it lies on the skin rather than in an intradermal or intraparenchymal location.[1]

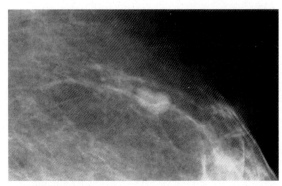

Fig MA 1-15
Intramammary lymph node. Typical well-defined, bean-shaped density in the superolateral quadrant.[1]

Ill-Defined Breast Masses

Condition	Imaging Findings	Comments
Carcinoma of the breast (Fig MA 2-1)	Distinct, irregular, central tumor mass from which dense spicules radiate in all directions. Spicules that reach the skin or muscle cause retraction and localized skin thickening.	This sunburst appearance is most commonly seen in scirrhous infiltrating ductal carcinoma. Associated malignant-type calcifications are common. A web-like pattern of spicules may be seen with invasive lobular carcinoma, which may be clinically obvious on palpation but difficult to detect on mammography.
Radial scar (sclerosing duct hyperplasia) (Fig MA 2-2)	Ill-defined lesion without a solid, dense, central tumor mass of a size corresponding to the length of the spicules. Characteristic lucent oval or circular areas at the center of the radiating structure. May contain coarse calcifications or microcalcifications.	Benign, rarely palpable lesion that often mimics carcinoma. It typically varies in appearance from one projection to another. Skin thickening and retraction over the lesion are infrequent. Because a precise mammographic diagnosis is difficult, biopsy and histologic examination usually are necessary to exclude malignancy.
Post-traumatic changes Fat necrosis (Fig MA 2-3)	Ill-defined, spiculated structure with no distinct central mass. Localized skin thickening and retraction may occur.	Nonsuppurative inflammatory response to trauma, including biopsy or surgery. Extensive fibrotic response may produce a spiculated mass resembling carcinoma; a mild response leads to the development of a thin-walled radiolucent oil cyst. A history of recent surgery or severe blunt trauma is helpful in excluding malignancy.
Hematoma (Fig MA 2-4)	May appear as an ill-defined lesion (more commonly a relatively well-defined mass or a diffuse increase in density).	Overlying skin thickening from edema and bruising may simulate carcinoma. Hematomas tend to resolve within 3–4 weeks.

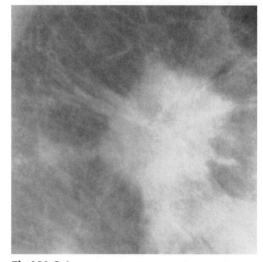

Fig MA 2-1
Breast cancer. Magnified coned view demonstrates an ill-defined, irregular mass with radiating spicules.

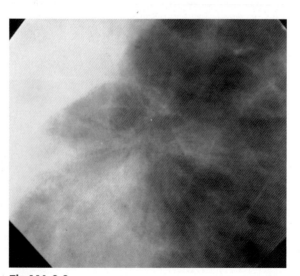

Fig MA 2-2
Radial scar. Note the absence of a central mass in this lesion, which was pathologically benign.[4]

Condition	Imaging Findings	Comments
Fibrocystic disease (Fig MA 2-5)	Various types of ill-defined lesions.	Focal fibrosis appears as dense tissue that is often irregularly marginated, may contain irregular microcalcifications, and may mimic carcinoma. In sclerosing adenosis, localized proliferation of lobules with surrounding fibrosis can simulate malignancy mammographically and even histologically.
Abscess (Fig MA 2-6)	Ill-defined mass often associated with skin thickening.	Abscesses tend to occur in lactating breasts, most often in the subareolar area.
Plasma cell mastitis (Fig MA 2-7)	Ill-defined mass with a prominent ductal pattern.	Ductal and periductal inflammatory process that typically occurs in the subareolar areas and tends to be bilateral. At times, the only manifestation may be an irregular, fan-shaped, subareolar density.
Hyalinized fibroadenoma	Ill-defined mass with radiating structures.	Myxoid degeneration rarely may result in retraction of the surrounding tissue to produce a lesion with radiating structures that changes with each projection. There may be associated coarse calcifications typical of fibroadenoma.

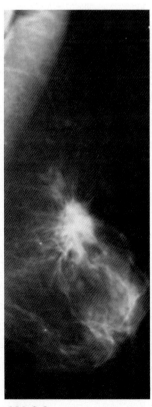

Fig MA 2-3
Fat necrosis. Mediolateral oblique view obtained 3 months after biopsy shows a dense, spiculated mass associated with architectural distortion and skin retraction and thickening.[1]

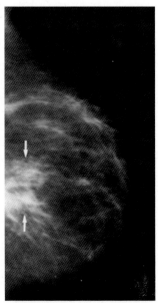

Fig MA 2-4
Hematoma. Ill-defined area of increased density (arrows) in the area of a lumpectomy performed 2 weeks previously.

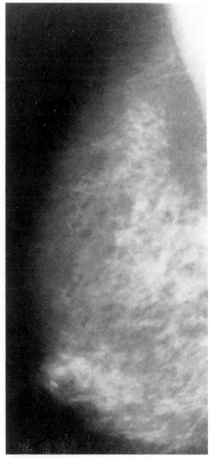

Fig MA 2-5
Fibrocystic disease. Ill-defined density indistinguishable from malignancy. Needle localization and biopsy revealed benign focal fibrosis.[3]

Condition	Imaging Findings	Comments
Granular cell myoblastoma (Fig MA 2-8)	Ill-defined stellate lesion.	Rare benign tumor that may produce a palpable lump suggestive of malignancy.

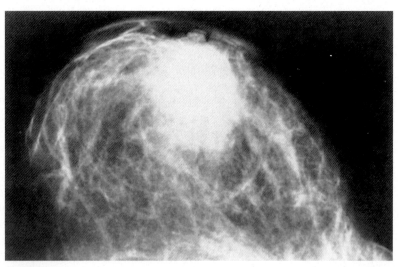

Fig MA 2-6
Abscess. Huge, dense, retroareolar mass with unsharp borders associated with nipple retraction and skin thickening over the areola.[5]

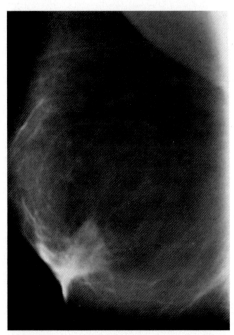

Fig MA 2-7
Plasma cell mastitis. Retroareolar triangle of increased density associated with nipple retraction.[1]

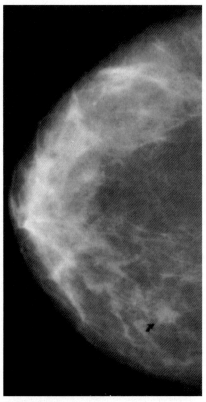

Fig MA 2-8
Granular cell myoblastoma. Ill-defined, low-density nodule (arrow) in an asymptomatic woman.[2]

Condition	Imaging Findings	Comments
Fibromatosis (Fig MA 2-9)	Ill-defined mass mimicking carcinoma.	Rare fibroblastic lesion that behaves in a locally invasive but nonmetastasizing manner. Breast involvement is thought to represent an extension from a lesion in the pectoralis fascia.
Pseudomass (summation shadows)	Ill-defined mass.	Overlapping glandular tissue may simulate a mass on one projection, but no similar mass is seen on an orthogonal view. Therefore, an area of asymmetric tissue must be identified on two views before it can be considered abnormal.

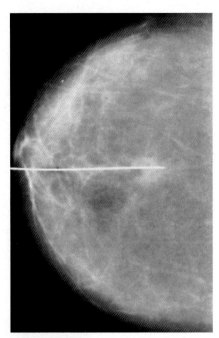

Fig MA 2-9
Fibromatosis. Craniocaudal view from a needle localization procedure shows an ill-defined, somewhat spiculated mass of medium density in the deep central portion of the left breast.[2]

Breast Calcifications

Condition	Imaging Findings	Comments
Carcinoma of the breast (Fig MA 3-1)	Calcification is extremely variable in distribution, size, form, density, and number. Malignant calcifications tend to form in clusters and are generally smaller, less dense, and more irregular than typical benign calcifications. In a single cluster, calcifications often vary in size, shape, and density.	Malignant calcifications can be detected mammographically in approximately 50% of cases. About 20% of breast carcinomas present only with calcification. Granular calcifications appear as tiny dot-like or somewhat elongated densities that are irregularly grouped close together in a cluster and resemble a stone crushed by a sledgehammer. *Casting calcification* refers to that formed in segments of irregular ductal lumen containing necrosis and debris from increased cellular activity.
Fibroadenoma (Fig MA 3-2)	Large, coarse, irregular but sharply outlined, dense calcifications.	As an old fibroadenoma undergoes myxoid degeneration, the soft-tissue component often regresses and is totally replaced by typical dense calcification. Peripheral eggshell-like calcification can occur rarely. In the early stages of calcification, a few punctate peripheral microcalcifications may develop that mimic malignancy and require biopsy. Rarely, granular or casting calcifications (or both) may be detected in a carcinoma arising in a fibroadenoma.
Cyst (Fig MA 3-3)	Thin rim of calcification.	Although almost invariably benign, a small retroareolar eggshell-like calcification rarely may be the result of bleeding in an intracystic carcinoma.

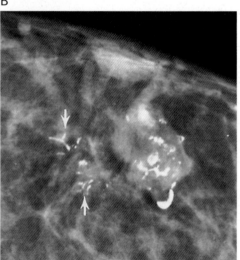
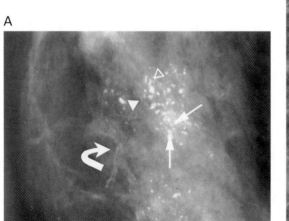

Fig MA 3-1
Carcinoma of the breast. (A) Numerous tiny calcific particles with linear (arrows), curvilinear (solid arrowhead), and branching (open arrowhead) forms characteristic of malignancy. Note the benign calcification in the wall of an artery, which is easily recognized by its large size and tubular distribution (curved arrow). (B) Magnification view in another patient shows a retroareolar tumor containing coarse calcifications. One centimeter medial to the tumor is a small cluster of calcifications (arrows) without a tumor shadow.[5]

Condition	Imaging Findings	Comments
Lobular-type calcifications (Fig MA 3-4)	Homogeneous, solid, sharply outlined, spherical densities. In large cavities, "milk of calcium" in the cystic fluid may settle to the dependent portion of the cavities and appear on upright lateral projections with a horizontal beam as crescent-shaped or elongated calcifications resembling a teacup seen from the side. On the craniocaudal projection with a vertical beam, these calcifications are less clearly seen and appear as poorly defined smudges.	This pattern of calcification in dilated ductules and lobules may be seen in such pathologic entities as sclerosing adenosis, atypical lobular hyperplasia, cystic hyperplasia, and blunt duct adenosis. Lobular-type calcifications may be numerous and scattered throughout much of the breast parenchyma. Milk of calcium secreted into the cyst fluid is seen in cystic hyperplasia; in sclerosing adenosis, extensive fibrosis compresses the lobules to produce multiple tiny dots of high density.
Fat necrosis Liponecrosis microcystica calcificans (Fig MA 3-5)	Single or multiple, small, smooth, ring-like calcifications. Typically dense, uniform calcification in the periphery with a lucent center.	May appear as solid, dense, spherical calcifications. Occasionally, irregular microcalcifications may be suspicious-looking enough to require biopsy.
Oil cyst (Fig MA 3-6)	Circumferential eggshell-like calcification surrounding a lucent mass.	Fatty acids precipitate as calcium soaps at the surface of the surrounding fibrous capsule, eventually forming a thin layer of calcification about the oil cyst.

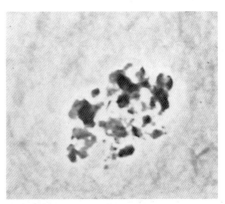

Fig MA 3-2
Fibroadenoma. Typical large and popcorn appearance of calcification in a degenerating lesion.

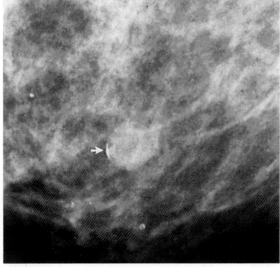

Fig MA 3-3
Cyst. A thin layer of calcification is seen in a portion of the cyst wall (arrow).[3]

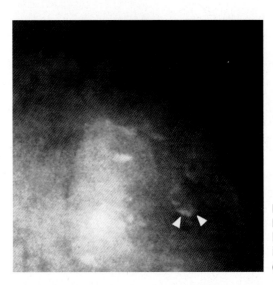

Fig MA 3-4
Lobular-type calcifications. Enlarged view of the upper breast in an asymptomatic woman shows "teacup" gravity-dependent calcifications of cystic lobular hyperplasia (arrowheads).[1]

Condition	Imaging Findings	Comments
Post–radiation therapy	Dense round or ring-like calcifications.	Dystrophic calcification identical to that of fat necrosis from trauma or biopsy. This appearance should not be confused with the lacy, linear, irregular microcalcifications that indicate recurrent carcinoma.
Plasma cell mastitis (secretory disease) (Fig MA 3-7)	Large, smooth, homogeneously dense calcifications that may be round, ovoid, linear, or needle-like with a branching pattern. The calcifications contain hollow centers if they are periductal in location.	Aseptic inflammation of the breast in which mucinous fluid fills the lobules and ducts and often extravasates into periductal connective tissue. Calcifications may be in the duct or periductal and tend to be multiple and bilateral. They can be differentiated from the malignant casting-type calcifications of intraductal carcinoma because of their high and uniform density, generally wider caliber, and tendency to follow the course of normal ducts and to be oriented toward the nipple.
Miscellaneous benign lesions Lipoma	Ring-like calcification (typical of fat necrosis), or a larger and coarser lesion.	Uncommon appearance that presumably reflects infarction or fat necrosis. The presence of a radiolucent mass with associated calcification should not suggest malignancy.

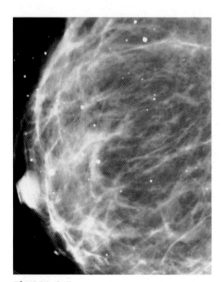

Fig MA 3-5
Liponecrosis microcystica calcificans. Multiple, round, dense calcifications with central lucencies. Most if not all of the calcifications lie in the subcutaneous fat.[5]

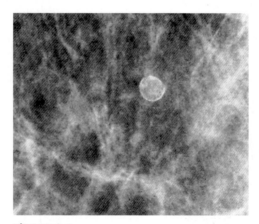

Fig MA 3-6
Oil cyst. Magnified image shows a circumlinear calcification surrounding a lucent fatty center.[2]

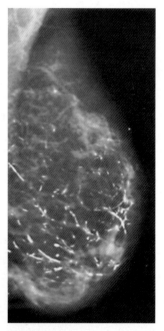

Fig MA 3-7
Plasma cell mastitis. Multiple, large, dense, needle-like intraductal secretory calcifications. Note their orientation toward the nipple.[1]

Condition	Imaging Findings	Comments
Intraductal papilloma (Fig MA 3-8)	Pattern varying from a few to a cluster of stippled calcifications simulating malignancy to a larger, denser, rounded calcification conforming to the walls of the duct.	Papillomas tend to become fibrotic or to infarct, possibly because these polypoid lesions may have a tenuous blood supply via their stalks.
Galactocele	Ring-like or eggshell-like calcification in the capsule.	Lucent or mixed-density mass that may contain a characteristic fat-fluid level when imaged with a horizontal beam.
Breast augmentation (Fig MA 3-9)	Round or cyst-like calcifications in multiple small nodules in dense breasts.	The nodular deposits may be related to fat necrosis and foreign body reaction or to the presence of silicone itself.
Arterial calcification (Fig MA 3-10)	Linear parallel streaks that may be discontinuous and follow a sinuous course.	Most commonly occurs as a result of atherosclerosis in elderly women or in patients with renal failure. Arterial calcification also may be more frequent in the breasts of patients with diabetes or hypertension.

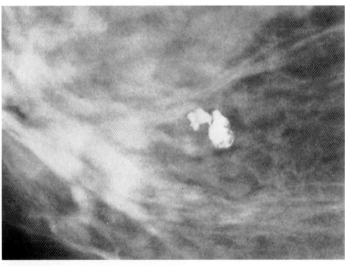

Fig MA 3-8
Intraductal papilloma. Totally calcified solitary lesion.[5]

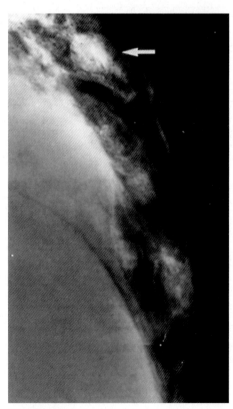

Fig MA 3-9
Breast augmentation. Multiple ring-like calcific densities (arrow) of various sizes throughout the breast.[2]

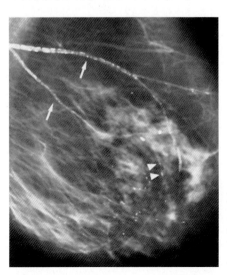

Fig MA 3-10
Arterial calcification. Well-developed vascular calcifications appear as parallel discontinuous bands (arrows). Early vascular calcifications are more isolated (arrowheads). Scattered secretory calcifications are also present.[1]

Condition	Imaging Findings	Comments
Skin calcifications (Fig MA 3-11)	Peripheral, well-demarcated, ring-like or spherical calcifications lying outside the breast parenchyma.	Very common. Sebaceous cyst calcifications are typically small and numerous and contain lucent centers. Other skin lesions that may calcify include nevi, hemangiomas, skin tags, and the dystrophic calcification associated with scarring.
Pseudocalcifications (Fig MA 3-12)	Various patterns.	Powders, creams, and ointments (especially those containing zinc oxide) appear as fine granular densities over the surface of the breast. Deodorants tend to produce larger, more clustered densities in the area of the axillary folds.

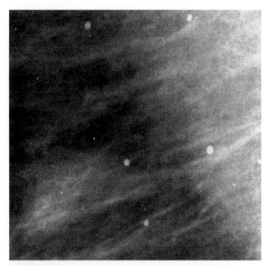

Fig MA 3-11
Sebaceous cysts. Magnification view shows several rounded calcifications containing central lucencies.[1]

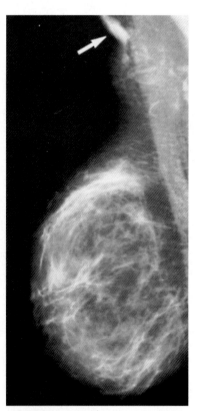

Fig MA 3-12
Pseudocalcifications. Calcific-like densities superimposed over the axillary folds (arrow) represent a deodorant artifact.[2]

Skin Thickening

Condition	Comments
Carcinoma of the breast (Figs MA 4-1 and MA 4-2)	Extension of tumor into lymphatic vessels can produce focal skin thickening and increased density of the subcutaneous tissue. In inflammatory carcinoma (1–2% of all breast malignancies), intense edema causes rapid enlargement and tenderness of the affected breast with diffuse skin thickening. The breast may become so dense that the internal architecture cannot be visualized.
Axillary lymphatic obstruction Metastases from breast carcinoma	Stagnation of fluid in the breast may make physical examination difficult. Resulting lymphedema produces increased mammographic density and a coarse reticular pattern. If no obvious malignancy is noted, one should closely check the axillary tail for direct extension of a small tumor and the area behind the nipple (extensive network of lymphatics permits early spread).

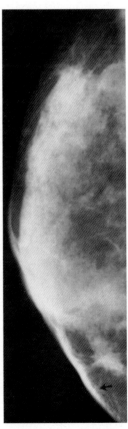

Fig MA 4-1
Infiltrating ductal carcinoma. Focal skin thickening (arrow) on the lower aspect of the breast. Beneath the thickening is a 1-cm spiculated mass that is tethering the skin.[2]

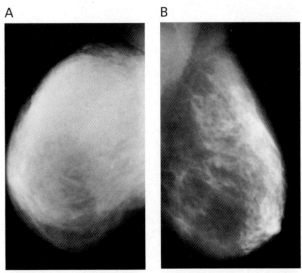

Fig MA 4-2
Inflammatory carcinoma. There is strikingly increased density of the left breast relative to the right and diffuse thickening of the skin. A large, rounded mass is noted in the upper outer quadrant.[2]

Condition	Comments
Metastases from non-breast primaries (Fig MA 4-3)	Advanced gynecologic malignancies (ovarian, uterine) rarely may block primary lymphatic drainage in the lesser pelvis, causing lymph flow through thoracoepigastric collaterals and overloading the axillary and supraclavicular lymphatic drainage.
Lymphoma	Lymphedema pattern may be secondary to lymphatic obstruction from malignant axillary nodes or the result of infiltration of the breast.
Postoperative axillary node removal or dissection	Edema of the breast may persist mammographically even when it is not obvious clinically. If axillary node dissection has been performed for metastatic disease (eg, melanoma) and skin thickening occurs, it may be impossible to determine whether this appearance represents metastatic involvement of the breast or impaired lymphatic drainage from surgery.
Radiation therapy (Fig MA 4-4)	Skin thickening and edema are most prominent during the first 6 months after treatment and gradually decline. If skin thickening and breast edema recur after the initial edema has resolved or decreased, recurrent carcinoma should be considered.

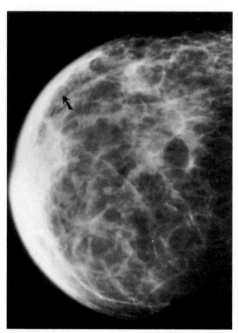

Fig MA 4-3
Metastatic melanoma. Marked skin thickening (arrow) is associated with a diffuse increase in the density of the interstitium.[2]

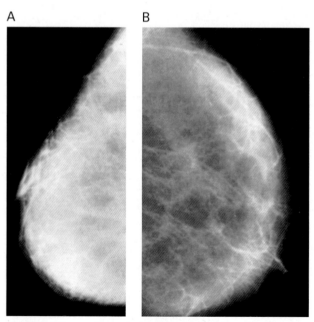

A   B

Fig MA 4-4
Radiation therapy. (A) Initial mammogram after lumpectomy and radiation therapy for a carcinoma in the lower inner quadrant of the breast. (B) Three years later, an oblique view shows marked skin thickening with diffusely increased density of the breast near the chest wall.[2]

Condition	Comments
Mastitis/breast abscess (Fig MA 4-5)	Focal or diffuse skin thickening that may be related to lactation, skin or nipple infection with extension into the breast, or hematogenous spread of infection.
Fat necrosis/interstitial hematoma (Fig MA 4-6)	Usually focal skin thickening, unless the trauma is severe or the hemorrhage is extensive. Clinical history is essential because post-traumatic changes with skin involvement may mimic locally advanced breast cancer.
Mediastinal blockage	May cause bilateral skin thickening. Underlying etiologies include Hodgkin's disease, advanced bronchial or esophageal carcinoma with mediastinal metastases, and advanced sarcoidosis.

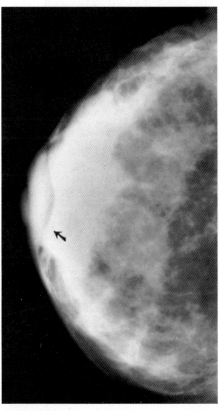

Fig MA 4-5
Mastitis with breast abscess. Prominent skin thickening over the areola (arrow) and diffuse skin thickening elsewhere. Generalized increased density in the area of the subareolar lactiferous ducts.[2]

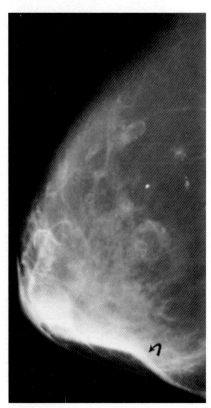

Fig MA 4-6
Fat necrosis. Mammogram obtained 6 months after severe blunt trauma to the breast shows skin thickening and retraction inferiorly (arrow) associated with multiple lucent masses with rim-like calcifications, typical of fat necrosis and oil cysts.[2]

Condition	Comments
Fluid overload state	Bilateral, diffuse skin thickening may develop in patients with cardiac failure, renal failure, cirrhosis, and hypoalbuminemia. The thickening occurs mostly in the dependent aspect of the breast. In a bedridden patient lying on one side, the skin thickening may be unilateral and involve only the dependent breast.
Chronic graft-versus-host disease (Fig MA 4-7)	Bilateral, diffuse skin thickening causing pruritus.

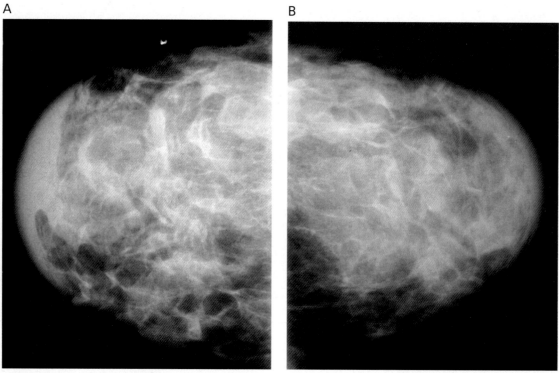

Fig MA 4-7
Chronic graft-versus-host disease. Craniocaudal mammograms of the right (A) and left (B) breasts show marked bilateral skin thickening. The periareolar skin of the right breast exceeds 1 cm in thickness. A screening mammogram obtained 3 years earlier showed no skin thickening.[6]

Sources

1. Reprinted from Handbook of Breast Imaging by ME Peters, DR Voegeli, and KA Scanlan (Eds) with permission of Churchill Livingstone, Inc, ©1989.

2. Reprinted from Atlas of Film-Screen Mammography by ES deParedes with permission of Urban and Schwarzenberg, ©1989.

3. Reprinted from Breast Imaging by DB Kopans with permission of JB Lippincott Company, ©1989.

4. Courtesy of Gunnar Cederbom, MD.

5. Reprinted from Teaching Atlas of Mammography by L Tabar and PB Dean with permission of Georg Thieme Verlag, ©1985.

6. Reprinted with permission from "Chronic Graft-Versus-Host Disease Causing Skin Thickening on Mammograms" by KA Scanlan and PA Propeck, *AJR Am J Roentgenol* (1995;165:555–556).

9

Fetal Ultrasound

Ultrasound Diagnosis of Fetal Anomalies

Condition	Imaging Findings	Comments
Central nervous system		
Anencephaly (Fig FUS 1-1)	Inability to identify normal brain tissue cephalad to the bony orbits or brainstem along with symmetric absence of the bony calvarium.	First congenital anomaly identified in utero with ultrasound. The diagnosis can be made as early as the 12th week of gestation and is typically made at the time of an attempted biparietal diameter determination for fetal age.
Encephalocele (Fig FUS 1-2)	Spherical fluid- or brain-filled sac extending through a defect in the bony calvarium.	Most commonly occurs in the occipital region in the midline (70%). Also can develop in the parietal, frontal, or nasal area.
Spina bifida (Figs FUS 1-3 and FUS 1-4)	Separation or outward splaying of posterior ossification centers on transverse and longitudinal scans. On sagittal scans, disappearance of a portion of the echoes representing the posterior elements of the vertebrae (also may be produced artifactually by transducer position), frequently with loss of overlying soft tissues.	Midline defect of the vertebrae, usually localized to the posterior arch, that results in exposure of the contents of the neural canal. Most common malformation of the central nervous system. Easily diagnosed if three or more vertebral segments are involved; may be difficult to detect if only one or two spinal segments are affected.
Meningocele/ myelomeningocele (Fig FUS 1-5)	Fluid- or neural-tissue–filled sac extending beyond the spinal canal and associated with spina bifida.	Most common in the lumbar and sacral regions. Associated with numerous intracranial anomalies, especially the Chiari II malformation.
Dandy-Walker malformation (Fig FUS 1-6)	Cystic mass in the posterior fossa associated with a defect in or agenesis of the vermis and separation of the cerebellar hemispheres.	Spectrum of disorders characterized by abnormal development of the cerebellum and fourth ventricle. Commonly associated with hydrocephalus.
Complete agenesis of corpus callosum (Fig FUS 1-7)	Increased separation of the lateral ventricles. Enlargement of the occipital horns and atria. Upward displacement of the third ventricle.	Although occasionally seen as an isolated lesion, agenesis of the corpus callosum frequently is associated with various other central nervous system malformations and syndromes.

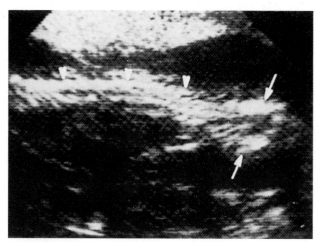

Fig FUS 1-1
Anencephaly. Long-axis image of a 14-week fetus demonstrates a poorly developed, small head (arrows) visualized in continuity with the fetal spine (arrowhead).[1]

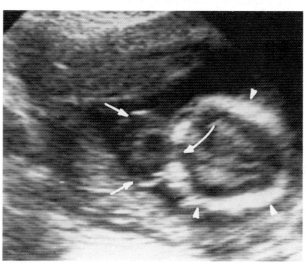

Fig FUS 1-2
Small occipital encephalocele. A complex mass (straight arrows) is seen posterior to a normally shaped head (arrowheads). There is a defect in the occipital bone of the calvarium in the posterior midline (curved arrow).[1]

Condition	Imaging Findings	Comments
Hydranencephaly (Fig FUS 1-8)	Large cystic mass filling the entire intracranial cavity with absence or discontinuity of the cerebral cortex and the midline echo. Brainstem typically bulges inside the cystic cavity.	Complete or nearly complete destruction of the cerebral cortex and basal ganglia with replacement by cerebrospinal fluid. Thought to be related to carotid artery occlusion in utero.

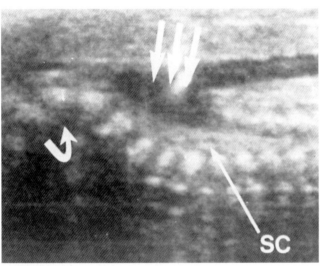

Fig FUS 1-3
Spina bifida. Sagittal scan of the spine shows a large spina bifida (triple arrow) and severe kyphoscoliosis (curved arrow). (SC, spinal cord.)[2]

Fig FUS 1-4
Spina bifida. Transverse scan of the fetal body shows absence of the soft tissue overlying the spine in the area of the defect (large arrows). Note the typical separation of the articular elements (small arrows).[2]

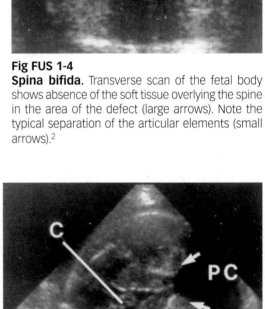

Fig FUS 1-5
Myelomeningocele. Longitudinal scan clearly shows the sac (M) extending beyond the spinal canal. (I, ischial ossification center; S, sacral promontory.)[3]

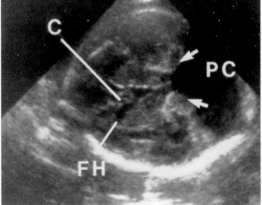

Fig FUS 1-6
Dandy-Walker malformation. Posterior fossa cyst (PC) with wide separation of the cerebellar hemispheres (arrows). (C, cavum septi pellucidi; FH, frontal horn.)[3]

Condition	Imaging Findings	Comments
Porencephaly (Fig FUS 1-9)	Intracranial cystic lesion communicating with the ventricular system. Generally, enlargement of the ipsilateral ventricle. Porencephaly is most commonly associated with cavitation of an intraparenchymal hematoma secondary to a postnatal subependymal bleed in a premature infant.	Local destruction of brain parenchyma by infarction or hemorrhage with subsequent necrosis of the destroyed area and gradual evacuation of contents into the adjacent ventricular lumen. Because the ischemic event is often more widespread than the resulting focal infarction, the hemisphere tends to be small and the ipsilateral ventricle large.
Holoprosencephaly (Fig FUS 1-10)	Spectrum of complex patterns that, in the most severe forms, includes a single ventricle and an array of facial deformities.	Complex developmental abnormality of the brain arising from failure of cleavage of the forebrain.
Choroid plexus cyst (Fig FUS 1-11)	Round hyperechoic area in the choroid plexus, most frequently at the level of the atrium of the lateral ventricle.	Common finding, probably of no clinical significance. Must be differentiated from hyperechoic choroid plexus papilloma.
Choroid plexus papilloma	Bright echogenic mass at the level of the atrium of one lateral ventricle.	Rare intracranial neoplasm that may be benign or malignant and causes severe hydrocephalus secondary to overproduction of cerebrospinal fluid.
Hydrocephalus (Fig FUS 1-12)	Variable pattern of ventricular enlargement.	Most common congenital forms are aqueductal stenosis (enlargement of the lateral and third ventricles but normal fourth ventricle), communicating hydrocephalus (generalized dilatation of the lateral, third, and fourth ventricles, although the fourth ventricular enlargement may be minimal and difficult to detect), and Dandy-Walker syndrome (associated posterior fossa cyst and defect in the cerebellar vermis).

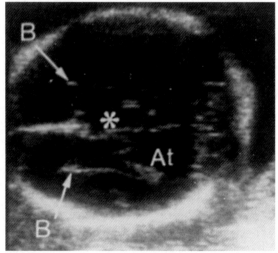

Fig FUS 1-7
Agenesis of the corpus callosum. Axial scan passing through the lateral ventricles demonstrates typical enlargement of the atria (At) as well as the widely separated bodies (B) and upward displacement of the third ventricle (*).[2]

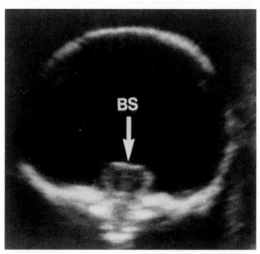

Fig FUS 1-8
Hydranencephaly. Typical appearance of the brainstem (BS) bulging inside an entirely fluid-filled intracranial cavity.[4]

Condition	Imaging Findings	Comments
Microcephaly	Suspected if the head perimeter is 3 SD below the mean for gestational age. If the head perimeter is 2 to 3 SD below the mean, suggestive signs include sloping forehead and dilatation of the lateral ventricles.	Clinical syndrome characterized by a head circumference less than the normal range and associated with abnormal neurologic findings and subnormal mental development. Causes include genetic defects, various prenatal infections, and drug or chemical exposures.

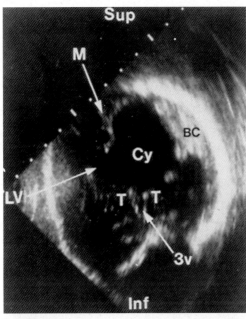

Fig FUS 1-9
Porencephaly. Coronal scan shows a large cystic cavity (Cy) occupying most of one hemisphere and amply communicating with the contralateral ventricle (LV). The hyperechoic area seen close to the parietal bone was found at birth to be a large blood clot (BC). (Inf, inferior; M, midline; Sup, superior; T, thalami; 3v, third ventricle.)[2]

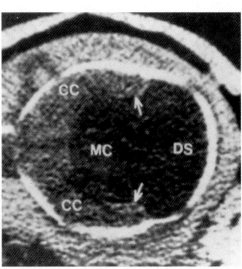

Fig FUS 1-10
Holoprosencephaly. Transverse axial scan shows a monoventricle (MC) communicating with the dorsal sac (DS). The line of demarcation (arrows) is the hippocampal ridge. The cerebral cortex (CC) is anteriorly displaced.[5]

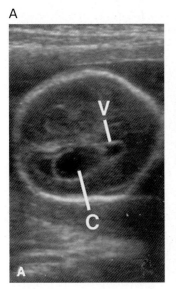
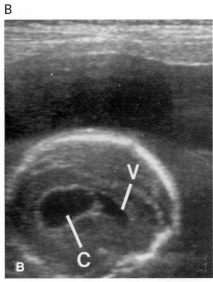

Fig FUS 1-11
Choroid plexus cyst. (A) Axial and (B) parasagittal scans show a cyst (C) so large that it expands the ventricle (V).[1]

Condition	Imaging Findings	Comments
Arachnoid cyst (Fig FUS 1-13)	Fluid-filled structure in the intracranial cavity (often impossible to distinguish from other cystic lesions).	Arachnoid cysts located on the surface of the brain and major fissures must be distinguished from porencephaly (which communicates with the ventricular system and is usually associated with ventriculomegaly and a shift in the midline) and brain tumors (which are usually inside the brain substance rather than located extra-axially). Posterior fossa arachnoid cysts must be differentiated from Dandy-Walker syndrome, in which there is a defect in the cerebellar vermis.
Face and neck Hypertelorism (Fig FUS 1-14)	Increased interorbital distance.	May occur as an isolated defect (cosmetic problem that may impair stereoscopic binocular vision) or be associated with a variety of other congenital malformations.

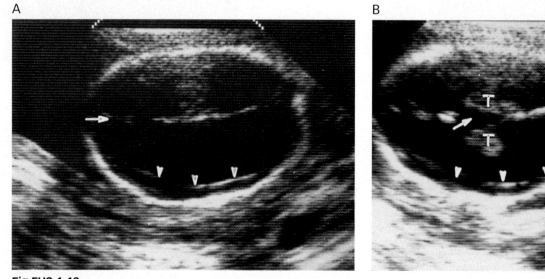

A   B

Fig FUS 1-12
Severe hydrocephalus secondary to aqueductal stenosis. (A) Transverse sonogram shows markedly dilated lateral ventricles (arrowheads) widely separated from the midline (arrow). (B) Transaxial view at a slightly lower level demonstrates a dilated third ventricle (arrow) between the thalami (T). The arrowheads denote the remaining cortical mantle.[1]

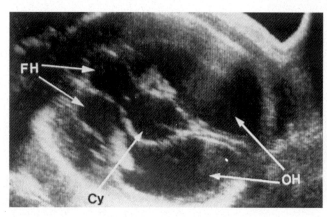

Fig FUS 1-13
Arachnoid cyst at the level of the interhemispheric fissure. There is an echo-spared area (Cy) at the midline with associated hydrocephalus. (FH, frontal horns; OH, occipital horns.)[2]

Condition	Imaging Findings	Comments
Hypotelorism (Fig FUS 1-15)	Decreased interorbital distance.	Associated with holoprosencephaly, microcephaly, and several chromosomal abnormalities (including trisomy 21 and trisomy 18).
Cyclopia (Fig FUS 1-16)	Single midline orbital fossa with a single or partially divided primitive eye.	Extreme form of hypotelorism that is usually associated with holoprosencephaly and a supraorbital proboscis.

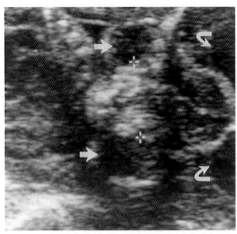

Fig FUS 1-14
Hypertelorism. Axial view through the orbits (arrows) demonstrates an increased interorbital distance between the calipers (+), which measured 23 mm compared with a normal of 18 mm for a fetus of this gestation age (29 weeks). The fetus also has hydrocephalus (curved arrows).[6]

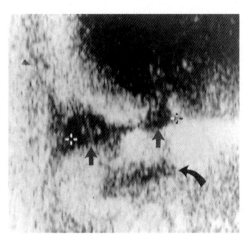

Fig FUS 1-15
Hypotelorism. Coronal view of the face of a fetus with holoprosencephaly demonstrates a decreased interorbital distance between the calipers (+), which measured 37 mm compared with a normal of 52 mm for a fetus of this gestational age (32 weeks). Asymmetric microphthalmos (arrows) is also evident. The curved arrow indicates the fetal mouth.[6]

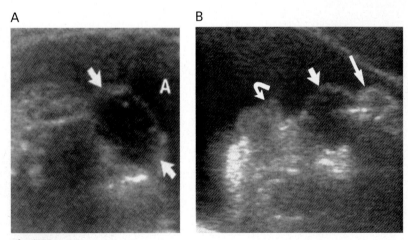

Fig FUS 1-16
Cyclopia. (A) Axial scan shows a solitary, midline, widened bony orbit (arrows) with a fused primitive globe. (A, anterior.) (B) Sagittal profile view of the fetal face demonstrates cyclopia (short straight arrow), midline proboscis cephalad to the fused orbit (long straight arrow), and the lips (curved arrow). The fetus also had holoprosencephaly.[7]

Condition	Imaging Findings	Comments
Cleft lip/cleft palate (Figs FUS 1-17 and FUS 1-18)	Various forms of midline and lateral defects involving the lip, palate, or both.	Most common congenital facial malformation (occurring in 1 of 700 live births in the United States).
Cystic hygroma (Fig FUS 1-19)	Asymmetric, thin-walled, multiseptate cystic mass involving the posterior neck bilaterally.	Anomaly composed of hugely dilated cystic lymphatic spaces. Up to 70% are found in fetuses with an abnormal karyotype (most commonly Turner's syndrome or trisomy 21). The development of associated fetal hydrops is nearly always fatal. A characteristic finding in cystic hygroma is a midline septation (representing the nuchal ligament), which permits differentiation of this entity from an occipital meningocele.
Abdominal wall Gastroschisis (Fig FUS 1-20)	Herniation of abdominal contents through a paraumbilical defect (usually on the right). The umbilical cord is normally connected to the abdominal wall, and the herniated organs float freely in the amniotic cavity (not covered by a membrane).	Herniation of visceral organs through a relatively small defect involving all layers of the anterior abdominal wall. Results from vascular compromise of either the umbilical vein or the omphalomesenteric artery.
Omphalocele (Fig FUS 1-21)	Large midline abdominal wall defect with herniated organs covered by a membrane that is continuous with the umbilical cord.	Unlike gastroschisis, the presence of a limiting membrane in omphalocele ordinarily prevents bowel from being exposed to amniotic fluid, so that it does not become thickened or matted. Furthermore, omphalocele is commonly associated with liver involvement, ascites, and cardiac and chromosomal abnormalities.

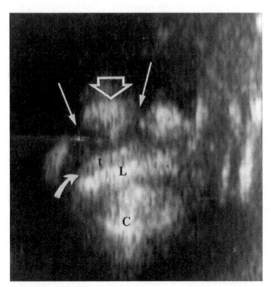

Fig FUS 1-17
Bilateral lateral cleft lip. Angled coronal image of the fetal face through the nose (open arrow) demonstrates bilateral clefts (arrows) through the upper lips extending into the nares. The mouth (curved arrow) is open. (C, chin; L, lower lip; t, tongue.)[6]

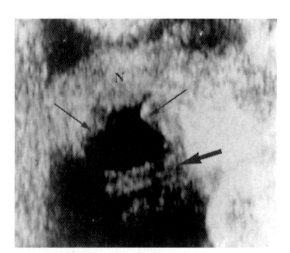

Fig FUS 1-18
Midline cleft lip. Coronal image shows a prominent medial cleft (thin arrows). The hypoechoic muscle of the lower lip is marked by the thick arrow. (N, nose.)[6]

Condition	Imaging Findings	Comments
Limb-body wall complex (body stalk anomaly) (Fig FUS 1-22)	Herniation of abdominal and thoracic contents through a large defect in the anterior abdominal wall.	Fatal malformation characterized by absence of the umbilicus and umbilical cord, with the placenta being directly attached to the herniated viscera. Complex anomaly with associated neural, gastrointestinal, genitourinary, and skeletal defects.

A   B

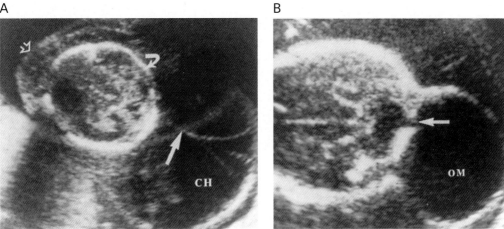

Fig FUS 1-19
Cystic hygroma versus occipital meningocele. (A) Axial plane image shows a huge cystic hygroma (CH) that extends from the fetal neck to envelop the fetal head (curved arrow). Note the characteristic midline septation (straight arrow) in the cystic hygroma that represents the nuchal ligament. The skin of the fetal scalp is markedly thickened because of hydrops (open arrow). (B) Axial plane image through the skull of another fetus shows an occipital meningioma (OM) as a cystic mass extending through a defect (arrow) in the occipital cranium. No septations are seen within the mass.[6]

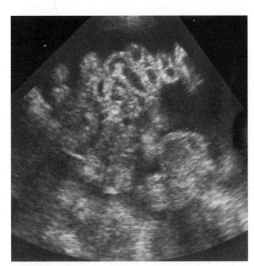

Fig FUS 1-20
Gastroschisis. Sonogram of a 37-week fetus shows mildly dilated, thickened small bowel loops floating in the amniotic fluid.[3]

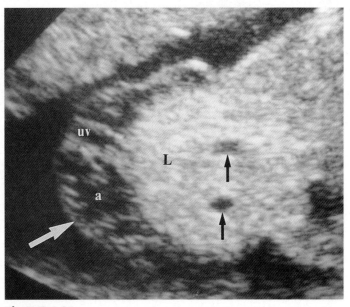

Fig FUS 1-21
Omphalocele. Axial plane image demonstrates an omphalocele containing liver (L). There is a highly visible covering membrane (large white arrow) that is outlined by amniotic fluid and fetal ascites (a). The liver is identified by its echotexture and blood vessels (small black arrows). The umbilical vein (uv) is part of the herniated mass.[8]

Condition	Imaging Findings	Comments
Congenital diaphragmatic hernia (Fig FUS 1-23)	Visualization of fluid-filled bowel at the level of the four-chamber view of the heart. Shift in position of the heart and mediastinum in the chest. Polyhydramnios is common (thought to be secondary to bowel obstruction).	Protrusion of the abdominal organs into the thoracic cavity through a diaphragmatic defect, most commonly on the left. Right diaphragmatic hernia is difficult to diagnose because of the similar echogenicity of liver and lung. A helpful hint is the identification of a fluid-filled gallbladder, which is frequently herniated into the chest. A major complication is ipsilateral pulmonary hypoplasia.
Gastrointestinal tract Esophageal atresia (Fig FUS 1-24)	Failure to visualize the stomach on serial examinations; associated with polyhydramnios.	More than 90% of cases of esophageal atresia cannot be diagnosed by ultrasound because gastric secretion or the occurrence of a tracheoesophageal fistula will allow visualization of some gastric distention.
Duodenal atresia (Fig FUS 1-25)	Characteristic double-bubble sign with associated polyhydramnios.	Most common type of congenital small bowel obstruction. The double-bubble sign reflects simultaneous distention of the stomach and the first portion of the duodenum.
Intestinal obstruction (atresia/stenosis) (Fig FUS 1-26)	Multiple distended, fluid-filled bowel loops. Polyhydramnios is seen with high small bowel obstructions (jejunal and duodenal).	Generally results from a vascular insult during fetal life rather than a disorder of embryogenesis. Differential diagnosis includes such causes of intra-abdominal anechoic lesions as duodenal atresia, hydronephrosis, ovarian cyst, and mesenteric cyst.

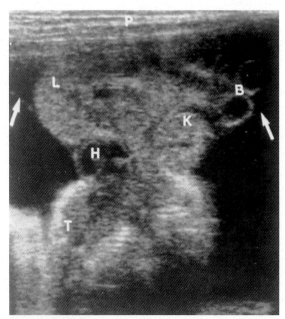

Fig FUS 1-22
Body stalk anomaly. Herniation of the viscera in proximity with the placenta. The condition was suspected because the infant was constantly apposed to one uterine wall. (B, bowel loops; H, heart; K, kidney; L, liver; P, placenta; T, thorax.)[10]

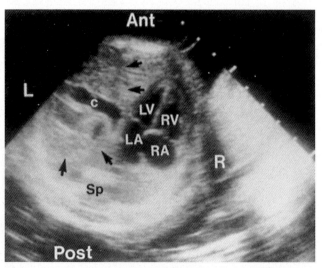

Fig FUS 1-23
Congenital diaphragmatic hernia. Transverse scan at the level of the heart shows a striking mediastinal shift with deviation of the heart to the right. The left hemithorax is occupied by a complex mass (arrows) with cystic components (c). (Ant, anterior; L, left; LA, left atrium; LV, left ventricle; Post, posterior; R, right; RA, right atrium; RV, right ventricle; Sp, spine.)[2]

Condition	Imaging Findings	Comments
Meconium peritonitis (Fig FUS 1-27)	Hyperechoic intra-abdominal mass with acoustic shadowing (representing calcium deposits); usually associated with ascites and polyhydramnios. Adhesions and calcifications tend to be more prominent than actual masses.	Peritoneal and inflammatory reaction secondary to intrauterine bowel perforation. In many cases, the perforation heals spontaneously; at times, an intense chemical reaction of the peritoneum leads to the formation of a dense mass with calcium deposits that eventually seals off the perforation.
Abdominal cysts (Fig FUS 1-28)	Anechoic, fluid-filled masses that may attain great size.	Diagnostic possibilities include mesenteric, choledochal, ovarian, urachal, and renal cysts; gut duplication cysts; and cystic teratoma.

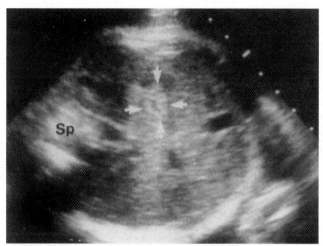

Fig FUS 1-24
Esophageal atresia. Transverse scan of the fetal abdomen shows nonvisualization of the normal stomach. The arrows point to the collapsed wall of the stomach. (Sp, spine.)[2]

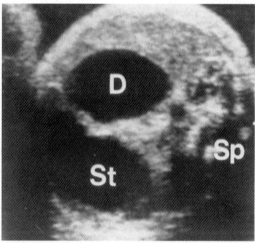

Fig FUS 1-25
Duodenal atresia. Transverse scan of the upper abdomen shows the typical double bubble. (D, dilated duodenal bulb; Sp, spine; St, stomach.)[2]

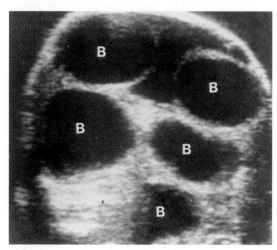

Fig FUS 1-26
Small bowel atresia. Transverse scan of the abdomen shows multiple dilated bowel loops (B). In the real-time examination, increased peristalsis was seen.[2]

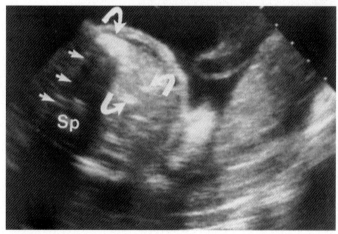

Fig FUS 1-27
Meconium peritonitis. Transverse scan shows multiple intra-abdominal calcifications (curved arrows). The largest calcification casts an acoustic shadow (small arrows). (Sp, spine.)[2]

Condition	Imaging Findings	Comments
Urinary tract		
Bilateral renal agenesis (Fig FUS 1-29)	Bilateral absence of fetal kidneys and bladder; associated with oligohydramnios.	An invariably fatal anomaly that can be an isolated finding or part of a syndrome. By 12 weeks, the fetal kidneys and bladder should be detectable in all fetuses. The adrenal glands, which are characteristically enlarged in this condition, may mimic the kidneys (sonolucent cortex, echogenic medulla) and produce a confusing appearance.
Multicystic dysplastic kidney disease (Fig FUS 1-30)	Paraspinous flank mass characterized by numerous cysts of variable sizes without identifiable communication or anatomic arrangement. No normal renal parenchyma. Oligohydramnios.	Most common neonatal renal mass. Usually unilateral, although it can be bilateral or segmental. The disorganized pattern of the cysts and the lack of renal parenchyma and reniform contour in multicystic kidney disease must be distinguished from the precise organization of symmetrically positioned fluid-filled spaces in hydronephrosis due to ureteropelvic junction obstruction.
Ureteropelvic junction obstruction (Fig FUS 1-31)	Spectrum of findings ranging from dilatation of the renal pelvis, infundibula, and calyces to a single fluid-filled structure (representing the dilated renal pelvis) with a thin surrounding rim of parenchyma.	Most common cause of neonatal hydronephrosis. In differentiating this condition from multicystic kidney disease, ureteropelvic junction obstruction is suggested by demonstration of renal parenchyma, nonspherical cystic lesions radiating from the renal pelvis, a dilated ureter or single large cyst, and visualization of communication of cysts with the renal pelvis.

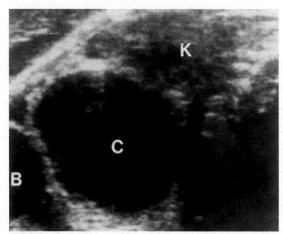

Fig FUS 1-28
Ovarian cyst. Oblique scan shows the large cystic lesion (C). The bladder (B) is the hypoechogenic image below the cyst. The kidney (K) is posterior to it.[2]

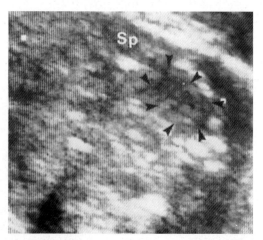

Fig FUS 1-29
Bilateral renal agenesis and severe oligohydramnios. The shadow (arrowheads) in the renal fossa was confused with a kidney. It corresponded to an adrenal gland. (Sp, spine.)[2]

Condition	Imaging Findings	Comments
Megaureter (Fig FUS 1-32)	Hypoechogenic intra-abdominal structure that can be traced back to the renal pelvis.	Causes include obstruction, vesicoureteral reflux, and sporadic idiopathic disease. Normal ureters are rarely visible sonographically in the fetus.

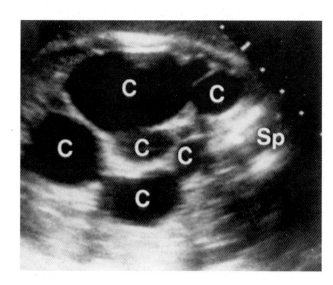

Fig FUS 1-30
Multicystic dysplastic kidney disease. Transverse scan shows multiple noncommunicating cystic structures (C). (Sp, spine.)[2]

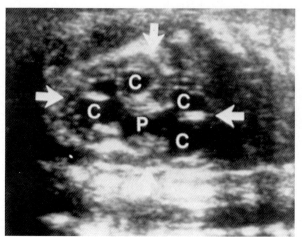

Fig FUS 1-31
Ureteropelvic junction obstruction. Longitudinal scan of the kidney of a fetus with unilateral hydronephrosis (arrows). Note that the cystic structures representing dilated renal calyces (C) communicate with the renal pelvis (P), which is an important clue in differentiating this entity from multicystic kidney disease.[2]

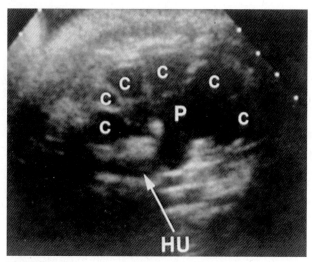

Fig FUS 1-32
Megaureter. Coronal scan shows the hydroureter (HU) associated with dilatation of the renal pelvis (P) and calyces (C).[2]

Condition	Imaging Findings	Comments
Posterior urethral valves (Fig FUS 1-33)	Dilatation of the urinary bladder and proximal urethra with thickening of the bladder wall, and dilatation and tortuosity of the ureters.	Low urinary tract obstruction that affects only male fetuses. The obstructing membrane-like valves are too small to be detected sonographically.
Infantile polycystic kidney disease (Fig FUS 1-34)	Bilaterally enlarged, echogenic kidneys with an absent fetal bladder and oligohydramnios.	Autosomal recessive disorder in which normal parenchyma is replaced by dilated collecting tubules. The typical hyperechogenic texture is attributed to multiple echo-producing interfaces related to the microscopic cystic structures that have replaced normal renal parenchyma. Ultrasound usually cannot demonstrate individual cysts because they are too small to be identified.
Prune-belly syndrome	Enlargement of the bladder with hydronephrosis and hydroureter associated with absence or hypoplasia of the abdominal muscles.	Rare condition occurring almost exclusively in males and thought to be related to urethral obstruction. The term *prune-belly* refers to the wrinkled appearance of the skin, which is due to absence or hypoplasia of the abdominal muscles.
Heart (Fig FUS 1-35)	Various appearances.	A broad spectrum of congenital heart diseases has been demonstrated by fetal ultrasound.

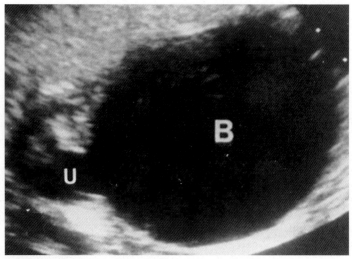

Fig FUS 1-33
Posterior urethral valves. The markedly dilated bladder (B), suggesting an outlet obstruction, is associated with dilatation of the proximal portion of the urethra (U).[2]

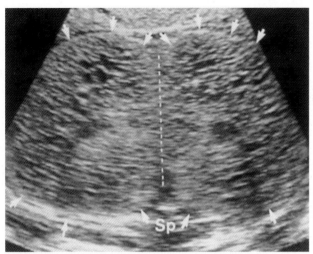

Fig FUS 1-34
Infantile polycystic kidney disease. Transverse scan shows multiple small cysts (arrows) in kidneys that fill the entire abdominal cavity. (Sp, spine.)[2]

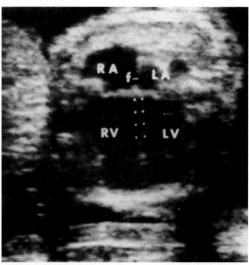

Fig FUS 1-35
Ventricular septal defect (white dots) in a fetus with tetralogy of Fallot. (f, foramen ovale; LA, left atrium; LV, left ventricle; RA, right atrium; RV, right ventricle.)[11]

Polyhydramnios

Condition	Comments
Idiopathic (Fig FUS 2-1)	In approximately 60% of cases of polyhydramnios, there are no abnormalities detectable in either the mother or the fetus.
Maternal factors (Fig FUS 2-2)	Approximately 20% of cases of polyhydramnios are associated with maternal diabetes mellitus. Proposed but unproven mechanisms include an increase in amniotic fluid osmolality resulting from increased glucose; fetal polyuria resulting from fetal hyperglycemia; and decreased swallowing by the large, well-fed fetus. Other underlying maternal factors associated with polyhydramnios include Rh incompatibility, preeclampsia, syphilis, and congestive heart failure.
Congenital fetal abnormalities Central nervous system	Represents almost half the fetal abnormalities associated with polyhydramnios. Anencephaly is by far the most common. Others include meningocele, encephalocele, cebocephaly, hydrocephaly, and hydranencephaly. Proposed underlying mechanisms include impaired fetal swallowing, polyuria due to lack of antidiuretic hormone, and transudation of fluid through the meninges.

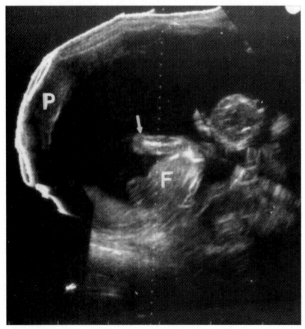

Fig FUS 2-1
Polyhydramnios. Sonogram of a fetus (F) with excessive amniotic fluid and a floating extremity (arrow). (P, placenta.)[12]

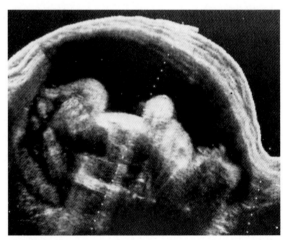

Fig FUS 2-2
Polyhydramnios. An excessive accumulation of amniotic fluid surrounds the fetus in a mother with diabetes mellitus.

Condition	Comments
Gastrointestinal	Represents approximately 30% of fetal anomalies occurring with polyhydramnios. Conditions include duodenal and esophageal atresia, annular pancreas compressing the duodenum, gastroschisis and omphalocele, diaphragmatic hernia, and esophageal compression by congenital goiter. The underlying mechanism appears to be gastrointestinal obstruction with diminished absorption of amniotic fluid.
Circulatory system	Fetal hydrops, cardiac dysrhythmias, myocardial disorders, coarctation and interruption of the fetal aorta, and fetofetal transfusion in monozygotic twins.
Miscellaneous abnormalities	Thanatophoric dwarfism and other short-limb dwarfs, trisomy 18, mesoblastic nephroma, congenital chylothorax, congenital pancreatic cyst, asphyxiating thoracic dystrophy, sacrococcygeal and cervical teratomas, multicystic dysplastic kidneys, and primary pulmonary hypoplasia.

Oligohydramnios

Condition	Comments
Urinary tract anomalies (Figs FUS 3-1 through FUS 3-3)	After the 18th to 20th week of gestation, fetal urine excretion is mainly or entirely responsible for amniotic fluid production. Therefore, oligohydramnios and even a total absence of amniotic fluid will develop in a fetus with renal failure or urethral obstruction, as in bilateral renal agenesis, bilateral multicystic kidneys, posterior urethral valves, and prune-belly syndrome.
Intrauterine growth retardation	Causes include congenital infection; fetal chromosomal abnormality or congenital malformation; maternal abuse of drugs, alcohol, or tobacco; and maternal illnesses such as cardiovascular disease, renal disease, anemia, and malnutrition.
Fetal distress	A decrease in amniotic fluid may be detected before evidence of a decrease in fetal growth.
Premature rupture of membranes	Most common cause of decreased amniotic fluid.
Postmaturity	Progressive decrease in amount of amniotic fluid as the fetus ages.
Idiopathic	An apparent decrease in the volume of amniotic fluid may occur without any fetal or maternal abnormality.

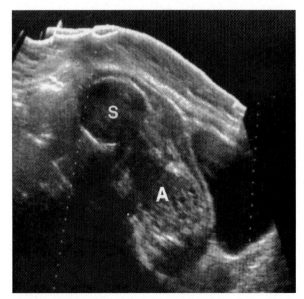

Fig FUS 3-1
Oligohydramnios. Absence of amniotic fluid. (A, fetal abdomen; S, fetal skull.)[12]

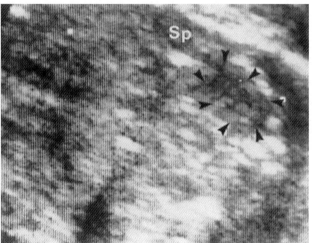

Fig FUS 3-2
Severe oligohydramnios associated with bilateral renal agenesis. The shadow (arrowheads) in the renal fossa that originally was confused with the kidneys was shown to correspond to an adrenal gland. (Sp, spine.)[2]

A

B

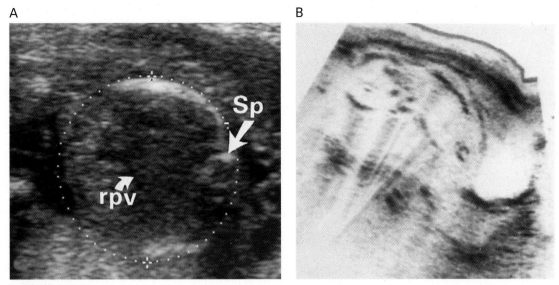

Fig FUS 3-3
Oligohydramnios associated with absent or poorly visualized stomach. (A) Transverse and (B) longitudinal images show poor visualization of the fluid-filled stomach, which probably resulted from paucity of amniotic fluid available for swallowing. (rpv, right portal vein; Sp, spine.)[3]

Fetal Ascites

Condition	Comments
Hydrops fetalis (Figs FUS 4-1 through FUS 4-3)	Intraperitoneal fluid is associated with some combination of pleural effusions, pericardial effusion, and skin edema.
Bladder outlet obstruction (especially posterior urethral valves)	Extravasation of urine into the peritoneal cavity may be secondary to transudation or associated with bladder rupture. Extreme amounts of urinary ascites can lead to atrophy of the abdominal wall muscles.
Bowel obstruction with perforation	Secondary to atresias, stenoses, or volvulus.
High-output heart failure	Most frequently due to Rh incompatibility, arteriovenous shunts, or placental tumors. Rare cardiac causes include dysrhythmias, coarctation or interruption of the aorta, and myocardial disorders.
Viral infection	Cytomegalovirus.
Twin-twin transfusion	In the "stuck-twin" syndrome that occurs secondary to intraplacental vascular shunting, one fetus ("recipient") is overtransfused and shows signs of high-output heart failure, hydrops, and polyhydramnios. The other twin ("donor") becomes anemic and severely growth retarded.

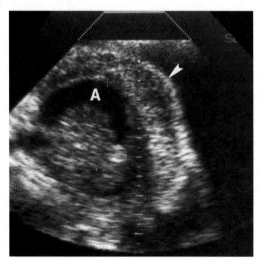

Fig FUS 4-1
Hydrops fetalis. Sonogram of the fetal abdomen shows edema of the abdominal wall (arrow) and fetal ascites (A).[12]

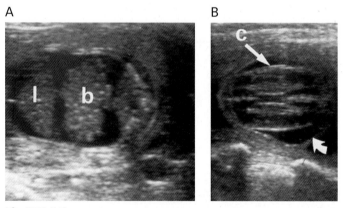

Fig FUS 4-2
Severe nonimmune hydrops fetalis in hypophosphatasia dwarfism. (A) Coronal view of the fetal abdomen shows ascites surrounding the liver (l) and bowel (b). (B) Transverse axial image of the fetal head shows massive scalp edema (curved arrow). Note the poorly mineralized calvarium (c) resulting from hypophosphatasia.[3]

Condition	Comments
Pseudoascites (Fig FUS 4-4)	A thin rim of lucent tissue is often observed along the anterior surface of the fetal abdominal cavity just beneath the skin. This appearance is thought to represent the hypoechoic anterior abdominal musculature (internal oblique, external oblique, and transversalis muscles) in the fetus. Unlike pseudoascites, true ascites surrounds bowel loops and frequently outlines the falciform ligament and umbilical vein; can be detected between the bony rib cage and viscera (liver and spleen); and can be confirmed by its presence in the peritoneal recesses of the fetal subhepatic space, flanks, or pelvis. Because of the insertion of the oblique muscles into the ribs, the lucent rim of pseudoascites fades posterolaterally and is not visualized between the dorsal ribs and liver.
Fetal death	Other definitive signs (eg, absent heart motion) generally are clearly evident.

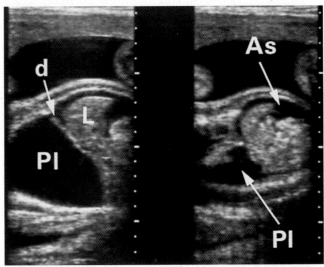

Fig FUS 4-3
Hydrops fetalis. Sagittal images of the fetal chest and abdomen show ascites (As) associated with a large pleural effusion (Pl). (d, diaphragm; L, liver.)[3]

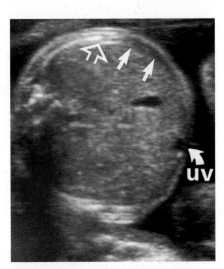

Fig FUS 4-4
Pseudoascites. The hypoechoic abdominal musculature (solid arrows) fades along the interface with the ribs (open arrow). Note that the hypoechoic pseudoascites does not outline the umbilical vein (uv).[3]

Multiple Gestations

Condition	Comments
Dichorionic, diamniotic (Figs FUS 5-1 and FUS 5-2)	All dizygotic twin pregnancies (because each conceptus implants separately in the uterus and develops its own amnion and chorion). Seen in approximately 33% of monozygotic twins if the division of the fertilized ovum occurs within 3 to 4 days after conception (two gestations implant separately). Sonographic findings include demonstration of a thick separating membrane between the two sacs; separate placentas (but in about 67% the placentas abut or are fused); twins of different sexes.
Monochorionic, diamniotic (Fig FUS 5-3)	Results from the division of the conceptus of a single fertilized ovum that occurs 4 to 7 days after conception (two amniotic cavities within a single chorionic cavity). Seen in approximately 67% of monozygotic twins. All monochorionic gestations are at increased risk for structural abnormalities (anencephaly, sacrococcygeal teratoma) as well as complications related to anastomoses across the common placenta (twin-twin transfusion syndrome, acardia).

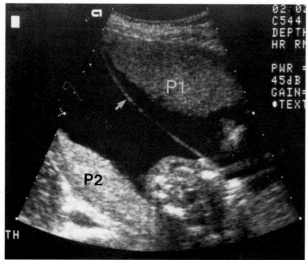

Fig FUS 5-1
Dichorionic gestation with two separate placentas. An anterior placenta (P1) is associated with one twin and a posterior placenta (P2) is seen with the other twin. The two sacs are separated by a thick membrane (arrow).[13]

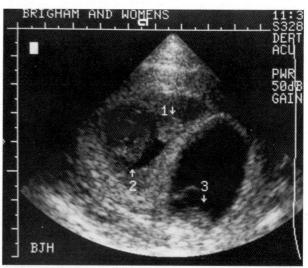

Fig FUS 5-2
Dichorionic triplet gestation. Two triplets lie in one chorionic cavity with a common placenta (1 and 2) and the third (3) in its own chorionic cavity with its own placenta.[14]

A
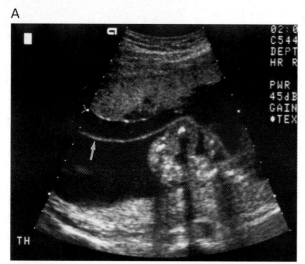

B
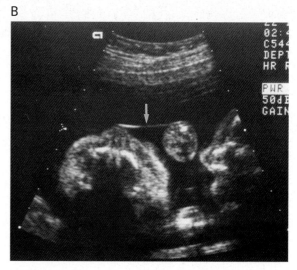

Fig FUS 5-3
Thin and thick dividing membranes. (A) Sonogram of a dichorionic, diamniotic twin gestation shows a thick dividing membrane (arrow). (B) Sonogram of a monochorionic, diamniotic twin gestation shows a thin dividing membrane (arrow).[15]

Condition	Comments
Monochorionic, monoamniotic	Rare condition in which the division of the conceptus of a single fertilized ovum occurs 8 days or more after conception. High mortality rate (complications of monochorionicity as well as subject to cord accidents from cord entanglement).
Conjoined twins (Fig FUS 5-4)	Rare condition that occurs when the conceptus of a single fertilized ovum incompletely divides 13 days or later after conception. The most common site of conjoining is across the thorax, but any portion can be involved (eg, abdomen, head, back). High mortality rate because of the high frequency of anomalies and the difficulty in surgically separating the common body parts.

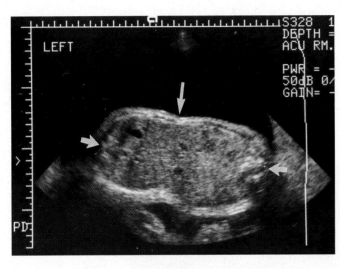

Fig FUS 5-4
Conjoined twins. Transverse sonogram shows conjoining of twins across the anterior abdomen (long arrow). The two fetal spines (short arrows) are seen posteriorly in each.[14]

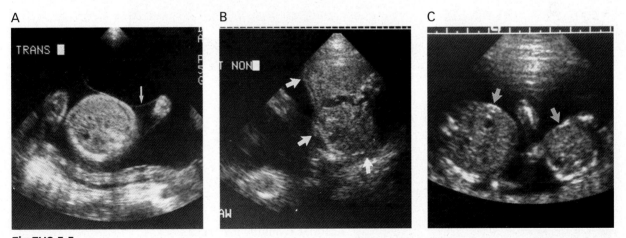

Fig FUS 5-5
Twin-twin transfusion syndrome. (A) Sonogram of a twin gestation with discrepant amniotic fluids. A diamniotic membrane (arrow) is draped over the donor twin with oligohydramnios.[14] (B) Severe oligohydramnios leads to a stuck twin, with the fetal abdomen (arrows) compressed against the uterine wall by the nonvisualized membrane.[14] (C) The two abdomens (arrows) of these discordant twins are obviously different in size.[15]

Condition	Comments
Twin-twin transfusion syndrome (Fig FUS 5-5)	Complication of monochorionic gestations (15% to 30%) in which there is unbalanced exchange of blood between the two fetuses across arterial to venous anastomoses in the common placenta. One fetus (donor twin) becomes anemic and growth retarded, whereas the other (recipient) becomes polycythemic and may develop high-output congestive heart failure. The mortality rate for both fetuses is 40% to 85%. Sonographic findings include discrepant amniotic fluid volumes (polyhydramnios around the recipient twin; oligohydramnios of the donor twin, which may appear to be "stuck" against the uterine wall by the invisible intervening membrane); discordant fetal sizes (small donor twin; normal or occasionally large recipient twin); and hydrops of the recipient twin (10% to 25% of cases).
Acardiac twinning (Fig FUS 5-6)	Rare complication of monochorionicity that results from large artery-to-artery and vein-to-vein placental anastomoses connecting the circulatory systems of the twins and leads to reversal of flow through the circulatory system of one twin. The reversed hemodynamics causes this twin to develop at most a rudimentary heart. On sonography, the "acardiac" twin has no beating heart, massive skin thickening and edema, and usually a two-vessel umbilical cord. The other twin (termed the "pump" because its heart supplies blood to both twins) may appear normal or have polyhydramnios and hydrops due to cardiac overload. Doppler can document the reversed direction of flow in the umbilical artery and vein of the acardiac twin.

A
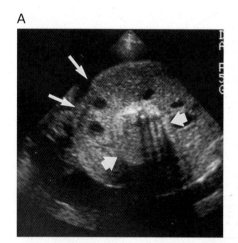

B
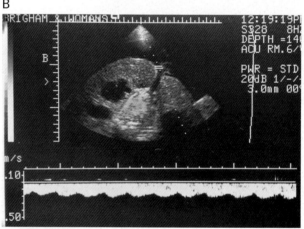

C
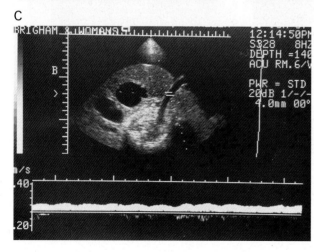

Fig FUS 5-6
Acardiac twins. (A) Transverse sonogram through the trunk of the acardiac twin shows massive skin thickening (arrows) around the abdomen (arrowheads). (B) Doppler study of the umbilical artery of the acardiac twin shows flow in the reverse direction, toward the fetus. (C) Doppler study of the umbilical vein shows reversed flow away from the fetus.[16]

Condition	Comments
Death of one twin (Fig FUS 5-7)	The sonographic appearance depends on the time of gestation when the demise occurs. Death in the first trimester results in resorption of the fetus and its sac within days or weeks and subsequently no evidence that there had been a twin gestation. A twin dying in the second trimester becomes macerated and compressed against the uterine wall ("fetus papyraceus," or paper-thin fetus). When the demise of one twin occurs in the third trimester, a macerated but identifiable dead fetus remains in utero.

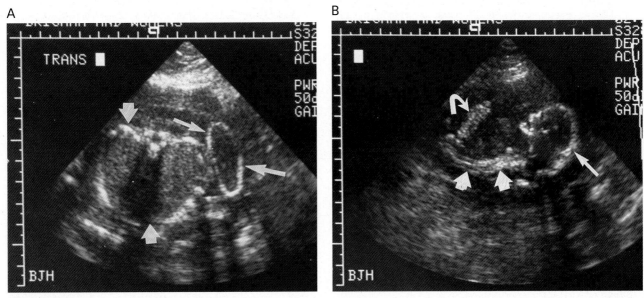

Fig FUS 5-7
Fetus papyraceus. (A) Sonogram of the paper-thin fetal head (long arrows) of a twin that died several months previously. The fetal remnants are compressed against the uterine wall by the live co-twin (short arrows). (B) Longitudinal scan of the compressed fetus shows the head (long arrow) and spine (short arrows). The thrombosed umbilical cord (curved arrow) extends from the fetus toward the uterine wall.[14]

Sources

1. Reprinted with permission from "The Prenatal Examination of the Fetal Cranium, Spine, and Central Nervous System" by ME Pasto and AB Kurtz, *Seminars in Ultrasound, CT and MR* (1984;5:170–193), Copyright ©1984, Grune and Stratton Inc.
2. Reprinted from *Prenatal Diagnosis of Congenital Abnormalities* by R Romero, G Pilu, P Jeanty, and JC Hobbins with permission of Appleton and Lange, ©1988.
3. Reprinted from *Ultrasonography in Obstetrics and Gynecology* by PW Callen with permission of WB Saunders Company, ©1988.
4. Reprinted with permission from "Antenatal Recognition of Cerebral Anomalies" by G Pilu, N Rizzo, LF Orsini et al, *Ultrasound in Medicine and Biology* (1986;12:319), Copyright ©1986, Pergamon Press Inc.
5. Reprinted with permission from "Alobar Holoprosencephaly: Ultrasonographic Prenatal Diagnosis" by RA Filly, DH Chinn, and PW Callen, *Radiology* (1984;151:455), Copyright ©1984, Radiological Society of North America Inc.
6. Reprinted with permission from "Ultrasound of the Fetal Face and Neck" by WE Brant, *The Radiologist* (1994;1:235–244).
7. Reprinted with permission from "Sonography of Facial Features of Alobar and Semilobar Holoprosencephaly" by JP McGahan, DA Nyberg, and LA Mack, *AJR Am J Roentgenol* (1990;154:143–148).
8. Reprinted with permission from "Sonographic Evaluation of the Fetal Abdominal Wall" by WE Brant, *The Radiologist* (1995;2:149–160).
9. Reprinted with permission from "Sonography of the Fetal Gastrointestinal System" by DH Mukuno, TG Lee, and HR Harnsberger et al, *Seminars in Ultrasound, CT and MR* (1984;5:194–209), Copyright ©1984, Grune and Stratton Inc.
10. Reprinted with permission from "Congenital Absence of the Umbilical Cord Resulting from Maldevelopment of Embryonic Body Folding" by CJ Lockwood, AL Scioscia, and JC Hobbins, *American Journal of Obstetrics and Gynecology* (1986;155:1049), Copyright ©1986, The CV Mosby Company.
11. Reprinted with permission from "Fetal Echocardiography: The Challenges of the 1980's" by GR Devore, *Seminars in Ultrasound, CT and MR* (1984;5:229–248), Copyright ©1984, Grune and Stratton Inc.
12. Reprinted from *Ultrasound Atlas of Disease Processes* by CA Krebs, VL Giyanani, and RL Eisenberg, with permission of Appleton & Lange, ©1993.
13. Reprinted with permission from "Sonography in Multiple Gestations" by CB Benson and PM Doubilet, *The Radiologist* (1994;1:147–154).
14. Reprinted with permission from "Sonography of Multiple Gestations" by CB Benson and PM Doubilet, *Radiology Clinics of North America* (1990;28:149–161).
15. Reprinted from "Fetal Twin Pregnancy" by CB Benson and PM Doubilet, by permission of Lippincott, *Obstetrical Ultrasound: A Practical Approach* by J McGahan and M Porto, eds. ©1994.
16. Reprinted with permission from "Doppler Demonstration of Reversed Blood Flow in an Acardiac Twin" by CB Benson, FR Bieber, and DR Genest et al, *Journal of Clinical Ultrasound* (1989;17:291–295).

Index

Note: Page numbers followed by *f* indicate figures.